PRINCIPLES OF CANCER BIOTHERAPY

Third revised edition

PRINCIPLES OF CANCER BIOTHERAPY

Third revised edition

Edited by

ROBERT K. OLDHAM

KLUWER ACADEMIC PUBLISHERS
DORDRECHT / BOSTON / LONDON

Library of Congress Cataloging-in-Publication Data

Principles of cancer biotherapy / edited by Robert K. Oldham. -- 3rd ed.
p. cm.
Includes bibliographical references and index.
ISBN 0-7923-3507-4 (hb : acid-free paper)
1. Cancer--Immunotherapy. 2. Biological response modifiers. 3. Biological products--Therapeutic use. I. Oldham, Robert K.
RC271.I45P75 1997
616.99'4061--dc21 97-2588

ISBN 0-7923-3507-4

Published by Kluwer Academic Publishers,
P.O. Box 17, 3300 AA Dordrecht, The Netherlands

Sold and distributed in North, Central and South America
by Kluwer Academic Publishers,
101 Philip Drive, Norwell, MA 02061, U.S.A.

In all other countries, sold and distributed
by Kluwer Academic Publishers Group,
P.O. Box 322, 3300 AH Dordrecht, The Netherlands.

Printed on acid-free paper

Printed in the Netherlands

TABLE OF CONTENTS

CONTRIBUTING AUTHORS

Paul G. Abrams, M.D.
NeoRx Corporation
Seattle, Washington
Chapter 15

Bharat B. Aggarwal, Ph.D.
Cytokine Research Section
M.D. Anderson Cancer Center
University of Texas
Houston, Texas
Chapter 4

Sharon Lea Aukerman, Ph.D.
Department of Cell Biology
M.D. Anderson Cancer Center
University of Texas
Houston, Texas
Chapter 2

Ernest C. Borden, M.D.
University of Maryland Cancer Center
Baltimore, Maryland
Chapter 11

Hazel B. Breitz, M.D.
NeoRx-Virginia Mason Chemical Research Unit
Seattle, Washington
Chapter 15

Jeffrey Crawford, M.D.
Duke University Medical School
Durham, Borth Carolina
Chapter 19

Robert O. Dillman, M.D., F.A.C.P.
Hoag Cancer Center
Newport Beach, California
and Clinical Professor of Medicine
Department of Medicine
University of California
Irvine, California
Chapter 12

Scott Ebbinghaus, M.D.
University of Alabama at Birmingham
Birmingham, Alabama
Chapter 22

George C. Fareed, M.D.
Chief of Medicine
Pioneers Memorial Hospital
Brawley, California
Chapter 8

Isaiah J. Fidler, D.V.M., Ph.D.
Department of Cell Biology
M.D. Anderson Cancer Center
University of Texas
Houston, Texas
Chapter 2

Kenneth A. Foon, M.D.
The University of Kentucky
Chandler Medical Center
Lucille P. Markey Cancer Center
Lexington, Kentucky
Chapter 14

Maryann Foote, Ph.D.
Amgen
Thousand Oaks, California
Chapter 19

Scott M. Freeman, M.D.
Department of Pathology and Laboratory Medicine
Tulane University Medical School
New Orleans, Louisiana
Chapter 21

Alan R. Fritzberg, Ph.D.
NeoRx Corporation
Seattle, Washington
Chapter 15

David Goldstein, M.D.
Centre for Immunology
Sydney, Australia
Chapter 11

Ann Jakubowski, M.D., Ph.D.
Memorial Sloan-Kettering Cancer Center
New York, New York
Chapter 20

Walter Lewko, Ph.D.
Cancer Therapeutics Inc.
Franklin, Tennessee
Chapter 10

Aizen J. Marrogi, M.D.
Department of Pathology and Laboratory Medicine
Tulane University Medical School
New Orleans, Louisiana
Chapter 21

Darryl Maher, M.D.
CSL Limited
Victoria, Australia
Chapter 19

Ernest Marshall, M.D.
The University of Texas
Galveston, Texas
Chapter 22

James Matcham
Amgen Inc., Cambridge, UK
Chapter 19

Georges Mathé, M.D., Ph.D.
Institut du Cancer et d'Immunogénétique
Groupe Hospitalier Paul-Brousse
Villejuif, France
Chapter 7

Rosemary Mazanet, M.D., Ph.D.
Amgen, Thousand Oaks, California
Chapter 19

Kapil Mehta, Ph.D.
Department of Bioimmunotherapy
M.D. Anderson Cancer Center
University of Texas
Houston, Texas
Chapter 4

George Morstyn, M.D., Ph.D.
Amgen
Thousand Oaks, California
and UCLA Medical School
Los Angeles, California
Chapter 19

Robert K. Oldham, M.D.
Biological Therapy Institute Foundation
Franklin, Tennessee
and Clinical Professor of Medicine
University of Missouri
Columbia, Missouri
Chapters 1 ,3, 5, 6, 9, 10, 14, 16, 18, 22, 23

Simone Orbach, M.D.
Institut du Cancer et d'Immunogénétique
Groupe Hospitalier Paul-Brousse
Villejuif, France
Chapter 7

Robert Radinsky, Ph.D.
Department of Cell Biology
M.D. Anderson Cancer Center
University of Texas
Houston, Texas
Chapter 2

John M. Reno, Ph.D.
NeoRx Corporation
Seattle, Washington
Chapter 15

Richard V. Smalley, M.D.
Synertron Inc.
Madison, Wisconsin
Chapter 9, 10, 11

Lynn E. Spitler, M.D.
Jenner Biotherapies, Inc.
San Ramon, California
Chapter 8, 13

Dianne Tomita
Amgen Inc.
Thousand Oaks, California
Chapter 19

Veronique Trillet-Lenoir, M.D.
Centre Hospitalier
Lyon Sud, France
Chapter 19

Paul L. Weiden M.D.
Virginia Mason Medical Center
Seattle, Washington
Chapter 15

Katharine A. Whartenby, Ph.D.
Department of Pathology and Laboratoy Medicine
Tulane University Medical School
New Orleans, Louisiana
Chapter 21

John R. Yannelli, Ph.D.
University of Kentucky
Lucille P. Markey Cancer Center
Lexington, Kentucky
Chapter 17

PREFACE

ROBERT K. OLDHAM, M.D.

The idea for the first edition of *Principles of Cancer Biotherapy* was formulated in the early 1980s. As the founding director of the Biological Response Modifiers Program for the National Cancer Institute from 1980-1984, I envisioned a textbook that would embody the principles of the then fledgling fourth modality of cancer treatment – biotherapy. Contributing authors were solicited in 1985, and the first edition came off the presses in 1987. *Principles* represented the first comprehensive textbook on the use of cancer biotherapy and summarized the work done in this field through 1986.

The second edition of *Principles* was published in 1991 about the time biotherapy was more broadly recognized as the fourth major cancer treatment method. Subsequent textbooks by DeVita, Hellman and Rosenberg [1] in 1991 and one by Mitchell [2] in 1993 confirmed the importance of this modality in cancer care.

This third edition is needed now as a result of the tremendous progress that has been made in the last five years using biologicals in cancer treatment. It is now generally agreed that biopharmaceuticals are producing major opportunities for new cancer therapies. Cancer biotherapy is now emerging as a more specific and selective form of systemic cancer treatment. Cancer growth control is becoming an effective method of treatment complementing cancer destruction as mechanisms of cancer treatment and 'cure'.

For years the chemical manipulation of small molecules has been pursued in drug development. We now have all the tools for the biological manipulation of natural substances for therapeutic use. In fact, as we better understand the interaction between biological molecules and their receptors, it is clear that biological manipulation and chemical manipulation will soon come together to bring molecular medicine to the bedside. Many biological molecules are large and have functions other than those mediated by their active sites. There is increasing evidence that drug development will focus on the interaction between the smaller active regions of these large biological molecules and their receptors. This opens up a broad field of molecular design for extending and improving the therapeutic activities of natural biological molecules. This has recently been extended to small molecules interacting with DNA/RNA (anti-sense). The 1990s will be an extraordinarily productive decade in the development of new anticancer drugs through chemical and biological manipulation of these natural molecules. Thus, the body itself has become the 'medicine cabinet' of the future.

In the 1990s and beyond into the next millennium, medicine will face extraordinary demands. While technology brings us tremendous opportunity, it also highlights problems in our medical care system. Most new technology is expensive and, as it comes from the laboratory to the clinic, is by its very nature untried and unproven. Our medical care system involves a private and government insurance reimbursement system that favors paying for marginally effective medical care of the past rather than innovative medical treatments of the future.

To more rapidly and efficiently exploit the opportunities in cancer biotherapy by the year 2000, patients, employers, insurers, universities, and government must come together and redefine the system of reimbursement to maximize the patient's opportunity for access to new and potentially effective cancer therapies. To simply reimburse for past ineffective or marginally effective treatment is not the answer. Provisions must be made to fund clinical research and afford these new approaches broader use at the bedside. We must develop methods to allow our patients access to the opportunities of the future, while maintaining solid support for effective therapies of the past. No longer is it acceptable to pay only for medical care that utilizes old technology, such as chemotherapeutic agents, that is approved but only marginally effective. Across the broad spectrum of human malignancies, most chemotherapeutic drugs are toxic and of limited medical value. We must support clinical research in its efforts to bring newer methods of cancer treatment to the clinic, methods that are less toxic and more effective.

I believe cancer biotherapy will ultimately replace much of what we utilize today in cancer treatment. In light of this view, I want to thank all the authors for their dedication to purpose in writing this third edition of *Principles*. This book summarizes an evolving science and a rapidly changing medical practice. As we near the millennium, it now becomes possible to envision a much more diversified system of cancer research and treatment that will afford greater opportunities for our patients. As indicated in some of the chapters in *Principles*, there is increasing evidence that our historical 'kill and cure'

R.K. Oldham (ed.), Principles of Cancer Biotherapy. 3rd ed., ix–x.

outlook in cancer treatment is in need of modification. Some forms of cancer biotherapy use the strategy of tumor growth stabilization and control through continued biological therapy over a longer period of time, akin to the use of insulin in the treatment of diabetes. These chapters illustrate some new methods of thinking and new strategies for the treatment and control of cancer. It is always difficult to move from past dogmas to future opportunities, but this third edition of *Principles of Cancer Biotherapy* illustrates why it is so important for researchers and clinicians to explore and apply these new opportunities in cancer biotherapy to the benefit of our patients.

REFERENCES

1. DeVita VT Jr, Hellman S, Rosenberg SA. *Biologic Therapy of Cancer.* J.B. Lippincott, 1991.
2. Mitchell MS. *Biological Approaches to Cancer Treatment.* McGraw-Hill, 1993.

CANCER BIOTHERAPY: GENERAL PRINCIPLES

ROBERT K. OLDHAM
Biological Therapy Institute Foundation, Franklin, Tennessee; and University of Missouri, Columbia, Missouri

The term biotherapy encompasses the therapeutic use of any biological substance, but more specifically it connotes the use of products of the mammalian genome. With modern techniques of genetic engineering, the mammalian genome represents the new 'medicine cabinet.' Biological response modifiers (BRM) are agents and approaches whose mechanisms of action involve the individual's own biological responses. Biologicals and BRM work through diverse mechanisms in the biotherapy of cancer. They may (a) augment the host's defenses through the administration of cells, natural biologicals, or the synthetic derivatives thereof as effectors or mediators (direct or indirect) of an antitumor response; (b) increase the individual's antitumor responses through augmentation or restoration of effector mechanisms, or decrease a component of the host's reaction that is deleterious; (c) augment the individual's responses using modified tumor cells or vaccines to stimulate a greater response, or increase tumor cell sensitivity to an existing biological response; (d) decrease transformation and/or increase differentiation or maturation of tumor cells; (e) interfere with growth-promoting factors produced by tumor cells; (f) decrease or arrest the tendency of tumor cells to metastasize to other sites; (g) increase the ability of the patient to tolerate damage by cytotoxic modalities of cancer treatment; and/or (h) use biological molecules to target and bind to cancer cells and induce more effective cytostatic or cytocidial antitumor activity.

While several of these approaches involve the augmentation or use of biological responses, an understanding of the biological properties or immune response molecules, growth and maturation factors, and other biological substances will assist in the development of specific molecular entities that can act on biological responses and/or act directly on tumor cells. Thus, one can visualize the development of biological approaches with response-modifying as well as direct cytolytic, cytostatic, growth-inhibiting (antiproliferative), or maturational effects on tumor cells.

Biotherapy is the fourth modality of cancer therapy and can be effective alone or in association with surgery, radiotherapy, and chemotherapy. To put biotherapy into perspective, it is important to dispel a historical misconception associated with immunotherapy: biotherapy can have activity on clinically apparent, even bulky, cancer, and treatment should not be restricted to situations where the tumor cell mass is imperceptible [59, 66]. Thus, the clinical trial designs for biotherapy can be similar to those used previously for other modalities of cancer treatment, as long as one measures both pharmacokinetics and the biological responses affected by these approaches [60]. Testing is continuing for biotherapy using the interferons, lymphokines and cytokines, growth and maturation factors, monoclonal antibodies and their immunoconjugates, vaccines, and cellular therapy [63].

HISTORICAL PERSPECTIVES

The use of chemical and biological compounds to modulate biological responses has been under active investigation for over 30 years. Although various chemicals, bacterial extracts, and viruses have been found to modulate immune responses in experimental animals, and, to a more limited extent, in humans, these 'nonspecific' immunomodulators have not been highly effective in clinical trials [66]. Molecular biologists have recently developed techniques for the isolation of genes and their subsequent translation into appropriate production systems. These methods make available virtually unlimited quantities of highly purified biological compounds for experimental and therapeutic use. As a result, several classes of biologicals are being evaluated in preclinical models and clinical trials (Table 1).

The continued investigation of nonspecific immunomodulators, as well as the recent advent of genetically

Table 1. Biologicals and BRM

Immunomodulators (chemicals, bacterial extracts, viruses, etc.)
Lymphokines/cytokines α, β, γ-interferon; IL-1-18; tumor necrosis factor (TNF); etc.
Growth/maturation factors (CSF, IL-2, EPO, etc.
Effector cells (cytotoxic and helper T cells, NK, and LAK cells, gene engineered cells, etc.)
Tumor-associated antigens and gene engineered cellular vaccines
Monoclonal antibodies
Immunoconjugates

R.K. Oldham (ed.), Principles of Cancer Biotherapy. 3rd ed., 1–15.

engineered biologicals, makes the need for predictive preclinical assays of biological activity and efficacy apparent [31]. *In vitro* assays of biological activity (bioassays) are generally used to define and quantitate the activity of a given biological substance. Subsequently, flow cytometry, immunoperoxidase staining, enzyme-linked immunosorbent assays (ELISA), radioimmunoassays (RIA), and variations of these methods allow the precise determination of levels of these molecules in appropriate fluids and tissues. Finally, there is the need to assess the *in vivo* activity of these materials in preclinical models to develop predictive assays for clinical efficacy and provide information useful in the rational selection of agents and the design of clinical trials [31, 49].

Given the variability in the biological behavior of cancer and its interface with the human outbred host, it is not surprising that trials of nonspecific and specific immunotherapy, as translated from artificially constructed animal models, have not been uniformly successful in cancer treatment [4, 31]. Naturally occurring cancers arise in a particular organ from one cell or a few cells under some carcinogenic stimulus. In humans, these initial foci of cancer cells may grow – and sometimes lie dormant – over very long periods of time (from 1% to 30% of the human life span) before there is clinical evidence of cancer. Dissemination of cells from the initial focus may occur at any time during the development of the primary tumor. Subsequently, growth and metastasis occur over periods of months to years from primary and secondary foci, causing complex biological interactions to occur.

In contrast, experimentally induced cancer is an artificial (even artifactual) situation. A short-duration, high-dose carcinogen may be used to induce cancer quickly so that experiments can proceed rapidly. In transplantable models, the tumor cells are injected into young, normal, syngeneic animals, thereby circumventing the influences of environmental or genetic factors that may be operative in the natural host during tumor development. Many of the experimental systems are models, transplantable tumors that have been maintained for decades, and therefore have only the most remote relevance to cancer in humans. The injection represents a single, instantaneous point source for a defined tumor load that has been manipulated *in vitro*. Regardless of whether that tumor load is 10 or 10^6 cells, it is being placed artificially in a single site and allowed to grow and metastasize from that selected single site. Thus, these transplantable cancers are simply not analogous to clinical cancer and the conclusions drawn from them are unlikely to be broadly applicable to human cancers [31].

The modern era of cancer treatment began in the 1950s with the recognition that most cancers were systemic problems. It became obvious that lymphatic and blood-borne metastases often occurred simultaneously with local growth and regional spread. The early success of alkylating-agent chemotherapy of lymphoma prompted a massive search for chemicals that might have cytolytic or cytostatic effects on cancer cells. More than one million compounds have been 'screened' for antitumor activity [11], and this effort has given clinicians less than 50 'approved and active' anticancer chemotherapy drugs. There is now widespread recognition that drugs in cancer treatment can effectively palliate and sometimes cure [19]. The development of three modalities (surgery, radiotherapy and chemotherapy) and their subsequent integration into what is now multimodal cancer treatment has been summarized [18, 20]. Between 1975 and 1985 a plateau was reached in cancer treatment. New surgical techniques (e.g., debulking, intra-operative methods for radiotherapy, and catheter isolation/infusion for chemotherapy) and new methods of radiotherapy (e.g., neutrons, protons, interstitial therapy, isotopes) continue to be developed, but these two modalities are primarily useful in local and regional cancer treatment. Chemotherapy continues to evolve, with new drugs and new combinations of drugs. There has been continued, but slow, progress in the treatment of highly replicative, drug-sensitive malignancies over the past 15 years. It is now apparent that further progress with chemotherapy will depend on a greater understanding of the metabolic processes of cancer cells and the differences between these and normal cells. In addition, there are the problems of drug resistance, selectivity of action, and drug delivery. Cancer cells are more like than unlike normal cells with respect to chemotherapy sensitivity. There is little evidence of selectivity in the delivery or effects of anticancer drugs. Many chemotherapeutic agents are highly cytolytic, but the problems of normal tissue toxicity, drug delivery, and tumor-cell resistance remain [19, 43]. Thus, cancer remains a systemic problem, and further systemic approaches are required for more effective treatment [20].

The scientific basis for biotherapy as the fourth modality of cancer treatment is now firm [21-23, 63, 65, 76, 77, 89]. Historically, there was an attempt to establish immunotherapy in this role. Whereas immunotherapy was reproducible under specific experimental protocols, it was not strikingly effective in animals bearing palpable tumors and did not translate well to patients. Given the observation that immunotherapy was more effective with small tumor burdens, investigators began to study both 'specific' and 'nonspecific' immunotherapy as treatment for minimal residual disease. Although it became widely accepted that the treatment of animals with minimal residual disease was analogous to the postsurgical treatment of cancer in humans, this analogy was often stretched beyond reason. Immunotherapy in young, normal, syngeneic animals was often begun on the day of the tumor transplant (or within 1 or 2 days), using a transplant of a very small number of tumor cells (1-1000) to a single site. In many of these studies, and in studies in which the tumor was surgically resected and no evident disease remained, the effects of immunotherapy were reasonably reproducible; the therapy was most beneficial when the tumor mass was less than 10^6 cells.

These experimental results produced a dogma that immunological manipulation or immunotherapy could work *only* when the tumor cell mass was imperceptible [4, 66]. This posed real problems for clinical immunotherapy, since the tumor cell mass at clinical diagnosis or after surgery is usually three orders of magnitude (or more) greater than 10^6 cells. Despite the obvious difficulties with the experimental models and the translation to humans, clinicians began immunotherapy trials in the 1970s. The results of initial, small, uncontrolled trials were often reported as positive. Larger, randomized, controlled studies were done to confirm the efficacy of a particular immunotherapeutic regimen in a particular type of cancer. Although some of the controlled studies were positive, most yielded marginal or negative results. Thus, immunotherapy had a poor image by the end of the 1970s [66, 101].

Immunotherapy failed to establish itself as a major mode of cancer treatment for several reasons. One important factor was the lack of definition and purity of immunotherapeutic agents. Many of the nonspecific approaches involved the use of complex chemicals, bacteria, viruses, and poorly defined extracts in an attempt to 'stimulate' the immune response. Thus, molecular definition of the actual stimulating entity was not available. Given the lack of analogy between model systems and humans, the poorly characterized reagents, and the problems of variability in experimental procedures, the lack of demonstrable clinical efficacy was predictable [66].

Immunotherapy is not an appropriate term for the modern use of biologicals and BRM in medicine. Biological control mechanisms should be envisioned on a much broader basis than the immune system. While immunotherapy remains a subcategory of biotherapy, growth and differentiation factors, the use of synthetically derived molecular analogs, and the pharmacological exploitation of biological molecules now involve a much broader range of approaches (Table 1) than those previously considered as immunotherapy [63].

Certain specific developments led to biotherapy becoming the fourth modality of cancer therapy. Advances in molecular biology have given scientists the capability to clone individual genes and produce significant quantities of highly purified genomic products as medicines. Unlike extracted and purified biological molecules, available in small quantities as semipurified mixtures, the products of cloned genes have a level of purity on a par with drugs. They can be analyzed alone or in combination as to their effects in cancer biology. In addition, recent progress in nucleic acid sequencing and translation, protein sequencing and synthesis, the isolation and purification of biological products, and mass cell culture has given the scientific community the opportunity to alter proteins at the nucleotide or amino acid level to manipulate then optimize their biological activity [39].

As a result of gene cloning, a major new approach in cancer treatment has evolved. Interleukin-2 can be used to stimulate the growth of a broad range of lymphocytes (T, NK, and LAK cells). This has given clinicians the ability to have large quantities of specific subclasses of effector cells for cancer treatment. Emerging evidence suggests that these effector cells can be helpful in the regional and systemic treatment of advanced, bulky cancer. It was the availability of Interleukin-2 that allowed this technology to prosper [78]. In addition, IL-2 is now being used as the T cell growth factor for gene engineered lymphocytes containing new genes to enhance their cancer treatment capacity [75, 95].

Another major technical advance was the discovery of hybridomas. A major limitation on the use of antibodies had been the inability to make reproducible high-titer, specific antisera and to define these preparations on a molecular basis. Immunoglobulin reagents can now be produced with the same level of molecular purity as cloned gene products and drugs. These antibodies are powerful tools in the isolation and purification of tumor-associated antigens, lymphokines/cytokines, and other biologicals, which can then be used in biotherapy. The advances in molecular biology and hybridoma technology have eclipsed previous techniques for the isolation and purification of biological molecules [58, 72].

Technical advances in instrumentation, computers, and computer software have been critically important in the isolation and purification of biological molecules. The construction of nucleotide or amino acid sequences to fit any biological message can now be considered possible. While this synthetic capability is currently limited to smaller gene products, techniques by which analysis and construction of nucleotide sequences will occur in an automated way, making enormously complex molecules possible to synthesize and manufacture, are rapidly becoming available.

PRECLINICAL MODELS

Biological activity in preclinical models

Central to the identification of biotherapy that might be useful in cancer patients is the recognition that, in the main, the challenge in humans is the eradication of metastases. Metastases can result from the dissemination of different subpopulations of cells within the primary neoplasm [30]. This may explain the observation that cells within a metastasis can be antigenically distinct from those that predominate in the parental tumor [30]. Metastases may also emanate from other metastases. The implications of cellular heterogeneity as it relates to the outcome of the specific immunotherapy are obvious. In addition, normal animals are not comparable to animals or humans bearing autochthonous neoplasms [31]. There may exist in animals and in humans specific or nonspecific defects important in the development of their autochthonous tumors. Corrections of such defects may require a form of biotherapy totally different from that required to assist the normal host in controlling a transplanted cancer.

Model screening criteria

Theoretically, an ideal procedure for screening new biologicals should employ a system of sequential and progressively more demanding protocols designed to select a maximum number of effective agents.

The term screening denotes a series of sequential assays through which promising agents are tested for therapeutic potential. For some biotherapies, a general screening procedure may be inappropriate. For example, the activity of a monoclonal antibody with antitumor specificity would not be detected by use of the general screen of biological activity. Design considerations for general screening in biotherapy have been extensively reviewed [31, 49]. A step-by-step approach to the screening of potential BRM was developed to define their effects on T-cell, B-cell, NK-cell, and macrophage functions. A progressive *in vitro* and then *in vivo* sequence allows the variables of dose, schedule, route, duration and maintenance of activity, adjuvanticity, and synergistic potential to be explored in an orderly fashion [31].

Models for testing efficacy

The preclinical evaluation of biotherapy efficacy requires the *in vivo* testing of agents in relevant model systems. The importance of using animals with primary autochthonous tumors to demonstrate therapeutic potential cannot be overemphasized. Although this concept has been frequently discussed, the ability to obtain significant numbers of animals bearing primary tumors in a reasonable time after initiation of a tumor by chemical or physical carcinogens remains a problem. Spontaneous neoplasms of unknown cause arise in aged rodents, but the use of these tumors as models is currently not practical.

The ultraviolet carcinogenesis model developed by Kripke and co-workers [31] has been used in screening. In this system, chronic exposure of mice to ultraviolet light results in the development of single or multiple skin neoplasms. These tumors are antigenic, and most are rejected when transplanted into normal, syngeneic recipients. However, the tumors grow progressively in immunologically deficient recipients or in syngeneic mice that have been exposed to low-dose, nontumorigenic ultraviolet radiation. The immune response of ultraviolet irradiated mice to a variety of exogenous antigens is normal, suggesting a mechanism involving suppressor cells with selectivity for antigens expressed on autochthonous ultraviolet radiation-induced tumors.

An ideal carcinogen-induced tumor system would be one in which the carcinogen is easily administered, is not highly toxic, has a short latent period, and is capable of reproducibly inducing palpable primary tumors, with metastases developing in over 50% of animals with primary tumors. The induction of mammary tumors in rats by *N*-nitro-*N*-methylurea appears to be a system with many of these characteristics [56]. It has been used as another model in biotherapy screening [31].

Evaluation of screening programs

Screening programs for chemotherapeutic agents were initiated in the mid-1950s, and attempts have been made to randomly examine thousands of compounds for antitumor activity [11]. Such large screening programs are empirically rather than rationally based, and are no longer appropriate [4, 5, 20, 31, 66]. Whether induced or transplantable animal tumor systems are valid models for testing therapeutic approaches for human cancer has been a controversial issue [31]. In patients, therapy successful against one type of cancer may not be successful against another type, or even for another patient with the same histological type of cancer. Unlike the model systems, in which treatment can be given with precise timing relative to the metastatic phase of a resected tumor or injected tumor cells, cancer diagnosis in humans is generally late, and micrometastases (and often macrometastases) have become well established before treatment can be initiated. Thus, screening programs can only provide tentative indications on agents and approaches of interest. The testing of biotherapy in an evolving, controlled screening system may help eliminate arbitrary decisions on the use of a given biological approach and ultimately may contribute to the development of novel approaches for the treatment of disseminated cancer [31]. While the idea of systematic screening was popular in the 1980s [31], very little in the way of rational screening is currently being done.

BIOTHERAPY: SPECIFIC AGENTS AND APPROACHES

Nonspecific immunomodulators

Since the early 1900s, immunotherapy with bacterial or viral products has been utilized with the hope of 'nonspecifically' stimulating the host's immune response [66]. These agents had been useful as adjuvants and as nonspecific stimulants in animal tumor models, but human trials have been disappointing. It is clear that in the animal tumor models specific requirements for immune stimulation are much better defined.

Perhaps purified viruses or specific chemicals (Table 2) will lead to the development of more effective adjuvants or stimulants of the immune response. Bacillus Calmette-Guerin (BCG) and other whole organisms were used early in immunotherapy. The use of a purified derivative of bacterial components, such as muramyl di or tripeptide, 'packaged' in liposomes as a method to stimulate macrophages to greater anticancer activity is a modern approach of greater promise. Such adjuvants may prove useful with genetically engineered or synthetic tumor-associated antigens, active specific immunotherapy, or immunoprophylaxis.

Multiple agents that appear capable of augmenting one or more immune functions already exist (Table 2). Several of these have been associated with prolongation of sur-

Table 2. Biologicals and biological response modifiers

Immunomodulating agents
Alkyl lysophospholipids (ALP)
Azimexon
BCG
Bestatin
Brucella abortus
Corynebacterium parvum
Cimetidine
Sodium diethyldithiocarbamate (DTC)
Endotoxin
Glucan
'Immune' RNAs
Krestin
Lentinan
Levamisole
Muramyldipeptide (MDP), tripeptide (MTP)
Maleic anhydride-divinyl ether (MVE-2)
Mixed bacterial vaccines (MBV)
Nocardia rubra cell wall skeleton (CWS)
Picibanil (OK432)
Prostoglandin inhibitors (aspirin, indomethacin)
Thiobendazole
Tuftsin
Interferons and interferon inducers
Interferons (α, β, γ)
Poly IC-LC
Poly A:U
GE-132
Brucella abortus
Tilorone
Viruses
Pyrimidinones
Thymosins
Thymosin alpha-1
Thymosin fraction 5
Other thymic factors
Lymphokines, cytokines, growth/maturation factors
Antigrowth factors
Chalones
Colony-stimulating factors (CSF)
Growth factors (transforming growth factor, TGF)
Lymphocyte activation factor [LAF-interleukin 1 (IL-1)]
Lymphotoxins (TNF, α, β LT)
Macrophage activation factors (MAF)
Macrophage chemotactic factor
Macrophage cytotoxic factor (MCF)
Macrophage growth factor (MGF)
Migration inhibitory factor (MIF)
Maturation factors
T-Cell growth factor ['TCGF' – interleukin 2 (IL-2)]
Interleukin 3-18, etc.
Thymocyte mitogenic factor (TMF)
Transfer factor
Transforming growth factors (TGF, α, β)

Table 2. (continued)

Antigens
Tumor-associated antigens
Molecular vaccines
Cell engineered cellular vaccines
Effector cells
Macrophages
NK cells
Cytotoxic T cells
LAK cells
T Helper cells
Miscellaneous approaches
Allogeneic immunization
Liposome-encapsulated biologicals
Bone-marrow transplantation and reconstitution
Plasmapheresis and *ex vivo* treatments (activation columns immunoabsorbents and ultrafiltration)
Virus infection of cells (oncolysates)

vival in prospectively randomized trials involving patients with a wide variety of malignancies (Table 3). Although some of these agents have produced modest clinical benefits, and do represent a potential method of immune augmentation, it is doubtful that they will have a major role in future cancer therapy. Great problems exist for most of the agents, including lack of chemical definition, low purity, and poor reproducibility from one lot to another. An additional problem has been the inability to define clearly a mechanism of action for these agents in humans. They are all nonspecific immune stimulants capable of augmenting a variety of functions in rodent systems, but the translation to humans has been difficult. The preclinical screening established by the Biological Response Modifiers Program (BRMP) of the National Cancer Institute was one mechanism to do this [31]. Data from this type of screening with subsequent phase I and phase II clinical data could have provided interesting insights and correlations [90, 96, 97]. Unfortunately, this approach has been abandoned. In addition, even though antitumor efficacy has been demonstrated with many of these agents in murine models, it has been demonstrated under ideal circumstances, which are rarely, if ever, available to the clinician.

Although many of these nonspecific immunstimulants have prolonged the survival of rodents, more knowledge is needed regarding the interrelationships and control mechanisms of the various aspects of the immune response. The ability to specifically control and manipulate immune responses with highly purified, defined molecules obtained by genetic engineering is in the immediate, foreseeable future. Thus, it seems probable that nonspecific immunotherapy as a sole modality will become obsolete, although adjuvants may find a role in active specific immunotherapy. For a contrasting view, please read Chapter 7 in this book.

Table 3. Studies of immunotherapy with random designs[a]

Specific cancer and type of immunotherapy	Positive studies	Equivocal studies	Negative studies
Leukemia			
BCG/AML			+
BCG/Cells/AML	+		+
MER/AML			+
CP/Cells/AML			+
All/Hodgkin's			
NHL/MM			
Lev/ALL			+
BCG/NHL	+		
Lev/MM		+	
Lung cancer			
IT BCG		+	+
IP BCG	+		+
IP BCG + Lev			+
IP CP		+	
Lev	+		+
Thy Fr V	+		
BCG/Cells		+	
TAA/Freund's adjuvant	+		
Breast cancer			
Poly A/Poly U	+		
BCG	+		+
Lev	+		
Colon cancer			
BCG		+	
MER	+		
CP			+
Lev	+		
Melanoma			
IL/BCG		+	
BCG/BCG + Cells	+		+
BCG		+	+
CP			+
Lev			+
Genitourinary cancer			
IC BCG/bladder	+		
BCG/prostate	+		
Gynecological cancer			
CP/cervix			+
CP/ovary	+		
BCG/ovary	+		
Other cancers			
Lev/H & N		+	
CP/H & N			+
BCG/cells/sarcoma			+
MER/neuroblastoma	+		

[a] Reference and abbreviations available in ref. 101.

Active specific immunotherapy

There has been a substantial effort to produce active immunization of autochthonous or syngeneic hosts with irradiated or chemically modified tumor cells in an attempt to use active specific immunotherapy (AST) [43]. Inherent is the assumption that tumor cells express immunogenic tumor-associated antigens (TAA). Treatment of tumor cells with a variety of unrelated agents, such as irradiation, mitomycin, lipophilic agents, neurominidase, viruses, or admixtures of cells with bacterial adjuvants, has produced nontumorigenic tumor cell preparations that are immunogenic upon injection into syngeneic hosts.

AST using BCG-tumor cell ('antigens') vaccines has been reevaluated using a syngeneic guinea pig hepatocarcinoma. The definition of several variables of vaccine preparation, such as a ratio of bacterial organisms to viable, metabolically active tumor cells, the procedures of tumor cell dissociation and cryobiologic preservation, and the irradiation attenuation of cells, has resulted in the development of an effective nontumorigenic vaccine. It has proven effective in both micro- and macrometastatic disease [44].

The nature of the anatomic alteration in metastatic nodules after AST was explored using a specific monoclonal antibody to assess vascular permeability within these tumor nodules [50, 51]. Immunohistologic analysis demonstrated significantly more antibody in tumors from vaccinated animals than in comparable tumors from unvaccinated guinea pigs. These data support the hypothesis that the anatomic characteristics of tumor foci restrict drug and antibody access, thus protecting tumors not only from immunotherapy but from other forms of treatment as well [42].

The regulation of the blood supply to neoplastic tissue may be unique in comparison to normal tissue. Tumor metastatic nodules may have a vascular 'barrier,' which contributes to a limitation in delivery for chemotherapeutic agents, monoclonal antibodies, and immune effector cells. Such vascular barriers may provide an environment in which some tumor cells survive bloodborne chemotherapeutic and biologic agents. Thus, solid tumor nodules may serve as 'pharmacologic sanctuaries,' allowing even drug-sensitive tumor cells to continue to grow [42-44].

Hanna and co-workers [44] demonstrated that strategically timed chemotherapy subsequent to immunotherapy can effectively double the number of survivors attainable with immunotherapy alone. This effect was not drug specific. These results suggest a new basis for AST in the treatment of solid tumors. Inflammatory disruption of anatomic barriers of metastatic nodules combined with strategically administered chemotherapy or biotherapy may prove useful in the design of future biotherapy trials in humans.

Another approach might involve the delivery of lymphokines and cytokines, such as tumor necrosis factor, lymphotoxins, macrophage cytotoxic factors, and activated complexes (such as those generated by plasma perfusion over protein A columns) to the tumor and its vascular bed. These substances are known to have powerful effects on tumor vasculature, something leading to tumor necrosis. This approach may, in addition, increase the access of antibody, immunoconjugates, drugs, and activated cells to the cancer nodule [42].

A major limitation of AST has been the availability of purified TAA. Whereas the present vaccine preparations must contain viable, nontumorigenic cells prepared from individual tumors, it is possible that in the future monoclonal antibody-defined or genetically engineered, purified TAA will prompt large-scale immunization. TAA purification and characterization followed by genetic engineering of the antigen for vaccine production is underway. Alternatively, synthetic peptide sequences of the active portion of TAA may prove useful in the near future. Even the combining site of antibody to TAA has recently been suggested as a potential vaccine. These technologies are now undergoing preclinical and clinical evaluation.

Thymic factors

It has been known for years that thymic extracts have immunological activity [37, 38]. Thymosin fraction 5 and thymosin alpha-1 have received the most attention in the laboratory and the clinic. Thymosin fraction 5 is an extract containing a variety of thymic polypeptides, and alpha-1 is a synthetic polypeptide component present in many thymic extracts. Thymic preparations have been shown to enhance and suppress immune responses in both intact and thymectomized animals. Many investigators have reported that the thymosins can correct selected immunodeficiency states, both natural and experimentally induced. There have also been reports that thymic factors can augment suppressed or depressed T-cell responses in patients with cancer. Studies in preclinical screening have demonstrated stimulation of T-cell activity [91], but clinical studies have not shown striking effects [25, 90, 91].

Recombinant DNA technology

Recombinant DNA technology, commonly referred to as genetic engineering, has provided us with the tool for the biosynthesis and subsequent mass production of a significant number of biologicals [27, 36]. This is highly relevant to lymphokines/cytokines as well as growth and maturation factors, and should revolutionize the treatment of cancer over the next 10 years. The process involves the incorporation (recombination) of a segment of a DNA molecule containing a desired gene into a vector, usually a plasmid, which in turn is inserted into a host organism, usually an *Escherichia coli*, although other bacteria, yeasts, insects, and mammalian cells have been utilized. The cells are cloned and the cells producing the desired protein or polypeptide are selected. This clone is mass produced using fermentation techniques, and the protein molecule is harvested and purified. The resultant product is a highly purified (95-99%) protein solution, and has a high specific activity (i.e., biological activity per weight of protein).

The relevant DNA can be obtained by a variety of methods. Once messenger RNA (mRNA) is isolated, complementary DNA (cDNA) can be produced through the use of reverse transcriptase. Alternatively, an artificial DNA molecule can be constructed once the nucleotide or amino acid sequence is known. This can be used to isolate the complementary sequence, which is then isolated and cloned. RNA molecules can also be used in cell-free systems to produce these biologicals. There are available over 200 restriction enzymes that can cut desired fragments of DNA and lead to their isolation. These enzymes can uniquely cleave a DNA molecule at specific, predictable sites relative to the nucleotide sequence. These fragments are then incorporated into the plasmid, and combine with plasmid DNA. Plasmids have a symbiotic relationship with selected bacteria inducing resistance to a variety of antibiotics, which allows for selection of engineered clones. A number of alpha interferons, as well as beta and gamma interferon, have been genetically engineered [24, 36, 98, 103]; interleukin-2 and -3, colony-stimulating factor, and tumor necrosis factor have been cloned [99]. The number of cloned biological products increases yearly (see Chapter 4). These biological products (Table 4) are rapidly being translated into high-quality pharmaceuticals for clinical testing [8].

Table 4. Clinical lymphokines/Cytokines

Colony-stimulating factors
Erythropoietin
Interferons: α, β, γ
Interleukins 1-18, etc.
Lymphotoxins: α, β (TNF)
Macrophage activating factors
Thymosins
Transfer factor(s)

Lymphokines/Cytokines

Lymphokines and cytokines are molecules secreted by a variety of cells. They provide one means through which the cells involved in the immune process communicate with one another and direct the overall process [37]. Lymphokines/cytokines with specific effects on cell proliferation have been identified and may prove useful as anticancer agents. Interleukins (IL) 1-18 are among the multiple lymphokines that appear to be involved in a cascade phenomenon leading to the induction of a variety of immune responses [79]. Other examples include multiple subclasses of colony-stimulating factors (CSF). The list of lymphokines/cytokines is long, and the po-

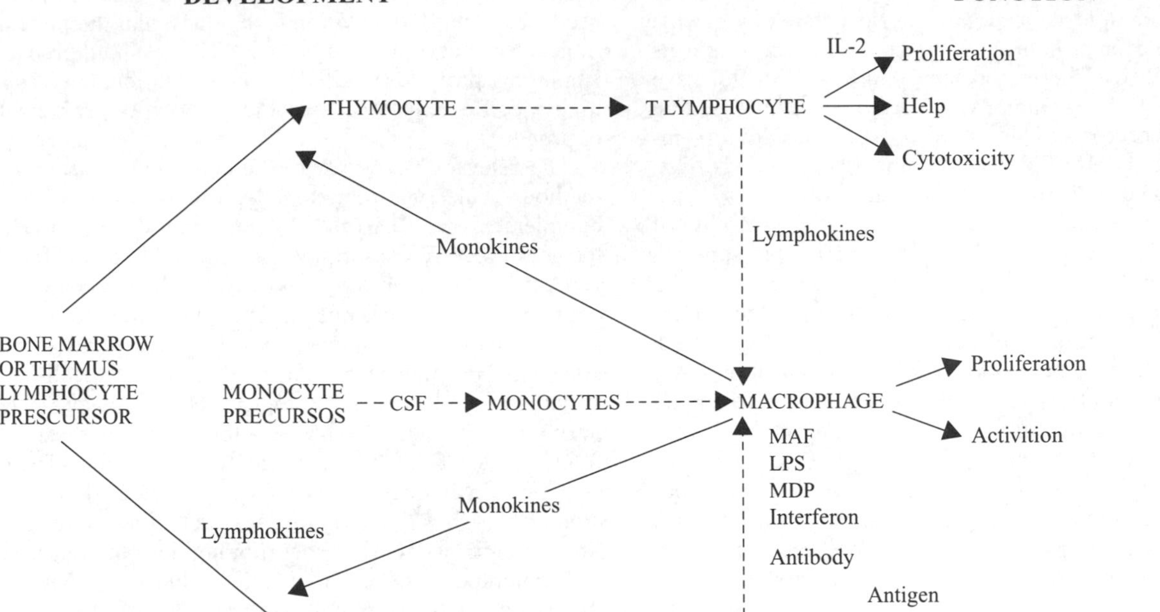

Figure 1. Immune response.

tential for therapeutic manipulation is great [68, 69]. The identification of these biological activities is the start of a process that should ultimately provide us with the knowledge and the tools to identify more accurately and control a number of immune responses. Physicians may then be able to manipulate the immune system (Fig. 1) intelligently, in favor of the host. Further, by selective activation and subsequent cloning *in vitro*, T-cell lines with specific cytotoxic capabilities can be obtained and utilized in autologous and allogeneic adoptive immunotherapy [16, 26, 86, 95, 104].

Many investigators have held the rather simplistic view that the immune system (Fig. 1) might be manipulated *in vivo* and corrected to better deal with the cancer problem. Evidence to date suggests that the pharmacologic use of biologicals, in rather high doses, is a more effective method for cancer treatment, with immunoactivation and immunomodulation, playing the dominant roles [64, 65].

Another specific use of lymphokines may be in the pharmacological regulation of tumors of the lymphoid system. Although many of these tumors are considered to be generally unresponsive to normal growth-controlling mechanisms mediated by lymphokines, it is possible that large quantities of pure lymphokines administered as medicinals, or the use of certain molecular analogs of these naturally occurring lymphokines, may be useful in the treatment of lymphoid malignancies. This hypothesis is suggested by the effectiveness of IL-2 with activated cells in the treatment of lymphoid malignancies. IL-2 can regulate chronic lymphocytic leukemia (CLL) almost as if they were normal lymphoid cells (R.K. Oldham, unpublished data).

The use of certain lymphokines/cytokines has been extended to other cancers, in that *in vitro* observations suggest an antiproliferative activity in some solid tumors. These antiproliferative effects might be maximized by testing the tumor cells of each patient to 'custom tailor' the treatment rather than giving these biologicals as general treatment, as has been done with anticancer drugs [65].

IL-1, originally known as lymphocyte activating factor, is a macrophage-derived cytokine that has an enhancing effect on murine thymocyte proliferation. Both IL-1 and viable macrophages are necessary for the initial step in activation of IL-2 (Fig. 2). Cloning of IL-1 and IL-2 has made large quantities of highly purified materials available for clinical studies.

Preclinical studies with IL-2 have been oriented around *in vitro* cell production protocols and induction or maintenance of antitumor T-cell effects *in vivo* [15, 16, 62, 65]. More recently, the use of IL-2 to activate peripheral blood cells has stimulated much interest [86, 104]. These activated cells are generally more cytotoxic against cancer cells than normal cells; however, their lineage can be T-cell or NK-cell (LAK cells) depending on the technique employed. This approach, though expensive and technically demanding, illustrates the rapidity with which developments in biotherapy are occurring [62, 65, 95].

A lymphotoxic product of antigen/mitogen-stimulated leukocytes was called lymphotoxin [85]. Lymphotoxin

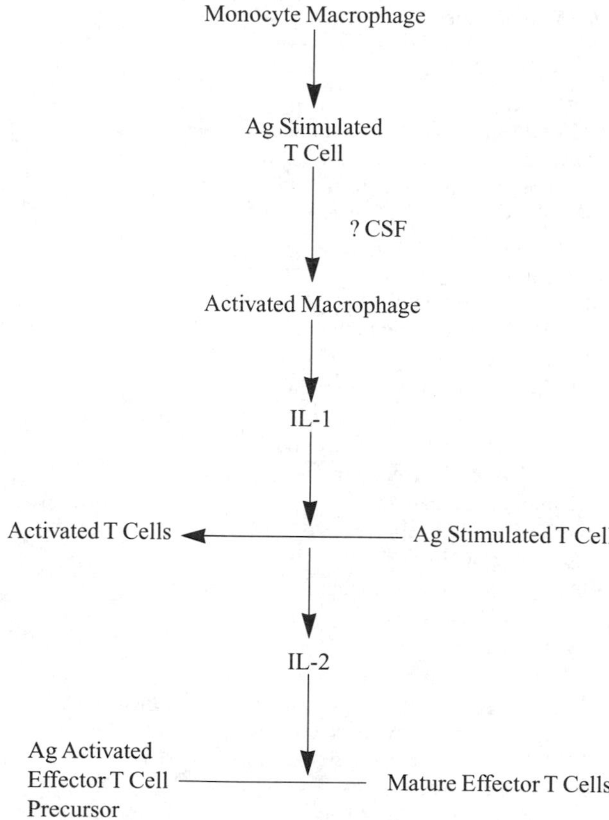

Figure 2. Model for interleukin stimulation of T-cell immune responses.

may be the principle effector of delayed hypersensitivity and, although conflicting data have been reported, may also be involved in the cytoxic reactions of T-cell-mediated lysis and NK- or K-cell lysis. Depending upon the type of tumor cell involved, the *in vitro* effect of lymphotoxin may be either cytolytic or cytostatic. Mouse tumor cells are frequently killed by homologous and heterologous lymphotoxins, whereas in other species reversible inhibition of tumor cell proliferation is more common [45].

Human lymphotoxin is of at least two species, alpha and beta [28, 35, 55, 81, 100]. Alpha lymphotoxin is tumor necrosis factor (TNF). Both have been cloned, and TNF has undergone rather extensive clinical trials [29, 93]. While some antitumor responses have been seen, the lymphotoxins have not been highly efficacious as single agents in the treatment of advanced human tumors and the toxicity of systemic administration has been unacceptable. Continued trials are underway combining lymphotoxins such as TNF with other lymphokine/cytokines and with chemotherapy. Targeted delivery of these molecules may prove more efficacious since they have high toxicity administered intravenously with what is probably minimal delivery to the tumor cell site [55]. Thus, intratumoral and regional perfusion studies with TNF have yielded positive results in patients with melanoma and sarcoma [17, 48, 54, 55, 83].

Combined treatments with lymphotoxin, administered locally or systemically, and other antitumor agents may be more valuable than lymphotoxin alone [84]. Lymphotoxin inhibits chemical- and radiation-induced neoplastic transformation [28]. Used as an adjunct to chemotherapy it may permit higher levels of effective but potentially carcinogenic agents to be used in cancer treatment with less risk of producing a second malignancy.

Lymphotoxin antitumor activity may be potentiated when it is given with other lymphokines such as interferon and IL-2 [6, 87, 92]. Lymphotoxins directly inhibit the growth of some tumor cells and also render these cells much more susceptible to NK-mediated lysis. Since interferon enhances the activity of NK cells, lymphotoxin and interferon given together or in sequence may result in more NK-mediated killing than is possible with either agent alone. There is now evidence that the combined use of various lymphokines may produce enhanced antiproliferative effects. Selective assays for lymphokine antiproliferative cocktails may prove useful in 'tailoring' such preparations for individual patients.

More than 100 biological molecules have already been described and named as lymphokines/cytokines (Table 5). Biologicals such as the interferons, lymphotoxins, TNF, CSF, IL-1-18 are now under evaluation (see Chapter 10). The studies require quantities of material sufficiently pure to exclude contributions by other factors and permit definitive evaluation of each lymphokine/cytokine. Larger-scale studies will require standardized preparations, in quantities best obtained through genetic engineering, using sensitive and rapid assay procedures to monitor production, purification, and bioavailability.

Interferons

Interferons are small, biologically active proteins with antiviral, antiproliferative, and immunomodulatory activities. Each interferon has distinctive capabilities in altering a variety of immunological and other biological responses. As a class, the interferons appear to have some growth-regulating capacity in that antiproliferative effects are measurable with *in vitro* assays and in animal model systems. The relative efficacy of the mixtures of natural interferons that occur after virus stimulation as compared to the cloned interferons remains to be precisely determined. There are more than 20 interferon molecules (and theoretically hundreds of recombinant hybrids therefrom), and attempts are underway to constitute mixtures of interferon for analysis. Efforts are underway altering individual interferon molecules in specific ways so the range of biological activities of the interferons as antiviral agents, as immunomodulating agents, and as antiproliferative agents may be very broad [61, 64].

In addition to antiviral and antiproliferative activity, the interferons have profound effects on the immune system. Low doses enhance antibody formation and lymphocyte

Table 5. Antigen-nonspecific mediators,[a] unrestricted by MHC

Helper factors
LAF (lymphocyte-activating factor, IL-1)
NMF (normal macrophage factor)
BAF (B-cell-activating factor)
TRF (T-cell-replacing factor)
MP (mitogenic protein)
TDF (thymus differentiation factor)
Transferrin
MF [mitogenic (blastogenic) factor]
NSF (nonspecific factor)
TDEF (T-cell-derived enhancing factor)
TEF (thymus extracted factor)
Complement components
DSRF (deficient serum-restoring factor)
Suppressor factors
Inhibitor(s) of DNA synthesis
AIM (antibody-inhibitory material)
IDA (inhibitor of DNA synthesis)
LTF (lymphoblastogenesis inhibition factor)
FIF (feedback inhibition factor)
MIFIF (Mif inhibition factor)
SIRS (soluble immune response suppressor)
IRF (immunoregulatory gamma-globulin)
Chalones
IF (interferons)
AFP (alpha-fetoprotein)
LDL (low-density lipoproteins)
CRP (C-reactive protein)
Fibrinogen degradation products
NIP (normal immunosuppressive protein)
LMWS (low-molecular-weight suppressor)
HSF (histamine-induced suppressor factor)
TCSF (T-cell suppressive factor)
Factors acting on inflammatory cells
MIF (migration inhibitory factor)
MCF (macrophage chemotactic factor)
MSF (macrophage slowing factor)
MEF (migration enhancement factor)
MAF (macrophage activating factor)
MFF (macrophage fusion factor)
PRS (pyrogen-releasing substance)
LIF (leukocyte inhibition factor)
NCF (neutrophil chemotactic factor)
PAR (products of antigenic recognition)
BCF (basophil chemotactic factor)
ECF (eosinophil chemotactic factor)
ESP (eosinophil stimulation promoter)
LCF (lymphocyte chemotactic factor)
LTF (lymphocyte trapping factor)
Factors acting on vascular endothelium
SRF (skin reactive factor)
TPF (thymic permeability factor)
LNPF (lymph node permeability factor)
LNAF (lymph node activating factor)
AIPF (anaphylactoid inflammation promoting factor)
IVPF (increased vascular permeability factor)

Table 5. (continued)

Factors acting on other cells
Interferons
TMIF (tumor cell migration inhibition factor)
OAF (osteoclast activating factor)
Fibroblast chemotactic factor
Pyrogens
FAF (fibroblast activating factor)
Growth-stimulating factors
BCGF (B-cell growth factor)
BCGF (B-cell differentiation factor)
MGF (macrophage growth factor)
MF [mitogenic (blastogenic) factor]
LIAF (lymphocyte-induced angiogenesis factor)
CSF (colony-stimulating factor)
TDF (thymus differentiation factor)
Thymopoietin, thymosin
TCGF (T-cell growth factor, IL-2)
IL-3 (interleukin 3)
EGF (epidermal growth factor)
Direct-acting factors
Lysosomal enzymes
CTF (cytotoxic factors)
MTF or MCF [macrophage toxic (cytotoxic) factor]
SMC (specific macrophage cytotoxin)
MCF (macrophage cytolytic factor)
ACT (adherent cell toxin)
Chromosomal breakage factors
Microbecidal factors
LT (lymphotoxin)
PIF (proliferation inhibitory factor)
CIF (cloning inhibition factor)
IDS (inhibitory of DNA synthesis)
Transforming factors
TNF (tumor necrosis factor)

[a] These names/factors are based on biological activity. Several may be the activity of single molecule.

blastogenesis, while higher doses inhibit these functions. Low to moderate doses may inhibit delayed hypersensitivity while enhancing macrophage phagocytosis and cytotoxicity, natural killer activity, and surface antigen expression. Interferons prolong and inhibit cell division (both transformed and normal cells). In addition, interferon stimulates the induction of several intracellular enzyme systems with resultant profound effect on macromolecular activities and protein synthesis. All of these functions have been documented in murine systems, but complete dose-response effects for all types of interferons in these cellular activities have not been thoroughly investigated in either the mouse or human.

We can draw some preliminary conclusions about interferon therapy for human cancer [9, 52, 64] (Tables 6 and 7). One is that the Cantell, lymphoblastoid, and recombinant alpha-interferons are surprisingly similar, both quantitatively and qualitatively, in their toxicity, antitumor

Table 6. Alpha interferon activity*

Active
Hairy-cell leukemia
Chronic myelogenous leukemia
Myeloproliferative disorders
Non-Hodgkin's lymphoma
Cutaneous T-cell lymphoma
Kaposi's sarcoma
Multiple myeloma
Melanoma
Renal-cell cancer
Bladder cancer (intravesical)
Inactive
Breast cancer
Colon cancer
Lung cancer
Prostate cancer
Acute myelogenous leukemia
Further study required
Chronic lymphocytic leukemia
Acute lymphocytic leukemia
Ovarian cancer (intraperitoneal)
Hodgkin's disease
Sarcomas
Brain tumors

*As a single agent.

efficacy, and other biologic effects. Second, objectively defined antitumor responses in phase I alpha-interferon trials (mostly involving leukemia, lymphoma, myeloma, Kaposi's sarcoma, melanoma, and renal cancer) have been observed in approximately 10% of all patients treated. That level of activity may not seem impressive, but it does compare favorably with an average response rate of 1-2% in phase I trials of recently developed chemotherapeutic agents. We should also note that very few responses in patients with tumors of the breast, colon, lung, or lower genitourinary system have been seen with alpha-interferon as a single agent. Overall, even though interferons have toxicities, they were more tolerable and less permanent than those observed in early-phase chemotherapy testing.

A third impression, suggested by increased response rates with higher alpha-interferon doses, is that interferons may produce their acute antitumor effect by a direct cytostatic action, rather than an indirect immunomodulatory mechanism. Finally, preliminary clinical experience with beta- and gamma-interferons indicates that both produce response rates and response patterns different from those obtained with alpha-interferon, even though gamma-interferon has exhibited higher specific activity in the preclinical studies.

With respect to cancer therapeutics, it is still unclear whether the interferons work primarily by their antiproliferative activity or through alterations of immune responses. Most of the current evidence with lymphoma supports a direct antiproliferative effect in that higher doses induce more responses, and patients failing in lower doses can be reinduced to response to higher doses [12, 34, 52, 61, 64, 67, 88]. What is clear from the current preclinical and clinical studies is that the interferons have antitumor activity even in bulky, drug-resistant cancers [94]. Clinical activity has been seen most reproducibly in several lymphomas and leukemias (Table 7), but responses in many other tumor types have been seen. The combination of alpha-interferon and 5-fluorouracil (and 'double modulation' adding folinic acid) has been encouraging in phase II trials in untreated patients with colorectal cancer, but not as salvage therapy [40, 41, 102]. The best dose, schedule, route of administration, and type of interferon need to be determined by further efficacy studies, and the use of interferon in combination with other anticancer agents is very promising [23, 52, 60].

Table 7. Hematologic malignancies: summary of responses to alpha-interferon*

Tumor type	Response rate (%)
Multiple myeloma	18-27
Chronic lymphocytic leukemia	0-77
Hairy-cell leukemia	80-90
Low-grade lymphoma	38-73
High-grade lymphoma	0-10
Kaposi's sarcoma	25-40
Chronic myelogenous leukemia	80-90

* Adapted from ref. 9.

Growth and maturation factors

Using technology similar to that employed for lymphokine/cytokines, scientists have recently cloned and produced a variety of growth and maturation factors. The clinical trials have focused mainly on erythropoietin and the colony-stimulating factors. The former is a drug now approved for use in refractory anemia, and GM-CSF and GCSF approved for the treatment of bone marrow dysplasia and chemotherapy-induced marrow suppression. Stimulating factors for platelet production are nearing approval. These factors are reviewed in later chapters, but it should be noted that they represent only the early beginnings of the very broad field of growth and maturation factors (See Chapter 18). It is now clear that a variety of biological substances up- and down-regulate growth of both normal and neoplastic cells. These substances may stimulate or inhibit growth and may change the maturation cycle of various normal and neoplastic cells. Contained within this broad category of factors are the tumor growth factors, colony-stimulating factors, and a variety of still to be defined factors important in the regulation of cell growth and maturation. Future therapeutic use of these factors may regulate growth and spread of cancer. Such a chronic growth restraining strategy may not 'cure' cancer; rather treatment may be more analogous to using insulin in diabetes. This is a field that is undergoing explosive growth and should be watched carefully over the coming decade for molecules with therapeutic activity.

Monoclonal antibodies

The advent of hybridoma technology in the late 1970s made available an important tool for the production of monoclonal antibodies for therapeutic trials [10]. These antibodies are now being produced in huge quantities and in highly purified form for cancer treatment. They will undoubtedly define a whole new range of antigens on the cell surfaces, which will improve our understanding of cell differentiation and of cancer biology. Major problems in understanding the biology of the cancer cell have been the difficulties of isolating, purifying, and characterizing tumor-associated antigens (TAA). The use of monoclonal antibody technology will improve the definition of the neoplastic cell surface and identify its differences from the normal counterpart. This will be of great value in cancer diagnosis and histopathologic classification, and will be useful in the imaging of tumor cell masses and in the therapy of cancer [1, 7, 13, 14, 32, 33, 46, 47, 50, 58, 70, 82]. Finally, antibodies may be useful reagents in treating certain immune deficiencies and in altering immune responses. The removal of T cells from bone marrow to improve bone marrow transplantation techniques is an example of using antibody as a BRM [58].

In spite of encouraging data from the use of antibodies and, especially, immunoconjugates to target toxic substances to cancer, the heterogeneity of cancer is an important consideration [2, 71-73, 80]. If a single antibody or a fixed combination of a few antibodies covering only a portion of the tumor cells is used, and if that preparation does not eliminate the true replicating cell population (stem cell) from the patient's tumor population, eventual outgrowth of viable, perhaps resistant cells is inevitable. Therefore, it seems logical to proceed with attempts to type human tumors and to deliver toxic substances to them utilizing 'cocktails' of antibodies sufficient to cover all the tumor cells suspected of replication in each patient. This type of approach may require a considerable amount of testing for each patient and a 'typing' of one or more tumors from each patient [3, 53, 57, 73, 74, 80]. Such approaches may be more individually designed than is easily approachable through the product development paradigm that has been used in the development of new anticancer drugs. If however, the spectrum of human tumor heterogeneity is great, the goal of the ideal antibody conjugated to the ideal toxic agent may not be achievable.

FUTURE PERSPECTIVES

How rapidly will biotherapy develop and what role will it have in cancer treatment in the next decade? It is certain that we now have much more powerful tools for improving cancer therapy in the future. We now have the techniques to decipher the major problems in cancer biology down to the genetic level. These techniques, along with the recognition that biotherapy can provide increased selectivity in cancer treatment, support the belief that new and highly effective approaches are near. Biotherapy provides an additional technique, which may work most effectively in combination with surgery or radiotherapy (to decrease the local and regional tumor) or with chemotherapy (to reduce the systemic tumor burden). It may work very effectively via antibodies in directing radioisotopes selectively to the tumor site, and with chemotherapy, toxins, and other cytostatic or cytotoxic molecules in directing the agent to the tumor bed, enhancing activity and selectivity.

The use of biotherapy is at an early stage. We have already seen that highly purified biologicals can be effective in patients with clinically apparent, even advanced, bulky cancer. Clinical studies with alpha-interferon have now demonstrated the responsiveness of radiation- and drug-resistant lymphoma, melanoma, and renal carcinoma. IL-2 with effector cells or alone (in high doses) produces partial and complete remissions in melanoma and kidney cancer. These results, along with the early clinical results using monoclonal antibody in selected cancers (lymphoma, melanoma, gastrointestinal and breast cancer), confirm the concept that we need not think of biotherapy as a tool that can be used only in patients with undetectable and minimal residual tumor burdens. While this modality may work best with minimal tumor burdens (a situation that is also true for chemotherapy), biotherapy can be used as a single modality in clinically apparent disease. It may be even more effective in multimodality treatment regimens. Biotherapy offers the hope for selective treatment to enhance the therapeutic/toxic ratio and lessen the problem of nonspecific toxicity, a major impediment to the development of more effective anticancer treatment. It is particularly encouraging to see a 10% response rate in phase I trials with alpha-interferon and 10-30% response rate with IL-2 in comparison with a 1-2% early response rate with new chemotherapeutic agents. In addition, very encouraging preliminary results are now being seen with combination biotherapy-chemotherapy trials (i.e., interferon – 5-fluorouracil in colon cancer).

This decade will provide many opportunities to pursue new approaches in cancer treatment. These approaches will employ new techniques in the laboratory and clinic, requiring special training and expertise. The medical oncologist of the 1970s and 1980s, trained in the administration of chemotherapy drugs, is not necessarily qualified to give biologicals for cancer treatment. Biotherapy uses biological substances that are often active on, or work in association with, the immune system. The tremendous diversity of this system is best understood by clinical immunologists and cell biologists who are well suited to assist in the translation of biotherapeutic approaches to the clinic.

Given these new techniques and new approaches, we must redesign many of the mechanisms for developmental therapeutics [59]. It may well be that the specificity of biologicals will require that biotherapy be developed in an individualistic fashion and applied to each patient in a specific way. This concept was conceptualized in 1977 by the Nobel laureate Sir Peter Medawar:

> 'The cure of cancer is never going to be found. It is far more likely that each tumor in each patient is going to present a unique research problem for which laboratory workers and clinicians between them will have to work out a unique solution.'

We must be prepared to change and adapt to the challenges and opportunities afforded by biotherapy in the years ahead.

REFERENCES

1. Abrams P, Oldham RK. Monoclonal antibody therapy of solid tumors. In: Foon KA, Morgan AC, Jr., eds. *Monoclonal antibody therapy of human cancer.* The Hague: Martinus Nijhoff, 1985: 103-120.
2. Abrams PG, Morgan AC, Schroff RW, et al. Monoclonal antibodies in cancer therapy: drug-antibody conjugates. In: *Localization and biodistribution studies of a monoclonal antibody in patients with melanoma.* Reisfeld and Sell (Eds.) Alan R. Liss, New York 27:233-236, 1985.
3. Avner BP, Liao SK, Avner B, et al. Therapeutic murine monoclonal antibodies developed for individual cancer patients. *J Biol Response Modif* 1989; 8(1):25-36.
4. Baldwin, RW. Relevant animal models for immunotherapy. *Cancer Immunol Immunother* 1976; 1:97-206.
5. Balkwill FR, Burke F. The cytokine network. *Immunol Today* 1989; 10(9):29-304.
6. Balkwill FR, Lee A, Aldam G, et al. Human tumor xenografts treated with recombinant human tumor necrosis factor alone or in combination with interferons. *Cancer Res* 1986; 46:3990-3993.
7. Bernhard MI, Foon KA, Oeltmann TN, et al. Guinea pig line 10 hepatocarcinoma model: Characterization of monoclonal antibody and *in vivo* effect of unconjugated antibody and antibody conjugated to diphtheria toxin A chain. *Cancer Res* 1983; 43:4420-4428.
8. Bollon AP, Barron EA, Berent SL, et al. Recombinant DNA techniques: isolation, cloning and expression of genes. In: Bollon AP, ed. Recombinant DNA products: Insulin interferon and growth hormone. Boca Raton, Fl.: *CRC Press*, 1984: 1-35.
9. Bonnem EM, Spregel RJ. Interferon-alpha: Current status and future promise. *J Biol Response Modif* 1984; 3:580.
10. Boss BD, Langman R, Trowbridge I, Dulbecco R, eds. *Monoclonal antibodies and cancer*. New York: Academic Press, 1983: 1-200.
11. Boyd MR. Status of the NCI preclinical antitumor drug discovery screen. *Prin Pract Oncol Suppl* 1989;3(10):1-12.
12. Bunn PA, Foon KA, Ihde DC, et al. Recombinant leukocyte A interferon: An active agent in advanced cutaneous T-cell lymphomas. *Ann Intern Med* 1984; 101:484-487.
13. Carrasquillo JA, Bunn PA Jr, Kennan AM, et al. Radioimmunodetection of cutaneous T-cell lymphoma with 111In-T101 monoclonal antibody. *New Engl J Med* 1986; 315:673-680.
14. Carrasquillo JA, Abrams PG, Schroff R, et al. Effect of antibody dose on the imaging and biodistribution of indium-111 9.2.27 anti-melanoma monoclonal antibody. *J Nucl Med* 1988; January, 29(1):39-47.
15. Cheever MA, Greenberg PD, Fefer A, Gillis S. Augmentation of the antitumor therapeutic efficacy of long-term cultured T lymphocytes by *in vivo* administration of purified interleukin-2. *J Exp Med* 1982; 155:968-980.
16. Cheever MA, Greenberg PD, Fefer A. Potential for specific cancer therapy with immune T lymphocytes. *J Biol Response Modif* 1984; 3:113-127.
17. Cumberlin R, DeMoss E, Lassus M, Friedman M. Isolation perfusion for malignant melanoma of the extremity: a review. *J Clin Oncol* 1985; 3:1022-1031.
18. DeVita VT. Progress in cancer management: keynote address. *Cancer* 1983; 51:2401-2409.
19. DeVita VT. The relationship between tumor mass and resistance to chemotherapy: implication for surgical adjuvant treatment of cancer. *Cancer* 1983; 51:1209-1220.
20. DeVita VT, Hellman S, Rosenberg SA, eds. *Important advances in oncology* 1989. New York: J.B. Lippincott, 1995: 1-118.
21. DeVita VT Jr, Hellman S, Rosenberg SA, eds. In: Biologic *Therapy of Cancer*, Second Edition. Philadelphia, J.B. Lippincott Company, 1995:295-327.
22. DeVita VT Jr, Hellman S, Rosenberg SA, eds. In: *Biologic Therapy of Cancer*, Second Edition. Philadelphia, J.B. Lippincott Company, 1995:329-345.
23. DeVita VT Jr, Hellman S, Rosenberg SA, eds. In: Biologic Therapy of Cancer, Second Edition. Philadelphia, J.B. Lippincott Company, 1995:427-433.
24. Devos R, Cheroutre H, Taya Y, et al. Molecular cloning of human immune interferon cDNA and its expression in eukaryotic cells. *Nucl Acids Res* 1982; 10:2487-2501.
25. Dillman RO, Beauregard JC, Mendelsohn J, et al. Phase I trials of thymosin fraction 5 and thymosin alpha-1. *J Biol Response Modif* 1982; 1:35-41.
26. Eberlein TJ, Rosenstein M, Spiess P, et al. Adoptive chemoimmunotherapy of a synergeneic murine lymphoma with long-term lymphoid cell lines expanded in T-cell growth factor. *Cancer Immunol Immunother* 1982; 13:5-13.
27. Emery AEH. Recombinant DNA technology. *Lancet* 1981; 2:1406-1409.
28. Evans CH, Lymphotoxin: an immunologic hormone with anticarcinogenic and antitumor activity. *Cancer Immunol Immunother* 1982; 12:181-190.
29. Feinberg B, Kurzrock R, Talpaz M, et al. A phase I trial of intravenously-administered recombinant tumor necrosis factor-alpha in cancer patients. *J Clin Oncol* 1988; 6:1328-1334.
30. Fidler IJ, Gersten DM, Hart IR. The biology of cancer invasion and metastasis. Adv Cancer Res 1978; 28:149-250.
31. Fidler IJ, Berendt M, Oldham RK. The rationale for and design of screening assays for the assessment of biological response modifiers for cancer treatment. *J Biol Response Modif* 1982; 1:15-26.

32. Foon KA, Bernhard MI, Oldham RK. Monoclonal antibody therapy: assessment by animal tumor models. *J Biol Response Modif* 1982; 1:277-304.
33. Foon KA, Schroff R, Bunn PA, et al. Effects of monoclonal antibody therapy in patients with chronic lymphocytic leukemia. *Blood* 1984; 64:1085-1093.
34. Foon KA, Sherwin SA, Abrams PG, et al. Treatment of advanced non-Hodgkin's lymphoma with recombinant leukocyte A interferon. *N Engl J Med* 1984; 311:1148-1152.
35. Gamm H, Lindemann A, Mertelsmann R, Herrmann F. Phase I trial of recombinant human tumour necrosis factor α in patients with advanced malignancy. *Eur J Cancer* 1991; 27:856-863.
36. Goeddel DV, Yelverton E, Ullrich A, et al. Human leucocyte interferon produce by *E. coli* is biologically active. *Nature* 1980; 287:411-416.
37. Goldstein AL, Chirigos MA, eds. *Lymphokines and thymic hormones; their potential utilization in cancer therapeutics. Progress in cancer research and therapy*, vol. 20. New York: Raven Press, 1981.
38. Goldstein AL, Chirigos MA. In: *Progress in cancer research and therapy*, vol. 20. New York: Raven Press, 1982: 1-324.
39. Gray PSW, Leung DW, Pennica D, et al. Expression of human immune interferon cDNA in *E. coli* and monkey cells. *Nature* 1982; 295:503-508.
40. Grem JL, Hoth D, Hamilton MJ, et al. An overview of the current status and future direction of clinical trials of 5-fluorouracil and folinic acid. *Cancer Treat Rep* 1987; 71:1249-64.
41. Grem JL, McAtee N, Murphy RF, et al. A pilot study of interferon alfa-2a in combination with fluorouracil plus high-dose leucovorin in metastatic gastrointestinal carcinoma. *J Clin Oncol* 1991; 9:1811-20.
42. Hanna MG, Key ME, Oldham RK. Biology of cancer therapy: some new insights into adjuvant treatment of metastatic solid tumors. *J Biol Response Modif* 1983; 4:295-309.
43. Hanna MG, Jr., Brandhorst JS, Peters LC. Active specific immunotherapy of residual micrometastasis: an evaluation of sources, doses and ratios of BCG with tumor cells. *Cancer Immunol Immunother* 1979; 7:165-174.
44. Hanna MG, Jr., Key ME. Immunotherapy of metastases enhances subsequent chemotherapy. *Science* 1982; 217:367-370.
45. Haranaka K. Macrophage Symposium 1987, *Tumor Necrosis Factor*. Japan, January 5-8, 1987.
46. Hwang KM, Foon KA, Cheung PH, et al. Selective antitumor effect on L-10 hepatocarcinoma cella of a potent immunoconjugate composed of the A chain of abrin and a monoclonal antibody to a hepatoma-associated antigen. *Cancer res* 1984; 44:4578-4586.
47. Hwang KM, Keenan AM, Frincke J, et al. Dynamic interaction of 111 indium-labeled monoclonal antibodies with surface of solid tumors visualized *in vivo* by external scintigraphy. *J Natl Cancer Inst* 1986; 76:849-855.
48. Kahn JO, Kaplan LD, Volberding PA, et al. Intralesional recombinant tumor necrosis factor-α for AIDS-associated Kaposi's sarcoma. A randomized, double-blind trial. *J Acquir Immune Defic Syndr* 1989; 2:217-223.
49. Kallman RF, ed. Rodent tumor models in experimental cancer therapy. New York: *Pergamon Press*, 1987: 1-310.
50. Key ME, Bernhard MI, Hoyer LC, et al. Guinea pig 10 hepatocarcinoma model for monoclonal antibody serotherapy: *In vivo* localization of a monoclonal antibody in normal and malignant tissues. *J Immunol* 1983; 139:1451-1457.
51. Key ME, Brandhorst JS, Hanna MC, Jr. Synergistic effects of active specific immunotherapy and chemotherapy in guinea pigs with disseminated cancer. *J Immunol* 1983; 130:2987-2992.
52. Kirkwood JM, Ernstoff MS. Interferon in the treatment of human cancer. *J Clin Oncol* 1984; 2:336-352.
53. Liao SK, Meranda C, Avner BP, et al. Immunohistochemical phenotyping of human solid tumors with monoclonal antibodies in devising biotherapeutic strategies. *Cancer Immunol Immunother* 1989; 28:77-86.
54. Lienard D, Ewalenko P, Delmitti JJ, et al. High-dose recombinant tumor necrosis factor alpha in combination with interferon gamma and melphalan in isolation perfusion of the limbs for melanoma and sarcoma. *J Clin Oncol* 1992; 10:52-60.
55. Mavligit GM, Zukiwski AA, Charnsargavej C. Regional biologic therapy: hepatic arterial infusion of recombinant human tumor necrosis factor in patients with liver metastases. *Cancer* 1992; 69:557-561.
56. McCormick DL, Adamowski CB, Fiks A, Moon RC. Lifetime dose-response relationships for mammary tumor induction by a single administration of *N*-methyl-*N*-nitrosourea. *Cancer Res* 1981; 41:1690-1694.
57. Ogden JR, Leung K, Kundra SA, et al. Immunoconjugates of doxorubicin and murine antihuman breast carcinoma monoclonal antibodies prepared via an n-hydroxysuccinimide active ester intermediate of cis-aconityl-doxorubicin: preparation and *in vitro* cytotoxicity. *Mol Biother* 1989; 1(3):170-174.
58. Oldham, RK. Monoclonal antibodies in cancer therapy. *J Clin Oncol* 1983; 1:582-590.
59. Oldham RK. Biologicals: new horizons in pharmaceutical development. *J Biol Response Modif* 1983; 2:199-206.
60. Oldham RK. Biologicals and biological response modifiers: new strategies for clinical trials. In: Finter NB, Oldham RK, eds. Interferons IV. Amsterdam: *Elsevier Science*, 1985: 235-249.
61. Oldham RK. Interferon: a model for future biological. In: Burke D, Cantell K, Gresser I, DeMaeyer E, Landy M, Revel M, Vilcek J, eds. Interferon VI. New York: *Academic Press*, 1985: 127-143.
62. Oldham RK. *In vivo* effects of interleukin 2. *J Biol Response Modif* 1984; 3:455-532.
63. Oldham RK. Biologicals and biological response modifiers: the fourth modality of cancer treatment. *Cancer Treatment Rep* 1984; 68:221-232.
64. Oldham RK. Biologicals for cancer treatment: interferons. *Hospital Pract* 1985; 20:72-91.
65. Oldham RK. Biotherapy: the fourth modality of cancer treatment. 1986; 4:91-99.
66. Oldham RK, Smalley RV. Immunotherapy: the old and the new. *J Biol Response Modif* 1983; 2:1-37.
67. Oldham RK, Smalley RV. The role of interferon in the treatment of cancer. In: Zoon KC, Noguchi PC, Lui T-Y, eds. Interferon: research, clinical application and regulatory consideration. Amsterdam: *Elsevier Science*, 1984: 191-205.
68. Oldham RK, Smalley RV. Biological and biological response modifiers. In: DeVita VT, Hellman S, Rosenberg

SA, eds. *Cancer: principles and practice of oncology*. Philadelphia: J.B. Lippincott, 1985; 2223-2245.

69. Oldham RK, Thurman GB, Talmadge JE, et al. Lymphokines, monoclonal antibodies and other biological response modifiers in the treatment of cancer. *Cancer* 1984; 54:2795-2810.
70. Oldham RK, Foon KA, Morgan AC, et al. Monoclonal antibody therapy of malignant melanoma: *In vivo* localization in cutaneous metastasis after intravenous administration. *J Clin Oncol* 1984; 2:1235-1242.
71. Oldham RK. Perspectives on the use of immunotoxins in clinical medicine. In: Immunoconjugates: antibody conjugates in radioimaging and therapy of cancer. Vogel C-W (Ed.), New York, *Oxford Univ. Press*, 281-289, 1987.
72. Oldham RK. Therapeutic monoclonal antibodies: effects of tumor cell heterogeneity. In: Therapeutic monoclonal antibodies: effects of tumor cell heterogeneity. S. Karger Ag. *Cancer Treatment Symposium* (Germany), 1988.
73. Oldham RK, Lewis M, Orr DW, et al. Adriamycin custom-tailored immunoconjugates in the treatment of human malignancies. *Mol Biother* 1988; 1(2):103-113.
74. Oldham RK, Lewis M, Orr DW, et al. Individually specified drug immunoconjugates in cancer treatment. Ceriani RL (Ed.) In: Breast cancer immunodiagnosis and immunotherapy. *Plenum Publishing*. 219-230, 1990.
75. Oldham RK. Gene therapy and cancer: Is it for everyone? *Cancer Investigation* 1992; 10(6):607-609.
76. Oldham RK. Cancer biotherapy: 1993 to the Millenium and more! *Cancer Biotherapy* 1993; 8(1):1-2.
77. Oldham RK. Cancer biotherapy: the first year. *Cancer Biotherapy* 1994; 9(3):179-181.
78. Oldham RK, Lewko W, Good R, et al. Growth of tumor derived activated T-cells for the treatment of cancer. *Cancer Biotherapy* 1994; 9(3):211-224.
79. Oppenheim JJ, Stadler BM, Siraganian RP, et al. Lymphokines: their role in lymphocyte responses properties of interleukin 1. *Fed Proc* 1982; 41:257-262.
80. Orr DW, Oldham RK, Lewis M, et al. Phase I trial of mitomycin-c immunoconjugate cocktails in human malignancies. *Mol Biother* 1989; 1(4):229-240.
81. Palladino MA, Shalaby MR, Kramer SM,et al. Characterization of the antitumor activities of human tumor necrosis factor-alpha, and the comparison with other cytokines: induction of tumor specific immunity. *J Immunol* 1987; 138:4023-4032.
82. Paranasivam G, Pearson JW, Bohn W, et al. Immunotoxins fo a human melanoma-associated antigen: comparison of gelonin with ricin and other a-chain conjugates. *Cancer Res* 1987; 47:3169-3173.
83. Pfreundschuh MG, Steinmetz HT, Tuschen R, et al. Phase I study of intratumoral application of recombinant human tumor necrosis factor. *Eur J Cancer Clin Oncol* 1989; 25:379-388.
84. Regenass U, Muller M, Curschellas E, Matter A. Antitumor effects of tumor necrosis factor in combination with chemotherapeutic agents. *Int J Cancer* 1987; 39:266-273.
85. Rosenau W. Lymphotoxin: properties, role and mode of action. *Int J Immunopharm* 1981; 3:1-8.
86. Rosenberg SA, Lotze MT, Muul LM,et al. Observations on the systemic administration of autologous lymphokine-activated killer cells and recombinant interleukin-2 to patients with metastatic cancer. *N Engl J Med* 1985; 313:1485-1492.
87. Schiller JH, Witt PL, Storer B, et al. Clinical and biologic effects of combination therapy with gamma-interferon and tumor necrosis factor. *Cancer* 1992; 69:562-571.
88. Sherwin SA, Knost JA, Fein S, et al. A multiple dose Phase I trial of recombinant leukocyte A interferon in cancer patients. *J Am Med Assoc* 1982; 248:2461-2466.
89. Smalley RV, Long CW, Sherwin SA, Oldham RK. Biological response modifiers: current status and prospects as anticancer agents. In: Herberman RB, ed. *Basic and clinical tumor immunology*. The Hague: Martinus Nijhoff, 1983: 257-300.
90. Smalley RV, Oldham RK. Biological response modifiers: preclinical evaluation and clinical activity. CRC *Crit Rev Oncol/Hematol* 1984; 1:259-280.
91. Smalley RV, Talmadge JA, Oldham RK, Thurman GB. The thymosins: preclinical and clinical studies with fraction V and alpha-1. *Cancer Treatment Rev* 1984; 11:69-84.
92. Smith JW, Urba WJ, Clark JW, et al. Phase I evaluation of recombinant tumor necrosis factor given in combination with recombinant interferon-gamma. *J Immunother* 1991; 10:355-362.
93. Spriggs DR, Sherman ML, Michie H, et al. Recombinant human tumor necrosis factor administered as a 24-hour intravenous infusion. A Phase I and Pharmacologic Study. *J Natl Cancer Inst* 1988; 80:1039-1044.
94. Stevenson HC, Ochs JJ, Halverson L, et al. Recombinant alpha interferon in retreatment of two patients with pulmonary lymphoma, dramatic responses with resolution of pulmonary complications. *Am J Med* 1984; 77:355-358.
95. Stevenson HC, eds. Adoptive cellular immunotherapy of cancer. New York: Marcel Dekker, 1989: 1-236.
96. Stringfellow DA, Smalley RV. Interferon inducers for clinical use. In: Finter N, Oldham RK, eds. *In vivo* application of interferons. Amsterdam: *Elsevier Science*, 1984.
97. Talmadge JE, Maluish AE, Collins M, et al. Immunomodulation and antitumor effects of MVE-2 in mice. *J Biol Response Modif* 1984; 3:634-652.
98. Taniguchi T, Mantei N, Schwarzstein M, et al. Human leukocyte and fibroblast interferons are structurally related. *Nature* 1980; 285:2848-2852.
99. Tanguichi T, Matsui H, Fujita T, et al. Structure and expression of cloned cDNA for human interleukin-2. *Nature* 1983; 302:305-310.
100. Taguchi T. Phase I study of recombinant human tumor necrosis factor (rHu-TNF:PT-050). *Cancer Detect Prev* 1988; 12:561-572.
101. Terry MD, Rosenberg SA, eds. Immunotherapy of cancer. New York: *Excerpta Medica*, 1982: 1-398.
102. Wadler S, Lembersky B, Atkins M, et al. Phase II trial of fluorouracil and recombinant interferon alfa-2a in patients with colorectal carcinoma: an Eastern Cooperative Oncology Group study. *J Clin Oncol* 1991; 9:1806-10.
103. Weissman C, Nagata S, Boll W, et al. Structure and expression of human alpha interferon genes. In: Miwa M, et al., eds. Primary and tertiary structure of nucleic acids and cancer research. Tokyo: *Japan Science Society Press*, 1982: 1-22.
104. West WH, Tauer KW, Yannelli JR, et al. Constant infusion recombinant interleukin-2 in adoptive immunotherapy of advanced cancer. *N Engl J Med* 1987; 316(15):898-905.

2

THE PATHOGENESIS OF CANCER METASTASIS: RELEVANCE TO BIOTHERAPY

ROBERT RADINSKY, SHARON L. AUKERMAN and ISAIAH J. FIDLER
Department of Cell Biology, The University of Texas M. D. Anderson Cancer Center, Houston, Texas

INTRODUCTION

Metastasis – the spread of malignant tumor cells from a primary neoplasm to distant parts of the body where they multiply to form new growths – is a major cause of death from cancer. The treatment of cancer poses a major problem to clinical oncologists, because by the time many cancers are diagnosed, metastasis may already have occurred, and the presence of multiple metastases makes complete eradication by surgery, radiation, drugs, or biotherapy nearly impossible (Table 1). Metastases can be located in different organs and in different locations within the same organ. These aspects significantly influence the response of tumor cells to therapy and the efficiency of anticancer drugs, which must be delivered to tumor foci in amounts sufficient to destroy cells without leading to undesirable side effects. Similarly, immune effector cells of current biotherapeutic regimens may have difficulty reaching or localizing in some metastatic sites.

Exacerbating the problems of treating metastatic disease is the fact that tumor cells in different metastases and in some instances even different regions within an individual metastatic lesion may respond differently to treatment. Although numerous promising anticancer drugs and biotherapeutic agents have been developed, their effectiveness is still hindered by the presence and accumulation of resistant cells within tumors. Tumor cell resistance to current therapeutic modalities is the single most important reason for the lack of success in treating many types of solid neoplasms. In part, the emergence of treatment-resistant tumor cells is due to the heterogeneous nature of malignant neoplasms. Indeed, this phenotypic diversity, which permits selected variants to develop from the parent tumor, implies not only that the primary tumor and metastases can differ in their response to treatment but also that individual metastases can differ markedly from one another.

Table 1. Limiting factors in cancer therapy

Limited range and efficacy of current modalities
Limited selectivity of available agents
Limited exploitable biochemical differences between normal and neoplastic cells
Limited drug distribution
Host toxicity
Metastatic disease
Intrinsic or acquired tumor cell resistance
Tumor cell heterogeneity
Tumor cell responses to organ-derived cytokines and growth factors

Insight into the molecular mechanisms regulating the pathobiology of cancer metastasis as well as a better understanding of the interaction between the metastatic cell and the host environment should provide a foundation for the design of new therapeutic approaches. Furthermore, the development of *in vivo* and *in vitro* models that will allow for the isolation and characterization of cells possessing metastatic potential within both primary tumors and metastases will be invaluable in the design of more effective and safe therapeutic modalities. In this chapter, we summarize data dealing with the biology of cancer metastasis with special emphasis on recent reports from our laboratories demonstrating that the organ microenvironment can profoundly influence the biologic behavior of metastatic tumor cells, including resistance to chemotherapy [44, 70, 252, 295], the production of degradative enzymes [50, 89, 183], angiogenesis [245-247], and cell proliferation [215, 216, 218, 219]. These data support the concept that the microenvironment of different organs can influence the biological behavior of tumor cells at different steps of the metastatic process and the development of biologic diversity in malignant neoplasms. These findings have obvious implications for the biotherapy of neoplasms in general and metastases in particular.

THE PATHOGENESIS OF CANCER METASTASIS

Although the phenomenon of cancer metastasis is a dynamic one that passes from beginning to end without interruption, it can, for descriptive purposes, be divided into a series of sequential processes (Fig. 1). Those malignant cells that eventually develop into established

R.K. Oldham (ed.), Principles of Cancer Biotherapy. 3rd ed., 16–38.

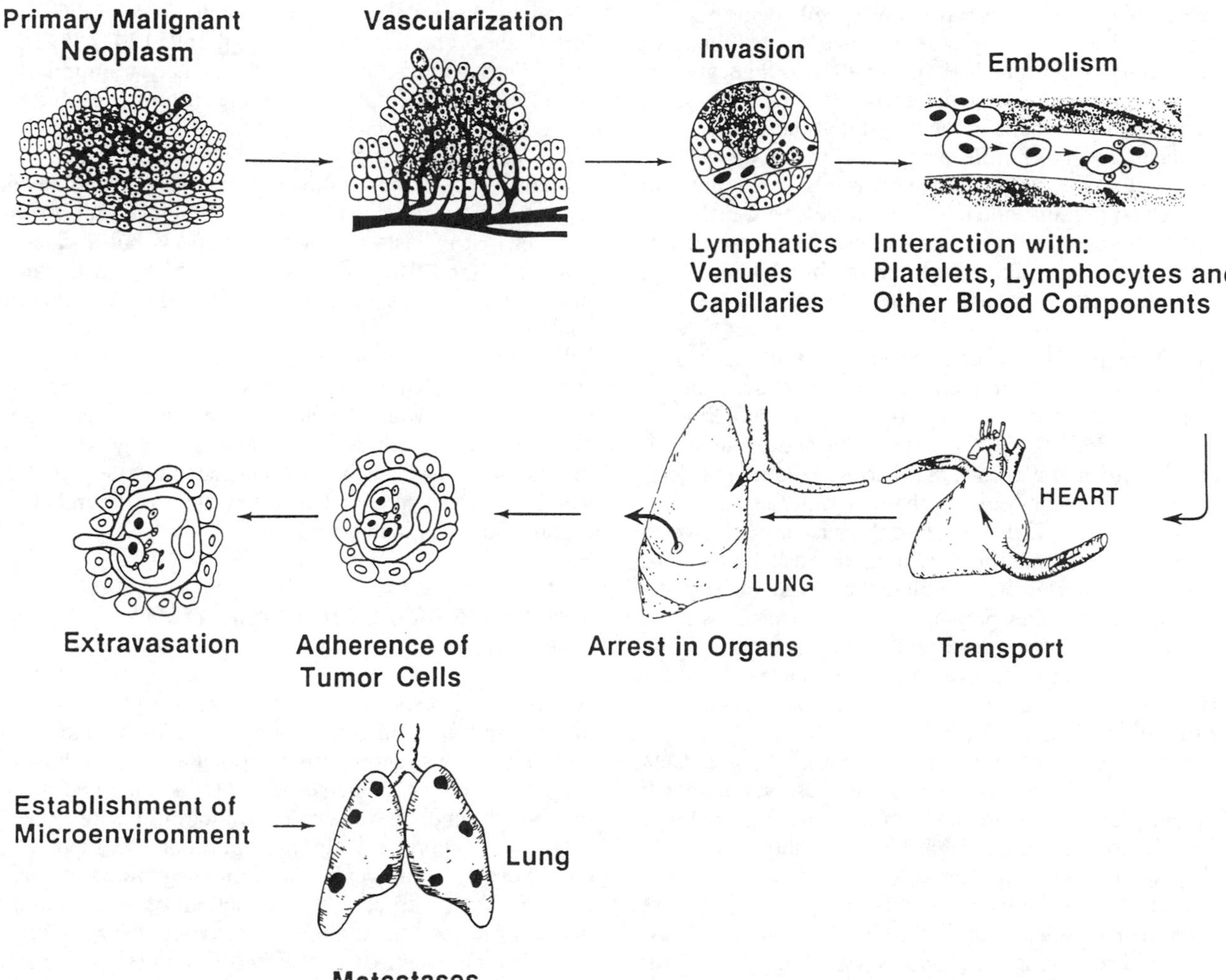

Figure 1. The pathogenesis of cancer metastasis.

metastases must survive a series of potentially lethal interactions with host homeostatic and immune mechanisms, the outcome of which is influenced by both host factors and the intrinsic properties of the tumor cells [reviewed in 56, 58, 60, 68, 105, 128, 187, 188, 214, 215].

The essential steps in the formation of a metastatic lesion may be briefly summarized as follows: (a) After the initial unicellular or multicellular transforming event, progressive growth of neoplastic cells is initially supported with nutrients supplied from the local microenvironment by simple diffusion. (b) Vascularization must occur next for a tumor mass to exceed approximately 2 mm in diameter. The synthesis and secretion of tumor angiogenesis factors play a key role in establishing a neocapillary network from the surrounding host tissue [62, 72, 73, 75].

(c) Local invasion of the surrounding host stroma by some tumor cells can occur by several mechanisms. Rapidly proliferating tumors may create mechanical pressure that pushes cells into areas of low resistance [206]. In contrast, tumors that grow within the major body cavities can shed cells that seed the mucosal or serosal surfaces of other organs, thereby establishing expansive secondary growths. Such routes of tumor cell dissemination are secondary in importance to spread of tumor cells via hematogenous or lymphatic channels. Tumor cell invasion of blood and lymphatic vessels is enhanced by the production of lytic enzymes such as lysosomal hydrolases and type IV collagenase from either tumor cells or host inflammatory cells [150, 151, 159, 256]. There also exists a strong correlation between the ability of tumor cells to bind to basement membrane components such as fibronectin and laminin and their metastatic capabilities [1]. In fact, fragments or peptides of laminin or fibronectin that contain the cell surface binding sites markedly inhibit metastasis [117, 118]. (d) Once the tumor breaches the stroma of the circulatory system, detachment and embolization of small tumor cell aggregates occurs, with most tumor cells being rapidly destroyed. Radiolabeling studies have shown that, for most tumors, fewer than 0.1% of tumor cells that enter the circulation survive to form metastases [57, 212]. Thus, the presence of tumor cells in the blood does not equate with metastasis and is of little prognostic value. Circulating tumor cells are unquestionably more susceptible to various host immune and nonimmune defenses, including blood turbulence and the trauma associated with arrest, transcapillary passage, and lysis by lymphocytes, monocytes, and natural killer (NK) cells [36, 63, 103, 157, 263].

(e) Once the tumor cells have survived the hostile environment of the circulation, they must arrest in the capillary beds of distant organs, either by adhering to capillary endothelial cells or by adhering to subendothelial basement membrane that may be exposed [145]. (f) Extravasation occurs next, probably by mechanisms similar to those that influence initial invasion. (g) Growth within the organ parenchyma and the development of second-order metastases complete the metastatic cascade. To grow in the organ parenchyma, the metastases must develop a vascular network and evade the host immune system. These metastases, when they have attained a certain size, may then give rise to additional metastases, the so-called metastasis of metastases.

For production of clinically relevant metastases, each of the steps of the metastatic process must be completed [68]. Failure to complete one or more steps (e.g., inability to invade host stroma, a high degree of antigenicity, inability to grow in a distant organ's parenchyma) eliminates the cells. Because few cells survive this arduous process to establish secondary foci, the development of metastases could represent the chance survival of a few tumor cells or could represent the selection from the parent tumor of a subpopulation of metastatic cells endowed with properties that enhance their survival. Data generated by our laboratory and many others strongly support the latter possibility. The first experimental proof for metastatic heterogeneity in neoplasms was provided in 1977 by Fidler and Kripke in their work with the murine B16 melanoma [66]. Using a modification of the fluctuation assay of Luria and Delbruck [155], they showed that different tumor cell clones, each derived from an individual cell isolated from the parent tumor, varied dramatically in their ability to produce pulmonary nodules following intravenous inoculation into syngeneic recipient mice. Control subcloning procedures demonstrated that the observed diversity was not a consequence of the cloning procedure [66]. The finding that preexisting tumor cell subpopulations proliferating in the same tumor exhibit heterogeneous metastatic potential has since been confirmed in numerous laboratories using a wide range of experimental animal tumors of different histories and histologic origins [reviewed in 56, 60, 110, 147, 207, 293]. In addition, studies using nude mice as models for metastasis of human neoplasms have shown that several human tumor lines and freshly isolated tumors also contain subpopulations of cells with widely differing metastatic properties [86, 143, 144, 169, 170, 180, 181, 251]. This demonstration of heterogeneity required that the tumor cells be implanted into the anatomically correct sites.

The data demonstrating metastatic heterogeneity in neoplasms and those showing that the outcome of metastasis is also dependent on host factors support the concept that metastasis is selective and is not a random process [58, 68, 105, 187-190, 214, 215]. Notwithstanding its implications for the value of current therapeutic strategies, the role of metastatic subpopulations of tumor cells in generating metastases offers a rational strategy for eventually combating this disease, whereas an entirely random process would be far less amenable to therapeutic manipulation. In other words, metastasis is governed by mechanisms that can be studied and ultimately understood in sufficient detail to allow the development of rational therapeutic interventions.

ORIGIN OF BIOLOGIC DIVERSITY IN NEOPLASMS

A substantial body of evidence, gained from studies on human and experimental animal neoplasms, now indicates that most neoplasms are populated by cells with different biologic characteristics. Cells obtained from individual tumors have been shown to differ with respect to many properties including morphology, metabolic characteristics, antigenic or immunogenic potential, growth rates, karyotypes, production of extracellular matrix proteins, sensitivity to destruction by NK or cytotoxic T lymphocytes, cell surface receptors for lectins, hormone receptors, drug and radiation sensitivities, invasiveness, and the ability to metastasize [33, 56, 60, 61, 64, 65, 67, 110, 147, 189, 293]. Biologic heterogeneity is not just confined to cells in primary tumors; it is equally prominent among the cells populating metastases.

Whether neoplasms are heterogeneous and contain subpopulations of tumor cells with different metastatic propensities is no longer at issue. The more interesting problem is to understand how this extensive cellular heterogeneity originates and is maintained and controlled. For example, do metastatic variants arise early or late in the development of malignant neoplasms? Once metastatic cells develop in a neoplasm, do they have a growth advantage over nonmetastatic cells so that, with the passage of time, metastatic cells constitute the majority of cells in a neoplasm? How is the proportion of metastatic cells to nonmetastatic cells regulated? Answers to some of these questions are now becoming available. They may help oncologists and surgeons make decisions critical to the timing and sequence of multimodality treatments for primary tumors and metastases.

Clinical observations of human neoplasms have suggested that spontaneous tumors tend to undergo a series of changes during the course of the disease. For example, a growth that initially appeared to be a benign tumor changes over a period of months or years into a malignant, lethal tumor. Extensive studies in murine mammary tumor systems led Foulds to describe this phenomenon of tumor evolution as 'neoplastic progression' [78-82]. Foulds defined tumor progression as 'acquisition of permanent, irreversible qualitative changes in one or more characteristics of a neoplasm.' This evolution of tumors is gradual, and tumor cells proceed toward increased autonomy from their host by changes in various properties over time. The acquisition or loss of various characteristics can be independent of each other. Moreover, because tumor progression can occur over periods of months or even years, the behavioral characteristics of a neoplasm in any given individual may vary at different stages of the disease. Because tumors progress in their host, it is not surprising that tumor progression is also influenced by host homeostatic factors, which serve as selection pressures [136, 189, 192-194, 210].

Some tumors originate from multiple transformed cells. In these tumors, the presence of diverse cellular populations may merely reflect the diverse parentages, although additional diversification is almost certainly necessary to explain the high degree of biologic heterogeneity. However, most human cancers probably result from the proliferation of a single transformed cell [3, 51, 54, 83, 175, 286, 287, 296], and the generation of biologic diversity in such tumors must therefore reflect a complex pattern of clonal diversification during tumor progression (Fig. 2) [78, 192-194].

Tumors of unicellular origin may exhibit metastatic heterogeneity at very early stages in their development. We base this conclusion on data generated by studies from this laboratory on the *in vivo* behavior of murine embryo fibroblasts transformed by an oncogenic virus [65]. Six colonies of BALB/c embryo fibroblasts, each derived from a single cell, were infected *in vitro* with mouse sarcoma virus and then propagated as individual cell lines. When viable cells from the clones were injected into the tail vein of BALB/c mice, the number of lung nodules produced by each clone differed markedly. Because the parent cell population was derived from a single, transformed cell, these data indicate that rapid phenotypic diversification occurs. Similarly, when the clones from two colonies (one of high and one of low experimental metastatic capacity) were subcloned and evaluated in the same manner, both clones exhibited metastatic heterogeneity. Interestingly, the clone with higher metastatic capacity exhibited a greater degree of variability than the clone with lower metastatic capacity. Thus, despite originating from a single cell, by the time of the first subcloning six weeks after initial transformation, the so-called 'clones' already contained subpopulations of cells with different metastatic properties. These data also demonstrate that the generation of metastatic heterogeneity in neoplasms does not require a prolonged latency period of months or even weeks, but that it can occur quite rapidly.

The origin of biological heterogeneity within and among cancer metastases

The cellular composition of different metastases in the same host is heterogeneous, both within a single metastasis (intralesional heterogeneity) and among different metastases (interlesional heterogeneity). This heterogeneity reflects two major processes: the selective nature of the metastatic process and the rapid evolution and phenotypic diversification of clonal tumor cell populations during progressive tumor growth (which itself results from the inherent genetic and phenotypic instability of many clonal populations of tumor cells) (Table 2).

Like primary neoplasms, metastases may have a unicellular or a multicellular origin [69, 128, 207, 264]. To determine whether individual metastases are clonal in their origin and whether different metastases can be produced by different progenitor cells, a series of ex-

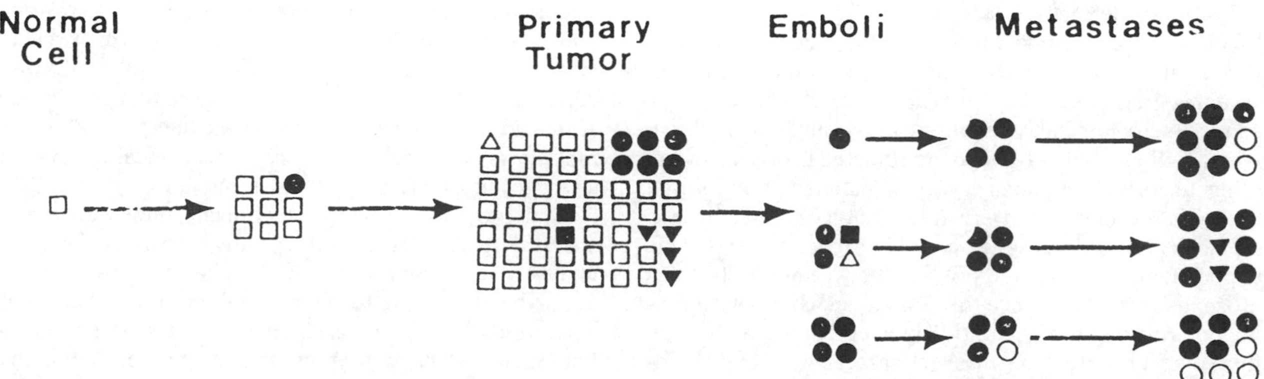

Figure 2. The generation of heterogeneity in primary tumors and their metastases. Often, tumors are of unicellular origin, but heterogeneity in any of a wide range of biologic properties can develop early. Metastases may result from the proliferation of a single cell in homotypic or heterotypic tumor emboli. Again, as with primary tumors, heterogeneity can develop quite rapidly.

Table 2. Possible mechanisms for the generation of biological heterogeneity within cancer metastases

A. Multicellular origin – Polyclonal
B. Unicellular origin – Monoclonal
  1. Genetic
    a. DNA repair alterations
    b. DNA replication infidelity
    c. DNA amplification
    d. Karyotypic alterations
      1. rearrangements – deletion, inversion, translocation
      2. breakage
      3. aneuploidy
    e. Changes in transcriptional or translational regulatory control
    f. Cell fusion
  2. Epigenetic
    a. Cellular interactions and communication
      1. Tumor cell – tumor cell
      2. Tumor cell – host cell
    b. Microenvironment
      1. Hormonal influences
      2. Growth factors
      3. Inducers of differentiation or apoptosis

periments was carried out utilizing the fact that x-irradiation of tumor cells induces random chromosome breaks and rearrangements that serve as 'markers.' Talmadge et al. [264] examined the metastases that arose from subcutaneously growing tumors produced by K-1735 mouse melanoma cells that had been x-irradiated to induce chromosomal damage. They reasoned that if a metastasis were derived from a single cell, all the chromosome spreads examined within an individual metastasis would exhibit the same karyotype. In contrast, if a metastasis had been formed from more than one progenitor cell, its constituent cells would exhibit different chromosomal arrangements, assuming, of course, that the different cells involved carried distinguishable karyotypic markers.

The cellular composition of 21 individual metastases was analyzed after cultivation of cells from individual solitary metastases. In 10 metastases, all the chromosomes were normal, making it impossible to establish whether they were of uni- or multicellular origin. In the other 11 lesions, unique karyotypic patterns of abnormal, marker chromosomes were found, suggesting that each metastasis originated from a single progenitor cell. This experiment, however, did not resolve whether metastases arose as a consequence of individual cells or homogeneous clumps (i.e., a multicellular embolus of cells with the same chromosome marker) surviving in the bloodstream, but it did establish that many metastases can originate from single cells. Moreover, the finding that different metastases are populated exclusively by cells with different chromosome markers indicates that different metastases can originate from different progenitor cells.

Subsequent experiments by Fidler and Talmadge [69] demonstrated that when heterogeneous clumps of two different K-1735 melanoma cell lines were injected i.v. to be arrested in the lung vasculature, the resultant metastases were all of unicellular origin. These results suggest that whether an embolus is homogeneous or heterogeneous, metastases can still originate from a single proliferating cell. Clonality of metastases has also been reported for different tumors, including mammary carcinoma, fibrosarcoma, and melanoma [115, 142, 198, 265].

Despite a clonal origin, most metastases undergo rapid diversification. We base this conclusion on experiments using B16 and K-1735 melanoma cell clones bearing identifiable biochemical or karyotypic markers. These studies demonstrated not only that the majority of metastases are of clonal origin but also that variant clones with diverse phenotypes are formed rapidly, thus generating significant cellular diversity within individual metastases [189, 197, 207, 262].

Collectively, these observations indicate that different metastases arise from different progenitor cells, a finding that can account for the well-documented differences in the behavior of individual metastases in the same patient, including differences in response to therapy. However, even within individual metastases of proven clonal origin, heterogeneity can develop rapidly to create significant intralesional heterogeneity.

HOST AND TUMOR INTERACTIONS IN PATHOGENESIS OF METASTASIS

In humans and in experimental rodent systems, numerous examples exist in which malignant tumors metastasize to specific organs [for review, see 105, 187, 188, 214, 215]. Two arguments have been advanced previously to explain organ-specific metastasis. In 1889, Paget [201] proposed that the growth of metastases is influenced by the interaction of particular tumor cells (the 'seed') with the unique organ's environment (the 'soil') and that metastases resulted only when the seed and soil were compatible. Forty years later, Ewing challenged Paget's seed and soil theory and proposed that the pattern of metastasis is controlled by purely mechanical factors that are a result of the anatomical structure of the vascular system [48]. In a review of clinical studies on organ-specific metastasis of some tumors, Sugarbaker concluded that common *regional* metastatic involvements could be attributed to anatomical or mechanical considerations such as efferent venous circulation or lymphatic drainage to regional lymph nodes but that *distant* organ metastases represent a unique pattern of organ specificity [259]. Experimental [105, 187, 188, 214, 215] and clinical [269] confirmation of this observation suggest that the microenvironment of each organ may influence the implantation, invasion, survival, and growth of particular tumor cells.

While the ability of some tumor cells to proliferate in the parenchyma of some organs is ultimately associated with the development of organ-specific metastasis, the mechanistic basis of this interaction remains largely unknown. The successful metastatic cell, referred to two decades ago as the 'decathlon champion' [59], must today be viewed also as a cell receptive to its environment [58, 214], i.e., during the metastatic cell's interaction with a number of host cells and systems, signals from endocrine, paracrine, or autocrine pathways, alone or in combination, could stimulate or inhibit tumor cell proliferation, with the eventual outcome dependent on the net balance of positive and negative regulators.

Models for human cancer metastasis

The design of an appropriate model for human cancer metastasis must use metastatic cells (the seed) that grow in a relevant organ environment (the soil). Many investigators have reported on the implantation of human tumor cells into the subcutis of nude mice, but in the majority of cases, the growing tumors failed to produce metastases [150]. In our laboratory, studies of primary human colon carcinomas (HCCs) showed that subcutaneous (s.c.) inoculation in nude mice was successful in initiating local tumors, but not metastasis [86]. Similarly, model systems developed in our laboratory with human colon carcinoma and human renal carcinoma contained heterogeneous populations of cells with different metastatic properties. This demonstration of heterogeneity required that the cells be implanted into the anatomically correct sites in athymic nude mice (orthotopic implantation) [58, 169, 170]. For example, HCC cells implanted into the spleen or cecum of nude mice produced exclusively hepatic and lymph node metastases (see below), whereas implantation of these same cancer cells at ectopic sites (e.g., subcutaneous or intramuscular) resulted in slow growth of primary tumors and only rarely in formation of metastases [58, 86, 87, 169, 170]. Similarly, implantation of human renal carcinoma cells (HRCC) into the kidney, but not other organs, of nude mice produced lung metastases [179, 180]. Thus, if a human tumor is biologically heterogeneous, some of its cells may possess a growth advantage, depending on whether it is transplanted to the skin, the cecum, the liver, or the kidney of nude mice. Recent data utilizing a genetically tagged HRCC population validates this concept [253]. Tumors grown in the orthotopic sites (kidney) were all populated by the same dominant clones, and each distant metastasis retained this clonality; in contrast, renal cell tumors growing subcutaneously showed a random pattern of clonal dominance [253]. The importance of orthotopic implantation of human neoplasms is also supported by results in other human tumor model systems, including melanoma (into the skin) [29], mammary carcinomas (into the mammary fatpad) [240], pancreatic carcinoma (into the pancreas) [266], lung cancer (into the bronchi [161], and prostate cancer (into the prostate) [255]. These studies illustrate the importance of anatomical compatibility of tumor cells with the organ environment in the design of a correct *in vivo* model for the analysis of human spontaneous metastasis.

The principle that specific organs support the growth of particular tumor cells was further demonstrated in numerous experiments utilizing radiolabeled tumor cells (rodent or human) [58, 105, 106, 187, 214]. In different model systems, tumor cells were shown to reach the microvasculature of many organs, but extravasation into the parenchyma and proliferation occurred in only specific organs [105, 187]. For example, two murine melanomas showed a remarkable difference in production of brain metastasis following intracarotid inoculation: some melanoma cells produced lesions only in the brain parenchyma, whereas the other cells produced only meningeal growths [233, 234]. Thus, the mere presence of viable tumor cells in a particular organ does not always predict that the cells will be able to proliferate and produce clinically relevant metastases.

Organ-derived growth factors

A mechanism for site-specific tumor growth involves interactions between receptive metastatic cells and the organ environment, possibly mediated by local growth factors (GFs). Although the involvement of particular peptide GFs is speculative in organ-specific metastasis, these factors are known to mediate the growth of normal and neoplastic cells [41]. Evidence supporting organ-specific GFs for metastatic cells has been obtained, in part, from experiments on the effects of organ-conditioned medium on the growth of particular neoplastic cells. The presence of stimulatory or inhibitory factors in a particular tissue correlated with the site-specific pattern of metastasis [for reviews, see refs. 105, 187, 188, 214, 215]. For example, lung-conditioned medium stimulated the *in vitro* growth of lung-colonizing K-1735 melanoma cells, and to a lesser degree, the growth of liver-colonizing M-5076 cells [179]. High lung-colonizing B16-F10 murine melanoma cells or high ovary-colonizing B16-O10 cells were growth-stimulated by lung- or ovary-conditioned medium, respectively, whereas extracts of other tissues were in each case found to be inhibitory [105, 187]. To date, only a few of these organ-derived growth factors have been isolated and purified to homogeneity. A potent growth-stimulatory factor was isolated from lung-conditioned medium [19, 188]. This transferrin-like factor stimulated epithelial tumor cell growth better than melanoma cell growth [19]. Other investigators have shown that stromal cells in the bone produce a factor that stimulates the growth of human prostatic carcinoma cells [21].

Conversely, a number of tissue-specific inhibitors have been isolated and purified. Transforming growth factor beta 2 (TGF-β2) was isolated and purified from kidney cell-conditioned medium [60]. Mammastatin, a physiologic mammary growth regulatory, was isolated from normal mammary cell conditioned media and found to selectively inhibit the growth of transformed human mammary cell lines in culture [47]. Finally, a growth inhibitory factor, amphiregulin, was isolated and found to be expressed in several normal tissues, including the placenta and ovary [205]. Together, this evidence suggests a role for organ-derived paracrine growth factors in the regulation of tumor cell proliferation. Once the new factors are purified to acceptable homogeneity, more definitive analyses of organ-specific paracrine factors involved in site-specific metastasis will be possible [106].

Different concentrations of hormones in individual organs, differentially expressed local factors, or paracrine growth factors may all influence the growth of malignant cells at particular sites [214, 215]. For example, specific peptide GFs are concentrated in distinct tissue environments. One example is insulin-like growth factor-I (IGF-I). IGF-I is synthesized in most mammalian tissue, its highest concentration being in the liver [297]. This GF stimulates cell growth by controlling cell cycle progression through G_1 [258]. A recent study demonstrated that carcinoma cells metastatic to the liver were growth stimulated by hepatocyte-derived IGF-I, correlating with IGF-I-receptor density on the metastatic versus nonmetastatic tumor cells; the correlation suggests a potential mechanism of selection in the process of liver colonization [154]. Another example is TGF-β. The principal sources of this peptide are the platelets and bone, suggesting they have roles in healing and remodeling processes [225, 226]. Many transformed cells produce increased levels of TGF-β and simultaneously lose their sensitivity to its growth inhibitory effects [226]. Interestingly, moderately or highly metastatic murine fibrosarcoma cells were growth-stimulated by TGF-β_1, while nonmetastatic and transformed cells of the identical lineage were growth inhibited, similar to the nontransformed parental cell lines [238]. Clonal stimulation or inhibition of human colon and renal carcinoma cells by TGF-β_1 has also been observed and correlated with differential expression of its receptors [52]. The mechanisms responsible for the observed altered GF responses are currently under investigation. At the least, these results indicate that the receptive metastatic cell (as compared to its nonmetastatic counterparts) may acquire altered responses to GF signals [for reviews, see 58, 105, 214, 215].

Tissue-specific repair factors

Host factors (autocrine or paracrine) that control organ repair and/or regeneration may also affect the proliferation of malignant tumor cells. It is interesting to speculate that metastatic cells may therefore proliferate in secondary organs that produce compatible GFs; that is, GFs similar to those involved in the cellular regulation of the normal tissue from which the primary tumor originated. For example, HCC cells utilize and respond to specific GFs that regulate normal colonic epithelium [92, 156, 158]. Some of these identical factors also regulate homeostasis and tissue renewal and repair in the liver (i.e., TGF-α and hepatocyte growth factor [HGF]) [162, 164]. Do these same factors and receptors participate in the regulation of HCC growth at the metastatic liver-specific site? There is evidence they do. For instance, subsequent to partial hepatectomy (60%), the liver undergoes rapid cell division termed regeneration. Recently, transplantation experiments in our laboratory using HCC cells were performed in nude mice that had been subjected to either partial hepatectomy (60%), nephrectomy, or control abdominal surgery [100]. Colon cancer cells implanted subcutaneously demonstrated accelerated growth in partially hepatectomized mice but not in nephrectomized or control mice. Conversely, HRCC established as micrometastases in the lungs of nude mice underwent significant growth acceleration following unilateral nephrectomy, but not hepatectomy [54, 100]. Consistent with these observations is the appearance during liver regeneration of factors in the peripheral blood that stimulate DNA synthesis in grafted hepatic parenchyma concomitant with DNA synthesis by the liver *in situ* [158]. As described above, the primary organ-specific site of the metastatic HCC is the liver, whereas the primary metastatic site of renal carcinoma is the lung. Thus, liver regeneration in the nude mouse stimulated the growth of HCC cells. Additionally, Van Dale and Galand [283] inoculated rat colon adenocarcinoma cells intraportally and showed a dramatic increase in the incidence and growth of tumor colonies in the liver of partially hepatectomized rats as compared to sham-operated controls.

Recently, TGF-α was described as a physiological regulator of liver regeneration by means of an autocrine mechanism [156]. TGF-α production by hepatocytes might also have a paracrine role, stimulating proliferation of adjacent nonparenchymal cells [158]. Furthermore, TGF-β may be a component of the paracrine regulatory loop, controlling hepatocyte replication at the late stages of liver regeneration [98]. Therefore, when normal tissues such as liver are damaged (possibly by invading tumor cells [187, 188]), growth factors are released to stimulate normal organ tissue repair, and these factors may also stimulate the proliferation of receptive malignant tumor cells. Hence, tumor cells that either originate from or have affinities for growth in a particular organ can respond to physiological signals that may produce organ-specific responses.

IMPLICATIONS OF TUMOR CELL-HOST INTERACTIONS FOR THE DESIGN OF THERAPEUTIC STRATEGIES

Even though great advances have been made in diagnosis, general patient care, surgical techniques, and local and systemic adjuvant therapies, most deaths from cancer are still due to metastases that are resistant to conventional therapies. Insight into the molecular mechanisms regulating the different and distinct steps of the metastatic process as well as a better understanding of the interaction between the metastatic cell and the host microenvironment should provide a foundation for new therapeutic approaches. This section will review new data from our laboratory and others supporting the premise that advances in the treatment of malignant cancers must involve strategies targeting the malignant cell in the context of its interaction with specific organ microenvironments.

Modulation of tumor cell multidrug resistance by the host microenvironment

A major challenge to oncologists is to design systemic therapy for metastatic disease. Two major factors influence the outcome of systemic therapy of cancer. The first is the heterogeneity of malignant neoplasms and their different metastases [67]. The second is host factors or *in vivo* conditions [58, 70, 209, 215, 253]. Although many cytotoxic effects of chemotherapeutic agents studied in a variety of tissue culture systems have revealed much about the intrinsic resistance of tumor cells to chemotherapy, other parameters that contribute to tumor-cell sensitivity and development of resistance may remain unknown because they are functional only *in vivo*.

Several intrinsic properties of tumor cells can render them resistant to chemotherapeutic drugs, including amplification of the *mdr*1 gene [14, 252], overexpression of the M_r 170,000 surface of P-glycoprotein (P-gp) [20, 31, 121, 122, 202, 227], overexpression of the M_r 22,000 calcium-binding cytoplasmic protein [102, 139], increased glutathione transferase levels [38], altered cellular calcium and calmodulin levels [178, 281], formation of double-minute chromosomes [5], increased activity of protein kinase C [195, 196], and inability of a drug to interfere with type II topoisomerase activity [88, 299].

Clinical studies have shown that after systemic chemotherapy, metastases in one organ may regress while those in another progress [248]. Similar organ-specific differences in the chemosensitivity of tumor cells have been reported by several authors. Pratesi et al. [209] investigated the antitumor efficacy of flavone acetic acid against human ovarian carcinoma cells xenografted into different organ sites in athymic nude mice. While tumors in the liver and subcutis were sensitive to the flavone, ascites and lung tumors were resistant. Smith et al. [250] demonstrated differential responses to cyclophosphamide of mouse tumor cells growing s.c. or in the lungs of syngeneic mice; specifically, tumors produced in the lungs were more sensitive than s.c. tumors of equal size. Staroselsky et al. [252] showed that a murine fibrosarcoma growing s.c. in syngeneic mice is more sensitive to doxorubicin (DXR) than the same tumor growing as lung metastases. Similarly, independent analyses demonstrated that both mouse and human colon carcinoma growing in the s.c. space were sensitive to DXR, whereas tumors growing in the cecal wall or as metastases in the liver and lung were not [44]. The observed differences in sensitivity to DXR were not attributable to differences in DXR distribution in the different tissues. These studies indicate that different host organ environments can influence the response of tumor cells and their metastases to systemic chemotherapy.

Since resistance of tumor cells to antineoplastic agents is one of the major obstacles in clinical management of this disease, a great deal of attention has been given to understanding the mechanisms controlling this phenomenon. Most of the present knowledge of drug resistance in tumor cells is derived from examining tumor cells growing in culture, but the relevance of culture conditions to the *in vivo* reality is uncertain. The nutritional status of cells [285], the presence of organ-specific growth factors and other signal-transducing agents [58, 215], the degree of oxygenation [173, 231, 273], pH [268], extent of the vascular network and its functionality [119, 120, 260, 261, 277, 285], local immunity [58], extracellular matrix components and encapsulation [183], cell-cell contact [70], and *in vivo* drug metabolism [44, 252, 295] can all contribute to the success or failure of cancer therapy.

Although DXR has not proved effective in the treatment of colon cancer in the clinical setting [127], it is useful experimentally for studying mechanisms of drug resistance in both *in vitro* and *in vivo* systems. DXR affects tumor cell growth by intercalating with DNA and by stabilizing DNA topoisomerase complexes (thus affecting DNA replication and protein synthesis), by formation of free radicals, and by reacting with membrane lipids and proteins [165, 176, 204, 231, 271]. Development of the multidrug resistant (MDR) phenotype in tumor cells is invariably associated with increased resistance to DXR, and this phenotype is most frequently associated with overexpression of the M_r 170,000 surface P-gp [14, 31, 120-122, 202, 227].

P-gp is a transmembrane transport protein that mediates the efflux of naturally occurring toxic products through an active transport mechanism [40, 101, 172, 280, 291]. The protein is physiologically expressed in cells of a variety of human tissues including cells of the proximal tubules, the luminal surface of colon mucosa, and the biliary canalicular surface of hepatocytes [28, 235]. Its expression in these excretory organs suggests that P-gp plays a physiological role in cell clearance of extrinsic or intrinsic toxins. Human tumors originating from these organ sites usually exhibit high levels of P-gp mRNA or protein [71, 95, 167, 242, 276], indicating that the signal for P-gp expression can be maintained during neoplastic transformation [242].

P-gp's are encoded by a small gene family, *mdr*, which consists of three members (*mdr*-1, *mdr*-2, *mdr*-3). Despite a high degree of homology, functional differences have been detected among the individual murine *mdr* genes

[32]; *mdr*-1 and *mdr*-3, but not *mdr*-2, are independently overexpressed in multidrug resistant cell lines of fibroblastic [32], lymphoid [220], and reticuloendothelial [114] origin. Transfection of either *mdr*-1 or *mdr*-3 but not *mdr*-2 [96], confers drug resistance. The *mdr*-1 and *mdr*-3 proteins appear to have overlapping but distinct substrate specificities [42].

Analyses of the mouse *mdr* gene transcripts in normal tissues have shown that the expression of the three genes is regulated in a tissue-specific manner [32], and that expression of *mdr*-1, but not *mdr*-2 or *mdr*-3, can be modulated in the endometrium during pregnancy [2, 32]. Although cell selection by exposure to various drugs may alter the normal pattern of *mdr* gene expression, the abundance of organ-specific factors regulating *mdr*-1 and *mdr*-3 expression in normal tissues may determine which of these two genes will be overexpressed in a multidrug-resistant derivative of a particular tissue type [220].

We therefore analyzed the mRNA and protein production of P-gp in both murine and human colon carcinoma cells growing in different organs of nude mice [44]. Our data demonstrated that mRNA expression of the *mdr*-1 gene and P-gp levels are significantly elevated in tumor cells harvested from lung, liver, and cecal tumors as compared with cells harvested from tumors growing s.c. and cells growing in culture [44, 295]. Interestingly, cultures established directly from lung metastases were initially resistant to DXR and showed elevated expression of *mdr*-1 mRNA transcripts and P-gp, but this resistance disappeared after 21 days in culture [44]. These results indicated that the drug resistance and accompanying elevated expression of *mdr*-1 in cells growing in the lung were dependent on interaction with the specific organ environment. Once removed from the lung, the cells reverted to a sensitive phenotype similar to parental cells [44].

The increased resistance to DXR in the colon cancer cells of lung metastases was not caused by the selection of resistant subpopulations. We based this conclusion on the results of crossover experiments. Once implanted into the subcutis of syngeneic mice, tumor cells from lung metastases produced tumors that were sensitive to DXR. In parallel studies, DXR-sensitive colon cancer cells from s.c. tumors became resistant to the drug when they were inoculated intravenously (i.v.) and grew in the lung parenchyma as metastases. Levels of mdr-1 mRNA-specific transcripts and P-gp were directly associated with the drug-resistant phenotype in these experiments. The P-gp antagonist verapamil could reverse this resistance to DXR [44].

In summary, these analyses illustrate that DXR sensitivity in colon cancer cells implanted into different organ sites in nude mice was modulated by the different organ environments. Although the organ-specific mechanism for upregulating *mdr*-1 and P-gp has yet to be elucidated, this environmental regulation of the MDR phenotype may explain many of the discrepancies between *in vivo* and *in vitro* studies designed to identify mechanisms of tumor cell resistance to chemotherapy. In any event, the models described in this section can be used to investigate molecular mechanisms that regulate the *in vivo* expression of the *mdr*-1 gene with special emphasis on designing new therapeutic strategies to target the molecules directly involved in the tumor cell acquisition of the MDR phenotype.

Organ-specific growth regulation of the metastatic cell

Successful metastasis depends in part on the interaction of favored tumor cells with a compatible milieu provided by a particular organ environment. Recent experimental evidence using different model systems suggests that paracrine stimulation of tumor cells by organ-derived GFs is one mechanism that determines the target organ preference of disseminated cancer cells [215]. Therefore, a modern interpretation of Paget's 1889 seed and soil hypothesis must take into account that organ-specific metastasis results from the proliferation of tumor cells differentially expressing growth factor receptors and that local GFs, organ-repair factors, or paracrine GFs stimulate the growth of malignant cells with receptors.

To distinguish the malignant potential of different Dukes' stage HCCs, our laboratory analyzed their growth in the liver parenchyma, the most common site of HCC metastasis [228]. A reproducible bioassay of hepatic metastasis was developed whereby tumor cells from HCC surgical specimens were inoculated into the spleens of nude mice [86, 87, 169, 170]. From this site, tumor cells gain access to the bloodstream and then reach the liver, where they proliferate into tumor colonies. The growth of HCC in the liver directly correlated with the metastatic potential of the cells, i.e., cells from surgical specimens of primary HCC classified as either modified Dukes' stage D (late stage) or liver metastases produced significantly more colonies in the livers of nude mice than cells from a Dukes' stage B HCC primary tumor (early stage) [169, 170]. Radioactive distribution analyses of both Dukes' stage B and D HCC cells demonstrated that shortly after intrasplenic injection, similar numbers of tumor cells reached the liver microvasculature [86, 87]. Thus, the mere presence of viable tumor cells in a particular organ does not always predict that the cells will proliferate to produce metastases.

These experiments stress that the sites of metastasis are determined not solely by the characteristics of the neoplastic cells, but also by the microenvironment of the host tissue. Experimental evidence to date strongly indicates that metastases result when the seed and soil are matched [58, 20]. Therefore, the production of HCC tumors in the livers of nude mice was determined by the ability of the HCC to proliferate in the liver parenchyma rather than by the ability of the cells to reach the liver [87].

To select and isolate metastatic subpopulations of HCC cells with increasing growth potential in the liver parenchyma from heterogeneous primary HCCs, cells were derived from a surgical specimen of a Dukes' stage

B2 primary HCC. These HCC cells were established in culture (KM12C) or injected into the subcutis, cecum, and spleen of nude mice [87, 169, 170]. Progressively growing tumors were then isolated and established in culture. Implantation of these four culture-adapted lines into the cecum or spleen of nude mice produced a few metastatic foci in the liver. HCC cells from these few liver metastases were expanded into culture and reinjected into the spleen of nude mice to provide a source for further cycles of selection. With each successive *in vivo* selection cycle, the metastatic ability of the isolated and propagated cells increased. Four cycles of intrasplenic selection yielded cell lines (KM12L4) with a very high metastatic efficiency as measured by the ability to proliferate in the liver parenchyma of nude mice. In analogous studies of a Dukes' stage D primary HCC, highly metastatic cell lines were isolated, but successive selection cycles for growth in the liver only slightly increased their metastatic properties [169, 170]. These results demonstrated that highly metastatic cells can be selected from early stage HCC and that orthotopic implantation of HCC cells in nude mice is a valid model for determining metastatic potential [87, 88, 169, 170, 213].

A mechanism that would explain the interaction between distinct HCC cells and the liver-specific environment could involve the proliferation of tumor cells differentially expressing certain growth factor receptors and their response to liver-specific paracrine growth factors or organ-repair factors. Indeed, highly metastatic HCC cells from Dukes' stage D or surgical specimens of liver metastases respond to mitogens associated with liver regeneration induced by hepatectomy in nude mice [58, 100]. Following partial hepatectomy, the liver undergoes rapid cell division. This process of liver regeneration involves quantitative changes in hepatocyte gene expression. TGF-α was recently shown to be one regulator of liver regeneration [98, 162, 191] and proliferation of normal colonic epithelial cells [156, 158]. TGF-α exerts its effect through interaction with the epidermal growth factor receptor (EGF-R), a plasma membrane glycoprotein that contains within its cytoplasmic domain a tyrosine-specific protein tyrosine kinase (PTK) activity. The binding of TGF-α to the EGF-R stimulates a series of rapid responses, including phosphorylation of tyrosine residues within the EGF-R itself and within many other cellular proteins, hydrolysis of phosphatidyl inositol, release of Ca^{2+} from intracellular stores, elevation of cytoplasmic pH, and morphological changes [284]. After 10 to 12 h in the continuous presence of EGF or TGF-α, cells are committed to synthesize DNA and to divide [236, 284].

EGF-Rs are present on many normal and tumor cells [236, 284]. Increased levels and/or amplification of EGF-R have been found in many human tumors and cell lines, including breast cancer [230], gliomas [11, 149], lung cancer [104], bladder cancer [10, 185], tumors of the female genital tract [98], the A431 epidermoid carcinoma [282], and colon carcinoma [97]. These results suggest a physiological significance of inappropriate expression of the EGF-R tyrosine kinase in abnormal cell growth control. Whether TGF-α can also regulate the proliferation of metastatic HCC cells in the liver or lymph nodes is unclear. We recently examined the expression and function of EGF-R in a series of HCC lines whose liver metastatic potential differed. The results demonstrated that the expression of EGF-R at the mRNA and protein levels directly correlated with the ability of the HCC cells to grow in the liver parenchyma and hence produce hepatic metastases [219]. The EGF-Rs expressed on metastatic HCC cells were functional based on *in vitro* growth stimulation assays using picogram concentrations of TGF-α and specific as shown by neutralization with anti-EGF-R or anti-TGF-α antibodies. Moreover, EGF-R-associated PTK activity also paralleled the observed EGF-R levels. Immunohistochemical analysis of the low metastatic parental KM12C HCC cells demonstrated heterogeneity in the EGF-R-specific staining pattern, with <10% of the cells in the population staining intensely for EGF-R, whereas the *in vivo* selected highly metastatic KM12L4 and KM12SM HCC cells exhibited uniform, intense staining. Western blotting confirmed the presence of higher EGF-R protein levels in the metastatic KM12L4 and KM12SM cells than in the low metastatic KM12C cells. Finally, isolation of the top and bottom 5% EGF-R-expressing KM12C cells by fluorescence-activated cell sorting (FACS) confirmed the association between levels of EGF-R on HCC cells and the production of liver metastases [219].

The binding of EGF to its receptor on KM12C cells and several metastatic variants was nonlinear on a Scatchard plot, indicating there were two classes of receptors: the binding affinity of the major class was more than a magnitude less than that of the minor class. Metastatic KM12L4 cells selected *in vivo* after intrasplenic injection into nude mice expressed >2.5-fold the parental KM12C levels of both high- and low-affinity EGF-R. Two classes of EGF-R have been detected in human squamous carcinoma A431 cells; high-affinity EGF-Rs constitute 5% to 10% of the total EGF binding capacity [124]. High-affinity EGF binding has been shown to play an important role in EGF/TGF-α signal transduction, explaining why the ID_{50} for EGF-stimulated cell proliferation (measured at 46 nM for human foreskin fibroblasts) is similar to the Kd for high-affinity binding but two orders of magnitude lower than the Kd for low-affinity binding [236, 284]. The demonstrated functionality of high-affinity-binding EGF-R is also important physiologically, since the level of EGF is extremely low, ranging from 20-27 μM in serum [112] and ranging from 1 to 5 ng/g in tissue [111]. Furthermore, treatment with Mab 108 (which binds to the high-affinity EGF-R) inhibits the growth of human tumor cells in culture and in nude mice [7]. Collectively, these data suggest that high-affinity EGF-R binding is the primary means for *in vivo* stimulation of cells by TGF-α [39, 236, 284].

We also observed a correlation between increased copy number of chromosome 7, EGF-R expression, and the ability of HCC to produce metastasis in the livers of nude mice. About 95% of KM12L4 cells had a chromosome 7/12 or 7/4 ratio >1.0 as compared with only 14% of KM12C cells, indicating a higher proportion of metastatic cells carried extra copies of chromosome 7. Gains of as many as 10 copies of particular chromosomes have been reported by fluorescent *in situ* hybridization (FISH) analyses in other solid tumors [254, 288]. Dukes' stage C HCC often exhibit additions of chromosomes 8 and 12 and a loss of chromosome 17 [129, 254, 288]. The correlation between chromosome copy number and the potential of HCC cells to produce liver metastasis may be direct and specific or indirect and nonspecific. Alternatively, the observed correlation may be a reflection of genetic instability, which can lead to any of a number of gene mutations or deletions on other chromosomes, which in turn may increase tumor cell proliferation and growth in the liver [129]. Several independent reports implicated gene sequences on chromosome 7 in the process of invasion and metastasis [27]. An increased copy number of chromosome 7, shown to be associated with high expression of the EGF-R, has been detected in advanced melanoma [140] and in cancer of the breast [230], bladder [232, 288], pancreas [141], and brain [109]. These data suggest that increases in chromosome 7 copy number, and thus in EGF-R expression, may increase metastatic propensity.

The analyses described show a direct correlation between EGF-R on variant cell lines isolated from HCC and ability to produce liver metastases in nude mice. These findings are likely to be more generalized because in our recent analysis of formalin-fixed paraffin-embedded colon carcinoma surgical specimens for EGF-R transcripts using a rapid colorimetric *in situ* mRNA hybridization (ISH) technique [217], we found that cell-surface hybridization with EGF-R-antisense hyperbiotinylated oligonucleotide probes in primary and metastatic colon carcinoma specimens directly correlated with immunohistochemistry and northern blot analyses. Moreover, unlike northern analyses, ISH showed intratumoral heterogeneity in EGF-R gene expression and identified particular cells expressing high levels of EGF-R in the tissues [217].

Collectively, these data suggest an involvement of the EGF-R in tumor progression and dissemination and indicate a potential use of this receptor as a target for therapy [for reviews, see 132, 163, 168]. Anti-EGF-R monoclonal antibodies (Mab), which block ligand binding, prevent the growth in culture of cells that are stimulated by EGF or TGF-α as well as the growth of human tumor xenografts bearing high levels of EGF-R [163, 168]. Recent studies have also indicated that anti-EGF-R Mab substantially enhance the cytotoxic effects of DXR or *cis*-diammine-dichloroplatinum on well-established xenografts [4, 53]. Furthermore, clinical trials with squamous cell carcinoma of the lung have demonstrated the capacity of the anti-EGF-R Mab to localize in such tumors and to achieve saturating concentrations in the blood for >3 days without toxicity [163]. Other therapeutic approaches targeting the EGF-R include strategies using EGF or TGF-α conjugated to toxins [203, 243], inhibitors of receptor dimerization [153], antisense RNA, PTK inhibitors preferential for the EGF-R [16, 84, 278], or receptor dominant-negative strategies [123, 222, 239]. These studies strongly support the premise that overexpressed EGF-Rs on malignant cells can be targeted for therapeutic intervention.

Organ-specific modulation of the invasive phenotype of metastatic carcinoma cells

As described thus far, the interaction of tumor cells with an organ environment can modulate their tumorigenic properties and metastatic behavior [58, 105, 215]. The implantation of HCC into the subcutis (ectopic site) or the wall of the cecum (orthotopic site) results in locally growing tumors [169, 170]. Metastasis to distant organs, however, was produced only by tumors growing in the wall of the cecum [169, 170]. This difference in production of distant metastasis directly correlated with the influence of the organ environment on the production of degradative enzymes by the HCC cells [183].

The ability of tumor cells to degrade connective-tissue extracellular matrix (ECM) and basement-membrane components is an essential prerequisite for invasion and metastasis [151, 160, 171, 190, 249, 256, 274, 275, 279]. Among the enzymes involved in degradation of the ECM are the metalloproteinases, a family of metal-dependent endopeptidases [256]. These proteinases are produced by connective tissue cells as well as many tumor cells and include enzymes with degradative activity for interstitial collagen, type IV collagen, type V collagen, gelatin, and proteoglycans. The Mr 72,000 type IV collagenase is a neutral metalloproteinase capable of degrading type IV collagen within the triple helical domain, resulting in one-fourth amino terminal and three-fourths carboxyterminal fragments from the intact molecule [55, 152]. The enzyme is mostly secreted into an extracellular milieu in a proenzymatic form [257].

Increased expression of the Mr 72,000 collagenase type IV has been demonstrated in HCC cells compared with that of normal mucosa cells [148], and the metastatic capacity of HCC cells from orthotopic sites in nude mice directly correlates with the production of this enzyme activity [169, 170, 183]. Thus, intracecal tumors (in nude mice) of metastatic HCC secreted high levels of 92-kDa and 68-kDa gelatinase activities, whereas HCC growing subcutaneously (not metastatic] did not produce or secrete the 68-kDa gelatinase activity [50, 183]. Moreover, histological examination of the HCC growing in the subcutis or cecum of nude mice revealed that mouse fibroblasts produced a thick pseudocapsule around the subcutaneous but not cecal tumors [50]. These differences suggested that the organ environment profoundly influenced the ability of metastatic cells to produce ECM-degradative enzymes.

Since recent analyses have demonstrated that the interaction of stromal fibroblasts can influence the tumorigenicity [15, 18, 26] and biological behavior of tumor cells [9, 12, 23, 30, 35, 137, 237], we investigated whether organ-specific fibroblasts could directly influence the invasive ability of HCC cells. Coculturing fibroblasts from skin, lung, and colon of nude mice with highly invasive and metastatic KM12SM HCC cells [50] showed that HCC cells adhered to and invaded through mouse colon and lung, but not skin fibroblasts. Moreover, nude mouse skin fibroblasts (ectopic environment), but not colon or lung fibroblasts (orthotopic environments) inhibited the production of 72-kDa type IV collagenases (gelatinases) by highly invasive and metastatic KM12SM HCC cells. This inhibition was due to a specific interaction between the HCC cells and skin fibroblasts. We based this conclusion on the data showing that nude mouse skin fibroblasts did not decrease the production of a 72-kDa type IV collagenase or the invasive capacity of the human squamous cell carcinoma A431 cells. These data, therefore, directly correlated with our studies showing that the KM12SM cells can grow in the wall of the cecum and the subcutis of nude mice, but are invasive only from the wall of the cecum [170, 171]. Moreover, HCC tumors in the subcutis did not produce type IV collagenase [183]. The present *in vitro* data directly correlate with the *in vivo* findings and suggest that fibroblasts populating the ectopic and orthotopic organs influence the invasive phenotype of HCC cells.

Mesenchymal cells such as fibroblasts play an essential role in the differentiation and biological behavior of both normal and neoplastic epithelial cells [18, 22, 26, 30, 34, 108]. Fibroblasts can produce factors that influence tumor cell growth, invasion, and metastasis [6], which ones depending on the stage of differentiation of the tumor cells [18, 26, 138, 267]. For example, in human melanoma, skin fibroblasts inhibited the *in vitro* growth of cells from nevi but stimulated the *in vitro* growth of invasive melanoma cells [30]. Similarly, the *in vitro* growth of normal rat prostate cells was inhibited by fibroblasts from the prostate whereas growth of prostate cancer cells was accelerated [22, 26]. While growth stimulation of human tumor cells by cultured fibroblasts has been well documented [15], the *in vitro* growth of human breast and colon carcinoma cells [174] or mouse breast carcinoma cells [46, 166] is enhanced by fibroblasts (or factors produced by fibroblasts) derived from the tissue of origin (orthotopic), but not by fibroblasts from ectopic tissues.

There are several mechanisms by which stromal cells and tumor cells interact and influence each other. Both *in vitro* and *in vivo* studies suggested that cell-to-cell contact is important [125, 126] and that at the epithelial cell junction, both cancer cells and fibroblasts have an altered capacity to synthesize basement membrane molecules [13]. Epithelial cells produce a variety of GFs that can influence fibroblast function, whereas fibroblasts produce ECM that can be tissue-specific [43, 223, 225]. GFs can induce and alter ECM gene expression [43, 225], and the ECM can, in turn, influence the type and level of GF, and even their receptor expression, in different cells [93]. Organ-specific ECM molecules have been shown to influence clonal growth of tumors [43, 298], probably by regulation of cell-cell adhesion and differentiation [107], maintenance of cell shape controlling response to hormones and GFs [94], and expression of tissue-specific proteins [43, 223, 225].

There is now increasing evidence that fibroblasts derived from different anatomical sites in the adult display functional phenotypic heterogeneity in their morphology, interaction with steroid hormones, growth capacity, and production of cytokines [9]. One possible regulator of metalloproteinase activity is the family of tissue inhibitor of metalloproteinases (TIMP), which can inhibit interstitial collagenase, stromelysin, and the 92-kDa type IV collagenase [137, 294]. TIMP-2 can also bind specifically to 72-kDa type IV collagenase [91, 257]. Furthermore, transfection of 3T3 fibroblasts with antisense DNA of TIMP resulted in the production of tumorigenic and metastatic cells [91]. In our study using anti-TIMP monoclonal antibodies, we did not observe TIMP expressed differently in HCC in the subcutis and the cecum. TIMPs can be separated from metalloproteinases by SDS-polyacrylamide gel electrophoresis [37, 91, 257], and latent forms of metalloproteinases are activated by SDS-polyacrylamide gel electrophoresis followed by a Triton X-100 treatment. As our data showed, low levels of type IV collagenolytic activity in s.c. tumors were caused by low production of the 92-kDa and 64-kDa type IV collagenases, not by TIMP inhibition of type IV collagenase.

The organ factors that modulate type IV collagenase production in the cecal wall and subcutis were also analyzed. Various GF and cytokines have been shown to modulate the level of cell-secreted metalloproteinases and serine proteinases. Production of collagenases in normal fibroblasts can be induced by various tissue factors, e.g., IL-1 [208], EGF, TGF-β, platelet-derived growth factor (PDGF) [25], and tumor-cell collagenase stimulatory factor [45]. Similarly, TGF-β induces synthesis of urokinase-type plasminogen activator in lung carcinoma cells [131] and increases production of the 72-kDa type IV collagenase in fibroblasts [200]. Welch et al. [292] found that TGF-β, at a concentration as low as 50 μg/mL, can maximally enhance the production of 92-kDa and 72-kDa type IV collagenases and heparinase in rat 13762NF mammary adenocarcinoma MTLn3 cells. Pretreatment of MTLn3 cells with TGF-β significantly enhanced lung colonization after the cells were injected into the tail vein of a rat [292]. In contrast, TGF-β can inhibit transcription of transin (rat stromelysin, matrix metalloproteinase-3 [130]), whose expression is correlated with the progression of squamous cell carcinoma [199]. In different organs, the normal stroma surrounding primary tumors of KM12 HCC cells may contain dissimilar levels of these or other growth factors, and this difference may affect the production and secretion of type IV collagenases, heparinases, and other tissue-degrading enzymes.

The exact mechanism by which nude mouse skin fibroblasts inhibit collagenase production by KM12SM cells was actively pursued by our laboratory. Since recombinant human IFN-α and IFN-γ have been shown to modulate the invasive capacity of human melanoma cells under *in vitro* conditions [116], we examined the effects of IFN-α, β, and γ on the production of gelatinase activity by KM12SM HCC cells. Whereas all the r-IFNs inhibited gelatinase production (68-kDa), only inhibition by IFN-β (fibroblast IFN) was significant [50].

We therefore investigated whether IFN-β or other IFNs could affect the production of gelatinase activity in other tumor cells or in normal cells, e.g., fibroblasts. To that end, we established a cell line from a surgical specimen of HRCC [90]. This cell line, designated KG-2, can be transplanted into nude mice, where it is tumorigenic in the subcutis (ectopic) and kidney (orthotopic). This tumor produces spontaneous metastasis to lung only from orthotopic implantation. KG-2 HRCC cells growing in the kidney and KG-2 lung metastases secrete higher levels of the 72-kDa gelatinase than do cells growing in the subcutis [89, 90]. Under culture conditions, the gelatinase level in the culture supernatants of KG-2 cells was increased by their cultivation with mouse kidney or lung fibroblasts, whereas the cocultivation of KG-2 cells with mouse skin fibroblasts resulted in a significant reduction of gelatinase activity similar to our results with HCC cells [50, 83]. Treatment with either IFN-β-serine or r-IFN-γ (but not IFN-α) decreased production of 72-kDa gelatinase and invasion through Matrigel by metastatic HRCC KG-2 cells [89]. The KG-2 cell invasion through Matrigel was induced by the conditioned media from human-kidney-fibroblast cultures [89]. Neither human IFN-α nor IFN-β was detected by immunoassays in the media conditioned by kidney fibroblasts. Although Matrigel could contain mouse IFNs, treatment with various amounts of anti-mouse IFN-α or -β monoclonal antibodies did not enhance KG-2 cell invasion through Matrigel. Thus, we concluded that the inhibition of invasion was directly caused by addition of r-IFNs [89].

Importantly, these inhibitory effects were independent of the antiproliferative activity of r-IFNs. For example, IFN-α produced the highest levels of cytostasis but did not significantly affect gelatinase production. Moreover, the r-IFNs did not modulate production of the 72-kDa gelatinase in normal human fibroblasts, suggesting that the action of r-IFNs on gelatinase production and invasion may be specific to certain types of cells, including those of HRCC. Shapiro et al. [241] suggested that the modification of metalloproteinase production in alveolar macrophages by IFN-γ occurs at a pretranslational level. We found an approximately 70% decrease in the 72-kDa gelatinase steady-state mRNA level in KG-2 HRCC cells treated with 100 U/ml of r-IFN-β-serine or r-IFN-γ, suggesting that the r-IFN-mediated inhibition of gelatinase production in KG-2 cells also occurred at a pretranslational level [89].

These laboratory findings are extremely relevant to the clinical setting where more than 20,000 new cases of HRCC are diagnosed each year in the United States [244]. Nearly half of these patients develop metastatic disease that is resistant to conventional therapy. In an effort to overcome this problem, several cytokines have recently been used to treat patients with metastatic HRCC [85, 135, 224]. The most prominent among these, the interferons (IFN-alpha, beta, or gamma) have been used as a single modality [85, 135, 224] or in combination with cytotoxic agents [77] or other cytokines [146]. The response of metastatic HRCC to IFNs has varied with the different treatment strategies. Overall, approximately 10% to 30% of metastatic HRCC respond to IFNs [77, 85, 135, 146, 224], but the responses have not been complete. Improvement in the use of IFNs for treatment of HRCC or any other neoplasm is dependent on a better understanding of the mechanisms by which IFNs regulate different functions of tumor cells, perhaps through the invasive phenotype.

Host-tumor interactions in the regulation of angiogenesis

Although tumors 1-2 mm in diameter can receive all nutrients by diffusion, further growth depends on the development of an adequate blood supply through angiogenesis [72, 73]. The induction of angiogenesis is mediated by several angiogenic molecules released by both tumor cells and host cells [62, 72-76]. Prevascular tumors are often local benign tumors, whereas vascular tumors are capable of metastasizing. Moreover, studies using light microscopy and immunohistochemistry concluded that the number and density of microvessels in different human cancers directly correlate with their potential to invade and produce metastasis [289, 290]. Not all angiogenic tumors produce metastasis, but the inhibition of angiogenesis prevents the growth of tumor cells at both the primary and secondary sites and thus can prevent the emergence of metastases [for review, see 62].

Inhibition of angiogenesis provides a novel and more general approach for treating metastases by manipulation of the host microenvironment. Endothelial cells in tumor blood vessels divide rapidly, whereas those in normal tissues do not [72-76]. The division of endothelial cells is induced by a variety of mitogens termed angiogenic factors, such as basic fibroblast growth factor (bFGF), IL-8, and vascular endothelial growth factor (VEGF) [for reviews, see 73, 76]. Systemic administration of antibodies to bFGF [113], VEGF [134], or angiogenin [197] has been shown to inhibit the *in vivo* (but not *in vitro*) growth of tumor cells, suggesting tumor growth may be inhibited indirectly by constraining angiogenesis. Treating neoplasms by targeting both the tumor cells (chemotherapy) and the organ environment (angiogenesis inhibitor) have been shown to produce additive or synergistic therapeutic effects in mice bearing the 3LL tumor [270, 272].

Recent data from our laboratory have demonstrated that the organ microenvironment can directly contribute to the induction and maintenance of the angiogenic factors bFGF [245] and IL-8 [247]. The production of these angiogenic factors by tumor cells or host cells (macrophages) or the release of bFGF from the ECM in the absence of angiogenesis inhibitors leads to growth of endothelial cells and hence vascularization [72-76]. Because the host microenvironment varies among different organs [105], we investigated whether bFGF expression (at the mRNA and protein levels) is influenced by the organ microenvironment. We implanted HRCC cells into the subcutis or the kidney-renal subcapsule (RSC) of nude mice [180, 181]. The HRCC tumors in the kidney were highly vascularized and produced a high incidence of systemic metastases. In contrast, the tumors in the subcutis of nude mice were poorly vascularized and produced few metastases. We detected 10 to 20 times the amount of bFGF mRNA in HRCC growing in the kidney as compared with HRCC growing in the subcutis. These differences were confirmed at the protein level. These data therefore demonstrate an association between the production of bFGF by tumor cells and vascularization [72-77] and the influence of a specific organ's microenvironment on bFGF expression level in HRCC cells [245]. Additionally, HRCC growing in the kidney produced lung metastases whereas HRCC cells growing in the subcutis did not. The differential expression of bFGF could have contributed to the invasive-metastatic phenotype of the HRCC growing in the kidney since bFGF can stimulate the activity of proteolytic enzymes such as tissue type and urokinase type plasminogen activator [211] and collagenase type IV [17], all of which are produced by the HRCC cells [89, 90, 229] (see previous section).

In patients, HRCCs produce various angiogenic factors including bFGF [24, 177, 184]. Reports indicate that the expression of bFGF in primary HRCC inversely correlates with survival [184], as do elevated levels of bFGF in the urine of patients [186]. In adults, physiological angiogenesis (wound healing) is regulated by the balance of positive and negative molecules. Several factors that downregulate or inhibit angiogenesis have already been incorporated into clinical trials, the most widely studied being IFN-α. Chronic daily administration of low-dose IFN-α has been shown to induce complete regression of life-threatening hemangiomas in infants [49] and highly vascular Kaposi's sarcoma [221]. The mechanisms responsible for this remarkable clinical outcome were not, however known.

To identify the mechanisms, we tested the ability of IFN-α to downregulate bFGF mRNA expression and protein production in multiple carcinoma cell lines [246]. In fact, IFN-α or IFN-β downregulated the steady-state mRNA expression and protein production of bFGF in HRCC cells by mechanisms independent of their antiproliferative effects. The inhibition of bFGF mRNA and protein production required long-term exposure (>4 days) of cells to IFNs. Moreover, once IFN was withdrawn, cells resumed production of bFGF [246]. These observations were consistent with the clinical experience that IFN-α must be given for many months to bring about involution of hemangiomas [49]. The incubation of human bladder, prostate, colon, and breast carcinoma cells with noncytostatic concentrations of IFN-α or IFN-β also downregulated bFGF production [246]. Since IFN-α and -β are constitutively produced by many host cells [101], their physiological role in limiting angiogenesis should be further investigated. It is especially relevant in patients with renal cancer, since bFGF is a major angiogenic molecule in renal tumors and its level in the serum is inversely correlated with survival [184]. Whether this is true for other neoplasms remains to be elucidated.

These results link together the findings from our laboratory, which showed that the invasive and angiogenic properties of human tumor cells are modulated by specific organ environments [50, 89, 90, 179, 180]. As described, the implantation of HRCC into the subcutis of nude mice yields not only localized noninvasive but also poorly vascularized tumors, whereas the implantation of the same cells into the kidney of nude mice results in highly vascularized and invasive neoplasms [58, 68]. These studies confirm the conclusion that the process of cancer metastasis is highly selective and is regulated by a number of different mechanisms [80, 90, 179, 180, 245]. This conclusion is contrary to the once-accepted idea that metastasis represents the ultimate expression of cellular anarchy. The view that cancer metastasis is selective implies that understanding the mechanisms that regulate the process will lead to better therapeutic intervention. The control of invasive potential by primary tumors or angiogenesis in metastases by known inhibitors is an excellent example of this principle.

CONCLUSIONS

A primary goal of cancer research is an increased understanding of the molecular mechanisms mediating the process of cancer metastasis. Analyses of cancer cells (the seeds) and the microenvironment (the soil) has increased our understanding of the biologic mechanisms mediating organ-specific metastasis. Insight into the molecular mechanisms regulating the pathobiology of cancer metastasis as well as a better understanding of the interaction between the metastatic cell and the host environment should produce a foundation for new therapeutic approaches. In this chapter, we summarized new experimental findings demonstrating that the host organ's microenvironment can profoundly influence the biologic behavior of metastatic tumor cells, including resistance to chemotherapy, the production of degradative enzymes, angiogenesis, and proliferation at the metastatic site. Each of these studies indicates that the production of clinically relevant metastases depends, in part, on the interaction of particular tumor cells with specific organ environments. Therefore, the successful metastatic cell whose complex phenotype helps make it the decathlon champion [59], must be viewed today as a cell receptive to its environment. The analyses presented herein add important evidence to support the concept that cancer metastasis is not a random process; it is a highly regulated process that can now be studied on the molecular level. This new knowledge should eventually lead to the design and implementation of more effective therapies for this dreaded disease, ones that will refine the use of all treatment modalities, including surgery, chemotherapy, radiotherapy and biotherapy.

REFERENCES

1. Albini A, Aukerman SL, Ogle RC, Noonan DM, Friedman R, Martin GR, Fidler IJ. The *in vitro* invasiveness and interactions with laminin of K-1735 melanoma cells. Evidence for different laminin-binding affinities in high and low metastatic variants. *Clin Exp Metastasis* 1989; 7:437-451.
2. Arceci RJ, Croop JM, Horwitz SB, Housman D. The gene encoding multidrug resistance is induced and expressed at high levels during pregnancy in the secretory epithelium of the uterus. *Proc Natl Acad Sci USA* 1988; 85:4350-4354.
3. Arnold A, Staunton CE, Kim HG, Gaz RD, Kronenberg HM. Monoclonality and abnormal parathyroid hormone genes in parathyroid adenomas. *N Engl J Med* 1988; 318:658-662.
4. Baselga J, Norton L, Masui H, Pandiella A, Coplan K, Miller Jr WH, Mendelsohn J. Antitumor effects of doxorubicin in combination with anti-epidermal growth factor receptor monoclonal antibodies. *J Natl Cancer Inst* 1993; 85:1327-1333.
5. Baskin F, Rosenberg RN, Dev V. Correlation of double-minute chromosomes with unstable multidrug cross-resistance in uptake mutants of neuroblastoma cells. *Proc Natl Acad Sci USA* 1981; 78:3654-3658.
6. Basset P, Bellocq JP, Wolf C, Stoll I, Hutin P, Limacher JM, Podhajcer OL, Chenard MP, Rio MC, Chambon P. A novel metalloproteinase gene specifically expressed in stromal cells of breast carcinomas. *Nature* 1990; 348:699-704.
7. Bellot F, Moolenaar W, Kris R, Mirakhur B, Verlaan I, Ullrich A, Schlessinger J, Felder S. High-affinity epidermal growth factor binding is specifically reduced by a monoclonal antibody, and appears necessary for early responses. *J Cell Biol* 1990; 110:491-502.
8. Benathan M, Frenk E. Melanocyte growth stimulation by lethally irradiated fibroblasts *in vitro*. *J Invest Dermatol* 1987; 89:323.
9. Benathan M, Pararas C, Frenk E. Modulatory growth effects of 3T3 fibroblasts on cocultivated human melanoma cells. *Anticancer Res* 1991; 11:203-208.
10. Berger MS, Greenfield C, Gullick WJ, Haley J, Downward J, Neal DE, Harris AL, Waterfield MD. Evaluation of epidermal growth factor receptors in bladder tumours. *Br J Cancer* 1987; 56:533-537.
11. Bigner SH, Humphrey PA, Wong AJ, Vogelstein B, Mark J, Friedman HS, Bigner DD. Characterization of the epidermal growth factor receptor in human glioma cell lines and xenografts. *Cancer Res* 1990; 50:8017-8022.
12. Biswas C. Collagenase stimulation in cocultures of human fibroblasts and human tumor cells. *Cancer Lett* 1984; 24:201-207.
13. Bouziges F, Simo P, Simon-Assman P, Haffen K, Kedinger M. Altered deposition of basement-membrane molecules in co-cultures of colonic cancer cells and fibroblasts. *Int J Cancer* 1991; 48:101-108.
14. Bradley G, Juranka PE, Ling V. Mechanism of multidrug resistance. *Biochim Biophys Acta* 1988; 948:87-128.
15. Brattain MG, Brattain DE, Sarrif AM, McRae LJ, Fine WD, Hawkins JG. Enhancement of growth of human colon tumor cell lines by feeder layers of murine fibroblasts. *J Natl Cancer Inst* 1982; 69:767-771.
16. Buchdunger E, Trinks U, Mett H, Regenass U, Muller M, Meyer T, McGlynn E, Pinna LA, Traxler P, Lydon NB. 4,5-Dianilinophtalimide: A protein-tyrosine kinase inhibitor with selectivity for the epidermal growth factor receptor signal transduction pathway and potent *in vivo* antitumor activity. *Proc Natl Acad Sci USA* 1994; 91:2334-2338.
17. Buckley-Sturrock A, Woodward SC, Senior RM, Grimm GL, Klagsbrun M, Davidson JM. Differential stimulation of collagenase and chemotactic activity in fibroblasts derived from rat wound repair tissue and human skin by growth factors. *J Cell Physiol* 1989; 138:70-78.
18. Camps JL, Chang SM, Hsu TC, Freeman MR, Hong SJ, Zhau HE, von Eschenbach AC, Chung LW. Fibroblast-mediated acceleration of human epithelial tumor growth *in vivo*. *Proc Natl Acad Sci USA* 1990; 87:75-79.
19. Cavanaugh PG, Nicolson GL. Purification and some properties of a lung-derived growth factor that differentially stimulates the growth of tumor cells metastatic to the lung. *Cancer Res* 1989; 49:3928-3933.
20. Chabner BA, Foji A. Multidrug resistance: P-glycoprotein and its allies - the elusive foes. *J Natl Cancer Inst* 1989; 81:910-913.
21. Chackal-Roy M, Niemeyer C, Moore M, Zetter BR. Stimulation of human prostatic carcinoma cell growth by factors present in human bone marrow. *J Clin Invest* 1989; 84:43-50.
22. Chang I, Chung LWK. Interaction between prostatic fibroblast and epithelial cells in culture: Role of androgen. *Endocrinology* 1989; 125:2719-2727.
23. Chew EC, Mok CH, Tsao SW, Liu WK, Riches DJ. Scanning electron microscopic study of invasiveness between normal and neoplastic cells and fibroblast in monolayer culture. *Anticancer Res* 1988; 8:275-280.
24. Chodak GW, Hospelhorn V, Judge SM, Mayforth R, Koeppen H, Sasse J. Increased levels of fibroblast growth factor-like activity in urine from patients with bladder or kidney cancer. *Cancer Res* 1988; 48:2083-2088.
25. Chua CC, Geiman DE, Keller GH, Ladda RL. Induction of collagenase secretion in human fibroblast cultures by growth promoting factors. *J Biol Chem* 1986; 260:5213-5216.
26. Chung LWK. Fibroblasts are critical determinants in prostatic cancer growth and dissemination. *Cancer Metastasis Rev* 1991; 10:263-275.
27. Collard JG, Roos E, La Riviere G, Habets GGM. Genetic analysis of invasion and metastasis. *Cancer Surveys* 1988; 7:691-710.
28. Cordon-Cardo C, O'Brien IP, Casals DD, Bertino JR,

Melamed MR. Expression of the multidrug resistance gene product (P-glycoprotein) in human normal and tumor tissues. *J Histochem Cytochem* 1990; 38:1277-1287.

29. Cornil I, Man MS, Fernandez B, Kerbel RS. Enhanced tumorigenicity, melanogenesis and metastasis of a human malignant melanoma observed after subdermal implantation in nude mice. *J Natl Cancer Inst* 1989; 81:938-944.
30. Cornil I, Theodorescu D, Man S, Herlyn M, Jambmrosie J, Kerbel RS. Fibroblast cell interactions with human melanoma cells affecting tumor cell growth are a function of tumor progression. *Proc Natl Acad Sci USA* 1991; 88:6028-6032.
31. Croop JM, Gros P, Housman DE. Genetics of multidrug resistance. *J Clin Invest* 1988; 81:1303-1309.
32. Croop JM, Raymond M, Haber D, de Vault A, Arceci RJ, Gros P, Housman DE. The three mouse multidrug resistance (*mdr*) genes are expressed in a tissue-specific manner in normal mouse tissues. *Molec Cell Biol* 1989; 9:1346-1350.
33. Crouch EC, Stone KR, Bloch M, McDivitt RW. Heterogeneity in the production of collagens and fibronectin by morphologically distinct clones of a human tumor cell line: Evidence for intratumoral diversity in matrix protein biosynthesis. *Cancer Res* 1987; 47:6086-6092.
34. Cunha GR, Chung LWK. Stromal-epithelial interaction: I. Induction of prostatic phenotype in urothelium of testicular feminized (TFm/y) mice. *J Steroid Biochem* 1981; 14:1317-1321.
35. Dabbous MK, Walker R, Haney LM, Custer LM, Nicolson GL, Wooley DE. Mast cells and matrix degradation at sites of tumor invasion in rat mammary adenocarcinoma. *Br J Cancer* 1986; 54:459-465.
36. Davey GC, Currie GA, Alexander P. Immunity as the predominant factor determining metastasis by murine lymphomas. *Br J Cancer* 1979; 40:590-596.
37. De Clerck YA. Purification and characterization of a collagenase inhibitor produced by bovine vascular smooth muscle cells. *Arch Biochem Biophys* 1988; 265:28-37.
38. Deffie AM, Alam T, Seneviratne C, Beenken SW, Batra JK, Shea TC, Henner WS, Goldenberg GJ. Multifactorial resistance to Adriamycin: Relationship of DNA repair, glutathione transferase activity, drug efflux, and P-glycoprotein in cloned cell lines of adriamycin-sensitive and -resistant P388 leukemia. *Cancer Res* 1988; 48:3595-3602.
39. Defize LHK, Boonstra J, Meisenhelder J, Kruijer W, Tertoolen LGJ, Tilly BC, Hunter T, van Bergen en Henegouwen PMP, Moolenaar WH, de Laat SW. Signal transduction by epidermal growth factor occurs through the subclass of high affinity receptors. *J Cell Biol* 1990; 109:2495-2507.
40. Deuchars KL, Ling V. P-glycoprotein and multidrug resistance in cancer chemotherapy. *Semin Oncol* 1989; 16:156-165.
41. Deuel TF. Polypeptide growth factors: Roles in normal and abnormal cell growth. *Annu Rev Cell Biol* 1987; 3:443-492.
42. Devault A, Gros P. Two members of the mouse *mdr* gene family confer multidrug resistance with overlapping but distinct drug specificities. *Molec Cell Biol* 1990; 10:1652-1663.
43. Doerr R, Zvibel I, Chiuten D, ET AL: Clonal growth of tumors on tissue-specific biomatrices and correlation with organ site specificity of metastases. *Cancer Res* 1989; 49:384-392.
44. Dong Z, Radinsky R, Fan D, Tsan R, Bucana CD, Wilmanns C, Fidler IJ. Organ-specific modulation of steady-state mdr gene expression and drug resistance in murine colon cancer cells. *J Natl Cancer Inst* 1994; 86:913-920.
45. Ellis SM, Nabeshima K, Biswas C. Monoclonal antibody preparation and purification of a tumor cell collagenase-stimulatory factor. *Cancer Res* 1989; 49:3385-3391.
46. Enami J, Enami S, Koga M. Growth of normal and neoplastic mouse mammary epithelial cells in primary culture: Stimulation by conditioned medium from mouse mammary fibroblasts. *Jpn J Cancer Res* 1983; 74:845-853.
47. Ervin PR, Kaminski MS, Cody RL, Wicha MS. Production of mammastatin, a tissue-specific growth inhibitor, by normal human mammary cells. *Science* 1989; 244:1585-1587.
48. Ewing J. Neoplastic diseases. Ed. 6. Philadelphia: W B Saunders, 1928.
49. Ezekowitz RAB, Mulliken JB, Folkman J. Interferon alfa-2a therapy for life-threatening hemangiomas of infancy. *N Engl J Med* 1992; 326:1456-1463.
50. Fabra A, Nakajima M, Bucana CD, Fidler IJ. Modulation of the invasive phenotype of human colon carcinoma cells by fibroblasts from orthotopic or ectopic organs of nude mice. *Differentiation* 1992; 52:101-110.
51. Failkow PJ. Clonal origin of human tumors. *Annu Rev Med* 1979; 30:135-143.
52. Fan D, Chakrabarty S, Seid C, Bell CW, Schackert H, Morikawa K, Fidler IJ. Clonal stimulation or inhibition of human colon carcinomas and human renal carcinoma mediated by transforming growth factor-β1. *Cancer Commun* 1989; 1:117-125.
53. Fan Z, Masui H, Altaws I, Mendelsohn J. Blockade of epidermal growth factor receptor function by bivalent and monovalent fragments of 225 anti-epidermal growth factor receptor monoclonal antibodies. *Cancer Res* 1993; 53:4322-4328.
54. Fearon ER, Hamilton SR, Vogelstein B. Clonal analysis of human colorectal tumors. *Science* 1987; 238:193-197.
55. Fessler L, Duncan K, Tryggvason K. Identification of the procollagen IV cleavage products produced by specific tumor collagenase. *J Biol Chem* 1984; 259:9783-9789.
56. Fidler IJ. The Ernst W. Bertner Memorial Award Lecture: The evolution of biological heterogeneity in metastatic neoplasms. In: Nicolson GL, Milas L, eds. *Cancer Invasion and Metastasis: Biologic and Therapeutic Aspects*. New York: Raven Press, 1984; 5-26.
57. Fidler IJ. Metastasis: Quantitative analysis of distribution and fate of tumor emboli labeled with ^{125}I-5-iodo-2'-deoxyuridine. *J Natl Cancer Inst* 1970; 45:773-782.
58. Fidler IJ. Special lecture: Critical factors in the biology of human cancer metastasis: Twenty-eighth G.H.A. Clowes Memorial Award Lecture. *Cancer Res* 1990; 50:6130-6138.
59. Fidler IJ. Tumor heterogeneity and the biology of cancer invasion and metastasis. *Cancer Res* 1978; 38:2651-2660.
60. Fidler IJ, Balch CM. The biology of cancer metastasis and implications for therapy. *Curr Probl Surg* 1987; 24:129-209.
61. Fidler IJ, Berendt MJ. The biological diversity of malig-

nant neoplasms. In: Mihich E, ed. *Biological Responses in Cancer*, vol 1. New York: Plenum Publishing Co, 1982; 269-299.

62. Fidler IJ, Ellis, LM. The implications of angiogenesis for the biology and therapy of cancer metastasis. *Cell* 1994; 79:185-188.
63. Fidler IJ, Gersten DM, Budman MB. Characterization *in vivo* and *in vitro* of tumor cells selected for resistance to syngeneic lymphocyte-mediated cytotoxicity. *Cancer Res* 1976; 36:3160-3165.
64. Fidler IJ, Hart IR. Biological diversity in metastatic neoplasms: Origins and implications. *Science* 1982; 217:998-1003.
65. Fidler IJ, Hart IR. The origin of metastatic heterogeneity in tumors. *Eur J Cancer* 1981; 17:487-494.
66. Fidler IJ, Kripke ML. Metastasis results from preexisting variant cells within a malignant tumor. *Science* 1977; 197:893-895.
67. Fidler IJ, Poste G. The cellular heterogeneity of malignant neoplasms: Implications for adjuvant chemotherapy. *Semin Oncol* 1985; 12:207-222.
68. Fidler IJ, Radinsky R. Genetic control of cancer metastasis (editorial). *J Natl Cancer Inst* 1990; 82:166-168.
69. Fidler IJ, Talmadge JE. The origin and progression of cancer metastases. *In*: Bishop JM, Rowley JD, Greaves M, eds. *Genes and Cancer*. New York: Alan R. Liss, Inc., 1984; 239-251.
70. Fidler IJ, Wilmanns C, Staroselsky A, Radinsky R, Dong Z, Fan D. Modulation of tumor cell response to chemotherapy by the organ environment. *Cancer Metastasis Rev* 1994; 13:209-222.
71. Fojo AT, Ueda K, Slamon DJ, Poplack DG, Gottesman MM, Pastan I. Expression of a multidrug resistance gene in human tumors and tissues. *Proc Natl Acad Sci USA* 1987; 84:265-269.
72. Folkman J. How is blood vessel growth regulated in normal and neoplastic tissue? G.H.A. Clowes Memorial Award Lecture. *Cancer Res* 1986; 46:467-473.
73. Folkman J. The role of angiogenesis in tumor growths. *Semin Cancer Biol* 1992; 3:65-67.
74. Folkman J. What is the evidence that tumors are angiogenesis-dependent? *J Natl Cancer Inst* 1990; 82:4-6.
75. Folkman J, Cotran R. Relation of vascular proliferation to tumor growth. *Int Rev Exp Pathol* 1976; 16:207-248.
76. Folkman J, Klagsburn M. Angiogenic factors. *Science* 1987; 235:444-447.
77. Fossa SD, De Garis ST, Heoer MS, Flokkmann A, Lien HH, Salveson A, Moe B. Recombinant interferon-α-2a with or without vinblastine in metastatic renal cell carcinoma. *Cancer* 1986; 57:1700-1704.
78. Foulds L. The experimental study of tumor progression. A review. *Cancer Res* 1954; 14:327-339.
79. Foulds L. The histologic analysis of mammary tumors of mice. I. Scope of investigations and general principles of analysis. *J Natl Cancer Inst* 1956; 17:701-712.
80. Foulds L. The histologic analysis of mammary tumors of mice. II. The histology of responsiveness and progression. The origins of tumors. *J Natl Cancer Inst* 1956; 17:713-754.
81. Foulds L. The histologic analysis of mammary tumors of mice. III. Organoid tumors. *J Natl Cancer Inst* 1956; 17:755-782.
82. Foulds L. The histologic analysis of mammary tumors of mice. IV. Secretion. *J Natl Cancer Inst* 1956; 17:783-802.
83. Friedman E, Sakaguchio K, Bale AE, Falchetti A, Streeten E, Zimering MB, Weinstein LS, McBride WO, Nakamura Y, Brandt ML. Clonality of parathyroid tumors in familial multiple endocrine neoplasia type I. *N Engl J Med* 1989; 321:213-218.
84. Fry DW, Kraker AJ, McMichael A, Ambroso LA, Nelson JM, Leopoid WR, Connors RW, Bridges AJ. A specific inhibitor of the epidermal growth factor receptor tyrosine kinase. *Science* 1994; 265:1093-1095.
85. Garnick MB, Reich SD, Maxwell B, Coval-Goldsmith S, Richie JP, Rudnick SA. Phase I/II study of recombinant interferon-γ in advanced renal cell carcinoma. *J Urol* 1988; 139:251-255.
86. Giavazzi R, Campbell DE, Jessup JM, Cleary KR, Fidler IJ. Metastatic behavior of tumor cells from primary and metastatic human colorectal carcinomas implanted into different sites in nude mice. *Cancer Res* 1986; 46:1928-1933.
87. Giavazzi R, Jessup JM, Campbell DE, Walker SM, Fidler IJ. Experimental nude mouse model of human colorectal cancer liver metastases. *J Natl Cancer Inst* 1986; 77: 1303-1308.
88. Glisson B, Gupta R, Hodges R, Ross W. Cross-resistance to intercalating agents in an epipodophyllotoxin-resistant Chinese hamster ovary cell line: Evidence for a common intracellular target. *Cancer Res* 1986; 46:1931-1941.
89. Gohji K, Fidler IJ Tsan R, Radinsky R, von Eschenbach AC, Tsuruo T, Nakajima M. Human recombinant interferons-beta and -gamma decrease gelatinase production and invasion by human KG-2 renal carcinoma cells. *Int J Cancer* 1994; 58:380-384.
90. Gohji K, Nakajima M, Dinney CPN, Fan D, Pathak S, Killion JJ, von Eschenbach AC, Fidler IJ. The importance of orthotopic implantation to the isolation and biological characterization of a metastatic human clear cell renal carcinoma in nude mice. *Int J Oncol* 1993; 2:23-32.
91. Goldberg GI, Marmer BL, Grant GA, Eisen AZ, Wilhelm S, He CS. Human 72-kilodalton type IV collagenase forms a complex with a tissue inhibitor of metalloproteinases designated TIMP-2. *Proc Natl Acad Sci USA* 1989; 86:8207-8211.
92. Goodland R, Wilson T, Lenton W, Gregory H, McCullagh K, Wright N. Intravenous but not intragastric urogastrone-EGF is trophic to the intestine of parenterally fed rats. *Gut* 1987; 28:573-582.
93. Gordon PB, Choi HU, Conn G, Ahmed A, Ehrmann B, Rosenberg L, Hatcher VB. Extracellular matrix heparan sulfate proteoglycans modulate the mitogenic capacity of acidic fibroblast growth factor. *J Cell Physiol* 1988; 140:584-592.
94. Gospodarowicz D, Greensburg G, Birdwell CR. Determination of cellular shape by the extracellular matrix and its correlation with the control of cellular growth. *Cancer Res* 1978; 38:4155-4171.
95. Gottesman MM, Pastan I. The multidrug transporter, a double-edged sword. *J Biol Chem* 1988; 263:12163-12166.
96. Gros P, Raymond M, Bell J, Housman D. Cloning and characterization of a second member of the mouse *mdr* gene family. *Mol Cell Biol* 1988; 8:2770-2778.
97. Gross ME, Zorbas MA, Daniels YJ, Garcia R, Gallick GE, Olive M, Brattain MG, Boman BM, Yeoman LC. Cellular growth response to epidermal growth factor in colon carcinoma cells with an amplified epidermal growth

factor receptor derived from a familial adenomatous polyposis patient. *Cancer Res* 1991; 51:1452-1459.

98. Grupposo PA, Mead JE, Fausto N. Transforming growth factor receptors in liver regeneration following partial hepatectomy in the rat. *Cancer Res* 1990; 50:1464-1469.
99. Gullick WJ, Marsden JJ, Whittle N, Ward B, Bobrow L, Waterfield MD. Expression of epidermal growth factor receptors on human cervical, ovarian, and vulvar carcinomas. *Cancer Res* 1986; 46:285-292.
100. Gutman M, Singh RK, Price JE, Fan D, Fidler IJ. Accelerated growth of human colon cancer cells in nude mice undergoing liver regeneration. *Invasion Metastasis*, in press.
101. Gutterman JU. Review: Cytokine therapeutics: Lessons from interferon-α. *Proc Natl Acad Sci USA* 1994; 91: 1198-1205.
102. Hamada H, Okochi E, Oh-hara T, Tsuruo T. Purification of the Mr 22,000 calcium-binding protein (sorcin) associated with multidrug resistance and its detection with monoclonal antibodies. *Cancer Res* 1988; 48:3173-3178.
103. Hanna N, Fidler IJ. The role of natural killer cells in the destruction of circulating tumor emboli. *J Natl Cancer Inst* 1980; 65:801-809.
104. Harris AL, Neal DE. Epidermal growth factor and its receptor in human cancer. *In*: Sluyser M, ed. *Growth Factors and Oncogenes in Breast Cancer*. Chichester, UK: Ellis Horwood, Ltd., 1987; 60-90.
105. Hart IR. 'Seed and Soil' revisited: Mechanisms of site-specific metastasis. *Cancer Metastasis Rev* 1982; 1:5-17.
106. Hart IR, Goode NT, Wilson RE. Molecular aspects of the metastatic cascade. *Biochim Biophys Acta* 1989; 989:65-84.
107. Hay ED. Cell-matrix interaction in the embryo: Cell shape, cell surface, and their role in differentiation. *In*: Trelstad RL, ed. *The Role of Extracellular Matrix in Development*. New York: Alan Liss, 1984; 1-31
108. Hayashi N, Cunha GR, Wong YC. Influence of male genital tract mesenchymes on differentiation of Dunning prostatic adenocarcinoma. *Cancer Res* 1990; 50:4747-4754.
109. Henn W, Blin N, Zang K. Polysomy of chromosome 7 is correlated with overexpression of the *erb*B oncogene in human glioblastoma cell lines. *Hum Genet* 1986; 74:104-106.
110. Heppner GH. Tumor heterogeneity. *Cancer Res* 1984; 44:2259-2265.
111. Hirata Y, Moore GW, Bertagna C, Orth DN. Plasma concentration of immunoreactive human epidermal growth factor (urogastrone) in man. *J Clin Endocrinol Metab* 1980; 40:440-444.
112. Hirata Y, Orth DN. Epidermal growth factor (Urogastrone) in human tissues. *J Clin Endocrinol Metab* 1979; 48:667.
113. Hori A, Sasada R, Matsutani E, Naito K, Sakura Y, Fujita T, Kozai Y. Suppression of solid tumor growth by immunoneutralizing monoclonal antibody against human basic fibroblast growth factor. *Cancer Res* 1991; 51:6189-6194.
114. Hsu SIH, Lothstein L, Horwitz SB. Differential overexpression of three *mdr* gene family members in multidrug resistant J774.2 cells. Evidence that distinct P-glycoprotein precursors are encoded by unique *mdr* genes. *J Biol Chem* 1989; 246:12053-12062.
115. Hu F, Wang RY, Hsu TC. Clonal origin of metastasis in B16 murine melanoma: A cytogenetic study. *J Natl Cancer Inst* 1987; 78:155-163.
116. Hujanen ES, Turpeenniemi-Hujanen T. Recombinant interferon alpha and gamma modulate the invasive potential of human melanoma *in vitro*. *Int J Cancer* 1991; 47:576-581.
117. Humphries MJ, Olden K, Yamada KM. A synthetic peptide from fibronectin inhibits experimental metastasis of murine melanoma cells. *Science* 1986; 233:467-470.
118. Iwamoto Y, Robey FA, Graf J, Sasaki M, Kleinman HK, Yamada Y, Martin GR. YIGSR, a synthetic laminin pentapeptide, inhibits experimental metastasis formation. *Science* 1987; 238:1131-1134.
119. Jain RK. Delivery of novel therapeutic agents in tumors: Physiological barriers and strategies. *J Natl Cancer Inst* 1989; 81:570-576.
120. Jain RK. Transport of molecules across tumor vasculature. *Cancer Metastasis Rev* 1987; 6:559-593.
121. Kanamaru H, Kakehi Y, Yoshida O, Nakanishi S, Pastan I, Gottesman MM. MDR1 RNA levels in human renal cell carcinomas: Correlation with grade and prediction of reversal of doxorubicin resistance by quinidine in tumor explants. *J Natl Cancer Inst* 1989; 81:844-849.
122. Kartner N, Riordan JR, Ling V. Cell surface P-glycoprotein associated with multidrug resistance in mammalian cell lines. *Science (Washington DC)* 1983; 221:1285-1288.
123. Kashles O, Yarden Y, Fischer R, Ullrich A, Schlessinger J. A dominant negative mutation suppresses the function of normal epidermal growth factor receptors by heterodimerization. *Mol Cell Biol* 1991; 11:1454-1463.
124. Kawamoto T, Sato JD, Le A, Polikoff J, Sato GH, Mendelsohn J. Growth stimulation of A431 cells by epidermal growth factor: Identification of high-affinity receptors for epidermal growth factor by an anti-receptor antibody. *Proc Natl Acad Sci USA* 1983; 80:1337-1341.
125. Kedinger M, Haffen K, Simon-Assmann P. Intestinal tissue and cell cultures. *Differentiation* 1986; 36:71-85.
126. Kedinger M, Simon-Assman P, Alexandre E, Haffen K. Importance of a fibroblastic support for in vitro differentiation of intestinal endodermal cells and for their response to glucocorticoids. *Cell Differentiation* 1987; 20:171-182.
127. Kemeny N. Role of chemotherapy in the treatment of colorectal carcinoma. *Semin Surg Oncol* 1987; 3:190-214.
128. Kerbel RS. Growth dominance of metastatic cancer cell: Cellular and molecular aspects. *Adv Cancer Res* 1990; 55:87-132.
129. Kern SE, Fearon ER, Tersmette KWF, Enterline JP, Leppert M, Nakamura Y, White R, Vogelstein B, Hamilton SR. Allelic loss in colorectal carcinoma. *JAMA* 1989; 261:3099-3103.
130. Kerr LD, Olashaw NE, Matrisian LM. Transforming growth factor beta 1 and cAMP inhibit transcription of epidermal growth factor- and oncogene-induced transin RNA. *J Biol Chem* 1988; 263:16999-17005.
131. Keski-Oja J, Blasi F, Leof EB, Moses HL. Regulation of the synthesis and activity of urokinase plasminogen activator in A549 human lung carcinoma cells by transforming growth factor-beta. *J Cell Biol* 1988; 106: 451-459.
132. Khazaie K, Schirrmacher V, Lichtner RB. EGF receptor in neoplasia and metastasis. *Cancer Metastasis Rev* 1993; 12:255-274.

133. Khokha R, Denhardt DT. Matrix metalloproteinases and tissue inhibitor of metalloproteinases: A review of their role in tumorigenesis and tissue invasion. *Invasion Metastasis* 1989; 9:391-405.
134. Kim KJ, Olson K, French T, Vallee B, Fett J. A monoclonal antibody to human angiogenin suppresses tumor growth in athymic mice. *Cancer Res* 1994; 54:4576-4579.
135. Kinney P, Triozzi P, Young D, Drago J, Behrens B, Wise H, Rinehart JJ. Phase II trial of interferon-β-serine in metastatic renal cell carcinoma. *J Clin Oncol* 1990; 8:881-885.
136. Klein G, Klein E. Immune surveillance against virus-induced tumors and nonrejectability of spontaneous tumors: Contrasting consequences of host-versus-tumor evolution. *Proc Natl Acad Sci USA* 1977; 74:2121-2125.
137. Khokha R, Waterhouse P, Yagel S, Lala PK, Overall CM, Norton G, Denhardt DT. Antisense RNA-induced reduction in murine TIMP levels confers oncogenicity on Swiss 3T3 cells. *Science* 1989; 243:947-950.
138. Knudson W, Biswas C, Toole BP: Interactions between human tumor cells and fibroblasts stimulate hyaluronate synthesis. *Proc Natl Acad Sci USA* 1984; 81:6767-6771.
139. Koch G, Smith M, Twentyman P, Wright K. Identification of a novel calcium-binding protein (CP22) in multidrug-resistant murine and hamster cells. *FEBS Lett* 1986; 195:275-279.
140. Koprowski H, Herlyn M, Balaban G, Parmiter A, Ross A, Nowell P. Expression of the receptor for epidermal growth factor correlates with increased dosage of chromosome 7 in malignant melanoma. *Somatic Cell Molec Genet* 1985; 11:297-302.
141. Korc M, Meltzer P, Trent J. Enhanced expression of epidermal growth factor receptor correlates with alterations of chromosome 7 in human pancreatic cancer. *Proc Natl Acad Sci USA* 1986; 83:5141-5144.
142. Korczak B, Robson IB, Lamarche C, Bernstein A, Kerbel RS. Genetic tagging of tumor cells with retrovirus vectors: Clonal analysis of tumor growth and metastasis *in vivo*. *Mol Cell Biol* 1988; 8:3143-3149.
143. Kozlowski JM, Fidler IJ, Campbell D, Xu Z, Kaighn ME, Hart IR. Metastatic behavior of human tumor cell lines grown in the nude mouse. *Cancer Res* 1984; 44:3522-3529.
144. Kozlowski JM, Hart IR, Fidler IJ, Hanna N. A human melanoma line heterogeneous with respect to metastatic capacity in athymic nude mice. *J Natl Cancer Inst* 1984; 72:913-917.
145. Kramer RH, Gonzalez R, Nicolson GL. Metastatic tumor cells adhere preferentially to the extracellular matrix underlying vascular endothelial cells. *Int J Cancer* 1980; 26:639-645.
146. Krigel RL, Padavic-Shaller KA, Rudolph AR, Konrad M, Bradley EC, Comis RL. Renal cell carcinoma: Treatment with recombinant interleukin-2 plus β-interferon. *J Clin Oncol* 1990; 8:460-467.
147. Leith JT, Dexter DL. *Mammalian tumor cell heterogenicity*. Boca Raton, FL: CRC Press, 1986.
148. Levy A, Cioce V, Sobel ME, Garbisa S, Grigioni WF, Liotta LA, Stetler-Stevenson WG. Increased expression of the 72 kDa type IV collagenase in human colonic adenocarcinoma. *Cancer Res* 1991; 51:439-444.
149. Libermann TA, Nusbaum HR, Razon N, Kris R, Lax I, Soreq H, Whittle H, Waterfield MD, Ullrich A, Schlessinger J. Amplification, enhanced expression and possible rearrangement of EGF receptor gene in primary brain tumours of glial origin. *Nature (London)* 1985; 313:144-147.
150. Liotta LA. Tumor invasion and metastases – Role of the extracellular matrix: Rhoads Memorial Award Lecture. *Cancer Res* 1986; 46:1-7.
151. Liotta LA, Thorgeirsson UP, Garbisa S. Role of collagenases in tumor cell invasion. *Cancer Metastasis Rev* 1982; 1:277-288.
152. Liotta LA, Tryggvason K, Garbissa S, Hart I, Foltz CM, Shafie S. Metastatic potential correlates with enzymatic degradation of basement membrane collagen. *Nature* 284:67-68, 1980
153. Lofts FJ, Hurst HC, Sterberg MJE, Gullick WJ. Specific short transmembrane sequences can inhibit transformation by the mutant *neu* growth factor receptor *in vitro* and *in vivo*. *Oncogene* 1993; 8:2813-2820.
154. Long L, Nip J, Brodt P. Paracrine growth stimulation by hepatocyte-derived insulin-like growth factor-1: A regulatory mechanism for carcinoma cells metastatic to the liver. *Cancer Res* 1994; 54:3732-3737.
155. Luria SE, Delbruck M. Mutations of bacteria from virus sensitivity to virus resistance. *Genetics* 1943; 28:491-511.
156. Malden L, Novak U, Burgess A. Expression of transforming growth factor alpha messenger RNA in normal and neoplastic gastrointestinal tract. *Int J Cancer* 1989; 43:380-384.
157. Mantovani A, Tagliabue A, Dean JH, Jerrells TR, Herberman RB. Cytolytic activity of circulating human monocytes on transformed and untransformed human fibroblast. *Int J Cancer* 1979; 23:28-31.
158. Markowitz SD, Molkentin K, Gerbic C, Jackson J, Stellato T, Willson JKV. Growth stimulation by coexpression of transforming growth factor-α and epidermal growth factor receptor in normal an adenomatous human colon epithelium. *J Clin Invest* 1990; 86:356-362.
159. Matrisian LM. The matrix-degrading metalloproteinases. *Bioessays* 1992; 14:455-463.
160. McDonnell S, Matrisian LM. Stromelysin in tumor progression and metastasis. *Cancer Metastasis Rev* 1990; 9:305-319.
161. McLemore TL, Liu MC, Blacker PC, Gregg M, Alley MC, Abbott BJ, Shoemaker RH, Bohlman ME, Litterst CC, Hubbard WC, Brennan RH, McMahon JB, Fine DL, Eggleston JC, Mayo JG, Boyd MR. Novel intrapulmonary model for orthotopic propagation of human lung cancers in athymic nude mice. *Cancer Res* 1987; 47:5132-5140.
162. Mead JE, Fausto N. Transforming growth factor α may be a physiological regulator of liver regeneration by means of an autocrine mechanism. *Proc Natl Acad Sci USA* 1989; 86:1558-1562.
163. Mendelsohn J. The epidermal growth factor receptor as a target for therapy with antireceptor monoclonal antibodies. *Semin Cancer Biol* 1990; 1:339-344.
164. Michalopoulos GK. Liver regeneration: Molecular mechanisms of growth control. *FASEB J* 1990; 4:176-187.
165. Mikkelsen RB, Lin PS, Wallach DF. Interaction of Adriamycin with human red blood cells: A biochemical and morphological study. *J Mol Med* 1977; 2:33-40.
166. Miller FR, McEachern D, Miller BE. Growth regulation of mammary tumor cells in collagen gel cultures by diffusible factors produced by normal mammary gland

epithelium and stromal fibroblasts. *Cancer Res* 1989; 49:6091-6097.

167. Mizoguchi T, Yamada K, Furukawa T, Hidaka K, Hisatsugu T, Shimazu H, Tsuruo T, Sumizawa T, Akiyama S. Expression of the *mdr*1 gene in human gastric antral carcinomas. *J Natl Cancer Inst* 1990; 82:1679-1683.
168. Modjtahedi H, Dean C. The receptor for EGF and its ligands: Expression, prognostic value and target for therapy in cancer (Review). *Int J Oncol* 1994; 4:277-296.
169. Morikawa K, Walker SM, Jessup JM, Fidler IJ. *In vivo* selection of highly metastatic cells from surgical specimens of different primary human colon carcinomas implanted into nude mice. *Cancer Res* 1988; 48:1943-1948.
170. Morikawa K, Walker SM, Nakajima M, Pathak S, Jessup JM, Fidler IJ. Influence of organ environment on the growth, selection, and metastasis of human colon carcinoma cells in nude mice. *Cancer Res* 1988; 48:6863-6871.
171. Moscatelli D, Rifkin DB. Membrane and matrix localization of proteinases: A common theme in tumor cell invasion and angiogenesis. *Biochim Biophys Acta* 1988; 948:67-85.
172. Moscow JA, Cowan KH. Multidrug resistance. *J Natl Cancer Inst* 1988; 80:14-20.
173. Moulder JE, Rockwell S. Tumor hypoxia: Its impact on cancer therapy. *Cancer Metastasis Rev* 1987; 5:313-341.
174. Mukaida H, Hirabayashi N, Hirai T, Iwata T, Saeki S, Toge T. Significance of freshly cultured fibroblasts from different tissues in promoting cancer cell growth. *Int J Cancer* 1991; 48:423-427,
175. Muleris M, Salmon RJ, Dutrillaux B. Chromosomal study demonstrating the clonal evolution and metastatic origin of a metachronous colorectal carcinoma. *Int J Cancer* 1986; 38:167-172.
176. Murphree SA, Cunningham LS, Hwang KM, Sartorelli AC. Effects of Adriamycin on surface properties of sarcoma 180 ascites cells. *Biochem Pharmacol* 1976; 25:1227-1231.
177. Mydlo JH, Heston WD, Fair WR. Characterization of a heparin-binding growth factor from adenocarcinoma of the kidney. *J Urol* 1988; 140:1575-1579.
178. Nair S, Samy TS, Krishan A. Calcium, calmodulin, and protein content of Adriamycin-resistant and -sensitive murine leukemia cells. *Cancer Res* 1986; 46:229-232.
179. Naito S, Giavazzi R, Fidler IJ. Correlation between the *in vitro* interaction of tumor cells with an organ environment and metastatic behavior *in vivo*. *Invasion Metastasis* 1987; 7:16-29.
180. Naito S, von Eschenbach AC, Giavazzi R, Fidler IJ. Growth and metastasis of tumor cells isolated from a human renal cell carcinoma implanted into different organs of nude mice. *Cancer Res* 1986; 46:4109-4115.
181. Naito S, Walker SM, Fidler IJ. *In vivo* selection of human renal carcinoma cells with high metastatic potential in nude mice. *Clin Exp Metastasis* 1989; 7:381-389.
182. Naito S, Walker SM, von Eschenbach AC, Fidler IJ. Evidence for metastatic heterogeneity of a human renal cell carcinoma. *Anticancer Res* 1988; 8:1163-1168.
183. Nakajima M, Morikawa K, Fabra A, Bucana CD, Fidler IJ. Influence of organ environment on extracellular matrix degradative activity and metastasis of human colon carcinoma cells. *J Natl Cancer Inst* 1990; 82:1890-1898.
184. Nanus DM, Schmitz-Drager BJ, Motzer RJ, Lee AC, Vlamis V, Cordon-Cardo C, Albino AP, Reuter VE. Expression of basic fibroblast growth factor in primary human renal tumors: Correlation with poor survival. *J Natl Cancer Inst* 1994; 85:1597-1599.
185. Neal DE, Marsh C, Bennet MK, Abel PD, Hall RR, Sainsbury JRC, Harris AL. Epidermal growth factor receptor in human bladder cancer: Comparison of invasive and superficial tumours. *Lancet* 1985; i:366-368.
186. Nguyen M, Watanabe H, Budson AE, Richie JP, Hayes DF, Folkman J. Elevated levels of an angiogenic peptide, basic fibroblast growth factor, in the urine of patients with a wide spectrum of cancers. *J Natl Cancer Inst* 1994; 86:356-361.
187. Nicolson GL. Cancer metastasis: Tumor cell and host organ properties important in metastasis to specific secondary sites. *Biochim Biophys Acta* 1988; 948:175-224.
188. Nicolson GL. Cancer progression and growth: Relationship of paracrine and autocrine growth mechanisms to organ preference of metastasis. *Exp Cell Res* 1993; 204:171-180.
189. Nicolson GL. Generation of phenotypic diversity and progression in metastatic tumors. *Cancer Metastasis Rev* 1984; 3:25-42.
190. Nicolson GL. Metastatic tumor cell interactions with endothelium, basement membrane, and tissue. *Curr Opin Cell Biol* 1989; 1:1009-1019.
191. Noji S, Tashiro K, Koyama E, Nohno T, Ohyama K, Taniguchi S, Nakamura T. Expression of hepatocyte growth factor gene in endothelial and Kupffer cells of damaged rat livers, as revealed by *in situ* hybridization. *Biochem Biophys Res Commun* 1990; 173:42-47.
192. Nowell PC. Chromosomal and molecular clues to tumor progression. *Semin Oncol* 1989; 16:116-127.
193. Nowell PC. The clonal evolution of tumor cell populations: Acquired genetic lability permits stepwise selection of variant sublines and underlies tumor progression. *Science* 1976; 194:23-28.
194. Nowell PC. Mechanisms of tumor progression. *Cancer Res* 1986; 46:2203-2207.
195. O'Brian CA, Fan D, Ward NE, Seid C, Fidler IJ. Level of protein kinase C activity correlates directly with resistance to Adriamycin in murine fibrosarcoma cells. *FEBS Lett* 1989; 246:78-82.
196. O'Brian CA, Ward NE. Biology of the protein kinase C family. *Cancer Metastasis Rev* 1989; 8:199-214.
197. Olsson L. Phenotypic diversity of malignant cell populations: Molecular mechanisms and biological significance. *Cancer Res* 1986; 3:91-114.
198. Ootsuyama A, Tanaka K, Tanooka H. Evidence by cellular mosaicism for monoclonal metastasis of spontaneous mouse mammary tumors. *J Natl Cancer Inst* 1987; 78:1223-1227.
199. Ostrowski LE, Finch J, Krieg P, Matrisian L, Patskan G, O'Connel JF, Phillips J, Slata TJ, Breathnach R, Bowden GT. Expression pattern of a gene for a secreted metalloproteinase during late stage of tumor progression. *Mol Carcinog* 1988; 1:13-19.
200. Overall CM, Wrana JL, Sodek J. Independent regulation of collagenase, 72-kDa progelatinase, and metalloendoproteinase inhibitor expression in human fibroblasts by transforming growth factor-beta. *J Biol Chem* 1989; 25:1860-1869.
201. Paget S. The distribution of secondary growths in cancer of the breast. *Lancet* 1889; 1:571-573.

202. Pastan I, Gottesman MM, Ueda K, Lovelace E, Rutherford AV, Willingham MC. A retrovirus carrying an MDR1 cDNA confers multidrug resistance and polarized expression of P-glycoprotein in MDCK cells. *Proc Natl Acad Sci USA* 1988; 85:4486-4490.
203. Phillips PC, Levow C, Catterall M, Colvin OM, Pastan, Brem H. Transforming growth factor-α-*Pseudomonas* exotoxin fusion protein (TGF-α-PE38) treatment of subcutaneous and intracranial human glioma and medulloblastoma xenografts in athymic mice. *Cancer Res* 1994; 54:1008-1015.
204. Pigram WJ, Fuller W, Hamilton LDH. Stereochemistry of intercalation: interaction of daunomycin with DNA. *Nature* 1971; 235:17-19.
205. Plowman GD, Green JM, McDonald VL, Neubauer MG, Disteche CM,Todaro GJ, Shoyab M. The amphiregulin gene encodes a novel epidermal growth factor-related protein with tumor-inhibitory activity. *Mol Cell Biol* 1981; 10:1969-1981.
206. Poste G. Experimental systems for analysis of the malignant phenotype. *Cancer Metastasis Rev* 1982; 1:141-199.
207. Poste G, Tzeng J, Doll J, Greig R, Rieman D, Zeidman I. Evolution of tumor cell heterogeneity during progressive growth of individual lung metastases. *Proc Natl Acad Sci USA* 1982; 79:6574-6578.
208. Postlethwaite AE, Lachman LB, Mainardi CL, Kang AH. Interleukin 1 stimulation of collagenase production by cultured fibroblasts. *J Exp Med* 1983:157:801-806.
209. Pratesi G, Manzotti C, Tortoreto M, Audisio RA, Zunino F. Differential efficacy of flavone acetic acid against liver versus lung metastases in a human tumour xenograft. *Br. J. Cancer* 1991; 663:71-74.
210. Prehn RT. Tumor progression and homeostasis. *Adv Cancer Res* 1976; 23:203-236.
211. Presta M, Maier JA, Ragnotti GJ. The mitogenic signaling pathway but not the plasminogen activator-inducing pathway of basic fibroblast growth factor is mediated through protein kinase C in fetal bovine aortic endothelial cells. *Cell Biol* 1989; 109:1877-1884.
212. Price JE, Aukerman SL, Fidler IJ. Evidence that the process of murine melanoma metastasis is sequential and selective and contains stochastic elements. *Cancer Res* 1986; 46:5172-5178.
213. Price JE, Daniels LM, Campbell DE, Giavazzi R. Organ distribution of experimental metastases of a human colorectal carcinoma injected in nude mice. *Clin Exp Metastasis* 1989; 7:55-68.
214. Radinsky R. Growth factors and their receptors in metastasis. *Semin Cancer Biol* 1991; 2:169-177.
215. Radinsky R. Paracrine growth regulation of human colon carcinoma organ-specific metastases. *Cancer Metastasis Rev* 1993; 12:345-361.
216. Radinsky R, Beltran PJ, Tsan R, Zhang R, Cone RD, Fidler IJ. Transcriptional induction of the melanocyte-stimulating hormone receptor in brain metastases of murine K-1735 melanoma. *Cancer Res* 1995; 55:141-148.
217. Radinsky R, Bucana CD, Ellis LE, Sanchez R, Cleary KR, Brigati DJ, Fidler IJ. A rapid colorimetric *in situ* messenger RNA hybridization technique for analysis of epidermal growth factor receptor in paraffin-embedded surgical specimens of human colon carcinomas. *Cancer Res* 1993; 53:937-943.
218. Radinsky R, Fidler IJ, Price JE, Esumi N, Tsan R, Petty CM, Bucana CD, Bar-Eli M. Terminal differentiation and apoptosis in experimental lung metastases of human osteogenic sarcoma cells by wild type *p53*. *Oncogene* 1994; 9:1877-1883.
219. Radinsky R, Risin S, Fan D, Dong Z, Bielenberg D, Bucana CD, Fidler IJ. Level and function of epidermal growth factor receptor predict the metastatic potential of human colon carcinoma cells. *Clinical Cancer Res* 1995; 1:19-31.
220. Raymond M, Rose E, Housman DE, Gros P. Physical mapping, amplification, and overexpression of the mouse *mdr* gene family in multidrug-resistant cells. *Molec Cell Biol* 1990; 10:1642-1651.
221. Real FX, Oettgen HF, Krown SE. Kaposi's sarcoma and the acquired immunodeficiency syndrome: Treatment with high and low doses of recombinant leukocyte interferon. *J Clin Oncol* 1986; 4:544-551.
222. Redemann N, Holzmann B, von Ruden T, Wagner EF, Schlessinger J, Ullrich A. Antioncogenic activity of signalling defective epidermal growth factor receptor mutants. *Mol Cell Biol* 1992; 12:491-498.
223. Reid LM, Abreu SL, Montgomery K. Extracellular matrix and hormonal regulation of synthesis and abundance of messenger RNAs in cultured liver cells. *In*: Arias IM, Jakoby WB, Popper H, Schachter D, Shafritz DA, eds. *The Liver: Biology and Pathobiology*, 2nd ed. New York: Raven Press, 1988; 717-737.
224. Rinehart JJ, Young D, LaForge J, Colburn D, Neidhart JA. Phase I/II trial of interferon-β-serine in patients with renal cell carcinoma: Immunological and biological effects. *Cancer Res* 1987; 47:2481-2485.
225. Roberts AB, Sporn MB, Assoian RK, Smith JM, Roche NS, Wakefield LM, Heine VI, Liotta LA, Falanga V, Kehr LJM. Transforming growth factor type B: Rapid induction of fibrosis and angiogenesis *in vivo* and stimulation of collagen formation *in vitro. Proc Natl Acad Sci USA* 1986; 83:4167-4171.
226. Roberts AB, Thompson NL, Heine U, Flanders C, Sporn MB. Transforming growth factor β: Possible roles in carcinogenesis. *Br J Cancer* 1988; 57:594-600.
227. Rothenberg M, Ling V. Multidrug resistance: Molecular biology and clinical relevance. *J Natl Cancer Inst* 1989; 81:907-910.
228. Russell AH, Tong D, Dawson LE, Wisbeck W. Adenocarcinoma of the proximal colon: Sites of initial dissemination and patterns of recurrence following surgery alone. *Cancer* 1984; 53:360-367.
229. Saiki I, Naito S, Yoneda J, Azuma I, Price JE, Fidler IJ. Characterization of the invasive and metastatic phenotype in human renal cell carcinoma. *Clin Exp Metastasis* 1991; 9:551-566.
230. Sainsbury JRC, Sherbert GV, Farndon JR, Harris AL. Epidermal growth factor receptors and oestrogen receptors in human breast cancer. *Lancet* 1986; i:364-366.
231. Sartorelli AC. Therapeutic attack of hypoxic cells of solid tumors: Presidential address. *Cancer Res* 1988; 48:775-778.
232. Sauter G, Haley T, Chew K, Kerschmann R, Moore D, Carroll P, Moch H, Gudat F, Mihatsch MJ, Waldman F. Epidermal growth factor receptor expression is associated with rapid tumor proliferation in bladder cancer. *Int J Cancer* 1994; 57:508-514.
233. Schackert G, Fidler IJ. Development of *in vivo* models for

studies of brain metastasis. *Int J Cancer* 1988; 41:589-594.

234. Schackert G, Fidler IJ. Site-specific metastasis of mouse melanomas and a fibrosarcoma in the brain or the meninges of syngeneic animals. *Cancer Res* 1988; 48: 3478-3483.

235. Schlaifer D, Laurent G, Chittal S, Tsuruo T, Soues S, Muller C, Charcasset JY, Alard C, Brousset P, Mazarolles C, Delsol G. Immunohistochemical detection of multidrug resistance-associated P-glycoprotein in tumor and stromal cells of human cancers. *Br J Cancer* 1990; 62:177-182.

236. Schlessinger J. Allosteric regulation of the epidermal growth factor receptor kinase. *J Cell Biol* 1986; 103:2067-2072.

237. Schor SL, Schor AM. Clonal heterogeneity in fibroblast phenotype: Implications for the control of epithelial-mesenchymal interactions. *BioEssays* 1987; 7: 200-204.

238. Schwarz LC, Gingras MC, Goldberg G, Greenberg AH, Wright JA. Loss of growth factor dependence and conversion of transforming growth factor-β1 inhibition to stimulation in metastatic H-ras-transformed murine fibroblasts. *Cancer Res* 1988; 48:6999-7003.

239. Selva E, Raden DL, Davis RJ. Mitogen-activated protein kinase stimulation by a tyrosine kinase-negative epidermal growth factor receptor. *J Biol Chem* 1993; 268: 2250-2254.

240. Shafie SM, Liotta LA. Formation of metastasis by human breast carcinoma cells (MCF-7) in nude mice. *Cancer Lett* 1980; 11:81-87.

241. Shapiro SD, Campbell EJ, Kobayashi DK, Welgus HG. Immune modulation of metalloproteinase production in human macrophages: Selective suppression of interstitial collagenase and stromelysin biosynthesis by interferon-γ. *J Clin Invest* 1990; 86:1204-1210.

242. Shen DW, Fojo A, Chin IE, Ronninson B, Richert N, Pastan I, Gottesman MM. Human multidrug resistant cell lines: Increased *mdr*1 expression can precede gene amplification. *Science* 1986; 232:643-645.

243. Siegall CB, FitzGerald DJ, Pastan I. Selective killing of tumor cells using EGF or TCGα-*Pseudomonas* exotoxin chimeric molecules. *Semin Cancer Biol* 1990; 1:345-350.

244. Silverberg BS, Lubera JA. Cancer statistics, 1989. *CA*, 1989; 39:3-4.

245. Singh RK, Bucana CD, Gutman M, Fan D, Wilson MR, Fidler IJ. Organ site-dependent expression of basic fibroblast growth factor in human renal cell carcinoma cells. *Am J Pathol* 1994; 145:365-374.

246. Singh RK, Gutman M, Bucana CD, Sanchez R, Llansa N, Fidler IJ. Interferons alpha and beta downregulate the expression of basic fibroblast growth factor in human carcinomas. *Proc Natl Acad Sci USA*, in press.

247. Singh RK, Gutman M, Radinsky R, Bucana CD, Fidler IJ. Expression of interleukin 8 correlates with the metastatic potential of human melanoma cells in nude mice. *Cancer Res* 1994; 54:3242-3247.

248. Slack NH, Bross JDJ. The influence of the site of metastasis on tumor growth and response to chemotherapy. *Br J Cancer* 1975; 32:78-86.

249. Sloane BF. Cathepsin B and cystatins: Evidence for a role in cancer progression. *Semin Cancer Biol* 1990; 1:137-152.

250. Smith KA, Begg AC, Denekamp J. Differences in chemosensitivity between subcutaneous and pulmonary tumors. *Eur J Cancer Clin Oncol* 1985; 21:249-256.

251. Spremulli EN, Scott C, Campbell DE, Libbey NP, Shochat D, Gold DV, Dexter DL. Characterization of two metastatic subpopulations originating from a single human colon carcinoma. *Cancer Res* 1983; 43:3828-3835.

252. Staroselsky A, Fan D, O'Brian CA, Bucana CD, Gupta KP, Fidler IJ: Site-dependent differences in response of the UV-2237 murine fibrosarcoma to systemic therapy with adriamycin. *Cancer Res* 1990; 40:7775-7780.

253. Staroselsky AN, Radinsky R, Fidler IJ, Pathak S, Chernajovsky Y, Frost P. The use of molecular genetic markers to demonstrate the effect of organ environment on clonal dominance in a human renal cell carcinoma grown in nude mice. *Int J Cancer* 1992; 51:130-138.

254. Steiner MG, Harlow SP, Colombo E, Bauer KD. Chromosomes 8, 12, and 17 copy number in Astler-Coller stage C colon cancer in relation to proliferative activity and DNA ploidy. *Cancer Res* 1993; 53:681-686.

255. Stephenson RA, Dinney CPN, Gohji K, Ordonez NG, Killion JJ, Fidler IJ. Metastatic model for human prostate cancer using orthotopic implantation in nude mice. *J Natl Cancer Inst* 1992; 84:951-957.

256. Stetler-Stevenson WG. Type IV collagenases in tumor invasion and metastasis. *Cancer Metastasis Rev* 1990; 9:289-303.

257. Stetler-Stevenson WG, Krutzsch HC, Wacher MP, Margulies IM, Liotta LA. The activation of human type IV collagenase proenzyme. *J Biol Chem* 1989; 264:1353-1356.

258. Stiles CD, Capone GT, Scher CD, Antoniades HN, Van Wyk JJ, Pledger WJ. Dual control of cell growth by somatomedins and platelet-derived growth factor. *Proc Natl Acad Sci USA* 1979; 76:1279-1283.

259. Sugarbaker EV. Patterns of metastasis in human malignancies. *Cancer Biol Rev* 1981; 2:235-278.

260. Susuki M, Hori K, Abe I. A new approach to cancer chemotherapy: Selective enhancement of tumor blood flow with angiotensin II. *J Natl Cancer Inst* 1981; 67:663-669.

261. Suzuki M, Hori M, Abe I, Sachiko S, Sato H. Functional characterization of the microcirculation in tumors. *Cancer Metastasis Rev* 1984; 3:115-126.

262. Talmadge JE, Benedict K, Madsen J, Fidler IJ. The development of biological diversity and susceptibility to chemotherapy in cancer metastases. *Cancer Res* 1984; 44:3801-3805.

263. Talmadge JE, Meyers KM, Prieur DJ, Starkey JR. Role of natural killer cells in tumor growth and metastasis: C57BL/6 normal and beige mice. *J Natl Cancer Inst* 1980; 65:929-935.

264. Talmadge JE, Wolman SR, Fidler IJ. Evidence for the clonal origin of spontaneous metastases. *Science* 1982; 217:361-363.

265. Talmadge JE, Zbar B. Clonality of pulmonary metastases from the bladder 6 subline of the B16 melanoma studied by Southern hybridization. *J Natl Cancer Inst* 1987; 78:315-320.

266. Tan MH, Chu TM. Characterization of the tumorigenic and metastatic properties of a human pancreatic tumor cell line (ASPC-1) implanted orthotopically into nude mice. *Tumour Biol* 1985; 6:89-98.

267. Tanaka H, Mori Y, Ishii H. Enhancement of metastatic capacity of fibroblast-tumor cell interaction in mice. *Cancer Res* 1988; 48:1456-1459.

268. Tannock IF, Rotin D. Acid pH in tumors and its potential for therapeutic exploitation. *Cancer Res* 1989; 49:4373-4384.
269. Tarin D, Price JE, Kettlewell MGW, Souter RG, Vass ACR, Crossley B. Mechanisms of human tumor metastasis studied in patients with peritoneovenous shunts. *Cancer Res* 1984; 44:3584-3592.
270. Teicher BA, Alvarez-Sotomayor E, Huang ZD. Antiangiogenic agents potentiate cytotoxic cancer therapies against primary and metastatic disease. *Cancer Res* 1992; 52:6702-6704.
271. Teicher BA, Holden SA, Al-Achi A, Herman TS. Classification of antineoplastic treatments by their differential toxicity toward putative oxygenated and hypoxic tumor subpopulations *in vivo* in the FSaIIC murine fibrosarcoma. *Cancer Res* 1990; 50:3339-3344.
272. Teicher BA, Holden SA, Ara G, Sotomayor E, Huang ZD, Chen YN, Brem H. Potentiation of cytotoxic cancer therapies by TNP-470 alone and with other antiangiogenic agents. *Int J Cancer* 1994; 57:920-925.
273. Teicher BA, Lazo JS, Sartorelli AC. Classification of antineoplastic agents by their selective toxicities toward oxygenated and hypoxic tumor cells. *Cancer Res* 1981; 41:73-81.
274. Testa JE, Quigley JP. The role of urokinase-type plasminogen activator in aggressive tumor cell behavior. *Cancer Metastasis Rev* 1990; 9:353-367.
275. Testa JE, Quigley JP. Reversal of misfortune: TIMP-2 inhibits tumor cell invasion. *J Natl Cancer Inst* 1991; 83:740-742.
276. Thorgeirsson SS, Huber BE, Sorell S, Fojo A, Pastan I, Gottesman MM. Expression of the multidrug-resistant gene in hepatocarcinogenesis and regenerating rat liver. *Science* 1987; 236:1120-1122.
277. Tozer GM, Lewis S, Michalowski A, Aber V. The relationship between regional variations in blood flow and histology in a transplanted rat fibrosarcoma. *Br J Cancer* 1990; 61:250-257.
278. Trinks U, Buchdunger E, Furet P, Kump W, Mett H, Meyer T, Muller M, Regenass U, Rihs G, Lydon N, Traxler P. Dianilinophtalimides: Potent and selective, ATP-competitive inhibitors of the EGF-receptor protein tyrosine kinase. *J Med Chem* 1994; 37:1015-1027.
279. Tryggvason K, Hoyhtya M, Salo T. Proteolytic degradation of extracellular matrix in tumor invasion. *Biochim Biophys Acta* 1987; 907:191-217.
280. Tsuruo T. Mechanisms of multidrug resistance and implication for therapy. *Jpn J Cancer Res* 1988; 79:285-296.
281. Tsuruo T, Iida H, Kawabara H, Tsukagoshi S, Sakurai Y. High calcium content of pleiotropic drug-resistant P388 and K562 leukemia and Chinese hamster ovary cells. *Cancer Res* 1984; 44:5095-5099.
282. Ullrich AL, Coussens L, Hayflick JS, Dull TJ, Gray A, Tam AW, Lee J, Yarden Y, Libermann TA, Schlessinger J, Downward J, Whittle ELV, Waterfield MD, Seeburg PH. Human epidermal growth factor receptor cDNA sequence and aberrant expression of the amplified gene in A431 epidermoid carcinoma cells. *Nature (London)* 1984; 309:418-425.
283. van Dale P, Galand P. Effect of partial hepatectomy on experimental liver invasion by intraportally injected colon carcinoma cells in rats. *Invasion Metastasis* 1988; 8:217-227.
284. van der Geer P, Hunter T, Lindberg RA. Receptor protein-tyrosine kinases and their signal transduction pathways. *Annu Rev Cell Biol* 1994; 10:251-337.
285. Vaupel P, Kallinowski F, Okunieff P. Blood flow, oxygen and nutrient supply, and metabolic microenvironment of human tumors: A review. *Cancer Res* 1989; 49:6449-6465.
286. Vogelstein B, Fearon ER, Kern SE, Hamilton SR, Preisinger AC, Nakamura Y, White R. Allelotype of colorectal carcinomas. *Science* 1989; 244:207-222.
287. Waghorne C, Thomas M, Lagarde A, Kerbel RS, Breitman ML. Genetic evidence for progressive selection and overgrowth of primary tumors by metastatic cell subpopulations. *Cancer Res* 1988; 48:6109-6114.
288. Waldman FM, Carroll PR, Kerschmann R, Cohen MB, Field FG, Mayall BH. Centromeric copy number of chromosome 7 is strongly correlated with tumor grade and labeling index in human bladder cancer. *Cancer Res* 1991; 51:3807-3813.
289. Weidner N, Carroll PR, Flax J, Blumenfeld W, Folkman J. Tumor angiogenesis correlates with metastasis in invasive prostate carcinoma. *Am J Pathol* 1993; 143:401-409.
290. Weidner N, Semple JP, Welch WR, Folkman J. Tumor angiogenesis and metastasis – correlation in invasive breast carcinoma. *N Engl J Med* 1991; 324:1-8.
291. Weinstein RS, Kuszak IR, Kluskens LF, Con JS. P-glycoprotein in pathology: The multidrug resistance gene family in humans. *Hum Pathol* 1990; 21:34-48.
292. Welch DR, Fabra A, Nakajima M. Transforming growth factor-beta stimulates mammary adenocarcinoma cell invasion and metastatic potential. *Proc Natl Acad Sci USA* 1990; 87:7678-7682.
293. Welch DR, Tomasovic SP. Implications of tumor progression on clinical oncology. *Clin Exptl Metastasis* 1985; 3:151-188.
294. Wilhelm SM, Collier IE, Marjer BL, et al. SV40-transformed human lung fibroblasts secrete a 92-kDa type IV collagenase which is identical to that secreted by normal human macrophages. *J Biol Chem* 1989; 264:17213-17221.
295. Wilmanns C, Fan D, O'Brian CA, Radinsky R, Bucana CD, Tsan R, Fidler IJ. Modulation of doxorubicin sensitivity and level of P-glycoprotein expression in human colon carcinoma cells by ectopic and orthotopic environments in nude mice. *Int J Oncol* 1993, 3:413-422.
296. Yunis JJ. The chromosomal basis of human neoplasia. *Science* 1983; 221:227-236.
297. Zarrilli R, Bruni CB, Riccio A. Multiple levels of control of insulin-like growth factor gene expression. *Mol Cell Endocrinol* 1994; 101:R1-R14.
298. Zvibel I, Halay E, Reid LM. Heparin and hormonal regulation of mRNA synthesis and abundance of autocrine growth factors: Relevance to clonal growth of tumors. *Mol Cell Biol* 1991; 11:108-116.
299. Zwelling LA, Michaels S, Erickson LC, Ungeleier RS, Nichols M, Kohn K. Protein-associated DNA breaks in L1210 cells treated with the DNA intercalating agents 4'-(9-acridinylamino)-methanesulfon-*m*-anisidide and Adriamycin. *Biochemistry* 20: 6553-6563, 1981.

DEVELOPMENTAL THERAPEUTICS AND THE DESIGN OF CLINICAL TRIALS

ROBERT K. OLDHAM
Biological Therapy Institute Foundation, Franklin, Tennessee; and University of Missouri, Columbia, Missouri

New techniques in biotechnology and the use of biological response modifiers in cancer treatment have made it apparent that there are differences in developmental therapeutics for biotherapy, in contrast to drug development. Over the past 25 years, more than one million chemicals have been tested as anticancer agents, but less than 50 have reached the clinic as commercial pharmaceuticals. Perhaps ten of these drugs can be classed as moderately effective; the rest are only marginally useful and all can be highly toxic. With the discovery of monoclonal antibodies and conjugates thereof, the exploitation of bioengineering to produce purified, characterized lymphokines/cytokines and other biologicals, and further information on the mechanism of action of these natural molecules, the rate of development for biological therapeutics has risen dramatically. Because of their selectivity and with their implicit biological diversity, new approaches are needed to efficiently bring biotherapy to the clinic. Previously, there have always been fewer promising agents (drugs) to test than patients who needed new

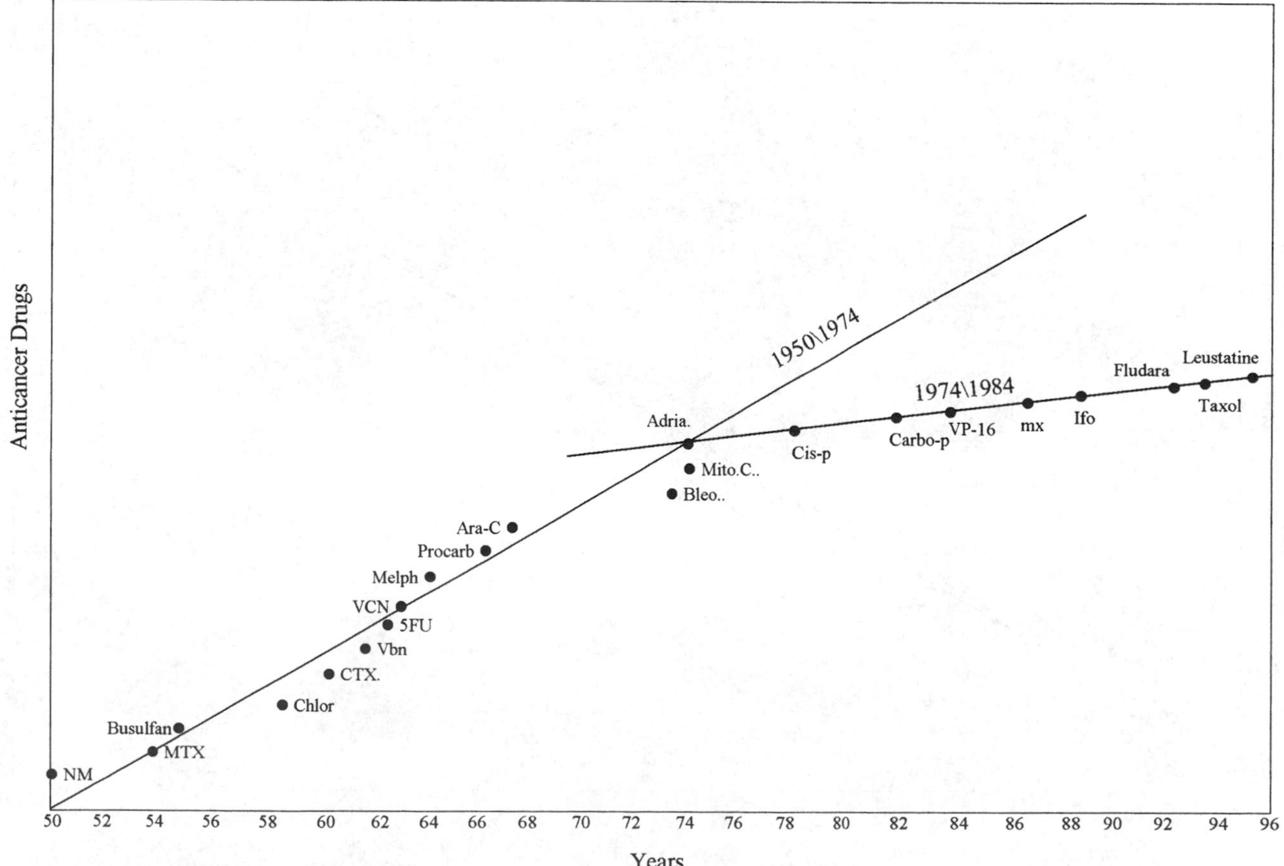

Figure 1. Drug development paradigm. NM, nitrogen mustard; MTX, methotrexate; Chlor, chlorambucil; CTX, cytoxan; Vbn, Velban; 5FU, 5-fluorouracil; VCN, vincristine; Melp, melphalan; Procarb, procarbazine; Ara-C, cytosine arabinoside; Bleo, bleomycin; Mito.C, mitomycin C; Adria, adriamycin; Cis-P, cisplatin; Leustatine; Mx, mitoxantrone; Ifo, ifosamide; Fludara, Fludaribine; Taxol.

R.K. Oldham (ed.), Principles of Cancer Biotherapy. 3rd ed., 39–50.

approaches. In fact, the drug development paradigm has been a slow and laborious mechanism of developmental therapeutics with each drug taking some 8-10 years to commercial approval, at a cost of 200 to 350 million dollars (Fig. 1). These extraordinary costs have resulted in only one to four anticancer drugs coming into the system annually. Far fewer have been approved for use in general medicine. VP-16, a recent drug approved for general use, entered clinical trials in 1972 and only became generally available in 1985; taking more than a decade to pass through our current system of drug development. On average, fewer than two drugs per year are approved for general use by oncologists. This expensive and slow paradigm reflects both the toxicity and marginal effectiveness of chemotherapeutic drugs and a bureaucratic regulatory system more fearful of criticism than a willingness to pursue opportunities for seriously ill patients [57, 58, 70].

More recently, a large number of biological substances and therapeutic options have been making their way to the clinic, increasing the difficulty of decisions as to the order and amount of preclinical and clinical testing. (Fig. 2). The current system for drug development is not sufficiently flexible, and needs major changes in direction and technique to optimize clinical testing and augment the translation of new biotherapeutic approaches to patients [6, 17, 42, 44, 48, 58, 63-69]

Although the concept of biotherapy is not new, the use of recombinant genetics to produce highly purified biologicals as medicinals dates from about 1980 [23]. A member of the alpha-interferon family was the first biological produced by recombinant methods to be used as an anticancer medicine in humans [81, 82]. In the few years since the first alpha-interferon molecule was prepared by recombinant methods, a large number of recombinant molecules have become available or are being prepared for testing in the clinic.

Historical aspects in the development of immunotherapy have been reviewed [62]. Before the 1980s, the term immunotherapy was considered to be synonymous with biological therapy by most investigators. However, it is now clear that there are many biological approaches that may affect cancer growth and metastases, yet are not with-

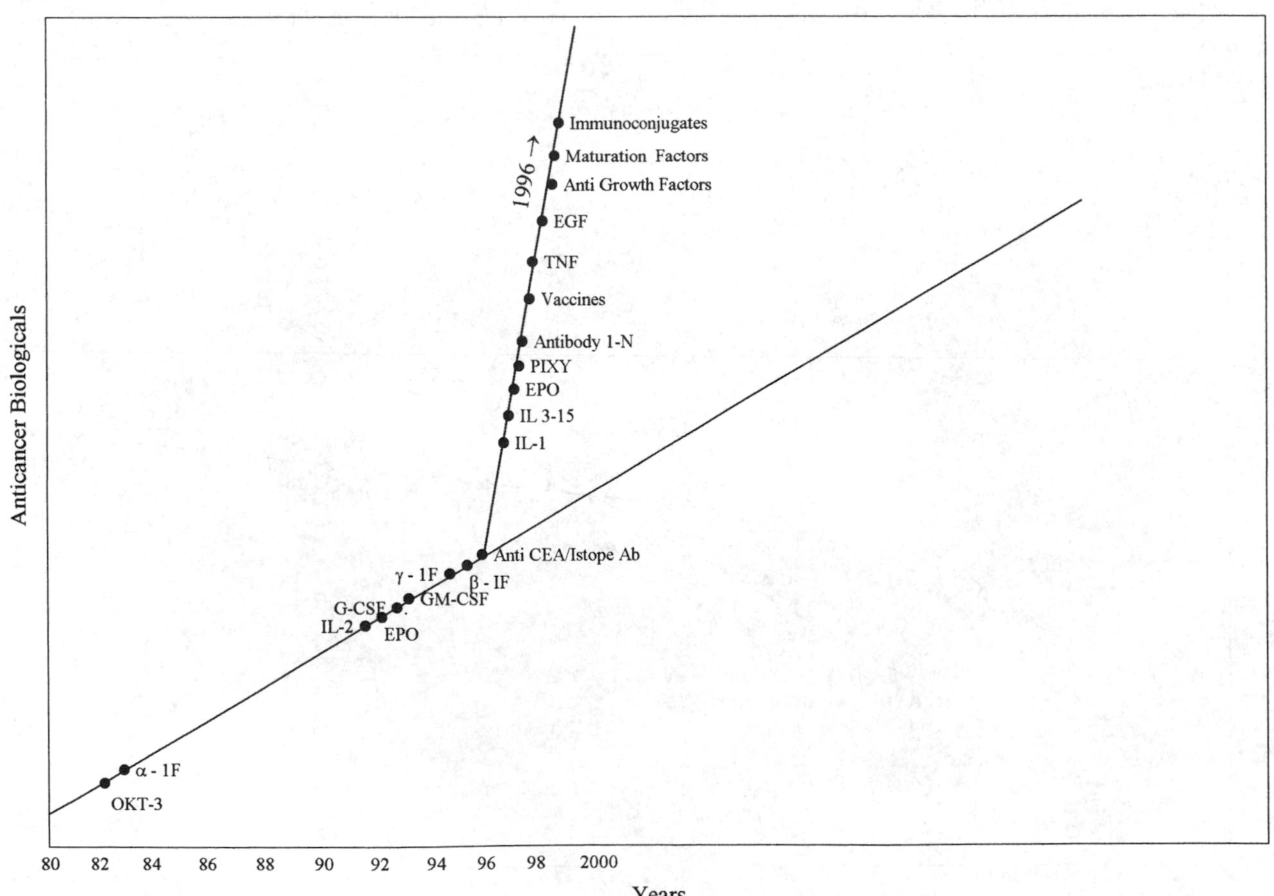

Figure 2. Development of biologicals. OK-T3, antibody to T-3 lymphocyte receptor; alpha IF, alpha-interferon; β IF, beta-interferon; γIF, gamma-interferon; IL-2, interleukin-2; TNF, tumor necrosis factor; EGF, epidermal growth factor; EPO, erythropoietin; G-CSF, granulocyte colony-stimulating factor; GM-CSF, granulocyte-macrophage colony stimulating factor; MoAb, monoclonal antibodies; IL-1, interleukin-1; IL-3, interleukin-3; IL-4-8, interleukins 4-8; Immuno, immunoconjugates; G&MF, growth and maturation factors; PIXY; hybrid growth factor.

in the immune system. Thus, biotherapy now refers to agents derived from biological sources and/or the use of agents that affect biological responses. The term biologicals describes agents extracted from or produced from biological materials. With biotechnology, this involves the use of recombinant genetics to isolate the gene, transfect it into an appropriate producer organism, and then isolate and purify the protein product. The types of materials that alter biological responses for the benefit of the patient have been called biological response modifiers (BRM). The use of biologicals and BRM in the treatment of cancer and other diseases can now be termed biotherapy (a term I initially used in 1984 to describe this fourth modality of cancer treatment) [71, 72]. As is always the case, nomenclature can be confusing and terms may be variously defined by different individuals. In the broadest sense, biotherapy includes blood products, transplanted organs, antibiotics (often derived by extraction from biological organisms and later synthesized), and a variety of other agents and approaches. However, in this chapter, the focus will primarily be on BRM, recombinant biologicals and gene engineered or activated cells being developed as medicinals.

Immunotherapy has had a checkered past. Kari Cantell said it well when describing some of the early interferon research: 'Much second class research was carried out with third class preparations slightly contaminated with interferon'[5]. In addition, there have been questionable approaches ('alternative medicine') used by certain practitioners, and even frank quackery by others who purported to deliver 'immunotherapy' as anticancer approaches. Even for the very dedicated scientists who have explored immunotherapy over the past several decades, there have been many pitfalls relating to the purity of their preparations, the source of the materials, and the assays and techniques by which their measurements were made.

Huge expenditures by the National Institute of Health (NIH) in the area of molecular biological and viral oncology over the last 20 years led to the current technology of 'genetic engineering.' In contrast to previous attempts to develop biological therapy, we now have techniques available that can isolate a single gene and use it in a biomanufacturing process to produce absolutely pure proteins identical to those found in the body. It is with these techniques that hundreds, and later thousands, of biological compounds and their synthetic analogs will be developed. Many of these biologicals will be candidates for use as medicinals. A major value of the research done thus far with interferon is that it may be viewed as a model for the development of other biological substances as medicinals [48, 63]. Interferon research in particular and biotherapy in general must be seen as a new challenge in developmental therapeutics, with agents to be tested appearing at a still accelerating rate. No longer can the historical drug development paradigm be used [42]. The methods used by the Food and Drug Administration [11], National Institutes of Health, and the pharmaceutical industry in the development of drugs must be drastically changed to a new paradigm that will accommodate the realities relevant to biologicals and their use in medicine [42, 58, 69, 73, 74].

DRUG DEVELOPMENT

The current process of drug development involves a very long and costly set of procedures [42, 67]. This includes the initial concept, extraction or synthesis, formulation, documentation of biological activity and purity, early studies in the laboratory and in experimental animals to determine the mechanism of action and toxicity, and compilation of all the preclinical data into an investigational new drug application (INDA). It costs several million dollars for a pharmaceutical company to file a single INDA. During preclinical development, companies make projections about the potential market size and profitability as justification for the investment. These projections are difficult, and are most accurate when related to an existing drug in a known market. It follows that predicting the market size for a totally new agent or new approach is much more difficult.

Subsequent to the INDA, further preclinical work on the mechanism of action and preclinical toxicology of a new drug is done. In addition, early-phase studies are begun in the clinic to determine biological activity in humans. Although the process is not uniform for all classes of pharmaceuticals, studies are termed 'phase I' when the dose of the drug is escalated to determine its biological activity and its toxicity. Based on the preclinical toxicology information in small animals and sometimes in primates, projections are made for the starting dose in humans. A low starting dose is selected to avoid severe toxicity in the initial patients in a phase I clinical trial. The rate of dose escalation in these trials and the acceptability of toxic side effects vary with the population at risk and are related to the seriousness of the disorder and the treatment alternatives for the patient. Because the starting doses are very low and because of phase I trial design using different patients at each dose level (to avoid cumulative toxicity), the chance of a therapeutic effect for the initial patients receiving a new agent is nearly zero. It is axiomatic that the phase I trials are designed to accumulate the maximum amount of clinical information with the least toxicity. Often, the end point for phase I trials is the achievement of a maximum tolerated dose (MTD), the dose at which side effects are unacceptable to the physician and the patient within the design of that clinical trial. These trials may require 100-500 patients to reach agreement on the MTD in two to four schedules and routes of administration. Once the MTD is established, subsequent investigators can be reasonably assured that the upper limit for the dose to be administered is well defined and that therapeutic activity will not be missed in later phase trials because of subtherapeutic doses.

Phase II studies are then conducted to determine the therapeutic activity of the new drug in various types of cancer. Patients with specific cancers are selected in order that these trials can be conducted in reasonably uniform patient groups. Based on the preclinical information and the clinical toxicology studies, as well as pharmacokinetic considerations, therapeutic doses are selected that represent the investigator's 'best guess' as to the therapeutically active dose range. In addition, schedule and route of administration must be considered. In phase II trials, it is often necessary to administer an agent at different doses by different routes (e.g., intramuscular, intravenous, subcutaneous, oral) and on different schedules (e.g., once a day, three times a day, 24-h infusion, etc.). Phase II trials are considered complete when a substantial body of data exists concerning the therapeutic activity of a new drug with reference to best dose, route of administration, and schedule for therapeutic efficacy. If one accepts classical criteria for cancer subtypes, over 100 histologic types of cancer exist. If one assumes a standard statistical criterion of at least 14 patients treated to look for one response so as not to miss a 20% response rate, then a new drug would need to be tested in a minimum of 1400 patients by each schedule and route to assure clinicians of its inactivity; and if one assumes three routes and five schedules must be tested, over 21,000 patients would need to participate just to prove a specific drug ineffective. More patients would be required to establish its optimal activity.

Following the completion of adequate phase I and phase II trials, phase III trials to compare a new agent with standard treatment are conducted. The extent of phase III trials depends on the treatment alternatives available. In the case of diseases for which other therapies are effective, such trials may need to be extensive, controlled, and employ random designs, sometimes with blinding of the study both to the physician and to the patient. Such phase III trials have produced an enormous literature on the subject of ethics, trial design, end points, and the assessment of efficacy [8, 16, 21, 28, 58, 69, 78, 79, 83, 84, 87]. If in such phase III trials a new agent proves therapeutically superior without unacceptable side effects, in comparison with or in addition to 'standard' therapy, the new agent is very likely to receive FDA approval. Where efficacious therapy with an approved drug is not available, fewer phase III data may be needed to gain approval.

Most drugs fail at the phase I/II level, being either too toxic or inactive. Drugs that complete phase II trials with acceptable toxicity and activity in at least one cancer have a greater than 80% chance of successfully passing phase III with eventual approval by the FDA. For this reason, it has been suggested that drugs should be approved for general use at the end of phase II to speed up the process of bringing new drugs to the clinic [70].

The final step in the commercial development of a new drug requires the filing of a new drug application (NDA). All the information available under the INDA and all of the data from the phase I, II, and III testing are made available to the FDA for review and consideration. Only the FDA is authorized to approve a new drug for sale in the United States; this usually involves defining the drug dose, route of administration, schedule, toxicity, and therapeutic activity in specific diseases (indications). After FDA approval, the company may begin to advertise the agent for the approved use only and the drug is available to the general medical community. Uses outside the specific FDA approval indication(s) are termed 'off label' uses.

The long time and enormous expenditure in the current drug development system have been justified as being in the public interest inasmuch as the FDA requires extensive testing so active agents with reasonable toxicities can be made available as medicinals. The definitions of reasonable toxicity and of therapeutic efficacy have been the subject of considerable debate, both in the general sense and relative to specific drugs. Often, the long-term effects and/or toxicities of approved drugs have prompted secondary revisions in the regulatory process, further lengthening and expanding the steps necessary for new drugs to be approved. This process would seem to be totally in the public interest. However, when viewed in another context, the process clearly has some exclusionary aspects [53, 58, 70]. The FDA defines a single standard for drug development in the United States. Marked differences exist between countries as to a regulatory body's role in drug development, and there are marked differences in the number of drugs available to patients in different countries. The regulatory agency of each country has its own view of what is in the public interest. Thus, there can be reasonable debate on which rules are the best for the development of new drugs. Finally, it is obvious that the long development times and the huge expenditures required effectively restrict competition in the area of drug development. Such restriction of competition gives major pharmaceutical firms a virtual monopoly on drug development. Although most pharmaceutical firms would undoubtedly say that they would prefer a lower cost for drug development, one may view the process as being in their best interests (barrier to entry), since it restricts competition from smaller firms that cannot marshal the resources to carry out these extensive and expensive studies [42, 58, 66, 67, 69, 70].

Thus, our drug development paradigm is highly restrictive. It has worked reasonably well over the past 30 years only because of public acceptance of a conservative regulatory structure and because of the small number of relatively toxic drugs that actually were available for clinical testing. The advent of biologicals will put great pressure on this paradigm. Indeed, the effective development of biologicals will require changes in the regulations and policies for the development of new pharmaceuticals [42, 58, 65, 69].

BIOLOGICALS AND BRM DEVELOPMENT

A process of developmental therapeutics similar to that described for chemicals (drugs) is now being applied to biopharmaceuticals. Historically, for new biologicals, the information on composition, formulation, and purity was often imprecise. In contrast to drugs, which are generally small, synthesized molecules with a chemical definition that is quite straightforward, biologicals have had a more variable developmental process. Preparing a biological for testing has involved extraction from a microorganism, from a fraction of a cell culture, or from a natural product (tree bark, root, or complex chemical mixture). Such extractions yielded complex mixtures with defined biological activity, where the precise chemical composition was unknown [62]. Biotechnology is now making available a range of biologicals (lymphokines/cytokines, monoclonal antibodies, antigens, growth and maturation factors) that are pure and well defined [42, 44].

Market size, the potential for profit, the need for a long development period of preclinical and clinical testing, and the large investment necessary to develop new therapeutic agents have defined the scope of drug development. The development and testing of new biologicals and BRM will require extensive procedural and regulatory changes if we are to be successful in bringing these agents to the clinic quickly and efficiently [42, 70]. Perhaps the most cogent example relates to the development of monoclonal antibodies. For years there have been sufficient data to indicate that monoclonal antibodies are eventually going to be very useful both diagnostically and therapeutically [9, 19, 26, 29, 38, 39, 41, 50, 60, 80, 86]. The problems of developing new monoclonal antibodies for therapy will be quite different from those previously encountered with drugs. The most striking of these problems relate to market size. Generally speaking, one looks at the population afflicted with a particular disease and makes the presumption that a new drug will be active in a certain percentage of patients with that disease. The percentage is often reasonably high and allows the market forecast to be applicable to a substantial number of patients. For example, the number of patients at risk per year with lung cancer is reasonably well defined, and once some evidence of clinical activity of a new drug in lung cancer is available, the market size for that drug can easily be calculated. For monoclonal antibodies, the situation may be very different. At the extreme is anti-idiotypic monoclonal antibody therapy. It has been demonstrated in preclinical models and, to a more limited extent, in humans that anti-idiotypic antibody can be made to the specific tumor antigen (idiotype) of the neoplastic cell [10, 22, 38, 52]. Such anti-idiotypic antibodies may be useful in controlling the growth of the neoplasm bearing that idiotype: direct regulatory effects intrinsic to the physiological function of the idiotype may serve as the target for a tumor-specific attack using anti-idiotypic monoclonal antibody with effector cells and/or as immunoconjugates with drugs, toxins, biologicals, or isotopes. However, a critical problem for the development of these reagents is market size; here, it is the individual patient with that particular neoplasm. Thus, the market size might be as small as one. Even with some cross-reactivity, these antibodies are expected to apply only to very small populations, much smaller than even the 'orphan drugs' envisioned by FDA policy. Obviously, pharmaceutical companies will not develop reagents of these kinds under existing guidelines [58].

A less extreme example relates to the development of monoclonal antibodies for tumor-associated antigens that may be restricted to subpopulations of cancer cells. Considerable heterogeneity exists within any one histologic type of cancer (between patients) and probably within a single patient's cancer [41, 51]. It may be that for any one cancer only a small portion of the patient population will have a particular antigen or array of antigens on the cancer cell surface. Therefore, a monoclonal antibody might be applicable only to 1%, 5%, or 10% of the patients with a particular type of neoplasm. Because of clonal heterogeneity, both between patients and in different clones within individual patients, there is the need to use multiple antibodies ('cocktails') in treatment [1, 34 ,56, 77]. Given the over 100 histologic types of cancer and the heterogeneity within each cancer type, market calculations may define very narrow applications [42, 50]. These considerations restrict market size to a level unapproachable given drug development costs under the current drug development paradigm.

Perhaps less obvious, but equally problematic, will be the development of other biologicals for treatment. For lymphokines and cytokines, there is already evidence of both antigen-specific and non-antigen-specific signals that may have growth regulatory effects (See Chapter 10). One can visualize, with an antigen-specific lymphokine, how the signal may relate to the specific antigen and be applicable in a single patient, or a very few patients (e.g., transfer factor, IgE suppressor factors). Less restricted, but still highly restricted compared with drug development, is the development of non-antigen-specific lymphokines (e.g., interferons, lymphotoxins, interleukins), which are active against certain classes of cells, thus making them clinically applicable only in selected populations [42, 44].

INTERFERONS: THE EARLY MODEL

Interferons represent models for new biological approaches in cancer treatment [44, 48, 63]. 'Natural' extracted interferons from stimulated white blood cells were used in initial clinical trials. The low purity, lot-to-lot variation, and expense of stimulating leukocytes to produce interferon, along with the difficulties in the extraction and purification methods, limited the clinical use of these materials. These preparations were typical of early forms of nonspecific immunotherapy [5, 62]. With the advent of increased interferon availability through recombinant genetics, and with the very high purity (greater than 98%) of these preparations, extensive trials were completed for alpha-interferon preparations which led to the approval of alpha-interferon as the first genetically engineered anticancer biopharmaceutical [30, 63].

The design of phase I biotherapy trials should differ markedly from those for drugs. The dose-response curve for these agents may be very broad (and sometimes multiphasic), with peak effects at different doses for each system responding to the biopharmaceutical. For example, the immunomodulatory activity of alpha-interferon can be seen at very low doses, whereas the anti-proliferative activity appears to be more reproducible at higher doses. In biotherapy there is a need to measure biological responses in the context of the clinical trials [27, 35, 37, 49, 82]. Since one may be administering the biological to stimulate a particular biological response, for which the dose-response curve may not be known a priori, one must perform studies with pharmacokinetics to assay serum availability, and also measure the desired biological effects to determine the optimal dose at which it might alter a particular biological response (optimal biological response modification, OBRM). Finally, schedule and route of administration have already proven important [30, 63]. The pharmacokinetics after intravenous and intramuscular administration differ for the alpha interferons [31], and there has been a variable lack of absorption of intramuscularly administered beta- and gamma-interferons [24, 61]. Thus, the proper design of phase I biotherapy trials must take into account appropriate measurements of bioavailability, pharmacokinetics, biological response modification, and toxicity, all in the context of escalating doses, to determine the dose-response curves for each of these properties. Responses to biologicals vary substantially between patients, and escalating doses in individual patients can yield valuable data.

Like most biologicals, the interferons may act through a diverse set of biological mechanisms. Cell surface receptors for their activity exist, and responses to the administration of biologicals are somewhat predetermined by the condition and biological receptor repertoire of the patient. This situation is in direct contradistinction to that of drugs, in which a totally new chemical is often administered to a patient in whom no standard biological response mechanism existed a priori. Thus, biologicals may be viewed in their physiologic role of correcting immunodeficiency states, as well as in the pharmacologic role of augmenting host responses and perhaps having direct antitumor effects.

Clearly, it was rational to test chemical drugs to MTD and to treat just below this dose in a 'kill or cure' approach to cancer therapy. Current evidence suggests the OBRM dose and the MTD dose should be determined in cancer biotherapy to properly design effective therapeutic trials. Once determined, to be sure biological effects and the highest dose tolerated are known, the design of therapeutic trials for biotherapy may differ greatly from classical chemotherapy studies.

BIOTHERAPY TRIAL STRATEGIES

Many strategies exist or can be envisioned for conducting clinical trials with new biologicals. Some of these strategies have already been utilized in the early-phase testing of the interferons [4, 20, 46, 47, 81]. Two underlying principles are apparent wherein biologicals and drugs differ: when biologicals are administered, patients already have physiologic mechanisms and receptors that respond to them; and biologicals are derivatives of natural products of the mammalian or human genome, and may be expected to have less acute and chronic toxicity than drugs at similar biologically effective doses. However, when high doses are used to exploit a certain action of a biological, acute toxicities may appear. These two considerations will not necessarily apply to those BRM that are well-defined chemical entities and behave more in the manner of drugs.

Empirical clinical testing

In many early interferon trials a set dose of a 'natural' interferon was given to a variety of patients with neoplastic or viral disorders [44, 49, 63]. The chosen dose was one expected, based on preclinical information or other clinical data, to be relatively nontoxic and yet to have sufficient biological effects to be therapeutically active. In this context, most early clinical trials with leukocyte interferon preparations were conducted at doses under 5 million units per day, although it became apparent later that doses up to 60 million units per day could be tolerated by the patients for a certain number of days. These trials were conducted as preliminary feasibility trials or pilot phase II trials to gain some information on the biological effects of the interferon preparations. Much of the information derived from them was anecdotal, but they yielded preliminary information about the biological effects and toxicities of alpha-interferons. Now that the development of biotherapy is proceeding more rapidly, other strategies are to be preferred.

Escalating dose trials using different groups of patients

Phase I trials for biologicals have been modeled after the standard phase I trial design used for drugs. Groups of patients (usually three to five) are treated with a particular dose of a new biological with a single route of administration [81]. These trials are begun with very low (probably subtherapeutic) doses based on preclinical information, and the schedule is designed to increase the dose gradually to levels where toxicity occurs [42, 61]. Generally, new patients are entered at each higher dose level after all the patients have been entered on the previous dose and have received at least several treatments. In this way, each patient group provides toxicity information before the higher dose is initiated in new patients. By utilizing different groups of patients at each dose level, cumulative toxicity for any one patient is avoided. Patients receive a predetermined number of doses at each dose level and then are followed. During this type of study, biological response modification and clinical toxicity are assessed [4, 35-37, 40]. Pharmacokinetics are also done in selected patients, so that the bioavailability can be determined [81].

The dose-escalation scheme can be a modified Fibonacci series, or some variation of this classical dose-escalation method. The considerations involved in dose-escalation methods dictated by drug toxicities do not necessarily apply to biologicals. Thus, some investigators have used much faster dose escalations for biologicals. Often, the dose escalation schedule is rather empirical, the one selected being based on the best guess of the investigators involved. This phase I drug development strategy is reasonable, and is based on historical data using new drugs, but it does have several potential disadvantages. Since each patient receives only a particular dose for a defined period of time, it is highly likely that a large percentage of the patients will receive subtherapeutic doses if antitumor effects are observed only at higher dose levels. If significant biological response modifying and clinical activities are both seen only at higher doses, similar underdosing will occur. Early clinical trials with biologicals have not produced severe cumulative toxicity. This clinical trial strategy, which was designed to avoid the cumulative toxic effects seen with drugs, may not be relevant to biotherapy. Since tolerance (tachyphylaxis) may develop for some effects (fever), entering different patients on progressively higher doses may expose patients to avoidable acute toxicities. Finally, the patients who are exposed to only one dose level are not individually assessed for biological response or for antitumor response over a wide dosage range. This could give them a greater opportunity for optimization of biological and therapeutic response [46]. This may be particularly true in the very-early-phase trials in which biological effects and antitumor effects are totally unknown.

Escalating-dose trials within individual patients

An alternative clinical trial strategy is the use of an escalating-dose trial within individual patients [45, 46, 61]. There are several variations of this theme, but each involves starting patients at a low dose and escalating the dose in each patient to determine the biological response modifying effects and toxicities over a broad dose range. This clinical trial strategy is very conservative of patients, in that studies in small numbers of patients can give a large amount of information over a broad dose range in each biotherapy trial. In the context of this dose escalation, pharmacokinetics and biological response modification can be measured in each patient.

It is important in such a clinical trial strategy that bioavailability studies be done and the information be available concomitantly with the study. Appropriate 'wash-out' periods between doses can be utilized so that the administered biological does not circulate in increasing quantities as the trial continues. For example, with the interferon trials, one can determine the serum level after each dose and administer the next dose when interferon is no longer detectable. This allows the patient to avoid the possibility of severe acute toxic effects based on cumulative serum levels. Obviously, biological and therapeutic effects can still be cumulative and must be monitored by appropriate clinical and biological measurements throughout this type of trial.

This strategy offers the possibility of low-, medium-, and high-dose therapy for the individual patient in the context of a single clinical trial. It maximizes the opportunity for the investigator to learn the optimal biological response modifying dose and the toxic dose, and perhaps to gain therapeutic information, all in the context of a single trial. Theoretically, rational maintenance regimens could be designed based on the observations made during the escalating dose trial for each patient.

For monoclonal antibody, this strategy may be particularly important, in that the delivery of the monoclonal antibody to the tumor site may be the most important consideration in developmental therapeutics [18, 26, 41, 50]. Giving a low dose and then progressively higher doses to the same patient, with subsequent determination of antibody localization, is a useful way of determining the correct dose for delivery of the antibody and/or its conjugates to the appropriate target organ in the context of a toxicity study. This trial design rationally ties targeting (delivery), toxicity, and therapeutic effects together in combined phase I/II studies in a manner perfectly appropriate for antibody and conjugates, in direct contradistinction to drug development [2, 3, 46].

In studies that employ escalating doses, a useful variation is to enter individual patients for a limited number of doses. With this trial design, the initial three or four patients may enter at the lowest dose level and progress through dose level 4 or 5, at which time the second group of patients may be entered at dose 3 and escalated upward in a manner that allows the second group to follow the first group in dosage escalation toward the MTD. A third group may be entered at dose level 6 and so on. This strategy allows one to avoid administering the full dose range to all patients, avoids most cumulative toxicity, and helps avoid subtherapeutic doses. It increases the patient's therapeutic opportunity without undue risk of toxicity. This strategy is most acceptable to patients and quite easy to describe in the informed consent [58].

Schedule

In the initial clinical trials, the schedule of administration is generally empirical or is based on preclinical observations. Once there is information on bioavailability, different schedules of administration can be designed rationally. Both the bioavailability of the molecule and its biological effects are relevant. There are some biologicals that have a very short serum half-life (measured in a few seconds to minutes) but may produce much longer lasting biological effects. It may be useful to compare the biological effects and toxicities of biologicals when administered under conditions of rather constant exposure as against intermittent exposure in order to gain a preliminary sense of which schedule is most relevant [25,61,85]. Once these data are available, schedules of administration for phase II studies can be more rationally designed. Many biologicals have short serum half-lives (e.g., interleukin-2, IL-2) and are best given by constant infusion [12-15, 55, 85].

Route

The route of administration and delivery of biotherapy to selected target organs is critical. There are data indicating that certain biologicals are inactivated, or poorly absorbed, when given intramuscularly or subcutaneously. For such biologicals intravenous administration is quite important. When data on bioavailability are not known from preclinical models, it is probably important to conduct early clinical trials with the intravenous route, since such trials can provide early data on serum pharmacokinetics and provide the best opportunity for broad biodistribution of the administered biological. It is important in phase I biotherapy trials to determine if serum levels are measurable and if biological effects are seen in the presence or absence of serum levels for agents given by any route of administration. There may be instances in which second mediators are involved, with useful biological effects occurring without apparent serum bioavailability.

Effusions may contain both tumor cells and reactive immunological elements, in which case the administration of a biological into a restricted space such as the thoracic or peritoneal cavity might be appropriate. There are indications that certain immunomodulators may be effective in this setting [43]. Patients with tumors that remain confined to a single compartment for a prolonged period of time may offer unique opportunities for biotherapy [59,75]. Ovarian cancer, with its propensity for remaining localized in the abdominal peritoneum, may be ideal for evaluating the antitumor activity of cells [59], biologicals, and BRM in a relatively closed space. Interleukin-2 with activated cells appears to be more active when infused into selected anatomical sites and visceral cavities where tumor is present [32, 75,]. It seems clear that targeting of monoclonal antibody and its conjugates may be improved by selective organ or region perfusion or infusion. Considerations for the design of early-phase trials in these spaces differ markedly from those using systemic administration.

Patient selection

Historically, patient selection for phase I drug trials has been broad, and patients bearing all tumor types have been entered into the trials. While this may be appropriate for drugs, and for selected lymphokines that act on immunological responses or may act in a general antiproliferative manner across a broad spectrum of tumors, it would not be appropriate for those biologicals that act more specifically. Thus, a lymphokine that acts on a very specific population of cells, such as lymphoid cells, may be more appropriately tested in patients with lymphoid tumors or with selected immunodeficiency states. And a monoclonal antibody that has been specifically designed to recognize a particular type of cancer can be appropriately tested only in patients with that type of cancer [33, 46].

In vitro determinations of specificity and activity may play a greater role in the selection of the patient populations for phase I biotherapy trials. The escalating-dose phase I trials, with the dose being escalated within individual patients, preselected on the basis of *in vitro* specificity and/or activity, appear to be most relevant and efficient for determining the distribution, biological effects, and toxicity of monoclonal antibodies. The same considerations may apply to certain lymphokines/cytokines, in which case selection as to activity may be on an individual patient basis. These trials may be more appropriately termed phase I/II trials. In fact, given the heterogeneity of cancer, both with respect to the specificity of recognition by antibody and with respect to activity by immunoconjugates and lymphokines/cytokines, *in vitro* determinations may play a major role in clinical trial design. Biological systems are diverse, and single patients may require specifically designed treatments when specificity and activity restrict the applicability of biotherapy. The design of early-phase clinical trials may need to be radically changed [42, 46, 58].

There has been much speculation concerning the types of patients most appropriate for trials with biologicals. Many believe that these agents should be tested primarily in the adjuvant setting, where the tumor burden is quite small and the biological responses to be modified are still healthy [62]. Although this sort of strategy may be optimal, it is also prohibitively expensive and very difficult to design. It would be virtually impossible to investigate a significant number of biologicals in phase I or II trials utilizing this type of clinical trial design. The number of patients required for trials in the adjuvant setting are enormous, in that the recurrence rate cannot be precisely predicted without a concurrent random control group. The lack of certainty for recurrence prompts ethical questions in designing phase I trials for these patients, since toxicity, dose, route, schedule, and therapeutic efficacy have not been determined.

For phase II trials, the uncertainty of recurrence requires that control patients be utilized to determine whether or not the experimental agent is effective in preventing recurrence. To carry out these types of trials for new biologicals would excessively limit the development of biotherapy. In addition, random-design trials prior to pilot phase II are difficult to envision, since the pilot studies often indicate effective dose, schedule, route, and responsive tumor types.

It has now been well demonstrated that certain biologicals have activity in patients with bulky and resistant disease [4, 13-15, 20, 44, 45, 49, 63, 76, 85]. Even though biotherapy may be more effective, as chemotherapy and radiotherapy are, when the tumor burden is small, that does not mean that it is totally ineffective in patients with bulky disease. Given the large number of biologicals available to the clinic, there is a need to develop methods of rapid clinical testing in early-phase trials, and this will necessitate testing in patients with apparent disease [42, 44, 62, 85]. Indeed, the initial clinical trials with interferon generally selected such patients with a good performance status and a reasonably normal immune system. These patients have shown evidence of biological response modification, and they have shown antitumor responses. Thus, such clinical trials can be used as indicators for biological activity of new agents [44, 49].

Patients with far advanced disease, protein malnutrition, and severe immunological defects should probably be excluded from trials with new biologicals. Furthermore, given the pyrexia produced by many of these agents, patients with severe cardiac disease and those with active central nervous system metastasis probably should also be excluded because of the stress on the cardiovascular system and/or seizure enhancement by the fever induced by interferon and similar biologicals [40, 85]. Thus, although biologicals can be, and are being, tested in patients with advanced disease, they are best assessed in patients with a Karnofsky performance status of 70% or better.

FUTURE PROSPECTS

Developmental therapeutics for biologicals and BRM have just begun. From the inception of this field in 1980 to the end of the 1990s, a great number of new approaches will be available in biotherapy [30, 44, 58, 85]. Unlike the field of drugs, where very large numbers of compounds are screened in a preclinical testing program and very few reach the clinic, a much higher percentage of the biologicals developed and tested in preclinical models will actually come to clinical trials. This is due to selection based on the known physiologic activities of biologicals as opposed to random testing of chemicals in drug development. The strategies for these clinical trials need to be cost efficient, advantageous to the patient, and scientifically interpretable to the clinician/scientist [51, 62]. Phase I strategies are most important in that they give the initial leads on which the design of early phase II and III trials are based. With proper selection clinical trial strategies, it is expected that new biologicals can be more effectively screened and evaluated as potential anticancer agents [46, 58].

Biotherapy is the fourth modality of cancer treatment [44, 45, 71, 72]. These agents and this technology have far broader applications in medicine than cancer therapeutics. Given the large number of cloned biologicals and the virtually unlimited number of recombinant molecules that can be produced therefrom, along with the great variety of monoclonal antibodies that can be produced through hybridoma technology, it is apparent that the coming decade will produce new challenges for those involved in developmental therapeutics. This tremendous expansion of agents and approaches available for cancer therapeutics will increase our opportunities and amplify our problems in the preclinical evaluation of these agents and their translation to the clinic. The numbers of biologicals to be evaluated and their selectivity call for new methods in the selection of the 'most likely to succeed.' Additionally, the methods used historically by pharmaceutical manufacturers and the regulations established by governmental agencies for approving anticancer drugs are inhibitory to the rapid development of biotherapy [42, 70]. Novel approaches will be necessary if these biologicals are to be effectively and rapidly translated to clinical trials [42, 51]. Immunomodulators, lymphokines/cytokines, gene engineered and/or activated cells, and monoclonal antibodies are being extensively evaluated in preclinical models and in phase I, II, and III clinical studies.

Alpha-interferon and IL-2 have antitumor effects, even in patients with bulky disease. This finding is likely to emerge for other forms of biotherapy [30, 44, 46, 54, 58, 85]. This should give pause to those who believe the immunological dogma that biotherapy can only be active in minimal residual disease. Like chemotherapy and radiotherapy, biotherapy may be more active with lesser tumor burdens, but the early data indicate that activity and hence selection of compounds for further study can be assessed in patients with advanced disease.

The potential for the use of biotherapy is great. We are on the threshold of a new era in cancer therapeutics. While many of these biological responses are general, some are quite specific. To develop biotherapy, we must begin to approach this new era in pharmaceutical research and to contemplate novel methods for the efficient and timely development of biotherapy rather than simply continuing in old paradigms (Fig. 3) [42, 58, 69, 70]. Some would still say no new treatment can be judged without randomized, clinical trials. Such trials are valid in searching for small differences between a new treatment and an ethically acceptable control (standard treatment). Whether placebo controls are even acceptable in cancer treatment is debatable; however, pilot studies without controls can be very useful even to the point of defining efficacy if the treatment effect is large and obvious. A recent and innovative '*n* of 1' trial also bears consideration in trials of biotherapy [25].

We must not just continue to simply do what has been done historically [58]. Development therapeutics for biologicals certainly represent the kind of science Lewis

Preclinical Testing (*in vitro*/animal model)

⇓

Phase I Clinical Trial

⇓

Phase II Clinical Trial

⇓

Phase III Clinical Trials

⇓

Unresponsive or poorly responsive neoplasm; less than partial responses

⇓

Partial responses to newer active single agents

⇓

Increased partial responses and rare complete responses to some single and combined agents

⇓

Increased complete responses to more effective combination therapy

⇓

Increased survival in complete responders with or without continued treatment during remission

⇓

A portion of long-term survivors are cured

Figure 3. Although radically different, chemotherapy and biotherapy share a systemic approach to cancer treatment. For those cancers that chemotherapy has been able to cure, reaching that goal required a sequence of steps in which new and increasingly more effective agents and combinations of agents had to be identified. Biotherapy can be expected to travel a similar path.

Thomas describes:

> 'It is hard to predict how science is going to turn out, and if it is really good science, it is impossible to predict. This is in the nature of the enterprise. If the things to be found are actually new, they are by definition unknown in advance, and there is no way of telling in advance where a really new line of inquiry will lead. You cannot make choices in this matter, selecting things you think you're going to like and shutting off the lines that make for discomfort. You either have science or you don't, and if you have it you are obliged to accept the surprising and disturbing pieces of information, even the overwhelming and upheaving ones, along with the neat and promptly useful bits. It is like that.'

REFERENCES

1. Avner B, Swindell L, Sharp E, et al. Evaluation and clinical relevance of patient immune responses to intravenous therapy with murine monoclonal antibodies conjugated to Adriamycin. *Molecular Biotherapy* 1991; 3(1):14-21.
2. Bernhard MI, Foon KA, Oeltman TN, et al. Guinea pig line 10 hepatocarcinoma model: characterization of monoclonal antibody and *in vivo* effect of unconjugated antibody and antibody conjugated to diphtheria toxin A chain. *Cancer Res* 1983; 43:4420-4428.
3. Bernhard MI, Hwang KM, Foon KA, et al. Localization of 111In- and 125I-labeled monoclonal antibody in guinea pigs bearing line 10 hepatocarcinoma tumors. *Cancer Res* 1983; 43:4429-4433.
4. Bunn PA, Jr., Foon KA, Ihde DC, et al. Recombinant leukocyte alpha interferon: an active agent in advanced cutaneous T-cell lymphomas. *Ann Intern Med* 1982; 101:484-487.
5. Cantell K. In: Burke D, Cantell K, DeMaeyer E, Landy M, Revel M, Vilcek J, eds. I*nterferon 1* New York: Academic Press, 1981.
6. Carter SK. The clinical trial evaluation strategy for interferons and other biological response modifiers – not a simple task [editorial]. *J Biol Response Modif* 1982; 1:101-105.
7. Cheever MA, Greenberg PD, Fefer A. Potential for specific cancer therapy with immune T lymphocytes. *J Biol Response Modif* 1984; 3:113-127.
8. Curran WJ, Reasonableness and randomization in clinical trials: fundamental law and governmental regulation [editorial]. *N Engl J Med* 1979; 300:1273-1274.
9. DeVita VT Jr, Hellman S, Rosenberg SA, eds. *Biologic Therapy of Cancer*, Second Edition. Philadelphia, J.B. Lippincott Company, 1995:553-607.
10. DeVita VT Jr, Hellman S, Rosenberg SA, eds. *Biologic Therapy of Cancer*, Second Edition. Philadelphia, J.B. Lippincott Company, 1995:553-565.
11. DeVita VT Jr, Hellman S, Rosenberg SA, eds. *Biologic Therapy of Cancer*, Second Edition. Philadelphia, J.B. Lippincott Company, 1995:879-890.
12. Dillman RO, Oldham RK, Barth NM, et al. Continuous interleukin-2 and tumor infiltrating lymphocytes as treatment of advanced melanoma. *Cancer* 1991; 68(1):1-8.
13. Dillman RO, Oldham RK, Tauer KW, et al. Continuous Interleukin-2 and lymphokine activated killer cells for advanced cancer: An NBSG trial. *Journal of Clinical Oncology* 1991; 9:1233-1240.
14. Dillman RO, Church C, Oldham RK, et al. Inpatient continuous infusion Interleukin-2 in 788 cancer patients: The NBSG Experience. *Cancer* 1993; 71:2358-2370.
15. Dillman RO. The clinical experience with Interleukin-2 in cancer therapy. *Cancer Biotherapy* 1994; 9(3):179-182.
16. Ellenberg SS. Studies to compare treatment regimens: the randomized clinical trial and alternative strategies. *J Am Med Assoc* 1982; 246:2481-2482.
17. Fidler IJ, Berendt M, Oldham RK. Rationale for and design of a screening procedure for the assessment of biological response modifiers for cancer treatment. *J Biol Response Modif* 1982; 1:15-26.
18. Foon KA, Bernhard KA, Oldham RK. Monoclonal antibody therapy: assessment by animal tumor models. *J Biol Response Modif* 1982: 1:277-304.

19. Foon KA, Schroff RW, Bunn PA, et al. Effects of monoclonal antibody serotherapy in patients with chronic lymphocytic leukemia. *Blood* 1984; 64:1085-1093.
20. Foon KA, Sherwin SA, Abrams PG, et al. Treatment of advanced non-Hodgkin's lymphoma with recombinant leukocyte alpha interferon. *N Engl J Med* 1984; 311:1148-1152.
21. Fost N. Consent as a barrier to research [editorial]. *N Engl J Med* 1979; 300:1272-1273.
22. Giardina SL, Schroff RW, Woodhouse CS, et al. Detection of two distinct malignant B-cell clones in a single patient using anti-idiotype monoclonal antibodies and immunoglobulin gene arrangement. *Blood* 1985; 66:1017-1021.
23. Goeddel D, Yelverton E, Ullrich A, et al. *Nature* (Lond) 1980; 287:411-416.
24. Gutterman JU, Rosenblum MG, Rios A, et al. Pharmacokinetic study of partially pure interferon in cancer patients. *Cancer Res.* 1984; 44:4164-4171.
25. Guyatt G, Sackett D, Taylor DW, et al. Determining optimal therapy – randomized trials in individual patients. *N Engl J Med* 1986; 314:889-892.
26. Hanna MG, Jr., Key ME, Oldham RK. Biology of cancer therapy: some new insights into adjuvant treatment of metastatic solid tumors. *J Biol Response Modif* 1983; 4:295-309.
27. Herberman RB, Thurman GB. Summary of approaches to the immunological monitoring of cancer patients treated with natural or recombinant interferons. *J Biol Response Modif* 1982; 2:548-562.
28. Horwitz RI, Feinstein AR. Improved observational method for studying therapeutic efficacy. *JAMA* 1981; 246:2455-2459.
29. Hwang KM, Foon KA, Cheung PH, et al. Selective antitumor effect of a potent immunoconjugate composed of the A chain of abrin and a monoclonal antibody to a hepatoma-associated antigen. *Cancer Res* 1984; 44:4578-4586.
30. Kirkwood JM, Ernstoff MS. Interferons in the treatment of human cancer. *J Clin Oncol* 1984; 2:336-352.
31. Knost JA, Sherwin SA, Abrams PG, et al. The treatment of cancer patients with human lymphoblastoid interferon: a comparison of two routes of administration. *Cancer Immunol Immunother* 1983; 15:144-151.
32. Lembersky B, Baldisseri M, Seski J, et al. Phase IB study of intraperitoneal (IP) interleukin-2 (IL-2) for refractory ovarian cancer (OC). *Proc Am Assoc Cancer Res* 1990; 31:277.
33. Lewko WM, Ladd PA, Pridgen D, et al. Tumor acquisition propagation and preservation: culture of human colorectal cancer. *Cancer* 1989; 64:1600-1608.
34. Liao SK, Meranda C, Avner BP, et al. Immunohistochemical phenotyping of human solid tumors with monoclonal antibodies in devising biotherapeutic strategies. *Cancer Immunol Immunother* 1989; 28:77-86.
35. Maluish AE, Leavitt R, Sherwin SA, et al. Effects of recombinant alpha interferon on immune function in cancer patients. *J Biol Response Modif* 1983; 2:470-481.
36. Maluish AE, Ortaldo JR, Sherwin SA, et al. Changes in immune function in patients receiving natural leukocyte interferon. *J Biol Response Modif* 1983; 2:418-427.
37. Maluish AE, Ortaldo JR, Conlon JC, et al. Depression of natural killer cytotoxicity following *in vivo* administration of recombinant leukocyte interferon. *J Immunol* 1983; 131:503-507.
38. Miller RA, Maloney DG, Warnke R, et al. Treatment of B cell lymphoma with monoclonal anti-idiotype antibody. *N Engl J Med* 1982; 306:517-522.
39. Nowinski RC, Tam MR, Goldstein LC, et al. Monoclonal antibodies for diagnosis of infectious disease in humans. *Science* 1983; 219:637.
40. Oldham RK. Toxic effects of interferon. *Science* 1982; 219:902.
41. Oldham RK. Monoclonal antibodies in cancer therapy. *J Clin Oncol* 1983; 1:582-590.
42. Oldham RK. Biologicals: new horizons in pharmaceutical development. *J Biol Response Modif* 1983; 2:199-206.
43. Oldham RK. Guest editorial: biological response modifiers. *J Natl Cancer Inst* 1983; 70:790-796.
44. Oldham RK. Biologicals and biological response modifiers; fourth modality of cancer treatment. *Cancer Treat Rep* 1984; 68:221-232.
45. Oldham RK. Biologicals and biological response modifiers: new approaches to cancer treatment. *Cancer Invest* 1985; 3:53-70.
46. Oldham RK. Biologicals and biological response modifiers: the design of clinical trials. *J Biol Response Modif* 1985; 4:117-128.
47. Oldham RK. Biologicals and biological response modifiers: New strategies for clinical trials. In: Finter NB and Oldham RK eds. *Interferons*, IV. Elsevier Science Publishers B.V. 1985:235-249.
48. Oldham RK. *Interferon*: A model for future biologicals. In: Burke D, Cantell K, Gresser I, De Maeyer E, Landy M, Revel M, Vilcek J, eds. Inf. VI. Academic Press, 1985: 127-143.
49. Oldham RK. Biologicals for cancer treatment: *Interferons*. Hospital Practice 1985; 20:72-91.
50. Oldham RK, Foon KA, Morgan AC, et al. Monoclonal antibody therapy of malignant melanoma: *in vivo* localization in cutaneous metastasis after intravenous administration. *J Clin Oncol* 1984; 2:1235-1242.
51. Oldham RK. Therapeutic monoclonal antibodies: effects of tumor cell heterogeneity. In: *Present status of nontoxic concepts in cancer therapy*. Cancer Symposium (Germany). Basel: Karger, 1986.
52. Oldham RK. Monoclonal antibody therapy. In: Chiao JW, ed. *Biological Response Modifiers and Cancer Research* Marcel Dekker, Inc. 1988; 40:3-16.
53. Oldham RK. Set my factors free. *Molecular Biotherapy*. 1990; 2(4):194-195.
54. Oldham RK. *Principles of Cancer biotherapy* New York: Marcel Dekker Inc. 1991.
55. Oldham RK, Dillman RO, Yannelli JR, et al. Continuous infusion interleukin-2 and tumor derived activated cells as treatment of advanced solid tumors. An NBSG trial. *Molecular Biotherapy* 1991; 3(2):68-73.
56. Oldham RK. Custom tailored drug immunoconjugates in cancer therapy. *Molecular Biotherapy* 1991; 3(3):148-162.
57. Oldham RK. The Cure. Pulse Publications, *Franklin*, TN, 1991.
58. Oldham RK. BioEthics: Opportunities, Risks and Ethics: The Privatization of Cancer Research. Media America, *Franklin*, TN, 1992.
59. Oldham RK, Greco FA. Brief intensive chemotherapy and second look laparotomy in advanced ovarian carcinoma. In: William CJ, Whitehouse M, eds. *Recent advances in clinical oncology*. London: Churchill Livingstone, 1982: 165-185.

60. Oldham RK, Morgan AC, Woodhouse CS, et al. Monoclonal antibodies in the treatment of cancer: preliminary observations and future prospects. *Med Oncol Tumor Pharmacother* 1984:1151-1162.
61. Oldham RK, Sherwin SA, Maluish A, et al. A phase I trial of immune interferon: a preliminary report. In: Goldstein AL, ed. *Thymic hormones and lymphokines*. New York: Plenum Press, 1984:497-506.
62. Oldham RK, Smalley RV. Immunotherapy: the old and the new. *J Biol Response Modif* 1983; 2:1-37.
63. Oldham RK, Smalley RV. The role of interferon in the treatment of cancer. In: Zoon KC, Noguci PD, Lui TY, eds. *Interferon*: research, clinical application and regulatory consideration. New York: Elsevier, 1984:191-206.
64. Oldham RK, Thurman GB, Talmadge JE, et al. Lymphokines, monoclonal antibodies and other biological response modifiers in the treatment of cancer. *Cancer* 1984; 54:2795-2810.
65. Oldham RK, Patient-funded cancer research. *N Engl J Med* 1987; 316:46-47.
66. Oldham RK. Drug development: who foots the bill? *Bio/technology* 1987; 5:648.
67. Oldham RK. Who pays for new drugs? *Nature* 1988; 332(28):795.
68. Oldham RK, Avent RA. Clinical research: who pays the bills? *Oncology Issues* 1989; 4(2):13-14.
69. Oldham RK. Clinical research in cancer: a time for consensus. *Pharm Exec* 1989; July.
70. Oldham RK. Regulatory hierarchies (editorial. *Mol Biother* 1988; 1(1):3-6.
71. Oldham RK. Biotherapy: the fourth modality of cancer treatment. Cancer: Perspective for Control Symposium. *J Cell Physiol Suppl* 1986; 4:91-99.
72. Oldham RK. Biotherapy: the fourth modality of cancer treatment. In: Mak TW, Sun TT, eds. Cancer: perspective for control symposium. New York: Alan R. Liss, 1986:91-99.
73. Oldham RK. The government-academic 'industrial' complex. *J Biol Response Modif* 1986; 5:109-111.
74. Oldham RK. The cure for cancer. *J Biol Response Modif* 1985; 4:111-116.
75. Oldham RK, Bartal AH, Yannelli JR, et al. Intra-arterial and intracavitary administration of lymphokine activated killer cells in patients with advanced cancer: feasibility and laboratory results. *Proc AACR* (abstr) 1988; 29:396.
76. Oldham RK, Lewko W, Good R, et al. Growth of tumor derived activated T cells for the treatment of cancer. *Cancer Biotherapy* 1994; 9(3):211-224.
77. Orr DW, Oldham RK, Lewis M, et al. Phase I trial of mitomycin-c immunoconjugate cocktails in human malignancies. *Mol Biother* 1989; 1(4):229-240.
78. Relman AS. The ethics of randomized clinical trials: two perspectives [editorial]. *N Engl J Med* 1979; 300:1272.
79. Schafer A. The ethics of randomized clinical trials. *N Engl J Med* 1982; 307:719-724.
80. Sears HF, Herlyn D, Steplewski Z, Koprowski H. Effects of monoclonal antibody immunotherapy on patients with gastrointestinal adenocarcinoma. *J Biol Response Modif* 1984; 3:138-150.
81. Sherwin SA, Knost JA, Fein S, et al. A multiple dose phase I trial of recombinant lymphocyte alpha interferon in cancer patients. *JAMA* 1982; 248:2461-2466.
82. Smalley RV, Oldham RK. Interferon as a biological response modifying agent in clinical trials. *J Biol Response Modif* 1983; 2:401-409.
83. Sylvester RJ, Pinedo J, De Pauw M, et al. Quality of institutional participation in multicenter clinical trials. *N Engl J Med* 1981; 305:852-855.
84. Weiss DG, Williford WO, Collins JF, Binham SF. Planning multicenter clinical trials; a biostatistician's perspective. *Controlled Clin Trials* 1983; 4:53-64.
85. West WH, Tauer KW, Yannelli JR, et al. Constant infusion recombinant interleukin-2 in adoptive immunotherapy of advanced cancer. *N Engl J Med* 1987; 316(15):898-905.
86. Vitetta ES, Krokick KA, Miyama-Inaba M, et al. Immunotoxins: a new approach to cancer therapy. *Science* 1983; 219:644-649.
87. Zelen M. A new design for randomized clinical trials. *N Engl J Med* 1979; 300:1242-1246.

RECOMBINANT ORGANISMS AS SOURCE OF CANCER BIOTHERAPEUTICS

KAPIL MEHTA[1] and BHARAT B. AGGARWAL[2]

[1] *Immunobiology and Drug Carriers Section, Department of Bioimmunotherapy and* [2] *Cytokine Research Laboratory, Department of Molecular Oncology, The University of Texas M. D. Anderson Cancer Center, Houston, Texas*

Abbreviations used. ADA, adenosine deaminase; AML, acute myeloid leukemia; bFGF, basic fibroblast growth factor; CML, chronic mylogenous leukemia; CSF, colony-stimulating factor; EGF, epidermal growth factor; EPO, erythropoietin; FDA, Food and Drug Administration; HIV, human immunodeficiency virus; IFN, interferon; IL, interleukin; LIF, leukemia inhibitory factor; MAb, monclonal antibody; PDGF, platelet-derived growth factor; PE, *Pseudomonas* exotoxin; PEG, polyethylene glycol; TGF, transforming growth factor; TNF, tumor necrosis factor.

INTRODUCTION

The last fifteen years have witnessed a tremendous rise in new biological treatments for cancer. These treatments, collectively referred to as 'biological therapy,'are primarily based on stimulating the natural host immune response against the cancerous cells. Biological therapies in combination with chemotherapy, surgery, or radiation therapy have started showing promise as effective means for treating cancer. New approaches in biological therapy have been possible mainly because of increased knowledge of the cellular immune system and especially to new developments in biotechnology. Recombinant DNA technology, for example, has made it possible to generate large amounts of many biological compounds for the first time. The novelty of recombinant technology is the precision and efficiency with which scientists can manipulate genes. The ability to isolate human genes and insert them into microorganisms which then produce human proteins, thereby serving as biological factories, has revolutionized the field of biological therapy.

Interferons have special significance to recombinant DNA technology as paradigm modifiers of immune response. The interest in the therapeutic potential of interferon against cancer and viral diseases has served as catalyst to the emerging recombinant DNA industry. Despite its great promise as an antiviral agent, the clinical application of interferon has been rather slow, mainly because of the lack of methods for producing adequate amounts of the protein. Interest in interferon beyond the field of virology began in the early 1960s, when workers began to recognize its growth-inhibitory and immune-activation properties. During the 1960s and early 1970s, reports of interferon's antiviral and antitumor activity in laboratory animals and humans stirred up this interest and several groups decided to purify human interferon for clinical use.

The first practical method of producing sufficient quantitites of interferon was developed by Cantell et al. [20]. They were able to isolate 100-200 mg of interferon from 1,000 liters of starting material that contained 2-5 kg of other contaminating proteins. The purified material had a specific activity of greater than 10^8 U/mg protein [50] and was sufficient for treating only a few patients [222], but the initial clinical results stimulated wider interest in expanding production of interferon for more extensive clinical trials. Enthusiasm intensified when interferon-alpha was successfully cloned and the purified recombinant protein became available [176, 177].

The first trial to test dose levels and side effects of the purified bacterial product in human beings began in 1981 [178, 86]. The availability of pure recombinant protein led researchers to crystallize interferon, the first step toward analysis of the protein's three-dimensional structure by X-ray crystallography. This permitted the production of individual molecular species of interferon free from other species and other proteins that are simultaneously induced in human cell cultures. By using this technique, our knowledge of the varied biological properties of interferons, previously determined with relatively crude preparations, has been confirmed and extended.

ISOLATION, CLONING AND EXPRESSION OF GENES

A gene is a defined region of a chromosome comprising a specific sequence or part of a long polynucleotide. It codes for some specific function or characteristic (phenotype) of a cell. The eukaryotic genome contains up to 10^9 nucleotides in 50,000 genes. To study the events in such a

R.K. Oldham (ed.), Principles of Cancer Biotherapy. 3rd ed., 51–77.

complex system,it is necessary to be able to isolate and study a single gene in a purified form. Molecular cloning provides a method for isolating a single discrete segment of DNA from a population of genes and amplifying the DNA segment to produce enough pure material for chemical, genetic, and biological analysis. Cloning and expression of foreign genes has permitted access to such complex biological mechanisms as RNA splicing, oncogene dynamics and antibody diversity. It has also been the foundation for the new biotechnology industry.

The organization of genes in higher organisms is more complex than in bacteria and viruses. The linear array of information in a complex gene contains one or more stretches of non-coding sequences, called introns. The remaining sequences which encode information for proteins, are called exons. When these genes produce a protein, the DNA is transcribed into a large RNA molecule from which the introns are removed; this mRNA molecule is then translated to produce the corresponding protein (Fig. 1).

The organization of bacterial genes is simpler. They do not produce the enzymes necessary for RNA splicing, so a eukaryotic gene containing introns, if introduced into a bacterial cell as in recombinant techniques, will not be properly expressed. This problem can be circumvented by making a DNA copy (cDNA) from the appropriate mRNA by using the enzyme reverse transcriptase (Fig. 2). Aa an alternative, the DNA can be fragmented at specific target sequences with the help of restriction endonucleases [198]; the DNA fragment that contains the gene of interest is inserted into the purified DNA genome of a self-replicating genetic element, generally a virus or a plasmid. A DNA fragment containing a human gene, for example, when inserted into such a virus or plasmid, can be joined in a test tube to the chromosome of a bacterial cell. Starting with only one such recombinant DNA molecule which can infect only a single cell, the normal replication mechanism of the virus can produce more than trillion identical molecules in less than a day, thereby amplifying the amount of the inserted human DNA fragment by the same factor, making it possible to infect millions of cells. The virus or plasmid used in this way is known as a cloning vector, and the DNA propagated by insertion into it is said to have been cloned.

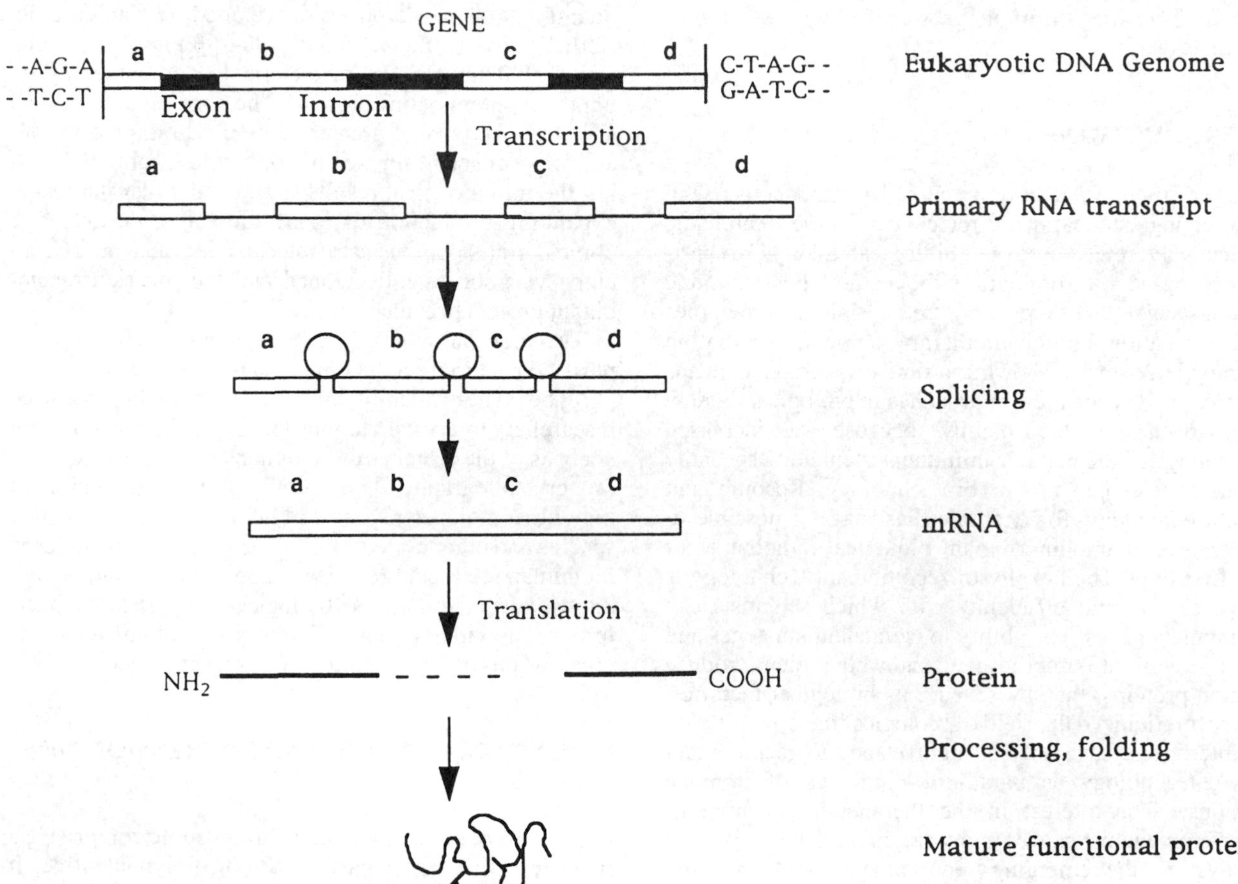

Figure 1. The organization of a Eukaryotic gene and processing of the RNA transcript.

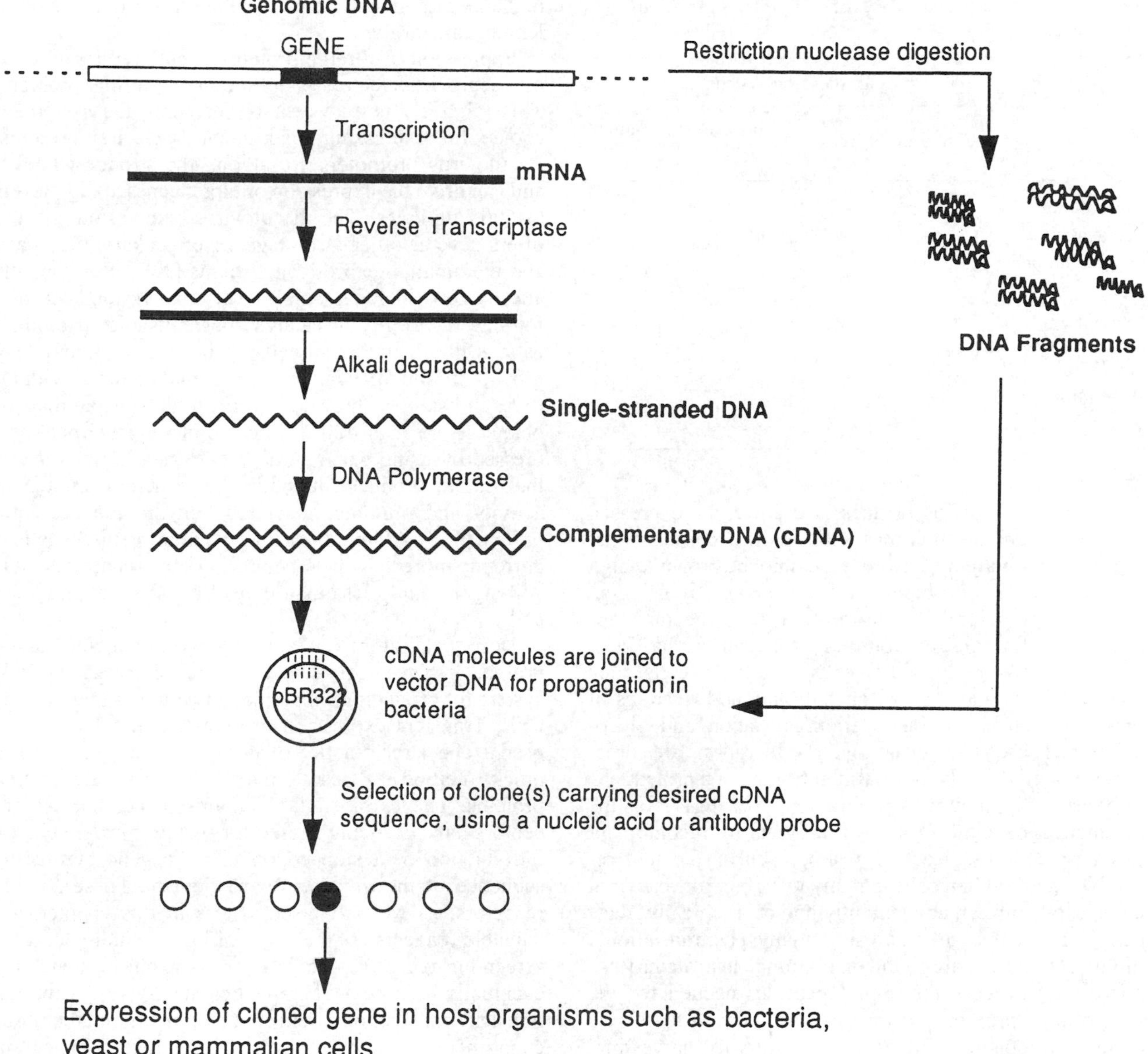

Figure 2. Gene cloning from mRNA or genomic DNA.

Cloning the gene or cDNA encoding a particular protein is only the first of many steps needed to produce a recombinant protein for medical and industrial use. Expression of foreign genes in a host organism requires vectors which contain specific control sequences governing transcription and efficient splicing of RNA. The most popular expression systems used for this purpose are the bacteria *Escherichia coli* and *Bacillus subtilis*, yeast, cultured insect cells and mammalian cells. The choice of expression system depends on the properties of the protein to be produced. Bacterial cells are most common and convenient host organisms. They are simple to grow, have short generation times, provide large yields, and are most cost-effective. In the case of *B. subtilis*, particularly the cells can be induced to secrete the product into culture medium that facilitates the purification of the cloned protein.

However, there are some disavantages of using bacterial cells for gene expression (Table 1). Though most proteins are expressed in large amounts in bacteria, some of them fail to fold properly, leading to formation of insoluble 'inclusion bodies.' Protein extracted from these inclusion bodies are sometimes biologically inactive. Small proteins can be refolded into their native form, but larger ones containing several cysteine residues, in general, stay inactive, most likely because of the improper

Table 1. Posttranslational processing of proteins in various expression systems

Event	Expression systems			
	Bacteria	Yeast	Insect cells	Mammalian cells
Proteolytic cleavage	+/-	+/–	+	+
Glycosylation	–	+	+	+
Secretion	+/–	+	+	+
Folding	+/–	+/–	+	+
Phosphorylation	–	+	+	+
Acylation	–	+	+	+
Amidation	–	–	+	+
% yield	1-5%	1%	30%	< 1%

formation of disulfide bridges. Moreover, the expressed foreign protein is sometimes toxic to the bacteria, so that the culture producing the protein cannot be grown to high cell density. This problem can be overcome by using an inducible promoter that is turned on to begin the transcription of the foreign gene only after the culture has been grown. Unlike eukaryotic cells, bacterial cells lack enzymes that catalyze posttranslational modifications of proteins such as phophorylation, acylation and glycosylation. These posttranslational modifications are sometimes essential for the normal functioning of a protein.

Yeast cells may be preferable to bacteria for the production of some proteins biological by recombinant DNA procedures. Yeast is a simple eukaryote that resembles mammalian cells in many ways but, like bacterial cells, can be grown conveniently and economically. Yeast cells are capable of catalyzing many posttranslational modifications that are found on mammalian proteins [99]. Also, they process the signal peptides needed for the secretion of protein and thus can be induced to secrete certain proteins into the growth medium for harvesting. Moreover, unlike bacteria, yeast cells do not have endotoxins. However, yeasts do produce active proteases that can degrade the foreign proteins, thereby reducing the yield of the final product. To overcome this problem, the construction of yeast strains with deleted protease genes is being attempted.

Until recently, the expression of a biologically active protein from a complex eukaryotic gene in large amounts was a problem. The problems with prokaryotic expression systems have already been described. Even in yeast (eukaryotic) expression systems, the low biological activity of complex eukaryotic proteins remains a common problem. Mammalian expression systems provide all the posttranslational modifications that may be necessary for full activity of eukaryotic proteins, but the yields from these systems are generally much lower than can be obtained from *E. coli* or yeast. Recently, protein yields as high as 10 mg/liter have been obtained by using mammalian expression systems [43], but this process is often lengthy and costly.

Expression of foreign proteins in cultured insect cells by baculovirus vectors is an alternative to this problem. This relatively new system is becoming the system of choice for expressing mammalian and viral proteins. Baculovirus promoters are among the strongest known and can drive the expression of target genes at high levels (1-500 mg/liter). The baculovirus expression system offers several other advantages over prokaryotic, yeast, and mammalian expression systems [139]. Some of the advantages include: high-level expression, correct folding, the ability to catalyze posttranslational modifications like mammalian cells (Table 1), quick and easy growth in monolayers or suspension cultures without CO_2, and safety – they do not infect humans, animals or plants. More than 400 different proteins have been expressed by using baculovirus vectors, and in most cases the protein produced is similar in structure, biological activity and immunological reactivity to the authentic protein [138]. Although the cost of culturing insect cells is currently more than that of culturing bacteria or yeast, it is still significantly less than that of culturing mammalian cells.

Despite the significant advantages of producing human proteins in heterologous host cells, in some cases the best system for producing a mammalian protein is mammalian cells. Transient expression in mammalian cells is often used to check the function of a newly cloned gene and as a quick method to assess the function of engineered proteins. The extracellular domains of cell-surface receptors have been engineered for secretion from cells by introduction of a stop codon into the gene before the sequence of the transmembrane domain. These soluble receptors, as we will discuss later in this chapter, are valuable reagents for the study of ligand binding and for screening receptor agonists or antagonists that may eventually be used as therapeutics themselves. Although transient transfections yield enough protein for laboratory experiments, stably integrated amplified genes in mammalian cells are necessary for large-scale production of proteins [1]. With this goal in mind, great improvements have been made in recent years in identification of appropriate promoters, vectors, transformation protocols and host cell systems. Table 2 lists some of the proteins that have been cloned, characterized and expressed by using various expression systems.

RECOMBINANT PROTEINS AS CANCER THERAPEUTICS

Biological therapy, as an alternative to the rigorous cytotoxic regimens used in the treatment of various malignant disorders, offers distinct and attractive advantages over conventional chemotherapy. Biological therapy is based on the principle of stimulating the body's own immune response against the disease. A perception of the

Table 2. Recombinant DNA-derived proteins relevant to treatment of cancer

Material produced*	Molecular weight (kDa)	mRNA (kb)	Reference
Interferon-α(IFN-α)	19-29	1.0-2.0	1, 176
Interferon-β (IFN-β)	20	0.7	229
Interferon-γ (IFN-γ)	20-25	1.2	78, 190
Interleukin-1-α(IL-1a)	17.5	2.1	1, 63
Interleukin-1-β (IL-1β)	17.5	1.6	1, 28
Interleukin-1 receptor antagonist	25	1.8	211, 212
Interleukin-2 (IL-2)	15-17	0.9	1
Interleukin-3 (IL-3)	15-17	1.0	1, 265
Interleukin-5 (IL-5)	18	0.9	1, 19
Interleukin-6 (IL-6)	21-26	1.3	1, 98
Interleukin-8 (IL-8)	8	1.8	1, 151
Interleukin-9 (IL-9)	25	1.9	189
Interleukin-10 (IL-10)	37	1.6	250
Interleukin-11 (IL-11)	23	1.5-2.5	173
Interleukin-12 (IL-12)	70	1.4, 2.4	82
Interleukin-13 (IL-13)	9-10	1.2	147
Interleukin 14 (IL-14)	53	1.8	7
Interleukin-15 (IL-15)	14-15	1.5-1.8	75
Tumor Necrosis Factor (TNF)	17	1.7	1, 159, 174
Lymphotoxin	20-25	1.3	1, 77, 160
Amphiregulin	9.0-9.8	1.4	207
Oncostatin M	20-36	2.0	140
Fas Ligand	38-42	2.0	225
Transforming Growth Factor-β (TGF-β)	11.5-12.5	5.8	1, 39
Thymosin α1	12		257
Epidermal Growth Factor (EGF)	6.4	4.2	1, 76
Platelet Derived Growth Factor (PDGF)	28	2.8 & 3.5	90
Fibroblast Growth Factor (Basic) (bFGF)	16	7.0	73
Fibroblast Growth Factor (Acidic) (aFGF)	16	4.2	73
Transforming Growth Factor-α (TGF-α)	5-20	4.5-4.8	40
Insulin like Growth Factor (IGF-I & II)	6.0	7.6 & 6.0	37
Hepatocyte Growth Factor (HGF)	82	6.0	157
Macrophage Colony-Stimulating Factor	45-90	4.2	1, 112
Granulocyte Colony-Stimulating Factor	19.6	1.6	1, 155, 217
GM-Colony Stimulating Factor	18-32	0.7	1, 263
Leukemia Inhibitory Factor (LIF)	32-45	4.2	1, 74
Stem Cell Factor (SCF)	36	6.0	1, 260
Erythropoietin (EPO)	34-36	1.6	1, 103
B cell growth factor	12	1.0, 1.7	206
Hepatitis B surface antigen	17		46, 248

* Space limitation permits only the use of commonly used names and abbreviations.

malignant cell as one whose differentiation has been blocked due to the lack, deficiency or mutation of some key element led to the emergence of a biological therapy. The strategy of biological therapy contrasts with the immediate cell death induced by cytotoxic drugs, where there is no attempt to restore homeostasis. Biological therapy may offer the opportunity to use relatively nontoxic agents, the body's own elements, to correct the underlying problem. Combining biological therapy with low-dose chemotherapy, radiation therapy or surgery may also be of particular value in the management of disorders resistant to conventional drug therapy.

It has long been recognized that the immune system plays a pivotal role in the patient's response to disease. Recently, therefore, cancer therapies have been directed at modulation of components of the immune system (Fig. 3). In particular, 'immune messengers' or cytokines may play a vital role in regulating host antitumor defense mechanisms. Knowledge of cytokines and their functions is expanding rapidly [2, 4, 10, 96, 100]. In the following section we will discuss the potential role of cytokines in the treatment of malignant disease.

Cytokines

In general, cytokines are low molecular weight (10-50 kDa) proteins secreted by cells of the immune system that bind with great specificity and affinity to receptors on target cells and regulate the proliferation, differentiation and metabolism of either the same cell (autocrine) or another cell (paracrine). Cytokines are different from endocrine hormones in that they are produced by any number of different cells rather than by specialized glands. Different cytokines exhibit considerable overlap in their biological activities. Because of the advent of recombinant DNA technology, cytokines have become available in highly pure form and in sufficient quantitites. This has accelerated the elucidation of *in vitro* and *in vivo* biological activities of these proteins and led to their rapid testing in the patients as therapeutic agents for the treatment of cancer. The cytokines that have been shown to have therapeutic potential in cancer include the interferons (IFNs), interleukins (ILs), colony- stimulating factors (CSFs), and tumor necrosis factors (TNF). Table 3 summarizes the clinical application of various re-

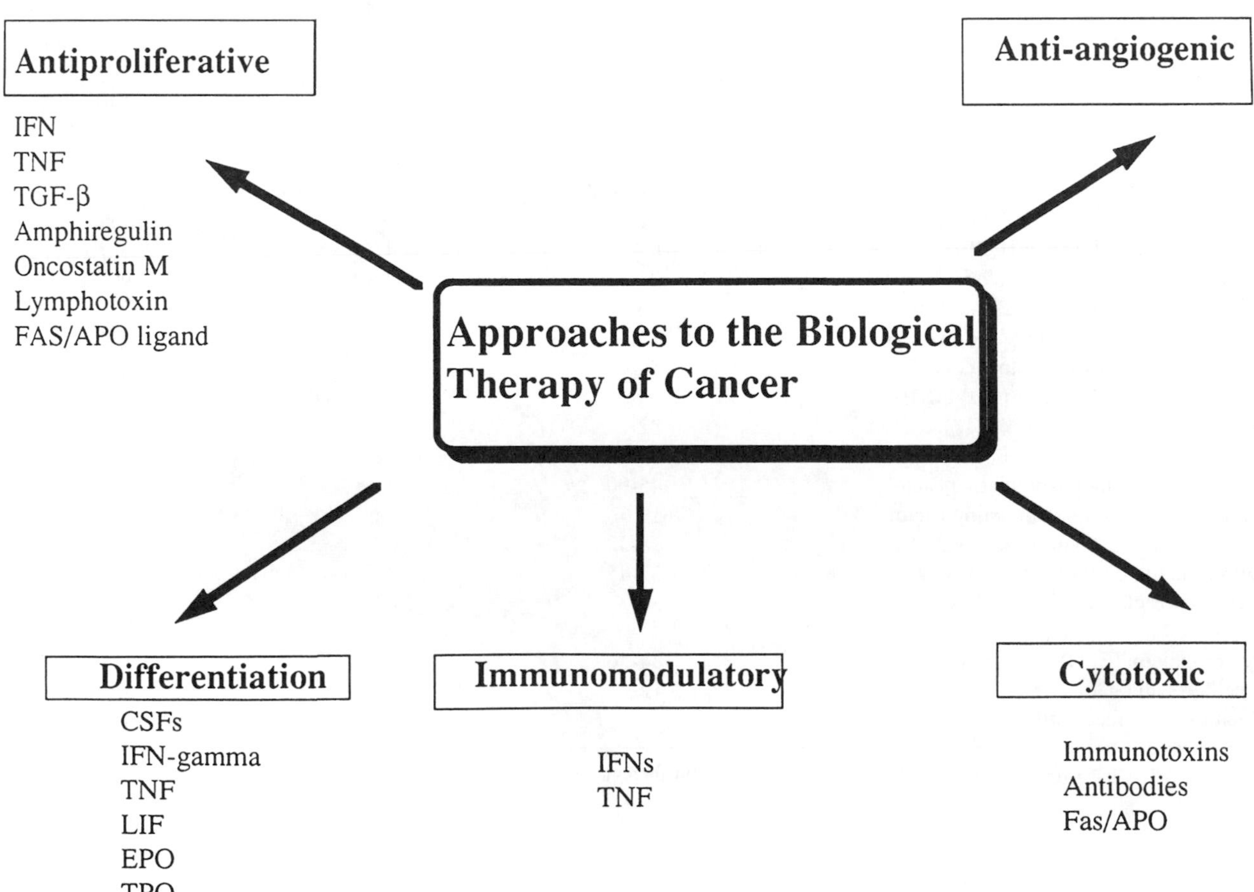

Figure 3. Model for recombinant DNA-derived protein therapeutics for cancer.

Table 3. Cytokines approved or in development for human use*

Cytokine	Target disease	Countries approved
r.Protein Biotherapeutics Approved by FDA for Human Use		
IFN-α	**Chronic myelogenous leukemia**	USA, Europe, Japan
	Hairy cell leukemia	USA, Europe, Japan
	AIDS-related Kaposi's sarcoma	USA
	Chronic non-A/non-B/C hepatitis	USA
	Condylomata acuminata	USA
	Lymphoma	
	Essential thrombocythemia	
	Melanoma	
	Certain solid tumors	
	Multiple myeloma	
	Acute hepatitis B	
IFN-β	**Renal cell carcinoma**	Europe
	Advanced solid tumors	
	Soft tissue carcinoma	
	Adult T cell leukemia	
IFN-γ	**Chronic granulomatous disease (CGD)**	USA
	Advanced solid tumors	
	Renal cell carcinoma	
	Adult T cell leukemia	
	Chronic myelogenous leukemia	
	Lepromatous leprosy	
IL-2	**Renal cell carcinoma**	Europe
	Metastatic melanoma	Japan, Europe
	Advanced malignancies	
G-CSF	**Non-myeloid malignancies associated with chemotherapy-induced myelosuppression**	USA
	Myelodysplastic syndromes	
	Severe chronic neutropenia (cyclic, idiopathic, congenital)	
	Acute myelogenous leukemia	
	Bone marrow transplantation	
GM-CSF	**Autologous bone marrow transplantation for non-Hodgkin's lymphomas, Hodgkin's disease, acute lymphocytic leukemia**	USA, Japan
	Allogeneic bone marrow transplantation for leukemias	
	Myelodysplastic syndromes/ Aplastic anemia	
	Cancer chemotherapy associated myelosuppression	
	Acute myelogenous leukemia	
	AIDS, anti-AIDS drug treatment	
	Associated myelosuppression	
EPO	**Anemia associated with**	
	– chronic renal failure	USA
	– malignancy, chemotherapy	
	– AIDS, AZT treatment	
	– rheumatoid arthritis	
	– anemia of prematurity	
	Autologous blood donation prior to surgery	
	Compensation of surgical blood loss	
	Hepatitis B hepatomas surface antigen	
r.Protein Biotherapeutics Currently under Clinical Trials		
IL-1α, β	Malignant disorders	
	Bone marrow transplantation	
	Severe aplastic anemia	
	Allotransplant patients	
IL-3	Advanced neoplasms	
	Secondary hematopoietic failure	
	Bone marrow recovery	
IL-4	Metastatic renal cell carcinoma	
	Metastatic breast carcinoma	
	Metastatic melanoma	
	Disseminated cancer	
	Advanced malignancies	
IL-6	Platelet deficiency	
TNF-α	Advanced neoplasms	
	Reduction of ovarian ascites	
M-CSF	Solid tumors	
	Breast cancer	
	Fungal infections	
	Acute myelogenous leukemia	
IL-1 receptor antagonist	AML, CML, sepsis, septic shock	

* Disease in bold indicates approved use of cytokine.

combinant cytokines currently being used for the treatment of malignant diseases.

Interferons

Interferons are a family of regulatory glycoproteins produced by many cell types in response to viral infections and a variety of mitogenic and antigenic stimuli. Three major classes of IFNs have been described: IFN-α and IFN-β, which share components of the same receptor and are referred to as type I; and IFN-γ, which uses a separate receptor system and is referred to as type II. Additional

IFNs have been discovered, but they are not well characterized [205]. Crude IFN was probably the first cytokine used in patients and was shown to delay recurrent growth of tumors in patients who had undergone surgery for osteogenic sarcoma [223]. Pharmacological doses of partially purified IFN-α were shown to bring regression of tumors in significant numbers of patients with metastatic breast cancer, low-grade lymphoma, or multiple myeloma [84]. In 1981, IFN-α was successfully cloned by two groups, and the purified protein was immediately tested in the clinic. This was the first study of a recombinant cytokine in patients with cancer and, for the most part, the biological activity seen with the partially pure natural form was reproduced with the recombinant DNA-derived form [85]. Treatment with IFN-α was also shown to induce remissions in some patients with well-differentiated B-cell tumors [222].

The most remarkable effects of recombinant IFN-α were observed in patients with hairy cell leukemia [187]. Treatment with partially purified or recombinant IFN-α suppressed peripheral blood cell production and rapidly increased platelet counts in these patients [86]. Their immune status improved and the number of hairy cells in the bone marrow and blood declined. These patients stopped having opportunistic infections and required no further platelet and erythrocyte transfusions. These studies led to the approval of IFN-α for treatment of hairy cell leukemia in June 1986 by the United States Food and Drug Administration (FDA), an action adopted by regulatory agencies from 31 other countries. The mechanisms of IFN-α action in the compromised survival of the patients with hairy cell leukemia are not known but may include differentiation, cell-cycle arrest and/or apoptosis.

Other B-cell neoplasms also show variable degrees of sensitivity to IFN-α [84, 85, 222]. In patients with multiple myeloma or low-grade lymphoma, the cytokine often has demonstrated a positive clinical impact on survival when combined with chemotherapy [142, 214, 216]. Clinical results with IFN-α in patients with chronic myelogenous leukemia (CML) have been rather interesting. During the chronic phase of CML, IFN-α treatment causes hematologic remission [86]. Approximately 75% of the patients in the benign phase of the disease achieve complete normalization of blood counts. Moreover, IFN-α had the astonishing capacity to suppress selectively the cells bearing the Philadephia chromosome, resulting in partial or complete restoration of the normal clone [228].

While showing great promise for leukemia, IFN-α therapy of solid tumors has been rather discouraging. Only 10-15% of patients with renal cell carcinoma or malignant melanoma undergo regression in response to IFN-α. However,the response of carcinoid tumors to the cytokine was encouraging. A majority of patients showed improvement in symptoms, and a smaller fraction experienced tumor regression [165]. Both squamous and basal cell carcinomas of the skin show sensitivity to IFN-α, as a single agent or in combination with retinoids [131, 180]. Mycosis fungoides, a malignancy of the T helper cells, is also sensitive to IFN-α alone or with other modalities including retinoids [108, 196]. Kaposi's sarcoma, an angioproliferative disease that commonly develops in individuals infected with human immunodeficiency virus (HIV), has responded well to IFN-α therapy: 40% of patients experienced significant regression of lesions [222]. This work led to the approval of IFN-α in the U.S. and 21 other countries for the treatment of AIDS-related Kaposi's sarcoma.

After isolation of its gene and 10 years' work identifying several of its biological activities, IFN-γ was tested in human subjects for a wide variety of diseases including cancer. It was found to have impressive effects against chronic granulomatous disease, leading to its approval by the FDA for human use [234]. More recently, IFN-β was approved for treatment of ambulatory patients with relapsing/remitting multiple sclerosis [3]. Clinical toxic effects associated with administration of IFNs and other cytokines are summarized in Table 4. The IFNs, like most other cytokines, are produced by the body to act locally. When used as a systemic pharmaceutical, they have certain toxic effects [222].

Table 4. Common toxic effects associated with administration of cytokines

Fever
Chills
Nausea
Vomiting
Headache
Anorexia
Fatigue
Myalgias
Arthralgias
Bone pain
Flush
Local erythema
Inflammation at the site of injection
Capillary leak syndrome
Granulocytopenia
Thrombocytopenia
Anemia
Hypotension
Liquid accumulation in the lung, spleen, kidneys
Reversible increase in body weight
Reversible increase in the serum creatinine
Oliguria
Malaise
Asthenia
Rigors
Diarrhea
Hepatocytotoxicity
Lethargy, depression
Mental confusion
EEG-abnormalities

Interleukins

The interleukins are a family of cytokines that are essential to both cellular and humoral immune responses. At least 18 different types have been described, many with potential antineoplastic activity.

Interleukin 1 (IL-1): IL-1 was originally described as an 'endogenous pyrogen' in 1940 because of its ability to cause fever when injected into animals. Two forms of IL-1 are now recognized: IL-1α is cell-associated and is involved in antigen presentation, whereas IL-1β, the predominant form, is readily secreted by macrophages. Though the two forms have limited amino acid homology, IL-1α and IL-1β bind to the same receptor and share several biological properties. Other cell types that produce IL-1 are endothelial cells, keratinocytes, neutrophils and B lymphocytes. Constitutive expression of IL-1 occurs in cells lining the external environment, i.e., skin and mucosal surfaces [41]. The cDNAs coding for both human IL-1s were reported in 1985 [28, 63]. Recombinant IL-1s induced fever, hepatic protein synthesis, production of prostaglandin E2, cartilage breakdown, bone resorption, and elevated ACTH and augmented the T lymphocyte response to antigens and mitogens [41]. Recombinant IL-1 exhibits cytostatic activity toward human melanoma tumor cells *in vitro* and direct cytotoxic effects against human melanoma cell line A375 [122]. Recently, recombinant IL-1 was shown to enhance the recovery of platelets in ovarian cancer patients following carboplatin therapy, suggesting a potential role for IL-1 in attenuating thrombocytopenia associated with chemotherapy [245].

Interleukin-2 (IL-2): IL-2 is a 15.5-kDa glycoprotein produced by peripheral blood lymphocytes and is a potent growth factor for activated T lymphocytes. It acts as a cofactor in development of cytotoxic T lymphocyte activity against tumors and has been shown to participate in tumoricidal activity by inducing the growth of natural killer (NK) cells and lymphokine-activated killer (LAK) cells [191]. Several cancers show sensitivity toward recombinant IL-2, both in animal models and in the patients. LAK cells are peripheral blood lymphocytes that can be generated *in vitro* by incubation with high doses of IL-2. They have the ability to kill tumor cells specifically while leaving normal cells unharmed. IL-2 has been used in combination with LAK cells to achieve more potent antitumor response [191-194]. In 1985, Rosenberg and associates published the results of their first study documenting tumor regression in patients with melanoma following administration of IL-2 and LAK cells [192]. An update of the results in 180 patients was published in 1991 [191]. Antitumor responses were seen in patients with advanced melanoma, renal cell cancer, colon cancer or non-Hodgkin's lymphoma.

Like LAK, tumor-infiltrating lymphocytes (TILs), the lymphoid cells that infiltrate solid tumors, can be grown *in vitro* in the presence of IL-2. These cells have unique lytic activity against autologous tumors. Treatment with TILs in combination with IL-2 was shown to mediate substantial tumor regression in some patients with advanced malignant melanoma [135]. Objective responses were observed that lasted for 3-14 months in 29% patients with renal cell cancer and 23% of those with melanoma. Further potential of IL-2 in cancer therapy has been demonstrated by using recombinant IL-2 in combination with other cytokines [193, 241]. For example, recombinant IL-2 in combination with IFN-α elicited a potent antitumor response in several animal tumor models [136]. The most significant antitumor activity seen with IL-2 therapy has been in malignant melanoma and renal cell carcinoma. Other tumors treated with IL-2 include glioma, bladder carcinoma, ovarian carcinoma, neuroblastoma, lung carcinoma, head and neck carcinoma, breast carcinoma, lymphoma, colon carcinoma and mesothelioma [96]. As shown in Table 4, IL-2 administration in patients is associated with a wide range of toxic effects, the most common being fluid retention, anemia, thrombocytopenia and hypotension [136]. IL-2 is the first cytokine that has been employed so widely in clinical trials. However, because of its toxic effects, its clinical use has been limited.

Interleukin-3 (IL-3): Recombinant IL-3 is a 15 – 17-kDa polypeptide that is known to stimulate mast cells, neutrophils, macrophages and megakaryocytes. No direct antitumor activity has been observed for IL-3, but this cytokine has a role in increasing platelet and neutrophil counts in patients with advanced malignancy [65]. Phase I and II clinical trials with recombinant IL-3 have been carried out in patients with advanced malignancy. A dose-dependent increase in platelet counts and substantial increases in the numbers of circulating neutrophils, eosinophils, monocytes and lymphocytes were observed in these patients [65]. Hematopoietic failure caused by prolonged chemotherapy, radiotherapy or infiltration of bone marrow by tumor cells could be restored by recombinant IL-3 treatment. The side effects of rIL-3 therapy in patients include fever, bone pain and headache [65]. Thus, recombinant IL-3 is a multilineage hematopoietic cytokine with promising effects on platelet and neutrophil counts.

Interleukin-4 (IL-4): IL-4 is a T cell-derived glycoprotein of 20 kDa. The gene for human IL-4 has been cloned [11]. The antitumor functions of IL-4 include increased T cell, NK cell and monocyte proliferation. IL-4 has also been shown to enhance the generation of cytotoxic T lymphocytes and to participate in induction of LAK cell activity, and to synergize with IL-2 in this activity [152]. Furthermore, IL-4 can stimulate the generation of TILs in human melanoma, increase the antigen-presenting ability of mouse and human monocytes and augment the expression of tumoricidal activity in murine macrophages. It appears to inhibit the release of TNF, IL-1 and IL-6 by human monocytes [233].

Interleukin-4 has been shown to exert potent antitumor activity against several transplantable tumors in a murine model. Using IL-4-transfected tumor cells, the potential of transfecting lymphokine genes into tumor cells as a method of cancer therapy has been demonstrated [68]. Because of its antitumor effects *in vitro* and in murine models, IL-4 may be useful in inhibiting the growth of solid tumors and B-cell lymphomas (Table 3).

Other interleukins: The number of known interleukins is still growing, and many have biological effects that have clinical implications in the treatment of cancer. IL-15 is a the most recently cloned member of this family [128] and has been shown to be a growth factor for T lymphocytes and TILs [86]. Like IL-2, it binds to the beta and gamma chains of the IL-2 receptor to exert its action [75]. Other important members of the interleukin family include IL-5, IL-6, IL-7 and IL-12. IL-5 is an 18-kDa product of T lymphocytes that has been cloned and shown to be a lineage-specific eosinophil growth and differentiation factor [19, 199]. Murine IL-5 induces antibody-dependent killing of tumor cells by blood eosinophils and enhances phagocytosis by eosinophils.

Interleukin-6, initially described as β_2-interferon, is a 19 – 28-kDa protein produced by a variety of cells, including mononuclear phagocytes, fibroblasts, keratinocytes and endothelial cells. The experimental data support a potential clinical role for IL-6. Its hematopoietic activity and thrombopietic activity, in particular, may make this cytokine a useful agent for inducing the recovery of bone marrow in patients with myelosuppression that usually follows aggressive chemotherapy regimens. The results of phase I clinical studies of IL-6 have recently been reported [256]. IL-7 is a 22 to 25-kDa glycoprotein that was originally characterized on the basis of its ability to promote the growth of precursor B lymphocytes [71]. Recombinant IL-7 induces the proliferation of both thymocytes and mature T cells and is known to activate macrophages for tumor cell killing. In human monocytes, IL-7 induces the expression of IL-8, IL-6, IL-1α, IL-1β and TNF-α. IL-12, a product of B cells and mononuclear phagocytes, has multiple effects on both T cells and NK cells. It induces IFN-γ production in T and NK cells and sustains the cell-mediated immune response [240].

Colony-Stimulating Factors

The colony-stimulating factors (CSF) are a family of glycoproteins that have the ability to induce proliferation and differentiation of progenitor hematopoietic cells and have effects on the functional status of their mature progeny. Multi-colony stimulating factor (IL-3), macrophage colony-stimulating factor (M-CSF), granulocyte colony-stimulating factor (G-CSF), granulocyte-macrophage colony-stimulating factor (GM-CSF), erythropoietin (EPO), stem cell factor (SCF), and leukemia inhibitory factor (LIF) are some of the clinically important members of this family (Table 2). All the known CSFs have been produced by recombinant DNA methods and tested in human subjects (Table 3). The potential for using hematopoietic growth factors in the treatment of disease is enormous. Their ability to control the production of blood cells has been realized, and the results of clinical trials to date suggest that the side effects of these growth factors are relatively minor [258]. Three recombinant hematopoietic growth factors, G-CSF (filgrastim), GM-CSF (Sargramostim), and EPO (epoetin alfa), are now commercially available for clinical use in the United States.

Extensive clinical and preclinical data on recombinant human G-CSF and GM-CSF indicate that both these cytokines are effective in accelerating neutrophil recovery and shortening the duration of neutropenia following chemotherapy with or without bone marrow transplantation [34, 57, 145, 161]. Administration of recombinant human G-CSF as an adjunct to cyclophosphamide, doxorubicin and etoposide chemotherapy for small cell lung carcinoma significantly reduced duration and severity of neutropenia and associated clinical sequelae [239]. Similarly, patients with transitional cell carcinoma of the bladder treated with methotrexate, vinblastin, doxorubicin and cisplatin experienced up to fourfold increases in neutrophil count on administration of G-CSF with few or no toxic effects [64]. GM-CSF may also exert antitumor effect by inducing tumoricidal activation of macrophages. Administration of GM-CSF has been shown to decrease the tumor burden in a murine Lewis lung carcinoma model [95].

Clinical trials of M-CSF have been performed in an attempt to ameliorate leukopenia. A phase I trial of M-CSF in patients with metastatic melanoma showed an increase in the number and function of circulating monocytes [12]. In a non-randomized, controlled study (32 patients with urinary tract malignancies) and a randomized controlled study (98 patients with gynecological malignancies), M-CSF administration reduced the period of post-chemotherapy leukopenia [150, 162].

Among the cytokines whose role can be predicted from *in vitro* studies, EPO is perhaps the best example. EPO is produced mainly by the kidneys and is responsible for regulating the production of erythrocytes. EPO acts on erythroid precursors in the bone marrow, spleen and fetal liver and stimulates the colony formation of the burst-forming unit-erythroid. When infused in mice, EPO markedly increases both peripheral blood erythrocytes levels and the number of erythroid progenitor cells present in bone marrow. These results led to the clinical trials with a human recombinant EPO, the findings suggested that EPO can reverse anemia in patients with end-stage renal cell disease. EPO produced dose-dependent increases in hematocrit and hemoglobin levels, and in most cases eliminated the need for regular blood tranfusions [48]. The major side effect reported is increased blood pressure. EPO also increases the ability of patients undergoing elective surgery to donate autologous blood [69]. Double-blind placebo-controlled studies with recombinant EPO suggested that it is an effective treatment for predialysis patients [130].

Stem cell factor (SCF) has recently been used in the clinic as a single agent following chemotherapy. SCF by itself appears to have limited efficacy and significant toxicity-mainly due to mast cell stimulation at higher doses. However, Tong et al. [236] showed that patients receiving CSF have an increase in primitive progenitor cells suugesting that SCF might be highly effective in combination with later acting hemopoietins. From these data it is clear that recombinant CSFs are effective in correcting hematopoietic disorders of various etiologies. Whether these mediators improve morbidity and mortality in patients will be decided by further clincal results. However, combinations of cytokines, for example, those with relatively restricted biological activity (EPO, G-CSF, M-CSF etc.) and those that have a broad range of action (SCF, IL-3, GM-CSF, IL-6 etc.), are likely to show more promising effects on hematopoiesis than any single cytokine alone [88].

Tumor Necrosis Factors

Tumor necrosis factor (TNF) is a proinflammatory cytokine that is produced primarily by mononuclear phagocytes in response to endotoxin. There are two forms of TNF; TNF-α is a cytotoxic factor with a molecular weight of 17-kDa, and TNF-β, also known as 'lymphotoxin,' has a molecular weight of 25-kDa and is released from stimulated lymphocytes. Both forms have been produced by recombinant DNA technology and appear to have antiproliferative, cytostatic and cytolytic effects against human tumor cells *in vitro* as well as *in vivo* when injected into nude mice [167]. TNF-α exerts synergistic effects with different cytokines, such as IFNs, IL-1, IL-2 etc., and can induce secretion of series of mediators, including IL-1, IL-6, prostaglandins etc. It has been implicated in both the generation and the cytotoxicity of LAK cells and cytotoxic T lymphocytes [26].

Based on these observations, a large number of phase I and II studies were initiated to investigate the antitumor properties of TNF-α. Unfortunately, in clinical settings the efficacy of TNF-α has been very limited, and its use is associated with serious toxic effects [94]. Of 127 eligible patients enrolled in nine different phase II protocols between 1988 and 1990 for the treatment of diverse malignancies, including breast, colon, gastric, pancreatic, endometrial, and bladder cancers, multiple myeloma and sarcomas, only one patient responded (response rate, 0.8%), whereas 13% experienced grade four or fatal toxic effects. Despite the initial disappointing results with TNF-α as an antitumor agent, investigators have continued working on new and improved approaches for its use. In a recent study, Lienard and co-workers [129] used an intra-arterial route to administer high doses of TNF-α in conjunction with melphalan, hyperthermia and IFN-γ. Of the 23 patients treated (19 with melanoma and four with sarcoma), all responded, 21 with complete remission and two with partial remission. Eleven of these patients were previously unresponsive to melphalan alone and one had failed to respond to cisplatin therapy. The toxic effects observed (neutropenia, hypotension, thrombocytopenia and kidney failure) were reversible. The overall rate of survival was 70% and of disease-free survival over 12 months, 76%.

These results suggested that further understanding of the mechanisms of TNF-α's antitumor action could help improve its clinical efficacy. For example, decreasing the agent's systemic toxicity without reducing its anticancer effects could lead to substantial therapeutic advantages. TNF-α mediates its effects by interacting with two different surface receptors, p55 and p75 [232]. Studies have suggested that TNF-α's interaction with p75 may be responsible for its systemic toxicity [92, 232]. Thus, mutant TNF molecules that interact with p55 but not p75 could induce antitumor effects with reduced systemic toxicity, permitting higher doses of TNF-α. Indeed, such mutant human TNF molecules that specifically bind to p55 have already been described and shown to exert cytotoxic effects against transformed cells *in vitro* [168]. In addition, concomitant use of drugs that are able to decrease TNF-α systemic toxicity could permit use of higher, more effective doses of this cytokine in cancer therapy. Combination regimens of TNF-α with other cytokines, concomitant use of TNF toxicity inhibitors and use of mutant TNF molecules may provide better clinical outcomes. Moreover, regional therapy with TNF-α requires further exploration in view of the fact that such regimens have already produced some very promising results [129].

Soluble cytokine receptors

Certain membrane receptors are enzymatically cleaved from the cell surface and released into the extracellular medium in the form of soluble fragments. Soluble receptors corresponding to the ligand-binding domains of many polypeptide hormones and cytokine receptors have been described (Table 5). The function of soluble receptors is not yet known [53, 89]. However, it is likely that this process represents an important mechanism for regulation of surface expression of such receptors and may determine the effects of cytokines and growth hormones on the target cells. For example, the cell growth, differentiation and immunomodulatory effects of cytokines are exerted in response to their binding to specific cell-surface receptors. The presence of soluble receptors in the biological milieu may thus promote direct binding of the ligand to the soluble receptor, neutralizing and preventing its action.

The *in vivo* relevance of soluble cytokine receptors is well illustrated by several viruses. Vaccinia and cowpox viruses encode a protein that displays homology with soluble IL-1 receptor and is able to bind IL-1β [219]. Furthermore, proteins that bind to TNF have been identified in the open reading frame of pox viral strains [215]. Herpes and myxoma viruses encode proteins that can effectively bind IL-8 and IFN-γ ligands, respectively [5, 244]. Such soluble receptors assist virus infection by suppressing host defense mechanisms. From the studies

Table 5. List of soluble receptors identified for various cytokines

Receptor	Reference
Proteolytic cleavage:	
IL-1R	89, 219
IL-2R	53
IL-4R (murine)	54
IL-6R	153, 156
IL-6R (gp 130)	153, 156, 158
TNFR	8, 66, 107
IFN-α R	163
IFN-γ R	164
NGFR	42
M-CSFR	44
Hergulin R	125
EGFR	83
EPOR	14, 154
PDGFR	235
Alternative splicing:	
IL-4R	149
IL-5R (murine)	227
IL-7R	70
LIFR	123
GM-CSFR	200
G-CSFR	59
EGFR	179
c-erbB3	110

on induction of antiviral soluble LDL receptors by IFNs, it seems that host organisms make use of a similar mechanism for the opposite role of controlling viral infection.

During the release of cell-surface receptors, it is usually the extracellular domain of the receptor that is shed; thus, soluble receptors act as inhibitors of cytokines. The soluble receptors may originate via two separate mechanisms, one involving alternate splicing in which a receptor gene lacks a transmembrane domain. As an aternative, the receptors can be shed from the cell surface as a result of activation of specific proteolytic enzyme or enzymes. The identity of enzymes involved in proteolytic cleavage of the receptors is not known; however, it is a highly regulated process and appears to be controlled by phosphatases and kinases [3]. The treatment of cells with ligand can also lead to down modulation of the receptors and their subsequent shedding.

The significance of soluble cytokine receptors as a therapeutic modality for treatment of cancer will be determined by further research and evaluation. Since soluble receptors can provide highly specific biological inhibitors for cytokines and growth factors, and because the majority of transformed cells require cytokines for their growth and survival, soluble receptors may have therapeutic potential as antagonists to cytokine action. For example, hematopoietic growth factors are known to maintain the viability of hematopoietic cells through the prevention of apoptosis [261]. Several investigators have reported that autocrine production of hematopoietic growth factors such as IL-1β [62, 79] or GM-CSF [268] supports the growth and survival of acute myeloid leukemia (AML) cells *in vitro*. In contrast, their soluble receptors and receptor antagonist could inhibit the growth of leukemic cells including AML [267], chronic myelocytic leukemia (CML) [49], and juvenile CML [203]. Receptor proteins for most of the cytokines have been cloned and expressed [1]. However, the information available on their therapeutic potential in cancer is very limited.

Like the soluble and membrane-bound forms of cytokine receptors, the cytokine ligands also exist in these two forms. For example, the cytokines IL-1, TNF, FGF, TGF-α, TGF-β and SCF have been reported to exist in both the soluble and membrane-bound forms. This process, commonly initiated by cell stimulation, may regulate the surface expression of such cytokines and play an important role in determination of cytokine activity.

Antibodies and conjugates

Antibodies are highly selective proteins that can bind to a single target among millions of irrelevant sites. Because of this specificity, the antibodies have been used extensively to target drugs, prodrugs, toxins and other agents to particular sites in the body. It is this use of antibodies as targeting devices that led to the concept of 'magic bullets,' a treatment that could effectively seek and selectively destroy tumor cells wherever they resided. The major problem in the therapeutic use of antibodies was their production in large quantities, but the development of 'monoclonal antibody' technology changed the situation dramatically [146]. Monoclonal antibodies (MAb) are already widely used for the diagnosis and treatment of cancer and for imaging of tumors for radiotherapy.

Despite the rapid progress being made in application of MAbs as therapeutic agents, their use has been limited because of their immunogenicity problem. MAbs are usually mouse proteins; when injected into patients they are eventually recognized as foreign proteins and cleared from the circulation. To overcome this problem, researchers set out to engineer fully 'humanized MAbs' that will be indistinguishable from natural proteins [21, 262]. Humanizing MAbs is a technology that uses recombinant DNA techniques to improve or change the function of these antibodies [184]. The first fully humanized MAb recognizes an antigen on the surface of human lymphocytes and is being evaluated as an immunosuppresant and for treatment of lymphoid tumors. Another potentially useful humanized MAb recognizes a growth factor receptor in large numbers on the surface of several breast tumor cells. This MAb successfully inhibited tumor cell growth in culture and is currently being evaluated in patients [255]. In the following section, we will briefly discuss the potential use of MAb-based immunotherapies that have been used for the treatment of malignant diseases. Detailed aspects of this approach will be discussed somewhere else in this book.

Monoclonal antibodies as agonists

Antibodies directed against cell-surface molecules on many types of tumor cells can act as ligands, resulting in powerful antitumor effects mediated by signal transduction [253]. For example, MAb 4D5 against *erb*B-2, when added to breast or ovarian carcinoma cells that overexpress *erb*B-2, induces a strong antiproliferative effect and is currently being evaluated in patients with these tumors [127, 264]. The erbB-2 protein product is a member of the EGF receptor family and is shown to act as a signaling receptor for a recently identified ligand, heregulin, in regulation of growth and differentiation of breast cancer and other cell types [33]. Similarly, ligation of Fas/APO-1 protein with an anti-Fas/anti-APO-1 MAb resulted in apoptosis (programmed cell death) of malignant cells. Using MAbs, the human Fas and APO-1 proteins were identified as cell-surface proteins of 200- and 48-kDa molecular mass, respectively, in two different laboratories. Both induced apoptosis in a variety of cell types upon binding. Subsequent isolation of cDNAs encoding the two proteins revealed that they were identical despite a difference in apparent molecular weight [101, 166]. Apoptosis triggered by the anti-Fas/APO-1 Mab has been successfully used for the treatment of mice bearing human hematopoietic tumors [238]. The clinical use of anti-Fas/APO-1 therapy for cancer treatmentwill be decided by further evaluation.

Besides negative signaling, Mabs have other potential uses in tumor therapy. Some MAbs can block interactions between tumor cells and neighboring cells, stroma, or matrix that are necessary for tumor growth or metastases. For example, injection of anti-CD44 MAb or its $F(ab')_2$ fragment one week after inoculation of human melanoma cells in mice with severe combined immunodeficiency (SCID) prevented metastases but not the development of primary tumor [58]. The antibody had no effect on growth of tumor cells *in vitro*. MAbs against growth factors or their receptors can also exert significant antitumor effects. For example, antibodies against IL-6 and IL-6 receptor were effective in the treatment of human myeloma in SCID mice [226] and produced transient responses in patients bearing IL-6-dependent tumors [113]. MAbs against the IL-2 receptor have been used to treat adult T-cell leukemia with some partial or complete remissions [254]. Thus MAbs selected against tumor surface antigens to exert either potent growth-inhibitory effects or host-tumor interactions should lead to new strategies for selecting the antitumor activity of MAbs.

Monoclonal antibodies-conjugated drugs

The clinical progress with conjugates of Mabs and cytotoxic drugs has been rather slow. An important factor that has limited the use of this approach for treatment of cancer is the relatively low potency of standard chemotherapeutic agents. The potency of these compounds is further reduced by their conjugation with MAbs [115]. However, a recent report that such a conjugate, BR96-doxorubicin (BR96-Dox), is highly effective in curing xenografted human carcinoma-bearing mice [237], has rejuvenated great interest in MAb-drug conjugates. BR96 is a chimeric monoclonal antibody that contains a framework region of human immunoglobulin and the binding region of a murine antibody. The antibody binds to an antigen that is expressed on the surface of many human carcinomas. Treatment of tumor-bearing athymic mice with BR96-Dox induced complete regressions and cures of xenografted human lung, breast, and colon carcinomas and cured 70% of mice with extensive metastases from a human lung carcinoma [237]. Clinical trials with BR96-Dox were recently initiated to determine its safety in patients. Similar results with MAb-vinblastine conjugates were reported years ago, but evaluation of this MAb-drug conjugate was discontinued because of unacceptable gastrointestinal toxic effects [9, 181].

Recently, several groups have concentrated their research on more potent immunotoxins conjugated with agents such as calicheamicins, maytansines and trichothecenes. Calicheamicin is a family of antibiotics that produce double-stranded DNA breaks; when conjugated with Mab CT-M-01, which recognizes PEM antigen and is located on the surface of human cancerous epithelial cells, and injected into breast carcinoma-xenografted mice, it significantly inhibited tumor growth and produced long-term tumor-free survivors [97]. Similarly, maytansinoids, which are 100 to 1,000-fold more potent than doxorubicin and vinblastine, when conjugated to Mab A7, which recognizes an antigen expressed on human colon cancer cell lines, showed high antigen-specific *in vitro* cytotoxicity against cancer cells and low systemic toxicity in mice [23]. Similar specificity and potency have been observed in MAb-trichothecenes conjugates (protein synthesis inhibitors) in terms of their tumor cell-killing ability [148].

More recently, Mabs have been used to deliver enzyme inhibitors to tumor cells. Thus, conjugation of Geninstein (an inhibitor of *Src* protooncogene family protein tyrosine kinases) to MAb B43, which recognizes the B cell-specific receptor CD19, selectively bound to B-cell precursor leukemia cells, inhibited CD19-associated tyrosine kinases and triggered rapid apoptotic cell death [243]. Treatment of B-cell precursor leukemia-xenografted SCID mice with less than one-tenth the maximum tolerated dose of B43-Geninstein resulted in more than 99.999% killing of human leukemia cells, which led to 100% long-term event-free survival from an otherwise invariably fatal leukemia of these mice [243]. It remains to be seen whether antibody-drug conjugates will be effective anti-cancer agents in clinical settings as well.

Immunotoxins

Immunotoxins are chimeric molecules in which antibodies or the ligand that interacts with the cell-surface molecules are coupled to toxins or their subunits (Fig. 4). The antibody or growth factor binds with high selectivity to the target cells. The toxins are derived from plants or bacteria. DNA sequences encoding the bacterial toxins; *Pseudomonas* exotoxin (PE) and diphtheria toxin and the plant toxins; ricin and gelonin have been cloned and expressed in *E. coli*, [172, 197]. The topic of immunotoxins is discussed in detail elsewhere in this book and, therefore, we will concentrate in this section on the therapeutic potential of recombinant immunotoxins only.

Initially, the toxins produced in bacteria were chemically linked to antibodies to make immunotoxins. In recent years, significant progress has been made in engineering recombinant immunotoxins by fusing the cell-binding ligand genes to modified toxin genes [172]. For example, a truncated form of *Pseudominas* exotoxin (PE40) has been produced by deleting the first 252 amino acids; this toxin has extremely low toxicity because of its inability to bind to cellular receptors [104]. However, when chemically conjugated to an antibody [56, 121] or the recombinant chimeric toxin generated by fusing the PE40 gene to DNA fragments encoding growth factors, antibody-binding sites, or other target-recognition elements, *Pseudomonas* exotoxin becomes highly specific and potent in killing target cells [171, 172]. The gene encoding this chimeric toxin is expressed in *E. coli*. Table 6 lists some of the recombinant immunotoxins that have been produced by fusing the PE40 gene to cDNAs encoding different targeting molecules. Anti-Tac(Fv)-PE40 is one such recombinant immunotoxin that was generated by fusing the truncated form of the *Pseudomonas exotoxin* (PE40) gene with the variable region of an antibody against the IL-2 receptor [25, 120]. This immunotoxin is highly toxic to cells from patients with adult T-cell leukemia and induced regression of IL-2 receptor-bearing carcinoma tumors in athymic mice [47, 118, 119]. TGF-α-PE40 recombinant chimera toxin targets PE40 to cells with EGF [47, 204]. Although many normal cells contain EGF receptors, tumor cells often have extremely large number of receptors because of amplification and overexpression of the EGF receptor gene [188]. When administered systemically, TGF-α-PE40 caused regression of subcutaneous epidermoid carcinoma and prostate carcinoma tumors in mice [172].

Interleukin-2-PE40 is a recombinant chimeric protein designed to deliver the toxin to cells with IL-2 receptors [133]. Normal resting lymphocytes do not express IL-2 receptors, but when they are activated with an antigen or IL-2, the receptors are induced. IL-2-PE40 has been shown to be highly toxic to activated mouse and rat T cells and had some therapeutic effect against mouse lymphoma [116]. Similarly, IL-6-PE40 chimeric toxin killed many human myeloma and hepatoma cell lines that express IL-6 receptors at high numbers and also several other carcinomas [116, 208, 209]. The first clinical trial of a

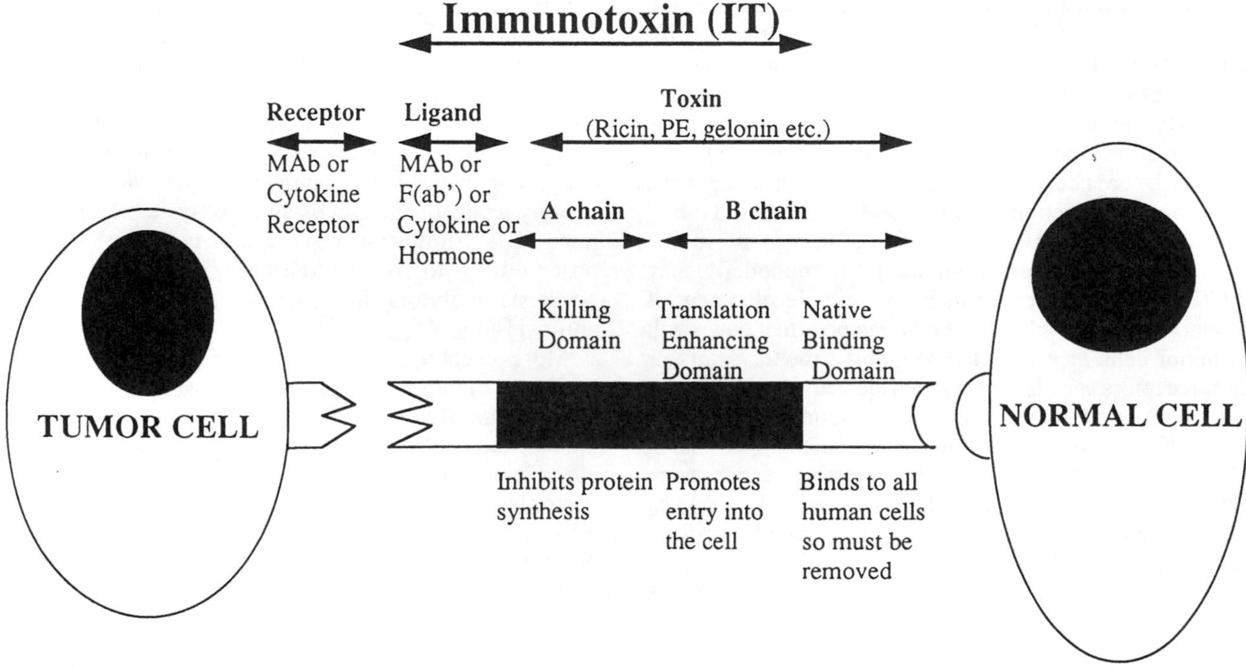

Figure 4. Schematic representation of immunotoxin.

Table 6. Recombinant toxins derived from *Pseudomonas* exotoxin

Immunotoxin	Target	Reference
PE40	–	
Anti-Tac (Fv)-PE40	human IL-2 receptor (leukemia)	25, 118-120
TGF-α-PE40	EGF receptor, epidermoid carcinomas adenocarcinomas, glioblastomas smooth muscle cells	47, 87, 204, 201
IL-2-PE-40	IL-2 receptor (leukemia)	116, 133
IL-6-PE40	IL-6 receptor myelomas, hepatomas, prostate	209-210
B3(dsFv)-PE38KDEL	many carcinomas	15, 16
e23(Fv)PE40	*erb*B2 lung, breast, ovary and stomach adenocarcinomas	13

genetically engineered immunotoxin (B3LysPE38) was initiated in April 1993 in breast and colon carcinoma patients. Some responses were evident, but toxic effects appeared to be greater in human patients than seen in mice and primates [213].

In contrast to *Pseudomonas exotoxin*-immunotoxins, the immunotoxins composed of ricin or its A subunit and MAbs have generally been constructed using chemical cross-linking reagents [67, 134]. Recombinant ricin-based chimera molecules have been difficult to produce, because the A chain of the plant toxins must be attached to the cell recognition domain by a disulfide bond, and disulfide-linked subunits are difficult to produce in bacteria [188]. Many reviews have already described the activities and properties of immunotoxins made with ricin and other plant toxins [67, 182, 198, 242, 249, 252]. Ricin-containing immunotoxins have been used to eliminate selected populations of lymphocytes. Vitetta, Uhr and associates have produced ricin conjugates of antibodies to B cell-specific antigens and shown such conjugates to cause complete regression of B-cell lymphomas in mice [60]. Significant antitumor activity of ricin A chain immunoconjugates has been observed against solid or ascites tumors in animal models [55, 80].

Because of encouraging results in preclinical studies, several ricin-containing immunoconjugates have been developed and approved for human trials, and two kinds of human trials have been conducted. The first involves the *ex vivo* treatment of harvested bone marrow to eliminate contaminating tumor cells prior to re-infusion in patients undergoing autologous bone marrow transplantation. The second kind of trial involves the parenteral administration of immunotoxins [182, 242, 249, 252]. Some patients with B-cell lymphoma responded to immunotoxin therapy [67]. Currently, an anti-CD22 dgA immunotoxin is being evaluated in phase II clinical studies in lymphoma patients.

The side effects observed with administration of immunotoxins are different from those of conventional chemotherapy; immunotoxins do not exert cytotoxic effects against normal rapidly dividing cells. Immunotoxins such as the bacterial toxins, *Pseudomonas exotoxin* and diptheria toxin, induce hepatotoxicity, whereas the ricin-based immunotoxins cause reversible vascular leak and myalgias [252]. Several groups of researchers are currently working on second- and third-generation immunotoxins to eliminate the immunogenicity and side effects of the first generation immunotoxins. Continued refinement in design of these pharmaceuticals may eventually prove useful in the treatment of cancer.

Monoclonal antibodies and radioimmunotherapy

The use of MAbs to deliver radioisotopes for treatment of certain cancers has yielded some encouraging results [81, 105, 106]. Some of the most promising of these results radioimmunoconjugates in bone marrow transplantation. In the treatment of leukemia, radioiodine-MAb conjugates ablate marrow safely, delivering up to fourfold more radiation to the marrow than to other normal tissues. Responses have been less frequent in solid tumors treated with radioimmunoconjugates in clinical trials [143, 144]. Objective tumor regressions, however, were seen in four patients with non-bulky disease who were treated with rhenium-186-labeled Mab NR-LU-10 [102]. Because of their size and high molecular weight, diffusion of MAbs within bulky tumors can be a problem, as illustrated by the results of a clinical trial that used radiolabeled anti-CD20 and anti-CD21 MAbs to treat patients with B-cell lymphomas [186, 202]. Among the most promising approaches to overcoming this problem is the use of genetically engineered, low molecular weight $F(ab')_2$, Fab and single-chain Fv fragments that may diffuse better at tumor sites. Early results of clinical trials employing humanized MAbs appear encouraging. In addition to reduced immunogenicity, $F(ab')_2$, Fab and Fvs, with their improved ability to penetrate tumors, may prove useful carriers for radiotherapy. Newer regimens combining radioantibody-based therapy with other treatment modalities may prove even more effective.

Chimeric proteins

One interesting aspect of recombinant DNA technology is the potential for producing of new proteins with novel properties. For example, the hybrid proteins formed by fusion of two or more genes (chimera) offer several advantages in terms of their stability, affinity, efficacy and pharmacology over the individual component proteins. A chimera protein formed by fusion of the IFN-γ and LT genes was shown to have better antiproliferative activity than IFN-γ or LT alone [51]. Similarly, PIXY321, a genetically engineered hybrid of the GM-CSF and IL-3 proteins exhibits greater colony-stimulating effects *in vitro* than the combination of GM-CSF and IL-3 [35]. In preclinical studies, PIXY321 has been shown to accelerate both neutrophil and platelet recovery in rhesus monkeys subjected to sublethal irradiation [259]. Because of the preclinical bservations, PIXY321 was tested in patients for its ability to ameliorate disease- or treatment-related bone-marrow suppression. The clinical results were encouraging and suggested that the hybrid protein elicits the biological effects of both its component cytokines [18, 245, 246, 247]. Thus, PIXY321 became the first recombinant fusion of two hematopoietins to enter the clinic. Early clinical experience has shown great potential in the prevention and treatment of hematopoietic sppression. The other recombinant fusion proteins have been made, including chimeric toxins constructed by fusion of genes encoding human cytokines and *Pseudomonas exotoxin* [24, 38, 224]. For example, IL-4-PE, a chimera of human IL-4 and *Pseudomonas exotoxin* proteins, is highly potent against many cancer cells [38], suggesting that it might be useful in the therapy of many cancers.

Generation of homologues and analogues of natural biotherapeutic proteins is another potentially important application of recombinant DNA technology. The technology involves alteration or deletion of key nucleotide sequences in the gene that will result in the modification of only a few amino acid sequences in the resultant protein, compared with the natural protein. Synthesis of novel human TNF-α, IFN-α and IFN-γ homologues has already been reported [6, 168]. All three of these homologues are distinct from their parent protein. Prolonged activity of insulin has been achieved by various substitutions that increase the isoelectric point. The prolonged activity seems to occur because the novel homologues precipitate when they encounter the neutral pH of the body [141]. These examples indicate an interesting way by which protein modifications can be exploited for therapeutic potential.

Furthermore, the ability afforded by newer techniques in recombinant DNA technology such as 'phage display' to correlate protein structure and function in a systematic way makes it possible to design novel drugs [27, 36, 137]. Such a technique could be used to design or even select a small peptide that binds to the receptor with the same affinity as the larger protein. And then, using computer modeling to display the molecular contacts between ligand and receptor, small nonprotein molecules that make the same contacts could be designed and synthesized. The end product would be a small organic molecule that could be produced more cheaply than the recombinant protein, yet would retain the full biological activity of the protein hormone. What's more, such molecules could be administered orally, eliminating the major disadvantage of most recombinant protein therapeutics, which must be delivered directly into the blood stream by injection.

Cancer vaccines

The issue of genetically engineered vaccines for cancer treatment will be discussed in detail in another part of this book. We will, therefore, focus in this section only on the novel aspects of vaccines that may have some potential as cancer therapeutics. The function of a vaccine is to give the immune system a boost, thus helping it recognize and destroy the 'non-self' antigens on the surface of cancer cells. Though the idea of inciting the immune system to fight cancer has been around for a long time, recent developments in biotechnology and better understanding of the immune-system network have caused an explosion of research and development in the field of cancer vaccines. Table 7 lists some cancer vaccines that are currently undergoing clinical trial.

Prior to the advent of recombinant DNA technology, two types of vaccines were used, inactivated vaccines (chemically killed derivatives of actual infectious agents) and attenuated vaccines (actual infectious organisms altered so that they do not multiply). However, these types of vaccines are potentially dangerous, as they can carry over the infectious contaminations. For example, a small number of children each year contract polio from their polio vaccinations. Thus, one of the most promising applications of recombinant DNA technology is the production of subunit vaccines, consisting solely of the surface protein to which the immune system responds and thus eliminating the risk of infection [17]. The arrival of

Table 7. Cancer vaccines under clinical trials

Immunogen	Target cancer	Reference
Recombinant vaccinia encoding for CEA	Colorectal, lung, breast	117
Gene therapy using patient's own cells	Renal cell, carcinoma, melanoma prostate, colorectal	32, 117, 226
Recombinant poxvirus encoding for MAGE antigen	Melanoma	249
Heat Shock Protein	Melanoma	126
Naked DNA	Lymphoma, cervical prostate, prostate, melanoma, renal, colorectal	126, 183, 269
Synthetic peptides	Melanoma, cervical	52, 175, 266
Synthetic antigens	Ovarian, breast, melanoma, colorectal	31, 126
Anti-idiotypic antibodies	Melanonoma, colorectal, gastric, ovarian	218, 231
Inactivated tumor cells with the cytokine IL-2	Colon	126
Recombinant antigens	Colorectal, lung prostate	45, 93, 218
Gene transfer	Melanoma	126

biotechnology in the late 1970s enabled targeting of specific cell-surface antigens, and monoclonal antibody technology permitted identification of tumor-associated antigens, their characterization and tissue distribution. The polymerase chain reaction (PCR) brought the technology of cloning and expressing gene products. These technologies jointly led to the development of the subunit vaccines of the 1990s.

The human melanoma antigen MAGE-1 was the first tumor-specific antigen identified [250]. Poxvirus containing the MAGE-1 gene is currently being evaluated as a candidate vaccine for treatment of melanoma and breast cancers in humans [126]. Similarly, the recombinant vaccinia virus containing carcinoembryonic antigen (CEA) is being evaluated for treatment of certain cancers. CEA is expressed on the surface of virtually all colorectal cancers, 70% of lung cancers, and 50% of breast cancers. Clinical results if these phase I trials of this vaccine in late-stage cancer patients were promising [117]. A recombinant fusion of a tumor-derived idiotype and GM-CSF, yielded a strongly immunogenic protein that was capable of inducing idiotype-specific antibodies and protected the recipient animals from challenge with an otherwise lethal dose of B-cell lymphoma [231]. These results can be applied not only to B-cell lymphoma but perhaps can be generalized to other classes of tumor antigens as well.

The discrete peptide fragments from certain tumor-specific oncoproteins (such as mutant p53 and the protein products of the *ras* and *HER-2/neu* genes) are rapidly progressing as potential vaccine candidates for cancer treatment [52, 266]. This strategy is based on the principle that intracellular proteins are degraded and presented back on the cell surface as small peptides in the groove of class I major histocompatibility complex (MHC) antigens. A nine amino acid peptide from the HER-2/neu oncoprotein was shown to be recognized by both breast and ovarian cytotoxic T lymphocytes, and this small peptide was able to induce a tumor-specific immune response [175]. It is now possible to isolate and custom synthesize tumor-specific immunogenic oncopeptides by using the patients's own mutation to prepare an autologous peptide vaccine that is selectively targeted to tumor cells containing the mutant gene product [266]. The ability of human oncopeptide vaccines to generate a peptide-specific $CD8^+$ cytotoxic T-lymphocyte response in animal models has formed the rationale for clinical trials of autologous peptide immunizations in patients with diverse epithelial malignancies (breast, lung, gastrointestinal) that are commonly accompanied by p53 and *ras* mutations [109]. It is likely that similar considerations will apply to other recently identified oncoproteins such as the product of the *BRCA*-1 gene in breast cancer.

Recently, there have been several attempts to generate tumor cell vaccines engineered to secrete various cytokines [29, 30, 100, 185]. The strategy seeks to alter the local immunologic environment of the tumor cell so as to enhance either the antigen presentation of tumor-specific antigens to the immune system or the activation of tumor-specific lymphocytes. Many cytokine genes have been introduced into tumor cells with varying effects on both tumorigenicity and immunogenicity. Some of these cytokines, when produced by tumor, induce a local inflammatory response that results in elimination of the injected tumor. The local inflammatory response is, in general, dependent on leukocytes other than classical T cells. Many cytokine genes have been introduced into tumor cells, including IL-1α, IL-2, IL-4, IL-5, IL-6, IL-7, IL-12, GM-CSF, IFN-α, IFN-γ and TNF-α [29, 169]. Preclinical data from various animal models suggest that tumor cells engineered to produce cytokines indeed provide a novel approach for tumor therapy [29, 170]. Clinical trials are currently in progress to assess the therapeutic efficacy of cytokine-transduced tumors as vaccines for the treatment of established solid tumors.

A remarkably straightforward and potentially useful approach in the field of cancer vaccines was recently developed. It involves the direct *in vivo* delivery of MHC-associated tumor antigens to provoke a tumor-directed immune response. This approach for treatment of diverse malignant diseases is currently under clinical investigation (Table 7). In essence, this approach is based on the ability of some viral and human 'naked DNA' genes to transfect certain cells without the need for elaborate genetic engineering maneuvers, sometimes using modified DNA/liposome complexes to deliver genes by direct injection at the tumor site or by systemic administration [183, 269]. For example, injection of naked DNA or mRNA transcripts encoding human CEA in mice has been shown to elicit strong cytotoxic T-lymphocytes and antibody responses against this antigen [31, 32]. The development of this simple and direct approach for *in vivo* gene therapy-based immunotherapy is an extremely important avenue for continued clinical and preclinical investigations.

Most tumor vaccines must be employed subsequent to the development of cancer. However, in some instances, for example, in those geographic areas in which human papilloma virus infection is highly endemic and thus rates of cervical carcinoma are high, it may be useful to vaccinate children prophylactically. Ultimately, as we discussed earlier in this chapter, development of multiple strategies that could be applied in synergy are most likely to yield beneficial results in cancer treatment and control. It remains to be seen what place the immunotherapy will have in this armamentarium. However, it is obvious that availability of recombinant DNA technology has made it possible to design vaccines on a molecular basis.

PROBLEMS UNIQUE TO RECOMBINANT BIOTHERAPEUTICS

The development of protein therapeutics by using recombinant DNA technology has presented many new and interesting challenges to pharmacologists and drug delivery scientists. Many of these biotherapeutics have multiple biological effects [4]; thus, an important priority in their development is the evaluation of their potency, pharmacological profile and toxic effects. One strategy to understand the potency and toxicity of anticancer agents is the use of appropriate animal models. However, many animal models that have been developed for testing conventional low molecular-weight drugs may not be useful for testing rDNA-derived therapeutic proteins. Species specificity of protein therapeutics further narrows down the choice for appropriate animal models. Certain *in vitro* biological properties of the interferons for example, did not translate to their efficacy in intact animals or in patients [220].

The lack of information on preclinical pharmacological behavior also limits a general analysis of the toxic effects of therapeutic proteins. For example, agents such as IFN-γ, IFN-α and IL-2 are produced in *E. coli* and are nonglycosylated. EPO, in contrast, is produced in Chinese hamster ovary cells and is glycosylated. Rats, dogs, hamsters and monkeys were used to study the toxicity of these agents. Comparison of results on gross morphology, histology, blood chemistry and hematology obtained from these studies demonstrated no general responses that might be attributed to the use of biotherapeutic proteins. The effects observed were primarily related to the known or anticipated biological effects of the agent and, as expected, occurred only in the species in which the agents were known to be biologically active.

Considering these results, it is apparent that toxicologic findings in animals essentially reflect the pharmacological effects of biotherapeutic agents. Therefore, the use of biotherapeutic agents in species in which they are active should be most informative. However, observations of the lack of toxic effects in other species may be important in addressing some concerns about nonspecific toxic effects. Cross-species activity may be seen for some if not all biological effects. For example, human IFN-α has pyrogenic activity in rabbits. Clearly, the pharmacological effects observed with materials that lack pronounced species specificity are likely to be more dependable, especially if different species have manifested the same toxicity profile. Similarly, human TNF was found to be less toxic in mice than in human subjects because one of the receptor subunits with which TNF interacts is species-specific and the other is not. In contrast, the pharmacological effects of agents like EPO are highly cell type and species specific.

There have been relatively few preclinical studies of the immunogenicity of recombinant therapeutic proteins. The useful information has come from the clinical studies. The generation of antibodies to proteins administered over long periods may result in formation of soluble immune complexes. These immune complexes can induce vascular and tissue injury, particularly glomerulonephritis [221]. As an alternative, immune complexes can elicit the release of inflammatory mediators from cells. However, to date there have been no examples of antibody responses to any recombinant therapeutic protein that have been shown to be attributable to pathologic effects.

Another potential problem that requires a mention is incorporation of the wrong amino acids when a high level of expression of recombinant proteins is enforced. Such errors are generally difficult to pinpoint, since current analytical methods for amino acid composition and sequence are not really amenable to detecting variations below 10% of the major constituents. It is conceivable that such altered sequences may resemble a toxic peptide or a protein with different biological functions. Also, the altered sequences in the protein may render them immunogenic and thus may provoke immunogenic responses.

Delivery of therapeutic proteins

The potential use of therapeutic proteins in medicine is severely limited because of their poor activity when administered orally. Proteins are rapidly degraded by proteolytic enzymes in the gastrointestinal tract and therefore have to be administered by injection. Moreover, proteins are generally characterized by short biological half-lives in the circulatory system, so that the repeated injections are generally needed. Even after intramuscular or subcutaneous administration, their bioavailability is often low because of their small size and the widespread distribution of proteolytic enzymes. In addition, most proteins pass through biological barriers rather poorly because of low diffusion and a low partition coefficient. These considerations have led to the development of different strategies to prolong the bioavailability of therapeutic proteins.

Conjugation of certain proteins to synthetic polymers can circumvent the problems of rapid clearance from the circulation, immunogenicity and instability. The general requirements of any polymer used for this purpose are that it be water-soluble, biocompatible, nonimmunogenic and devoid of biological activity. Zoladex® and Nafarelin®, the decapeptide agonists of luteinizing hormone releasing hormone (LHRH), have been formulated in slow-releasing polymer base and used effectively in clinical studies [61, 91]. Attempts have also been made to stabilize the proteins against degradation at the site of injection as well as in the circulation, but these studies are still preliminary in nature [124].

Covalent conjugation of certain proteins with water soluble polyethylene glycol (PEG) enhances their solubility and permits the design of stable formulations suitable for clinical use. This is particularly important for recombinant proteins produced in *E. coli* that are usually recovered as insoluble refractile bodies, and unlike many of their native counterparts, are not glycosylated. For example, conjugation of both IL-2 and IFN-β with PEG increased their solubility, and aqueous solutions were stable for long periods of time [111]. PEGylation of TNF-α alters its pharmacokinetics and reduces its *in vivo* toxicity [111]. G-CSF conjugated to PEG has a four times slower clearance rate in rats than unmodified G-CSF. In addition, PEG-G-CSF administration exerted a sustained biological effect on peripheral blood neutrophils [230]. PEGylated adenosine deaminase (ADA), an enzyme unrelated to cancer, is now approved for use as replacement therapy for severe combined immunodeficiency diseases that are due to inherited ADA deficiency. Patients who received PEG-ADA did not develop neutralizing antibodies to ADA activity [22].

The key factor with any drug delivery system is to achieve adequate concentrations of the drug at the desired sites while avoiding significant concentrations at sites that mediate toxic effects. Novel delivery systems such as liposomes may prove to be useful in achieving this. The ability of IFN-γ to stimulate the tumoricidal activity of monocytes was increased 1,000-fold by its encapsulation in liposomes [114]. Encapsulation of TNF-α in liposomes ameliorated the systemic toxicity of this cytokine in dogs [132]. Delivery can also be modified by a combination of the biotherapeutic protein with an antibody [43]. For example, the *in vivo* clearance of human IFN-α in rats is threefold slower when it is combined with a specific MAb [195]. However, it remains to be seen whether such delivery systems will confer any advantages to biotherapeutic proteins *in vivo* in terms of local delivery, reduced toxicity or altered pharmacokinetics.

CONCLUSIONS

It is clear that recombinant DNA technology has brought a revolution in the field of cancer therapeutics. The dream of biological therapy, thought to have a great potential for cancer, can now be realized. The ability to manufacture cancer drugs by using genetically engineered organisms has given rise to a novel biotechnology industry within the last decade that has earned as much as 10 billion dollars. The revolution has been not only in the industrial sector; but also in the academic sector. It has enabled scientists to discover new molecules, redesign molecules for lower toxicity and more efficacy, and investigate the pathology of disease at the molecular level. This technology, however, has given rise to new set problems in the area of drug manufacturing and delivery. One of the major problems in the manufacturing area is ensuring that the recombinant biological product is identical or very similar to the natural counterpart. Another problem is the rapid degradation of proteins in the circulation and their short circulating half-lives which restrict oral delivery of biotherapeutic proteins and may require continuous injection.

It is now possible to design from the crystal structures of the ligand and the receptor small molecules that can mimic these large proteins and thus may help to overcome delivery problems. Some of these problems might be circumvented by directly injecting the gene for a given protein: although this approach seems attractive, it also suffers from the delivery and organ/cell-specificity problems. Treatment with antisense DNA and RNA to inhibit the expression of oncogenes in tumor cells and the new technologies based on viral vectors for the delivery of vaccines and genes may find widespread application in the near future. Many of these approaches work effectively in the test tube, and the main challenge now is to translate these laboratory techniques into commercially viable processes.

ACKNOWLEDGEMENTS

The authors thank Ms. Katherine Hale for critical editorial review of this article. Research was supported in part by Clayton Foundation.

REFERENCES

1. Aggarwal BB, Gutterman JU eds. Human Cytokines: Handbook for Basic and Clinical Research, Boston (USA), *Blackwell Scientific Publications*, 1992.
2. Aggarwal BB, Pocsik E. Cytokines: From clone to clinic. *Arch Biochem Biophys* 1992; 292: 335-359.
3. Aggarwal BB, Puri R. Common and uncommon features of cytokines and cytokine receptors: an overview. In: Human Cytokines: Their Role in Disease and Therapy (Aggarwal BB, Puri R, eds), *Blackwell Science*, 1994: pp3-24.
4. Aggarwal BB, Puri R (eds). Human cytokines: Their role in disease and therapy. *Blackwell Science*, 1994
5. Ahuja SK, Murphy PM. Molecular piracy of mammalian interleukin-8 receptor type B by herpes virus saimiri. *J Biol Chem* 1993; 268: 20691-20694.
6. Alton K, Stabinsky Y, Richards R, et al. Production, characterization and biological effects of recombinant DNA derived human IFN-α and IFN-γ analogues. In: *The Biology of Interferon System* (De Maeyer E, Schellekens H, eds), Elsevier, North Holland 1983; pp119-127.
7. Ambrus JL, Pippin J, Joseph A, et al. Identification of a cDNA for a human high molecular weight B-cell growth factor. *Proc Natl Acad Sci USA* 1993; 90: 6330-6334.
8. Andus T, Gross V, Holstege A, et al. High concentrations of soluble tumor necrosis factor receptors in ascites. *Hepatology* 1992; 16: 749-755.
9. Apelgren LD, Zimmerman DL, Briggs SL, Bumol TF. Antitumor activity of the monoclonal antibody-vinca alkaloid immunoconjugate LY203725 in a nude mouse model of human ovarian cancer. *Cancer Res* 1990; 50: 3540-3544.
10. Arai K, Lee F, Miyajima A, et al. Cytokines: Coordinators of immune and inflammatory responses. *Annu Rev Biochem* 1990; 59: 783-836.
11. Arai N, Nomura D, Villaret D, et al. Complete nucleotide sequence of the chromosomal gene for human interleukin 4 and its expression. *J Immunol* 1989; 142: 274-282.
12. Bajorin DF, Cheung NKV, Houghton AN. Macrophage colony stimulating factor: biological effects and potential applications for cancer therapy. *Semin Hematol* 1991; 28: 42-48.
13. Batra JK, Kasprzyk PG, Bird RE, Pastan I, King RC. Recombinant anti-erbB2 immunotoxins containing *Pseudomonas exotoxin. Proc Natl Acad Sci USA* 1992; 89: 5867-5871.
14. Baynes RD, Reddy GK, Shih YJ, Skikne BS, Cook JD. Serum form of the erythropoietin receptor identified by a sequence-specific peptide. *Blood* 1993; 82: 2088-2095.
15. Brinkmann U, Pai LH, FitzGerald DH, Willingham MC, Pastan I. B3(Fv)-PE38KDEL, a single chain immunotoxin that causes complete regression of human carcinoma in mice. *Proc Natl Acad Sci USA* 1991; 88: 8616-8620.
16. Brinkmann U, Reiter Y, Jung SH, Lee B, Pastan I. A recombinant immunotoxin containing a disulfide-stabalized Fv fragment. *Proc Natl Acad Sci USA* 1993; 90: 7538-7542.
17. Brown F. From Jenner to genes-the new vaccines. *Lancet* 1990; 335: 587-590.
18. Broxmeyer HE, Benninger L, Cooper S, Huge N, Benjamin RS, Vadhan-Raj S. Effects of *in vivo* treatment with PIXY321 on proliferation kinetics of bone marrow and blood myeloid progenitor cells in patients with sarcoma. *Exp Hematol* 1995; 23: 335-340.
19. Campbell HD, Tucker WQJ, Hort Y, et al. Molecular cloning, nucleotide sequence, and expression of gene encoding human eosinophil differentiation factor (IL-5). *Proc Natl Acad Sci USA* 1987; 84: 6629-6633.
20. Cantell K, Hirvonen S, Mogensen KT, Pyhala L. Human leukocyte interferon: production, purification, stability, and animal experiments. *Monograph*. 1977; 3: 35-139.
21. Carter P, Presta L, Gorman CM, et al. Humanization of anti-p185^{HER2} antibody for human cancer therapy. *Proc Natl Acad Sci USA* 1992; 89: 4285-4289.
22. Chaffee S, Mary A, Stiehm ER, Girault D, Fischer A, Hershfield MS. IgG antibody response to ethylene glycol-modified adenosine deaminase in patients with ADA deficiency. *J Clin Invest* 1992; 89: 1643-1651.
23. Chari RVJ, Martell BA, Gross JL, et al. Immunoconjugates containing novel maytansinoids: promising anticancer drugs. *Cancer Res* 1992; 52: 127-131.
24.. Chaudhary VK, FitzGerald DJ, Adhaya S, Pastan I. Activity of a recombinant fusion protein between transforming growth factor-alpha and *Pseudomonas* toxin. *Proc Natl Acad Sci USA* 1987; 84: 4538-4542.
25. Chaudhary VK, Queen C, Junghans RP, Waldman TA, FitzGerald DJ, Pastan I. A recombinant immunotoxin consisting of two antibody variable domains fused to *Pseudomonas exotoxin*. *Nature* 1989; 339: 394-396.
26. Chong CF, Scuderi P, Grimes WJ, et al. Tumor tragets stimulate IL-2 activated killer cells to produce IFN-gamma and TNF. *J Immunol* 1989; 142: 2133-2139.
27. Clackson T, Hoogenbbom HR, Griffiths AD, Winter G. Making antibody fragments using phage display libraries. *Nature* 1991; 352: 624-628.
28. Clark BD, Collins KL, Gandy MS, Webb AC, Auron PE. Genomic sequence for human interleukin-1 beta gene. *Nucleic Acid Res* 1986; 14: 7897-7914.
29. Colombo MP, Forni G. Cytokine gene transfer in tumor inhibition and tumor therapy: where are we now? *Immunol Today* 1994; 15: 48-51.
30. Colombo MP, Modesti A, Parmiani G, Forni G. Local cytokine availability elicits tumor rejection and systemic immunity through granulocyte-T lymphocyte cross talk. *Cancer Res* 1992; 52: 4853-4857.
31. Conry RM, LoBugilio A, Wright M, et al. Characterization

of a messenger RNA polynucleotide vaccine vector. *Cancer Res* 1995; 55: 1397-1400.

32. Conry RM, LoBuglio AF, Kantor J, et al. Immune response to a carcinoembryonic antigen polynucleotide vaccine. *Cancer Res* 1994; 54: 1164-1168.
33. Coussens L, Yang-Feng TL, Liau YC, et al. Tyrosine kinase recptor with extensive homology to EGF receptor shares chromosomal location with *neu* oncogene. *Science* 1985; 230: 1132-1139.
34. Crawford J, Ozer H, Stoller R. Reduction by granulocyte colony stimulating factor of fever and neutropenia induced by chemotherapy in patients with small cell lung cancer. *N Engl J Med* 1991; 325: 164-170.
35. Curtis BM, Williams DE, Broxmeyer HE, et al. Enhanced hematopoietic activity of a human granulocyte/macrophage colony stimulating factor-interleukin-3 fusion protein. *Proc Natl Acad Sci USA* 1991; 88: 5809-5813.
36. Cwirla SE, Peters EA, Barrett RW, Dower WJ. Peptides on phage: a vast library of peptides for identifying ligands. *Proc Natl Acad Sci USA* 1990; 87: 6378-6382.
37. Daughaday WH, Rotwein P. Insulin-like growth factors I and II. Peptide, messenger ribonucleic acid and gene structures, serum, and tissue concentrations. *Endocr Rev* 1989; 10: 68-91.
38. Debinski W, Puri RK, Kreitman RJ, Pastan I. A wide range of human cancers express interleukin-4 receptors that can be targeted with chimeric toxin composed of IL-4 and *Pseudomonas exotoxin. J Biol Chem* 1993; 268: 14065-14070.
39. Derynck R. The physiology of transforming growth factor-b. *Adv Cancer Res* 1992; 58: 27-52.
40. Derynck R, Jarrett JA, Chen EY, et al. Human transforming growth factor-beta cDNA sequence and expression in tumor cell lines. *Nature* 1985; 316: 701-705.
41. Dinarello CA. The interleukin-1 family: 10 years of discovery. *FASEB* J 1994; 8: 1314-1325.
42. DiStefano PS, Johnson EM. Identification of a truncated form of nerve growth factor receptor. *Proc Natl Acad Sci USA* 1988; 85: 270-274.
43. Dorai H, McCartney JE, Hudziak RM, Tai M-S, Laminet AA, Houston LL, Huston JS, Oppermann H. Mammalian cell expression of a single chain Fv (sFv) antibody protein and their C-terminal fusions with interleukin-2 and other effector domains. *Biotechnology* 1995,12: 890-897.
44. Downing JR, Rousesel MF, Sherr CJ. Ligand and protein kinase C downmodulate the colony stimulating factor 1 receptor by independent mechanism. *Mol Cell Biol* 1989; 9: 2890-2896.
45. Dranoff G, Mulligan C. Gene transfer as cancer therapy. *Adv Immunol* 1995; 58: 417-454.
46. Edman JC, Halliwell RA, Valenzuela P, Goodman HM, Rutter WJ. Synthesis of hepatitis B surface and core antigens in *E. coli. Nature* 1981; 291: 503-506.
47. Edwards GM, DeFeo-Jones D, Tai JY, et al. Epidermal growth factor receptor binding is affected by structural determinants in the toxin domain of transforming growth factor-alpha-*Pseudomonas* exotoxin fusion protein. *Mol Cell Biol* 1989; 9: 2860-2867.
48. Eschbach JW, Egrie JC, Downing MR, Browne JK, Adamson JW. Correction of the anemia of end-stage renal disease with recombinant human erythropoietin. *N Engl J Med* 1987; 316: 73-78.
49. Estrov Z, Kurzrock R, Wetzler M, et al. Suppression of chronic myelogenous leukemia colony growth by IL-1 receptor antagonist and soluble IL-1 receptors: a novel application for inhibitors of IL-1 activity. *Blood* 1991; 78: 1476-1484.
50. Fantes KH, Allen GJ. Specific activity of pure human interferons and a non-biological method for estimating the purity of highly purified interferon preparations. *Interferon Res* 1981; 1: 465-472.
51. Feng GS, Gray PW, Shepard HM, Taylor MW. Antiproliferative activity of a hybrid protein between interferon-γ and tumor necrosis factor-β. *Science* 1988; 241: 1501-1503.
52. Fenton RG, Taub DD, Kwak LW, Smith MR, Longo DL. Cytotoxic T cell response and *in vivo* protection against tumor cells harboring activated *ras* proto-oncogenes. *J Natl Cancer Inst* 1993; 85: 1294-1302.
53. Fernandez-Botran R. Soluble cytokine receptors: their role in immunoregulation. *FASEB* J 1191; 5: 2567-2574.
54. Fernadez-Borton R, Vitetta ES. A soluble, high affinity interleukin-4 binding protein is present in the biological fluids of mice. Proc Natl Acad Sci USA 1990; 87: 4202-4206.
55. FitzGerald DJ, Bjorn MJ, Ferris R, et al. Antitumor activity of an immunotoxin in nude mouse model of human ovarian cancer. *Cancer Res* 47: 1407-1410.
56. FitzGerald DJ, Pastan I. A recombinant immunotoxin consisting of two antibody variable domains fused to Pseudomonas exotoxin. *Nature* 1989; 339: 394-397.
57. Fletcher FA, Williams DE. Recent progress in the discovery and invention of novel hematopoietic cytokines. Crit Rev Oncol Hematol 1992; 13: 1-15.
58. Fujiwara K, Yoshino T, Miyake K, Ohara N, Akagi T. Expression of lymphocyte adhesion molecule (CD44) in malignant lymphomas. Relevance to primary site, histological subtype and clinical stage. *Acta Med Okayama* 1993; 47: 215-222.
59. Fukunaga R, Seto Y, Mizushima S, Nagata S. Three different mRNAs encoding human granulocyte colony-stimulating factor receptor. *Proc Natl Acad Sci USA* 1990; 87: 8702-8706.
60. Fulton RJ, Uhr JW, Vitetta ES. *In vivo* therapy of the BCL1 tumor: effect of immunotoxin valency and deglycosylation of the ricin A chain. *Cancer Res* 1988; 48; 2626-2631.
61. Furr BJA, Hutchinson FG. A biodegradable delivery system for peptides: preclinical experience with the gonadotropin-releasing hormone agonist Zoladex. *J Controlled Release* 1992; 21: 117-128.
62. Furukawa Y, Ohata M, Miura Y, Saito M. Interleukin-1 production by monocytic leukemia cells and its role in coagulation abnormalities. *Leuk Res* 1991; 15: 1133-1137.
63. Furutani Y, Notake M, Fukui T, et al. Complete nucleotide sequence of the gene for human interleukin-1 alpha. *Nucleic Acid Res* 1986; 143: 3167-3179.
64. Gabrilove J, Jakubowski A, Grous J, et al. Initial results of a study of rhG-CSF in cancer patients. *Exp Hematol* 1987; 15: 461-465.
65. Ganser A, Lindemann A, Seipelt G, et al. Clinical effects of recombinant interleukin-3. *Am J Clin Oncol* 1991; 14: 51-63.
66. Gatanaga T, Hwang C, Kohr W, et al. Purification and characterization of an inhibitor (soluble TNF receptor) for TNF and lymphotoxin obtained from the serum infiltrates of human cancer patients. *Proc Natl Acad Sci USA* 1990; 87: 8781-8784.

67. Ghetie MA, Vitetta ES. Recent developments in immunotoxin therapy. *Curr Opin Immunol* 1994; 6: 707-714.
68. Golumbek PT, Lazenby AJ, Levitsky HI, et al. Treatment of established renal cell cancer by tumor cells engineered to secrete interleukin-4. *Science* 1991; 254: 713-716.
69. Goodnough LT, Rudnick S, Price TH, et al. Increased preoperative collection of autologous blood with recombinant human erythropoietin therapy. *N Engl J Med* 1989; 321: 1163-1168.
70. Goodwin R, Friend D, Ziegler SF, et al. Cloning of the murine and human interleukin receptors: demonstration of a soluble form and homology to a new receptor superfamily. *Cell* 1990; 60: 941-951.
71. Goodwin RG, Lupton S, Schmierer A, et al. Human interleukin-7: molecular cloning and growth factor activity on human and murine B-lineage cells. *Proc Natl Acad Sci USA* 1989; 86: 302-306.
72. Gorman CM. Mammalian cell expression. *Curr Opin Biotech* 1990; 1: 36-43.
73. Gospodarowicz D. Fibroblast growth factor. *Crit Rev Oncog* 1989; 1: 1-26.
74. Gough NM, Gearing DP, King JA, et al. Molecular cloning and expression of the human homologue of the murine gene encoding myeloid leukemia inhibitory factor. *Proc Natl Acad Sci USA* 1988; 85: 2623-2627.
75. Grabstein KH, Eisenman J, Shanebeck K, et al. Cloning of a novel T cell growth factor that interacts with the β chain of the interleukin-2 receptor. *Science* 1994; 264: 965-968.
76. Gray A, Dull TJ, Ullrich A. Nucleotide sequence of epidermal growth factor cDNA predicts a 128,000-molecular weight protein precursor. *Nature* 1983; 303: 722-725.
77. Gray PW, Aggarwal BB, Benton C, et al. Cloning and expression of cDNA for human lymphotoxin, a lymphokine with tumor necrosis factor activity. *Nature* 1984; 312: 721-724.
78. Gray PW, Goeddel DV. Structure of the human immune interferon cDNA. *Nature* 1982; 298: 859-863.
79. Griffin JD, Rambaldi A, Vallenga E, Young DC, Ostapovicz D, Cannistra SA. Secretion of interleukin-1 by acute myeloblastic leukemia cells *in vitro* induces endothelial cells to secrete colony stimulating factors. *Blood* 1987; 70: 1218-1221
80. Griffin TW, Richardson C, Houston LL, LePage D, Bogden A, Raso V. Antitumor activity of intraperitoneal immunotoxins in a nude mouse model of human malignant mesothelioma. *Cancer Res* 1987; 47: 4266-4270.
81. Grossbard ML, Press OW, Appelbaum FR, Bernstein ID, Nadler LM. Monoclonal antibody-based therapies of leukemia and lymphoma. *Blood* 1992; 80: 863-878.
82. Gubler U, Chua AO, Schoenhaut DS, et al. Coexpression of two distinct genes is required to generate secreted, bioactive cytotoxic lymphocyte maturation factor. *Proc Natl Acad Sci USA* 1991; 88: 4143-4147.
83. Gunther N, Betzel C, Weber W. The secreted form of the epidermal growth factor receptor. *J Biol Chem* 1990; 265: 22082-22085.
84. Gutterman JU, Blumenshein GR, Alexanian R, et al. Leukocyte interferon-induced tumor regression in human metastatic breast cancer, multiple myeloma, and malignant lymphoma. *Ann Intern Med* 1980; 93: 399-406.
85. Gutterman JU, Fine S, Quesada J, et al. Recombinant leukocyte A interferon: pharmacokinetics, single-dose tolerance, and biological effects in cancer patients. *Ann Intern Med* 1982; 96: 549-556.
86. Gutterman JU. Cytokine therapeutics: lessons from interferon alpha. *Proc Natl Acad Sci USA* 1994; 91: 1198-1205.
87. Hall WA, Merill MJ, Walbridge S, Youle RJ. Epidermal growth factor receptors on ependymomas and other brain tumors. *J Neurosurg* 1990; 72: 641-646.
88. Han ZC, Caen JP. Cytokines acting on committed hematopoietic progenitors. *Clin Hematol* 1994; 7: 65-89.
89. Heaney ML, Golde DW. Soluble hormone receptors. *Blood* 1993; 82: 1945-1948.
90. Heldin C-H. Structural and functional studies on platelet derived growth factor. *EMBO* J 1992; 11: 4251-4259.
91. Heller J. Polymers for controlled parenteral delivery of peptides and proteins. *Adv Drug Deliv Rev* 1993; 10: 163-204.
92. Heller RA, Song K, Fan N, et al. The p70 tumor necrosis factor receptor mediates cytotoxicity. *Cell* 1992; 70: 47-56.
93. Hellstrom I, Hellstrom KE. Anti-idiotypic antibodies as tumor vaccines. In: *New Generation Vaccines* (Woodrow GC, Levine MM, eds), Marcel Dekker, Inc., New York 1990; pp863-870.
94. Hersch EM, Metch BS, Muggia FM, et al. Phase II studies of recombinant tumor necrosis factor alpha in patients with malignant disease: a summary of the Southwest Oncology Group experience. *J Immunother* 1991; 10: 426-431.
95. Hill ADK, Redmond HP, McCarthy J, Croke DT, Grace PA, Bouchier-Hayes D. Antineoplastic effects of granulocyte macrophage colony stimulating factor. *Br J Surg* 1992; 79: 459 (Abstr).
96. Hill ADK, Redmond HP, Croke DT, Grace PA, Bouchier-Hayes D. Cytokines in tumor therapy. *Br J Surg* 1992; 79: 990-997.
97. Hinman LM, Hamann PR, Wallace R, Menedez TA, Durr FE, Upeslacis J. Preparation and characterization of monoclonal antibody conjugates of the calicheamicins: a novel and potent family of antitumor antibiotics. *Cancer* Res 1993; 53: 3336-3342.
98. Hirano T, Yasukawa K, Harada H, et al. Complementary DNA for a novel human interleukin (BSF-2) that induces B-lymphocytes to produce immunoglobulin. *Nature* 1986; 324: 73-76.
99. Hitzeman RA, Chen CY, Hagie FE, Lugovoy JM, Singh A. Yeast: an alternative organism for foreign protein production. In: *Recombinant DNA Products* (Bollon, AP ed), CRC Press, 1983; pp 47-65.
100. Hock H, Dorsch M, Kunzendorf U, et al. Vaccination with tumor cells genetically engineered to produce different cytokines: effectivity not superior to a classical adjuvant. *Cancer Res* 1993; 53: 714-716.
101. Itoh N, Yonehara S, Ishii A, et al. The polypeptide encoded by the cDNA for the human cell surface antigen Fas can mediate apoptosis. *Cell* 1991; 66: 233-243.
102. Jacobs AJ, Fer M, Su FM, et al. A phase I trial of a Rhenium 186-labeled monclonal antibody administered intraperitoneal in ovarian carcinoma: toxicity and clinical response. *Obstet Gynecol* 1993; 82: 586-593.
103. Jacobs K, Shoemaker C, Rudersdorf R, et al. Isolation and characterization of genomic and cDNA clones of human erythropoietin. *Nature* 1985; 313: 806-810.
104. Jinno Y, Chaudhary VK, Kondo T, Adhya S, FitzGerald D, Pastan I. Mutational analysis of domain I of Pseudomonas exotoxin. *J Biol Chem* 1988; 263: 13203-13207.

105. Jurcic JC, Scheinberg DA, Houghton AN. Monoclonal antibody therapy of cancer. In: *Cancer Chemotherapy and Biological Response Modifiers Annual 14*, (Pinedo HM, Longo DL, Chabner BA, eds), Elsevier Medical Publishers, Amsterdam 1993; pp129-149.
106. Jurcic JG, Scheinberg DA. Recent developments in the radiotherapy of cancer. *Curr Opin Immunol* 1994; 6: 715-721.
107. Kalinkowich A, Engelmann H, Harpaz N, et al. Elevated serum levels of soluble tumor necrosis factor in patients with HIV infection. *Clin Exp Immunol* 1992; 89: 351-355.
108. Kaplan EH, Leslie WT. Cutaneous T-cell lymphomas. *Curr Opin Oncol* 1993; 5: 812.
109. Karp JE, Broder S. New directions in molecular medicine. *Cancer Res* 1994; 54: 653-665.
110. Katoh M, Yazaki Y, Sugimura T, Terada M. C-*erbB3* gene encodes secreted as well as transmembrane receptor tyrosine kinase. *Biochem Biophys Res Commun* 1993; 192: 1189-1197.
111. Katre NV. The conjugation of proteins with polyethylene glycol and other polymers: altering properties of proteins to enhance their therapeutic potential. *Adv Drug Deliv Rev* 1993; 10: 91-114.
112. Kawasaki ES, Ladner MB, Wang AM, et al. Molecular cloning of a complementary DNA encoding human macrophage-specific colony stimulating factor (CSF-1). *Science* 1985; 230: 291-296.
113. Klein B, Wijdenes J, Xang XG, et al. Murine anti-interleukin-6 monoclonal antibody therapy for a patient with plasma cell leukemia. *Blood* 1991; 78: 1198-1204
114. Koff WC, Paige C, Gutterman J, Fidler IJ. Efficient activation of human blood monocytes to a tumoricidal state by liposomes containing human recombinant gamma interferon. *Cancer Immunol Immunther* 1985; 19: 85-89.
115. Koppel GA. Recent advances with monoclonal antibody drug targeting for the treatment of human cancer. *Bioconjug Chem* 1990; 1: 13-23.
116. Kozak RW, Lorberboum GH, Jone L, et al. IL-2-PE40 prevents the development of tumors in mice injected with IL-2 receptor expressing EL4 transfectant tumor cells. J *Immunol* 1990; 145: 2766-2771.
117. Kreeger KY. Cancer immunotherapies: an old idea sparks new studies, industry interest. *The Scientist* 1995; 9: 1.
118. Kreitman RJ, Bailon P, Cahudhary VK, FitzGerald DJ, Pastan I. Recombinant immunotoxins containing anti-Tac(Fv) and derivatives of *Pseudomonas exotoxin* produce complete regression in mice of interleukin-2 receptor-expressing human carcinoma. *Blood* 1994; 83: 426-434.
119. Kreitman RJ, Chang CN, Hudson DV, Queen C, Bailon P, Pastan I. Anti-Tac(Fab)-PE40, a recombinant double chain immunotoxin which kills interleukin-2 receptor bearing cells and induces complete remission in an *in vivo* tumor model. *Int J Cancer* 1994; 57: 856-864.
120. Kreitman RJ, Chaudhary VK, Waldman T, Willingham MC, FitzGerald DJ, Pastan I. The recombinant immunotoxin anti-Tac (Fv)-Pseudomonas exotoxin 40 is cytotoxic towards peripheral blood malignant cells from patients with adult T cell leukemia. *Proc Natl Acad Sci USA* 1990; 87: 8291-829
121. Kreitman RJ, Hansen HJ, Jones AL, FitzGerald D, Goldenberg DM, Pastan I. Pseudomonas exotoxin-based immunotoxin containing the antibody LL2 or LL2 Fab' induce regression of subcutaneous human B-cell lymphoma in mice. *Cancer Res* 1993; 53: 819-825.
122. Lachman LB, Dinarello CA, Llansa LD, Fidler IJ. Natural and recombinant human interleukin-1 is cytotoxic for human melanoma cells. *J Immunol* 1986; 136: 3098-3102.
123. Layton MJ, Cross BA, Metcalf D, Ward LD, Simpson RJ, Nicola NA. A major binding-protein for human leukemia inhibitory factor in normal mouse serum: identification as a soluble form of the cellular receptor. *Proc Natl Acad Sci USA* 1992; 89: 8616-8620.
124. Lee VHL. Peptide and protein drug delivery: opportunities and challenges. *Pharm Int* 1986; 208-212.
125. Leitzel K, Teramoto Y, Sampson E, et al. Elevated soluble c-erb-2 antigen levels in the serum and effusions of a proportion of a breast cancer patients. *J Clin Oncol* 1992; 10: 1436-1443.
126. Lewis R. End of century marks dawn of clinical trial era for cancer vaccines. *The Scientist* 1995; 9: 15.
127. Lewis GD, Figari L, Fendly B, Carter P, Gorman C, Shepard M. Differential responses of human tumor cell lines to anti-p185^{HER2} monoclonal antibodies. *Cancer Immunol Immunother* 1993; 37: 255-263.
128. Lewko WM, Smith TL, Bowman DJ, Good RW, Oldham RK. Interleukin-15 and the growth of tumor derived activated T cells. *Cancer Biother* 1995; 10: 13-16.
129. Lienard D, Ewalenko P, Delmotte JJ, et al. High dose recombinant tumor necrosis factor alpha in combination with interferon gamma and melphalan in isolation perfusion of the limbs for melanoma and sarcoma. *J Clin Oncol* 1992; 10: 52-60.
130. Lim VS, DeGowin RL Zavala D, et al. Recombinant human erythropoietin treatment in pre-dialysis patients. *Ann Intern Med* 1989; 110: 108-118.
131. Lippman SM, Parkinson DR, Itri LM, et al. 13-Cis retinoic acid and interferon a-2a: effective combination therapy for advanced squamous cell carcinoma of the skin. *J Natl Cancer Inst* 1992; 84: 235-241.
132. Lodato RF, Feig B, Akimaru K, Soma GI, Klostergaard J. Hemodynamic evaluation of recombinant human tumor necrosis factor (TNF), TNF-$_{SAM2}$ and liposomal TNF$_{SAM2}$ in an anesthetized dog model. *J Immunother* 1995; 17: 19-29.
133. Lorberboum GH, FitzGerald DJ, Chaudhary VK, Adhya S, Pastan I. Cytotoxic activity of an interleukin 2-Pseudomonas exotoxin chimeric protein produced in *Escherichia coli*. *Proc Natl Acad Sci USA* 1988; 85: 1922-1926.
134. Lord MJ, Roberts LM, Robertus JD. Ricin: structure, mode of action, and some current applications. *FASEB J* 1994; 8: 201-208.
135. Lotze MT, Custer MC, Bolton ES, Wiebke EA, Kwakami Y, Rosenberg SA. Mechanisms of immunological anti-tumor activity: lessons from the laboratory and clinical application. *Hum Immunol* 1990; 28: 198-207.
136. Lotze MT, Matory YL, Rayner AA. Clinical effects and toxicity of interleukin-2 in patients with cancer. *Cancer* 1986; 58: 2764-2772.
137. Lowman HB, Bass S, Simpson S, Wells JA. Selecting high affinity binding proteins by monovalent phage display. *Biochemistry* 1991; 30: 10832-10838.
138. Luckow VA. Recombinant DNA *Technology and Applications* (Prokop A, Bajpai RK, Ho CS eds), 1991; pp97-152.
139. Luckow VA, Summers MD. Trends in the development of baculovirus expression vectors. *Biotechniques* 1988; 6: 47-55.
140. Malik N, Kallestad JC, Gunderson NL, et al. Molecular

cloning, sequence analysis, and functional expression of a novel growth regulator, oncostatin M. *Mol Cell Biol* 1989; 9: 2847-2853.

141. Markussen J, Diers I, Engesgaard A, et al. Soluble, prolonged acting insulin derivatives. II Degree of protraction and crystallizability of insulins substituted in positions A17, B8, B27 and B30. *Protein Eng* 1987; 1: 215-223.
142. McLaughlin P, Cabanillas, F, Hagemeister FB, et al. CHOP-Bleo plus interferon for stage IV low-grade lymphoma. *Ann Oncol* 1993; 4: 205-211.
143. Meredith RF, Khaxaeli MB, Lui T, et al. Dose fractionation of radiolabeled antibodies in patients with metastatic colon cancer. *J Nucl Med* 1992; 33: 1648-1653.
144. Meredith RF, Khazaeli MB, Plott WE, et al. Phase I trial of iodine-131 chimeric B72.3 (human IgG4) in metastatic colorectal cancer. *J Nucl Med* 1992; 33: 23-29.
145. Miller L. Current status of G-CSF in support of chemotherapy and radiotherapy. *Oncology* 1993; 7: 67-88.
146. Milstein C. Monoclonal antibodies (review). *Sci Am* 1980; 243: 66-74.
147 Minty A, Chalon P, Derocq JM, et al. Interleukin 13 is a new human lymphokine regulating inflammatory and immune responses. *Nature* 1993; 362: 248-250.
148. Morgan AC, Comezoglu FT, Manger R, Jarvis B, Abrams PJ, Sivam G. Immunoconjugates of a protein-synthesis-inhibiting drugs. In: Therapeutic Monoclonal Antibodies (Borrebaeck C, Larrick J, eds), Stockton Press, NY 1990: pp143-158.
149. Mosley B, Beckman MP, March CJ, et al. The murine interleukin-4 receptor: a molecular cloning and characterization of secreted and membrane-bound forms. *Cell* 1989; 59: 335-348.
150. Motoyshi K, Takaku F. Human monocytic colony stimulating factor, phase I/II clinical studies. In: *Hematopoietic Growth Factors in Clinical Applications*. (Metelsmann R, Hermann F, eds), Marcel Dekker, NY, 1990; pp 161-175.
151. Mukaida N, Shiroo M, Matsushima K. Genomic structure of the human monocyte-derived neutrophil chemotactic factor IL-8. *J Immunol* 1989; 143: 1366-1371.
152. Mule JJ, Smith CA, Rosenberg SA. Interleukin 4 (B cell stimulatory factor 1) can mediate the induction of lymphokine activated killer activity directed against fresh tumor cells. *J Exp Med* 1987; 166: 792-798.
153. Mullberg J, Schooltink H, Stoyan T, et al. The soluble interleukin-6 receptor is generated by shedding. *Europ J Immunol* 1993; 23: 473-480.
154. Nagao M, Masuda S, Abe S, Ueda M, Sasaki R. Production and ligand-binding characteristics of the soluble form of murine erythropoietin receptor. *Biochem Biophys Res Commun* 1992; 188: 888-897.
155. Nagata S, Tsuchiya M, Asano S, et al. Molecular cloning and expression of cDNA for human granulocyte colony-stimulating factor. Nature 1986; 319: 415-418.
156. Nakajima T, Yamamoto S, Cheng M, et al. Soluble interleukin-6 receptor is released from receptor-bearing cell lines *in vitro*. *Japan J Cancer Res* 1992; 83: 373-378.
157. Nakamura T, Nishizawa T, Hagiya M, et al. Molecular cloning and expression of human hepatocyte growth factor. *Nature* 1989; 342: 440-443.
158. Narazaki M, Yasukawa K, Saiton T, et al. Soluble form of IL-6 signal transducing receptor component gp130 in human serum processing a potential to inhibit signals through membrane anchored gp130. *Blood* 1993; 82: 1120-1126.
159. Nedwin GE, Jarrett-Nedwin J, Smith D, et al. Structure and chromosomal localization of the human lymphotoxin gene. *J Cell Biochem* 1985; 29: 171-182
160. Nedwin GE, Naylor SL, Sakaguchi AY, et al. Human lymphotoxin and tumor necrosis factor genes: structure, homology and chromosomal localization. *Nucleic Acid Res* 1985; 13: 6361-6371.
161. Nemunaitis J, Rabinowe SN, Singer JW, et al. Recombinant granulocyte-macrophage colony stimulating factor after autologous bone marrow transplantation for lymphoid cancer. *N Engl J Med* 1991; 324: 1773-1778.
162. Niskanen E. Hematopoietic growth factors in clinical hematology. *Ann Med* 1991; 23: 615-624.
163. Novick D, Cohen B, Rubinstein M. Soluble interferon-alpha receptor molecules are present in body fluids. *FEBS Lett* 1993; 314: 445-448.
164. Novick D, Engelmann H Rubinstein M, Wallach D. Soluble cytokine receptors are present in normal huamn urine. *J Exp Med* 1989; 170: 1409-1414.
165. Obreg K, Norheim I, Lind E. Treatment of malignant carcinoid tumors with human leukocyte interferon: long term results. *Cancer Treat Rev* 1986; 70: 1297-1304.
166. Oehm A, Behrmann I, Falk W, et al. Purification and molecular cloning of the APO-1 cell surface antigen, a member of the tumor necrosis factor/nerve growth factor receptor superfamily; sequence identity with the Fas antigen. *J Biol Chem* 1992; 267: 10932-10937.
167. Old LJ (ed). Tumor necrosis factor and related cytotoxins. *CIBA Foundation Symp*. 1987; vol 131.
168. Ostade XV, Vandenabeele P, Everaerdt B, et al. Human TNF mutants with selective activity on the p55 receptor. *Nature* 1993; 361: 266-269.
169. Ostrand-Rosenberg S. Tumor immunotherapy: the tumor cell as an antigen-presenting cell. *Curr Opin Immunol* 1994; 6: 722-727.
170. Pardoll D. Cancer Vaccines. *Immunol Today* 1993; 14: 310-316.
171. Pastan I, FitzGerald DJ. Recombinant toxins for cancer treatment. *Science* 1991; 254: 1173-1177.
172. Pastan I, Chaudhary V, FitzGerald DJ. Recombinant toxins as novel therapeutic agents. *Annu Rev Biochem* 1992; 61: 331-354.
173. Paul SR, Bennet F, Calvetti JA, et al. Molecular cloning of a cDNA encoding interleukin 11, a stromal cell-derived lymphpoietic and hematopoietic cytokine. *Proc Natl Acad Sci USA* 1990; 87: 7512-7516.
174. Pennica D, Nedwin GE, Hayflick JS, et al. Human tumor necrosis factor: precursor structure, expression and homology to lymphotoxin. *Nature* 1984; 312: 724-729.
175. Peoples GE, Goedegebuure PS, Smith R, Linehen DC, Yoshino I, Eberlein TJ. Breast and ovarian cancer-specific cytotoxic T lymphocytes recognize the same HER1/neu-derived peptide. *Proc Natl Acad Sci USA* 1995; 92: 432-436.
176. Pestka S. The human interferons-from protein purification and sequence to cloning and expression in bacteria: before, between and beyond. *Arch Biochem Biophys* 1983; 221: 1-37.
177. Pestka S. The purification and manufacture of human interferons. *Sci Am* 1983; 249: 36-43.
178. Pestka S, Langer JA, Zoom KC, Samuel CE. Interferons and their actions. *Annu Rev Biochem* 1987; 56: 727-777.

179. Petch L, Harris J, Raymond VW, Blasband A, Lee DC, Earp HS. A truncated secreted form of the epidermal growth factor receptor is encoded by an alternatively spliced transcript in normal rat tissue. *Mol Cell Biol* 1990; 10: 2973-2982.
180. Peters K, Vejlsgaard GL. Basal cell and squamous cell carcinoma and Kaposi's carcinoma. *Curr Opin Oncol* 1992; 4: 380-385.
181. Petersen BH, DeHerdt SV, Schneck DW, Bumol TF. The human immune response eto KS1/4-desacetylvinblastin (LY256787) and KS1/4-desacetylvinblastin hydrazide (LY203728) in single and multiple dose clinical studies. *Cancer Res* 1991; 51: 2286-2290.
182. Pietersz GA, McKenzie IFC. Antibody conjugates for the treatment of cancer. *Immunol Rev* 1992; 129: 57-80.
183. Plautz GE, Yang ZY, Wu BY, Gao X, Huang L, Nabel GJ. Immunotherapy of malignancy by *in vivo* gene transfer into tumors. *Proc Natl Acad Sci USA* 1993; 10: 4645-4649.
184. Pluckthun A. Antibodies from *Escherichia coli*. *Nature* 1990; 347: 497-498.
185. Porgador A, Tzehoval E, Katz A, et al. Interleukin 6 gene transfection into Lewis lung carcinoma tumor cells suppresses the malignant phenotype and confers immunotherapeutic competence against parental metastatic cell. *Cancer Res* 1992; 52: 3679-3686.
186. Press OW, Eary JF, Appelbaum FR, et al. Radiolabeled antibody therapy of B cell lymphoma with autologous bone marrow support. *New Engl J Med* 1993; 329: 1219-1224.
187. Quesada JR, Hersh E.M, Manning J, et al. Treatment of hairy cell leukemia with recombinant α-interferon. *Blood* 1986; 68: 493-497.
188. Ramakrishnam S, Bjorn MJ, Houston LL. Recombinat ricin A chain conjugated to monoclonal antibodies: improved tumor cell inhibition in the presence of lysosomotropic compounds. *Cancer Res* 1989; 49: 613-617
189. Renauld JC, Druez C, Kermouni A, et al. Expression cloning of the murine and human interleukin 9 receptor cDNAs. *Proc Natl Acad Sci USA* 1992; 89: 5690-5694.
190. Rinderknecht E, O'Connor BH, Rodriguez H. Natural human interferon gamma. *J Biol Chem* 1984; 259: 6790-6797.
191. Rosenberg SA. Immunotherapy and gene therapy of cancer. *Cancer Res* 1991; 51: 5074s-5079s.
192. Rosenberg SA, Lotze MT, Muul LM, et al. Observations on the systemic administration of autologous lymphokine activated killer cells and recombinant interleukin-2 of high dose IL-2 alone. *N Engl J Med* 1985; 313: 1485-1490.
193. Rosenberg SA, Lotze MT, Yang JC, et al. Combination therapy with interleukin-2 and alpha-interferon for treatment of patients with advanced cancer. *J Clin Oncol* 1989; 7: 1863-1874.
194. Rosenberg SA, Spiess P, Lafreniere RA. A new approach to the adoptive immunotherapy of cancer with tumor infiltrating lymphocytes. *Science* 1986; 233: 1318-1321.
195. Rosenblum MG, Unger BW, Gutterman JU, Hersh EM, David GS, Frincke JM. Modification of human leukocyte interferon pharmacology with a monoclonal antibody. *Cancer Res* 1985; 45: 2421-2424.
196. Ross C, Tingsgaard P, Jorgensen H, Vejlsgaard GL. Interferon treatment of cutaneous T-cell lymphoma. *Eur J Haematol* 1993; 51: 63-72.
197. Ramakrishnan S, Bjorn MJ, Houston LL. Recombinant ricin A chain conjugated to monoclonal antibodies: improved tumor cell inhibition in the presence of lysosomotropic compounds. *Cancer Res* 1989; 49: 613-617.
198. Sambrook J, Fritsch EF, Manatis T. Molecular Cloning: A Laboratory Manual. *Cold Spring Harbor Laboratory Press*, 1989; pp 5.30-5.90.
199. Sanderson CJ. The biological role of interleukin-5. *Int J Cell Cloning* 1990; 8 (suppl.1): 147-153.
200. Sasaki K, Chiba S, Mano H, Yazaki Y, Hirai H. Identification of a soluble GM-CSF binding-protein in the supernatant of a human choriocarcinoma cell line. *Biochem Biophys Res Commun* 1992; 183: 252-257.
201. Scambia G, Panici PB, Battaglia F, et al. Receptors for epidermal growth factor and steroid hormones in primary lyrangeal tumors. *Cancer* 1991; 67: 1347-1351.
202. Sceinberg DA, Straus DJ, Yeh SD, et al. A phase I toxicity, pharmacology, and dosimetery trial of monoclonal antibody OKB7 in patients with non-Hodgkin's lymphoma: effect of tumor burden and antigen expression. *J Clin Oncol* 1990; 8: 792-803.
203. Schiro R, Longoni D, Rossi V, et al. Suppression of juvenile chronic myelogenous leukemia colony growth by IL-1 receptor antagonist. *Blood* 1994; 83: 460-465.
204. Seigall CB, Xu YH, Cahudary VK, Adhya S, Fitzgerald D, Pastan I. Cytotoxic activities of a fusion protein compromised of TGF*a* and *Pseudomonas* exotoxin. *FASEB J* 1989; 3: 2647-2652
205. Sen GC, Lengyel P. The interferon system. *J Biol Chem* 1992; 267: 5017-5020.
206. Sharma S, Mehta S, Morgan J, Maizel A. Molecular cloning and expression of a human B-cell growth factor gene in *E. coli*. *Science* 1985; 235: 1489-1492.
207. Shoyab M, Plowman GD, McDonald VL, Bradley JG, Todaro GJ. Structure and function of human amphiregulin: a member of the epidermal growth factor family. *Science* 1989; 243: 1074-1076.
208. Siegall CB, FitzGerald DJ, Pastan I. Cytotoxicity of IL6-PE40 and derivatives on tumor cells expressing a range of interleukin 6 receptor levels. *J Biol Chem* 1990; 265: 16318-16323.
209. Siegall CB, FitzGerald DJ, Pastan I. Selective killing of IL6 receptor bearing myeloma cells using recombinant IL6-Pseudomonas toxin. *Curr Top Microbiol Immunol* 1990; 166: 63-69.
210. Siegall CB, Kreitman RJ, FitzGerald DJ, Pastan I. Antitumor effects of interleukin-6 Pseudoman exotoxin chimeric molecules against the human hepatocellular carcinoma. *Cancer Res* 1991; 51: 2831-2836.
211. Sims JE, Acres RB, Grubin CE, et al. Cloning of the interleukin-1 receptor from human T-cells. *Proc Natl Acad Sci USA* 1989; 86: 8946-8950.
212. Sims JE, March CJ, Cosman D, et al. cDNA expression cloning of the IL-1 receptor, a member of the immunoglobulin superfamily. *Science* 1988; 241: 585-589.
213. Skolnick AA. First immunotoxin therapy for many common solid tumors enters phase I clinical trial. *JAMA* 1993; 270: 2280.
214. Smalley RV, Andersen JW, Hawkins MJ, et al. Interferon alpha combined with cytotoxic chemotherapy for patients with non-Hodgkin's lymphoma. *N Engl J Med* 1992; 327: 1336-1341.
215. Smith CA, Davis T, Anderson D, et al. A receptor for

human tumor necrosis factor defines an unusual family of cellular and viral proteins. *Science* 1990; 248: 1019-102
216. Solal-Celigny P, Lepage E, Brousse N, et al. Recombinant interferon alfa-2b combined with a regimen containing doxorubicin in patients with advanced follicular lymphoma. *N Engl J Med* 1993; 329: 1608-1614.
217. Souza LM, Boone TC, Gabrilove J, et al. Recombinant human granulocyte colony-stimulating factor: effects on normal and leukemic myeloid cells. *Science* 1986; 232: 61-65.
218. Spitler LE. Cancer vaccines: the interferon analogy (editorial). *Cancer Biother* 1995; 10: 1-3.
219. Spriggs MK, Hruby DE, Maliszewski CR, et al. Vaccinia and cowpox viruses encode a novel secreted interleukin-1 binding protein. *Cell* 1992; 71: 145-152.
220. Stebbing N, Weck PK. Preclinical assessment of biological properties of recombinant DNA derived interferons. In: *Recombinant DNA Products*: insulin, interferon, and growth hormone (Bollon AP, ed), CRC Press, Boca Raton, FL 1984; pp75-114.
221. Stills HF, Bullock BC, Clarkson TB. Increased atherosclerosis and glomerulonephritis in cynomolgus monkeys given injections of BSA over an extended period of time. *J Pathol* 1983; 113: 222-234.
222. Strander H. Interferon treatment of human neoplasia. *Adv Cancer Res* 1986; 46: 1-265.
223. Strander H, Cantell K, Jakobsson PA, Nilsonn U, Soderberg G. Exogenous interferon therapy of osteogenic sarcoma. *Oerhop Scand* 1975; 45: 958-959.
224. Strom TB, Anderson PL, Rubin-Kelley VE, Williams DP, Kijokawa T, Murphy JR. Immunotoxins and cytotokine toxin fusion proteins. *Semin Immunol* 1990; 2: 467-479.
225. Suda T, Takahashi T, Golstein P, Nagata S. Molecular cloning and expression of the Fas ligand, a novel member of the tumor necrosis factor family. *Cell* 1993; 75: 1169-1178.
226. Suzuki H, Yasukawa K, Saito T, et al. Anti-human IL-6 receptor antibody inhibits human myeloma growth *in vivo*. *Eur J Immunol* 1992; 22: 1189-1193.
227. Takaki S, Tominaga A, Hitoshi Y, et al. Molecular cloning and expression of the murine interleukin-5 receptor. *EMBO J* 1990; 9: 4367-4374.
228. Talpaz M, Kantarjian HM, McCredie K, Trujillo JM, Keating MJ, Gutterman JU. Hematological remission and cytogenetic improvement induced by recombinant human interferon alpha in chronic myelogenous leukemia. *N Engl J Med* 1986; 314: 1065-1069.
229. Tanaguchi T, Ohno S, Fujii-Kuriyama Y, Murmatsu M. The nucleotide sequence of human fibroblast interferon cDNA. *Gene* 1980; 10: 11-15.
230. Tanaka H, Satake IR, Ishikawa M, Matsuki S, Asano K. Pharmacokinetics of recombinant human granulocyte colony stimulating factor conjugated to polyethylene glycol in rats. *Cancer Res* 1991; 51: 3710-3714.
231. Tao MH, Levy R. Idiotype/granulocyte-macrophage colony stimulating factor fusion protein as a vaccine for a B-cell lymphoma. *Nature* 1993; 362: 755-758.
232. Tartaglia LA, Goeddel DV. Two TNF receptors. *Immunol Today* 1992; 13: 151-153.
233. TeVelde AA, Huijbens RJF, DeVries JE, Figdor CG. Interleukin 4 inhibits secretion of IL-1, tumor necrosis factor and IL-6 by human monocytes. *Blood* 1990; 76: 1392-1398.
234. The International Chronic Granulomatous Disease Comparative Study Group. *N Engl J Med* 1991; 324: 509-516.
235. Tiesman J, Hart CE. Identification of a soluble receptor for platelet-derived growth factor in cell-conditioned medium and human plasma. *J Biol Chem* 1993; 268: 9621-9628.
236. Tong J, Gordon MS, Srour EF, et al. *In vivo* administration of recombinant human stem cell factor expands the number of hematopoietic stem cells. *Blood* 1993; 82: 784-791.
237. Trail PA, Willner D, Lasch SJ, et al. Cure of xenografted human carcinomas by BR96-doxorubicin conjugates. *Science* 1993; 261: 212-214.
238. Trauth BC, Klas C, Peters AMJ, et al. Monoclonal antibody-mediated tumor regression by induction of apoptosis. *Science* 1989; 245: 301-305.
239. Trillet-Lenoir V, Green J, Manegold C, et al. Recombinant granulocyte colony stimulating factor reduces the infectious complications of cytotoxic chemotherapy. *Eur J Cancer* 1993; 29A: 319-324.
240. Trinchieri G. Interleukin-12 and its role in generation of Th1 cells. *Immunol Today* 1993; 14: 335-338.
241. Truitt GA, Brunda MJ, Levitt D, Anderson TD, Sherman MI. The therapeutic activity in cancer of interleukin-2 in combination with other cytokines. *Current Surv* 1989; 8: 875-889.
243. Uckun FM, Evans WE, Forsyth CJ, et al. Biotherapy of B-cell precursor leukemia by targeting Geninstein to CD19-associated tyrosine kinases. *Science* 1995; 267: 886-891.
242. Uckun FM, Frankel A. The current status of immunotoxins: an overview of experimental and clinical studies as presented at the 3rd International Symposium on Immunotoxicins. *Leukemia* 1993; 7: 341-348.
244. Upton C, Mossman K, McFadden G. Encoding of a homolog of the IFN-gamma receptor by myxoma virus. *Science* 1992; 258: 1369-1372.
245. Vadhan-Raj S, Kudelka AP, Garrison L, et al. Effect of interleukin-1 on carboplatin-induced thrombocytopenia in patients with recurrent ovarian cancer. *J Clin Oncol* 1994; 12: 707-714.
246. Vadhan-Raj S, Papadopoulous NE, Burgess MA, et al. Effects of PIXY321, a GM-CSF/IL-3 fusion protein, on chemotherapy-induced multilineage myelosuppression in patients with sarcoma. *J Clin Oncol* 1994; 12: 715-724.
247. Vadhan-Raj S. PIXY321 (GM-CSF/IL-3 fusion protein) biology and early clinical development. *Stem Cells* 1994; 12: 253-261.
248. Valezuela P, Medina A, Rutter WJ, Ammerer G, Hall BD. Synthesis and assembly of hepatitis B virus surface antigen particles in yeast. *Nature* 1982; 298: 347-350.
249. Vallera DA. Immunotoxins: will their clinical promise be fulfilled? *Blood* 1994; 83: 309-314.
250. Van Der Bruggen P, Traversari C, Chomez P, et al. a gene encoding an antigen recognized by cytolytic T lymphocytes on a human melanoma. *Science* 1991; 254: 1643-1647.
251. Vieira P, deWaal Malefyt R, Dang W, et al. Isolation and expression of human cytokine synthesis inhibitory factor (CSIF/IL-10) cDNA clones: homology to Epstein Barr virus open reading frame BCRF1. *Proc Natl Acad Sci USA* 1991; 88: 1172-1176.
252. Vitetta ES, Thrope PE, Uhr JW. Immunotoxins: magic bullets or misguided missiles. *Immunol Today* 1993; 14: 252-259.
253 . Vitetta ES, Uhr JW. Monoclonal antibodies as agonists: an

expanded role for their use in cancer therapy. *Cancer Res* 1994; 54: 5301-5309.

254. Waldmann TA, Goldman CK, Bongiovanni KF, et al. Therapy of patients with human T-cell lymphotropic virus I-induced adult T cell leukemia with anti-Tac, a monoclonal antibody to the receptor for interleukin-2. *Blood* 1988; 72: 1805-1816.
255. Watson, J (ed). *Recombinant DNA in medicine and industry.* 1992; 453-471.
256. Weber J, Yang JC, Topalian SL, et al. Phase I trial of subcutaneous interleukin-6 in patients with advance malignancies. *J Clin Oncol* 1993; 11: 499-506.
257. Wetzel R, Heyneker HL, Goeddel DV, et al. Production of biologically active N- desacetylthymosin in *E. coli* through expression of a chemically synthesized gene. *Biochemistry* 1980; 19: 6096-6104.
258. Whetton AD. The biology and clinical potential of growth factors that regulate myeloid cell production. *Trends Pharmacol Sci* 1990; 11: 285-289.
259. Williams DE, Dunn JT, Park LS, FriedenEA, Seiler FR, Farese AM, Mac Vittie TJ. GM-CSF/IL-3 fusion protein promotes neutrophil and platelet recovery in sublethally irradiated rhesus monkeys. *Biotechnol Ther* 1993; 4: 17-29.
260. Williams DE, Eisenman J, Baird A, et al. Identification of a ligand for the c-kit protooncogene. *Cell* 1990; 63: 167-174.
261. Williams GT, Smith CA, Spooncer E, Dexter TM, Taylor DR. Hematopoietic colony stimulating factors promote cell survival by suppressing apoptosis. *Nature* 1990; 343: 76-79.
262. Winter G, Milstein C. Man-made antibodies. *Nature* 1991; 349: 293-299.
263. Wong GG, Witek J, Temple PA, et al. Human GM-CSF: molecular cloning and the complementary DNA and purification of the natural and recombinant proteins. *Science* 1985; 228: 810-815.
264. Xu F, Lupu R, Rodriguez GC, et al. Antibody induced growth inhibition is mediated through immunologically and functionally distinct epitopes on the extracellular domain of the *erb*B-2R gene product p185. *Int J Cancer* 1993; 53: 401-408.
265. Yang YC, Ciarletta AB, Temple PA, et al. Human IL-3 (multi-CSF): identification by expression cloning of a novel hematopoietic growth factor related to human IL-3. *Cell* 1986; 47: 3-10.
266. Yanuck M, Carbone DP, Pendleton CD, et al. A mutant p53 tumor suppressor protein is a target for peptide-induced CD8+ cytotoxic T cells. *Cancer Res* 1993; 53: 3257-3261.
267. Yin M, Gopal V, Banavali S, Gartside P, Preisler H. Effects of IL-1 receptor antagonist on acute myeloid leukemia. *Leukemia* 1992; 6: 898-901.
268. Young DC, Wagner K, Griffin JD. Constitutive expression of the granulocyte macrophage colony stimulating factor gene in acute myeloblastic leukemia. *J Clin Invest* 1987; 79: 100-106.
269. Zhu N, Leggitt D, Liu Y, Debs R. Systemic gene expression after intravenous DNA delivery into adult mice. *Science* 1993; 261: 209-211.

CURRENT CONCEPTS IN IMMUNOLOGY

ROBERT K. OLDHAM
Biological Therapy Institute Foundation, Franklin, Tennessee; and University of Missouri, Columbia, Missouri

The main function of the immune system is to protect the host from certain death due to numerous potential pathogens present in the environment. The development and maintenance of immunity is dependent on a complex and highly sophisticated defense organization functionally divided into the innate and adaptive immune systems.

Innate immunity provides the first line of defense against most pathogens. Phagocytes, including neutrophils and monocytes/macrophages, and natural killer cells are the most important cell types participating in this form of immunity. In addition, several soluble factors, including the complement cascade, lysozyme, and acute-phase reactants, reinforce the physical barriers that prevent most infectious organisms from penetrating the body. These factors also promote the activation of the inflammatory reaction that contains the injury caused by an invasive infectious agent. These cells and factors are able to accomplish this function because their activity does not depend on a prior encounter with the antigen in the microbial agent or tumor cells, and they lack the fine specificity of the cells and humoral factors of the adaptive immune system.

Specificity and memory are two cardinal features of the adaptive immune system. The main cellular components are the T and B lymphocytes. Each clone of these cell populations has an extraordinary and unique antigen specificity via the expression of genetically programmed antigen-specific receptors on the cell surface. The adaptive immune system has the ability to differentiate between foreign and self molecules and in this way most destructive reactions against the host's own tissues are prevented. When the immune system loses its capacity to differentiate self from nonself, autoimmunity develops.

The innate and adaptive systems communicate with each other directly by cell-cell interactions and through soluble mediators termed cytokines. For example, macrophages are important not only in innate immunity but also in specific immune responses since they can present the antigen and activate T and B cells. In turn, T cells regulate macrophages, B cells, and natural killer cell activity through the synthesis and release of cytokines. Some of the cytokines also behave as messengers that mediate the communication between cells of the immune system and other organs of the body, such as the central nervous and endocrine systems.

This chapter presents a summary of the structure and function of the immune system with emphasis in those areas relevant to the defense against tumors and to cancer biotherapy. The following sections will briefly describe the characteristics and functions of the major cells and mechanisms that control immune responses and the clinical methodologies for assessing the general state of immunocompetence.

CURRENT CONCEPTS OF IMMUNITY

All the major cells of the immune system, that is, monocytes/macrophages, B and T lymphocytes, natural killer cells, polymorphonuclear cells, etc., originate in the bone marrow from pluripotent stem cells [63]. Although the exact mechanisms and mediators involved are not completely understood, it is now accepted that stem cells under the influence of growth and differentiation factors such as erythropoietin, colony-stimulating factors, and interleukins differentiate into two main progenitors: stem cells that have the potential to originate erythrocytes, eosinophils, platelets, granulocytes and monocytes/macrophages (GEMM-CFC); and stem cells that are the precursors for mature lymphoid cells (L-CFU) [37, 47, 65, 86, 116, 119] (Fig. 1).

We now know many of the factors that induce proliferation of the committed stem cells. Most of these cytokines have been purified, sequenced, and are currently produced by recombinant techniques [37, 47, 65, 86, 116, 119, 146]. The availability of these recombinant cytokines has contributed significantly to defining and characterizing their biological activities (Fig. 1).

Four separate colony-stimulating factors (CSFs) have been recognized. They are interleukin 3 (IL-3; multi-CSF), granulocyte-macrophage colony-stimulating factor (GM-CSF), monocyte-colon-stimulating factor (M-CSF) and granulocyte-stimulating factor (G-CSF) [37, 119]. These factors, together with interleukin 1 (IL-1), interleukin 4 (IL-4), interleukin 5 (IL-5), and interleukin 6 (IL-6), are essential for the proliferation and differentiation of committed stem cells, such as GEMM-CFC, GM-CFC, and L-CFU. For example, IL-3 and GM-CSF are required to induce GEMM-CFC to differentiate into granulocyte/monocyte-colony forming cells (GM-CFC), while M-

R.K. Oldham (ed.), Principles of Cancer Biotherapy. 3rd ed., 78–92.

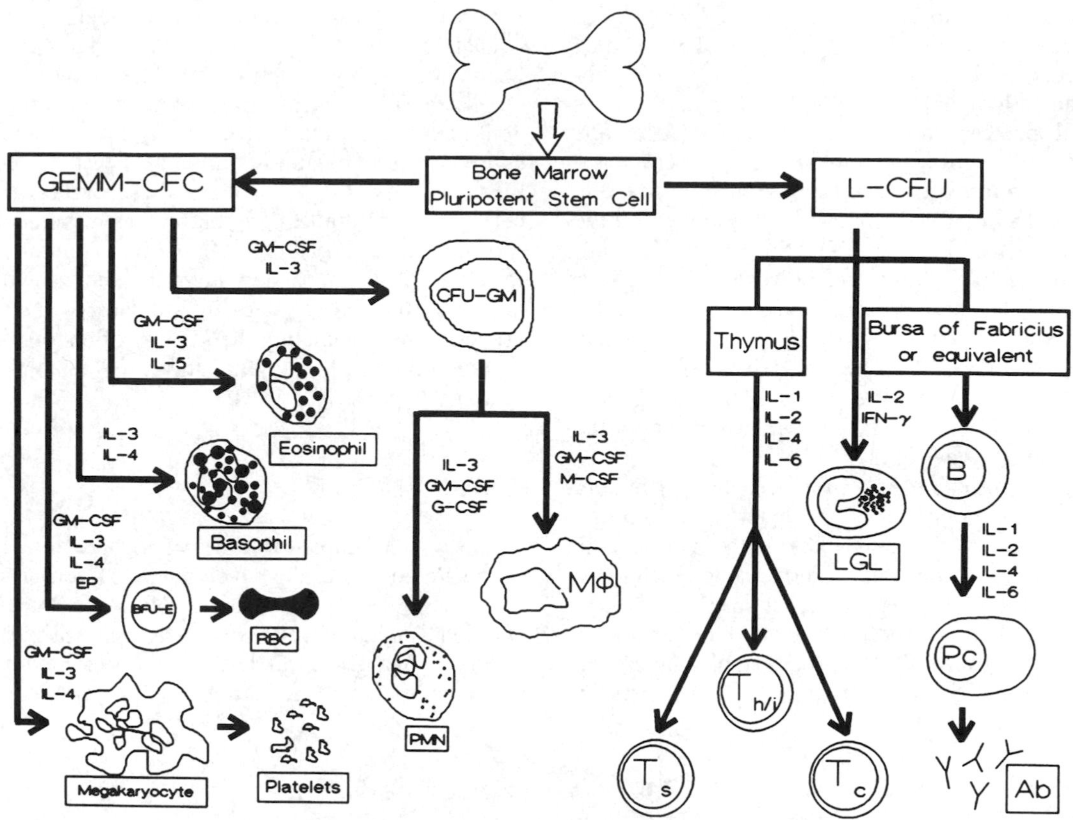

Figure 1. Origin of the cells of the immune system. All te cells of the immune system are derived from the multipotential stem cell in the bone marrow. Proliferation, maturation, and differentiation of the different cell lineages are driven by a multitude of cytokines. GEMM-CFC, granulocyte/erythroid/megakaryocyte/monocyte colony-forming cell; L-CFU, lymphocyte colony-forming unit; CFU-GM, granulocyte/monocyte colony-forming unit; B, B lymphocyte; $T_{h/i}$, T helper inducer; T_s, T suppressor, T_c, T cytotoxic; Mo, macrophage; LGL, large granulate lymphocyte; Pc, plasma cell; Ab, antibody; PMN, polymorphonuclear cell; EP, erythropoietin; BFU-E, burst-forming unit – erythroid; RBC, red blood cell; GM-CSF, granulocyte/monocyte colony-stimulating factor; G-CSF, granulocyte colony-stimulating factor; M-CSF, monocyte colony-stimulating factor; IL-1, interleukin 1; IL-2, interleukin 2; IL-3, interleukin 3; IL-4, interleukin 4; IL-6, interleukin 6; IFN-γ, interferon-γ.

CSF, GM-CSF, and IL-3 are necessary for GM-CFC to differentiate into precursors of the monocytic lineage (Fig. 1) [37, 86, 119]. Some of these cytokines act on targeted cell lineages; for example, IL-5 regulates eosinophilic maturation and B-cell activity while erythropoietin (EP) has its predominant effects on committed erythroid cells (B-CFU) (Fig. 1). Macrophages, activated T lymphocytes, fibroblasts, and endothelial cells are the major sources of GM-CSF, G-CSF, M-CSF, IL-1, IL-3, IL-5, and IL-6 [16, 37, 45, 47, 55, 65, 86, 98, 116, 119, 146].

Some of these cytokines (i.e., C-CSF, GM-CSF) are already approved for the treatment of patients with chronic severe neutropenia associated with cancer chemotherapy, AIDS, bone marrow transplantation, myelodysplasia, and aplastic anemia [27, 37]. Others, such as platelet growth activation factors are in clinical trials.

Lymphocyte-precursors originating from the L-CFU migrate to the thymus where they differentiate into mature T lymphocytes. This cell population is comprised of several subpopulation, including T helper/inducer ($T_{h/I}$) lymphocytes, which modulate the activity of virtually all other cell types of the immune system (Fig. 1), T-cytotoxic (T_c) lymphocytes, which are the effectors of the cytotoxic responses against tumors, foreign tissues, virus-infected cells, etc and T-suppressor (T_s) lymphocytes, which are involved in the down-regulation of the immune response. In addition to T lymphocytes, the bone marrow lymphocyte-precursor cells also give rise to natural killer cells (NK), which are involved in the defense against tumors, and B lymphocytes (B), which after maturing in the bursa of Fabricius (in birds) or bursa equivalent (bone marrow in humans), migrate to peripheral tissues, where in response to antigens they differentiate into antibody-producing plasma cells (Fig. 1).

Mature lymphoid cells circulate in blood, from where they populate peripheral lymphoid tissues, such as the paracortical areas of the lymph nodes and the periarteriolar sheaths of the spleen, the skin, and the mucosal linings of the digestive, respiratory, and genitourinary tracts. The migration of circulating B and T lymphocytes into specific lymphoid tissues appears to be governed by complementary adhesion molecules present on lymphocytes and on endothelial cells of high endothelial venules (HEV) and postcapillary venules (homing receptors, specialized adhesion molecules) [125, 141]. The expression of some specialized adhesion molecules by endothelial cells is induced by cytokines produced at the inflammatory sites. For example, the intracellular adhesion molecule 1 (ICAM-1), which serves as a receptor for the leukocyte-function-associated antigen-1 (LFA-1) molecule present on leukocytes [5, 22, 120], is induced by IL-1 in endothelial cells. The rapid increase in these surface proteins facilitates the adhesion of leukocytes to the endothelium, thus accelerating the initial stages of the inflammatory reaction (Fig. 2).

In addition to traffic to and from secondary lymphoid organs, a small number of lymphocytes travel through most non-lymphoid tissues of the body. This traffic pattern is designed to optimize the interaction of foreign antigens with the appropriate receptor specificities in T and B cells and to assure the fast development of a specific immune response. This process is also facilitated by migration of antigen presenting cells (APC) from the peripheral tissues to local lymph nodes [125]. Following cognative interaction (i.e., involving antigen and class II histocompatibility complex molecules) between APC and T cells and T-B cell cooperation, lymphocyte proliferation and maturation take place, with the generation and subsequent recirculation of antigen specific effector and memory cells (Fig. 3). During these events, lymphoid cells secrete a number of cytokines, such as transforming growth factor β (TGF-β), IL-1, IL-6, tumor necrosis factor α (TNF-α), and platelet-derived growth factor (PDGF), that affect the inflammatory and healing processes by modulating the activity of endothelial cells and fibroblasts, thus linking the inflammatory and the immune response (Fig. 2) [135].

T LYMPHOCYTES

T cells which comprise 70-80% of all circulating lymphocytes, are central to the development of normal immune responses. They play a critical role in cellular immune reactions, including delayed-type hypersensitivity (DTH), resistance against certain bacteria, viruses and tumor, and as effector cells mediating the rejection of organ

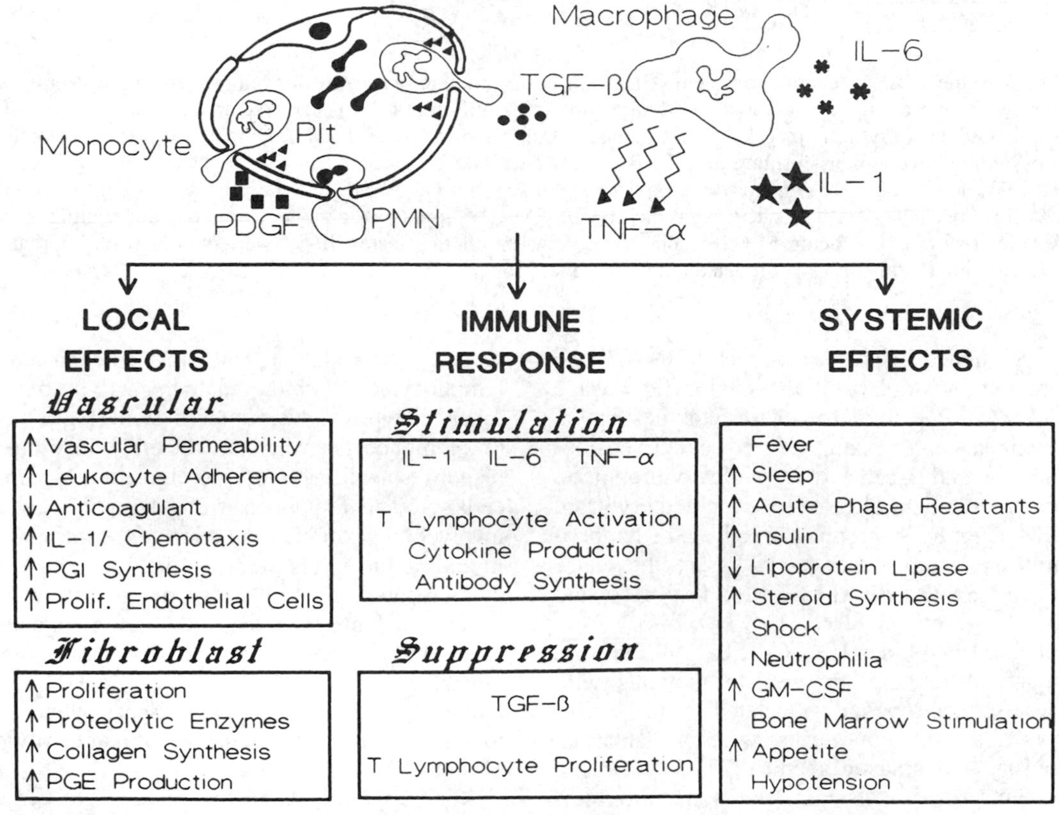

Figure 2. Cytokine participation in inflammatory and immune responses. Early mononuclear cell recruitment is induced by platelet-derived transforming growth factor β (TGF-β). Activated macrophages produce additional TGF-β and other cytokines, including interleukin 1 (IL-1), tumor necrosis factor α (TNF-α), and interleukin 6 (Il-6), that have local and systemic effects as well as effects on the immune response. PDGF, platelet-derived growth factor; PMN, polymorphonuclear cell; Plt, platelets.

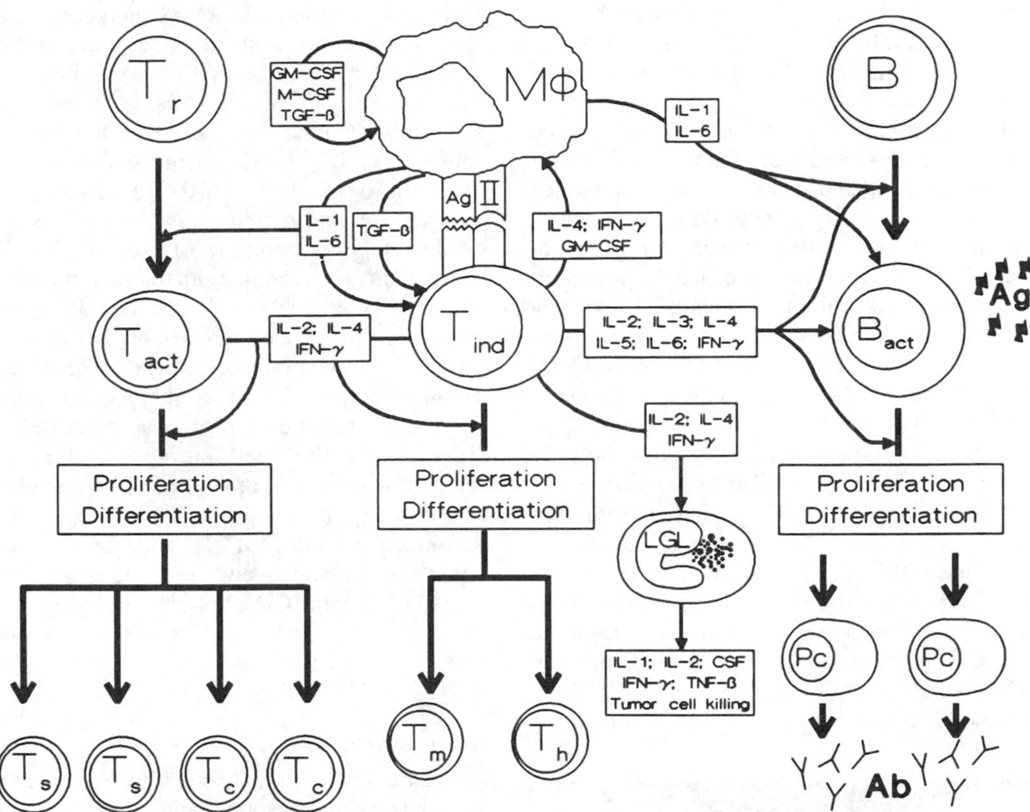

Figure 3. Simplified scheme of the lymphokine cascade and its role in the modulation of immune response. Various cytokines with unique and overlapping biological activities are produced during the immube response. These cytokines act in concert to tegulate the activation, profileration and maturation of cells participating in the specific and nonspecific arms of the immune system. Mo, macrophage; T_r, T activated lymphocyte, T_{ind}, T inducer; T_m, T memory; T_h, T helper; B B cell; T_s, T suppressor, T_c, T cytotoxic, Pc, plasma cell; LGL, large granular lymphocyte; IL-1, interleukin 1; IL-2, interleukin 2; IL-3, interleukin 3; IL-4, interleukin 4; IL-5, interleukin 5; IL-6, interleukin 6, CSF, colony-stimulating factor; TNF-β, tumor necrosis factor β/lymphotoxin; IFN-γ, interferon-γ, TGF-β, transforming growth factor β; GM-CSF, granulocyte/monocyte colony-stimulating factor; M-CSF, monocyte colony-stimulating factor; Ag, antigen; Ab, antobody; II, class II histocompatibility complex molecules.

transplants [2, 58]. T cells also have important regulatory function, due to their ability to produce cytokines that act on other T cells, B cells and macrophages, and by directly interacting with other lymphocytes [18, 72, 82, 122, 123, 127]. In general terms, the functions of T cells can be divided into regulatory and effector categories. The positive and negative regulatory functions are mediated by different lymphocyte subsets. The positive signals are associated with the helper/inducer subpopulation of T cells ($T_{h/I}$) and the negative with the suppressor T-cell subpopulations (T_s) [2, 19, 104, 114, 115, 136]. The effector category includes the cytotoxic (killer) T cells (T_c) reactive against virally infected cells and foreign histocompatibility antigens, and the sensitized $T_h(T_{DTH})$ cells, mediating delayed hypersensitivity reactions [23, 99, 100].

T cell subpopulations can be identified by immunofluorescence or flow cytometry with the use of specific monoclonal antibodies (mAb), which react with specific surface markers. Recently, an International Nomenclature Subcommittee examined a large number of mAb directed to leukocyte antigens and clustered them into groups of antibodies with the same reactivities (clusters of differentiation or CD), and a number was assigned to each group [49]. This nomenclature is now in widespread use. Helper/inducer T lymphocytes bear the CD4 marker, while cytotoxic/suppressor T cells are recognized by the presence of the CD8 marker [41 ,49, 104, 105]. Other mAb, which recognize the T3 portion of the T-cell antigen receptor complex (CD3), and others that recognize the receptor for sheep erythrocytes or E-rosette receptor (CD2), react with virtually all T cells and are widely used for the determination of total T-cell numbers [41, 49, 104, 105]. In human peripheral blood, there are twice as many CD4 as CD8, a proportion that is altered in many diseases including immunodeficiencies and cancer. Recently, two mAb, called 4B4 and 2H4, have been used to further divide the CD4+lymphocytes into helper-inducer (CDw29+) and suppressor-inducer (CD45+) $T_{h/I}$ subpopulations, respectively [74, 75]. Furthermore, the use of the Leu 15 mAb (which reacts with suppressor, but not cytotoxic T cells) in combination with CD8 mAb provides distinction of T-cytotoxic from T-suppressor lymphocyte subpopulations [61].

The T-cell antigen receptor (TCR) has been isolated and characterized [1, 12]. It is a disulfide-linked heterodimer composed of an α and β polypeptide chain, each containing a constant and a variable (antigen binding) region somewhat similar to the structure of immunoglobulins (Fig. 4). In a small number of T cells present in peripheral blood (0.5-10% T cells), thymus, epidermis, and gut epithelium, a different type of T-cell receptor consisting of two distinct polypeptide chains (γ and δ) has been recognized [101]. The majority of these cells do not express CD4 or CD8 on the cell surface and their functions are not completely understood, but they are believed to represent a mature functional lineage of lymphocytes that can be activated by triggering through the γ/δ receptor.

Both α/β and γ/δ receptors are non-covalently associated with the CD3 molecular complex, which is composed of at least four polypeptide chains, γ,δ,ε,and ζ one of which (the γ chain) has a long intracytoplasmic portion with several phosphorylation sites [12]. It is believed that the CD3 complex is involved in mediating signal transduction during the interaction of antigen with the specific binding site in the α/β receptor (Fig. 4) [12].

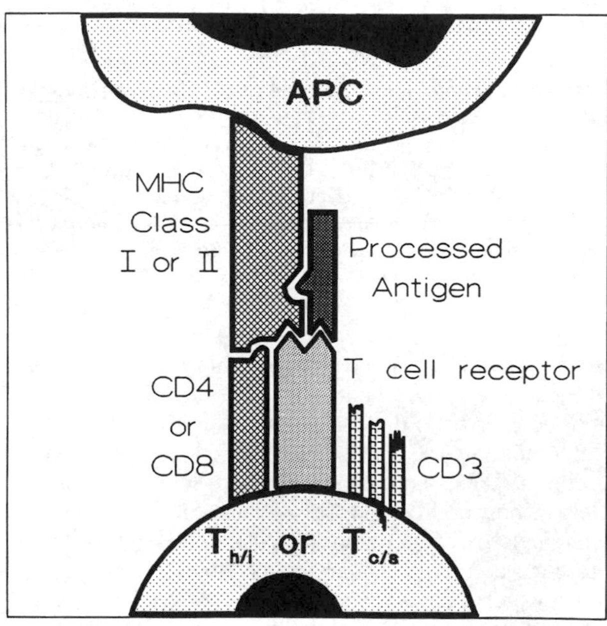

Figure 4. The current model for T-cell antigen recognition. Antigen-presenting cells (APC) incorporate, process, and express the modified antigen in conjunction with MHC molecules for presentation to T cells. The interaction of T helper ($T_{h/i}$) cells with APC is class II restricted, that is, it occurs when the antigen is presented to the $T_{h/i}$ cell together with class II molecules that interact with the T-cell receptor and CD4 molecules respectively. Class I restriction occurs between APC expressing class I and the T-cell receptor in $CD8_+$ ($T_{c/s}$) cells. In both cases the delivery of the transduction signal for cell activation appears mediated by the CD3 molecular complex.

Antigen recognition by T cells requires that the antigen be presented to the T cells in association with the appropriate major histocompatibility complex (MHC) molecules [32] (Fig. 4). T-helper cells recognize antigen in the context of class II MHC molecules expressed by antigen-presenting cells and B cells (class II restriction), while T-suppressor and most cytotoxic T cells recognize antigen in association with class I molecules (class I restriction). Recent work has demonstrated that CD4 molecules present on T cells bind with low affinity to certain invariable regions in the class II molecules. These findings support the theory that a complex involving the TCR α/β-CD3 and CD4 or CD8 molecules is formed on the surface of the T cells during antigen recognition (Fig. 4). In this situation, the specificity is determined by the variable region of the α/β receptor, the reaction is stabilized by binding of CD4 and CD8 to class II or Class I molecules, respectively, and the activation signal is transduced by the CD3 complex [69, 117].

T-HELPER CELLS

T-helper cells have been first described as the T lymphocyte subpopulation that 'helps' B lymphocytes mount an optimal antibody response and 'induces' the generation of cytotoxic T cells. These T cells recognize processed antigen presented by macrophages or other APC in the context of Class II (DR) products (Fig. 4). The induction of lymphoid cell proliferation upon stimulation by mitogens or antigens is characterized by two distinct phases: competence and progression. The activating signals (competence signals) cause the resting T cells to move from G_9 into the early G_1 phase of the cell cycle. During this 'competence stage,' binding of antigens to the TCR/CD3 (TCR complex) induces the generation of intracellular signals, such as increases in intracellular free calcium, membrane depolarization, generation of diacylglycerol (DG) and phosphatidyl inositol (PI) turnover, activation of protein kinase C (PKC), and changes in the levels of cAMP, cGMP, protein phosphorylation, and express of *c-fos, c-myc,* and other proto-oncogenes (13,102,103,118,121,137]. These events (some of which are triggered by IL-1) lead to the expression of specific genes [including interleukin 2 and IL-2 receptor (IL-2R)] critical for the progression phase [6, 137]. During the progression stage, binding of IL-2 to its high-affinity receptor is a critical event leading to passage of competent T cells from early G_1 through the other phases of the cell cycle, culminating in cell proliferation [6, 7, 29]. Other changes noted during activation are increased numbers of interleukin 1 receptors (IL-IR), de novo expression of Class II molecules, and acquisition of transferrin receptors (TR) to ensure incorporation of iron, since this element is essential for cell division [83].

The rate of T-cell proliferation is tightly regulated by

the transient expression of IL-2R and the limited production of IL-2. The high-affinity IL-2R (HA-IL-2R), a heterodimer consisting of an α chain (p55) associated with a β chain (p70), is rapidly internalized in the presence of the ligand and is widely recognized as the IL-2R species that mediates the biological responsiveness to IL-2 [20, 57, 106, 107, 129, 133, 138]. Small numbers of α-chain (MW 55 kD) molecules are normally expressed by resting CD4+ T cells. Normally, IL-2R expression lasts for about 1 week, and IL-2 production for 2 or 3 days.

Antigen-activated CD4 T-cells release a number of cytokines including IL-2, gamma-interferon (IFN-γ), colony-stimulating factors (CSFs), B-cell growth factors (IL-4, IL-5, IL-6), etc. [24, 38, 40, 48, 50, 53, 80, 81, 87, 95, 96, 128, 144] (Fig. 3). These cytokines, in turn, induce activation, proliferation and differentiation of other antigen-specific T and B cells resulting in a specific immune response and the production of memory T cells (Fig. 3).

Although no human counterparts have yet been described, there are two well-defined subpopulations of murine $T_{h/I}$ lymphocytes, termed TH1 and TH2 [76]. These subpopulations are characterized by the secretion of different sets of cytokines, leading to different functional properties [76]. Although some cytokines such as GM-CSF, TNF-α, and IL-3 are produced by both cell types, TH1 but not TH2 clones produce IL-2, γ-interferon, and lymphotoxin (TNF-β) [76]. In contrast, TH2 but not TH1 cells synthesize IL-4, IL-5 and IL-6. TH2 cells induce growth and immunoglobulin (Ig) secretion of B cells in response to specific antigens and polyclonal activators. These functions require not only IL-4 and IL-5 synthesis but also TH2-B cell-cell interactions. In addition, IL-4 is essential for IgE production, and IL-5 appears to play a role in B-cell hyperactivation observed in mice prone to develop a severe lupus-like auto-immune syndrome.

The function of TH1 cells has not been well defined yet, but they appear to be involved in proliferation (but no Ig synthesis) of B cells, induction of T-cell activity, and generation of cells participating in the late phase of delayed hypersensitivity reactions. It has been postulated that immune responses characterized by predominant activation of TH1 cells may result in strong induction of macrophage-mediated cytotoxic reactions induced by IFN-α and TNF-β and increased expression of Fc receptors for IgG2a in macrophages. Thus, these responses would result in effective killing of target cells with intracellular viral or parasite infections and strong DTH reactions. In contrast, activation of TH2 cells should lead to immune responses characterized by high levels of antibody production. Clearly many, if not all, normal immune responses probably involve the participation of both cell types [76].

T-SUPPRESSOR CELLS

T-suppressor cells suppress (down-regulate) T cell activity, antibody production by B cells, DTH, contact sensitivity, cytolytic T-cell function, proliferation of T cells, and immune responses against tumors [2, 19, 115]. The T_s cells are activated during normal responses to a variety of antigens, thereby providing a safety mechanism that continuously controls the magnitude of the immune response. Although T-suppressor cells are antigen-specific, they are also able to bind antigen in the absence of accessory cells or specific products of the MHC. T-suppressor cells appear to be selectively activated when the antigen is presented in certain routes, that is, intravenously or orally, or when administered in very low doses (low zone tolerance). T-cell induced suppression might be mediated directly by T_s cell or by antigen-specific and non-antigen-specific soluble factors released by them (TSF). It has been postulated that T_s factors consist of an antigen-binding portion and an I-J molecule (28kD) that binds to the acceptor cell through the antigen molecule and an I-J binding site [73]. Suppressor T cells inhibit tumor immunity in some experimental systems and might play an adverse role in human cancer [115].

T-CYTOTOXIC CELLS

T-cytotoxic cells were originally described as the effector cells of specific cell-mediated cytotoxicity against allografts, virus-infected cells, bacteria, tumor cells, etc. These cells are derived from a radiosensitive cell population. The T_c lymphocytes also interact with the antigen (most commonly a foreign cell, tumor cells, or virus-infected cells) through the T-cell receptor [58, 78]. The interaction of specific cytotoxic T cells with the target structure results in lysis of the latter. 'Killing' of a target cell, including tumor cells, consists of a number of mechanisms that can be divided in three phases [35, 36, 143]. Initially, binding between target and effector cells must take place. The majority of cytotoxic T cells are CD8+ and therefore recognize the antigen in the context of MHC 1 molecules (class I restriction) [32]. In addition, they can also recognize foreign class I antigens alone, indicating that they can be effective in the destruction of allogeneic transplanted tissues. A small percentage (10%) of cytotoxic T cells bearing the CD4+ phenotype recognize antigens in association with class II molecules and might play a role in lysis of virus-infected cells [36].

The second phase ('programming for lysis') involves the reorganization of cytoplasmic organelles, including polarization of the microtubule organizing center and tubulin and actin. This leads to an increased area of contact between the target and effector cells, leading to an increase in the efficiency of the cytolytic process. This is followed by reorientation of the cytoplasmic granules into the binding region, fusion to the membrane, and release of lytic molecules (perforins) contained in those granules.

The presence of Ca^{2+} is the limiting factor in this phase, since polymerization of the perforin molecules on the membrane of the target cell with channel formation does not occur in the presence of Ca^{2+} chelators [42, 43, 71, 78]. The granules also contain other factors known to mediate cytotoxic and cytostatic effects on tumor cells, such as estearases and proteoglycans [97]. The third phase includes the delivery of the lethal hit and death of the target cell. Following interaction with the cytotoxic T cell, disturbances in the ion concentrations and DNA fragmentation and blebbing occur, culminating in target-cell disintegration. Interestingly, cytolytic cells are resistant to the cytolytic mechanisms that they generate, and in this way each effector Tc may kill more than one target cell.

B LYMPHOCYTES

B cells are responsible for humoral immunity, and, like T cells, are present in peripheral blood where they represent about 10-20% of the circulating lymphocyte pool. After activation, B cells mature into specific antibody-secreting cells or plasma cells [52, 140, 145]. Mature B cells express surface immunoglobulins (Ig) with identical specificity to the antibodies (Ab) they secrete [140]. The majority of peripheral blood B cells express both IgM and IgD, while most B lymphocytes present in body tissues express IgG, IgA, and IgE. Most B cells also express Class II molecules in the cell membrane. These molecules participate during the physical cell-cell interaction that takes place during T-B cell cooperation. In addition, receptors for the Fc portion of IgG, the third component of complement (C3b), IL-2 and a number of markers (CD19,CD20,CD21,CD22, etc.) have also been found on the surface of mature B lymphocytes [52, 140, 145].

The process of activation and maturation of B lymphocytes into plasma cells involves the interaction of antigens with the specific immunoglobulins on the surface of B lymphocytes, which triggers cell activation and proliferation. The cooperation between B cells and $T_{h/I}$, macrophages, and other accessory cells, a process requiring identity of Class II products of the MHC among these cells, is necessary to induce optimal B lymphocyte responses. However, binding of antigen to B cells is necessary but not sufficient to initiate antibody production. Nonspecific maturation and differentiation factors (i.e., cytokines) mainly produced by $T_{h/I}$ cells are also involved in the activation and progression of mature B cells into antibody-forming cells [53, 140]. Among these factors are IL-1 (produced by macrophages and other accessory cells), IL-2, IL-4, IL-5, IL-6, IFN-γ and other factors secreted by activated T lymphocytes [17, 21, 24, 40, 45, 48, 53, 55, 81, 86, 87, 96, 98, 140]. Several of these cytokines, including IL-1 and IL-4 are also produced by B cells [21, 53]. Most of the circulating B lymphocytes are in the resting state (G_0 phase of the cell cycle), but they become activated after interaction with the specific antigen or antigen-presenting cells in the presence of IL-4 and IL-1, progressing to the G_1 phase of the cell cycle. Activated B cells, which express IL-2R after interaction with these ligands, undergo cell division in the presence of IL-2. Differentiation of proliferating B cells into plasma cells is mediated by IFN-γ, IL-4, IL-5 and IL-6 [24, 40, 2, 86, 87]. Alternatively, proliferating cells may return to the resting state and remain as memory B lymphocytes (Fig. 3).

During the maturation process, they not only increase their rate of Ig synthesis and actively secrete Ig, but they also switch the class of heavy chains that carry the variable region of Ig involved in antigen recognition [53, 140]. It has been demonstrated that a single clone of proliferating B cells may switch at any division. Not all the proliferating clones mature into secreting plasma cells. Some return to the resting state and remain as long-lived memory cells [140].

MONOCYTES AND MACROPHAGES

Monocytes are large cells (15-30 μm in diameter) that comprise about 20-30% of peripheral blood mononuclear cells (PBMC). They originate in the bone marrow from monoblasts, circulate in peripheral blood as monocytes, and then enter various tissues where they are termed resident tissue macrophages (Fig. 1). The large degree of heterogeneity that exists within the macrophage population is believed to represent different stages of the maturational process and environmental conditions at the tissue level, rather than distinct macrophage subpopulations [62]. Monocytes/macrophages can be identified by a number of methods, including morphology, ingestion of particles (such as latex), histochemical staining of cytoplasmic enzymes (such as nonspecific estearase), and by flow cytometry with a number of mAb that recognize markers present on their membrane (i.e., CD11, CD14, etc.) [49, 126]. A large number of receptors and surface molecules have also been identified on their cell surface, including receptors for the Fc portion of immunoglobulins (Fc receptors) and complement receptors.

Monocytes/macrophages play a critical role in the defense against bacterial and other infections by ingesting and killing the attacking microorganisms [62, 134]. They have also been shown to be very effective in destroying neoplastic cells and removing dead or injured cells (scavenger function). In addition, monocyte/macrophages are critical for the development of normal immune responses since they process and present antigen dendritic cells to T lymphocytes and secrete cytokines that play a major role in the initiation of specific immune responses, such as IL-1 and IL-6 [10, 11, 17, 21, 45, 55, 62, 98, 113, 130] (Fig. 3).

Monocytes/macrophages have been shown to secrete more than a hundred different molecules which mediate their functions. These products include (a) enzymes with bactericidal capacities, such as lysozyme and lysosomal hydrolases, neutral proteases (e.g., collagenase and plasminogen activator); (b) arachidonic acid metabolites (e.g., prostacyclin, prostaglandin E_2, and leukotrienes), which have profound effects in the regulation of the immune response; (c) reactive oxygen metabolites (e.g., superoxide, O_2 radical, and H_2O_2), which are important mediators in macrophage-mediated cytotoxicity; (d) complement components; (e) coagulation factors; and (f) cytokines, which in turn exert a multiplicity of regulatory actions including playing a critical role in antigen presentation to T cells [10, 11, 17, 21, 45, 55, 62, 98, 113, 130, 134] (Fig. 3).

Antigen-presenting cells, which include dendritic cells, Langerhans cells, veiled cells, interdigitating cells, and others in addition to macrophages, are characterized by their ability to process and present antigen to T cells in conjunction with MHC Class molecules, as well as cytokine production, resulting in T-cell activation. Macrophages incorporate antigens nonspecifically by phagocytosis or by binding of immune complexes to the Fc receptors. In contrast, activated B lymphocytes bind antigen via the specific antigen receptor, and dendritic cells are likely to process antigen directly in the cell membranes. These short peptides (8-24 amino acids) are then linked to the antigen cleft in the class II molecules and returned to the cell membrane for interaction with the $T_{h/s}$ cells [32] (Fig. 4).

NATURAL KILLER CELLS

Natural killer cells were first discovered by Oldham and co-workers [88]. Later studies defined their ability to bind and lyse sensitive tumor and virus-infected normal cells without the need of previous sensitization [31, 64, 92, 132]. These cells, which constitute approximately 15% of peripheral blood lymphocytes, are a relatively homogeneous cell type identified as large granular lymphocytes (LGL). LGL are nonphagocytic, express receptors for the Fc portion of IgG (FcR-positive), and have a high cytoplasm to nucleus ratio, indented nucleus, and a few discrete azurophilic granules in the cytoplasm [92, 132].

Several monoclonal antibodies have helped define the surface markers and the phenotype of natural killer cells. Some human NK cells express the following T-cell markers: E-receptors for sheep erythrocytes (CD2), CD8 (a marker present in suppressor/cytotoxic T cells), and after activation, they express T10 (a marker present in thymocytes and activated T cells) [49, 64, 92, 132].

NK cell function is regulated by stimulatory and inhibitory mechanisms. The generation and function of NK cells are regulated mainly by IFN-α, IFN-γ, IL-2 and IL-4 [64]. IL-2 and IFNs increase the lytic activity of mature NK cells, promote the recruitment and activation of nonlytic cells, and induce proliferation of precursors and mature cells either *in vivo* or *in vitro* [132]. In addition to their nonspecific cytotoxic activity against tumor cells, NK cells may exert a regulatory role in specific immune responses mediated by T and B cells because of their ability to produce a variety of cytokines including IFN-α and γ, IL-2, IL-1, CSF, and TNF-α [64, 92, 132].

Natural killer cell appear to play an important role in the resistance to growth and metastasis of malignant tumors [89]. Results obtained using several *in vivo* experimental models suggest that NK cells are of paramount importance during the early stages of tumor development. For example, NK-sensitive clones of tumor cell lines take longer to develop into palpable tumors when injected in the footpads of syngeneic hosts than NK-insensitive clones with similar doubling times [4, 39, 51]. Furthermore, selective depletion of natural killer cells in experimental animals has been correlated with increased frequency of spontaneous tumor metastasis.

LYMPHOKINE-ACTIVATED KILLER CELLS

The lymphokine-activated killer phenomenon (LAK) was originally defined as the ability of PBMC incubated for several days *in vitro* in the presence of IL-2 to lyse freshly isolated tumor cells and NK-resistant targets, such as the HL-60 cell line [33, 34, 84, 109, 111, 142]. The LAK phenomenon, which is not MHC restricted [93], can be mediated by cells expressing markers present in both T and NK cell populations. For example, the presence of cell populations with LAK activity expressing CD16 (Leu ll, an NK marker) and/or CD56 (Leu19, a marker present in both T_c and NK cells) has been reported in short-term cultures. Most of the LAK activity in long-term cultures stimulated with IL-2 and anti-CD3 was observed in the CD3+ CD16-; CD3- CD16+; CD3+ CD4- CD8-; CD16- and CD3- CD56+ cell populations. On the contrary, the CD3+ CD4+ or CD3+ CD8+ populations present in these cultures exhibited a significantly lower level of LAK activity [85].

Interleukin-2 mediated induction of LAK cells can be enhanced by the addition of IL-1α or -1β, probably by rendering LAK precursors more susceptible to the activity of IL-2 [14]. Interestingly, recent evidence indicates that the generation of LAK cells is dependent upon the expression of the p70/75 (intermediate affinity) IL-2 binding protein in the cell membrane. The expression of p70 occurs in the absence of the p55 (low affinity, Tac) IL-2 binding protein, which is critical for the expression of high-affinity IL-2R in activated T lymphocytes [94]. In addition to their remarkable tumoricidal activity, LAK cells are able to secrete IL-1α, IL-1β, IFN-γ, TNF-α, and TNF-β (lymphotoxin) [56].

Experiments in murine models have clearly established the *in vivo* antitumor activity of the cells mediating LAK activity (i.e., LAK cells) when administered in conjunction with high doses of IL-2 [59, 60, 77, 112]. Based on these observations, a number of clinical trials in advanced cancer patients have been completed [110, 139, 16].

CLINICAL ASSESSMENT OF IMMUNE COMPETENCE

In vivo

Delayed type hypersensitivity (DTH)

DTH is a test of cell-mediated immunity based on the response against a test antigen after it is injected intradermally, or applied topically to the skin (Table 1). Reddening and induration of the test site occur in 8-12h, reaches a peak at 48-72h, and thereafter slowly subsides. The DTH lesion is characterized by the accumulation of mononuclear cells in the subcutaneous and deep and superficial dermis [8]. It should be stressed that DTH reactions are complex immunological phenomena requiring the participation of effector T lymphocytes as well as monocytes/macrophages as accessory cells. Thus, a deficit of T cells or monocyte/macrophages, or the presence of certain serum inhibitory factors that impair T cell or monocyte/macrophage activity, or active suppressor cells, could lead to impaired DTH reactivity.

Antigens used in DTH testing can be divided into two classes: recall antigens and neoantigens (an antigen to which the subject has never been previously exposed). One of the most commonly used neoantigens is 2,4-dinitrochlorobenzene (DNCB), which has been used extensively in cancer patients. Among the recall antigens, tuberculin (PPD), mumps, tricophytin, and candida have been the most commonly used [8]. In general, several recall antigens are studied simultaneously to ensure that a patient will have been exposed to at least one or more of them. The interpretation of skin tests can vary widely between studies, since antigen concentration, reader variability, patient's prior exposure to the antigen, boosting effects of repeated antigen administration, time course of the reaction, and definition of a positive reaction are all variables that can influence the final assessment of a positive or negative response.

Of the available agents, only DNCB has been a consistently useful skin test agent. However, DNCB is an awkward reagent to employ, as repeated testing will clearly yield anamnestic responses. Thus, only the original test on an individual can provide clear information on the responsiveness to a neoantigen.

Table 1. Selected immunologic tests

Parameter	Test
T Cells	
Total and subpopulations	Flow cytometry
Responses to antigens	Cell proliferation elicited by PHA, Con A, MLR
	Delayed-type hypersensitivity
Cytokine production	Bioassays/RIA/ELISA
T-Receptor gene rearrangement	Southern blot analysis
Cytotoxicity	Release of radiolabeled compounds from target cells
B Cells	
Total number	Flow cytometry
Surface Ig	Flow cytometry
Ig gene rearrangements	Southern blot analysis
Serum immunoglobulins	Serum electrophoresis
Serum Ig classes	Nephelometry, RID
Reticuloendothelial system: monocytes, macrophages	
Cytokine production	Bioassays, RIA, ELISA
Phagocytosis	
Chemotaxis	
Tumor cell killing	Cytotoxicity *in vitro*
Activation	Production of oxygen radicals

HUMORAL IMMUNITY

The testing of the levels of total and different classes of Ig, as well as the primary or secondary antibody responses to a variety of antigens in the sera of cancer patients, has been used as an indication of the existence of alterations of immunoregulatory processes or of defects in the production of Ig. Quantitation of the levels of Ig is usually measured by the single radial immunodiffusion method or by nephelometry [67, 68]. Among the antigens used to elicit primary and secondary antibody responses are brucella endotoxin, salmonella extract, hemocyanin, etc. Antigens have been divided into T-cell dependent or T-cell-independent depending upon whether or not $T_{h/I}$ cells are required for maximal antibody production by B cells.

RETICULOENDOTHELIAL SYSTEM

The *in vivo* phagocytic cell function can be assessed by measuring the rate of clearance from the bloodstream after intravenous injection of a variety of materials including colloidal gold, bacterial proteases, lipid emulsions, or aggregated human albumin labeled with radioactive iodine [79, 124]. Another technique that has been used to study reticuloendothelial function is the Rebuck skin window. In this procedure, a microabrasion of the skin surface is made, followed by application of a cover slip to the raw area, and assessment of the accumulation of macrophages onto the coverslip [46].

In vitro

Immune cell quantitation

The accuracy in the quantitation of the levels of the different cells and cell subsets involved in the immune response has improved dramatically with the advent of the monoclonal antibody technology. It is possible to accurately estimate the numbers of monocytes/macrophages, $T_{h/I}$, T_c, and T_s lymphocytes, LGL, B lymphocytes, granulocytes, etc. with the use of flow cytometry using mAb that recognize specific markers in the surfaces of individual cell types [49].

Lymphoproliferative responses

This is one of the most widely applied tests for the determination of lymphocyte function. It is based on the property of lymphocytes to undergo blast transformation and proliferate in response to mitogenic or antigenic stimulation [66]. The most commonly used mitogens include phytohemagglutinin (PHA) and concanavalin A (Con A), which primarily stimulate T cells, and pokeweed mitogen (PWM), which stimulates both T and B cells. Whereas mitogens nonspecifically activate broad subpopulations of cells, antigens activate specifically sensitized antigen-reactive clones. The assay can be performed with whole blood but most laboratories usually first isolate PBMC (from whole blood, lymph nodes, or tumor specimens) by density-gradient fractionation on Ficoll-Hypaque followed by incubation with the appropriate mitogen at various concentrations. Seventy-two hours later cultures are pulsed with radiolabeled [^{3}H]thymidine, which is incorporated into the cellular DNA. Cells are then harvested and the radioactivity quantitated in a liquid scintillation counter and expressed as counts per minute (cpm). A similar technique has been extensively employed to measure proliferative responses to antigenic stimulation. In these studies, mitogen is replaced by the specific antigen under study and longer incubation periods are usually required [66]. Antigen responses are usually lower in magnitude that those observed with mitogens, since they represent the activation of specific T-cell clones, rather than most lymphocytes as is the case with mitogens.

Another proliferative response widely used is mixed leukocyte reaction (MLR). This test is based in the ability of T cells to proliferate in response to alloantigenic stimulation (that is cells expressing different MHC antigens). This is the *in vitro* correlate of *in vivo* graft rejection, and is usually performed by incubating PBMC obtained from the patient (responder cells) with irradiated PBMC obtained form one or more histoincompatible individuals (stimulator cells) for 6 days. Response is measured by [^{3}H]thymidine incorporation as described above [66].

Cytotoxicity

Cytotoxic reactions mediated by antigen-specific T cells, NK cells, antibody-dependent killer cells, lymphokine-activated killer cells (LAK), and activated macrophages are measured most commonly in microcytotoxicity assays [9, 30]. In general, target cells are labeled with a radioactive element able to bind to some intracytoplasmatic structure, which is released to the media when the cell dies. ^{51}Cr is the most popular label. Fixed numbers of labeled target cells are incubated in microtiter plates with different numbers of effector cells. The assays last for 4 or 18 h, after which the supernatants are collected and the radioactivity counted. The extent of radioactivity present in the supernatants is in direct relationship with the amount of killing. The results are expressed as percent cytotoxicity [9, 31].

Lymphokine production

As the roles of some of the soluble mediators in the immune response have become clearer, assays have been developed for their quantitation in the clinical setting [28]. For example, the measurement of IL-2 is based on (a) the fact that T lymphocytes produce IL-2 in response to mitogenic and antigenic stimulation and (b) the ability of IL-2 to induce lymphocyte proliferation and maintain *in vitro* T cell lines (called IL-2 dependent cell lines). The first step is the generation of cell culture supernatants containing IL-2 by incubating PBMC with mitogens (usually PHA or Con A) for 24-48 h. The IL-2 content in these supernatants is then determined by their ability to support the *in vitro* growth of an IL-2 dependent T-cell line, as assessed by [^{3}H]thymidine incorporation after 24-48 h of culture [30]. Most recently the concentrations of a variety of cytokines, including IL-1, IL-2, IL-4, IL-6, GM-CSF, TNF-α, IFN-γ, etc., are measured in tissue culture supernatants and serum using commercially available immunoassays [radioimmunoassay (RIA) and/or ELISA], which employ specific monoclonal antibodies.

Immunoglobulin production

Immunoglobulin production can be assessed *in vitro* by exposing a suitable effector cell population (e.g., PBMC) to either a polyclonal B-cell mitogen (e.g., PWM) or specific antigen and following a period of incubation, detecting the immunoglobulin produced. Secreted Ig can be detected either in the culture supernatants by using ELISA or radial immunodiffusion (RID) techniques, or the number of Ig-producing cells can be assessed using hemolytic plaque assays, in which red blood cells are coated with antigen against which the antibody generated reacts. In the presence of complement the red cells are lysed and the number of resulting 'plaques' can be easily determined [25].

Phagocytic cell function

Both mononuclear (e.g., monocytes/macrophages) and polymorphonuclear (PMN; e.g., granulocytes) leukocytes exhibit phagocytic activity. Well-established techniques exist for the assessment of monocyte phagocytosis, hemotaxis (motility), and response to lymphokines (e.g., migration inhibition factors, MIF) [25, 70, 108]. Established techniques also exist for the assessment of monocyte/macrophage cytotoxicity [54]. In general PBMC or peripheral monocytes/macrophages, isolated by adherence to plastic, are used as effector cells. Various tests are also available to measure PMN functions, including tests of phagocytic cell activity, bactericidal capacity, and the ability to take up and reduce nitroblue tetrazolium dye (NBT) [3]. Prior to the performance of the procedures, PMN must be separated from PBMC using density-gradient fractionation or elutriation.

Immunoregulatory cell functions

These assays are technically difficult to perform and are not usually part of the routine assessment of immune competence. Three broad classes of immunoregulatory cell assays have been utilized:

1. Coculture assays. In these assays effector cells (e.g., B cells, T cells) are exposed to a polyclonal activator (e.g., PWM, MLR) in the absence or presence of test cells. The test-cell population might induce either enhancement (e.g., increases in antibody production or enhanced MLR responses) or reduction (suppression) of the response of the effector cells [136].
2. Mitogen-induced suppressor T-cell activity. In this system suppressor cells are generated from resting T cells by exposing them to a polyclonal T-cell lectin such as Con A. Con A induced suppressor cells are then added in coculture to an effector-cell assay as described above [114].
3. Adherent suppressor cells. The presence of suppressor monocytes can be assessed by either a positive or negative effect. In the former situation, removal of adherent cells (e.g., monocytes) leads to augmentation of effector cell function (e.g., lymphoproliferative responses to mitogens), while in the latter case, readdition of adherent cells leads to suppression of the response [131].

Quality control of in vitro *assays*

In practice, it has been difficult to standardize lymphoproliferative or cytolytic assays to insure the universal validity and reproducibility of results. A number of conditions affect the comparability of *in vitro* assays as performed in different laboratories such as assay incubation time, presence or absence of physiological buffers and/or serum supplementation, choice of methodology to prepare the responder cell population (i.e., purified lymphocytes or unfractionated mononuclear cells), and the purity and/or concentrations of mitogen/antigen, or radioactive label.

In addition, various *in vivo* confounding variables, such as the influence of concurrently administered drugs, or seasonal and/or diurnal effects, provide further sources of assay variability. A number of procedures have been employed in an attempt to minimize interassay variability such as the use of cryopreserved reference lymphocyte preparations [44, 90] or indices based on results from a panel of reference lymphocytes [15]. Nevertheless, because of the inherent variability of *in vitro* assays, only limited successes have been achieved in clinical trials to date. Indeed, neither appropriate guidelines for interpreting the results of clinical trials employing immunorestorative agents nor statistically significant end points upon which to select appropriate sample sizes for such clinical trials currently exist [91].

ACKNOWLEDGMENT

Dr. Susana A. Serrate-Sztein (National Institutes of Health, Bethesda, Maryland) and Dr. Marcelo B. Sztein (University of Maryland School of Medicine, Baltimore, Maryland) contributed much of this chapter in the 2nd edition, but were unable to undertake the 3rd edition revisions.

I would especially like to acknowledge the assistance of Dr. Richard S. Schulof, who co-authored this chapter in the 2nd edition, but died in an accident during the preparation of the 3rd edition.

REFERENCES

1. Allison JP, Lanier LL. Structure, function and serology of the T-cell antigen receptor complex. *Annu Rev Immunol* 1987; 5: 503-540.
2. Asherson GL, Colizzi V, Zembala M. An overview of T-suppressor cell circuits. *Annu Rev Immunol* 1986; 4: 37-68.
3. Baehner RL, Boxer LA, Davis J. The biochemical basis of nitroblue tetrazolium reduction in normal human and chronic granulomatous disease polymorphonuclear leukocytes. *Blood* 1976; 48: 309-313.
4. Barlozzari T, Reynolds CW, Herberman RB. *In vivo* role of natural killer cells: involvement of large granular lymphocytes in the clearance of tumor cells in anti-asialo GM1-treated rats. *J Immunol* 1983; 131: 1024-1027.
5. Bevilacqua MP, Pober JS, Mendrick DL, Cotran RS, Jr. Identification of an inducible endothelial-leukocyte adhesion molecule. *Proc Natl Acad Sci USA* 1987; 84: 9238-9242.
6. Bich Thuy LT, Dukovich M, Peffer NJ, et al. Direct activation of human resting T cells by IL 2: The role of an Il 2 receptor distinct from the Tac protein. *J Immunol* 1987; 139: 1550-1556.
7. Bierer BE, Mentzer SJ, Greenstein JL, Burakoff SJ. The role of functional cell surface antigens in T cell activation. *Year Immunol* 1986; 2: 39-59.
8. Buckley, CE III (1986). Delayed hypersensitivity skin testing. In: Rose NR, Friedman H, Fahey JL, eds. *Manual of clinical laboratory immunology*. Washington, D.C.: American Society for Microbiology, 259-273.
9. Carpenter CB, Lymphocyte-mediated cytotoxicity. In: Rose NR, Friedman H, Fahey JL, eds. *Manual of clinical laboratory immunology*. Washington, D.C.: American Society of Microbiology, 304-307.
10. Ceuppens JL, Baroja ML, Lorre K, et al. Human T cell

activation with phytohemagglutinin. The function of IL-6 as an accessory signal. *J Immunol* 1988; 141: 3868-3874.
11. Chiu CP, Moulds C, Coffman RL, et al. Multiple biological activities are expressed by a mouse interleukin 6 cDNA clone isolated from bone marrow stromal cells. *Proc Natl Acad Sci USA* 1988; 85: 7099-7103.
12. Clevers H, Alarcon B, Wileman T, Terhorst C. The T cell receptor/CD3 complex: a dynamic protein ensemble. *Annu Rev Immunol* 1988; 6: 629-662.
13. Crabtree GR. Contingent genetic regulatory events in T lymphocyte activation. *Science* 1989; 243: 355-361.
14. Crump WL 3d, Own Schaub LB, Grimm EA. Synergy of human recombinant interleukin 1 with interleukin 2 in the generation of lymphokine-activated killer cells. *Cancer Res* 1989; 49: 149-153.
15. Dean JH, Connor R, Herberman RB, et al. The relative proliferation index as a more sensitive parameter for evaluating lymphoproliferative responses of cancer patients to mitogens and alloantigens. *Int J Cancer* 1977; 20: 359-370.
16. Dillman RO, Oldham RK, Tauer KW, et al. Continuous interleukin-2 and lymphokine activated killer cells for advanced cancer: an NBSG trial. *Journal of Clinical Oncology* 1991; 9: 1233-1240.
17. Dinarello CA. Interleukin-1 and its biologically related cytokines. *Adv Immunol* 1989; 44: 153-206.
18. Dinarello CA, Mier JW. Lymphokines. *N Engl J Med* 1987; 317: 940-945.
19. Dorf ME, Benacerraf B. Suppressor cells and immunoregulation. *Annu Rev Immunol* 1984; 2: 127-157.
20. Dukovich M, Wano Y, Le thi BT, et al. A second human interleukin-2 binding protein that may be a component of high-affinity interleukin-2 receptors. *Nature* 1987; 327: 518-522.
21. Durum SK, Schmidt JA, Oppenheim JJ. Interleukin 1: an immunological perspective. *Annu Rev Immunol* 1985; 3: 263-287.
22. Dustin ML, Springer TA. Lymphocyte function-associated antigen-1 (LFA-1) interaction with intercellular adhesion molecule- (ICAM-1) is one of at least three mechanisms for lymphocyte adhesion to cultured endothelial cells. *J Cell Biol* 1988; 107: 321-331.
23. Dvorak HF, Galli SJ, Dvorak AM. Cellular and vascular manifestations of cell-mediated immunity. *Hum Pathol* 1986; 17: 122-137.
24. Falkoff RJ, Butler JL, Dinarello CA, Fauci AS. Direct effects of a monoclonal B cell differentiation factor and of purified interleukin 1 on B cell differentiation. *J Immunol* 1984; 133: 692-696.
25. Fauci AS, Pratt KR. Activation of human B lymphocytes. I. Direct plaque-forming cell assay for the measurement of polyclonal activation and antigenic stimulation of human B lymphocytes. *J Exp Med* 1976; 144: 674-684.
26. Gallin JI, Quie PG. *Leukocyte chemotaxis: methods, physiology and clinical implications*. New York: Raven Press, 1978.
27. Ganser A, Ottmann OG, Erdmann H, et al. The effect of recombinant human granulocyte-macrophage colony-stimulating factor on neutropenia and related morbidity in chronic severe neutropenia. *Ann Intern Med* 1989; 111: 887-892.
28. Gearing AJ, Johnstone AP, Thorpe R. Production and assay of the interleukins. *J Immunol Methods* 1985; 83: 1-27.
29. Geller RL, Gromo G, Inverardi L, et al. Stepwise activation of T cells. Role of the calcium ionophore A23187. *J Immunol* 1987; 139: 3930-3934.
30. Gillis S. Interleukin 2: biology and biochemistry. *J Clin Immunol* 1983; 3: 1-13.
31. Goldfarb RH, Serrate SA. Natural killer cells. In: Yoshida T, ed. *Investigation of Cell-Mediated Immunity*. New York: Churchill-Livingston, 1985: 65-80.
32. Grey Hm, Sette A, Buus S. How T cells see antigen. *Sci Am* 1989; 261: 56-64.
33. Grimm EA, Mazumder A, Zhang HZ, Rosenberg SA. Lymphokine-activated killer cell phenomenon. Lysis of natural killer-resistant fresh solid tumor cells by interleukin 2-activated autologous human peripheral blood lymphocytes. *J Exp Med* 1982; 155: 1823-1841.
34. Grimm EA, Owen Schaub LB, Loudon WG, Yagita M. Lymphokine-activated killer cells. Induction and function. *Ann NY Acad Sci* 1988; 532: 380-386.
35. Gromo G, Geller RL, Inverardi L, Bach FH. Signal requirements in the step-wise functional maturation of cytotoxic T lymphocytes. *Nature* 1987; 327: 424-426.
36. Gromo G, Inverardi L, Geller RL, et al. The stepwise activation of cytotoxic T lymphocytes. *Immunol Today* 1987; 8: 259-261.
37. Groopman JE, Molina JM, Scadden DT. Hematopoietic growth factors. Biology and clinical applications. *N Engl J Med* 1989; 321: 1449-1459.
38. Han X, Itoh K, Balch CM, Pellis NR. Recombinant interleukin 2 (RIL-4) inhibits interleukin 2-induced activation of peripheral blood lymphocytes. *Lymphokine Res* 1988; 7: 227-235.
39. Hanna N, Fidler IJ. Role of natural killer cells in the destruction of circulating tumor emboli. *J Natl Cancer Inst* 1980; 65: 801-809.
40. Harada N, Matsumoto M, Koyama N, et al. T cell replacing factor/interleukin 5 induces not only B-cell growth and differentiation, but also increased expression of interleukin 2 receptor on activated B-cells. *Immunol Lett* 1987; 15: 205-215.
41. Haynes BF. Human T lymphocyte antigens as defined by monoclonal antibodies. *Immunol Rev* 1981; 57: 127-161.
42. Henkart PA. Mechanism of lymphocyte-mediated cytotoxicity. *Annu Rev Immunol* 1985; 3: 31-58.
43. Henkart PA, Millard PJ, Reynolds CW, Henkart MP. Cytolytic activity of purified cytoplasmic granules from cytotoxic rat large granular lymphocyte tumors. *J Exp Med* 1984; 160: 75-93.
44. Herberman RB, Thurman GB. Approaches to the immunological monitoring of cancer patients treated with natural or recombinant interferons. *J Biol Response Modif* 1983; 2: 548-562.
45. Hirano T, Taga T, Yamasaki K, et al. A multifunctional cytokine (IL-6/BSF-2) and its receptor. *Int Arch Allergy Appl Immunol* 1989; 88: 29-33.
46. Hong R. Immunodeficiency. In: Rose NR, Friedman H, Fahey JL, eds. *Manual of clinical laboratory immunology*. Washington, D.C.: American Society for Microbiology, 1986: 702-722.
47. Horiguchi J, Sariban E, Kufe D. Transcriptional and post-transcriptional regulation of CSF-1 gene expression in human monocytes. *Mol Cell Biol* 1988; 8: 3951-3954.
48. Howard M, Farrar J, Hilfiker M, et al. Identification of a T cell-derived B cell growth factor distinct from interleukin 2. *J Exp Med* 1982; 155: 914-923.

49. IUIS-WHO Nomenclature Subcommittee. Announcement. *J Immunol* 1985; 134: 659-660.
50. Johnson HM. Modulation of the immune response by interferons and their inducers. In: Mihick E, ed. Immunological approaches to cancer therapeutics. New York: *Wiley*, 1982; 241-256.
51. Kawase I, Urdal DL, Brooks CG, Henney CS. Selective depletion of NK cell activity *in vivo* and its effect on the growth of NK-sensitive and NK-resistant tumor cell variants. *Int J Cancer* 1982; 29: 567-574.
52. Kehrl JH, Muraguchi A, Butler JL, et al. Human B cell activation, proliferation and differentiation. *Immunol Rev* 1984; 78: 75-96.
53. Kishimoto T. Factors affecting B-cell growth and differentiation. *Annu Rev Immunol* 1985; 3: 133-157.
54. Kleinerman ES, Schroit AJ, Fogler WE, Fidler IJ. Tumoricidal activity of human monocytes activated *in vitro* by free and liposome-encapsulated human lymphokines. *J Clin Invest* 1983; 72: 304-315.
55. Koj A. The role of interleukin-6 as the hepatocyte stimulating factor in the network of inflammatory cytokines. *Ann NY Acad Sci* 1989; 557: 1-8.
56. Kovacs EJ, Beckner SK, Longo DL, et al. Cytokine gene expression during the generation of human lymphokine-activated killer cells: Early induction of interleukin 1β by interleukin 2. *Cancer Res* 1989; 49: 940-944.
57. Kumar A, Moreau JL, Baran D, Theze J. Evidence for negative regulation of T cell growth by low affinity interleukin 2 receptors. *J Immunol* 1987; 138: 1485-1493.
58. Kupfer A, Singer SJ. Cell biology of cytotoxic and helper T cell functions: immunofluorescence microscopic studies of single cells and cell couples. *Annu Rev Immunol* 1989; 7: 309-337.
59. Lafreniere R, Rosenberg SA. Adoptive immunotherapy of murine hepatic metastases with lymphokine activated killer (LAK) cells and recombinant interleukin 2 (RIL 2) can mediate the regression of both immunogenic and nonimmunogenic sarcomas and an adenocarcinoma. *J Immunol* 1985; 135: 4273-4280.
60. Lafreniere R, Rosenberg SA. Successful immunotherapy of murine experimental hepatic metastases with lymphokine-activated killer cells and recombinant interleukin 2. *Cancer Res* 1985; 45: 3735-3741.
61. Landay A, Gartland GL, Clement LT. Characterization of a phenotypically distinct subpopulation of Leu-2+ cells that suppresses T cell proliferative responses. *J Immunol* 1983; 131: 2757-2761.
62. Lasser A. The mononuclear phagocytic system: a review. *Hum pathol* 1983; 14: 108-126.
63. Lipton JN, Nathan DJ. Interactions between lymphocytes and macrophages in hematopoiesis. In: Golde DW, Takaku F, eds. *Hematopoietic stem cells*. New York: Marcel Dekker, 1980: 145-202.
64. Lotzova E, Herberman RB. *Immunobiology of natural killer cells*. Boca Raton, FL: CRC Press, 1986.
65. Lu L, Welte K, Gabrilove JL, et al. Effects of recombinant human tumor necrosis factor alpha, recombinant human gamma-interferon, and prostaglandin E on colony formation of human hematopoietic progenitor cells stimulated by natural human pluripotent colony-stimulating factor, pluripoietin alphà, and recombinant erythropoietin in serum-free cultures. *Cancer Res* 1986; 46: 4357-4361.
66. Maluish AE, Strong DM. Lymphocyte proliferation. In: Rose NR, Friedman H, Fahey JL, eds. *Manual of clinical laboratory immunology*. Washington, D.C.: American Society of Microbiology, 1986: 274-281.
67. Mancini G, Carbonara AO, Heremans JF. Immunochemical quantitation of antigens by single radial immunodiffusion. *Immunochemistry* 1965; 2: 235-254.
68. Meriney DK. Methodology of immunologic assays relating to humoral components. In: Grieco MH, Meriney DK, eds. *Immunodiagnosis for clinicians*. Chicago: Year Book Medical Publishers, 1983: 19-39.
69. Meuer SC, Acuto O, Hercent T, Schlossman SF, Reinherz EL. The human T-cell receptor. *Annu Rev Immunol* 1984; 2: 23-50.
70. Michel RH, Pancake SJ, Noseworthy J, Karnovsky ML. Measurement of rates of phagocytosis: the use of cellular monolayers. *J Cell Biol* 1969; 40: 216-224.
71. Millard PJ, Henkart MP, Reynolds CW, Henkart PA. Purification and properties of cytoplasmic granules from cytotoxic rat LGL tumors. *J Immunol* 1984; 132: 3197-3204.
72. Miyajima A, Miyatake S, Schreurs J, et al. Coordinate regulation of immune and inflammatory responses by T cell-derived lymphokines. *FASEB* J 1988; 2: 2462-2473.
73. Moller G. Concanavalin-A-activated lymphocytes suppress immune responses *in vitro* but are helper cells *in vivo*. *Scand J Immunol* 1985; 21: 31-34.
74. Morimoto C, Letvin NL, Boyd AW, et al. The isolation and characterization of the human helper inducer T cell subset. *J Immunol* 1985; 134: 3762-3769.
75. Morimoto C, Letvin NL, Distaso JA, et al. The isolation and characterization of the human suppressor inducer T cell subset. *J Immunol* 1985; 134: 1508-1515.
76. Mosmann TR, Coffman RL. TH1 and TH2 cells: different patterns of lymphokine secretion lead to different functional properties. *Annu Rev Immunol* 1989; 7: 145-173.
77. Mule JJ, Shu S, Rosenberg SA. The antitumor efficacy of lymphokine-activated killer cells and recombinant interleukin 2 *in vivo*. *J Immunol* 1985; 135: 646-652.
78. Muller Eberhard HJ. The molecular basis of target cell killing by human lymphocytes and of killer cell self-protection. *Immunol rev* 1988; 103: 87-98.
79. Munthe-Kaas AC, Kaplan G. Endocytosis by macrophages. In: Carr I, Daems WT, eds. The reticuloendothelial system: a comprehensive treatise. New York: *Plenum*, 1980: 19-55.
80. Nagler A, Lanier LL, Phillips JH. The effects of IL-4 on human natural killer cells. A potent regulator of IL-2 activation and proliferation. *J Immunol* 1988; 141: 2349-2351.
81. Nakanishi K, Malek TR, Smith KA, et al. Both interleukin 2 and a second T cell-derived factor in EL-4 supernatant have activity as differentiation factors in IgM synthesis. *J Exp Med* 1984; 160: 1605-1621.
82. Nathan CF. Secretory products of macrophages. *J Clin Invest* 1987; 79: 319-326.
83. Neckers LM, Cossman J. Transferrin receptor induction in mitogen-stimulated human T lymphocytes is required for DNA synthesis and cell division and is regulated by interleukin 2. *Proc Natl Acad Sci* USA 1983; 80: 3494-3498.
84. Ochoa AC, Gromo G, Alter BJ, et al. Long-term growth of lymphokine-activated killer (LAK) cells: role of anti-CD3, beta-IL 1, interferon-gamma and -beta. *J Immunol* 1987; 138: 2728-2733.

85. Ochoa AC, Hasz DE, Rezonzew R, et al. Lymphokine-activated killer activity in long-term cultures with anti-CD3 plus interleukin 2: Identification and isolation of effector subsets. *Cancer Res* 1989; 49: 963-968.
86. OGarra A, Umland S, DeFrance T, Christiansen J. 'B-cell factors' are pleiotropic. *Immunol Today* 1988; 9: 45-54.
87. OGarra A, Warren DJ, Sanderson CJ, et al. Interleukin-4 (B cell growth factor-II/eosinophil differentiation factor) is a mitogen and differentiation factor for preactivated murine B lymphocytes. *Curr Top Microbiol Immunol* 1986; 132: 133-141.
88. Oldham RK. Natural killer cells: history and significance. *J Biol Response Modif* 1982; 1: 217-231.
89. Oldham RK. NK cells: artifact to reality, an odyssey in biology. *Can Metas Rev* 1983; 2: 232-336.
90. Oldham RK, Gail MH, Baker MA, et al. Immunological studies in a double blind randomized trial comparing intrapleural BCG against placebo in patients with resected stage I non-small cell lung cancer. *Cancer Immunol Immunother* 1982; 13: 164-173.
91. Oldham RK, Weese JL, Herberman RB, et al. Immunological monitoring and immunotherapy in carcinoma of the lung. *Int J Cancer* 1976; 18: 739-749.
92. Ortaldo JR, Herberman RB. Heterogeneity of natural killer cells. *Annu Rev Immunol* 1984; 2: 359-394.
93. Ortaldo JR, Mason A, Overton R. Lymphokine-activated killer cells. Analysis of progenitors and effectors. *J Exp med* 1986; 164: 1193-1205.
94. Owen-Schaub L, Yagita M, Tsudo M, et al. Evidence for distinct IL-2 receptors in induction versus maintenance of LAK function. *Ann NY Acad Sci* 1988; 532: 480-481.
95. Paetkau V, Bleackley RC, Riendeau D, et al. Toward the molecular biology of IL-2. *Contemp Top Mol Immunol* 1985; 10: 35-61.
96. Palacios R, Henson G, Steinmetz M, McKearn JP. Interleukin-3 supports growth of mouse pre-B-cell clones *in vitro*. *Nature* 1984; 309: 126-131
97. Pasternack MS, Verret CR, Liu MA, Eisen HN. Serine esterase in cytolytic T lymphocytes. *Nature* 1986; 322: 740-743.
98. Perlmutter DH. IFNβ2/IL-6 is one of several cytokines that modulate acute phase gene expression in human hepatocytes and human macrophages. *Ann NY Acad Sci* 1989; 557: 332-342.
99. Platt JL, Grant BW, Eddy AA, Michael AF. Immune cell populations in cutaneous delayed-type hypersensitivity. *J Exp Med* 1983; 158: 1227-1242.
100. Poulter LW, Seymour GJ, Duke O, et al. Immunohistological analysis of delayed-type hypersensitivity in man. *Cell Immunol* 1982; 74: 358-369.
101. Raulet DH. The structure, function, and molecular genetics of the gamma/delta T cell receptor. *Annu Rev Immunol* 1989; 7: 175-207.
102. Reed JC, Alpers JD, Nowell PC, Hoover RG. Sequential expression of proto-oncogenes during lectin-stimulated mitogenesis of normal human lymphocytes. *Proc Natl Acad Sci USA* 1986; 83: 3982-3986.
103. Reed JC, Prystowsky MB, Kern JA, et al. Regulation of proto-oncogene expression during lymphocyte activation and proliferation. In: Gupta S, Paul WE, Fauci AS, eds. *Advances in experimental medicine and biology*. New York: Plenum Press, 1986: 249-262.
104. Reinherz EL, Schlossman SF. Current concepts in immunology: regulation of the immune response – inducer and suppressor T-lymphocyte subsets in human beings. *N Engl J Med* 1980; 303: 370-373.
105. Reinherz EL, Schlossman SF. The characterization and function of human immunoregulatory T lymphocyte subsets. *Immunol Today* 1981; 2: 69-73.
106. Robb RJ, Greene WC, Internalization of interleukin 2 is mediated by the beta chain of the high-affinity interleukin 2 receptor. *J Exp Med* 1987; 165: 1201-1206.
107. Robb RJ, Rusk CM, Yodoi J, Greene WC. Interleukin 2 binding molecule distinct from the Tac protein: analysis of its role in formation of high-affinity receptors. *Proc Natl Acad Sci USA* 1987; 84: 2002-2006.
108. Rocklin RE, Meyers OL, David JR. An *in vitro* assay for cellular hypersensitivity in man. *J Immunol* 1970; 104: 95-102.
109. Rosenberg SA, Eberlein TJ, Grimm EA, et al. Development of long-term cell lines and lymphoid clones reactive against murine and human tumors: a new approach to the adoptive immunotherapy of cancer. *Surgery* 1982; 92: 328-336.
110. Rosenberg SA, Lotze MT, Muul LM, et al. Observations on the systemic administration of autologous lymphokine-activated killer cells and recombinant interleukin-2 to patients with metastatic cancer. *N Engl J Med* 1985; 313: 1485-1492.
111. Rosenberg SA, Mule JJ. Immunotherapy of cancer with lymphokine-activated killer cells and recombinant interleukin-2. *Surgery* 1985; 98: 437-444.
112. Rosenberg SA, Mule JJ, Spiess PJ, et al. Regression of established pulmonary metastases and subcutaneous tumor mediated by the systemic administration of high-dose recombinant interleukin 2. *J Exp Med* 1985; 161: 1169-1188.
113. Rosenblum MG, Donato NJ. Tumor necrosis factor α: A multifaceted peptide hormone. *CRC Crit Rev Immunol* 1989; 9: 21-44.
114. Sakane T, Green I. Human suppressor T cells induced by concanavalin A: suppressor T cells belong to distinctive T cell subclasses. *J Immunol* 1977; 119: 1169-1178.
115. Schatten S, Granstein RD, Drebin JA, Greene MI. Suppressor T cells and the immune response to tumors. *CRC Crit Rev Immunol* 1984; 4: 335-379.
116. Schlick E, Hartung K, Stevenson HC, Chirigos MA. Secretion of colony-stimulating factors by human monocytes and bone marrow cells after *in vitro* treatment with biological response modifiers. *J Leukocyte Biol* 1985; 37: 615-627.
117. Schwartz RH. T-lymphocyte recognition of antigen in association with gene products of the major histocompatibility complex. *Annu Rev Immunol* 1985; 3: 237-261.
118. Shipp MA, Reinherz EL. Differential expression of nuclear proto-oncogenes in T cells triggered with mitogenic and non-mitogenic T3 and T11 activation signals. *J Immunol* 1987; 139: 2143-2148.
119. Sieff CA. Hematopoietic growth factors. *J Clin Invest* 1987; 79: 1549-1557.
120. Smith CW, Rothlein R, Hughes BJ, et al. Recognition of an endothelial determinant for CD 18-dependent human neutrophil adherence and transendothelial migration. *J Clin Invest* 1988; 82: 1746-1756.
121. Smith KA. Dissection of the molecular events occurring during T cell cycle progression. In: Gupta S, Paul WE, and Fauci AS, eds. *Advances in experimental medicine and*

biology. New York: Plenum Press, 1986: 125-128.
122. Smith KA. The interleukin 2 receptor. *Adv Immunol* 1988; 42: 165-179.
123. Smith KA. Interleukin-2: inception, impact, and implications. *Science* 1988; 240: 1169-1176.
124. Spencer RP, Pearson HH. *Radionuclide studies of the spleen*. Cleveland: CRC Press, 1975.
125. Springer TA, Dustin ML, Kishimoto TK, Marlin SD. The lymphocyte function-associated LFA-1, CD2, and LFA-3 molecules: cell adhesion receptors of the immune system. *Annu Rev Immunol* 1987; 5: 223-252.
126. Springer TA, Unkeless JC. Analysis of macrophage differentiation and function with monoclonal antibodies. *Contemp Top Immunobiol* 1984; 13: 1-31.
127. Taniguchi T. Regulation of cytokine gene expression. *Annu Rev Immunol* 1988; 6: 439-464.
128. Te Velde AA, yard BA, Klomp JP, et al. Modulation of phenotypic and functional properties of human peripheral blood monocytes by interleukin-2 (IL-4). *Agents Actions* 1989; 26: 199-200.
129. Teshigawara K, Wang HM, Kato K, Smith KA. Interleukin 2 high-affinity receptor expression requires two distinct binding proteins. *J Exp Med* 1987; 165: 223-238.
130. Tosato G, Pike SE. Interferon-beta 2/interleukin 6 is a co-stimulant for human T lymphocytes. *J Immunol* 1988; 141: 1556-1562.
131. Tracey DE. Macrophage mediated injury. In: Rose NR, Siegel BV, eds. *The reticuloendothelial system: a comprehensive treatise*. New York: Plenum Press, 1983: 77-101.
132. Trinchieri G, Perussa B. Human natural killer cells: biologic and pathologic aspects. *Lab Invest* 1984; 50: 489-513.
133. Tsudo M, Kozak RW, Goldman CK, Waldmann TA. Demonstration of a non-Tac peptide that binds interleukin 2: a potential participant in a multichain interleukin 2 receptor complex. *Proc Natl Acad Sci* USA 1986; 83: 9694-9698.
134. Unanue ER. Antigen-presenting function of the macrophage. *Annu Rev Immunol* 1984; 2: 395-428.
135. Wahl SM, McCartney-Francis N, Mergenhagen SE. Inflammatory and immunomodulatory roles of TGF-β. *Immunol Today* 1989; 10: 258-261.
136. Waldmann TA, Broder S. Suppressor cells in the regulation of the immune response. *Prog Clin Immunol* 1977; 3: 155-199.
137. Weiss A, Imboden JB. Cell surface molecules and early events involved in human T lymphocyte activation. *Adv Immunol* 1987; 41: 1-38.
138. Weissman AM, Harford JB, Svetlik PB, et al. Only high-affinity receptors for interleukin 2 mediate internalization of ligand. *Proc Natl Acad Sci* USA 1986; 83: 1463-1466.
139. West WH, Tauer KW, Yannelli JR, et al. Constant-infusion recombinant interleukin-2 in adoptive immunotherapy of advanced cancer. *N Engl J Med* 1987; 316: 898-905.
140. Whitlock C, Denis K, Robertson D, Witte O. *In vitro* analysis of murine-B-cell development. *Annu Rev Immunol* 1985; 3: 213-235.
141. Woodruff JJ, Clarke LM, Chin YH. Specific cell-adhesion mechanisms determining migration pathways of recirculating lymphocytes. *Annu Rev Immunol* 1987; 5: 201-222.
142. Yang SC, Owen Schaub L, Grimm EA, Roth JA. Induction of lymphokine-activated killer cytotoxicity with interleukin-2 and tumor necrosis factor-alpha against primary lung cancer targets. *Cancer Immunol Immunother* 1989; 29: 193-198.
143. Young JD, Liu C. Multiple mechanisms of lymphocyte mediated killing. *Immunol Today* 1988; 9: 140-144.
144. Zlotnik A, Fischer M, Roehm N, Zipori D. Evidence for effects of interleukin 4 (B cell stimulatory factor 1) on macrophages: enhancement of antigen presenting ability of bone marrow-derived macrophages. *J Immunol* 1987; 138: 4275-4279.
145. Zola H. The surface antigens of human B lymphocytes. *Immunol Today* 1987; 8: 308-310.
146. Zucali JR, Broxmeyer HE, Gross MA, Dinarello CA. Recombinant human tumor necrosis factors alpha and beta stimulate fibroblasts to produce hemopoietic growth factors *in vitro*. *J Immunol* 1988; 140: 840-844.

THERAPEUTIC APPROACHES TO CANCER-ASSOCIATED IMMUNE SUPPRESSION

ROBERT K. OLDHAM*

The Biological Therapy Institute Foundation, Franklin, Tennessee; and University of Missouri, Columbia, Missouri

It is now well established that many cancer patients exhibit *in vivo* and *in vitro* evidence of immune suppression, which often correlates with tumor-cell burden, stage of disease, and prognosis. Cancer-associated immune suppression appears to be a direct result of the presence of disease, or follows treatment for it, rather than being an antecedent or predisposing condition. However, the precise role that nonspecific and/or specific antitumor immunity plays in the control of human cancer remains controversial. Indeed, there is some evidence that suggests that the development of certain antitumor immune responses may lead to augmented tumor cell growth rather than tumor regression [314,442,443].

The clinical relevance of the relative state of general immunocompetence in determining whether or not a patient can be cured of cancer also remains controversial. A case in point is the dissociation between immunodeficiency and curability of patients with Hodgkin's disease. Despite the well-recognized immune suppression associated with this malignancy, and the immunosuppressive therapies used to treat patients (e.g., lymphoid irradiation and steroid-containing combination chemotherapy), it is one of the most curable of all cancers. Such a discrepancy suggests that unique biological properties of malignant cells, rather than the general immune competence of the patient, are the more critical factors in determining the curability of cancer.

Even though the precise relationship between the general state of immune competence and cancer curability has not been established, investigators have administered a variety of agents to cancer patients including biologicals, vitamins, hormones, and drugs, hoping that the reversal or prevention of immune suppression might translate into prolonged disease-free remissions and improved patient survival. This chapter will review the multifactorial basis of cancer-associated immune suppression and the therapeutic strategies that have been utilized. The sections on immune suppression will focus exclusively on the general assessment of immunity, and not specific antitumor immunity. The sections on therapy of immune suppression will be limited to those biological response modifiers (BRMs), both chemical and biological, that were administered either to restore depressed immunity to normal, or to prevent the deterioration of immune competence due to surgery, radiation therapy, or chemotherapy. BRMs that have been employed as adjuvants along with tumor cell or tumor antigen vaccines (e.g., BCG) to boost specific anti-tumor immune responses, or whose primary mechanisms of action are by activating effector cells directly, such as interferons and/or interferon inducers (e.g., poly I-poly C, ampligen), muramyl dipeptide and cogeners, or interleukin-2 and other interleukins (e.g., tumor necrosis factor), will not be covered, nor will more 'traditional' whole organisms from the older literature [e.g., *Bacillus Calmette-Guerin* (BCG), *Corynebacterium parvum*, or mixed bacterial vaccine].

IMMUNOSUPPRESSION AND CANCER

It is clear that preexisting immunodeficiency plays a permissive role in the development of certain cancers, such as malignant lymphoma or Kaposi's sarcoma [427]. Patients with primary (e.g., Wiscott-Aldrich syndrome, at ataxia-telangiectasia) or secondary (e.g., acquired immune deficiency syndrome, AIDS) immunodeficiency syndromes in which defects in cell-mediated immunity predominate and patients receiving immunosuppressive drugs following organ transplantation all exhibit an increased incidence of Burkitt's and non-Burkitt's lymphoma, Kaposi's sarcoma, and a variety of other tumors not otherwise commonly seen. In several instances, following the cessation of immunosuppressive therapies, cancer regressions have been noted, suggesting that when immunocompetence is restored, control of tumor growth may occur. Patients with primary (e.g., Bruton's-type agammaglobulinemia) and secondary (e.g., chronic lymphocytic leukemia) immunodeficiency syndromes in which defects in humoral immunity predominate also exhibit an increased incidence of malignancies including skin cancer, primary brain neoplasms, sarcomas, carcinomas, and leukemias [184,262,428].

* Dr. Robert K. Oldham revised this chapter from the Second Edition due to lack of available time from Drs. Oates, Goldstein and Sztein to prepare the revision.

R.K. Oldham (ed.), Principles of Cancer Biotherapy. 3rd ed., 93–140.

Since the malignancies associated with underlying immunodeficiency states are not common in the general population in comparison with lung, breast, and gastrointestinal cancer, it would appear that most adult malignancies do not reflect underlying immunodeficiency. It is more likely that a combination of genetic factors, chronic immune system stimulation (possibly as a result of recurrent infections), the presence of infectious carcinogenic agents (e.g., viruses), chronic chemical carcinogenesis, and other undefined factors leads to the high incidence of certain cancers in patients with primary or secondary immunodeficiency states. There is evidence to indicate that certain carcinogens – for example, asbestos – can suppress immune functions such as NK activity [469]. However, for the majority of common cancers, the overwhelming evidence suggests that immunodeficiency arises *secondarily* as a consequence of cancer and the therapies used to treat it; that is, *cancer itself is an immunosuppressive disease*. Cancer-associated immunodeficiency is further influenced by other factors, including age and genetic background, as well as environmental factors, such as nutritional status, stress, and infections. For example, nutritional status is frequently impaired in patients with head and neck cancer [93], which accounts for many of the immunodeficiencies reported in these patient populations such as decreased T cell numbers. A recent report of patients with locally advanced breast cancer has suggested that stress-related factors are associated with a sustained depression of NK-cell activity and predict a worse prognosis [330]. Thus, it is the balance of many different endogenous and exogenous factors that ultimately contributes to the overall immune deficiency state of cancer patients.

Multifactorial basis of immunodeficiency in cancer patients

Because of subtle variations in methodologies employed by different investigators, it is often difficult (and sometimes impossible) to directly compare the results of *in vitro* and *in vivo* immunologic assays from different studies. Nevertheless, a number of general conclusions have been reached concerning cancer-associated immune suppression. No single explanation, or generally agreed-upon concept, has emerged to explain the immunodeficiency. Rather, there is a complex set of interactions involving a number of different mechanisms. This multifactorial basis of immunodeficiency is outlined in simplified form in Fig. 1. The scheme is equally applicable to T-, B-, NK-, or phagocytic effector-cell immune mechanisms.

Five major factors each play a role in determining the immune responsiveness of cancer patients: (a) the proportions and absolute numbers of circulating, tissue-derived, or intratumoral effector cells; (b) the intrinsic functional capabilities of the effector cells on a per-cell basis; (c) the influence of immunoregulatory helper and suppressor cells; (d) the influence of local systemic-circulating and immunomodulatory soluble factors; and (e) the influence of systemic treatment. In Fig. 1, it is shown schematically how the relative contributions of these five factors modulate immune responsiveness of cancer patients as assessed with *in vitro* and *in vivo* assays.

Effector cell numbers and function

Any basic immune response reflects both the number (or relative proportion) of effector cells present and the intrinsic functional capability of the effector cells. Thus, impaired immunity can result purely from a deficiency in absolute numbers (or proportions) of effector cells that

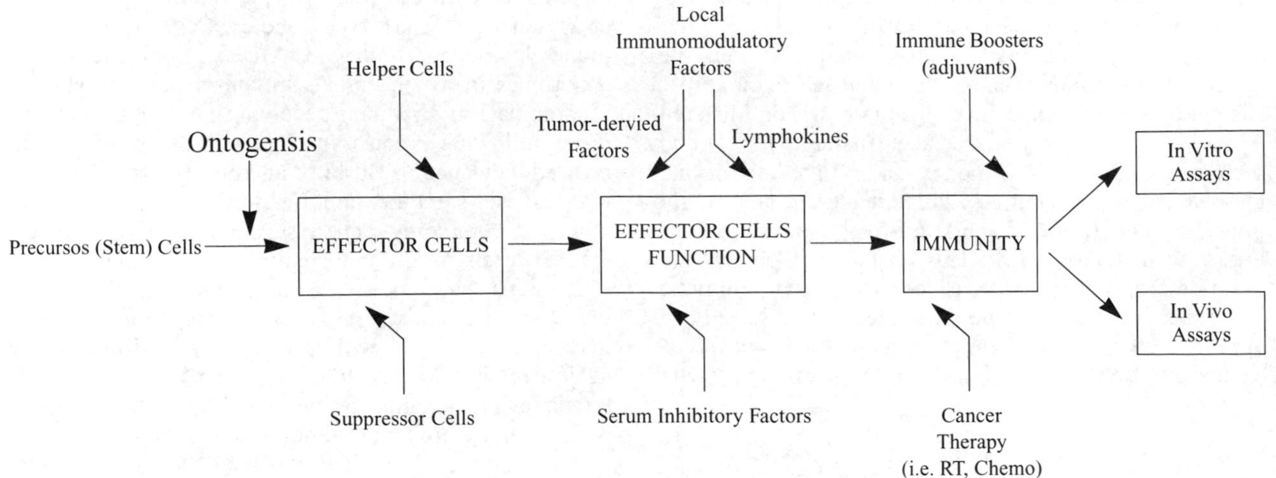

Figure 1. Multifunctional basis of immunodeficiency in cancer patients.

otherwise exhibit normal function on a per-cell basis, from effector cells that exhibit intrinsic functional defects despite normal cell numbers, or from a combination of both decreased cell numbers and impaired function of the individual cells.

The primary immunodeficiency syndromes, such as the DiGeorge syndrome, ataxia-telangiectasia, and severe combined immunodeficiency syndrome (SCID), are examples of immune deficiency resulting from defective ontogenesis of the immune system. However, since the development of the immune system occurs during fetal and neonatal life, defects in ontogeny are not a consideration in the immune deficiency of cancer patients. Cancer patients do, however, often exhibit lymphocytopenia and decreased T-cell numbers [80, 109, 110, 227, 315, 349, 382, 397, 405, 408, 416, 452, 481, 524, 599, 597, 600], which contribute to their overall state of immunodeficiency. In contrast to primary immunodeficiency states, the effector cell abnormalities detected in cancer patients arise secondarily, probably as a result of the suppressive effects of cancer-derived factors on effector cell production and/or survival.

When PBMC is used as the source of effector cells in a lymphocyte or monocyte function assays, it cannot be established whether a depressed functional immune response results from a decreased proportion of effector cells within the PBMC mixture, from intrinsic functional defects of the effector cells themselves, from the presence of excessive suppressor cell activity, or from a combination of abnormalities in cell proportions, functions, and immunoregulation. There is considerable evidence indicating that cancer patients exhibit depressions in mitogen and antigen-induced proliferative assays [80, 100, 104, 110, 111, 155, 189, 192, 216, 261, 310, 315, 339, 349, 363, 382, 405, 408, 444, 457, 468, 524, 599, 597, 627] and in cytolytic activity [30, 108, 136, 163, 164, 287, 336, 360, 445, 484, 540, 568, 580, 591, 595] using PBMC as effector cells. In some cancers, for example, head and neck cancer [433] and Hodgkin's disease [508], it has been possible using purified T cells to document intrinsic functional T-cell defects. Studies in cancer patients have shown an impaired ability of T cells to produce the lymphokine IL-2 [208, 350, 383] following activation by mitogens; but that spontaneous IL-2 production (reflecting possible stimulation due to circulating tumor antigens) is increased [257]. However, in Hodgkin's disease, although IL-2 production and/or IL-2R expression of PBMC has been reported to be low [52, 389, 534, 634], the abnormality in T-cell lymphoproliferation does not appear to be related to defects in the IL-2 system [52].

Peripheral blood monocytes and polymorphonuclear leukocytes isolated from patients with a variety of cancers also exhibit depressed functional activity [32, 78, 112, 150, 190, 224, 482, 531, 580]. NK-cell activity is also frequently depressed in cancer patients [136, 175, 445, 591]. At the local level, NK activity may be more impaired than other lymphocyte functions such as LPRs [17].

Thus, many studies now suggest that intrinsic functional defects of effector cells contribute, at least in part, to the immunodeficiency of cancer.

Immunoregulatory cells

The intrinsic functional capabilities of T, B, NK, and phagocytic cells are modulated by interactions with a variety of immunoregulatory cells. The T- and B-cell functions can be influenced either positively or negatively, depending upon the relative balance between $T_{n/I}$ and $T_{c/s}$ cells, respectively [589]. Once again, both absolute numbers (or proportions) and immunoregulatory function per cell are considerations in determining the overall influence of immunoregulatory cells on effector cell function.

Another important immunoregulatory cell is the monocyte/macrophage. Most normal immune responses require the presence of monocytes/macrophages as accessory cells for optimal processing of antigen and appropriate activation of effector lymphocytes. In many disease states, including cancer, monocytes/macrophages exhibit suppressor-cell activity rather than helper-cell activity [589]. It is likely that such 'suppressor' cells may develop in cancer patients to release factors capable of suppressing tumor growth as their primary action and thus that the suppression of immune reactivity is an 'innocent bystander' effect. The influence of monocytes/macrophages is dependent upon cell numbers (or proportions) and their state of activation. In general, an excess in the proportion of monocytes/macrophages relative to effector lymphocytes results in suboptimal immune response. However, although monocytosis is seen in advanced cancer patients, it has not been generally possible to correlate the degree of monocyte-mediated suppression with the degree of monocytosis [589].

There is considerable evidence for immune suppression mediated by activated monocytes/macrophages in cancer patients [5, 29, 31, 54, 86, 211, 213, 214, 274, 281, 359, 503, 571, 581, 589]. For example, monocyte-mediated suppression of lymphocyte-proliferative functions have been demonstrated in Hodgkin's disease [171, 193, 207, 366, 496, 584] as well as in patients with lung cancer [5, 211, 274], breast cancer [213, 274], malignant melanoma [393], colorectal cancer [29, 213, 571], head and neck cancer [31, 54, 603], bladder cancer [214], and a variety of other malignancies [86, 589]. Monocyte-mediated suppression of cytolytic effector-cell activity has also been demonstrated in cancer patients [14, 18, 134, 168, 250, 251, 589], including NK-cell activity [268] and autologous T-cell-mediated anti-tumor cytotoxic responses [168, 503]. In comparative studies, it has been demonstrated that such suppressor-cell activity is of greater magnitude at the local level (i.e., intratumoral, TIL cells and in draining lymph nodes) than in the systemic circulation [14, 18, 134, 250, 251].

The contribution of suppressor lymphocytes to the generation of cancer-associated immunodeficiency is less certain and still somewhat controversial. Several studies that identified helper and suppressor T-cells on the basis of the presence of surface Fc receptors for IgM (Tμ cells) or IgG (Tγ cells), respectively, have suggested that the $T_{h/I}/T_{c/s}$ ratio is depressed in cancer patients [225, 292, 579]. However, more recent studies using monoclonal antibodies to detect surface antigens indicate that the relative proportion SOF $T_{h/I}$ and $T_{c/s}$ cells are preserved in most untreated cancer patients unless they have extremely widespread disease [143, 221, 291, 339, 504]. Few reports have focused on functional aspects of suppressor lymphocyte activity in cancer patients. Definitive conclusions are lacking, although such activity has been reported in patients with Hodgkin's disease [240, 523] and various solid tumors [168, 258, 259, 309, 586]. Inducible suppressor T-cell activity has generally [113, 201, 258, 506] but not always [569] been found to be depressed in cancer patients.

Immunomodulatory factors

It is now well established that, in normal immune reactions, the influence of immunoregulatory cells is mediated at least in part by the local release of cytokines such as IL-1 by monocytes, and IL-2 and γ-interferon by helper T cells. In a variety of disease states including cancer, there may be a deficiency in the production of cytokines by cells that normally produce them [176, 208, 228, 350, 383, 490, 598, 625, 633].

The release in cancer patients of a variety of immunomodulatory factors produced by monocytes/macrophages and/or the tumor cells themselves has been described. Immunosuppressive factors, for example, the E series of prostaglandins, are released in excessive quantity from both monocytes/macrophages [5, 29, 31, 54, 86, 171, 193, 207, 393, 420, 495, 571] and tumor cells [77, 153, 154, 243, 286, 388, 571], which could suppress cytolytic activities [388] and proliferative functions [134] of TIL cells as well as of circulating lymphocytes. However, prostaglandins alone do not mediate the complete suppressor cell activity of monocytes [29, 31, 171, 495, 571]. Monocyte-derived toxic oxygen metabolites, for example, hydrogen peroxide [366], and other as yet undefined mediators also appear to play a role. Increased monocyte production of prostaglandins has been shown to directly impair lymphocyte proliferative and cytolytic functions [153, 154] as well as the phagocytic function of monocytes themselves [167]. A variety of other factors have been identified that are shed by tumor cells and modulate both local as well as systemic immune responses. These include tumor-associated glycoproteins [476] and lipids [215]. For example, various melanoma-associated gangliosides have been shown to both up-regulate and down-regulate lymphocyte responses to IL-2 [252]. Thus, it has been suggested that the unique tumor-antigen-associated phenotype of each individual tumor (based on the proportion of various immune-suppressing and augmenting factors released by it) determines whether the individual tumor will exhibit immune stimulation or suppression. In this regard, a recent report has demonstrated that whereas primary melanomas stimulate autologous lymphocyte responses, metastatic melanomas suppress immune responsiveness [554].

It is also apparent that a number of different substances with immunosuppressive properties can be detected in the blood of patients with cancer. Many investigators have shown that serum from cancer patients is immunosuppressive in that it suppresses mitogen and antigen responsiveness of lymphocytes from normal donors [11, 60, 105, 181, 200, 206, 248, 453, 458, 517, 526, 546]. Cancer serum inhibitory factors include acute-phase reactants, such as α_1-acid glycoprotein [37, 553], α-globulins [256], C-reactive protein [415], and immune complexes [36, 284]. A serum factor in young cancer patients has been reported to inhibit serum thymic-hormone bioactivity [131]. Circulating immune complexes have been shown to produce immunosuppressive effects by a variety of mechanisms including (a) blocking of B-cell differentiation and antibody production [475, 563]; (b) stimulating the production of anti-idiotype antibody which then interferes with the immune response to the original antigen [475, 563]; (c) inducing suppressor T-cells [114]; (d) reducing IL-2 levels [455]; and (e) blocking Fc receptors on effector cells [185]. Theoretically, the quantitative removal of tumor antigens, antitumor antibodies, and/or immune complexes could lead to a specific or nonspecific stimulation of the immune system, leading to an increase in general immune competence as well as in specific antitumor immune responsiveness. This has formed the basis for therapeutic trials with extracorporeal treatment of cancer with immobilized staphylococcal protein A [365, 392] and for attempts at plasma ultrafiltration. The mechanism of antitumor activity of such approaches has still not been defined. However, plasmapheresis has been associated with increased LPRs and antitumor immune responses [510, 512], probably due to removal of immunosuppressive serum factors.

In conclusion, it is clear that the state of immunocompetence of an individual cancer patient is dependent upon a number of complex interactions among effector cells, immunoregulatory cells, and local and systemic immunomodulatory factors. A simplified explanation for the immunosuppression of cancer is that products released from the malignant cells themselves lead to (a) activation of suppressor cells (e.g., monocytes/macrophages); (b) impaired effector cell production and survival; and (c) direct inhibition of effector cell function. In assessing the state of immune competence with *in vitro* and *in vivo* assays, the underlying basis of immunodeficiency may or may not be identified. For example, with *in vivo* tests to assess DTHS responses, and with *in vitro* assays using PBMC, it is impossible to establish the etiology of depressed reactivity among the various possible mechanisms.

Immunosuppression and tumor cell burden

In newly diagnosed, untreated cancer patients, the degree of immunodeficiency generally parallels the extent of disease. The most reasonable explanation for such an association is that the release of tumor-derived immunosuppressive factors relates directly to the tumor cell burden. Immune parameters of which impairment correlates with extent of disease include DTHS to recall antigens as well as to DNCB, blood effector cell levels (e.g., T-lymphocyte levels), lymphocyte functions, including proliferative responses to mitogens and antigens, cytotoxic activity, phagocytic cell activity, serum immunoglobulin levels, and primary antibody responses to a variety of immunizing antigens. Whereas quite early cancer is associated with only subtle abnormalities of immune competence, more advanced disease, particularly after treatment, leads to abnormalities in all measurable immune parameters.

Solid tumors

Delayed-type hypersensitivity (DTHS)

Many reports have confirmed that as the extent of disease increases, the incidence of positive DTHS reactions decreases. For example, in one large study of 234 patients with various types of cancer, patients without metastases exhibited positive reactions to DNCB (83%) more often than those with regional metastases (67%) or with distant metastases (41%) [435]. Similar findings using both DNCB as well as recall antigens have been noted in a wide variety of solid tumor-bearing patients, including those with breast cancer [2, 80, 81, 160, 315, 324, 540], gastrointestinal cancer [81, 600], head and neck cancer [405, 539, 599], lung cancer [8, 249, 380, 614], renal cancer [92, 385], gynecologic cancer [614], urologic cancer [40, 91, 499], malignant melanoma [159, 444], sarcomas [159], and primary brain cancers [90, 346].

The incidence of positive DTHS responses varies according to type of cancer. For example, patients with localized head and neck cancer had a much lower reactivity (42%) than patients with sarcomas (73%) and lung cancer (80%) [81]. This result has been explained, at least in part, by the alcohol intake and general state of malnutrition associated with head and neck cancer patients [59, 340]. In another study, it was found that the correlation between DNCB reactivity and clinical status was more pronounced in patients with squamous-cell carcinomas of the head and neck than in those with sarcomas or melanomas [615]. These findings suggest that although DNCB reactivity generally correlates with extent of disease, the relationships are modified depending upon the particular type of cancer.

It has been easy to demonstrate the marked degree of impairment in DTHS reactions found in patients with metastatic cancer; however, it has been much more difficult to discern relative differences in reactivity of patients with similar stages of disease whose tumors differ in size, regional lymph-node involvement, or local invasiveness. For example, in one report of patients with head and neck cancer, DTHS skin responses to recall antigens were impaired to a greater extent in cases with larger primaries, or if lymph nodes were involved [405]. Other studies using DNCB have failed to duplicate these findings [110, 599]. In addition, no correlation between lymph-node involvement and impairment of DNCB reactivity was found in patients with breast cancer [540]. No significant differences could be detected among stage I melanoma patients based on the depth of invasion (Clark level) of the primary lesion [474]. However, an inverse relationship between DNCB reactivity and local invasiveness has been found in patients with primary resectable colorectal cancer [600]. Among 181 patients, 20% of Dukes A patients were DNCB-negative, compared with 40% of Dukes B and 60% of Dukes C patients [600]. Thus, depending upon the particular cancer, subtle differences in DTHS reactivity as a function of tumor size or invasiveness may or may not be apparent.

Lymphoproliferative responses (LPRs)

An exhaustive literature has accumulated in which various *in vitro* lymphoproliferative assays were employed to assess the state of immune competence of cancer patients. In general, PBMC were the responder cells, and T-cell mitogens (e.g., PHA, Con A) were used to induce blastogenic transformation. Many reports have documented an inverse correlation between PHA response and stage of disease for patients with a variety of solid tumors. For example, among 179 patients with gastric carcinoma, 87% with stage I-II, 49% with stage II, and only 24% with stage IV disease could exhibit morphological evidence for blastogenic transformation of PBMC following exposure to PHA [408]. A study of 154 patients with carcinoma of the lung revealed that lymphoproliferative responses were significantly decreased in patients with stage III disease, but not in those with stages I and II [597]; other studies have reported similar results [111, 155, 216, 457]. Depressed LPRs to alloantigens in mixed leukocyte culture (MLR) were observed in 46% of patients with small (TINOMO) stage I lung cancers [104]. Depressed mitogenic responsiveness has been correlated with advancing stage of disease in breast cancer [261, 349, 363, 540, 617], and, in one study, lymphocyte responses to PHA were impaired in earlier stages of disease than was DTHS reactivity [540]. Similar inverse correlations between stage of disease and LPRs have been noted in colorectal cancer [189, 600], malignant melanoma [192, 310, 524], and head and neck cancer [110, 405, 599]. One of the most consistent findings in head and neck cancer has been the correlation between impaired reactivity to PHA and size of primary tumor, although clinical involvement of regional lymph nodes was not associated with further impairment.

Although many reports have documented that LPRs generally decrease with advancing stage in solid tumor patients, this finding has not been universal. For example, lack of correlation between blastogenic responses and disease stage has been reported in patients with breast cancer [80, 315, 339, 468], malignant melanoma [100, 192, 444], and colorectal cancer [382]. These reported inconsistencies have probably resulted from differences in techniques and quality control procedures for assays with a great deal of inherent variability. Nevertheless, the same general conclusion holds for *in vitro* LPRs and DTHS skin testing, namely, that there tends to be an inverse correlation between immune reactivity and tumor burden and/or stage of disease. However, the correlation for LPRs may be stronger for some cancers (lung cancer, head and neck cancer) than for others (breast cancer, malignant melanoma).

Immune cell quantitation

There is presently a wide variety of monoclonal antibody reagents available to quantitate blood, organ, and intratumoral levels of various immune effector cells; however, most of the preliminary observations concerning lymphocyte quantitation and cancer were made using more primitive assay methods. The quantitation of lymphocytes in the peripheral blood of cancer patients has been studied as a measure of immunocompetence since the early 1920s, when lymphocytopenia was found to be common in patients with malignancies [632]. Other studies found an inverse correlation between total lymphocyte count and stage of disease in breast [416], lung [597], and head and neck cancer [599].

The observation that human T lymphocytes could be easily identified by a binding reaction to sheep red blood cells to form E rosettes (E-RFC), coupled with the emerging recognition of the importance of T cells in immune responsiveness, led to numerous studies on cancer patients. Using E-rosette techniques, the percentage of circulating T cells has been determined for patients with a wide variety of solid tumors and correlated with clinical stage of disease. For example, a decrease in the percentage of E-RFC was found in patients with disseminated melanoma, but not in those with melanoma confined to the primary site [524]. In two studies of more than 300 women with breast cancer, there was a decreased percentage of E-RFC in all stages except locally advanced disease [349, 620]. Among patients with cervical carcinoma, there was a significant depression in the percentage of T cells in association with invasive, but not preinvasive, conditions [452]. T-cell levels quantitated before surgery were decreased in 60% of 50 colorectal cancer patients, in both percentages and absolute numbers [227]. Inverse correlations between absolute circulating T cells and tumor stage have also been reported in patients with lung cancer [597], colorectal cancer [600], head and neck cancer [110, 405], and bladder cancer [109]. Other studies have not found such a correlation [80, 315, 382, 397, 408]. In general, however, as with the *in vitro* assays of T-cell functions, peripheral blood T-cell numbers tend to decrease in association with more advanced stages of cancer.

Although assessments of B cells, monocytes, and $T_{n/I}$ and $T_{c/s}$ ratios have been performed less frequently in cancer patients, in general, B-cell numbers have paralleled T-cell numbers [291, 339, 382, 481, 562], whereas absolute monocyte counts tend to increase with advancing disease [339]. T-cell subset abnormalities have been found in some patients with malignant melanoma [291], head and neck cancer [143, 225], and lung cancer [575, 618]. T-cell subset abnormalities were more pronounced in lung lavage cells than in PBMC from patients with lung cancer [177], suggesting that such perturbations occur first at a local level before systemic abnormalities become detectable. In general, abnormalities of the $T_{n/I}$ and $T_{c/s}$ ratios are found in patients with advanced or progressive disease.

Cytolytic functions

The measurement of nonspecific lymphocyte-mediated cytotoxicity has been employed with increasing frequency as part of the general assessment of immune competence in patients with solid cancers. In general, cytotoxic activity (most often NK activity) was depressed in cancer patients, particularly those with metastatic disease, but clear correlations have not been identified between impaired function and clinical stage of disease [287, 549, 591, 336]. For example, 31% of 51 patients with solid tumors had depressed NK activity of PBMC, compared with 7% of normal donors [591]. When patients with metastatic disease were considered separately, this number increased to 50%. On the other hand, in one study of patients with clinically localized breast cancer, a wide range of NK activity comparable to that seen in healthy individuals was observed [164]. Among 83 women with primary untreated breast cancer, however, one-third exhibited poor NK activity [136]. No decrease in NK activity could be detected in 72 patients with metastatic lung cancer prior to treatment [484]. Other studies in early lung cancer show similar NK activity of PBMC to that observed in nonsmoker normal control donors [311]. Additional studies in patients with small-cell lung cancer and stage I and II malignant melanoma have found an inverse correlation between NK activity and amount of clinically detected tumor [175]. Similarly, NK-cell activity was more likely to be depressed in stage II breast cancer than in stage I disease [330].

A large study of 247 cancer patients showed that circulating NK cell numbers, assessed by monoclonal antibody methods, were significantly reduced in patients with colon, lung, and breast cancer, but not in those with melanoma or sarcomas [30]. In contrast, in oral squamous-cell cancer, NK cell numbers were increased, possibly due to release of a tumor-derived soluble factor [166]. In a comparative study, NK-cell activity was higher in bronchoalveolar lavage cells of lung cancer patients than in those of control donors [437], but tumor-infiltrating lymphocytes exhibited depressed NK activity [13]. Thus, a depression of NK cell numbers could explain the depressed NK function reported in some, but not all, cancer patients. Other cytotoxic cell functional assays, such as antibody-dependent cellular cytotoxicity (ADCC) [108, 163, 360, 568, 595] and monocyte-mediated cytotoxicity [580], have been employed using PBMC from solid tumor patients, but little data are available, and correlations between functional activity and clinical stage of disease are lacking.

The relationship between NK activity and other measures of immunocompetence has been explored. A lack of association was found between DTHS reactivity to PPD and NK activity [445]. A comparison between TIL activity and PBMC revealed that TIL expressed diminished NK activity compared with PBMC [247]. In one study, although PBMC exhibited depressed NK activity, proliferative responses to PHA and in MLR were maintained [445]. This suggested that cytolytic and proliferative effector-cell mechanisms represent distinct functional entities.

Antibody formation
A variety of humoral immune abnormalities have been found to occur in association with solid tumors. A large study of 984 patients with nonhematopoietic cancers found no general trends, but did find increases in serum IgG and IgA in males with skin and lung tumors, increases in IgM in males with sarcomas and females with melanoma, decreases in IgM in patients with ovarian cancer, and increases in IgA in patients with oral, gastrointestinal, and uterine cancers [260]. Increased IgA has also been demonstrated in head and neck cancer [348, 605] and prostate cancer [6], but to date, no correlations have been observed between serum immunoglobulin level and clinical stage of disease. In a study of breast cancer and malignant melanoma, IgG and IgA levels were elevated, but there were no differences between patients with primary disease and those with metastases [125]. IgA has also been found to be elevated in all three stages of uterine cancer, with an elevation of IgG in stage I and a decrease in IgM in stage III [438]. Circulating IgE levels were low in patients with a variety of neoplasms in their early stages [269], and a marked decrease in the prevalence of allergy has been noted in patients with lung, breast, skin, gastrointestinal, urologic, and gynecologic cancers [172].

The serologic response to several different B-cell immunogens has also been studied in solid-tumor patients. Patients with nonlymphomatous malignancies were found to exhibit decreased specific antibody responses to *Salmonella* extract [325]. Patients with stage III squamous-cell lung cancer exhibited deficits in IgG and IgA production following immunization with *Helix pomatia* hemocyanin, a T-cell-dependent antigen [271]. A significant impairment in the ability of certain patients with solid tumors to produce both IgM and IgG antibody in response to primary challenge with monomeric *S. Adelaide* flagellin has been reported [325]. Both complete and incomplete primary antibody responses to heat-killed *Brucella* were reduced in patients with breast and lung cancer [593]. However, precise kinetic data for humoral antibody production in most patients with solid tumors are lacking, as are correlations between humoral immunity and extent of disease.

Phagocytic cell function
Other impairments of immune responsiveness in solid-tumor patients have been documented. For example, the inflammatory response of patients with advanced cancer is associated with a reduced capacity to mobilize monocytes [32, 150, 186, 190, 596]. Reticuloendothelial function in patients with breast and colorectal cancer is depressed [152]. Depressed monocyte chemotaxis has been correlated with disease stage for a variety of tumor types [78, 224, 531]. A detailed evaluation of monocyte function in 90 solid-tumor patients revealed abnormalities in patients with malignant melanoma, breast cancer, colorectal cancer, and head and neck cancer, but no consistent correlations could be identified between tumor type, monocyte defect, and clinical stage of disease [580]. Another study revealed increased monocyte phagocytosis and decreased mitogen reactivity in untreated patients with advanced colorectal cancer [482]. Polymorphonuclear leukocytes from patients with low-stage breast or colon cancer were found to exhibit subnormal cytotoxic activity, whereas those from patients with advanced disease exhibited greater-than-normal activity [102]. Thus, the precise role and relationship between phagocytic cell function and tumor burden are still not clear.

Correlations among immune cell numbers and function
A number of studies have attempted to find correlations between *in vitro* and *in vivo* abnormalities of immune cell numbers and function. For example, both *in vitro* PHA responses and *in vivo* DNCB reactivity were normal in patients with early bladder cancer, but significantly impaired in patients with advanced disease [109]. Similar correlations have been seen in patients with lung cancer [461] and breast cancer [397]. In contrast, in a study of 48 patients with lung cancer, LPRs were more often suppressed than were skin test responses [8], and no correlations between DNCB reactivity and *in vitro* immune functions were found in patients with head and neck cancer [238].

It has also not been possible to identify any consistent association between alterations in effector-cell numbers and function. For example, whereas a depression in absolute T-cell counts paralleled the depression of *in vitro* LPRs in patients with head and neck cancer [599] and urologic cancer [112], no such correlations were seen in patients with lung or breast cancer [275]. In this last study, sophisticated regression analyses were performed. It was concluded that although some cancer patients have depressed LPRs in association with low levels of T cells, others have depressed functional activity with completely normal T-cell levels.

Hematopoietic malignancies

Reed's report in 1902 that patients with Hodgkin's disease (HD) failed to react to tuberculin skin tests even if they were known to have had active tuberculosis [456] led to a vast number of immunologic studies for this malignancy. Many of the immune abnormalities first reported – for example, alterations of absolute lymphocyte counts, impairments of T-cell LPRs, and the presence of suppressor monocytes/macrophages – were subsequently also found in patients with a variety of other cancers. Even though the primary immune defects described in untreated patients with HD involve T-cell immunity, other defects have also been documented [289, 472] including impaired *in vitro* B-cell production of antibodies, phagocytic cell function, and NK-cell activity [178].

The clinical relevance of the T-cell immunodeficiency in patients with HD has been recognized for many years. Patients with HD have an increased susceptibility to infections associated with defective T-cell immunity, including *Pneumocystis carinii* pneumonia and viral infections such as herpes simplex, herpes zoster, and cytomegalovirus [22, 472]. In most of these studies, however, it has been difficult to assess the role of the treatment for HD (radiation therapy, chemotherapy) in exaggerating the T-cell immune deficiencies, since many of the infectious complications occurred only during or after the completion of therapy.

A number of studies have now attempted to correlate defects in T-cell functions with depression in T-cell numbers in untreated patients with HD [76, 117, 246, 502]. In general, no such relationships could be identified, although lymphocytopenia patients were more likely to exhibit impaired LPRs. There is an easily identifiable correlation between defects in immune responsiveness and clinical stage of disease, in that most immune abnormalities are more readily apparent in patients with advanced stages of disease (III and IV) than in those with localized disease (i.e., stages I and II). The immune abnormalities include cutaneous anergy, lymphocytopenia, and depressed T-cell LPRs. In one study, of the patients with stage I and/or II HD, 40% exhibited lymphocytopenia, 11% impaired reactivity to DNCB, and 46% impaired PHA responses [502]. In contrast, of the patients with stage III or IV disease, 63% exhibited lymphocytopenia, 33% impaired reactivity to DNCB, and 89% impaired PHA responses.

Immune deficiencies have also been shown to correlate with lymphoma subtype and extent of disease in the non-Hodgkin's lymphomas. These include impaired *in vitro* LPRs to mitogens [12, 234] and impaired *in vivo* DTHS responses [12]. In general, patients with high-grade lymphomas exhibit more profound abnormalities than those with more favorable histologies [283].

It has been very difficult to relate the extent of immunodeficiency to tumor burden in patients with cancers involving the bone marrow (e.g., leukemia, multiple myeloma) since, with the exception of multiple myeloma, staging systems based on tumor cell burdens do not exist. However, a wide variety of *in vitro* as well as *in vivo* abnormalities have been documented in patients with lymphoid and nonlymphoid leukemias [220, 231]. Furthermore, a spectrum of intrinsic functional abnormalities has been identified in B cells and also purified T-cell populations of patients with chronic lymphocytic leukemia and multiple myeloma [258, 270]. Both of these diseases are often associated with profound depressions of normal serum immunoglobulin levels and impaired ability to mount primary humoral immune responses.

Prognostic implications of immunosuppression

Since immunodeficiency generally correlates with the stage and extent of disease, and since stage and extent of disease are the most important prognostic indicators for any particular cancer, it is logical that the general state of immunocompetence and prognosis should be closely related. The potential importance for correlating immunocompetence and prognosis at the time of diagnosis or at the onset of therapy is obvious. Assessment of immune status could, in theory, help to select patients with a poor prognosis who might require more aggressive therapy than usual, or adjuvant therapy even if all disease appeared to be surgically excised. In a now classic study, it was observed that patients who could be sensitized to DNCB and freed of disease by surgery had a good prognosis, whereas those who were apparently freed of disease by surgery but could not react to DNCB had a poor prognosis and relapsed within 6 months to 1 year [615]. The DNCB responses of patients in the poor-prognosis group were identical to those of patients who were found to be inoperable at surgery. The two groups of patients were otherwise comparable with regard to type of tumor, extent of disease, and all other usual clinical prognostic factors. This report formed the basis for a number of subsequent studies attempting to correlate immunodeficiency with prognosis for previously untreated patients with solid tumors and hematopoietic malignancies. In many of the more recent studies, a battery of *in vitro* and *in vivo* immunologic assays has been employed in an attempt to identify multiple immune defects that could more accurately predict prognosis than single defects.

Solid tumors

Since 1970, there have been numerous attempts to correlate impaired DTHS skin reactions with prognosis. Associations between impaired DNCB reactivity and disease recurrence have been observed in lung cancer [327], head and neck cancer [238, 347, 483], gastrointestinal cancer [82], and breast cancer [160]. A number of reports have suggested that patients with or without metastases but without reactivity to DNCB have a poor prognosis [84, 91, 161, 290, 326, 347, 436]. Lack of reactivity to common skin test recall antigens has also been correlated with poor prognosis in breast [160, 349], lung [15, 267, 280, 327], gastrointestinal [382], urologic [364], and head and neck cancer [538, 599], although this has not been a universal finding [59, 315, 324, 380, 391, 426, 442, 494]. Several studies have subcharacterized patients with identical clinical stages of disease on the basis of impaired skin test reactivity to define further the relationship between anergy and prognosis. Such correlations have been found, for example, in patients with stage I [19] or stage III and IV [323] malignant melanoma, and in limited-disease small-cell lung cancer [280]. However, in another detailed study of 202 accurately staged patients with breast cancer, although DNCB-negative patients had a worse overall survival, when survival distributions of DNCB-positive and -negative patients with either primary operable or advanced breast cancer were compared separately, significant differences were not seen [315]. Thus, studies to date have yielded conflicting conclusions concerning the correlation between impaired *in vivo* immunity and prognosis.

Associations between poor prognosis and impaired *in vitro* LPRs have also been reported. For example, among 44 surgically resected Dukes B and C colon cancer patients, 90% of those with diminished PHA responses subsequently suffered recurrence [426]. In 35 stage I non-small-cell cancer patients tested postoperatively, those with depressed MLR had a shorter disease-free interval, and MLR was a better predictor of outcome than PHA response [104]. A similar study found that PHA and MLR both gave similar prognostic information [212], but other studies of breast cancer and malignant melanoma have not produced such correlations [100, 192, 315, 468, 488]. On serial monitoring of postsurgical patients with stage I or II non-small-cell lung cancer, clinical relapse was usually antedated by a decline in PHA responsiveness of PBMC along with the development of indomethacin-sensitive suppressor cells [85].

Studies correlating absolute lymphocyte counts or absolute T-cell levels with prognosis have provided conflicting results. Lack of correlations between absolute T-cell counts and prognosis has been reported in breast [315, 397], gastrointestinal [408], and lung cancer [147]. Several recent studies, each involving more than 150 breast cancer patients, found that high absolute circulating lymphocyte levels were associated with a poor prognosis [481, 521]. This contrasts with the generally held view that low lymphocyte counts are associated with a large tumor burden and a poor prognosis. In addition, a follow-up study in breast cancer patients indicated that a low pretreatment lymphocyte count with a steady rise after surgery carried a good prognosis, and vice versa [522]. On serial monitoring, a decrease in absolute T-cell levels has been associated with subsequent relapse in patients with lung cancer [147] and malignant melanoma [56]. High T-cell numbers have been associated with higher chemotherapy response rates for patients with lung cancer [631].

The use of multiparameter immunological assessments has not generally improved the ability to assess prognosis for previously untreated solid tumor patients, including those with head and neck [186, 238], breast [35, 141, 315, 349], gastrointestinal [382, 600], or lung cancer [138, 334], malignant melanoma [192, 562], or osteogenic sarcoma [509]. However, some investigators have developed predictive indices based on multiple immunological parameters. For example, in one study, an integrated score of immunocompetence based on various *in vivo* and *in vitro* assays showed that the recurrence of breast cancer was significantly higher in suboptimal (61%) as opposed to optimal (28%) responders [3]. Similarly, an immunological staging system based on absolute lymphocyte counts and serum immunoglobulin level was found capable of predicting the outcome off stage III head and neck cancer patients in 86% of cases [293]. However, in a report using logistic regression methodology, it was demonstrated that only the level of complement binding activity, which may reflect levels of circulating immune complexes, correlated with the likelihood of responding to induction chemotherapy [494]. No associations could be determined between response to chemotherapy and abnormalities of a variety of other immune parameters, including lymphoproliferative responses, NK activity, lymphocyte subset numbers and percentages, and serum immunoglobulin levels.

Hematopoietic malignancies

Among the hematopoietic malignancies, most attention has focused on correlating defects in T-cell immunity with prognosis in HD. In one early study, the ability to develop DTHS to PPD following BCG immunization was associated with an improved 3-year median survival compared to nonconverters [532]. In subsequent studies, no relationships were found between depressions of DTHS reactions to recall antigens, or of PHA responses, and prognosis [117, 132, 630]. However, several more recent reports suggest that there is a correlation between extent of immune dysfunction and prognosis. In 33 untreated patients with HD, a lymphocyte score based on decreases in T-cell numbers, increases in spontaneous DNA synthesis of PBL, and depressions in mitogen responses correlated with response to treatment [63]. A detailed analysis of 35 untreated patients using logistic regression methods concluded that a general assessment of immunocompetence provides better prognostic information than that derived from a combination of stage B symptoms and histopathology [170]. Another study comparing a wide range of immune parameters with prognosis in 47 untreated patients with HD concluded that the prognostic information supplied by age and LPR in MLR exceeded the predictive value of any combination of clinical parameters [582].

Relationships between immunocompetence and prognosis have also been reported for a variety of other hematopoietic tumors. For example, in acute leukemia, patients with showed DTHS skin reactivity and, to a lesser degree, *in vitro* blastogenic responses to mitogens exhibited the best overall survival, outranking such prognostic variables as age, type of leukemia, and absolute blast cell count [232, 233]. In chronic lymphocytic leukemia, both cell-mediated and humoral immune functions have been found to correlate with prognosis [64, 130]. While DTHS was only moderately decreased, diminution in antibody responses and PHA responses correlated with the duration of disease, status of therapy, degree of lymphocytosis, and immunoglobulin levels [130]. A correlation has been reported between depressed absolute circulating NK-cell levels and poor prognosis in patients with large-cell lymphoma [39]. Patients with high-grade lymphomas who have high levels of serum IL-2R have been shown to have more advanced disease [446] and a worse prognosis [592]. However, in this instance, the IL-2R is synthesized by the tumor cells so that serum levels parallel tumor cell bulk. Nevertheless, the predictive value of soluble IL-2R was superior to that of other markers that reflected tumor cell bulk such as lactic dehydrogenase level (LDH) or clinical stage [446].

Perioperative immunosuppression

Although it is perhaps not universally recognized, the operative procedure and its associated general anesthesia result in a variety of transient immunological defects that can persist for several weeks after surgery. During operative procedures under general anesthesia for a variety of benign and malignant conditions, patients exhibit inhibition of skin reactivity to DNCB [556] and DTHS recall antigens [527], suppression of circulating T-cell levels [299], diminished LPRs to PHA and other mitogens [49, 51, 285, 418, 464, 465, 477, 527], and depressed NK activity [336, 493, 498, 558, 559]. Patients with cancer appear more likely to experience these periods of postsurgical immunosuppression than do patients who undergo surgery for benign conditions. Among the conditions associated with the greatest degree of postoperative immunosuppression are intraabdominal and intrathoracic procedures, blood transfusions, and longer operating times [477].

Perioperative blood transfusion

Several studies have suggested that perioperative blood transfusion, possibly by inducing a greater degree of immunosuppression, results in an adverse effect on prognosis for postoperative patients with colorectal cancer [244], breast cancer [560], non-small-cell lung cancer [557], prostate cancer [226], and soft-tissue sarcoma [473]. However, three recent studies in breast cancer [590], colorectal cancer [612], and lung cancer [296] have not confirmed initial reports. Thus, it has not been conclusively proven that perioperative blood transfusions worsen the prognosis of patients with cancer. It is possible that the requirement for transfusion is a marker for other risk factors such as advanced stage of disease, need for more extensive operation, or greater blood loss during surgery, thus accounting for the worse prognosis following surgery.

The precise mechanisms for postoperative immune suppression have not been fully defined. Among the considerations are the immunosuppressive effects of surgical stress [135], or of the anesthetic agents themselves [556], a relative decrease in circulating T-cell levels compared with other cell types [199, 198], and/or the generation of suppressor cells [493, 390]. In nonsurgical patients, chronic blood transfusion is associated with depressed $T_{n/I}/T_{c/s}$ ratios and impaired NK activity. Theoretically, the associations between perioperative blood transfusion and earlier cancer recurrence, and between prolongation of renal allograft survival and transfusion, may be attributed to a transfusion-induced immune suppression resulting from a graft-versus-host reaction mediated by transfused T-lymphocytes. Although the precise mechanisms to explain perioperative immune suppression have not yet been defined, this well-documented abnormality has nevertheless formed the basis for a number of therapeutic trials in which various putative immunorestorative agents have been administered as surgical adjuvants.

Radiation therapy-induced immunosuppression

The immunological effects of external-beam radiation therapy have been delineated in detail. Radiation therapy to a variety of portals, including mediastinal [146, 298, 335, 402, 542], pelvic [70, 335, 407, 449, 542], head and neck [196, 273, 335, 402, 417, 528, 538, 604], lymphoid [182, 203, 471], and breast [34, 209, 335, 449, 478, 570, 609] portals, results in similar acute and chronic changes characterized by a generalized lymphocytopenia involving primarily a depletion of circulating T cells as well as marked depressions in various T-cell functions such as *in vitro* LPRs to mitogens and antigens and *in vivo* DTHS reactions [290].

The depression of T-cell numbers and function occurs progressively with radiotherapy. The magnitude of immune depression reflects both the dose of radiation received and the volume of tissue, blood, lymph, or bone marrow included within the radiation portals. This acute immune suppression is short-lived, and substantial recovery is apparent within 3 weeks of cessation of therapy. However, most patients show a modest chronic depression in both numbers and functions of T cells, which may last for years following the completion of radiotherapy.

A number of other observations have been made concerning the mechanism of functional immune impairment following radiation therapy. Mediastinal irradiation for treatment of localized lung cancer has been associated with a decrease in proliferative responses of purified peripheral blood T cells, suggesting that radiation directly impairs their functional capabilities [504]. Several studies have assessed the effects of radiotherapy on T-cell subset proportions. Although there was a drop in the absolute numbers of both helper and cytotoxic/suppressor T-cells following mediastinal irradiation, the drop in cytotoxic/suppressor T-cells was greater, so that treatment resulted in a significant increase in the $T_{h/I}/T_{c/s}$ ratio [504]. These observations are consistent with *in vitro* functional data indicating that suppressor T-cells are more radiation-sensitive than helper T cells [202, 432]. In contrast, radiotherapy for patients with breast cancer [276, 431], head and neck cancer [272, 626], and Hodgkin's disease [440, 471] has been associated with a relative increase in the proportion of T cells bearing surface antigens and/or Fc receptors (IgG) of cytotoxic/suppressor cells, leading to a decrease in the $T_{h/I}/T_{c/s}$ ratio. Indeed, in postradiotherapy patients with breast cancer [431] and Hodgkin's disease [203], helper T-cell levels remained low for years after irradiation.

Several studies have assessed the influence of therapeutic irradiation on suppressor cell function. They indicate that radiation therapy can activate suppressor monocytes [68, 73, 342] as well as increase the sensitivity of lymphocytes to the suppressive effects of prostaglandins [342].

External-beam radiotherapy, such as pelvic [219, 407, 449, 542, 543] or chest wall [69, 449, 542, 543, 570, 609] radiotherapy, has also been associated with a decrease in B-cell and NK-cell numbers and functions in many, but not all, reports. Mediastinal irradiation more severely depressed NK activity than treatment to nonmediastinal sites [362], possibly reflecting the relatively large volume of blood and/or lymph node volume included within the mediastinal radiation portal, leading to damage of NK cells, or their more radiation-sensitive precursor cells. However, within 3-4 months following the completion of radiotherapy, NK-cell activity returned to pretreatment levels, which then persisted for at least 2 years [72]. There was a partial recovery in B-cell function, which remained below pretreatment levels for 12-18 months after completion of therapy [479, 544]. Reports concerning the effects of radiotherapy on absolute blood monocyte levels have been conflicting [570, 602]. Other immunological parameters have not been significantly affected. For example, radiotherapy did not produce changes in serum immunoglobulin levels or neutrophil function [219]. However, the ability of monocytes to differentiate into macrophages was impaired in breast cancer patients treated by radiotherapy [561], and absolute monocyte levels increased after treatment [570], whereas pelvic radiotherapy produced a decrease in both monocyte numbers and functions in patients with colorectal cancer [602].

In the earlier literature it was not possible to correlate the extent of radiotherapy-induced immunosuppression with relapse or survival [146, 397, 504, 509, 608]. In general, however, patients who exhibited skin reactivity to DNCB prior to radiotherapy had a better prognosis than those who did not [84]. In two more recent studies of patients who received primary radiation therapy for breast cancer [543, 608] and/or cervical cancer [543], those who exhibited the greatest postradiotherapy depressions of LPRs to mitogens or antigens had the shortest survival [608]. Several studies on postradiotherapy patients with lung cancer have serially assessed the immune status of those who responded transiently to treatment but relapsed at a later date [146, 147]. Lung cancer patients who responded clinically to radiotherapy showed some improvement of absolute T-cell levels in the months following cessation of treatment, whereas those who progressed did not show such partial recovery [146]. In addition, for postradiotherapy patients with locally advanced non-small-cell lung cancer, there was a gradual and progressive decrease in T-cell and helper T-cell percentages, and in the $T_{h/I}/T_{c/s}$ ratio that preceded relapse [504].

Chemotherapy-induced immunosuppression

It has been much more difficult to assess the effects of cancer chemotherapy than of radiation therapy on immune responsiveness. In part, this is due to the fact that a wide variety of different cancer chemotherapy drugs are available for clinical use, many of which can be administered by a variety of routes and doses, either alone or in combination with other drugs. The majority of anticancer drugs produce a dose-dependent pancytopenia, which itself is immunosuppressive because of the associated granulocytopenia. In addition, most, if not all, cancer chemotherapy drugs exhibit immunosuppressive properties as assessed with conventional *in vivo* and *in vitro* assays. This includes the alkylating agents, antimetabolites, and antitumor antibiotics.

The direct immunosuppressive effects of cancer chemotherapy drugs probably reflect their biochemical interactions with effector cells, as well as with immunoregulatory cells. Any drug that interferes with DNA, RNA, or protein synthesis should inhibit the proliferative activity of the cells responsible for immune reactions. For example, both alkylating agents, which act at the level of the DNA template, and antimetabolites, which act on enzymes involved in DNA synthesis, should in theory impair proliferative activities of lymphocytes. The immunosuppressive effects of single drugs and combination chemotherapy regimens result from a summation of effects on the various cell types involved in generating immune responses.

Cancer chemotherapy may lead to profound depressions of cellular as well as humoral immunity [223, 229, 235]. Newly acquired DTHS and primary humoral immune responses appear to be more sensitive to drug-induced immunosuppression than are secondary responses. Less often, the administration of selective drugs, for example, cyclophosphamide (CTX), at low doses can lead to a temporary enhancement of immune responsiveness due to preferential inhibitory effects on suppressor cells.

Traditionally, it has been felt that intermittent chemotherapy schedules of administration using single or multiple drugs tend to be associated with relatively little effect on DTHS responses and with transient depressions of lymphocyte numbers, *in vitro* LPRs, antibody responses, and inflammatory responses, with at least some recovery several weeks after discontinuation of treatment [232, 454]. In contrast, continuous therapy, if given in adequate doses, has been shown to lead to a progressive decline in all phases of immune reactivity [183, 229, 232, 361, 454], which is reversible after the cessation of administration of drug(s). In several more recent studies, however, it has been demonstrated that intermittent combination chemotherapy regimens lead to cumulative depressions of lymphocyte numbers and functions over months to years [344, 545], which may or may not be reversible. These changes include depressions of absolute T- and B-cell levels, depression in the $T_{n/I}/T_{c/s}$ ratio, and depressions of LPRs to mitogens and antigens.

Another phenomenon that has been described is the recovery or transient rebound overshoot of immune responsiveness after a single cycle of chemotherapy [87, 118, 222]. Rebound is found in patients who are responding clinically to treatment. Patients whose immune functions remain suppressed either have not responded clinically to treatment or are at high risk for relapse compared with those who exhibit recovery to levels above those pretherapy. It has been suggested that the rebound overshoot in immune reactivity following chemotherapy may be due to a reduction in monocyte suppressor cell function [87]. The effect can result from a transient, chemotherapy-induced decrease in relative numbers of monocytes/macrophages, from a reduction in suppressor cell function on a per-cell basis, or from a combination of both. Recovery of suppressor monocyte/macrophage function is responsible for the eventual decline in immune function following drug-induced rebound overshoot.

Antimetabolites

All of the antimetabolites commonly used for treating cancer patients, including thiopurines such as 6-mercaptopurine (6-MP) and 6-thioguanine (6-TG), antifolates such as MTX, fluorinated pyrimidine analogs such as 5-fluorouracil (5-FU), cytosine arabinoside (Ara-C), and DTIC (5-[3-3-dimethyl-1-triazeno]-imidazole-4-carboxamide) are immunosuppressive in humans. 6-MP has been one of the most extensively studied agents [229, 235, 328]. Azathioprine, a nitroimidazole derivative of 6-MP, is a potent immunosuppressive drug, and has found more use in clinical transplantation than as a cancer chemotherapy drug [373]. 6-MP, 6-TG, MTX, and 5-FU have all been shown to preferentially depress primary antibody responses and the development of new DTHS reactivity [235, 373, 375, 376]. However, 5-FU treatment restored DTHS to recall antigens such as PPD, mumps, and trichophytin [67, 375], but caused a transient decrease of *in vitro* LPRs to PHA and PPD [401]. Intravenous 5-FU produced a rapid (within 1-2 days) decrease in absolute T- and B-lymphocyte levels, which returned to baseline over the ensuing 1-3 weeks [169]. Ara-C has been shown to partially suppress primary and secondary antibody responses [376]. Although both MTX and Ara-C abolished established DTHS to recall antigens, Ara-C was much more potent in inhibiting DNCB reactivity [376]. *In vitro* MTX did not affect the phagocytic or cytolytic activities of human neutrophils [279]. DTIC has been considered only weakly immunosuppressive in humans, based on studies in patients with malignant melanoma in which only a minority of treated patients exhibited depressions in antibody production to typhoid vaccine or in DTHS reactions to primary sensitization [95]. More recent studies with DTIC have indicated that treatment is associated with a cumulative decrease of T-cell numbers, but no change in B-cell numbers [57]. A normalization of $T_{n/I}$ cell numbers occurred after cessation of treatment.

Alkylating agents

The alkylating agents comprise a variety of drugs including cyclophosphamide (CTX), nitrogen mustard (HN2), chlorambucil (CLB), thiotepa (TT), and busulfan (BS). These compounds have found widespread clinical use, particularly for the treatment of leukemias and lymphomas. Their antiproliferative effects also extend to normal host hematopoietic precursor cells of all lineages, including lymphoid precursors. In animals, these agents are potent immunosuppressants of antibody formation [489].

Recent clinical interest has focused on the novelty of CTX as an immunomodulatory agent [38, 158, 223, 229, 235, 354, 412]. The immunologic effects of CTX and other oxazaphosphorines such as mafosfamide have recently been reviewed [239]. Phosphoramide mustard and 4-hydroxy CTX are considered to be the major active metabolites and mediators of the antitumor effects of CTX. Administration of oral daily CTX maintenance therapy to patients with lymphomas did not result in interference with the development of normal humoral and cell-mediated immune response to keyhole limpet hemocyanin. Other studies have revealed that prolonged oral therapy with CTX can produce lymphopenia and suppress *in vitro* LPRs to PHA. CTX administered intravenously at conventional doses for 7 days inhibited the production of primary antibody responses, but did not significantly interfere with DTHS. Low intravenous doses of CTX (100-600 mg/m^2) preferentially decreased circulating B-cell numbers. Doses from 200 to 600 mg/m^2 selectively depleted cytotoxic/suppressor T cells, leading to a transient increase in the $T_{n/I}/T_{c/s}$ ratio, whereas higher doses affected all T-cell subsets equally. Intravenous administration of conventional doses of CTX for 5 days has been shown to depress established DTHS by 7-10 days after the cessation of therapy, at a time when the peripheral white blood cell count was at its nadir.

Perhaps the most intriguing aspect of CTX-induced immune changes has been the elucidation of the selective immunopotentiating effects of CTX [158, 354]. For example, in a study of 22 patients with metastatic cancer, CTX pretreatment significantly augmented the development of DNCB reactivity as well as DTHS to new antigens [45], even though absolute lymphocyte counts fell within 1-2 days and did not recover for 21 days [48]. The T-cell, B-cell, and T-cell subset numbers were all affected equally. Lymphoproliferative responses to mitogens and alloantigens also fell significantly within a day, but recovered to pretreatment levels by day 3; some cases exhibited rebound overshoot by day 7. Inducible T-cell suppressor cell activity was also diminished within 1 day after CTX administration; however, in contrast to LPRs, suppressor-cell activity remained significantly impaired on day 3 and only partially recovered by day 7. Thus, between 3 and 7 days after intravenous administration of CTX, there appears to be a preferential impairment of nonspecific T-cell-mediated suppressor cell activity, which could account for the augmented DTHS noted in CTX-treated patients. Most recently, a single intravenous low dose (300 mg/m^2) of CTX was shown to inhibit the generation of inducible suppressor cell activity in cancer patients for up to 19 days without affecting lymphoproliferative responses to T-cell mitogens or the $T_{n/I}/T_{c/s}$ ratio [47]. This CTX dose (300 mg/m^2) 3 days prior to immunotherapy has been employed clinically in a variety of circumstances in an attempt to abrogate suppressor cell activity, for example, as an adjunct to active specific immunotherapy with a melanoma tumor cell vaccine [44], and in combination with low-dose intravenous IL-2 [374]. Although the mechanism by which CTX augments the immune response has not yet been elucidated, the leading hypothesis, at present, is an abrogation of suppressor-cell function, with blockage of the subset of helper T-cells that is the inducer of suppressor cells, that is, CD4+, 2H4+ T-cells [158].

It is clear that CTX is not the only cytotoxic drug that can augment immune responsiveness. In animals, a variety of agents including thio-tepa, mitomycin, adriamycin, 5-FU, vincristine, and MTX could augment the development of DTHS to an antigen given 4 days later [354].

Antitumor antibiotics

Surprisingly, clinical information concerning the immunosuppressive effects of this class of anticancer drugs that includes such widely employed drugs as adriamycin (ADR), daunomycin (DNR), mitomycin (MTC), and bleomycin (BLEO) is limited. However, in animal models, these agents affect a variety of immune cells, in particular, macrophages and immunoregulatory cells [158, 370], suggesting that they should exert a spectrum of immunomodulatory effects in humans. On the other hand, ADR has been shown to augment both monocyte- and lymphocyte-mediated cytotoxicity of human PBMC [20, 21, 308]. Following a single intravenous dose (25 mg/m^2), PBL from cancer patients showed an increase in lymphocyte cytotoxicity as well as an increase in $T_{c/s}$ levels [20]. In cancer patients, intravenously administered ADR has been shown to produce a rapid but reversible lymphocytopenia of both T and B cells [169]. *In vitro*, ADR has been shown to impair phagocytic function of human polymorphonuclear leukocytes [585], whereas similar effects were not seen with a variety of other drugs, including MT, VCR, 5-FU, and cisplatin. In addition, ADR has also been shown to inhibit granulocyte degranulation and release [101]. Some evidence has been provided that low doses of ADR can also augment both T- and B-cell mediated immune responses [158]. Thus, it now appears as if ADR, like CTX, can exhibit a variety of immunomodulatory activities.

Vinca alkaloids

The vinca alkaloids, vincristine (VCR) and vinblastine (VLB), possess a unique mechanism of antitumor activity involving drug-induced microtubular dysfunction leading to mitotic arrest. VCR has been shown to depress granulocyte aggregation, lysozyme release, and chemotaxis [101, 536]. However, there remains a substantial lack of studies concerning the immunomodulatory effects of these agents in humans. They are often administered in conjunction with steroids as treatment for hematopoietic cancers, making it impossible to define their selective immunosuppressive effects. Not unexpectedly, they inhibit human LPRs *in vitro*, and they should exert similar effects *in vivo*. Both VCR and VLB have not been particularly immunosuppressive in humans [230]. Vindesine, a new semisynthetic vinca alkaloid, was devoid of immunosuppressive activity in preliminary clinical trials [462].

Other drugs

Other frequently employed anticancer drugs, such as cisplatin, nitrosoureas (BCNU, CCNU) and taxol also exhibit varying degrees of immunomodulatory activity when incubated *in vitro* with human PBMC [536], but clinical data are sparse. Single intravenous doses of cisplatin have been associated with a rapid depression of LPRs, with recovery in 1-2 days, whereas a single dose of CCNU leads to depressed PHA responsiveness for up to 6 weeks, in the absence of changes in T- and B-cell proportions. Long-term therapy with CCNU has been associated with cumulative depressions of absolute levels of both and T cells [57]. The reduction of T-lymphocyte levels was due mainly to a depletion of $T_{n/I}$ cells. One dose of methyl-CCNU did not markedly affect antibody production to a variety of antigens of DTHS reactions to recall antigens in resected patients with malignant melanoma [46].

Hormones

Hormonal agents such as tamoxifen (TAM) and medroxyprogesterone acetate (MPA) are used widely in the treatment of breast cancer. Both estrogen and progesterone receptors have been identified in human lymphocytes [127, 139]. There is considerable experimental and clinical evidence suggesting that hormones can modulate immune mechanisms [124, 402, 413]. Long-term treatment of patients with TAM has not produced significant immunosuppression [278, 492], whereas MPA depressed LRPs as well as the $T_{n/I}$ $T_{c/s}$ ratio of treated patients [492].

Combination chemotherapy

When multiple cancer chemotherapy drugs are administered together, it is impossible to predict what effects their interactions will have on their individual immunosuppressive properties. Nevertheless, at the present time, most cancer chemotherapy regimens include a combination of drugs. A number of recent studies have begun to define the immunological consequences of combination chemotherapy as currently used for the treatment of patients with advanced disease, as well as for patients treated in the adjuvant setting.

A comparison of intravenous doses of single drugs, namely ADR and 5-FU, with combinations such as COBAM (CTX, VCR, BLEO, ADR, MTX) or DOMF (DTIC, VCR, methyl-CCNU, 5-FU x 5) revealed that both the single agent and multiagent regimens produced a rapid drop (within several days) in the percentage and absolute numbers of circulating B and T cells, which was more pronounced for the combined drug regimens [169]. Such decreases were transient, and either a partial or complete recovery (with or without rebound) to baseline levels was then observed over the 1 or 2 weeks after drug administration [169]. Similar acute effects of multiagent chemotherapy regimens have been noted with respect to functional immune parameters such as *in vitro* LPRs [87], B-cell activation [254], reticuloendothelial cell function [151], and cytotoxic cell (NK) activity [89, 485]. In general, there has not been a good correlation between the depressions in immune cell numbers and functions. In addition, it has been found that if immune functions such as LPR are markedly depressed prior to administration of chemotherapy, for example, in patients with advanced breast cancer, then no further reductions are noted following treatment [282]. The temporal difference in effects of combination chemotherapy on lymphocyte numbers versus functions probably reflects the combined influences of chemotherapy on effector cells, as well as on immunoregulatory cell functions.

Cyclic combination chemotherapy can result in cumulative immunosuppressive sequelae [344, 430, 545]. Three similar studies have all involved patients receiving cyclic adjuvant chemotherapy for breast cancer who did not exhibit evidence of immune suppression before treatment. Serial immune assessments revealed that cyclic chemotherapy was associated with a marked initial (within a month) decrease in T- and B-lymphocyte numbers, and then gradual progressive further decreases [545], the same being observed in $T_{n/I}$ $T_{c/s}$ ratios [430]. There was also a rapid initial decrease in functional immune parameters, such as *in vitro* LPRs to antigens, with stabilization or some improvement over the ensuing year of treatment. In general, the functional immunological parameters tended to normalize during or, more often, within several months of stopping chemotherapy, whereas the abnormalities of immune cell numbers were still apparent 1 year after cessation of treatment [344]. Thus, it appears that prolonged administration of cyclic combination chemotherapy results in cumulative impairments of immune cell numbers and functions, some of which are long-lasting [480, 545]. In contrast, a study of 75 patients who received adjuvant chemotherapy with CTX and ADR, or MTX and 5-FU with or without local radiotherapy, failed to show any changes in NK activity over time after initiation of treatment [330]. In none of these series could it be established that depressed immune parameters, either before or after therapy, could predict on an individual patient basis who was more likely to relapse.

Immune status of patients in clinical remission

A number of studies have evaluated the immune status of patients in remission following the successful treatment of their cancer. In general, there tends to be improvement and/or normalization of immune cell numbers and function for patients who achieve clinical remission following chemotherapy or radiation therapy. Nevertheless, some immunologic impairments persist for years after completion of successful treatment. Thus, in many cases, it may be extremely difficult to dissociate the chronic immunologic consequences of therapy from the presence of persistent immune defects while in clinical remission.

Solid tumors

Patients surgically cured of their cancers generally have a restoration of immune cell numbers and function after the perioperative periods [49, 51, 285, 299, 418, 465, 464, 477, 493, 527]. Although patients in clinical remission following potentially curative radiation therapy may have some normalization of immunity, it does not usually become apparent until years after the completion of treatment [407].

In nonrandomized trials of irradiated patients with cervical cancer, T- and B-cell numbers were found to normalize at 5 years after therapy, whereas defects in LPRs and DTHS reactivity persisted despite the maintenance of clinical remission [219]. Similar long-term defects in immune cell numbers and functions have been observed in irradiated patients with head and neck [273, 417, 525, 555, 601, 626] and breast cancer [478, 544, 570]. Selective decreases of helper T-cell numbers of in the $T_{n/I}$ $T_{c/s}$ ratio were noted on long-term follow-up [196, 219, 478]. Finally, as discussed previously, it has also become apparent that adjuvant chemotherapy for breast cancer results in cumulative depressions of both lymphocyte numbers and functions [344, 430, 545].

Hematopoietic malignancies

Much important information concerning the long-term effects of chemotherapy and radiation therapy in cured patients has resulted from studies of children who received maintenance chemotherapy for acute lymphoblastic leukemia and of adult patients with HD. In acute lymphoblastic leukemia patients who remained in clinical remission for 1-3 years after completion of chemotherapy, immune competence was found to recover. Those patients destined to relapse showed a subsequent deterioration in immune status, which was detectable some months before clinical relapse [195, 232, 514]. The immune status of patients with HD in long-term clinical remission after treatment with chemotherapy or radiation therapy has also been evaluated in detail. At the completion of radiotherapy, DNCB reactivity was lost in almost all patients who were initially sensitive. However, many patients regained their DTHS responses during the first year after discontinuation of chemotherapy [7, 117, 466] or radiotherapy [182, 467]. NK-cell activity also improved following successful therapy for HD [178].

Several studies have shown that, following the completion of successful MOPP chemotherapy, patients in remission from HD exhibited gradual improvements of *in vitro* T-cell functions [7, 466]. In contrast, other studies have revealed a persistent depression of LPRs at 1-10 years after the completion of treatment, with no evidence for recovery [61, 62, 107, 171, 207, 467], along with a preferential chronic depletion of $T_{n/I}$ cells [203, 319, 440, 466, 471]. In some of these studies, patients had received radiation therapy, which was felt possibly to contribute to the prolonged immune deficiency [182, 203, 440, 471]. Several authors have argued, however, that patients with HD in prolonged clinical remission continue to manifest immune abnormalities as a reflection of their underlying disease [61, 62, 107, 171, 319]. For example, persistent defects in T-cell functions were more severe in irradiated patients with HD than in similarly treated patients with testicular cancer [62, 471]. Although some improvements were noted on serial immune assessments following discontinuation of treatment, there have been no correlations between the status of immunity during clinical remission and likelihood of relapse [466, 467]. It has been suggested that an increased sensitivity of T-cells to the inhibitory effects of suppressor cells may account for the persistent depressions of T-cell functions in cured HD patients [584].

TREATMENT OF CANCER-ASSOCIATED IMMUNODEFICIENCY

The term immunotherapy was introduced to clinical oncology two decades ago following the independent observations that *Bacillus Calmette-Guerin* (BCG) administration could prolong the survival of patients with acute lymphoblastic leukemia [355] and induce regressions of injected as well as noninjected malignant melanoma lesions [387]. Since these reports, a wide variety of chemicals and biologicals have been administered to immunosuppressed cancer patients in the hope of reconstituting or boosting host immune mechanisms (Table 1). A broader term, biotherapy, is now being used since there are many biological substances that stimulate cells outside of those from the immune system. These stimulations with colony stimulating factors, growth and maturation factors may have secondary effects on cancer and immune function.

Table 1. Biological response modifiers with immunorestorative properties

Chemicals	Biologicals
Azimexone	Bestatin
Cimetidine	FK-565
Copovithane	IMreg-1
Coumarin	ImuVert
DTC	Interleukin 1-15
Ibuprofen	Interferon gamma
Indomethacin	Lentinan
Interferon inducers	OK-432
Isoprinosine	Retinoids
Levamisole	T-Cell reconstituting factor
NPT 15392	(SR 270258)
Oxyphenbutazone	Thymic factors
Piroxicam	Transfer factor
Ranitidine	Tuftsin

Immunorestorative agents

Chemicals

Levamisole, an orally active synthetic phenylimidazole, 2, 3, 5, 6-tetrahydro-6-phenyl-imidazol[2, 1-6]thiazole, is the levo isomer of tetramisole, a potent, broad-spectrum antihelminthic agent introduced in 1966 [564]. The demonstration in mice that tetramisole could augment the protective effect of a *Brucella* vaccine [460] led to widespread clinical investigation of the immunomodulatory activity of both tetramisole and levamisole. In various animal models, and also following *in vitro* incubation with effector cells from human donors, levamisole has been found to increase both T-cell numbers and functions (e.d., LPR), if initially depressed [450, 627], as well as phagocytic and chemotactic activities of polymorphonuclear leukocytes and monocytes [121]. Its immunorestorative mechanism of action is currently unknown. It has been shown to induce thymic factor-like activity, which has been attributed to the presence of a sulfur atom in its structure [204]. Levamisole, which contains an imidazole ring, may function like imidazole in affecting enzymes that control cyclic nucleotide levels in lymphoid precursors of lymphocytes. Both imidazole and levamisole, which themselves are not mitogenic, elevate cyclic GMP levels in lymphocytes *in vitro* and enhance their proliferative responses to mitogens or foreign antigens [121].

Only a limited number of dose- and schedule-seeking trials for cancer patients have been performed with levamisole. In general, it has been administered intermittently, using two or three daily doses every 1-2 weeks [9]. The drug is well absorbed, and a single oral dose of 150 mg produces a peak plasma level in 2 h (0.49 + 0.05 μg/ml), which is the concentration required for *in vitro* activity. The plasma half-life of levamisole is 4 h. It is widely distributed and can be detected in all tissues and fluids, with the highest levels in liver and kidneys. It is excreted primarily in the urine, most of it by 24 h, although much of the excreted product has already undergone extensive metabolic changes.

A number of side effects of levamisole have been reported [547]. In studies on 3900 patients with a variety of diseases (including rheumatic and inflammatory diseases and cancer), reactions included idiosyncratic or allergic ones, such as a rash or febrile influenza-like illness, sensorineural reactions such as alterations of taste and smell, and gastrointestinal symptoms. Rashes and fever resulted in the cessation of levamisole treatment in 7% and 1.5% of cases, respectively, but were quickly reversible. The major serious side effects have been agranulocytosis and/or neutropenia and, less commonly, thrombocytopenia, which have been observed in between 0.2% and 2% of all treated patients. Agranulocytosis could not be related to dose or schedule of administration, and was always spontaneously reversible following discontinuation of treatment [9]. The incidence of side effects in various clinical trials has varied from insignificant to major, requiring interruption of therapy in up to 21% of cases [419].

Isoprinosine (IPS), a synthetic antiviral agent, is a complex of inosine and the *p*-acetamidobenzoate (PacBA) salt of *N, N*-dimethylamino-1-propanol (DIP) is a 1:3 molar ratio [121, 204]. In early clinical trials with rhinovirus-infected humans, IPS increased the titers of circulating antiviral antibody, suggesting it had B-cell immunomodulatory activity [533]. Subsequent *in vivo* studies in animal models and *in vitro* studies with human PBMC have indicated that IPS enhances T-cell functions such as LPR to mitogens and alloantigens [121, 204, 386]. Helper T cells appear to be the main target for the drug in humans. IPS has also been shown to induce the appearance of T-cell surface markers in mouse prothymocytes, similar to that of thymic factors, as well as increase the proportions of various T-cell subpopulations following incubation with human PBMC. *In vitro*, IPS at a concentration of 100 μg/ml restored LPRs, NK activity, and monocyte chemotaxis of PBMC isolated from cancer patients [574]. Because the immunomodulatory activity of IPS is similar to that of a variety of thymic factors, it has been classified as a thymomimetic drug.

Although IPS has been investigated clinically in several different viral diseases (including human immunodeficiency virus [HIV] infections), only a limited number of studies have been performed with cancer patients [121, 564]. Extensive tolerance and safety studies have been conducted in which IPS was administered orally for periods of 1 week to 2 years at doses of 1-8 g/day. Minimal side effects have been noted, including transient rises in serum and urine uric acid levels and, occasionally, transient nausea associated with higher daily dosages. Following oral or intravenous administration to rhesus monkeys, the inosine moiety of IPS is rapidly metabolized, with a half-life of less than 4 h.

The presence of a purine moiety in IPS suggests that inosine itself may be the active molecule responsible for its immunorestorative activity. It is possible that the availability of inosine and its metabolic products is responsible for an optimization of DNA synthesis during cell proliferation, a requirement for most T-cell immune responses.

Azimexone (BM 12.531) is an orally active aziridine dye, 2-[2-cyanaziridinyl-(1)-2-[2-carbamoylaziridinyl-(1)]-propane, which has been found to increase the number of cytotoxic autoreactive cells. It exhibits antitumor activity in animal models [58, 121, 204] and exerts a variety of immunomodulatory effects on T cells, monocytes, phagocytic cells, and NK cells. Azimexone has exhibited immunorestorative activity in various animal models of infectious diseases. *In vitro* studies using PBL from advanced cancer patients revealed that azimexone at various concentrations (0.2-10 μg/ml) enhanced the LPR to PHA with a maximal effect at 0.2 μg/ml. Other studies have indicated that azimexone also enhances the percentage of activated T lymphocytes *in vitro*.

In a limited number of clinical studies performed to date, the only significant side effect observed with intravenous administration has been a dose-dependent self-limiting hemolysis [422]. Oral absorption of azimexone is almost complete, and the serum half-life is 6 h.

Histamine receptor antagonists

Cimetidine *N'*-cyano-*N*-methyl-*N'*-2-[(5-methyl-imidazol-4-yl)methylthio:]ethylguanidine] is a histamine type II receptor antagonist widely used for the treatment of gastrointestinal ulcers. A growing body of evidence has suggested that suppressor T cells that possess histamine receptors (H2 type) may play an important immunoregulatory role in normal immunologic responses [94, 165, 409]. The rationale for administering H2 blockers to cancer patients is based on the observation that cimetidine could abrogate *in vitro* histamine-induced suppressor T-cell activity using human PBL. Histamine has been shown to suppress human LPRs to mitogens, and cimetidine might block the inhibition. Recently, results of *in vitro* preclinical testing with cimetidine have been summarized [358]. It has been shown to augment LPRs and IL-2 production of PBMC from cancer patients to mitogens and alloantigens [162, 317, 358]. *In vitro* cimetidine also enhances NK-cell activity of PBMC from cancer patients, probably through its inhibitory effects on suppressor cells [173]. No effects have been seen on transformation of peripheral blood monocytes to macrophages [187]. Cimetidine has been employed in ai phase I/II study [552] and in combination with coumarin [351, 565, 566]. Varying degrees of antitumor activity have been noted in patients with malignant melanoma [565, 566] and renal cancer [351] treated with the combination of cimetidine plus coumarin. The mechanism of antitumor activity has not been established but the doses used are approximately 2x that for treatment of ulcers.

Nonsteroidal anti-inflammatory and antipyretic agents (NSAID)

Indomethacin and ibuprofen are prototype inhibitors of prostaglandin synthesis. A large number of *in vitro* studies using PBMC from patients with solid tumors and HD have suggested that (a) the depressed LPRs of cancer patients result, at least in part, from the immunosuppressive effects of prostaglandins released by activated monocytes/macrophages, and (b) indomethacin is capable of abrogating the suppressor cell influence. In addition, it has been shown *in vitro* that indomethacin also acts directly on T cells of patients with malignant melanoma to augment mitogen responsiveness [567]. It has been postulated that this direct immunomodulatory action results from specific pharmacologic effects such as alteration of intracellular cyclic AMP levels. Finally, a correlation has been observed between tumor spread and content of prostaglandin E2 of the tumor [43]. These observations have formed the basis for administering prostaglandin inhibitors to cancer patients [103, 441, 616].

NPT 15392

Studies with IPS suggested that the inosine moiety might be responsible for its immunomodulatory activity on LPRs. Subsequently, a number of purines with inosine-like structures were synthesized, one of which is NPT 15392 (9-erythro-2-hydroxy-3-nonylhypoxanthine) [174, 204, 628]. In animals, NPT 15392 has exhibited effects on T-cell and monocyte/macrophage functions and T-cell differentiation similar to those of the parent compound [174]. Toxicological studies have shown that it is nontoxic at oral doses up to 35 mg/day. This drug has recently entered clinical trials in cancer patients [628].

DTC, sodium diethyldithiocarbamate (Immunothiol), was developed as a result of preliminary studies with levamisole in an attempt to synthesize a chemically defined sulfur-containing compound that would be la more potent immunorestorative agent than the parent compound [204, 459]. DTC is a chelating agent in use for the treatment of heavy-metal poisoning. In animal models, it exhibits a variety of immune-augmenting effects on T-cell dependent immune responses as well as on the induction of T-cell differentiation. No significant toxicity has been noted following long-term administration. Clinical trials have recently been started in cancer patients and in patients with HIV disease.

Coumarin (1, 2 benzopyrone) has been reported to exhibit immunomodulatory activity [53, 635]. Unlike warfarin, coumarin is devoid of anticoagulant activity. In cancer patients, coumarin administration was reported to enhance LPRs to PHA but did not effect T-cell numbers [53]. *In vitro* coumarin has augmented HLA DR expression and NK activity [635]. It has been administered in combination with cimetidine to patients with malignant melanoma [565, 566] and renal cancer [351] with varying degrees of antitumor activity reported. The mechanism of antitumor activity of the combination has not been established.

Copovithane (BAYi7433) is a copolymer of 1, 3-bis(methyl amino carboxy)-2 methylene propane carbamate, has exhibited antitumor activity in a variety of pre-clinical models [500]. A phase I trial in advanced cancer patients using weekly intravenous dosing revealed minimal fatigue, and occasional nausea and proteinuria, as the only side effects, some antitumor effects, and some improvements in $T_{n/I}/T_{c/s}$ and *in vitro* toxicity responses and LPRs [255].

Biologicals

Thymic factors

A functioning thymus gland is an essential requirement for the normal development and maintenance of cell-mediated immunity [191]. The thymus is responsible for the normal maturation of all the various subclasses of T-lymphocytes, including various effector cells, as well as immunoregulatory cells. The thymus exerts its influence during the ontogenesis of the immune system of releasing, in situ from its epithelial stroma, a variety of differentiating factors that induce the maturation of resident pre-T stem cells (thymocytes) into mature T cells, which ultimately circulate in the peripheral blood and lymph. It is now well established that the thymus gland is an endocrine organ and that at least several of its locally released differentiating factors are also secreted into the bloodstream. Thymic hormone-like bioactivity has been demonstrated in the blood of animals and humans. This activity decreases following thymectomy, as well as with age, in parallel to the physiological age-dependent involution of the thymus. More recent evidence also indicates that the presence of the thymus is important well into adulthood in order to maintain immune T-cell mechanisms.

A number of factors with thymic hormone-like activity have been prepared from thymus tissue and blood, and these are in varying stages of characterization [191, 505]. The best studied are thymosin fraction 5 (TF5), thymosin α_1 (Tα_1), prothymosin α (Pro Tα), thymostimulin (TP-1), thymulin (FTS-Zn), thymopoietin (TP), thymic humoral factor (THF), and thymic factor x (TFX). These agents all exhibit a broad spectrum of immunorestorative effects on T-cell numbers and functions in animal models and humans. In some bioassays, many of the well-characterized thymic preparations have identical, or even opposite, effects. An increasing number of thymic factors have been employed therapeutically in treating a variety of diseases – predominantly cancer and HIV disease.

The well-characterized thymic preparations are listed in Table 2 [191, 210, 505]. Among the thymic factors that have been administered to cancer patients are TF5, Tα_1, TP-1, THF, and TFX. Both TF5 and TP-1 are partially purified extracts of calf thymus glands. They include a mixture of different biologically active as well as inactive polypeptides. The purification procedures for TF5 and TP-1 are similar but not identical. TF5 consists of 10 major – and at least 30 minor – polypeptides on analytical isoelectric gel focusing with molecular weights ranging from 1000 to 15,000. The first biologically active polypeptide isolated from TF5 is Tα_1. Biologically active Tα_1 has a molecular mass of 3108 daltons. It has been synthesized by classical chemical, solid-phase, and recombinant DNA techniques, but only the chemically synthesized material has been employed in clinical trials. Thymopoietin, THF, and TFX are purified thymic peptides with molecular weights ranging from 3220 to 5562. TP-5 is a biologically active synthetic pentapeptide that represents amino acids 32-36 of thymopoietin. In contrast to all other thymic preparations, thymulin (FTS-Zn) has usually been isolated from pig blood rather than thymus tissue. Although thymulin, Tα_1, and thymopoietin are all detectable in the blood, only thymulin levels drop significantly following thymectomy, and are restored by thymic grafts.

None of the well-characterized thymic peptides exhibit any significant homology with the other characterized peptides. However, a 50% homology has recently been identified between a 35 amino acid region of Tα_1 and that of the p17 core protein of the AIDS retrovirus (HIV) [491].

Thymic factors, which have been administered to more than 1000 cancer patients, have shown minimal toxicity. The purified preparations that have been administered by intramuscular or subcutaneous injection have not produced any significant side effects [191, 505]. Partially purified bovine preparations, such as TF5, have produced rare (less than 1%) allergic reactions and erythema and/or pain at the sites of injection in about one-third of treated patients. However, potentially immunizing treatment schedules, such as daily injections for 1 week followed by 3 weeks of rest, and reinstitution of treatment, have been associated with a high (10%) incidence of anaphylactoid-like reactions. As a single agent, TF5 has exhibited minimal antitumor activity in patients with renal cancer in one study [507] and none in another [149].

Table 2. Chemical properties of thymic hormones

Name	Chemical properties
Thymosin fraction 5 (TF5)	Heat-stable, acidic Peptides MW 1000-15,000
Thymosin α_1 (Tα_1)	Peptide of 28 residues, MW 3108
Prothymosin α (Proα)	113 Amino acids, MW 13,500
Thymosin α_9	Acidid peptide, MW 2000, pl 3.5
Thymosin α_{11} (T α_{11})	Peptide of 35 residues, 28 residues identical To Tα_1
Thymosin β_3 (T β_3)	Peptide of 49 residues, MW 5700, 43 residues Identical to Tβ_4
Thymosin β_4 (Tβ_4)	Peptide of 43 residues, MW 4963
Thymic factor X (TFX)	Mixture of peptides; active compound is a peptide, MW 4200
Thymostimulin (TS/TP-1)	Mixture of peptides
Thymulin (FTS-Zn)	Nonapeptide, MW 857,
Thymic humoral factor (THF)	Peptide MW 3200
Thymopoietin (TP)	Peptide of 49 residues, MW 5562

T-Cell reconstituting factor (pre-albumin; SR 270258)
This is a highly purified protein fraction isolated from human serum that has been shown to exhibit immunomodulatory effects on T-cell numbers and functions [394]. In preliminary phase I/II trials, no unexpected toxicities have been observed following SQ administration.

TsIF is a thymic isolate, distinct from other thymic factors and cytokines, that induces immature bone marrow cells to differentiate into competent suppressor T cells. It has a molecular mass of 75,000 daltons as determined by gel filtration and high-performance liquid chromatography. Recent studies in mice indicated that TsIF administration suppresses the development of autoimmune disease in lupus-rheumatoid arthritis-prone animals [371].

Transfer factor

In 1955 it was demonstrated in humans that the transfer of DTHS to streptoccal M substance and tuberculin could be accomplished by administration of a suspension of leukocytes disrupted by either distilled water or repeated freeze-thaw cycles [322]. The substance (or substances) responsible for this transfer was resistant to RNAase and DNAase and was termed *transfer factor*. This initial work was extended using dialyzable human leukocyte extracts from patients sensitized to various antigens [25], including skin allograft antigens [537]. The crude dialyzable preparation has subsequently been shown to enhance LPRs *in vitro* [24, 156]. The further chemical characterization of transfer factor has been hampered by the lack of a unique biological assay to monitor final purification. Preliminary fractionation studies of human leukocyte extracts capable of transferring DTHS responses have indicated that transfer factor is probably a low-molecular-weight material (approximately 1000) with the electrophoretic mobility of slow γ-globulin but with no reactivity to anti-immunoglobulin antisera. Its possible composition, that is, a short polypeptide chain joined with a three- or four-base segment of RNA, has been difficult to verify. Unlike other nonspecific immunorestorative BRMs, transfer factor appears to exert antigen-specific immune-restorative effects.

Despite the lack of readily reproducible *in vitro* or *in vivo* assays, the effects of transfer factor have been studied following subcutaneous administration to patients with a variety of immunodeficiency diseases, including cancer [384].

Interleukins

Many of the BRMs currently being synthesized by recombinant DNA techniques are products of lymphocytes (lymphokines), monocytes (monokines), or other cells (cytokines). Various interferons and interleukins have been purified to homogeneity produced by genetic engineering to make large quantities available for clinical trials. Various other cytokines are undergoing active clinical investigation. The characteristics and results of clinical trials with these materials are discussed elsewhere in this book. It is noteworthy, however, that of the lymphokines IL-2 has the potential to act as an immunorestorative agent [205]. The perioperative administration of low-dose recombinant α-interferon has also recently been shown to prevent the postoperative impairment of NK activity, but not of IL-2 production [513].

Retinoids

Considerable interest has recently been focused on the influence of vitamin A (retinol) and its natural and synthetic derivatives ('retinoids') on the growth and differentiation of neoplastic cells. Although retinoids have been administered to cancer patients primarily as chemopreventive agents [79, 337], accumulated evidence also indicates that they have beneficial effects on the host immune system. For example, in animals they have been shown to restore PHA responsiveness, to induce augmentation of cytotoxic and helper T-cell numbers and functions, and to inhibit prostaglandin synthesis by host tumor-activated macrophages. However, the role that altered immune mechanisms play in the chemopreventative action of retinoids, such as 13-*cis*-retinoic acid, remains unclear.

FK-565 [heptanoyl-8-D-Glu-(L)*meso*-α_1-A_2pm(L) AlaOH] is a heptanoyl tripeptide analogue of FK-156, a biologically active acylpeptide isolated from fermentation products of *Streptomyces*. Preclinical studies in mice have shown that FK-565 augments NK-cell activity and macrophage functions as well as T-cell functions both *in vitro* and *in vivo* [551]. However, in animals, mitogen-induced IL-2 production is decreased [4]. Clinical trials in cancer patients are underway.

Bestatin [(2*S*, 3*R*)-3-amino-2-hydroxy-4-phenylbutanoyl-L-leucine] is a low-molecular-weight immunomodifier found in supernatants of *Streptomyces olivoreticuli* [356]. It is a competitive inhibitor for the enzymes aminopeptidase B and leucine aminopeptidase. These enzymes are associated with the outer membranes of most mammalian cells, including lymphocytes. In animal models, bestatin augmented both humoral as well as cell-mediated immune responses [65, 74], particularly in immunosuppressed mice. Macrophage activation, but not NK activity, was also observed both *in vitro* and *in vivo* [550]. It has also been shown to enhance T-cell numbers and cytotoxic functions following *in vitro* incubation with human lymphocytes, but it has not significantly influenced LPRs [74]. It has been shown to augment phagocytic cell function *in vitro*.

Bestatin has now been chemically synthesized and is available for clinical trials. The drug has been well tolerated in cancer patients at daily doses of 30 mg for up to 2 years [65, 74, 400, 629].

Tuftsin is a naturally occurring tetrapeptide (Thr-Lys-Pro-Arg), found normally in human and animal plasma, and represents residues 289-292 of the heavy chain of γ-globulin [121, 157, 395]. It is released enzymatically from a protein carrier (Leukokinin) and is capable of activating various functions (particularly phagocytosis) of polymorphonuclear leukocytes and monocytes/macrophages, T-cell cytolytic activity, and IL-2 production at physiologic concentrations [137, 356]. It has also been shown to enhance antibody production to thymic-dependent as well as thymic-independent antigens in animals and Ia-suppression. It has also been able to reduce tumor necrosis factor in animals [624].

Lentinan is a purified polysaccharide obtained from the extracts of the edible mushroom *Lentinus edodes* [71, 404]. Chemically, lentinan is a β-(1, 3)-glucan with some β-(1, 6)-glucoside side chains. It has a molecular weight of about 500,000. Evidence has been presented that lentinan is a T-cell adjuvant, but a variety of immunomodulatory activities have been observed [119, 356]. In animal models, it has been shown to augment antibody production only in the presence of T cells. It has also been shown to augment a variety of cytotoxic effector-cell mechanisms following administration to animals and to trigger production of various kinds of serum factors including IL-1, CSF, and IL-3 [119]. *In vitro*, it activates monocytes/macrophages and NK-cell activity of PBMC from cancer patients but does not enhance LPRs or LAK-like cytotoxicity [288].

OK-432 is a heat-killed substrain of *Streptococcus pyogenes* that has been studied extensively in Japan. OK-432 predominantly acts by augmenting NK-cell activity [410, 588, 594], as well as augmenting macrophage [294] and T-cell [245] cytotoxicity. It has also been shown to induce various cytokines such as interferon, IL-1, and IL-2 [264, 399, 486]. A variety of phase I, II, and III studies have been performed in cancer patients in which it has been administered intradermally [115, 217, 369, 594], intramuscularly [217], or intralesionally [588]. The major toxicities have been fevers and local inflammatory reactions at injection sites.

ImuVert is prepared from the bacterium *Serratia marcesseus*. Its primary components are vescicles derived from the bacterial membrane and ribosomes [607]. It augments natural killer-cell activity and has antitumor cell activity in animals. It is currently in clinical trials in patients with malignant gliomas and other cancers.

Imreg-1 is a natural, leukocyte-derived immunomodulator containing two low-molecular-weight peptides: a dipeptide (tyrosine-glycine) and a tripeptide (tyrosine-glycine-glycine). *In vitro* Imreg-1 enhances the production of various cytokines, including IL-2 [194]. Clinical trials to date have been limited to patients with HIV disease.

Treatment of cancer-associated immunosuppression: phase I and II studies

Most of the agents described in the preceding section have already been employed therapeutically in patients with cancer. Of the chemical BRMs, levamisole has been by far the most exhaustively studied, whereas among the biologicals, the interleukins have received the most attention. No organized approach has been employed for the clinical evaluation of the immunorestorative BRMs. In general, a small phase I or phase II study to assess the tolerability and immunomodulatory effects of the agent in advanced cancer patients has been followed by phase III trials with random experimental designs in which survival was the end point and immunological monitoring was minimal, or even omitted. Thus, it has been difficult to make any firm conclusions concerning the immunorestorative properties of these agents in cancer patients.

A number of preliminary small-scale phase I and II studies have indicated that levamisole [121, 331, 379, 396, 611], isoprinosine [121, 386, 439], azimexone [58, 422], bestatin [74, 316, 357, 400, 613, 629], OK-432 [578, 594], retinoids [367], NPT 15392 [628], DTC [459], coumarin [53], various thymic factors [191, 505], lentinan [265], cimetidine [317, 358, 463, 552], and transfer factor [537] could improve T-cell, NK-cell, or B-cell numbers and/or functions in advanced cancer patients with pretreatment abnormalities. In general, however, the effects have not been striking. When administered to patients *without* immunodeficiencies, however, therapy was often followed by a deterioration of immune competence. In several reports, no immunomodulatory effects of levamisole were observed on T-cell numbers or functions [242, 611]. A recent study of patients with colorectal cancer suggests that the major *in vivo* effect of levamisole is augmentation of monocyte chemotaxis [197]. Of the thymic factors, THF and TFX have been employed predominantly in patients with infectious complications, and reports have been mostly anecdotal, TF5, Tα_1, THF, and TP-1 are currently being prepared by pharmaceutical companies, and large quantities are available for more extensive clinical trials. Cimetidine has increased an *in vivo* local graft-versus-host reaction of advanced cancer patients [552]. However, in other studies, it had no effects on immune cell numbers or functions, or on DTHS [345]. Similarly indomethacin has been of only limited utility in restoring immunity in advanced cancer patients [241]. The administration of cimetidine or ranitidine to advanced cancer patients has been associated with improvements in performance status [98]. In one study, treatment with the combination of coumarin plus cimetidine increased the percentage of monocytes and of DR+ monocytes of treated patients [352].

Multiple single and repetitive doses of TF5 and Tα_1 [529] were studied following subcutaneous or intramuscular injection, and detailed immunological studies were performed. No clear-cut dose or schedule of administration could be identified as optimal. Overall, of the patients treated with a single dose of TF5 or Tα_1, 28.4% and 18.3%, respectively, of abnormal immune parameters were improved following treatment, whereas 16% of initially normal responses became abnormal. Most of the responses occurred within 24 h and did not persist for more than 72 h. In this study, an optimal immunorestorative dose of TF5 could not be identified, but a dose of 1.2 mg/m^2 of Tα_1 was associated with substantial improvement in 46% of the initially abnormal immune parameters [148].

Another approach to identifying the clinical effectiveness of putative immunorestorative agents has been to evaluate their immunologic effects in phase I/II studies using homogeneously immunosuppressed patients with similar cancers who were either untreated or were in clinical remission following successful therapy.

Chemicals

Hodgkin's disease
HD has been chosen because of the well-documented abnormalities of T-cell immunity that are present prior to treatment and that persist in patients during clinical remission. Levamisole has been shown *in vitro* to enhance T-cell proportions [50, 451] among PBMC of HD patients. Treatment of patients with HD in remission for less than 2 years after the completion of radiotherapy resulted in improvement in T-cell percentages and functions [329]. Twenty patients in remission were treated with 150 mg daily for 3 consecutive days and every 2 weeks, for 3-6 months. The proportion of patients exhibiting positive skin tests increased from 13% to 48%; DTHS reactions and PHA responses also increased [50]. Continuation of treatment beyond 3 months led to a slight but consistent decline of these parameters.

Solid tumors
A pilot study has been performed with levamisole in surgically resected patients with malignant melanoma and squamous-cell carcinoma of the head and neck [62]. Patients treated with levamisole (150 mg orally twice a week) for 6 months exhibited improvements in absolute circulating T-cell levels, and only 1 of 8 melanoma patients treated with levamisole relapsed. Based on these results, large-scale phase III were designed, the results of which have been reported as negative in one and marginally positive in the others [448, 535].

Chronic lymphocytic leukemia
Patients with this disease have been treated with levamisole [26]. No effects on immune cell numbers or functions were seen, and levamisole administration was associated with a high rate (46%) of clinical and hematologic adverse reactions.

Biologicals

Hodgkin's disease
In one study, nineteen consecutive untreated patients with HD received TP-1 at a dose of 1 mg/kg daily for 7 days, and immunological monitoring was performed prior to treatment and again on day 8 [353]. A majority of untreated patients exhibited depressed T-cell percentages as well as depressed DTHS and LPRs to PHA. The mean T-cell percentage increased significantly, from 47% to 55.7% (normal is 58.9%) following treatment with TP-1, whereas the mean PHA response improved but did not totally normalize. Similarly, DTHS responses to recall antigens were positive in 53% of patients before therapy, and in 95% after therapy. The patients most likely to respond to TP-1 were the most lymphopenic, for whom an *in vitro* enhancing effect of TP-1 was observed on T-cell percentages and LPRs of PBMC prior to therapy. In a similar study, 15 patients with HD (in remission and off therapy for at least 1 year) were treated with 50 mg TP-1 by daily intramuscular injections for 60 consecutive days [332]. For patients with initially depressed T-cell numbers, including depressed helper ($T_{n/I}$) cell numbers, reconstitution to normal occurred within 30 days after the onset of therapy, but returned to pretreatment levels after the discontinuation of therapy. There was also a significant increase in NK activity, but *in vivo* DNCB reactivity did not become positive in any patient who had been negative prior to treatment. In a more recent report from the same group, 19 patients in remission for at least 6 months were randomized to receive TP-1 at 50 mg IM daily, every other day for 35 days, or no treatment [333]. Patients who received TP-1 were then maintained on TP-1 twice weekly. Before treatment, patients exhibited depressed percentages and absolute numbers of circulating T cells and $T_{n/I}$ cells. Following 5 weeks of daily TP-1, the proportions and numbers of all T-cell subpopulations increased significantly, while alternate-day treatment was not as effective. Maintenance TP-1 therapy did not produce any further improvements in T-cell or B-cell numbers or proportions. PBMC from some patients also exhibited improvements in mitogen-induced lymphokine production (e.g., IL-2, IFN-γ), but the improvements were not statistically significant overall. No significant changes were observed in a variety of serum markers including neopterin and β2-microglublin. It was concluded that TP-1 has the potential to expand the T-cell pool, and, in particular, $T_{n/I}$ cells, in patients with HD in remission, but that intensive (daily) induction therapy is required. In this small sample, no conclusions could be established between immune reconstitution and likelihood for relapse or development of second malignancies or other infections. Large-scale clinical trials were recommended to answer these questions.

Malignant melanoma
TP-1 has been studied in a novel random-design trial involving 32 patients with localized stage I malignant melanoma who were rendered disease-free following surgery [55]. Subjects were selected from a cohort of 211 postsurgical patients who were monitored at 3-month intervals in the first 2 years after surgery. In prior work, it was demonstrated that patients who developed low circulating T-cell levels were at high risk for relapse. Patients who either exhibited presurgical depressions of total T-cell numbers or on serial monitoring developed a depression of absolute circulating T cells to less than $1000/mm^3$ were considered eligible for random assignment to one of three treatment arms: TP-1 alone (25 mg IM once a week, 8 patients); chemotherapy alone (DTIC, 200 mg/m^2 intravenously for 5 days, repeated monthly, 8 patients); or no further therapy (16 patients). In the 8 patients who received TP-1, T-cell numbers began increasing within 3 days after the first injection, and weekly immunological monitoring revealed that levels returned to normal and were maintained at that level. Only inconsistent effects on T-cell functions were seen in the group that received TP-1, and no changes were observed

in any parameter in patients who were untreated or who received chemotherapy. Overall survival was better for the TP-1 group, but the improvement was not statistically significant.

On the basis of these results, two random-design, large-scale, phase III trials were initiated with TP-1 in early-stage melanoma patients. One multicenter United Kingdom trial is accruing 160 patients [403]. In this study, TP-1 administration (50 mg IM, twice a week) is begun before surgery in an attempt to prevent any transient surgery-related immunosuppression. After surgery, TP-1 is continued once weekly for a total of 6 months. However, in contrast to the pilot study, no prescreening is being performed to select patients with low T-cell numbers.

Chronic lymphocytic leukemia (CLL)

Patients with Cll have also been treated with TP-1 [318]. TP-1 significantly increased $T_{n/I}$-cell proportions, leading to an improvement in the $T_{n/I}/T_{c/s}$ ratio accompanied by an increase in LPRs to PHA and helper-cell function. In this study, the *in vitro* incubation of purified T-cells with TP-1 did not produce modifications of subset proportions or of immune functions. In contrast, *in vitro* incubation of T-cells with $T\alpha_1$ from patients with stable-phase CLL led to an increase in T-cell proportions and an improvement in T-cell functions [42].

Phase II/III surgical adjuvant studies

Chemicals

Lung cancer

The vast majority of large-scale phase III surgical adjuvant studies have been performed with levamisole. Two randomized, double-blind trials in patients with non-small-cell lung cancer have been reported [10, 16]. In the first trial, a fixed dose of levamisole was administered preoperatively for 3 days, and then for 3 days every 2 weeks [10]. Treatment was continued for 2 years or until relapse. Among 211 patients, although there was no difference in overall survival, levamisole treatment was associated with a reduction in distant metastases and in cancer deaths. When analyzed on the basis of adequacy of drug dosage, it was found that the greatest benefit of levamisole was seen with patients who received a daily dose of 2.1 mg/kg or more. The second study was designed as a confirmatory trial, and a weight-related dose of levamisole was employed, with a schedule identical to that in the original study [16]. Nevertheless, among the 217 evaluable patients, overall survival was decreased in those who received levamisole, because of non-cancer-related deaths in the perioperative period.

Gastrointestinal cancer

A number of surgical adjuvant trials of levamisole and other agents have been performed on patients with gastrointestinal malignancies. Recent evidence has indicated that levamisole is a useful and important new postoperative adjuvant therapy for patients with resected colon cancer treated with 5-FU.

In the early 1980s, results of several small-scale trials were reported that suggested that levamisole could prevent perioperative immune suppression. A British report in 1979 first indicated that the administration of levamisole on 3 postoperative days could accelerate the recovery of antitumor immunity (in an LMI assay) but not LPRs to PHA [623]. In a Japanese trial of 50 patients with colon cancer, 15 were treated with levamisole at a dose of 150 mg daily for 2 consecutive days, every other week, beginning 3 days before surgery. Treatment with levamisole appeared to prevent the postoperative depression of LPRs to PHA, as compared with a control group of patients, but did not affect DNCB reactivity [519]. A Belgian colorectal trial used levamisole (150 mg for 3 days every 2 weeks) in a matched group of patients operated on by the same surgeon. In both the overall group and the 40 patients with Dukes B2 and C cancers, survival was prolonged with levamisole [587]. Improved survival of resected patients was reported in a broad trial of 177 patients with various gastrointestinal cancers treated with levamisole [377]. There was also improvement in DTHS reactions and *in vivo* LPRs. Similar results from the Japanese literature have been reported for patients with advanced gastric cancer treated with levamisole [378].

An interesting recent report of a randomized trial involving 181 resected patients with gastric cancer showed an increase in median survival for patients who received cimetidine [572].

Phase III levamisole trials in colon cancer

Within the past several years, results of a series of phase III trial results have been reported, in which levamisole was administered alone, or in combination with adjuvant chemotherapy in patients with resected colorectal cancer [23, 33, 123, 266, 320, 321, 381, 516, 622].

A large-scale trial that was designed to compare treatment with levamisole to surgery only reported by the European Organization for Research and Treatment of Cancer (EORTC) Gastrointestinal Tract Cancer Cooperative Group [23]. This double-blind placebo-controlled trial involved 297 patients with Dukes C colon cancer. Levamisole dosage was based on body weight and ranged from 100 to 250 mg/day for 2 consecutive days each week for a period of 1 year. Treatment was started as soon as possible after surgery, usually within 2 weeks. With a median follow-up time of 3 years, no benefit was seen in disease-free survival for patients who received levamisole. Although the proportion of patients alive at 5 years was 51% in the levamisole group versus 39% in the placebo group, this difference was not statistically significant.

Other large-scale trials have now convincingly demonstrated that postoperative adjuvant therapy with levamisole plus 5-FU impacts significantly on survival of patients with colon cancer [266, 320, 321, 381]. Thus, levamisole plus 5-FU is now considered standard adjuvant treatment for resected Dukes C colon cancer.

The mechanism by which the combination of levamisole plus 5-FU led to improved survival in these trials has not been elucidated, and it is not clear that levamisole acts as an immunorestorative agent and/or whether it acts directly on tumor cells to enhance the antitumor activity of 5-FU.

Gynecologic and urologic cancer

Positive surgical adjuvant studies have been reported with levamisole in postoperative patients with cervical cancer [447] and bladder cancer [530].

Malignant melanoma

Only one study has focused on assessing in detail the immunorestorative effects of levamisole in patients with locally advanced malignant melanoma following surgical resection [277]. Levamisole was administered at 150 mg/twice weekly. No improvements were noted in T-cell numbers, or in LPRs to mitogens or antigens.

A large-scale phase III trial with levamisole involved 203 postsurgical patients with malignant melanoma. No improvement in either relapse rates or overall survival was noted in patients who received levamisole [535]. In stage I patients, there was a trend in favor of levamisole regarding time-to-recurrence and survival. More recently, a large study involving 548 patients with completely resected malignant melanoma having a poor prognosis (Clark levels 3, 4, or 5, greater than 0.75 mm, satellite lesions, in-transit metastases, or regional lymph node metastases) revealed that patients treated postoperatively with levamisole (2.5 mg/kg orally on 2 consecutive days weekly for 3 years) survived significantly longer than those who received either no postoperative therapy or weekly BCG, or a combination of BCG alternating with levamisole [448]. Median follow-up time for this trial was 5.1 years. In a randomized trial involving 156 stage I Clark level 3, 4, and 5 patients, there was a trend for a delay in appearance of distant metastases in patients receiving levamisole (30 months versus 9 months for patients receiving placebo), but overall survival was not significantly improved [338].

Head and neck cancer

A large, placebo-controlled randomized trial involving 134 patients did not reveal improvement in survival or immune competence for patients who received levamisole as an adjuvant [601].

Biologicals

Lung cancer

Several studies have focused on the effects of transfer factor administered as an adjuvant to surgery. A tumor antigen-specific preparation, prepared from household contact family members with positive reactivity to lung cancer antigen, was administered to 28 resected patients with non-small-cell lung cancer twice by subcutaneous injection. Treatment was associated with a significant improvement in a variety of specific as well as non-specific immune parameters, including DTHS reactions and LPRs to PHA [180]. In a randomized study of 63 postoperative patients with non-small-cell lung cancer (some of whom received mediastinal radiotherapy), those who received transfer factor from normal donors beginning 1 month after surgery and continuing every 3 months showed a significant improvement in survival at 2 years compared with nontreated patients [302].

Head and neck cancer

The impact of preoperative perilesional therapy with OK-432 was studied in 13 patients [588]. Treatment was associated with less pronounced decreases in NK activity of PBMC, and higher NK activity in draining lymph nodes, than in patients treated by surgery alone.

Malignant melanoma

TP-1, transfer factor [96], isoprinosine [439], and TF5 [505] have been administered to postoperative patients with malignant melanoma. Each of these trials involved random treatment assignments and varying degrees of immune monitoring. No adjuvant effects could be demonstrated in these small studies. The trial with TF5 was complicated by the fact that only 45 patients were allocated to treatment with either a low dose (4 mg/m^2) or high dose (40 mg/m^2) administered subcutaneously, concurrently with BCG, with or without DTIC chemotherapy. Results of a large-scale, randomized, double-blind phase III trial were recently reported that involved 168 resected patients with high-risk stage I and stage II malignant melanoma [372]. Therapy (normal donor transfer factor or placebo) was initiated within 90 days of resection and continued for 2 years. With a median follow-up period of 25 months, patients who received placebo exhibited a trend for improved disease-free survival and overall survival. Thus, this large-scale trial has indicated that normal donor transfer factor is not an effective postsurgical adjuvant therapy for malignant melanoma.

Treatment of radiotherapy-induced immunosuppression

Although a number of clinical trials using immunorestorative BRMs in irradiated patients have been reported, little information is available concerning whether or not treatment can prevent and/or reverse radiotherapy-induced immunosuppression.

Chemicals

Levamisole

Of the putative chemical immunorestorative agents, levamisole has been most extensively evaluated as an adjunct to radiation therapy. Since the larger trials have focused almost exclusively on survival as an end point, very little information has been obtained concerning its immunorestorative properties.

Several of the smaller trials have included serial immune monitoring. In a study involving 57 patients with colorectal cancer treated with surgery and radiation therapy, levamisole at a dose of 150 mg/day for 2 consecutive days every other week, beginning concurrently with postoperative radiation therapy, enhanced LPRs to PHA as compared with an untreated control group [321]; no effects were observed on DNCB reactivities. In a randomized double-blind study involving 71 postoperative patients with stage II breast cancer, 38% of those who received levamisole (2.5 mg/kg/day on 2 consecutive days, twice weekly, beginning with the initiation of radiation therapy) exhibited improvement in DTHS to at least three recall antigens, as compared with only 19% of those given a placebo [303]. Similar results were noted in an earlier trial using DNCB reactivity [470]. Thus, such studies suggested that levamisole may improve some aspects of T-cell functions in irradiated patients.

A number of large-scale cooperative group trials have now demonstrated that levamisole administration does not improve the survival of patients treated with radiotherapy. Four separate negative trials have been reported involving patients with non-small-cell lung cancer (NSCLC). The Southeastern Cancer Study Group reported that levamisole was without significant clinical benefit in ai large randomized, placebo-controlled trial of 251 patients undergoing radiotherapy for inoperable non-small-cell lung cancer [312]. In this study, levamisole was administered at a dose of 2.4 mg/kg twice weekly beginning at the initiation of radiotherapy. The median survival of patients treated with levamisole was shorter than that of those who received placebo. Negative results have also been reported in a SWOG similar trial [619]. The Radiation Therapy Oncology Group (RTOG) has recently reported results of two separate randomized, placebo-controlled trials, one involving 74 patients with resected NSCLC and positive lymph nodes [237], and a second involving 285 patients with unresectable tumors [429]. Levamisole (2.5 mg/kg on days 1 and 2, weekly) or placebo was initiated at the beginning of radiation therapy and continued for up to 2 years. Accrual to the first trial was terminated prematurely when survival data became available from the second study indicating a worse survival (9 months versus 12 months). Thus, it appears to be conclusively established that levamisole combined with radiation therapy has no benefit in the treatment of NSCLC. Another study in postradiotherapy patients with squamous-cell lung cancer employed levamisole in combination with BCG so as to make interpretation difficult [434].

In the randomized trial involving 71 stage II breast cancer patients treated with radiotherapy postoperatively, those who received levamisole exhibited a slight prolongation of disease-free survival [303]. Among postmenopausal patients, levamisole significantly increased both disease-free and overall survival, and the levamisole group showed fewer distant metastases as the first sign of recurrence. In another trial involving 150 patients randomized to postoperative radiotherapy, chemotherapy, or both with or without levamisole, patients receiving radiotherapy plus levamisole exhibited improved disease-free and overall survival [305, 306]. These results are in contrast to two other similar studies. In a randomized but not double-blind study, levamisole treatment was associated with an increased recurrence rate [140]. In a more recent report involving 198 patients with resectable axillary node-positive disease, levamisole, when begun following completion of postoperative radiotherapy, had no effect on either disease-free or overall survival [573]. Nearly a third of patients treated with levamisole had to terminate therapy prematurely because of toxicity (primarily leukopenia, skin rash, nausea, fever, and mucosal infection). It has been argued that differences in patient characteristics led to these discordant results.

In head and neck cancer, three recent reports from the same Italian group have indicated that radiotherapy led to a decrease in both T-cell numbers and functions (LPRs), and that treatment with levamisole accelerated the restoration of T-cell counts, compared to patients who received placebo [27, 28, 414]. With a median follow-up of 30 months, there was some improvement in disease-free interval for patients who received levamisole. Another similar trial failed to demonstrate an improvement in survival for patients with head and neck cancer treated with levamisole [406].

Isoprinosine

In a double-blind, placebo-controlled trial designed to evaluate the immunorestorative effects of isoprinosine following radiotherapy, one-half of 106 irradiated patients with breast, head and neck, or uterine cancers were randomly assigned to receive isoprinosine or placebo in discontinuous courses for 5 months. After 3 months of treatment, 64% of the isoprinosine-treated patients exhibited evidence of improvement of DTHS and *in vitro* functional tests, whereas only 23% of placebo-treated patients did [386]. No correlations have yet emerged between immune reconstitution and clinical status, but follow-up is continuing.

Prostaglandin antagonists

The nonsteroidal anti-inflammatory drug oxyphenbutazone was found to improve survival of patients with stage III cervical cancer when administered during radiation therapy [616]. This trial involved 160 patients. Thirty of 73 patients with stage III disease were treated with 100 mg oxyphenbutazone 3 times daily. Treatment was associated with an improved survival, but no studies were performed to assess the drug's effect on immune responsiveness.

Biologicals

Thymic factors
Several clinical trials with TF5 and $T\alpha_1$ have indicated that thymic factors may accelerate the reconstitution of T-cell functions following radiation therapy to head and neck or mediastinal portals. The first clinical trial involved 75 patients with localized but unresectable head and neck cancer [606]. Patients were randomly assigned to receive TF5 (60 mg/m^2) subcutaneously) in a loading dose (daily for 10 days, then twice weekly) schedule or no further therapy. Treatment with TF5 began concurrently with the initiation of radiotherapy and continued for a year or until relapse. TF5 administration did not prevent, nor could it restore, the marked T-cell lymphocytopenia that followed radiotherapy. Patients treated with TF5 exhibited a prolongation of disease-free survival, but of only borderline statistical significance.

Similar findings have been reported with $T\alpha_1$ in postradiotherapy patients with non-small-cell lung cancer [501]. This study was a double-blind, random-design trial involving 42 patients with localized, unresectable disease who had just completed a course of radiotherapy to the primary tumor and mediastinum. Patients who received mediastinal radiation were chosen specifically as the study population, based on an *in vitro* study, indicating that TF5 could increase T-cell proportions of PBMC from patients who had received mediastinal radiation to other portals [297]. Patients whose disease regressed or remained stable at the completion of radiotherapy were randomized to receive $T\alpha_1$ (900 μg/m^2 subcutaneously) either by a loading dose (daily for 14 days, then twice a week) or on a twice-weekly schedule; treatment began within a week after completion of radiotherapy. All patients exhibited a marked depletion in absolute circulating T-cell levels and in T-cell LPRs at the completion of radiation therapy. Serial immunological monitoring revealed that the patients who received $T\alpha_1$ had a complete normalization of T-cell function in MLR, which became apparent following 7 weeks of treatment. However, only patients treated on the twice-weekly schedule maintained normal $T_{n/I}/T_{c/s}$ ratios throughout the study period. The $T\alpha_1$ administration, however, did not influence absolute circulating T-cell numbers or T-cell subset numbers, and all treated patients remained lymphocytopenia over the 15-week follow-up period. These results were interpreted to indicate that more intensive schedules of $T\alpha_1$ administration are optimal for inducing restoration of T-cell functions, whereas less intensive schedules are optimal for maintaining immune balance of T-cell subsets.

In a recent study, lymphopenic patients with Hodgkin's disease in remission after receiving subtotal or total nodal irradiation with or without combination chemotherapy were randomized to receive either TP or TP-5. Both the thymic hormone and the synthetic were capable of inducing increases in both Tind as well as T c/s cells without changing the $T_{n/I}/T_{c/s}$ ratio. This was explained as a nonspecific effect on all lymphocytes. Such changes were only observed in patients with severe lymphopenia (<1000/mm^3). In addition, there was a significant decrease in the incidences of herpes virus infections compared to patients not receiving treatment.

Transfer factor
In a randomized, double-blind trial involving 100 patients with nasopharyngeal carcinoma, transfer factor (derived from young adults with a proven history of infectious mononucleosis and from normal blood donors with high anti-Epstein-Barr virus capsid antigen antibody levels) was administered for 18 months in conjunction with radiotherapy [188]. This trial was based on the association of Epstein-Barr virus with nasopharyngeal cancers. No significant effects of transfer factor were noted on disease-free and overall survival. Immune competence studies were not performed.

A recent study was reported involving 111 patients with NSCLC who had surgery followed by radiotherapy [99]. Twenty-six patients received transfer factor (normal donor) bimonthly beginning after RT was completed. Increased DTHS and a lower relapse rate were observed in patients who received transfer factor, but the small sample size of this trial precludes any definitive interpretations.

In a small randomized, placebo-controlled trial of 47 patients receiving radiotherapy with or without chemotherapy for Hodgkin's disease, DTHS skin responses were markedly enhanced in 22 patients who received transfer factor (prepared from normal donor buffy coat cells), but no improvements were noted in a variety of other immunologic parameters, nor in the prevention of infection, including varicella/zoster [218].

T-cell reconstituting factor
A pilot clinical trial has been performed in which this factor (pre-albumin or SR 27025) was administered by SQ injection (2 mg/m^2 TIW) for a month to 11 patients who had just completed radiotherapy for a variety of locally advanced solid tumors. A variety of immune parameters were followed serially and compared to those of five patients randomized not to receive treatment. Treatment produced a generalized lymphocytosis involving both $T_{n/I}$ and $T_{c/s}$ cell numbers, but no effects were noted on DTHS or LPRs at the dose and schedule employed [122].

Retinoids
Therapeutic and immune restorative effects of vitamin A have been evaluated in a randomized trial of 42 patients undergoing radiation therapy for inoperable cervical carcinoma [368]. Vitamin A palmitate was administered orally at a daily dose of 1.5x10^6 IU on days 1-5, 8-12, 16-20, and 23-27, and radiotherapy began on day 22 for 8 weeks. Vitamin A was well tolerated, although most of the 21 treated patients developed scaling of the skin. Serial immunological assessments were performed on some of the patients. No effects were found on DTHS reactivity, in

that only about 50% of patients reacted in both the treatment and control groups. Vitamin A treatment increased *in vitro* LPRs (albeit to a low degree) from pretreatment values, whereas the control patients showed no change or decrease in LPRs during radiation treatment. Thus, it was concluded that vitamin A administered concurrently with radiation could prevent the radiation-induced depression of at least one T-cell function.

Bestatin
Several studies have explored the *in vivo* effects of bestatin in irradiated cancer patients [66, 71, 75, 404]. In a prospective randomized trial, the clinical efficacy of bestatin was evaluated in 151 evaluable patients who had completed a course of local radiotherapy for bladder cancer. Patients were randomly assigned to receive 10 mg bestatin orally, 3 times daily, for at least 1 year, or no further treatment. The recovery of LPRs to PHA and PPD proceeded at an accelerated rate for 9 months in the bestatin-treated patients [75]. Patients treated with bestatin exhibited a greater percentage of circulating T cells after 1 month of treatment, but levels declined to control values within 3 months. Similar transient changes were noted in NK-like activity. It was concluded that the schedule or dose of bestatin was not optimal, and that either higher doses or intermittent schedules require evaluation. A recent update of the trial has shown that the bestatin-treated patients exhibited an improvement in disease-free survival compared to the radiotherapy-only group, but no improvement in overall survival [71]. The disease-free survival benefit was more apparent in patients with earlier stages of disease.

OK-432
A large multicenter trial in Japan randomized 382 patients with cervical cancer, stratified by presence or absence of surgery and clinical stage, to radiotherapy with or without intradermal OK-432 starting concurrently at 2-day intervals with the initiation of radiation treatment [115], and continuing biweely for 2 years. Patients who received OK-432 exhibited a decrease in 3-year recurrence rate, a more rapid restoration in DTHS to PHA, a-polysaccharide antigen, and peripheral blood lymphocyte counts than the control patients.

Combined-modality studies with chemotherapy

Three major problems in combined-modality studies (Table 3) have made it difficult to draw conclusions concerning the influence of putative immunorestorative agents on chemotherapy-induced immunosuppression: (a) the changing and varied combination chemotherapy regimens available for clinical use; (b) the lack of well-defined doses and schedules of administration for the immunorestorative agents; and (c) the almost universal omission of detailed serial immunologic assessments of patients receiving treatment. For the most part, these studies have emphasized conventional chemotherapy parameters as their end point, that is, tumor regression rates and overall patient survival, on the assumption that if improvements were noted in patients who received an immunorestorative agent, they would result from undefined immunomodulatory effects on the immune response.

Advanced disease

Three broad approaches are feasible for the treatment of advanced cancer patients with combined chemotherapy-immunorestorative therapy. The putative immuno-restorative agent could be administered concurrently with chemotherapy, following the completion of chemotherapy when clinical remission has been achieved, or during maintenance chemotherapy if it is continued. All three approaches have been applied, and most studies have employed levamisole and/or thymic factors.

Chemicals

Levamisole
This compound has been evaluated in several large-scale clinical trials as an adjunct to conventional chemotherapy, with mixed results. In general, levamisole has been administered as either 150-200 mg or 2.5 mg/kg on 2 consecutive days each week between chemotherapy courses. Serial immunological studies have usually not been performed. In 82 patients with metastatic colorectal cancer, survival of those receiving 5-FU and levamisole was significantly greater than those receiving 5-FU alone [83]. Improvements in response rates and/or survival have also been seen in patients receiving levamisole in addition to combination chemotherapy for advanced breast cancer [304, 307, 541]. In one study, an improvement in DNCB reactivity was noted with levamisole treatment; however, negative reports have also appeared concerning breast cancer [106, 421], colorectal cancer [97], non-small-cell lung cancer [116, 142], and malignant melanoma [133]. A recent report in 669 patients with non-small-cell lung cancer indicated that patients who received combination chemotherapy along with levamisole plus warfarin plus tranexamic acid survived longer than those receiving chemotherapy alone [515].

Levamisole has also been evaluated as an adjunct to maintenance chemotherapy for a variety of hematologic malignancies. Improvements in survival from the start of maintenance chemotherapy have been noted in patients receiving levamisole in cases of multiple myeloma [487] and acute lymphoblastic leukemia [424, 425]. Thus, levamisole does appear to have potential as an adjunct to maintenance chemotherapy for patients with hemato-poietic cancers; however, no effects were observed when levamisole was administered concurrently with intensive induction chemotherapy for ANLL [583].

Isoprinosine has been administered concurrently with intravenous 5-FU at various doses without any observable antitumor effects [129].

Table 3. Summary of combined modality studies designed to treat chemotherapy-induced immunosuppression

	Cancer types	Outcome	References
Advanced disease			
Chemicals			
Levamisole	Colon	+	83
		–	97
	Breast	+	304,307,541
		–	421,106
	Non-small-cell lung	+	515
		–	116,142
	Melanoma	–	133
	Multiple myeloma	+	487
	Acute lymphoblastic leukemia	+	425,424
	Acute myeloblastic leukemia	–	583
Isoprinosine	Colon	–	129
Azimexone	Breast	+	121,313
Piroxicam	Non-small-cell lung	+	88
Cimetidine	Ovarian	+	301
Biologicals			
Thymostimulin	Gastrointestinal	+	520
	Melanoma	–	55
	Small-cell lung	+	343
	Non-small-cell lung	–	145,341
Thymosin Fr. 5	Small-cell lung	+	128
		–	518,497
	Non-small-cell lung	–	41
OK-432	Non-small-cell lung	+	610
Lentinan	Gastric	+	548,253
Bestatin	Acute nonlymphoblastic leukemia	+	411
Adjuvant treatment			
Chemicals			
Levamisole	Colon	+	123,321,320
		–	266,381
	Breast	+	306,305
		–	196,295
	Gastric	+	398
	Ovarian	–	300
Biologicals			
Thymostimulin	Breast	+	263
Transfer factor	Non-small-cell lung	+	179
OK-432	Non-small-cell lung	+	610

Azimexone has been administered to ten patients with breast cancer after remission was induced by chemotherapy (CTX, MTX, 5-FU, VCR, prednisone) to assess whether it could ameliorate the immunosuppressive effects of treatment. Detailed weekly serial immunological assessments, performed while patients were receiving 100-mg weekly intravenous injections, revealed that chemotherapy-induced immunosuppression was markedly reversed during azimexone administration. Significant increases in peripheral blood lymphocyte counts and *in vitro* LPRs were noted without change in T- or B-cell percentages [121, 313].

Prostaglandin inhibitors

It has been demonstrated that the concurrent administration of nonsteroidal anti-inflammatory drugs can prevent some aspects of chemotherapy-induced immune suppression [88].

Cimetidine

Recently, a study of the immunomodulatory effects of cimetidine was performed in patients with advanced ovarian cancer who received concurrent chemotherapy (cisplatin, ADR, CTX) [301]. Treatment with chemotherapy produced a decrease in CD4 cell counts and in IL-

2 production of PBL, which was significantly improved in patients who received concurrent cimetidine.

Biologicals

Thymic factors

Two studies performed in the late 1970s with TP-1 and TF5 suggested both a rationale and role for the use of thymic factors in conjunction with combination chemotherapy [520]. Although overall response rates were not altered by TF5, its administration at a high dose (60 mg/m^2) led to a significant improvement in overall median survival [126]. Improved survival was limited to patients who had exhibited pretreatment depressions of total T-cell levels below 775/mm^3 and serum HS glycoprotein levels below 60.5 mg/dl. Although serial immunological assessments were not performed, it was concluded that, whereas TF5 had no detectable direct antitumor effects, its administration to immunosuppressed patients may have improved survival by ameliorating the immune defects due to the presence of tumor, and exacerbated by the chemotherapy.

These two reports culminated in the performance of a number of confirmatory trials, as well as a variety of other studies in which TF5 and TP-1 were administered concurrently with combination chemotherapy for patients with solid tumors, generally small-cell or NSCLC [41, 55, 145, 341, 343, 497, 518]. In only one of these studies did the administration of thymic factors improve the overall response rate to the chemotherapy and survival [343]. Although this trial involved very small patient numbers, the favorable effects of TP-1 on both myelotoxicity and survival indicate that further studies should be performed adding TP-1 to conventional chemotherapy.

In a randomized trial involving 91 of patients with small-cell lung cancer [497, 518], TF5 (60 mg/m^2 subcutaneously, twice weekly) had no effect on survival when combined with chemotherapy, compared to chemotherapy alone (CTX, ADR, VCR alternating with VP-16, cisplatin). An analysis based on pretreatment immune function, total white blood cell count, and absolute lymphocyte count revealed no difference in survival distributions. These results could not confirm the prior reported study [128]. However, this latter trial differed from the original study in that it used different chemotherapy regimens and included prophylactic chest and whole-brain radiotherapy for patients who responded to chemotherapy. Thus, no firm conclusions can be reached regarding the role of TF5 as an adjunct to chemotherapy for small-cell lung cancer.

Several different trials in patients with advanced non-small-cell lung cancer treated with combination chemotherapy with or without TF5 [41] or TP-1 [145, 341] and in metastatic melanoma patients treated with TP-1 [55] failed to find improvements in survival for patients treated with thymic factors. In one of the lung cancer trials, only immunosuppressed patients were considered eligible for study; however, no significant immunorestorative effects were noted in the TP-1-treated patients except transient mild improvement in absolute T-cell levels. *In vitro* LPRs to mitogens remained suppressed following treatment, and no improvements in DTHS were observed.

Thus, follow-up combined modality studies with TF5 and TP-1 have not provided evidence that thymic factors could either prevent chemotherapy-induced immunosuppression or improve survival.

Lentinan

In small studies, administration of lentinan in combination with tegafur [548] or 5-FU and mitomycin [253] to patients with advanced gastric cancer has been reported to improve patient survival.

Bestatin

In a randomized controlled trial of 101 patients with ANLL, patients over 50 years of age who received bestatin along with induction chemotherapy exhibited a better remission duration and survival than the chemotherapy-only group [411].

Adjuvant chemotherapy

Adjuvant chemotherapy has become an accepted treatment modality for patients with breast cancer. Evidence is also accumulating that postsurgical adjuvant chemotherapy for other solid tumors (such as colorectal cancer and non-small-cell lung cancer) may also improve patient survival. The acute and chronic immunosuppressive effects of contemporary adjuvant chemotherapy regimens have recently been evaluated [344, 430, 545].

Chemicals

Levamisole

In a randomized trial of 135 postoperative breast cancer patients with positive axillary nodes, patients received L-phenylalanine mustard with levamisole (150 mg for 3 days every 2 weeks) or placebo for up to 2 years [295]. No significant effects of levamisole were noted, although trends for improved survival were seen in postmenopausal patients and in those with four or more positive lymph nodes. In a study involving 120 postoperative patients with stage III breast cancer treated by either radiotherapy or adjuvant chemotherapy (ADR, CTX, VCR), there was a high incidence of toxicity (primarily transient agranulocytosis), requiring discontinuation of levamisole in 22 of 59 patients [196]. Follow-up is continuing on this trial. In a study comparing postoperative radiation therapy and adjuvant chemotherapy (vincristine, adriamycin, and cyclophosphamide), levamisole administered concurrently appeared to improve both disease-free, as well as overall, survival for patients who received chemotherapy alone or combined radiation therapy plus chemotherapy [306]. Improvements were also noted in various immune parameters in the levamisole treatment group [305].

Although this trial involved 150 patients, the multiple randomizations made it difficult to analyze.

In other recent studies, levamisole was shown to improve the survival of resected patients with gastric cancer treated with MIT and tegafur [398], but there was a deleterious effect of levamisole in a trial of 140 patients with ovarian cancer who received adjuvant chemotherapy following maximal surgical reduction of tumor [300].

Biologicals

Transfer factor

The administration of transfer factor, prepared from leukocytes from household contacts, has been reported to improve survival for stage I and II patients with resected non-small-cell lung cancer who were treated further with a variety of adjuvant combination chemotherapy regimens [179].

OK-432

In a trial of 311 patients, OK-432 was shown to improve survival of patients with resected stage I, II and III non-small-cell lung cancer when combined with 3-drug combination chemotherapy, compared to chemotherapy [610].

Thymic factors

Recently, results of a randomized trial were reported, in which 51 patients received adjuvant CMF chemotherapy with or without TP-1 (50 mg/m^2 IM daily x 2 weeks, then twice weekly for a minimum of 3 months) following radical mastectomy for breast cancer [263]. Although details of the patients' clinical characteristics were not discussed, patients who received TP-1 exhibited a significant decrease in the incidence of infections (mostly cystitis, conjunctivitis, and mucositis), and an increase in $T_{h/I}/T_{c/s}$ compared to the control (no treatment) group. There was also a lower incidence of myelotoxicity in the TP-1 treated patients. These results require confirmation with a large-scale trial.

CURRENT STATUS OF THERAPEUTIC ALTERATIONS FOR CANCER-ASSOCIATED IMMUNE SUPPRESSION

The results with levamisole in combination with 5-FU as adjuvant therapy for Dukes C colon cancer have provided strong evidence that drugs with immunorestorative properties can play an important role in the treatment of human cancer. What has been learned about the reversibility or prevention of cancer-associated immunosuppression? All of the agents discussed in this chapter, at least in small phase I and II studies, appear to have the capability of improving immune cell numbers and/or functions in immunosuppressed patients. The large-scale phase III surgical adjuvant trials for the most part have provided only limited information concerning whether or not perioperative immunosuppression could be prevented. Part of this relates to the fact that it is extremely difficult – and probably impossible – to perform adequate quality control assays of immunity in multiple different institutions participating in the same large-scale trial. Nevertheless, the promising results with levamisole plus 5-FU indicate a new role for this drug as adjuvant therapy for patients with advanced resectable colorectal cancer. However, the mechanism by which levamisole improved survival was not addressed, and it is not clear whether the drug exerted its effects as a result of immunomodulation or by other, as yet undefined, mechanisms. Several smaller studies in patients with GI cancers suggested that certain aspects of T-cell immunity (i.e., LPRs) could be maintained during the perioperative period by treatment with levamisole. However, if perioperative immunosuppression is only transient, then it may not be appropriate to continue administration of a putative immunorestorative drug like levamisole for up to 2 years, as has been routinely done.

Studies with levamisole, TF5, Tα_1, bestatin, and vitamin A have suggested that various immunorestorative agents could ameliorate radiotherapy-induced depression of T-cell numbers or functions, or accelerate the reconstitution of immunity following radiotherapy. In no case, however, did treatment totally normalize both T-cell numbers and functions, and so efficacy can be considered partial at best. In several clinical trials, levamisole has not improved survival in irradiated patients with non-small-cell lung cancer. Preliminary analysis of the trial in postradiotherapy patients with non-small-cell lung cancer has suggested that Tα_1 can improve overall patient survival when used as an adjunct to radiotherapy. However, the mechanism by which Tα_1 improved survival is not known. In addition to accelerating the reconstitution of T-cell dependent immunity, it is possible that thymic factors can protect bone marrow stem cells from the myelotoxic effects of radiotherapy or chemotherapy [263]. Such a mechanism has been proposed to explain the lower incidence of myelotoxicity in breast cancer patients who received TP-1 along with adjuvant CMF chemotherapy [263].

Because radiation therapy results in a uniform and marked depression of immune cell numbers and functions, patients who have received this treatment are ideal candidates for studies of the immunorestorative effects of BRMs. Several of the newer BRMs are being evaluated using this clinical model. However, it must be recognized that if putative immunorestorative agents are administered concurrently with radiation, their effects on immunity might be negated to some degree. An agent could exert a beneficial effect during radiation treatment only if it provided a direct protective action on immune cells from the deleterious effects of radiation.

Although a number of large-scale clinical trials have been performed with patients receiving concurrent chemotherapy, there are only very limited data concerning the prevention of chemotherapy-induced immunosuppression. Several studies have suggested that levamisole may have a role as a therapeutic adjunct for patients with hematopoietic malignancies who are receiving maintenance chemotherapy, yet the mechanism by which levamisole exerts its effects remains unknown. Although none of the immunorestorative agents have proven effective when administered concurrently with intensive combination chemotherapy for patients with advanced metastatic cancers, their potential role in patients treated with adjuvant chemotherapy remains to be explored. The promising adjuvant studies with levamisole in combination with 5-FU for patients with colorectal cancer and those with TP-1 in combination with adjuvant CMF chemotherapy for breast cancer will hopefully stimulate the design and performance of new similar trial with other adjuvant chemotherapy regimens.

The success or failure of future studies with BRMs will be determined primarily, if not exclusively, by the selection of suitable phase II and III clinical models for study and by the avoidance of confounding variables or inadequate sample sizes, which could lead to uninterpretable results. It is likely that a two-phased approach will be necessary to evaluate BRMs with immunorestorative properties: focusing initially on phase I/II, single-institution pilot studies to establish the pharmacokinetics and immunomodulatory potential of the agent, and then on properly stratified, large-scale phase III randomized trials performed by a cooperative cancer group to establish clinical efficacy using the optimal immunomodulatory dose and schedule and an appropriate patient population.

Since the ultimate confirmation of any new cancer therapy depends upon the performance of well-designed, large-scale, phase III trials, the most promising BRMs must be evaluated according to protocols that are technically feasible for multi-institution trials, and with improved survival as the major end point.

ACKNOWLEDGMENT

Dr. Richard Schulof co-authored this chapter in the 2nd edition, but died in an accident during the preparation of the 3rd edition.

REFERENCES

1. Addison I, Baggage J, Gandossini M, Souhami R. Assessment of host defense against infection during chemotherapy of Hodgkin's disease. *Cancer Chemother Pharmacol* 1978; 1: 129-133.
2. Adler A, Stein JA, Ben-Efraim S. Immunocompetence, immunosuppression, and human breast cancer, II. Further evidence of initial immune impairment by integrated assessment effect of nodal involvement (N) and of primary tumor size (T). *Cancer* 1980; 45: 2061-2073.
3. Adler A, Stein JA, Ben-Efraim S. Immunocompetence, immunosuppression, and human breast cancer. III. Prognostic significance of initial level of immunocompetence in early and advanced disease. *Cancer* 1980; 45: 2074-2083.
4. Ahmed K, Turk JL. Effect of anticancer agents neothramycin, aclacinomycin, FK-565 and FK-156 on the release of interleukin-2 and interleukin-1 *in vitro*. *Cancer Immunol Immunother* 1989; 28: 87-92.
5. Alberola V, Gonzalez-Molina A, Trenor A, et al. Mechanism of suppression of the depressed lymphocyte response in lung cancer patients. *Allergol Immunopathol (Madr)* 1985; 13: 213-219.
6. Albin RJ, Gordon MJ, Soane WA. Levels of immunoglobulins in the serum of patients with carcinoma of the prostate. *Neoplasma* 1972; 19: 57-60.
7. Alexopoulos LG, Wiltshaw E. Immunological monitoring during chemotherapy for advanced Hodgkin's disease. *Cancer* 1978; 42: 2631-2640.
8. Alsabti EA. *In vivo* and *in vitro* assays of incompetence in bronchogenic carcinoma. *Oncology* 1979; 36: 171-175.
9. Amery WK, Butterworth BS. The dosage regimen of levamisole in cancer: Is it related to efficacy and safety? *Int J Immunopharmacol* 1983; 5: 1-9.
10. Amery WK, Cosemans J, Gooszen HC, et al. Four-year results from double-blind study of adjuvant levamisole treatment in resectable lung cancer. In: Terry WD, Rosenberg SA, eds. *Immunotherapy of human cancer*. New York: Elsevier/North-Holland, 1982: 123-133.
11. Amlot PL, Anger A. Binding of phytohaemagglutinin to serum substances and inhibition of lymphocyte transformation in Hodgkin's disease. *Clin Exp Immunol* 1976; 26: 520-527.
12. Anderson TC, Jones SE, Sochnlen BJ, et al. Immunocompetence and malignant lymphomas: Immunologic status before therapy. *Cancer* 1981; 48: 2702-2709.
13. Anderson TM, Ibayashi Y, Tokuda Y, et al. Natural killer activity of lymphocytes infiltrating human lung cancers following preoperative systemic recombinant interleukin-2. *Arch Surg* 1987; 122: 12; 1446-1450.
14. Anderson TM, Ibayashi Y, Holmes EC, Golub SH. Modification of natural killer activity of lymphocytes infiltrating human lung cancers. *Cancer Immunol Immunother* 1987; 25: 65-68,
15. Anthony HM, Templeman GH, Madsen KE, Mason MK. The prognostic significance of DHS skin tests in patients with carcinoma of bronchus. *Cancer* 1974: 1901-1906.
16. Anthony HM. Yorkshire trial of adjuvant therapy with levamisole in surgically treated lung cancer. In: Terry WD, Rosenberg SA, eds. *Immunotherapy of human cancer*. New York: Elsevier/North-Holland, 1982: 135-440.
17. Aparicio-Pages NM, Verspaget HW, Pena SA, Lamers CB. Impaired local natural killer-cell activity in human colorectal carcinomas. *Cancer Immunol Immunother* 1989; 28: 4, 301-304.
18. Aparicio-Pages NM, Verspaget HW, Pena SA, Lamers CBHW. Impaired local natural killer cell activity in human colorectal carcinomas. *Cancer Immunol Immunother* 1989; 28: 301-304.
19. Aranha GV, McKhann CF, Simmons RL, Grage TB. Recall skin test antigens and the prognosis of stage I melanoma. *J Surg Oncol* 1976; 11: 13-16.
20. Arinaga S, Akiyoshi T, Tsuji H. Augmentation of the generation cell mediated cytotoxicity after a single dose of adriamycin in cancer patients. *Cancer Res* 1986; 46: 4213-4216.

21. Arinaga S, Akiyoshi T, Tsuji H. Augmentation of the cell-mediated cytotoxic response induced in mixed cell culture by adriamycin. *Jpn J Cancer Res* 1985; 76: 414-419.
22. Armstrong D, Chmel M. Infectious complications of Hodgkin's disease. In: Lacher MJ, ed. *Hodgkin's disease*. New York: Wiley, 1976: 267-290.
23. Arnaud JP, Buyse M, Nordlinger B, et al. Adjuvant therapy of poor prognosis colon cancer with levamisole: Results of an EORTC double-blind randomized clinical trial. *Br J Surg* 1989; 76: 284-289.
24. Ascher MS, Schneider WJ, Valentine FT, Lawrence HS. *In vitro* properties of leukocyte dialysates containing transfer factor. *Proc Natl Acad Sci USA* 1974; 74: 1178-1182.
25. Ashorn RG, Vandenbard AA, Acott KM, Krohn KJ. Dialysable leukocyte extracts (transfer factor) augment non-specifically keyhole limpet haemocyanin and horseshoe crab haemocyanin skin reactivity in immunized human recipients. *Scand J Immunol* 1976; 23: 161-167.
26. Aymard JP, Janot C, Thibaut G, et al. Levamisole in chronic lymphocytic leukaemia: A prospective study of 15 patients. *Acta Haematol* (Basel) 1984; 71: 316-321.
27. Balaram P, Remani P, Padmanabhan TK, Vasudevan DM. Role of levamisole immunotherapy as an adjuvant to radiotherapy in oral cancer: Immune responses. *Neoplasma* 1988; 35: 6; 617-625.
28. Balaram P, Padmanabhan TK, Vasudevan DM. Role of levamisole immunotherapy as an adjuvant to radiotherapy in oral cancer. II. Lymphocyte subpopulations. *Neoplasma* 1988; 35: 2; 235-242.
29. Balch CM, Doughtery PA, Cloud GA, Tilden AB. Prostaglandin E_2-mediated suppression of cellular immunity in colon cancer patients. *Surgery* 1984; 95: 71-77.
30. Balch CM, Tilden AB, Dougherty PA, Cloud GA. Depressed levels of granular lymphocytes with natural killer (NK) cell function in 247 cancer patients. *Ann Surg* 1983; 198: 192-199.
31. Balch CM, Dougherty PA, Tilden AB. Excessive prostaglandin E2 production by suppressor monocytes in head and neck cancer patients. *Ann Surg* 1982; 196: 645-650.
32. Balm FA, Drexhage HA, von Blomberg M, et al. Mononuclear phagocytic function in head and neck cancer. *Cancer* 1984; 54: 1010-1015.
33. Bancewicz J, Calman K, MacPherson SG, et al. Adjuvant chemotherapy and immunotherapy for colorectal cancer; preliminary communication. *J R Soc Med* 1980; 73: 197-199.
34. Baral E, Blomgren H, Petrini B, Wasserman J. Blood lymphocytes in breast cancer patients following radiotherapy and surgery. *Int J Radiat Oncol Biol Phys* 1977; 2: 289-295.
35. Baral E, Blomgren H, Petrini B, et al. Prognostic relevance of immunologic variables in breast carcinoma. *Acta Radiol Ther Phys Biol* 1977; 16: 417-426.
36. Baseler MW, Maxim PE, Veltri RW. Circulating IgA immune complexes in head and neck cancer, nasopharyngeal carcinoma, lung cancer, and colon cancer. *Cancer* 1987; 59: 1727-1731.
37. Baskies AM, Chretien PB, Weiss JF, et al. Serum glycoproteins in cancer patients: First report of correlations with *in vitro* and *in vivo* parameters and cellular immunity. *Cancer* 1980; 45: 3050-3060.
38. Bast RC, Reinherz EL, Maven C, et al. Contrasting effects of cyclophosphamide and prednisolone on the phenotype of human peripheral blood leukocytes. *Clin Immunol Immunopathol* 1983; 28: 101-114.
39. Baumann MA, Milson TJ, Patrick CW, et al. Correlation of circulating natural killer cell count with prognosis in large cell lymphoma. *Cancer* 1986; 57: 2309-2312.
40. Bean MA, Schelhammer PS, Her HW, et al. Immunocompetence of patients with transitional cell carcinoma as measured by DNCB skin tests and *in vitro* lymphocyte function. *Natl Cancer Inst Monogr* 1978; 49: 111-114.
41. Bedikian AY, Patt YZ, Murphy WK, et al. Prospective evaluation of thymosin fraction V immunotherapy in patients with non-small cell lung cancer receiving vindesine, doxorubicin, and cisplatin (VAP) chemotherapy. *Am J Clin Oncol* 1984; 7: 399-404.
42. Benkovic B, Burek B, Jaksic B, Vitale B. Modulation of chronic lymphocytic leukemia (CLL) lymphocyte phenotypes by *in vitro* incubation with alpha-1 thymosin. *Blood Cells* 1987; 12: 2; 441-455.
43. Bennett A, Berstock A, Harris M, et al. Prostaglandins and their relationship to malignant and benign breast tumors. In: Sammuelsson B, Ramuell PW, Paoletti R, eds. *Advances in prostaglandin and thromboxane research vol 6*. New York: Raven Press, 1980: 595-599.
44. Berd D, Macguire HC Jr, Mastrangelo MJ. Induction of cell-mediated immunity to autologous melanoma cells and regression of metastases after treatment with a melanoma cell vaccine preceded by cyclophosphamide. *Cancer Res* 1986; 46: 2572-2577.
45. Berd D, Mastrangelo MJ, Enstron PF, et al. Augmentation of the human immune response by cyclophosphamide. *Cancer Res* 1982; 42: 4862-4866.
46. Berd D, Wilson EJ, Bellet RE, Mastrangelo MJ. Effect of 1-(2-chlorethyl)-3-(4-methyl-cyclohexyl)-1-nitrosourea adjuvant therapy on the immune response of patients with malignant melanoma. *Cancer Res* 1979; 39: 4472-4476.
47. Berd D, Mastrangelo MJ. Effect of low dose cyclophosphamide on the immune system of cancer patients: Reduction of T-suppressor function without depletion of the CD8+ subset. *Cancer Res* 1987; 47: 3317-3321.
48. Berd D, Maguire HC, Mastrangelo MJ. Impairment of concanavalin A-inducible suppressor activity following administration to patients with advanced cancer. *Cancer Res* 1984; 44: 1275-1280.
49. Berenbaum MC, Fluck PA, Hurst NP. Depression of lymphocyte responses after surgical trauma. *Br J Exp Pathol* 1973; 54: 597-607.
50. Berenyl E, Kavai M, Szabolcsi M, Szegedi G. Levamisole in the treatment of Hodgkin's disease. *Acta Med Acad Sci Hung* 1979; 36: 177-185.
51. Bergman S, Borgstrom S, Tarnik A. Lymphocyte response to phytohaemagglutinin following cholecystectomy. *Acta Pathol Microbiol Scand* 1969; 75: 363-366.
52. Bergmann L, Mitrou PS, Demmer-Dieckmann M, et al. Impaired T- and B-cell functions in patients with Hodgkin's disease. *Cancer Immunol Immunother* 1987; 25: 59-64.
53. Berkarda B, Bouffard-Eyaboglu H, Derman U. The effect of coumarin derivatives on the immunological system of man. *Agents Actions* 1983; 13: 50-52.
54. Berlinger NT. Deficient immunity in head and neck cancer due to excessive monocyte production of prostaglandins. *Laryngoscope* 1984; 94(11, Pt.1): 1407-1410.
55. Bernengo MG, Fra P, Lisa F, Meregilli M, Zina G.

Thymostimulin therapy in melanoma patients: Correlation of immunologic effects with clinical course. *Clin Immunol Immunopathol* 1983; 28: 311-324.
56. Bernengo MG, Lisa F, Meregalli M, et al. The prognostic value of T-lymphocyte levels in malignant melanoma. A five year follow-up. *Cancer* 1983; 52: 1841-1898.
57. Bernengo MG, Lisa F, Meregalli M, Doveil GC. Changes in T- and B-lymphocyte subpopulations before, during and after chemotherapy for malignant melanoma. *Int J Tissue React* 1984; 6: 505-511.
58. Bicker U. Immunomodulation by 2-cyanaziridine derivatives. In: Serrou B, Rosenfeld C, Daniels JC, Saunder JP, eds. Current concepts in human immunology and cancer immunomodulation. Amsterdam: *Elsevier Biomedical*, 1982: 521-534.
59. Bier J, Nicklisch U, Platz H. The doubtful relevance of nonspecific immune reactivity in patients with squamous-cell carcinoma of the head and neck region. *Cancer* 1983; 52: 1165-1172.
60. Bjorkholm M, Wedelin C, Holm G, et al. Lymphocytotoxic serum factors and lymphocyte functions in untreated Hodgkin's disease. *Cancer* 1982; 50: 2044-2048.
61. Bjorkholm M, Holm G, Mellstedt H. Persisting lymphocyte deficiencies during remission in Hodgkin's disease. *Clin Exp Immunol* 1977; 28: 389-393.
62. Bjorkholm M, Holm G, Mellstedt H. Immunologic profile of patients with cured Hodgkin's disease. *Scand J Hematol* 1977; 18: 361-368.
63. Bjorkholm M, Holm G, Mellsted H, Johansson B. Immunodeficiency and prognosis in Hodgkin's disease. *Acta Med Scand* 1975; 198: 275-279.
64. Block JB, Haynes HA, Thompson WL, Neiman PE. Delayed hypersensitivity in chronic lymphocytic leukemia. *J Natl Cancer Inst* 1969; 42: 973-980.
65. Blomgren H, Edsmyr F, Esposti PL, et al. Influence of bestatin, a new immunomodifier, on human lymphoid cells. In: Serrou B, Rosenfeld C, Daniels JC, Saunders JP, eds. Current concepts in human immunology and cancer immunomodulation. Amsterdam: *Elsevier Biomedical*, 1982: 593-610.
66. Blomgren H, Edsmyr F, Esposti PL, Naslund I. Immunological and haematological monitoring in bladder cancer patients receiving adjuvant bestatin treatment following radiation therapy. A prospective randomized trial. *Biomed Pharmacother* 1984; 38: 143-149.
67. Blomgren SE, Wolberg WH, Kisken WA. Effect of fluoropyrimidines on delayed cutaneous hypersensitivity. *Cancer Res* 1965; 25: 977-979.
68. Blomgren H, Wasserman J, Rotstein S, et al. Possible role of prostaglandin-producing monocytes in the depression of mitogenic response of blood lymphocytes following radiation therapy. *Radiother Oncol* 1984; 1: 255-261.
69. Blomgren H, Baral E, Edsmyr F, et al. Natural killer activity in peripheral blood lymphocyte populations following local radiation therapy. *Acta Radiol Oncol* 1980; 2: 139-143.
70. Blomgren H, Wasserman J, Littbrand B. Blood lymphocytes after radiation therapy of carcinoma of prostate and urinary bladder. *Acta Radiol Ther Phys Biol* 1974; 13: 357-367.
71. Blomgren H, Naslund I, Esposti PL, et al. Adjuvant bestatin immunotherapy in patients with transitional cell carcinoma of the bladder. Clinical results of a randomized trial. *Cancer Immunol Immunother* 1987; 25: 1; 46.
72. Blomgren H, Strender LE, Petrini B, Wasserman J. Changes of the spontaneous cytotoxicity of the blood lymphocyte population following local radiation therapy for breast cancer. *Eur J Cancer Clin Oncol* 1982; 18: 637-643.
73. Blomgren H, Wasserman J, Baral E, Petrini B. Evidence for the appearance of non-specific suppressor cells in the blood after local irradiation therapy. *Int J Radiol Oncol Biol Phys* 1978; 4: 249-253.
74. Blomgren H, Strender LE, Edsmyr F. Bestatin treatment and the peripheral lymphocyte population in cancer patients. *Recent Results Cancer Res* 1980; 75: 133-138.
75. Blomgren H, Edsmyr F, von Stedingk L-V, Wasserman J. Bestatin treatment enhances the recovery of radiation-induced impairments of the immunological reactivity of the blood lymphocyte population in bladder and cancer patients. *Biomed Pharmacother* 1986; 40: 50-54.
76. Bobrove AM, Fuks Z, Strober S. Quantitation of T- and B-lymphocytes and cellular immune function in Hodgkin's disease. *Cancer* 1975; 36: 169-179.
77. Bockman RS. Prostaglandins in cancer: a review. *Cancer Invest* 1983; 1: 485-493.
78. Boetcher DA, Leonard EJ. Abnormal monocyte chemotactic response in cancer patients. *J Natl Cancer Inst* 1974; 52: 1091-1098.
79. Bollag W, Matta A. From vitamin A to retinoids in experimental and clinical oncology: achievements, failures, and outlook. *Ann NY Acad Sci* 1981; 359: 9-23.
80. Bolton PM, Teasdale C, Mander AM, et al. Immune competence in breast cancer: relationships of pretreatment immunologic tests to diagnosis and tumor stage. *Cancer Immunol Immunother* 1976; 1: 251-258.
81. Bolton PM, Mander AM, Davidson JM, et al. Cellular immunity in cancer: comparison of delayed hypersensitivity skin tests in three common cancers. *Br J Med* 1975; 3(5974): 18-20.
82. Bone G, Appleton DR, Venebles CW. The prognostic value of the cutaneous delayed hypersensitivity response to 2, 4-dinitrochlorobenzene in gastrointestinal cancer. *Br J Cancer* 1974; 29: 403-406.
83. Borden EC, Davis TE, Crowley JJ, et al. Interim analysis of trial of levamisole and 5-fluorouracil in metastatic colorectal carcinoma. In: Terry WD, Rosenberg SA, eds. *Immunotherapy of human cancer*. New York: Elsevier/North-Holland, 1982: 231-235.
84. Bosworth JL, Ghossein NA, Brooks TL. Delayed hypersensitivity in patients treated by curative radiotherapy. Its relation to tumor response and short-term survival. *Cancer* 1975; 36: 353-358.
85. Braun DP, Nisius S, Hollinshead A, Harris JE. Serial immune testing in surgically resected lung cancer patients. *Cancer Immunol Immunother* 1983; 15: 114-120.
86. Braun DP, Harris JE, Rugenstein M. Relationships of arachidonic acid metabolism to indomethacin-sensitive immunoregulatory function and lymphocyte PGE sensitivity in peripheral blood mononuclear cells of disseminated solid-tumor cancer patients. *J Immunopharmacol* 1984; 6: 227-236.
87. Braun DP, Harris JE. Effects of combination chemotherapy on immunoregulatory cells in peripheral blood of solid-tumor cancer patients: Correlation with rebound

overshoot immune function recovery. *Clin Immunol Immunopathol* 1981; 20: 193-214.

88. Braun DP, Harris JE. Modifications of the effects of cytotoxic chemotherapy on the immune responses of cancer patients with a non-steroidal, anti-inflammatory drug, piroxicam. (Abstr.) *Proc Am Soc Clin Oncol* 1985; 4: 223.
89. Brenner BG, Friedman G, Margolese RG. The relationship of clinical status and therapeutic modality to natural killer cell activity in human breast cancer. *Cancer* 1985; 56: 1543-1548.
90. Brooks WH, Caldwell HD, Mortara RH. Immune responses in patients with gliomas. *Surg Neurol* 1974; 2: 419-423.
91. Brosman S, Elhilali M, Vescura C, Fahey J. Immune response in bladder cancer patients. *J Urol* 1979; 121: 162-169.
92. Brosman S, Hausman M, Shacks SJ. Studies on the immune status of patients with renal adenocarcinoma. *J Urol* 1975; 114: 375-380.
93. Browder JP, Cretien PB. Immune reactivity in head and neck squamous carcinoma and relevance to the design of immunotherapy trials. *Sem Oncol* 1977; 4: 4; 431-439.
94. Brown AE, Badger AM, Poste G. The effects of cimetidine on immune cell function and host response to tumors. In: Serrou B, Rosenfeld C, Daniels JC, and Sanders JP, eds. Current concepts of human immunology and cancer immunomodulation. Amsterdam: *Elsevier Biomedical*, 1982: 513-519.
95. Bruckner HW, Mokyr MB, Mitchell MS. Effect of imidazole-4-carboxamide-5-(3, 3-dimethyl-1-triazeno) on immunity in patients with malignant melanoma. *Cancer Res* 1974; 34: 181-183.
96. Bukowski RM, Deodhar S, Hewlett JS, Greenstreet R. Randomized controlled trial of transfer factor in stage II malignant melanoma. *Cancer* 1983; 51: 269-272.
97. Buroker TR, Moertel CG, Fleming TR, et al. A controlled evaluation of recent approaches to biochemical modulation or enhancement of 5-fluorouracil therapy in colorectal carcinoma. *J Clin Oncol* 1985; 3: 1624-1631.
98. Burtin C, Noirot C, Scheinmann P, et al. Clinical improvement in advanced cancer disease after treatment combining histamine and H2-antihistaminics (rantidine or cimetidine). *Eur J Cancer Clin Oncol* 1988; 24: 2, 161-167.
99. Busutti L, Blotta A, Mastrorilli M, et al. Transfer factor adjuvant therapy in non-small-cell lung carcinoma (NSCLC) after surgery and radiotherapy. *J Exp Pathol* 1987; 3: 4, 565-568.
100. Butterworth C, Oon CJ, Westbury G, Hobbs JR. T-lymphocyte response in patients with malignant melanoma. *Eur J Cancer* 1977; 10: 639-646.
101. Cairo MS, Mallett C, Vande Ven C, et al. Impaired *in vitro* polymorphonuclear function secondary to the chemotherapeutic effects of vincristine, adriamycin, cyclophosphamide, and actinomycin D. *J Clin Oncol* 1986; 5: 798-804.
102. Cameron DJ. A comparison of the cytotoxic potential in polymorphonuclear leukocytes obtained from normal donors and cancer patients. *Clin Immunol Immunopathol* 1983; 28: 115-124.
103. Cameron DJ, O'Brien P, Majeski JA. Effects of *in vivo* treatment with ibuprofen on macrophage function in breast and colon cancer patients. *J Clin Lab Immunol* 1986; 20: 1, 23-28.
104. Cannon GB, Dean JH, Herberman RB, et al. Association of depressed postoperative lymphoproliferative responses to alloantigens with poor prognosis in patients with stage I lung cancer. *Int J Cancer* 1980; 25: 9-17.
105. Carmignani G, Belgrano E, Puppo P, Cornaglia P. T-lymphocyte-inhibiting factors in renal cancer: Evaluation of differences between arterial and renal venous blood levels of E-rosette-forming cells. *J Urol* 1978; 120: 673-675.
106. Carpenter JT Jr, Smalley RV, Raney M, et al. Ineffectiveness of levamisole in prolonging remission or survival of women treated with cyclophosphamide, doxorubicin, and 5-fluorouracil for good-risk metastatic breast carcinoma: A Southeastern Cancer Study Group Trial. *Cancer Treat Rep* 1986; 70: 9; 1073-1079.
107. Case DC, Hansen JA, Corrales E, et al. Depressed *in vitro* lymphocyte responses to PHA in patients with Hodgkin's disease in continuous long remissions. *Blood* 1977; 49: 771-778.
108. Catalona WJ, Ratliff TL, McCool RE. Discordance among cell-mediated cytolytic mechanisms in cancerous patients: importance of the assay system. *J Immunol* 1979; 122: 1009-1014.
109. Catalona WJ, Tarpley JL, Potvin C, Chretien PB. Host immunocompetence in genitourinary cancer: Relationship to tumor stage and prognosis. *Natl Cancer Inst Monogr* 1978; 49: 105-110.
110. Catalona WJ, Chretien PB. Abnormalities of quantitative dinitrochlorobenzine sensitization in cancer patients: Correlation with tumor stage and histology. *Cancer* 1973; 31: 353-356.
111. Catalona WJ, Sample WF, Chretien PB. Lymphocyte reactivity in cancer patients: Correlation with tumor histology and clinical stage. *Cancer* 1973; 31: 65-71.
112. Catalona WJ, Tarpley JL, Potvin C, Chretien PB. Correlations among cutaneous reactivity to DNCB, PHA-induced lymphocyte blastogenesis and peripheral blood E-rosettes. *Clin Exp Immunol* 1975; 19: 327-332.
113. Catalona WJ, Ratliff TL, McCool R. Concanavalin-A-activated suppressor cell activity in peripheral blood lymphocytes of urologic cancer patients. *J Natl Cancer Inst* 1980; 65: 553-557.
114. Caulfield MJ, Luce KJ, Proffitt MR, Cevy J. Induction of idiotype-specific suppressor T-cells with antigen/antibody complexes. *J Ex Med* 1983; 157: 1713-1725.
115. Cervical Cancer Immunotherapy Study Group. Immunotherapy using the streptococcal preparation OK-432 for the treatment of uterine cervical cancer. *Cancer* 1987; 60: 2394-2402.
116. Chahinian AP, Goldberg J, Holland JF, et al. Chemotherapy vs. Chemoimmunotherapy with levamisole or *Corynebacterium parvum* in advanced lung cancer. *Cancer Treat Rep* 1982; 66: 1291-1297.
117. Chang TC, Statzman L, Sokal JE. Correlation of delayed hypersensitivity responses with chemotherapeutic results in advanced Hodgkin's disease. *Cancer* 1975; 36: 950-955.
118. Cheema AR, Hersh EM. Patient survival after chemotherapy and its relationship to *in vitro* lymphocyte blastogenesis. *Cancer* 1971; 28: 851-855.
119. Chihara G, Hamuro J, Maeda YY, et al. Antitumor and metastasis-inhibitory activities of lentinan as an immuno-

modulator: An overview. *Cancer Detect Prev Suppl* 1987; 1: 423-443.
120. Chirhara G. The antitumor polysaccharide lentinan: an overview. In: Aoki T, Urushizaki I, and Tsubara E, eds. Manipulation of host defense mechanisms. *Excerpta Medica* 1981: 1-16.
121. Chirigos MA, Mastrangelo MJ. Immunorestoration by chemicals. In: Milhich E, ed. *Immunological approaches to cancer therapeutics*. New York: Wiley, 1982: 191-239.
122. Chisesi T, Capnist G, Rancan L, et al. The effect of thymic substances on T-circulating cells of patients treated for Hodgkin's disease. *J Biol Regul Homeost Agents* 1988; 2: 4, 193-198.
123. Chlebowski RT, Nystrom S, Reynolds R, et al. Long-term survival following levamisole or placebo adjuvant treatment of colorectal cancer: a Western Cancer Study Group trial. *Oncology* 1988; 45: 3, 141-143.
124. Clemens LE, Siiteri PK, Stities DP. Mechanism of immunosuppression of progesterone of natural lymphocyte activation during pregnancy. *J Immunol* 1979; 122: 5; 1978-1985.
125. Cochran AJ, Mackie RM, Grant RM, et al. An examination of the immunology of cancer patients. *Int J Cancer* 1976; 18: 298-309.
126. Cohen MH, Chretien PB, Johnston-Early A, et al. Thymosin fraction V prolongs survival of intensively treated small-cell lung cancer patients. In: Terry WD, Rosenberg SA, eds. *Immunotherapy of human cancer*. New York: Elsevier/North-Holland, 1982: 141-145.
127. Cohen JHD, Danel L, Cordier G, et al. Sex steroid receptors in peripheral T-cell: Absence of androgen receptors to OKT8-positive cells. *J Immunol* 1983; 131: 2767-2771.
128. Cohen MH, Chretien PB, Indo DC, et al. Thymosin fraction V and intensive combination chemotherapy prolonging the survival of patients with small-cell lung cancer. *JAMA* 1979; 241: 1813-1815.
129. Colozza M, Tonato M, Belsanti V, et al. 5-Fluorouracil and isoprinosine in the treatment of advanced colorectal cancer: A limited phase I, II evaluation. *Cancer* 1988; 62: 1049-1052.
130. Cone L, Uhr JW. Immunological deficiency disorders associated with chronic lymphocyte leukemia and multiple myeloma. *J Clin Invest* 1964; 43: 2241-2249.
131. Consolini R, Cei B, Cini P, et al. Circulating thymic hormone activity in young cancer patients. *Clin Exp Immunol* 1986; 66: 1; 173-180.
132. Corder MP, Young RC, Brown RS, DeVita VT. Phytohemagglutinin-induced lymphocyte transformation: The relationship to prognosis of Hodgkin's disease. *Blood* 1972; 39: 595-601.
133. Costanzi JJ, Fletcher WS, Balcerzak SP, et al. Combination chemotherapy plus levamisole in the treatment of disseminated malignant melanoma. A Southwest Oncology Group Study. *Cancer* 1984; 53: 833-836.
134. Cozzolino F, Torcia M, Carossino AM, et al. Characterization of cells from invaded lymph nodes in patients with solid tumors. *J Exp Med* 1987; 166: 303-318.
135. Cullen BF, Van Belle G. Lymphocyte transformation and changes in leukocyte count. Effect of anesthesia and operation. *Anesthesiology* 1975; 43: 563-569.
136. Cunningham-Rundles S, Filippa A, Braun DW, et al. Natural cytotoxicity of peripheral blood lymphocytes and regional lymph node cells in breast cancer in women. *J Natl Cancer Inst* 1981; 67: 585-590.
137. Dagan S, Tzehoval E, Fridkin M, Feldman M. Tuftsin and tuftsin conjugates potentiate immunogenic processes: effects and possible mechanisms. *J Biol Response Mod* 1987; 6: 6, 625-636.
138. Dalbow MH, Concannon JP, Eng CP, et al. Lymphocyte mitogen stimulation studies for patients with lung cancer: evaluation of prognostic significance of preirradiation therapy studies. *J Lab Clin Med* 1977; 90: 295-302.
139. Danel L, Sonweine G, Monier JC, Saez S. Specific estrogen binding sites in human lymphoid cells and thymic cells. *J Steroid Biochem* 1983; 18: 5; 559-563.
140. Danish Breast Cancer Cooperative Group. Increased breast cancer recurrence rate after adjuvant therapy with levamisole. *Lancet* 1980; 2: 824-827.
141. Das SN, Khanna NN, Khanna S. A multiparametric observation of immune competence in breast cancer and its correlation with tumor load and prognosis. *Ann Acad Med Singapore* 1985; 14: 374-381.
142. Davis S, Mietlowski W, Rohweder JJ, et al. Levamisole as an adjuvant to chemotherapy in extensive bronchogenic carcinoma. A Veterans Administration Lung Cancer Group study. *Cancer* 1982; 50: 646-651.
143. Dawson DE, Everts EC, Vetto RM, Burger DR. Assessment of immunocompetent cells in patients with head and neck squamous-cell carcinoma. *Ann Otol Rhinol Laryngol* 1985; 94: 342-345.
144. DeBoer KP, Braun DP, Harris JE. Natural cytotoxicity and antibody-dependent cytotoxicity in solid-tumor cancer patients: Regulation by adherent cells. *Clin Immunol Immunopathol* 1982; 23: 133-144.
145. Del Giacco GS, Cengiarotti L, Mantovani G, et al. Advanced lung cancer treated with combination chemotherapy with or without thymostimulin. In: Byrom NA, Hobbs JR, eds. *Thymic factor therapy Serono Symposium Publications*: New York Raven Press, 1982: 321-328.
146. Dellon AL, Potvin C, Chretien PB. Thymus-dependent lymphocyte levels during radiation therapy for bronchogenic and esophageal carcinoma: correlations with clinical course in responders and nonresponders. *Am J Roentgenol Radiat Ther Nucl Med* 1975; 123: 500-511.
147. Dellon AL, Potvin C, Chretien PB. Thymus-dependent lymphocyte levels in bronchogenic carcinoma: correlations with histology, clinical stage, and clinical course after surgical treatment. *Cancer* 1975; 35: 687-694.
148. Dillman RO, Beauregard JC, Zavanelli MI, et al. *In vivo* immune restoration in advanced cancer patients after administration of thymosin fraction V or thymosin alpha-*1*. *J Biol Response Mod* 1983; 2: 139-147.
149. Dimitrov NV, Arnold D, Munson J, et al. Phase II study of thymosin fraction 5 in the treatment of metastatic renal cell carcinoma. *Cancer Treat Rep* 1985; 69: 137-138.
150. Dizon QS, Southam CM. Abnormal cellular response in skin abrasion in cancer patients. *Cancer* 1963; 16: 1288-1292.
151. Domellof L. Athlin L, Berghem L. Effects of long-term combination chemotherapy on the reticuloendothelial system. *Cancer* 1984; 53: 2073-2078.
152. Donoran AJ. Reticuloendothelial function in patients with cancer: initial observations. *Am J Surg* 1967; 111: 230-238.
153. Droller MJ, Schneider MU, Perlmann P. A possible role of prostaglandins in the inhibition of natural and antibody-dependent cell-mediated cytotoxicity against tumor cells.

Cell Immunol 1978; 39: 165-177.

154. Droller MJ, Perlmann P, Schneider MU. Enhancement of natural and antibody-dependent lymphocyte cytotoxicity by drugs which inhibit prostaglandin production by tumor target cells. *Cell Immunol* 1978; 39: 154-164.
155. Ducos J, Mingueres J, Colombio P, et al. Lymphocyte response to PHA in patients with lung cancer. *Lancet* 1970; 1: 111-112.
156. Dupont B, Ballon M, Hansen JA, et al. Effects of transfer factor therapy on mixed lymphocyte culture reactivity. *Proc Natl Acad Sci* USA 1974; 71: 867-871.
157. Edelman GM, Cunningham BA, Gall WE, et al. The covalent structure of and entire gamma G immunoglobulin molecule. *Proc Natl Acad Sci* USA 1969; 63: 78-85.
158. Ehrke MJ, Mihich E, Berd D, Mastrangelo MJ. Effects of anticancer drugs on the immune system in humans. *Sem Oncol* 1989; 16: 3; 230-253.
159. Eilber FR, Nizze HA, Morton DL. Sequential evaluation of general immune competence in cancer patients: Correlation with clinical course. *Cancer* 1975; 35: 660-665.
160. Eilber FR, Morton DL. Impaired immunologic reactivity and recurrence following cancer surgery. *Cancer* 1970; 25: 362-367.
161. Eilber FR, Morton DL, Ketcham AS. Immunologic abnormalities in head and neck cancer. *Am J Surg* 1974; 128: 534-538.
162. Eisenthal A, Monselise J, Zinger R, Adler A. The effect of cimetidine on PBL from healthy donors and melanoma patients: Augmentation of T-cell responses to TCGF mitogens and alloantigens and of TCGF production. *Cancer Immunol Immunother* 1986; 21: 2; 141-147.
163. Eremin O, Ashby J, Franks D. Killer (K) cell activity in human normal lymph node, regional tumor lymph node, and inflammatory lymph node. *Int Arch Allergy Appl Immunol* 1977; 54: 210-220.
164. Eremin O, Ashby J, Stephens JP. Human natural cytotoxicity in the blood and lymphoid organs of healthy donors and patients with malignant disease. *Int J Cancer* 1978; 21: 35-41.
165. Ershler WB, Hacker MP, Burroughs BJ, et al. Cimetidine and the immune response. *In vivo* augmentation of nonspecific and specific immune response. *Clin Immunol Immunopathol* 1983; 26: 10-17.
166. Eskinazi DP, Perna JJ, Mihail R. Mononuclear cell subsets in patients with oral cancer. *Cancer* 1987; 60: 376-381.
167. Estervez ME, Ballart IJ, Diez RA, et al. Normalization of monocyte candidacidal deficiency by cyclooxygenase inhibitors in Hodgkin's disease. *Cancer* 1985; 55: 2774-2778.
168. Eura M, Maehara T, Tsutomo I, Ishikawa T. Suppressor cells in the effector phase of autologous cytotoxic reactions in cancer patients. *Cancer Immunol Immunother* 1988; 27: 147-153.
169. Ezdinli EZ, Simonson KL, Smith RA. Comparison of the effects of single vs. multiple agent chemotherapy on lymphocytes assayed by the rosette techniques. *Cancer* 1978; 42: 2234-2243.
170. Faguet GB, Davis HC. Survival in Hodgkin's disease: The role of immunocompetence and other major risk factors. *Blood* 1982; 59: 938-945.
171. Fisher RI, Bostick-Bruton F. Depressed T-cell proliferative responses in Hodgkin's disease: Role of monocyte-mediated suppression via prostaglandins and hydrogen peroxide. *J Immunol* 1982; 129: 1770-1774.
172. Fisherman EW. Does the allergic diathesis influence malignancy? *J Allergy* 1960; 31: 74-78.
173. Flodgren P, Sjogren HO. Influence *in vitro* on NK and K-cell activities by cimetidine and indomethacin with and without simultaneous exposure to interferon. *Cancer Immunol Immunother* 1985; 19: 28-34.
174. Florentin I, Kraus L, Mathé G, Hadden JW. *In vivo* study in mice of the immunopharmacological properties of NPT-15392. In: Serrou B, Rosenfeld C, Daniels JB, Saunders JP, eds. *Current concepts of human immunology and cancer* Amsterdam: Elsevier Biomedical, 1982: 463-469.
175. Forbes JT, Greco FA, Oldham RK. Human natural cell-mediated cytotoxicity: II. Levels in neoplastic disease. *Cancer Immunol Immunother* 1982; 11: 147-153.
176. Ford RJ, Tsao J, Kouttab NM, et al. Association of an interleukin abnormality with the T-cell defect in Hodgkin's disease. *Blood* 1984; 64: 386-392.
177. Fracchia A, Pacetti M, Barberis M, et al. Determination of T-lymphocyte subpopulations in patients with lung cancer. A comparison between lung lavage and peripheral blood by monoclonal antibodies and flow cytometry. *Respiration* 1987; 51: 3, 161-169.
178. Frydecka I. Natural killer-cell activity during the course of disease in patients with Hodgkin's disease. *Cancer* 1985; 56: 2799-2803.
179. Fujisama T, Yamaguchi Y, Kimura H, et al. Adjuvant immunotherapy of primary resected lung cancer with transfer factor. *Cancer* 1984; 54: 663-669.
180. Fujisawa T, Yamaguchi Y, Kimura H. Transfer factor in restoration and cell-mediated immunity in lung cancer patients. *Jpn J Surg* 1983; 13: 304-311.
181. Fuks Z, Strober S, Kaplan HS. Interaction between serum factors and T-lymphocytes in Hodgkin's disease. *N Eng Med* 1976; 295: 1273-1278.
182. Fuks Z, Strober W, Bobrove AM, et al. Long-term effects of radiation on T- and B-lymphocytes in peripheral blood of patients with Hodgkin's disease. *J Clin Invest* 1976; 58: 803-814.
183. Garay GE, Pavlovsky S, Sasiain MC, et al. Immunocompetence and prognosis in children with acute lymphoblastic leukemia: Combination of two different maintenance therapies. *Med Pediatr Oncol* 1976; 2: 403-415.
184. Gatti RA, Good RA. Occurrence of malignancy in immunodeficiency disease: a literature review. *Cancer* 1971; 28: 89-98.
185. Geffner JR, Serebrinsky G, Isturiz MA. Normal human serum restores the expression of Fc8 receptors in immune complex: blocked human mononuclear cells. *Immunology* 1986; 59: 239-243.
186. Gilbert HA, Kagan AR, Miles J, et al. Delayed hypersensitivity in patients treated by curative radiotherapy. Its relation to tumor response and short-term survival. *J Surg Oncol* 1978; 10: 73-77.
187. Giulivi A, Cilano L, Roncoroni L, et al. Effects of cimetidine on *in vitro* transformation of peripheral monocytes to macrophages in healthy volunteers and cancer patients. *Int J Immunopharmacol* 1986; 8: 5; 517-523.
188. Goldenberg GJ, Brandes LJ, Lau WH, et al. Cooperative trial of immunotherapy for nasopharyngeal carcinoma with transfer factor from donors with Epstein-Barr virus antibody activities. *Cancer Treat Rep* 1985; 69: 761-767.

189. Goldrosen MH, Han T, Jung D, et al. Impaired lymphocyte blastogenic response in patients with colon adenocarcinoma: effects of disease and age. *J Surg Oncol* 1977; 9: 229-234.
190. Goldsmith HS, Levin AG, and Southam CM. A study of cellular responses in cancer patients by quantitative and qualitative Rebuck tests. *Surg Forum* 1965; 16: 102-104.
191. Goldstein AL, Low TLK, Thurman GB, et al. Thymosins and other hormone-like factors of the thymus gland. In: Mihich E, ed. *Immunological cancer therapeutics*. New York: Wiley, 1982: 137-190.
192. Golub SH, Rangel DM, Morton D. *In vitro* assessment of immunocompetence in patients with malignant melanoma. *Int J Cancer* 1977; 20: 873-880.
193. Goodwin JS, Messner RP, Bankhurst AD, et al. Prostaglandin-producing suppressor cells in Hodgkin's disease. *N Engl J Med* 1977; 297: 963-968.
194. Gottlieb AA, Farmer JL, Matzura CT, et al. Modulation of human T-cell production of migration inhibitory lymphocytes by cytokines derived from human leukocyte dialysates. *J Immunol* 1984; 132: 1, 256-260.
195. Green AA, Borella L. Immunologic rebound after cessation of long-term chemotherapy in acute leukemia. II. *In vitro* response to phytohemagglutinin and antigens by peripheral blood and bone marrow lymphocytes. *Blood* 1973; 42: 99-110.
196. Grohn P, Heinonen E, Klefstrom P, Tarkkanen J. Adjuvant postoperative radiotherapy, chemotherapy and immunotherapy in stage III breast cancer. *Cancer* 1985; 54: 670-674.
197. Groveman DS, Borden EC. *In vitro* and *in vivo* effects of levamisole on monocyte chemotaxis in normal donors and patients with colorectal carcinoma. *J Biol Response Mod* 1983; 2: 167-174.
198. Grzelak I, Olszewski WL, Engeset A. Decreased suppressor cell activity after surgery. *J Clin Lab Immunol* 1985; 16: 201-205.
199. Grzelak I, Olszewski WL, Engeset A. Suppressor cell activity in peripheral blood in cancer patients after surgery. *Clin Exp Immunol* 1983; 51: 149-156.
200. Guiliano AE, Rangel D, Golub SH, et al. Serum-mediated immunosuppression in lung cancer. *Cancer* 1979; 43: 917-924.
201. Gupta S, Cunningham-Rundles S. Deficient concanavalin-A-induced suppressor cell activity in women with untreated breast cancer. *J Clin Lab Immunol* 1982; 9: 159-161.
202. Gupta S, Good RA. Subpopulations of human T-lymphocytes: II. Effect of thymopoietin, corticosteroids, and irradiation. *Cell Immunol* 1977; 34: 10-18.
203. Haas GS, Halperin E, Doseretz D, et al. Differential recovery of circulating T-cell subsets after nodal irradiation for Hodgkin's disease. *J Immunol* 1984; 132: 1026-1030.
204. Hadden JW. Chemically-defined immunotherapeutic drugs under development for the treatment of cancer. In: Serrou B, Rosenfeld C, Daniels JC, and Saunders JP, eds. Current concepts in human immunology and cancer immunomodulation Amsterdam: *Elsevier Biomedical*, 1982: 439-448.
205. Hadden JW. Recent advances in the preclinical and clinical immunopharmacology of interleukin-2: emphasis on IL-2 as an immunorestorative agent. *Cancer Detect Prev* 1988; 12: 537-552.
206. Hadjipetrou-Kourounakis L, Manikou H, Tsougranis A. Restoration of immunosuppression in lung cancer by normal sera. *J Clin Lab Immunol* 1985; 16: 149-153.
207. Haim N, Meidav A, Samuelly B, et al. Prostaglandin-related and adherent cell suppressor system in apparently cured Hodgkin's disease patients. *J Biol Response Mod* 1984; 3: 219-225.
208. Hakim AA. Peripheral blood lymphocytes from patients with cancer lack interleukin-2 receptors. *Cancer* 1988; 61: 4, 689-701.
209. Halili M, Bosworth J, Romney S, et al. The long-term effect of radiotherapy on the immune status of patients cured of a gynecologic malignancy. *Cancer* 1976; 37: 2875-2878.
210. Hall HRS, Goldstein AL. The endocrine thymus. In: Becker KC, ed. *Principles and practice of endocrinology and metabolism*. New York Lippincott, 1990.
211. Han T, Takita H. Indomethacin-mediated enhancement of lymphocyte response to mitogens in healthy subjects and lung cancer patients. *Cancer* 1980; 46: 2416-2420.
212. Han T. Studies of correlation of lymphocyte response to phytohemagglutinin with the clinical and immunologic status in chronic lymphocytic leukemia. *Cancer* 1973; 31: 280-285.
213. Han T, Nemoto T, Ledesma EJ, Bruno S. Enhancement of T-lymphocyte response to mitogens by indomethacin in breast and colorectal cancer patients. *Int J Immunopharmacol* 1983; 5: 11-15.
214. Herr HW. Adherent suppressor cells in the blood of patients with bladder cancer. *J Urol* 1981; 126: 457-460.
215. Hakim AA. Lipid-like agent from human neoplastic cells suppresses cell-mediated immunity. *Cancer Immunol Immunother* 1980; 8: 1330.
216. Han T, Takita H. Immunologic impairment in bronchogenic carcinoma: A study of lymphocyte response to phytohemagglutinin. *Cancer* 1972; 30: 616-620.
217. Hanaue H, Kim DY, Machimura T, et al. Hemolytic streptococcus preparation Ok-432: Beneficial adjuvant therapy in recurrent gastric carcinoma. *Tokai J Exp Clin Med* 1987; 12: 4, 209-214.
218. Hancock BW, Bruce L, Sokol RJ, Clark A. Transfer factor in Hodgkin's disease: A randomized clinical and immunological study. *Eur J Cancer Clin Oncol* 1988; 24: 5; 929-933.
219. Hancock BW, Bruce L, Whitham MD, Ward AM. The effects of radiotherapy on immunity in patients with cured localized carcinoma of the cervix uteri. *Cancer* 1984; 53: 884-887.
220. Harris J, Copeland D. Impaired imunoresponsiveness in tumor patients. *Ann NY Acad Sci* 1974; 230: 56-85.
221. Harris JE, DeBoer KP, Vahey AC, Braun DP. The measurement of leukocyte subsets in the peripheral blood of cancer patients using monoclonal antibody reagents. *Med Pediatr Oncol* 1982; 10: 185-194.
222. Harris JE, Stewart THM. Recovery of mixed lymphocyte reactivity (MLR) following cancer chemotherapy in man. In: Schwartz MR, ed. *Proceedings of the Sixth Leukocytes Culture Conference*. New York: Academic Press, 1979: 555-580.
223. Haskell CM. Immunologic aspects of cancer chemotherapy. *Ann Rev Pharmacol Toxicol* 1977; 17: 179-195.
224. Hausman MS, Brossman SA, Snyderman R, et al. Defective monocyte function in patients with genitourinary carcinoma. *J Natl Cancer Inst* 1975; 55: 1047-1054.

225. Hayashi Y, Nishida T, Yoshida H, et al. Peripheral T-gamma lymphocyte population in head and neck cancer. *Cancer Immunol Immunother* 1984; 17: 160-164.
226. Heal JM, Chuang C, Blumberg N. Perioperative blood transfusions and prostate cancer recurrence and survival. *Am J Surg* 1988; 156: 374-379.
227. Hernandez JL, Sanz M, Crisi CD, et al. Lymphocyte subpopulations in colorectal cancer-postoperative evaluation. *Allergy Immunopathol* 1978; 6: 339-344.
228. Hersey P, Bindon C, Czerniecki M, et al. Inhibition of interleukin-2 production by factors released from tumor cells. *J Immunol* 131: 2837-2842.
229. Hersh EM, Gutterman JU, Mavligit GM, Reed RC. Immunologic aspects of chemotherapy. In: Cancer Chemotherapy-Fundamental Concepts and Recent Advances 1975; pp 279-294; *Yearbook medical*, Chicago.
230. Hersh EM. Vinca alkaloids. In: Sartorelli AC, Johns DG, eds. *Antineoplastic and immunosuppressive agents, part I.* New York: Springer Verlag, 1974: 601-602.
231. Hersh EM, Gutterman JU, Mavligit GM. Immunotherapy of leukemia. *Med Clin North Am* 1976; 60: 1019-1042.
232. Hersh EM, Gutterman JU, Mavligit GM, et al. Serial studies of immunocompetence of patients undergoing chemotherapy for acute leukemia. *J Clin Invest* 1974; 54: 401-408.
233. Hersh EM, Whitecan JP Jr, McCredie JB, et al. Chemotherapy, immunocompetence, immunosuppression and prognosis in acute leukemia. *N Engl J med* 1971; 285: 1211-1216.
234. Hersh EM, Irwin WS. Blastogenic responses of lymphocytes from patients with untreated and treated lymphomas. *Lymphology* 1969; 2: 150-160.
235. Hersh EM. Immunosuppressive agents. In: Sartorelli AC, Johns DG, eds. *Antineoplastic and immunosuppressive agents, part I.* New York: Springer Verlag, 1974: 555-576.
236. Hersh EM, Oppenheim J. Inhibition of *in vitro* lymphocyte transformation during chemotherapy in man. *Cancer Res* 1979; 27: 98-105.
237. Herskovic A, Bauer M, Seydel G, et al. Postoperative thoracic irradiation with or without levamisole in non-small-cell lung cancer: results of a radiation therapy oncology group study. *Int J Radiation Oncology Biol Phys* 1988; 14: 1; 37-42.
238. Hilal EY, Wanebo HJ, Pinsky CM, et al. Immunologic evaluation and prognosis in patients with head and neck cancer. *Am J Surg* 1977; 134: 68-73.
239. Hilgard P, Pohl J, Stekar J, Voegeli R. Oxazaphosphorines as biological response modifiers: experimental and clinical perspective. *Cancer Treat Rev* 1985; 12: 155-162.
240. Hillinger SM, Herzig GP. Impaired cell-mediated immunity in Hodgkin's disease mediated by suppressor lymphocytes and monocytes. *J Clin Invest* 1978; 61: 1620-1627.
241. Hirsh B, Johnson JT, Rabin BS, Thearle PB. Immunostimulation of patients with head and neck cancer. *In vitro* and preliminary clinical experience. *Arch Otolaryngol* 1983; 109: 298-301.
242. Hirshaut Y, Pinsky CM, Frydecka I, et al. Effect of short-term levamisole therapy on delayed hypersensitivity. *Cancer* 1980; 45: 362-366.
243. Hoagland JG, Scoggin S, Giavazzi R, et al. Tumor-derived suppressor factors (TDSFs) in normal and neoplastic colon and rectum. *J Surg Res* 1986; 40: 5, 467-474.
244. Hodgson WJB, Lowenfels AB. Blood transfusion and recurrence rates in colonic malignancy. *Lancet* 1982; 2: 1047.
245. Hojo H, Hashimoto Y. Cytotoxic cells induced in tumor-bearing rats by a streptococcal preparation (OK-432). *Gann* 1981; 72: 62-69.
246. Holm G, Mellstedt H, Bjorkholm M, et al. Lymphocyte abnormalities in untreated patients with Hodgkin's disease. *Cancer* 1976; 37: 751-762.
247. Holmes EC. Immunology of tumor-infiltrating lymphocytes. *Ann Surg* 1985; 201: 158-163.
248. Holmes E, Sibbitt WL, Bankhurst AD. Serum factors which suppress natural cytotoxicity in cancer patients. Int *Arch Allergy Appl Immunol* 1986; 80: 39-43.
249. Holmes EC, Golub SH. Immunologic defects in lung cancer patients. *J Thoracic Cardiovasc Surg* 1976; 71: 161-168.
250. Hoon DSB, Bowker RJ, Cochran AJ. Suppressor-cell activity in melanoma-draining lymph nodes. *Cancer Res* 1987; 47: 1529-1533.
251. Hoon DSB, Korn EL, Cochran AJ. Variations in functional immunocompetence of individual tumor-draining lymph nodes in humans. *Cancer Res* 1987; 47: 1740-1744.
252. Hoon DS, Irie RF, Cochran AJ. Gangliosides from human melanoma immunomodulate responses of T-cells to interleukin-2. *Cell Immunol* 1988; 111: 2, 410-419.
253. Horiguchi M, Saito A, Sonoda H. A gastric cancer showing marked improvement (stage IV) with lentinan immunotherapy and 5-FU, MMC-chemotherapy. *Gan To Kagaku Ryoho* 1988; 15: 6, 1973-1977.
254. Horrino N. Impaired PWM-induced polyclonal B-cell activation in patients with malignancies treated with various intermittent combination chemotherapies including doxorubicin. *Cancer* 1982; 50: 659-667.
255. Hortobagyi GN, Hersh EM, Papadopoulos EJ, et al. Initial clinical studies with copovithane. *J Biol Response Mod* 1986; 5: 319-329.
256. Hsu CC, Logerfo P. Correlation between serum alpha globulin and plasma inhibitory effect of PHA-stimulated lymphocytes in colon cancer patients. *Proc Soc Exp Biol Med* 1972; 139: 575-578.
257. Huang AT, Mold NG, Fisher Sr, et al. A prospective study of squamous head and neck carcinoma. *Cancer* 1987; 59: 1721-1726.
258. Hubbard GW, Wanebo H, Fukuda M, Pace R. Defective suppressor-cell activity in cancer patients: A defect in immune regulation. *Cancer* 1981; 47: 2177-2184.
259. Ninneman JL. Melanoma-associated immunosuppression through B-cell activation of suppressor T-cells. *J Immunol* 1978; 120: 1573-1579.
260. Hughes NR. Serum concentrations of gamma G, gamma A and gamma M immunoglobulins in patients with carcinoma, melanoma, and sarcoma. *J Natl Cancer Inst* 1971; 46: 1015-1028.
261. Humphrey LJ, Humphrey MA, Singla O, Volenec FJ. Immunologic responsiveness of patients with cancer: relationship to tumor type, stage and prognosis. *Ann Surg* 1981; 193: 574-578.
262. Hyman GA. Increased incidence of neoplasia in association with chronic lymphocytic leukemia. *Scand J Haematol* 1969; 6: 99-104.
263. Iaffaioli RV, Frasci G, Tortora G, et al. Effect of thymic extract 'thymostimulin' on the incidence of infections and myelotoxicity during adjuvant chemotherapy for breast cancer. *Thymus* 1988; 12: 69-75.

264. Ichimura O, Suzuki S, Saito M, et al. Augmentation of interleukin-1 and interleukin-2 production by OK-432. *Int J Immunopharmacol* 1985; 7: 263-270.
265. Inagaki T, Morise K, Matsunaga H. Effects of endoscopic intratumoral injection of lentinan in patients with gastric cancer. *Gan To Kagaku Ryoho* 1988; 15: 2, 319-324.
266. Intergropu 5-FU/levamisole study positive; untreated arms stopped, clinical alert sent. Clin Trials – *Clin Cancer Lett* 1989; October.
267. Israel L, Mugica J, Chahinian PH. Prognosis of early bronchogenic carcinoma: Survival cures of 451 patients after resection of lung cancer in relation to the results of preoperative tuberculin skin test. *Biomed Exp* 1973; 19: 68-72.
268. Itoh K, Pellis NR, Balch C. Monocyte-dependent serum-borne suppressor of induction of lymphokine-activated killer cells in lymphocytes from melanoma patients. *Cancer Immunol Immunother* 1989; 29: 57-62.
269. Jacobs D, Houri M, Landon J, Merret TG. Circulating levels of immunoglobulin E in patients with cancer. *Lancet* 1972; 2: 1059-1061.
270. Jacobson DR, Zolla-Pazner S. Immunosuppression and infection in multiple myeloma. *Sem Oncol* 1986; 13: 3; 282-290.
271. Jansen HM, The TH, deGast GC, et al. The primary immune response of patients with different stages of squamous-cell bronchial carcinoma. *Thorax* 1978; 33: 755-760.
272. Jenkins VK, Ray P, Ellis HN, et al. Lymphocyte response in patients with head and neck cancer: effect of clinical stage and radiotherapy. *Arch Otolaryngol* 1976; 102: 596-600.
273. Jenkins VK, Griffiths CM, Ray P, et al. Radiotherapy and head and neck cancer. Role of lymphocyte response and clinical stage. *Arch Otolaryngol* 1980; 106: 414-418.
274. Jerrells TR, Dean JH, Richardson GL, et al. Role of suppressor cells in depression of *in vitro* lymphoproliferative responses of lung cancer and breast cancer patients. *J Natl Cancer Inst* 1978; 61: 1001-1009.
275. Jerrells TR, Dean JH, Herberman RB. Relationship between T-lymphocyte levels and lymphoproliferative responses to mitogens and alloantigens in lung and breast cancer patients. *Int J Cancer* 1978; 21: 282-290.
276. Job G, Pfeundschuh M, Bauer M, et al. The influence of radiation therapy on T-lymphocyte subpopulations defined by monoclonal antibodies. *Int J Radiat Oncol Biol Phys* 1984; 10: 2077-2081.
277. Joensun H, Nordman E, Toivanen A. Long-term effect of levamisole on the immune functions in melanoma patients. *Strahlenther Onkol* 1986; 162: 12, 753-756.
278. Joensun H, Toivanen A, Nordman E. Effect of tamoxifen on immune function. *Cancer Treat Rep* 1986; 7: 3, 381-382.
279. Johnson JD, Summersgill JT, Raff MJ. The *in vitro* effects of methotrexate on the phagocytosis and intracellular killing of *Staphylococcus aureus* by human neutrophils. *Cancer* 1986; 57: 2343-2345.
280. Johnston-Early A, Cohen MH, Fossieck BE, et al. Delayed hypersensitivity skin testing as a prognostic indicator in patients with small-cell lung cancer. *Cancer* 1983; 52: 1395-1400.
281. Jondal M, Merrill J, Ullberg M. Monocyte-induced human natural killer cell suppression followed by increased cytotoxic activity during short-term *in vitro* culture in autologous serum. *Scand J Immunol* 1981; 14: 555-563.
282. Jones KD, Whitehead RH, Grimshaw D, Hughes LE. Lymphocyte response to PHA and patient response to chemotherapy in breast cancer. *Clin Oncol* 1980; 6: 159-166.
283. Jones SE, Griffith K, Dombrowski P, Gaines JA. Immunodeficiency in patients with non-Hodgkin's lymphomas. *Blood* 1977; 49: 335-344.
284. Jose DG, Seshadri R. Circulating immune complexes in neuroblastoma: direct assay and role in blocking specific cellular immunity. *Int J Cancer* 1974; 13: 824-838.
285. Jubert AV, Lee ET, Hersh EM, McBridge CM. Effects of surgery, anesthesia and intraoperative blood loss on immunocompetence. *J Surg Res* 1973; 15: 399-403.
286. Jung TT, Berlinger NT, Juhn SK. Prostaglandins in squamous-cell carcinoma of the head and neck: a preliminary study. *Laryngoscope* 1985; 95: 307-312.
287. Kadish AS, Doyle AT, Steinhaur EH, Ghossein NA. Natural cytotoxicity and interferon production in human cancer: deficient natural killer activity and normal interferon production in patients with advanced disease. J *Immunol* 1981; 127: 1817-1822.
288. Kaneko T. Effects of lentinan on cytotoxic functions of human lymphocytes. *Immunopharmacol Immunotoxicol* 1988; 10: 2, 157-163.
289. Kaplan HS. *Hodgkin's disease*. Cambridge Mass: Harvard University Press, 1980.
290. Kaplan HS. *Hodgkin's disease*. Cambridge, Mass. Harvard University Press, 1980.
291. Karavodin LM, Guilliano AE, Golub SH. T-lymphocyte subsets in patients with malignant melanoma. *Cancer Immunol Immunother* 1981; 11: 251-254.
292. Kaszubowski PA, Husky G, Tung KS, Williams RC Jr. T-lymphocyte subpopulations in peripheral blood and tissues of cancer patients. *Cancer Res* 1980; 40: 4684-4657.
293. Katz AE. Immunobiologic staging of patients with carcinoma of the head and neck. *Laryngoscope* 1983; 93: 445-463.
294. Kawaguchi T, Suematsu M, Koizumi HM, et al. Activation of macrophage function by intraperitoneal administration of the streptococcal anti-tumor agent OK-432. *Immunopharmacology* 1983; 6: 1077-1089.
295. Kay RG, Mason BH, Stephans EJ, et al. Levamisole in primary breast cancer: A controlled study in conjunction with L-phenylalanine mustard. *Cancer* 1983; 51: 1992-1997.
296. Keller SM, Groshen S, Martini N, Kaiser LR. Blood transfusion and lung cancer recurrence. *Cancer* 1988; 62: 606-610.
297. Kenady DE, Chretien PB, Potvin C, et al. Effect of thymosin *in vitro* on T-cell levels during radiation therapy. *Cancer* 1972; 39: 642-652.
298. Kerman RH, Stefani SS. Phytohemagglutinin stimulation of lymphocytes in lung cancer patients. *Oncology* 1977; 34: 10-12.
299. Kerman RH, Smith R, Stefani SS. Active T-rosette forming cells in the peripheral blood of cancer patients. *Cancer Res* 1976; 36: 3274-3280.
300. Khoo SK, Whitaker SV, Jones IS, Thomas DA. Levamisole as adjuvant to chemotherapy of ovarian cancer. Results of a randomized trial and 4-year follow-up. *Cancer* 1984; 54: 986-990.

301. Kikuchi Y, Kizawa I, Oomori K, et al. Effects of cimetidine on interleukin-2 production by peripheral blood lymphocytes in advanced ovarian carcinoma. *Eur J Cancer Clin Oncol* 1988; 24: 7, 1185-1190.

302. Kirsh MM, Orringer MB, McAuliffe S, et al. Transfer factor in the treatment of carcinoma of the lung. *Ann Thorac Surg* 1984; 38: 140-145.

303. Klefstrom P, Holsti P, Grohn P, et al. Levamisole in the treatment of stage II breast cancer. Five-year follow-up of a randomized double-blind study. *Cancer* 1985; 55: 2753-2757.

304. Klefstrom P. Combination of levamisole immunotherapy and polychemotherapy in advanced breast cancer. *Cancer Treat Rep* 1980; 64: 65-72.

305. Klefstrom P, Nuortio L, Taskinen E. Post-operative radiation therapy and adjuvant chemoimmunotherapy in breast cancer. Aspects of timing and immune competence. *Acta Radiol* [Oncol] 1986; 25: 3; 161-166.

306. Klefstrom P, Grohn P, Heinonen E, et al. Adjuvant post-operative radiotherapy, chemotherapy, and immunotherapy in stage III breast cancer. II. Five-year results and influence of levamisole. *Cancer* 1987; 60: 5, 936-942.

307. Klefstrom P, Holsti P, Grohn P, Heinonem E. Combination of levamisole immunotherapy with conventional treatments in breast cancer. In: Terry WD, ed. Proceedings of Second International Conference on Immunotherapy of Cancer. Bethesda, Md: 19 : 4128-4130.

308. Kleinerman ES, Zwelling LA, Schwartz R, et al. Effect of L-phenylalanine mustard, adriamycin and actinomycin D, and 4'-(9-acridinylamino) methanesulfon-m-anisidide on naturally occurring human spontaneous monocyte-mediated cytotoxicity. *Cancer Res* 1982; 42: 1692-1695.

309. Koba F, Akiyoshi T, Tsuji H. Natural killer-cell activity in the perigastric lymph nodes from patients with gastric carcinoma or benign lesions. *J Clin Lab Immunol* 1987; 23: 4; 191-195.

310. Kova J, Ninger E, Zemanov D, Lauerov P. A prospective study of lymphocyte responses to phytohemagglutinin in melanoma (lack of prognostic value of correlation with minimal tumor burden). *Neoplasma* 1980; 27: 575-582.

311. Kratikanont P, deShazo RD, Banks DE, Chapman Y. Cytotoxic cell function in bronchogenic carcinoma. *Chest* 1098; 92: 1, 90-94.

312. Kraus S, Comas F, Perez C, et al. Treatment of inoperable non-small-cell carcinoma of the lung with radiation therapy, with or without levamisole. *Am J Clin Oncol* 1984; 7: 405-412.

313. Kreienberg R, Boerner D, Melchert F, and Lemmell EM. Reduction of the immunosuppressive action of chemotherapeutics in patients with mammary carcinoma by Azimexon. *J Immunopharmacol* 1983; 5: 49-64.

314. Kripke ML. Immunoregulation of carcinogenesis: Past, present, and future. *J Natl Cancer Inst* 1988; 80: 722-727.

315. Krown S, Pinsky CM, Wanebo HJ, et al. Immunologic reactivity and prognosis in breast cancer. *Cancer* 1980; 46: 1746-1752.

316. Kumano N, Suzuki S, Oizumi K, et al. Imbalance of T-cell subsets in cancer patients and its modification with bestatin, a small molecular immunomodifier. *Tohoku J Exp Med* 1985; 147: 125-133.

317. Kurosu Y, Tanaka N, Furusho Y, Morita K. Cimetidine-mediated augmentation of lymphocyte responses to phytohemagglutinin in gastric cancer patients. *Jpn J Clin Oncol* 1989; 19: 1; 56-61.

318. Lauria F, Raspadori D, Tura S. Effect of a thymic factor on T-lymphocytes in B-cell chronic lymphocytic leukemia: *In vitro* and *in vivo* studies. *Blood* 1984; 64: 667-671.

319. Lauria F, Foa R, Gobbi M, et al. Increased proportion of suppressor/cytotoxic (OKT8+) cells in patients with Hodgkin's disease in long-lasting remission. *Cancer* 1983; 52: 1385-1388.

320. Lauria JA, Moertel CG, Fleming TR, et al. Surgical adjuvant therapy of large-bowel carcinoma: An evaluation of levamisole and the combination of levamisole and fluorouracil. *J Clin Oncol* 1989; 7: 1447-1456.

321. Laurie J, Moertel C, Fleming T, et al. Surgical adjuvant therapy of poor prognosis colorectal cancer with levamisole alone or combined levamisole and 5-fluorouracil (5-FU) (Abstract). *Proc ASCO* 1986; 5: 81.

322. Lawrence HS. The transfer in humans of delayed skin sensitivity to streptococcal M substance and to tuberculin with disrupted leukocytes. *J Clin Invest* 1955; 34: 219-230.

323. Lee ET, Ishmael R, Bottomley RH, Murray JL. An analysis of skin tests and their relationship to recurrence and survival in stage III and stage IV melanoma patients. *Cancer* 1982; 49: 2336-2341.

324. Lee YT. Delayed cutaneous hypersensitivity, lymphocyte count, and blood tests, in patients with breast carcinoma. *J Surg Oncol* 1984; 27: 135-140.

325. Lee AKY, Rowley M, MacKay IR. Antibody-producing capacity in human cancer. *Br J Cancer* 24: 454-463.

326. Lee YT, Sparks FC, Eilber FR, Morton DL. Delayed cutaneous hypersensitivity and peripheral lymphocyte counts in patients with advanced cancer. *Cancer* 1975; 35: 748-755.

327. Leibler GA, Concannon JP, Magorern GJ, et al. Immunoprofile studies for patients with bronchogenic carcinoma. *J Thorac Cardiovasc Surg* 1977; 74: 506-518.

328. Levin RH, Landy M, Frei E. The effect of 6-mercaptopurine on immune response in man. *N Engl J Med* 1964; 271: 16-22.

329. Levo Y, Rotter V, Ramot B. Restoration of cellular immune response by levamisole in patients with Hodgkin's disease. *Biomedicine* 1975; 23: 198-200.

330. Levy S, Herberman R, Lippman M, d'Angelo T. Correlation of stress factors with sustained depression of natural killer cell activity and predicted prognosis in patients with breast cancer. *J Clin Oncol* 1987; 5: 3; 348-353.

331. Lewinski UH, Mavligit GM, Hersh EM. Cellular immune modulation after a single high dose of levamisole. *Cancer* 1980; 46: 2185-2194.

332. Liberati AM, Bragia M, Edwards BS, et al. Immunorestorative properties of thymostimulin (TS) in patients with Hodgkin's disease in clinical remission. *Cancer Immunol Immunother* 1985; 19: 136-141.

333. Liberata AM, Ballatori E, Fizzotti M, et al. A randomized trial to evaluate the immunorestorative properties of thymostimulin in patients with Hodgkin's disease in complete remission. *Cancer Immunol Immunother* 1988; 26: 87-93.

334. Liberata AM, Voekel JG, Borden EC, et al. Influence of non-specific immunologic factors on prognosis in advanced bronchogenic carcinoma. *Cancer Immunol Immunother* 1982; 13: 140-144.

335. Lichtenstein A, Zighelboim J, Dorey R, et al. Comparison of immune derangements in patients with different

malignancies. *Cancer* 1980; 45: 2090-2095.

336. Lin CC, Kuo YC, Huang WC, Lin CY. Natural killer-cell activity in lung cancer patients. *Chest* 1987; 92: 6, 1022-1024.
337. Lotan R. Effects of vitamin A and its analogs (retinoids) on normal and neoplastic cells. *Biochim Biophys Acta* 1980; 605: 33-91.
338. Loutfi A, Shakr A, Jerry M, et al. Double-blind randomized prospective trial of levamisole/placebo in stage I cutaneous malignant melanoma. *Clin Invest Med* 1987; 10: 4, 325-328.
339. Ludwig CU, Hartmann D, Landmann R, et al. Unaltered immunocompetence in patients with nondisseminated breast cancer at the time of diagnosis. *Cancer* 1985; 55: 1673-1678.
340. Lundy J, Raaf JH, Deakins S, Wanebo HJ. The acute and chronic effects of alcohol on the human immune system. *Surg Gynecol Obstet* 1975; 141: 212-218.
341. Luzi G, Troopea F, Seminara R, et al. Clinical and immunological evaluation in non-resectable lung cancer patients treated with thymostimulin. In: Byrom NA, Hobbs JR, eds. *Thymic factor therapy*. New York: Raven Press, 1984: 309-320.
342. Maca RM, Panje WR. Indomethacin-sensitive suppressor-cell activity in head and neck cancer patients pre- and post-irradiation therapy. *Cancer* 1982; 50: 483-489.
343. Macchiarini P, Danesi R, Del Tacca M, Angeletti CA. Effects of thymostimulin on chemotherapy-induced toxicity and long-term survival in small-cell lung cancer patients. *Anticancer Res* 1989; 9: 1; 193-196.
344. Mackay JR, Goodyear MD, Riglar C, et al. Effect on immunologic and other indices of adjuvant cytotoxic chemotherapy including melphalan in breast cancer. *Cancer* 1984; 53: 2619-2627.
345. Maguire LC, Roszman TL, Lackey S. Failure of cimetidine as an immunomodulator in cancer patients and normal subjects. *South Med J* 1985; 78: 1078-1080.
346. Mahaley MS Jr, Brooks WH, Roszman TL, et al. Immunobiology of primary intracranial tumors. I. Studies of the cellular immunity of brain tumor patients. *J Neurosurg* 1977; 46: 467-476.
347. Maisel RH, Ogura JH. Dinitrochlorobenzene skin sensitization and peripheral lymphocyte count: predictors of survival in head and neck cancer. *Ann Otol Rhinol Laryngol* 1976; 85: 517-522.
348. Mandel MA, Dvorak K, Decasse JJ. Salivary immunoglobulins in patients with oropharyngeal and bronchopulmonary cancer. *Cancer* 1973; 31: 1408-1413.
349. Mandeville R, Lamoureux G-T, Poisson SL, Poisson R. Biological markers and breast cancer: a multiparameter study. II. Depressed immune competence. *Cancer* 1982; 50: 1280-1288.
350. Mantovani G, Floris C, Maccio A, et al. Role of interleukin-2 (IL-2) in cancer-related immune deficiency: *In vitro* response to IL-2, production of IL-2, and IL-2 receptor expression in patients with advanced cancer. *Cancer Detect Prev* 1988; 12: 149-159.
351. Marshall ME, Mendelsohn L, Butler K, et al. Treatment of metastatic renal cell carcinoma with coumarin (1, 2-benzopyrone) and cimetidine: a pilot study. *J Clin Oncol* 1987; 5: 6; 862-866.
352. Marshall ME, Riley LK, Rhoades J, et al. Effects of coumarin (1, 2-benzopyrone) and cimetidine on peripheral blood lymphocytes, natural killer cells, and monocytes in patients with advanced malignancies. *J Biol Response Mod* 1989; 8: 1, 62-69.
353. Martelli MF, Velardi A, Rambotti P, et al. The *in vivo* effect of a thymic factor (thymostimulin) in immunologic parameters of patients with untreated Hodgkin's disease. *Cancer* 1982; 50: 490-497.
354. Mastrangelo MJ, Berd D, Maguire H Jr. Cell-mediated immunity: The immunoaugmenting effects of cancer chemotherapeutic agents. *Sem Oncol* 1986; 13: 2; 186-194.
355. Mathé G, Amiel JL, Schwarzenberg L, et al. Active immunotherapy for acute lymphoblastic leukemia. *Lancet* 1969; 1: 697-699.
356. Mathé G. Do tuftsin and bestatin constitute a biopharmacological immunoregulatory system? *Cancer* Detect Prev Suppl 1987; 1: 445-455.
357. Mathé G, Umezawa H, Misset JL, et al. Immunomodulating properties of bestatin in cancer patients. A phase II trial. *Biomed Pharmacother* 1986; 40: 10, 379-382.
358. Mavligit GM. Immunologic effects of cimetidine: potential uses. *Pharmacotherapy* 1987; 7: 120S-124S.
359. Mavligit GM, Raphael LS, Calvo DB III, Wong WL. Indomethacin-induced monocyte-dependent restoration of local graft-versus-host reaction among cells from cancer patients. *J Natl Cancer Inst* 1980; 65: 317-320.
360. McCredie JA, Macdonald HR. Antibody-dependent cellular cytotoxicity in cancer patients: Lack of prognostic value. *Br J Cancer* 1980; 41: 880-885.
361. McGeorge MB, Russel EC, Mohanakumar T. Immunologic evaluation of long-term effects of childhood ALL chemotherapy: Analysis of *in vitro* NK- and K-cell activities of peripheral blood lymphocytes. *Am J Hematol* 1982; 12: 19-27.
362. McGinnes K, Florence J, Penny R. The effect of radiotherapy on the natural killer (NK) cell activity of cancer patients. *J Clin Immunol* 1987; 7: 3, 210-217.
363. Menconi E, Barzi A, Greco M, et al. Immunological profile of breast cancer patients in early of advanced disease. *Experimentia* 1979; 35: 820-822.
364. Merrin C, Han T. Immune responses in bladder cancer. *J Urol* 1974; 111: 170-172.
365. Messerschmidt GL, Henry DH, Snyder HW Jr, et al. Protein A immunoadsorption in the treatment of malignant disease. *J Clin Oncol* 1988; 6: 2; 203-212.
366. Metzher Z, Hoffeld JT, Oppenheim JJ. Evidence for the involvement of monocyte-derived toxic oxygen metabolites in the lymphocyte dysfunction of Hodgkin's disease. *Clin Exp Immunol* 1981; 46: 313-320.
367. Micksche M, Cerni C, Kokron K, et al. Stimulation of the immune response in lung cancer patients by vitamin A. *Oncology* 1977; 34: 234-239.
368. Micksche M, Colot M, Kucera H. Radioimmunotherapy in advanced cervical cancer. In: Dubois JB, Serrou B, Rosenfeld C, eds. *Immunopharmacologic effects of radiation therapy*. New York: Raven Press, 1981: 499-518.
369. Mihich E. Biological response modifiers in cancer therapeutics: Potentialities and limitations. *Cancer Detect Prev* 1988; 12: 531-535.
370. Mihich E, Ehreke MJ, Ishizuka M. Immunomodulation by antibiotics. In: Mihich E, Sakurai Y, eds. *Biological responses in cancer, vol 3: immunomodulation by anti-cancer drugs*. New York: Plenum Press, 1985: 71-73.
371. Miller HC, Vito C. Action of a thymic cytokine TsIF in

reversing the autoimmune disease state of the MRL/1pr mouse. *Mol Biother* 1989; 1: 4, 213-217.

372. Miller LL, Spitler LE, Allen RE, Minot DR. A randomized, double-blind, placebo-controlled trial of transfer factor as adjuvant therapy for malignant melanoma. *Cancer* 1988; 61: 1543-1549.

373. Miller FR, Kataoka T. Interactions of antimetabolites with tumors and the immune system. In: Mihich E, Sakurai Y, eds. *Biological responses in cancer, vol 3: immunomodulation by anti-cancer drugs.* New York: Plenum Press, 1985: 33-69.

374. Mitchell MS, Kempf RA, Harel W, et al. Effectiveness and tolerability of low-dose cyclophosphamide and low-dose intravenous interleukin-2 disseminated melanoma. *J Clin Oncol* 1988; 6: 3; 409-424.

375. Mitchell MS, Defonti RC. Immunosuppression by 5-fluorouracil. *Cancer* 1970; 26: 884-889.

376. Mitchell MS, Wade ME, Deconti RC, et al. Immunosuppressive effects of cytosine arabinoside and methotrexate in man. *Ann Int Med* 1969; 70: 535-547.

377. Miwa H, Orita K. Immunotherapy of gastrointestinal cancer patients with levamisole. *Acta Med Okayama* 1979; 33: 29-42.

378. Miwa H, Orita K. Cancer immunotherapy with levamisole. *Acta Med Okayama* 1978; 32: 239-245.

379. Miwa H, Orita K. Reactivating effect of levamisole on cell-mediated immunity in gastrointestinal cancer patients. *Acta Med Okayama* 1977; 31: 325-329.

380. Modini C, Ziparo V, Cicconetti F, et al. Role of delayed cutaneous hypersensitivity reaction in classifying patients with bronchial carcinoma. *Tumori* 1985; 71: 277-281.

381. Moertel CG, Fleming TR, MacDonald JS, et al. Levamisole and fluorouracil for adjuvant therapy of resected colon carcinoma. *N Engl J Med* 1990; 322: 6; 352-358.

382. Moertel CG, Ritts RE, O'Connell MJ, Silvers A. Nonspecific immune determinants in the patient with unresectable gastrointestinal carcinoma. *Cancer* 1979; 43: 1483-1492.

383. Monson JR, Ramsden C, Guillou PJ. Decreased interleukin-2 production in patients with gastrointestinal cancer. *Br J Surg* 1986; 73: 6; 483-486.

384. Monte JE, Bukowski RM, James RE, et al. A critical review of immunotherapy of disseminated renal adenocarcinoma. *J Surg Oncol* 1982; 21: 5-8.

385. Morales A, Eidinger D. Immune reactivity in renal cancer. *J Urol* 1976; 115: 510-513.

386. Morin A, Ballet J, Touraine J, Hadder JW. Current status of isoprinosine. In: Serrou B, Rosenfeld C, Daniels JC, Saunders JP, eds. *Current concepts in human immunology and cancer immunomodulation.* Amsterdam: Elsevier Biomedical, 1982: 479-489.

387. Morton DL, Eilber FR, Malmgren RA, Wood WC. Immunological factors which influence response to immunotherapy in malignant melanoma. *Surgery* 1970; 68: 158-164.

388. Mukherji B, Guha A, Loomis R, Ergin MT. Cell-mediated amplification and down regulation of cytotoxic immune response against autologous human cancer. *J Immunol* 1987; 138: 1987-1991.

389. Mukhopadhyaya R, Advani SH, Gangal SG. Functional evaluation of T-lymphocytes from peripheral blood and spleens in Hodgkin's disease. *Br J Cancer* 1987; 56: 800-802.

390. Munster AM. Post-traumatic immunosuppression is due to activation of suppressor T-cells. *Lancet* 1976; 1: 1329.

391. Munzarova M, Mechl Z, Kovarik J, Kolcova V. Skin tests with autologous cholesteryl hemisuccinate-treated tumor cells, DNCB and PPD and their relationship to prognosis in malignant melanoma patients. *Neoplasma* 1988; 35: 2, 229-234.

392. Murphy RM, Colton CK, Yarmush ML. Staphylococcal protein A adsorption in neoplastic disease: Analysis of physiochemical aspects. *Mol Biother* 1989; 1: 4, 186-207.

393. Murray JL, Kollmorgen GM. Inhibition of lymphocyte response by prostaglandin-producing suppressor cells in patients with melanoma. *J Clin Immunol* 1983; 3: 268-276.

394. Murray JL, Reuben JM, Smith TL, et al. A pilot clinical trial of the toxicity and immunorestorative effects of T-cell reconstituting factor (SR 270258) in immunosuppressed cancer patients. *J Biol Response Mod* 1987; 6: 1, 56-68.

395. Najjar VA. Biochemistry and physiology of tuftsin – Thr-Lys-Pro-Arg. In: Sbarra S, Strauss R, eds. *The reticuloendothelial system.* New York: Plenum Press, 1980: 45-71.

396. Nathanson SD, Zamfirescu PL, Portaro JK, et al. Acute effects of orally administered levamisole on random monocyte motility and chemotaxis in man. *J Natl Cancer Inst* 1978; 61: 301-306.

397. Nemoto T, Han T, Minowada J, et al. Cell-mediated immune status of breast cancer patients: evaluation by skin tests, lymphocyte stimulation and counts of rosette-forming cells. *J Natl Cancer Inst* 1974; 53: 641-645.

398. Niimoto M, Hattori T, Ito I, et al. Levamisole as post-operative adjuvant immunochemotherapy for gastric cancer. A randomized controlled study of the MMC + Tegafur regimen with or without levamisole. Report I. *Cancer Immunol Immunother* 1984; 18: 13-18.

399. Noda T, Asano M, Yoshie O, et al. Interferon-γ induction of human peripheral blood mononuclear cells by OK-432, a killed preparation of Streptococcus pyogenes. *Microbiol Immunol* 1985; 30: 81-88.

400. Noma T, Yoshimura N, Yata J. Depressed lymphocyte functions of cancer patients and their correlation by bestatin (product of *Streptomyces olivereticuli*). In: Serrou S, Rosenfeld C, Daniels JC, Saunders JP, eds. *Current concepts in human immunology and cancer immunomodulation.* Amsterdam: Elsevier Biomedical, 1982: 611-616.

401. Nordman E, Saarimaa H, Tolvanen A. The influence of 5-fluorouracil on cellular and humoral immunity in cancer patients. *Cancer* 1978; 41: 64-69.

402. Nordman E, Tolvanen A. Effects of irradiation of the immune function in patients with mammary, pulmonary or head and neck carcinoma. *Acta Radiol Oncol Radiat Phys Biol* 1978; 17: 3-9.

403. Norris RW, Byrom NA, Nagvekar NM, et al. Thymostimulin plus surgery in the treatment of primary truncal malignant melanoma: Preliminary results of a U.K. multicentre clinical trial. In: Byrom NA, Hobbs JR, eds *Thymic factor therapy*. New York: Raven Press, 1984: 341-348.

404. Oka S. A review of clinical studies of bestatin. Recent results. *Cancer Res* 1980; 75: 126-132.

405. Olivari A, Pradier R, Feierstein H, et al. Cell-mediated immune response in head and neck cancer patients. *J Surg Oncol* 1976; 8: 287-294.

406. Olivari AJ, Glait HM, Guardo A, et al. Levamisole in

squamous-cell carcinoma of the head and neck. *Cancer Treat Rep* 1979; 63: 983-990.

407. Onsrud M. Whole pelvic irradiation in stage I endometrial carcinoma: changes in numbers and reactivities of some blood lymphocyte subpopulations. *Gynecol Oncol* 1982; 13: 283-292.
408. Orita K, Miwa H, Fukuda H, et al. Preoperative cell-mediated immune status of gastric cancer patients. *Cancer* 1976; 38: 2343-2348.
409. Osband M, Shen Y, Schlesinger M, et al. Successful tumor immunotherapy with cimetidine in mice. *Lancet* 1981; 1: 636-638.
410. Oshimi K, Kano S, Takaku F, Okumura K. Augmentation of mouse natural killer cell activity by a streptococcal preparation OK-432. *J Natl Cancer Inst* 1980; 65: 1265-1269.
411. Ota K, Kurita S, Yamada K, et al. Immunotherapy with bestatin for acute non-lymphocytic leukemia in adults. *Cancer Immunol Immunother* 1986; 23: 1; 5-10.
412. Ozer H. Effects of alkylating agents on immunoregulatory mechanisms. In: Mihich E, Sakurai Y, eds. *Biological responses in cancer, vol 3: immunomodulation by anti-cancer drugs.* New York: Plenum Press, 1985: 95-129.
413. Paavonen T, Anderson LC, Adlercrentz H. Estradiol enhances human B-cell maturation via inhibition of suppressor T-cells in pokeweed mitogen-stimulated cultures. *J Exp Med* 1981; 154: 1935-1945.
414. Padmanabhan TK, Balaram P, Vasudevan DM. Role of levamisole immunotherapy as an adjuvant to radiotherapy in oral cancer. I. A three-year clinical follow-up. *Neoplasma* 1987; 34: 5, 627-632.
415. Paik YK, Kimura L, Yanagihora E, et al. Inhibition of the phytohemagglutinin stimulation of leukocytes by C-reactive protein. *J Reticuloendothel Soc* 1972; 11: 420.
416. Papatestas AE, Kark AE. Peripheral lymphocyte counts in breast carcinoma: an index of immune competence. *Cancer* 1978; 34: 2014-2017.
417. Papenhausen PR, Kukwa A, Croft CB, et al. Cellular immunity in patients with epidermoid cancer of the head and neck. *Laryngoscope* 1979; 89: 538-549.
418. Park SK, Brody JL, Wallace HA, Blakemore WS. Immunosuppressive effect of surgery. Lancet 1971; 1: 53-55.
419. Parkinson DR, Cano PO, Jerry LM, et al. Complications of cancer immunotherapy with levamisole. *Lancet* 1977; i: 1129-1132.
420. Passwell J, Lavanon M, Davidsohn J, Ramot B. Monocyte PG E2 secretion in Hodgkin's disease and its relation to decreased cellular immunity. *Clin Exp Immunol* 1983; 51: 61-68.
421. Paterson AHG, Natting M, Takata L, et al. Chemoimmunotherapy with levamisole in metastatic breast carcinoma: a controlled clinical trial. *Cancer Clin Trials* 1980; 3: 5-10.
422. Patt YZ, Hersh EM, Reuben J, et al. A phase-I study of intravenous azimexon therapy in human cancer. J Biol *Response Mod* 1986; 5: 4; 313-318.
423. Pauwels R, Van der Straeter M. Delayed hypersensitivity in patients with bronchial carcinoma. *Scand J Resp* 1975; 56: 160-164.
424. Pavlovsky S, Muriel FS, Garay G, et al. Chemoimmunotherapy with levamisole in acute lymphoblastic leukemia. *Cancer* 1981; 48: 1500-1507.
425. Pavlovsky S, Garay G, Sackman MF, Svarch E. Levamisole therapy during maintenance of remission in patients with acute lymphoblastic leukemia. In: Terry WD, ed. *Proceedings of Second International Conference on Immunotherapy of Cancer.* Amsterdam: Elsevier/North-Holland, 1980: 47-54.
426. Payne JE, Meyer JH, Macpherson JG, et al. The value of lymphocyte transformation in carcinoma of the colon and rectum. *Surg Gynecol Obstet* 1980; 150: 687-693.
427. Penn I. Tumors of the immunocompromised patient. *Annu Rev Med* 1988; 39: 63-73.
428. Penn I. Occurrence of cancer in immune deficiency. *Cancer* 1974; 34: 858-866.
429. Perez CA, Bauer M, Emami BN, et al. Thoracic irradiation with or without levamisole (NSC #177023) in unresectable non-small-cell carcinoma of the lung: A phase III randomized trial of the RTOG. *Int J Radiation Oncology Biol Phys* 1988; 15: 6, 1337-1346.
430. Petrini B, Wasserman J, Blomgren H, Rotstein S. T-helper/suppressor ratios in chemotherapy and radiotherapy. *Clin Exp Immunol* 1983; 53: 255-256.
431. Petrini B, Wasserman J, Glas U, Blomgren H. T-lymphocyte subpopulations in blood following radiation therapy for breast cancer. *Eur J Cancer Clin Oncol* 1982; 18: 921-924.
432. Petrini B, Wasserman J, Biberfeld G, et al. The effect of *in vitro* irradiation on PHA-mediated cytotoxicity and lymphocytes with receptors for the Fc pat of Ig. *J Clin Lab Immunol* 1979; 2: 333-336.
433. Pierri I, Cordone G, Rogna S, et al. T-lymphocyte phenotype and functions in patients with head and neck cancer. *Laryngoscope* 1985; 95: 577-581.
434. Pines A. BCG plus levamisole following irradiation of advanced squamous bronchial carcinoma. *Int J Radiation Oncology Biol Phys* 1980; 6: 1041-1042.
435. Pinsky CM, El-Domeiri A, Caron AA, et al. Delayed hypersensitivity reactions in patients with cancer. In: Mathé G, Weiner R, eds. *Recent results in cancer research*, pp. 37-41.
436. Pinsky CM, Wanebo H, Mike V, Oettgen H. Delayed cutaneous hypersensitivity reactions and prognosis in patients with cancer. *Ann NY Acad Sci* 1976; 276: 407-410.
437. Pitchenik AE, Guffee J, Stein-Streilein J. Lung natural killer and interleukin-2 activity in lung cancer. A pulmonary compartment of augmented natural killer activity occurs in patients with bronchogenic carcinoma. *Am Rev Respir Dis* 1987; 136: 6, 1327-1332.
438. Plesnicar S. Immunoglobulins in carcinoma of the uterine cervix. *Acta Radiol* 1972; 11: 37-47.
439. Pompidou A, Soubrane C, Cour V, et al. Immunological effects of isoprinosine as a pulse immunotherapy in melanoma and ARC patients. *Cancer Detect Prev Suppl* 1987; 1: 457-462.
440. Posner MR, Reinherz E, Lane H, et al. Circulating lymphocyte populations in Hodgkin's disease after mantle and para-aortic irradiation. *Blood* 1983; 61: 705-708.
441. Powles TJ, Dady DJ, Williams J, et al. Use of inhibitor of prostaglandin synthesis and patients with breast cancer. In: Sammuelsson B, Ramwel PW, Paoletti R, eds. *Advances in prostaglandin and thromboxane research*, vol 6. New York: Raven Press, 1980: 511-516.
442. Prehn RT, Prehn LM. The flip side of tumor immunity. *Arch Surg* 1989; 124: 102-106.
443. Prehn RT, Prehn LM. The autoimmune nature of cancer. *Cancer Res February* 15, 1987: 927-932.

444. Pritchard DJ, Ritts RE Jr, Taylor WF, Miller GC. A prospective study of immune responsiveness in humans. I. Assessment of initial pretreatment status with stage of disease. *Cancer* 1978; 41: 2165-2173.
445. Pross HF, Baines MG. Spontaneous human lymphocyte-mediated cytotoxicity against tumor target cells: I. The effect of malignant disease. *Int J Cancer* 1976; 18: 593-604.
446. Pui C-H, Ip SH, Kung P, et al. High serum interleukin-2 receptor levels are related to advanced disease and a poor outcome in childhood non-Hodgkin's lymphoma. *Blood* 1987; 70: 3; 624-628.
447. Pulay TA, Csomor S. Effect of levamisole treatment on immunological parameters and the early course of cervical cancer. *Neoplasia* 1980; 29: 81-86.
448. Quirt I, Shelley W, Bodurtha A, et al. Adjuvant levamisole improves survival and disease-free survival in patients with poor prognostics with malignant melanoma. (Abstr.) *Proc ASCO* 1986; 5: 130.
449. Raben M, Walch N, Galili U, Schlesinger M. The effect of radiation therapy on lymphocyte subpopulations in cancer patients. *Cancer* 1976; 37: 1417-1421.
450. Ramot B, Biniaminov M, Shoham C, Rosenthal E. The effect of levamisole on E-rosette-forming cells *in vivo* and *in vitro* in Hodgkin's disease patients. *N Engl Med* 1976; 194: 809-811.
451. Ramot B, Rosenthal E, Biniaminov M, Ben-Bassat I. Effect of levamisole, thymic humoral factor, and indomethacin on E-rosette formation of lymphocytes in Hodgkin's disease. *Isr J Med Sci* 1981; 17: 232-235.
452. Rand RJ, Jenkins DM, Bulmer R. T and B lymphocyte subpopulations in pre-invasive and invasive carcinoma of the cervix. *Clin Exp Immunol* 1977; 30: 421-428.
453. Rangel DM, Golub SH, Morton DL. Demonstration of lymphocyte blastogenesis-inhibiting factors in sera of melanoma patients. *Surgery* 1977; 82: 224-232.
454. Rapson NT, Cornbleet MA, Chessells JM, Hardisity RM. Immunosuppression and serious infections in children with acute lymphoblastic leukemia: a comparison of the three chemotherapy regimens. *Br J Hematol* 1980; 45: 41-52.
455. Ravikumar T, Steele G, Rodrick M, et al. Effects of tumor growth on interleukins and circulating immune complexes. *Cancer* 1984; 53: 1373-1378.
456. Reed DM. On the pathological changes in Hodgkin's disease with special references to its relation to tuberculosis. *Johns Hopkins Hosp Rep* 1902: 10: 133-198.
457. Rees JC, Rossio JL, Wilson HG, et al. Cellular immunity in neoplasia. Antigen and mitogen responses in patients with bronchogenic carcinoma. *Cancer* 1975; 36: 2010-2015.
458. Remacle-Bonnet MM, Rommier GJ, Luc C, et al. Nonspecific suppressive and cytostatic activities mediated by human colonic carcinoma tissue or cultured cell extract. *J Immunol* 1978; 121: 44-52.
459. Renoux G, Renoux M. DTC. A summary of current status. In: Serrou B, Rosenfeld C, Daniels JC, Saunder JP, eds. *Current concepts in human immunology and cancer immunomodulation.* Amsterdam: Elsevier Biomedical 1982: 575-584.
460. Renoux G, Renoux M. Effect immunostimulant d'un imidothiazole dans l'immunization des souris contre l'infecction par *Brucella abortus*. *C R Acad Sci* (Paris) 1971; 272; 349-350.
461. Ress JC, Rossio HL, Wilson HE, et al. Cellular immunity in neoplasia. Antigen and mitogen response in patients with bronchogenic carcinoma. *Cancer* 1975; 36: 2010-2015.
462. Retsas S, Thomas C, Hobbs JR. The effect of vindesine therapy on the *in vitro* immune response of patients with advanced malignant melanoma. *Clin Oncol* 1981; 7: 33-37.
463. Richtsmeier WJ, Eisele D. *In vivo* anergy reversal with cimetidine in patients with cancer. *Arch Otolaryngol Head Neck Surg* 1986; 112: 10; 1074-1077.
464. Riddle PR. Disturbed immune reactions following surgery. *BR J Surg* 1967; 54: 882-886.
465. Riddle PR, Berenbaum MC. Postoperative depression of the lymphocyte response to phytohemagglutinin. *Lancet* 1967; 1: 746-748.
466. Rijswijk REN, Sybesma JPH, Kater L. A prospective study of the changes in the immune status before, during and after multiple agent chemotherapy for Hodgkin's disease. *Cancer* 1983; 51: 637-644.
467. Rijswijk REN, Sybesma JPH, Kater L. A prospective study of the changes in immune status following radiotherapy for Hodgkin's disease. *Cancer* 1984; 53: 62-69.
468. Roberts MM. Lymphocyte transformation in breast cancer. *Br J Surg* 1970; 57: 381.
469. Robinson BW. Asbestos and cancer: human natural killer cell activity is suppressed by asbestos fibers but can be restored by recombinant interleukin-2. *Am Rev Respir Dis* 1978; 139: 4, 897-901.
470. Rojas AF, Feirstan JN, Glait HM, Olivari AJ. Levamisole action in breast cancer. In: Terry WD, Windhorst D, eds. *Immunotherapy of cancer: present status on trials in man.* New York: Raven Press, 1978: 635-646.
471. Romagnani S, Maggi E, Del Prete G, et al. Short- and long-term effects of radiation on T-cell subsets in peripheral blood of patients with Hodgkin's disease. *Cancer* 1980; 46: 2590-2595.
472. Romagnani S, Ferrini PLR, Ricci M. The immune derangement in Hodgkin's disease. *Semin Oncol* 1985; 22: 41-55.
473. Rosenberg SA, Seipp CA, White DE, Wesley R. Perioperative blood transfusions are associated with increased rates of recurrence and decreased survival in patients with high-grade soft-tissue sarcomas of the extremities. *J Clin Oncol* 1985; 3: 5; 698-709.
474. Roses DF, Campion JF, Harris MN, Gumport SL. Malignant melanoma. Delayed hypersensitivity skin testing. *Arch Surg* 1979; 114: 35-38.
475. Rossen RD, Morgan AC. Blockage of the humoral immune response: Immune complexes in cancer. *Cancer Immunol* 1980; 210-280.
476. Roth JA, Osborne BA, Ames RS. Immunoregulatory factors derived from human tumors. II. Partial purification and further immunobiochemical characterization of a human sarcoma-derived immunosuppressive factor expressing HLA-DR and immunoglobulin-related determinants. *J Immunol* 1983; 130: 303-308.
477. Roth JA, Golub SH, Grimm EA, et al. Effects of operation on immune response in cancer patients: Sequential evaluation of *in vitro* lymphocyte function. *Surgery* 1976; 79: 47-51.
478. Rotstein S, Blomgren H, Petrini B, et al. Long-term effects on the immune system following local radiation

for breast cancer. I. Cellular composition of the peripheral blood lymphocyte population. *Int J Radiat Oncol Biol* Phys 1985; 11: 921-925.
479. Rotstein S, Blomgren H, von Stedingk LV, et al. Long-term effects on the immune system following local irradiation for breast cancer. Pokeweed mitogen-induced immunoglobulin secretion by blood lymphocytes and serum immunoglobulin levels. *Eur J Surg Oncol* 1985; 11: 137-141.
480. Rotstein S, Blomgren H, Nilsson B, et al. Prognostic value of various immunological tests in breast cancer patients treated with adjuvant postoperative chemotherapy. *Chemotherapy* 1984; 3: 227-231.
481. Rotstein S, Blomgren H, Petrini, et al. Blood lymphocyte counts with subset analysis in operable breast cancer. *Cancer* 1985; 56: 1413-1419.
482. Ruco LP, Procopio A, Valtieri M, et al. Increased monocyte phagocytosis and decreased lymphocyte mitogen reactivity in colorectal cancer patients. *Appl Pathol* 1983; 1: 149-156.
483. Ryan RE Jr, Neel HB, Ritts RE. Correlation of pre-operative immunologic test results with recurrence in patients with head and neck cancer. *Otolaryngol Head Neck Surg* 1980; 88: 58-63.
484. Saijo N, Shimizu E, Irimajiri N, et al. Analysis of NK activity and ADCC in healthy volunteers and in patients with primary lung carcinoma and metastatic pulmonary tumors. *J Cancer Reg Clin Oncol* 1982; 102: 195-214.
485. Saijo N, Shimizu E, Shibuya M, et al. Effect of chemotherapy on natural killer (NK) activity and antibody-dependent cell-mediated cytotoxicity in carcinoma of the lung. *Br J Cancer* 1982; 46: 180-189.
486. Saito M, Ebina T, Koi M, et al. Induction of interferon-gamma in mouse spleen cells by OK-432, a preparation of *Streptococcus pyogenes*. *Cell Immunol* 1982; 68: 187-192.
487. Salmon SE, Hunt A, Bonnet JD, et al. Alternating combination chemotherapy and levamisole improves survival in multiple myeloma: A Southwest Oncology Group study. *J Clin Oncol* 1983; 1: 453-461.
488. Sample WF, Gertner HR, Chretien PB. Inhibition of phytohemagglutinin-induced *in vitro* lymphocyte transformation by serum from patients with carcinoma. *J Natl Cancer Inst* 1971; 46: 1291-1297.
489. Santos GW, Owens AH, Sensenbrenner LL. Effects of selected cytotoxic agents on antibody production in man: A preliminary report. *Ann NY Acad Sci* 1964; 114: 404-423.
490. Santos LB, Yamada FT, Scheinberg MA. Monocyte and lymphocyte interaction in patients with advanced cancer. Evidence for deficient IL-1 production. *Cancer* 1985; 56: 1553-1558.
491. Sarin PS, San DK, Thornton AH, et al. Neutralization of HTLV-III/LAV replication by antiserum to thymosin-alpha-one. *Science* 1986; 232: 1135-1137.
492. Scambia G, Panici PB, Mancuso S, et al. Effects of antiestrogen and progestin on immune functions in breast cancer patients. *Cancer* 1988; 61: 2214-2218.
493. Schantz SP, Romsdahl MM, Babcock GF, et al. The effect of surgery on natural killer cell activity in head and neck cancer patients: *In vitro* reversal of a postoperatively suppressed immunosurveillance system. *Laryngoscope* 1985; 95: 588-594.
494. Schantz SP, Savage HE, Racz T, et al. Immunologic determinants of head and neck cancer response to induction chemotherapy. *J Clin Oncol* 1989; 7: 7, 857-864.
495. Schlechter GP, Wahl LM, Oppenheim JJ. Suppressor monocytes in human disease: a review. *Adv Exp Med Biol* 1979; 121B, 283-298.
496. Schechter GP, Soehlen F. Monocyte-mediated inhibition of lymphocyte blastogenesis in Hodgkin's disease. *Blood* 1978; 52: 261-271.
497. Scher HI, Shank B, Chapman R, et al. Randomized trial of combined modality therapy with and without thymosin fraction V in the treatment of small cell lung cancer. *Cancer Res* 1988; 48: 1663-1670.
498. Schindler L, Leroux M, Zimmerman GF, et al. Reversal of defective lymphoproliferation in postoperative patients with colon cancer. *J Cancer Res Clin Oncol* 1987; 113: 2, 166-170.
499. Schlelhammer PF, Bracken RB, Bean M, et al. Immune evaluator with skin testing. A study of testicular, prostatic, and bladder neoplasms. *Cancer* 1976; 38: 149-156.
500. Schlumberger HD. BAY I 7433: a synthetic polymer with antitumor activity. In: Hersh EM, Cirigos MA, Mastrangelo, MJ, eds. *Augmenting agents in cancer therapy*. New York: Raven Press, 1981: 373-390.
501. Schulof RS, Lloyf MJ, Cleary PA, et al. A randomized trial to evaluate the immunorestorative properties of thymosin-alpha-one in patients with lung cancer. *J Biol Response Mod* 1985; 4: 147-158.
502. Schulof RS, Bockman RS, Garofalo JA, et al. Multivariate analysis of T-cell functional defects and circulating serum factors in Hodgkin's disease. *Cancer* 1981; 48: 964-973.
503. Schulof RS, Michitsch RW, Livingston PO, Gupta S. Monocyte-mediated suppression on lymphocyte cytotoxic activity for cultured autologous melanoma cells. *Cell Immunol* 1981; 57: 529-532.
504. Schulof RS, Chorba TC, Cleary PA, et al. T-cell abnormalities after mediastinal irradiation for lung cancer. The *in vitro* influence of synthetic thymosin alpha-1. *Cancer* 1985; 55: 974-983.
505. Schulof RS. Thymic peptide hormones: Basic properties and clinical applications in cancer. *CRC Critical Rev Oncol Hematol* 1985; 3: 309-376.
506. Schulof RS, Lee BJ, Lacher MJ, et al. Concanavalin-A-induced suppressor cell activity in Hodgkin's disease. *Clin Immunol Immunopathol* 1980; 16: 454-462.
507. Schulof RS, Lloyd MJ, Ueno WM, et al. Phase II trial of thymosin fraction 5 in advanced renal cancer. *J Biol Response Mod* 1984; 3: 151-159.
508. Schulof RS, Lacher MJ, Gupta S. Abnormal phytohemagglutinin-induced T-cell proliferative responses in Hodgkin's disease. *Blood* 1981; 57: 607-613.
509. Sears HF, Simon R, Rosenberg SA. Longitudinal studies of cellular immunity of patients with osteogenic sarcoma during chemoimmunotherapy. *Cancer Treat Rep* 1980; 64: 589-597.
510. Seder RH, Katz AE, Keggins JJ, et al. Plasma exchange in six patients with advanced cancers of the head and neck. *J Clin Apheresis* 1985; 2: 238-249.
511. Seder RH, Katz AE, Keggins JJ, et al. Plasma exchange in six patients with advanced cancers of the head and neck. *J Clin Apheresis* 1985; 2: 238-249.
512. Seder RH, Vaughn CW, Oh S-K, et al. Tumor regression and temporary restoration of immune response after plasmapheresis in a patient with recurrent oral cancer. *Cancer* 1987; 60: 318-325.

513. Sedman PC, Ramsden CW, Brennan TG, et al. Effects of low-dose perioperative interferon on the surgically induced suppression of antitumor immune response. *Br J Surg* 1988; 75: 976-981.
514. Sen L, Borella L. Expression of cell surface markers on T- and B-lymphocytes after long-term chemotherapy of acute leukemia. *Cell Immunol* 1973; 9: 84-95.
515. Serdengecti S, Buyukunal E, Molinas N, et al. Overall survival results of non-small cell lung cancer patients: Chemotherapy alone versus chemotherapy with combined immunomodulation. *Chemioterapia* 1988; 7: 2; 122-126.
516. Sertoli MR, Guarneri D, Rubagotti A, et al. Adjuvant immunochemotherapy in colorectal cancer. *Dukes C. Oncology* 1987; 44: 2; 78-81.
517. Shafir M, Bekesi JG, Papatestas A, et al. Preoperative and postoperative immunological evaluation of patients with colorectal cancer. *Cancer* 1980; 46: 700-705.
518. Shank B, Scher H, Hilaris BS, et al. Increased survival with high-dose multified radiotherapy and intensive chemotherapy in limited small cell carcinoma of the lung. *Cancer* 1985; 56: 2771-2778.
519. Shiraki S, Mori H, Kadomoto N, et al. Adjuvant immunotherapy of carcinoma colli with levamisole. Prevention of immunological depression following surgical therapy and radiotherapy. *Int J Immunopharmacol* 1982; 4: 73-80.
520. Shoham J, Theodore E, Brenner HJ, et al. Enhancement of the immune system of chemotherapy-treated cancer patients by simultaneous treatment with thymic extract, TP-1. *Cancer Immunol Immunother* 1980; 9: 173-180.
521. Shukla HS, Hughes LE, Whitehead RH, Newcombe RG. Long-term (5-11 years) follow-up of general immune competence in breast cancer. I. Pretreatment levels with reference to micrometastasis. *Cancer Immunol Immunother* 1986; 21: 1-5.
522. Shukla HS, Hughes LE, Whitehead RH, Newcomb RG. Long-term follow-up of general immune competence in breast cancer. II. Sequential pre- and post-treatment levels: A 10-year study. *Cancer Immunol Immunother* 1986; 21: 6-11.
523. Sibbit WL, Bankhurst AD, Williams RC. Studies of cell subpopulations mediating mitogen hyporesponsiveness in patients with Hodgkin's disease. *J Clin Invest* 1978; 61: 55-63.
524. Silverman NA, Alexander JC, Potvin C, Chretien PB. *In vitro* lymphocyte reactivity and T-cell levels in patients with melanoma: correlations with clinical and pathological stage. *Surgery* 1976; 79: 332-339.
525. Silverman NA, Alexander JC, Potvin C, Chretien PB. Effect of nonthymic irradiation on cellular immunocompetence. *Surg Forum* 1975; 26: 345-346.
526. Sinclair T, Ezdinli EZ, Boonlayangoor P, et al. Rosette and blastogenesis inhibition by plasma from Hodgkin's disease and other malignancies. Positive correlation in stage I and II Hodgkin's disease. *Cancer* 1983; 51: 238-244.
527. Slade MS, Simmons RL, Yunis E, Greenberg LJ. Immunodepression after major surgery in normal patients. *Surgery* 1975; 78: 363-372.
528. Slater JM, Ngo E, Lau BHS. Effect of therapeutic irradiation on the immune response. *Am J Roentgenol Radium Ther Nucl Med* 1976; 126: 313-320.
529. Smalley RV, Talmadge J, Oldham RK, Thurman GB. The thymosins: Preclinical and clinical studies with fraction V and alpha-1. *Cancer Treat Rev* 1984; 11: 69-84.
530. Smith RB, Dekernion J, Baron B, et al. Levamisole in the treatment of non-invasive and invasive bladder cancer: a preliminary report. *J Urol* 1978; 119: 347-349.
531. Snyderman R, Siegler HF, Meadew R. Abnormalities of monocyte chemotaxis in patients with melanoma: Effects of immunotherapy and tumor removal. *J Natl Cancer Inst* 1977; 58: 37-41.
532. Sokal JE, Aungst CW. Response to BCG vaccination and survival in advanced Hodgkin's disease. *Cancer* 1969; 24: 128-134.
533. Soto A, Hall T, Reed S. Trial of antiviral action of isoprinosine against rhinovirus infection of volunteers. *Antimicrob Agent Chemother* 1973; 3: 332-334.
534. Soulillou JP, Douillard JU, Vie H, et al. Defects in lectin-induced interleukin-2 (IL-2) production by peripheral blood lymphocytes of patients with Hodgkin's disease. *Eur J Cancer Clin Oncol* 1985; 21: 935.
535. Spitler LE, Sagebiel R. A randomized trial of levamisole versus placebo as adjuvant therapy in malignant melanoma. *N Engl J Med* 1980; 303: 1143-1147.
536. Spreafico F, Vecchi A. The imunomodulatory activity of certain cancer chemotherapeutic agents. In: Mihich E, Sakurai Y, eds. *Biological responses in cancer, vol. 3:* immunomodulation by anti-cancer drugs. New York: Plenum Press, 1985: 131-149.
537. Steele G, Wang BS, Mannick JA. Immune RNA and transfer factor. In: Mihich E, ed. *Immunological approaches to cancer therapeutics.* New York: Wiley, 1982: 257-276.
538. Stefani S, Kerman R, Abbate J. Serial studies of immunocompetence in head and neck cancer patients undergoing radiation therapy. *Am J Roentgenol Radium Ther Nucl Med* 1976; 126: 880-886.
539. Stefano S, Kerman R, Abbate J. Serial studies of immunocompetence in head and neck cancer patients undergoing radiation therapy. *Am J Roentgenol* 1976; 126: 880-886.
540. Stein JA, Adler A, Efraim SB, Maor M. Immunocompetence, immunosuppression and human breast cancer. *Cancer* 1976; 38: 1171-1187.
541. Stephens EJW, Wood HF, Mason B. Levamisole as adjuvant to cyclic chemotherapy in end-stage mammary carcinoma. *Recent Results Cancer Res* 1978; 68: 139-145.
542. Stratton JA, Byfield PE, Byfield JE, et al. A comparison of the acute effects of radiation therapy, including or excluding the thymus, or the lymphocyte subpopulations of cancer patients. *J Clin Invest* 1975; 56: 88-97.
543. Stratton JA, Fast PE, Weintraub I. Recovery of lymphocyte function after radiation therapy for cancer in relationship to prognosis. *J Clin Lab Immunol* 1982; 7: 147-153.
544. Strender LE, Blomgren H, Wasserman J, et al. Influence of adjuvant radiation therapy in breast cancer on PWM-induced Ig secretion by blood lymphocytes *in vitro*. *Anticancer Res* 1983; 3: 41-45.
545. Strender LE, Blomgren H, Petrini B, et al. Immunologic monitoring in breast cancer patients receiving postoperative adjuvant chemotherapy. *Cancer* 1981; 48: 1996-2002.
546. Sugden PJ, Lilleyman JS. Impairment of lymphocyte transformation by plasma from patients with advanced Hodgkin's disease. *Cancer* 1980; 45: 899-905.
547. Symoens J, Veys E, Mielants W, Pinals R. Adverse

reactions to levamisole. *Cancer Treat Rep* 1978; 62: 1721-1730.

548. Taguchi T. Clinical efficacy of lentinan on patients with stomach cancer: Endpoint results of a four-year follow-up survey. *Cancer Detect Prev Suppl* 1987; 1: 333-349.
549. Takusugi M, Ramseyer A, Takasugi J. Decline of natural non-selective cell-mediated cytotoxicity in patients with tumor progression. *Cancer Res* 1977; 37: 413-418.
550. Talmadge JE, Lenz BF, Pennington R, et al. Immunomodulatory and therapeutic properties of bestatin in mice. *Cancer Res* 1986; 46: 9; 4505-4510.
551. Talmadge JE, Lenz B, Schneider M, et al. Immunomodulatory and therapeutic properties of FK-565 in mice. *Cancer Immunol Immunother* 1989; 28: 93-100.
552. Talpaz M, Medina JE, Patt YZ, et al. The immune restorative effect of cimetidine administration *in vivo* on the local graft-vs-host reaction of cancer patients. *Clin Immunol Immunopathol* 1982; 24: 155-160.
553. Tamura K, Shibata Y, Matsuda Y, Ishida N. Isolation and characterization of an immunosuppressive acidic protein from ascitic fluids of cancer patients. *Cancer Res* 1981; 41: 3244-3252.
554. Taramelli D, Mazzocchi A, Clemente C, et al. Lack of suppressive activity of human primary melanoma cells on the activation of autologous lymphocytes. *Cancer Immunol Immunother* 1988; 26: 1, 61-66.
555. Tarpley JL, Potvin C, Chretien PB. Prolonged depression of cellular immunity in cured laryngopharyngeal cancer patients treated with radiation therapy. *Cancer* 1975; 35: 638-644.
556. Tarpley JL, Twomey PL, Catalona WJ, Cretien PB. Suppression of cellular immunity by anesthesia and operation. *J Surg Res* 1977; 22: 195-201.
557. Tartter PI, Burrows L, Kirshner P. Perioperative blood transfusion adversely affects prognosis after resection in stage I (subset No) non-oat cell lung cancer. *J Thorac Cardiovasc Surg* 1984; 88: 659-662.
558. Tartter PI, Martinelli G. Lymphocyte subsets, natural killer cytotoxicity, and perioperative blood transfusion for elective colorectal cancer surgery. *Cancer Detect Prev* (Suppl) 1987; 1: 571-576.
559. Tartter PI, Martinelli G, Steinberg B, Barron D. Changes in peripheral T-cell subsets and natural killer cytotoxicity in relation to colorectal cancer surgery. *Cancer Detect Prev* 1986; 9: 3-4, 359-364.
560. Tartter PI, Burrows L, Papatestas AE, et al. Perioperative blood transfusion has prognostic significance for breast cancer. *Surgery* 1985; 97: 225-230.
561. Taylor SA, Gordon MY, Currie GA, Shepherd VB. Irradiation and monocyte function in patients with breast cancer. *Int J Rad Oncol* 1979; 5: 2063-2067.
562. Thatcher N, Palmer MK, Swindell R, Crowther D. Lymphocyte function related to survival curves in patients with metastatic melanoma were evaluated immunologically prior to chemoimmunotherapy. *Med Pediatr Oncol* 1978; 4: 49-70.
563. Theofilopoulos A, Dixon FJ. The biology and detection of immune complexes. *Adv Immunol* 1979; 28: 89-220.
564. Thienpont D, Vanparjis OFJ, Racymakers AHM, et al. Tetramasole (R8299): A new potent broad spectrum anthelmintic. *Nature* 1966; 209: 1084-1086.
565. Thornes RD, Lynch G, Sheehan MV. Cimetidine and coumarin therapy of melanoma. *Lancet* 1982; 2: 328.
566. Thornes RD, Lynch G. Combination of cimetidine with other drugs for the treatment of cancer. *N Engl J Med* 1983; 308: 591.
567. Tilden AB, Balch CM. Immune modulatory effects of indomethacin in melanoma patients are not related to prostaglandin E2-mediated suppression. *Surgery* 1982; 92: 528-532.
568. Ting A, Terasaki PI. Depressed lymphocyte-mediated killing sensitized targets in cancer patients. *Cancer Res* 1974; 34: 2694-2698.
569. Toge T, Hamamoto S, Itagaki E, et al. Concanavalin-A-induced and spontaneous suppressor cell activities in peripheral blood lymphocytes and spleen cells from gastric cancer patients. *Cancer* 1983; 52: 1624-1631.
570. Toivanen A, Granberg I, Nordman E. Lymphocyte subpopulations in patients with breast cancer after postoperative radiotherapy. *Cancer* 1984; 54: 2919-2923.
571. Tom BH, Macek CM, Subramanian C, et al. *In vitro* expression of suppressogenic and enhancing activities in human colon cancer cells. *J Biol Response Mod* 1984; 3: 435-444.
572. Tonnesen H, Knigge U, Bulow S, et al. Effect of cimetidine on survival after gastric cancer. *Lancet* 1988; 29: 2(8618), 990-992.
573. Treurniet-Donker AD, Meischke-de Jongh ML, van Putten WLJ. Levamisole as adjuvant immunotherapy in breast cancer. *Cancer* 1987; 59: 1590-1593.
574. Tsang KY, Fudenberg HH, Pan JF, et al. An *in* vitro study on the effects of isoprinosine on immune responses in cancer patients. *Int J Immunopharmacol* 1983; 5: 481-490.
575. Tsuyuguchi I, Shiratsuchi H, Fukuoka M. T-lymphocyte subsets in primary lung cancer. *Jpn J Clin Onco*l 1987; 17: 1, 13-17.
576. Uchida A, Kolb R, Micksche M. Generation of suppressor cells for natural killer activity in cancer patients after surgery. *J Natl Cancer Inst* 1982; 68: 735-741.
577. Uchida A, Mickskche M. Generation of suppressor cells f or natural killer (NK) activity in cancer patients after surgery. *Cancer Immunol Immunother* 1981; 10: 203-210.
578. Uchida A, Hoshino T. Clinical studies on well-mediated immunity in patients with malignant disease. I. Effects of immunotherapy with OK-432 on lymphocyte subpopulation and phytomitogen responsiveness *in vitro*. *Cancer* 1980; 45: 476-483.
579. Umeda T, Yokoyama H, Kobayashi K, et al. Subsets of T-lymphocytes of patients with malignancies of the urogenital tract. *Cell Mol Biol* 1979; 25: 95-99.
580. Unger SW, Bernhard MI, Pace RC, Wanego HJ. Monocyte dysfunction in human cancer. *Cancer* 1983; 51: 669-674.
581. Uracz W, Mytar B, Zembala M, et al. Activated monocytes in gastric cancer patients. II. Suppressor and cytostatic activity *in vitro*. *J Cancer Res Clin Oncol* 1982; 104: 307-313.
582. Van Rijswijk REN, DeMeijer A, Bob Sybesma JPH, Kater L. Five-year survival in Hodgkin's disease. The prospective value of immune status at diagnosis. *Cancer* 1986; 57: 1489-1496.
583. Van-Stolen K, Wiernick PH, Schiffer CA, Schimpff SC. Evaluation of levamisole as an adjuvant to chemotherapy for treatment of ANLL. *Cancer* 1983; 51: 1576-1580.
584. Vanhaelen CPJ, Fisher RI. Increased sensitivity of T-cells to regulation by normal suppressor cells persists in long-term survivors with Hodgkin's disease. *Am J Med* 1982; 72: 385-390.

585. Vaudaux P, Kiefer B, Forni M, et al. Adriamycin impairs phagocytic function and induces morphologic alterations in human neutrophils. *Cancer* 1984; 59: 400-410.
586. Venkataraman M, Rao DS, Levin RD, Westerman MP. Suppression of B-lymphocyte function by T-lymphocytes in patients with advanced lung cancer. *J Natl Cancer Inst* 1985; 74: 37-41.
587. Verhaegen H, DeCree J, DeCock W, et al. Levamisole therapy in patients with colorectal cancer. In: Terry WD, Rosenberg SA, eds. *Immunotherapy of human cancer.* New York: Elsevier/North-Holland, 1982: 225-229.
588. Vinzenz K, Matejka M, Watzek G, et al. Modulation of NK activity in regional lymph nodes by preoperative immunotherapy with OK-432 in patients with cancer of the oral cavity. *Cancer Detect Prev Suppl* 1987; 1: 463-475.
589. Von Roenn J, Harris JE, Braun DP. Suppressor cell function in solid-tumor cancer patients. *J Clin Oncol* 1987; 5: 1; 150-159.
590. Voogt PJ, van de Velde CJH, Brand A, et al. Perioperative blood transfusion and cancer prognosis: Different effects of blood transfusion on prognosis of colon and breast cancer patients. *Cancer* 1987; 59: 836-843.
591. Vose BM, Vanky F, Argrov S, Klein E. Natural cytotoxicity in man: Activity of lymph node and tumor-infiltrating lymphocytes and regional lymphocytes. *Eur J Immunol* 1977; 7: 753-757.
592. Wagner DK, Kiwanuka J, Edwards BK, et al. Soluble interleukin-2 receptor levels in patients with undifferentiated and lymphoblastic lymphomas: correlation with survival. *J Clin Oncol* 1987; 5: 8, 1262-1274.
593. Wagner V, Janku O, Wagnerora M, et al. The production of complete and incomplete antibodies in patients with neoplastic disease. *Neoplasma* 1972; 19: 75-87.
594. Wakasugi H, Kasahara T, Minato N, et al. *In vivo* potentiation of human natural killer cell activity by a streptococcal preparation: interferon and interleukin-2 participation in the stimulation with OK-432. *J Natl Cancer Inst* 1982; 69: 807-812.
595. Waller CA, Gill BG, Machennon IC. Enhancement of lymphocyte-mediated cytotoxicity after tumor resection in patients with colorectal cancer. *J Natl Cancer Inst* 1980; 65: 223-230.
596. Walter RJ, Danielson JR. Defective monocyte chemotaxis in patients with epidermoid tumors of the head and neck. *Arch Otolaryngol* 1985; 11: 530-540.
597. Wanebo HJ, Rao B, Miyazawa N, et al. Immune reactivity in primary carcinoma of the lung and its relation to prognosis. *J Thorac Cardiovasc Surg* 1976; 72: 339-347.
598. Wanebo HJ, Pace R, Hargett S, et al. Production of and response to interleukin-2 in peripheral blood lymphocytes of cancer patients. *Cancer* 1980; 57: 656-662.
599. Wanebo HJ, Jun M, Strong E, Oettgen HF. T-cell deficiency in patients with squamous-cell cancer of head and neck. *Am J Surg* 1975; 130: 445-451.
600. Wanego HJ, Rao B, Attiyeh F, et al. Immune reactivity in patients with colorectal cancer: assessment of biological risk by immunoparameters. *Cancer* 1980; 45: 1254-1263.
601. Wanebo HJ, Hilal EY, Strong EW, et al. Adjuvant trial of levamisole in patients with squamous cancer of the head and neck: a preliminary report. *Cancer Res* 1978; 68: 324-333.
602. Wanebo HJ. Observations on the effects of adjuvant radiation on immune tests of patients with colorectal cancer and head and neck cancer. In: Dubois JB, Serrou B, Rosenfeld C, eds. *Immunopharmacologic effects of radiation therapy.* New York: Raven Press, 1980: 241-252.
603. Wanego HJ, Riley T, Katz D, et al. Indomethacin-sensitive suppressor-cell activity in head and neck cancer patients. *Cancer* 1988; 61: 462-474.
604. Wara WM, Phillips TL, Wara DW, et al. Immunosuppression following radiation therapy for carcinoma of the nasopharynx. *Am J Roentgenol Radium Ther Nucl Med* 1975; 123: 482-485.
605. Wara WM, Wara DW, Philips TL, Amman AJ. Elevated IgA in cancer of the nasopharynx. *Cancer* 1975; 35: 1313-1315.
606. Wara WM, Neely MH, Amman AJ, Wara DW. Biological modification of immunologic parameters in head and neck cancer patients with thymosin fraction V. In: Goldstein AL, Chirigos MA, eds. *Lymphokines and thymic hormones: their potential utilization in cancer therapeutics.* New York: Raven Press, 1981: 257-262.
607. Warren RP, McCall CA, Urban RW. Augmentation of natural killer cell activity by ImuVert: a biological response modifier derived from *Serratia marcescens*. *Mol Biother* 1989; 1: ; 3, 145-151.
608. Wasserman J, Wallgren A, Blomgren H, et al. Prognostic relevance of post-irradiation lymphocyte reactivity in breast cancer patients. *Cancer* 1986; 58: 348-351.
609. Wasserman J, Blomgren H, Petrini B, et al. Effect of radiation therapy and *in vitro* x-ray exposure on lymphocyte subpopulations and their functions. *Am J Clin* Oncol 1982; 5: 195-208.
610. Watanabe Y, Takashi I. Clinical value of immunotherapy for lung cancer by the streptococcal preparation OK-432. *Cancer* 1984; 53: 248-253.
611. Webster DJ, Whitehead RH, Richardson G, Hughes LE. Levamisole: A double-blind immunological study. *Anticancer Res* 1982; 2: 29-32.
612. Weiden PL, Bean MA, Schultz P. Perioperative blood transfusion does not increase the risk of colorectal cancer recurrence. *Cancer* 1987; 60: 870-874.
613. Wells SA Jr, Burdick JF, Christiansen C, et al. Demonstration of tumor-associated delayed cutaneous hypersensitivity reactions in lung cancer patients and in patients with carcinoma of the cervix. *Natl Cancer Inst Monogr* 1973; 37: 197-203.
614. Wells SA Jr, Burdick JF, Christiansen C, et al. Demonstration of tumor-associated delayed cutaneous hypersensitivity reactions in lung cancer patients and in patients with carcinoma of t he cervix. *Natl Cancer Inst Monogr* 1973; 37: 197-203.
615. Wells SA Jr, Burdick JF, Joseph WL, et al. Delayed cutaneous hypersensitivity reactions to tumor cell antigens and to nonspecific antigens. *J Thorac Cardiovasc Surg* 1973; 66: 557-562.
616. Weppelmann B, Monkemeir D. The influence of prostaglandin antagonists on radiation therapy of carcinoma of the cervix. *Gynecol Oncol* 1984; 17: 196-199.
617. Wesse J, Oldham RK, Tormey DC, et al. Immunologic monitoring in carcinoma of the breast. *Surg Gynecol Obstet* 1977; 145: 209-218.
618. Wesselius LJ, Wheaton DL, Manahan-Wahl LJ, et al. Lymphocyte subsets in lung cancer. *Chest* 1987; 91: 5; 725-729.
619. White JE, Chen T, Reed R, et al. Limited squamous-cell carcinoma of the lung: a Southwest Oncology Group

randomized study of radiation with or without doxorubicin and with or without levamisole immunotherapy. *Cancer Treat Rep* 1982; 66: 113-120.
620. Whitehead RH, Thatcher J, Teasdale C, et al. T- and B-lymphocytes in breast cancer: stage relationship and abrogation of T-lymphocyte depression by enzyme treatment *in vitro*. *Lancet* 1976; 1: 330-333.
621. Wilkins SA Jr, Olkowskii ZL. Immunocompetence of cancer patients treated with levamisole. *Cancer* 1977; 39: 487-493.
622. Windle R, Bell PR, Shaw D. Five-year results of a randomized trial of adjuvant 5-fluorouracil and levamisole in colorectal cancer. *Br J Surg* 1987; 74: 7, 569-572.
623. Windle R, Wood RFM, Bell PRF. The effect of levamisole on post-operative immunosuppression. *Br J Surg* 1979; 66: 507-509.
624. Wleklik MS, Luczak M, Najjajr VA. Tuftsin-induced tumor necrosis activity. *Mol Cell Biochem* 1987; 75: 2, 169-174.
625. Wolf GT, Lovett EJ III, Peterson KA, et al. Lymphokine production and lymphocyte subpopulations in patients with head and neck squamous carcinoma. *Arch Otolaryngo*l 1984; 110: 731-735.
626. Wolf GT, Amendola BE, Diaz R, et al. Definite vs. adjuvant radiotherapy. Comparative effects on lymphocyte subpopulations in patients with head and neck squamous carcinoma. *Arch Otolaryngol* 1985; 111: 716-726.
627. Wybran J, Govaerts P. Levamisole and human lymphocyte surface markers. *Clin Exp Immunol* 1977; 27: 319-321.
628. Wybran J, Serrou B, Belpomme D, et al. Immunomodulating of T-cell and NK function by NPT-15392 in cancer patients. A cooperative study by the tumor immunology group. In: Serrou B, Rosenfeld C, Daniels JC, Saunders JP, eds. *Current concepts in human immunology and cancer immunomodulation*. Amsterdam: Elsevier Biomedical, 1982: 471-478.
629. Yokoyama H, Umeda T, Kobayashi K, et al. Restoration of E-rosette formation by bestatin in patients with bladder cancer. *C Cancer Res Clin Oncol* 1980; 98: 195-201.
630. Young RC, Corder MP, Haynes HA, DeVita VT. Delayed hypersensitivity in Hodgkin's disease. *Am J Med* 1972; 52: 63-72.
631. Zabbe C, DeWitte JD, Lozach P, et al. Predictive value of T-cell subset derangements in lung cancer. *Med Oncol Tumor Pharmacother* 1986; 3: 2; 83-85.
632. Zacharski LR, Linman JW. Lymphocytopenia: its causes and significance. *Mayo Clin Proc* 1971; 46: 168-173.
633. Zamkoff KW, Reeves WG, Paolozzi FP, et al. Impaired interleukin regulation of the phytohemagglutinin response in Hodgkin's disease. *Clin Immunol Immunopathol* 1985; 35: 111-124.
634. Zamkoff KW, Reeves WQ, Paolozzi FP, et al. Impaired interleukin regulation of the phytohemagglutinin response in Hodgkin's disease. *Clin Immunol Immunopathol* 1985; 35: 111.
635. Zanker KS, Blumel G, Lange J, et al. Coumarin in malignant melanoma patients: an experimental and clinical study. *Drug Exp Clin Res* 1984; 10: 767-774.

NON-SPECIFIC EXOGENOUS IMMUNOMODULATOR IN ONCOLOGY

G. MATHÉ and S. ORBACH-ARBOUYS
Institut de Cancérologie et d'Immunologie 6 rue Minard – BP 60, 92133 Issy-les-Moulineaux Cedex, and Hôpital Suisse de Paris, 10 rue Minard, 92130 Issy-les-Moulineaux, France

A few decades of cancer chemotherapy practice [41] have shown that it can, alone or combined to other means of tumor treatments (surgery and radiotherapy), cure a remarkable proportion of malignant neoplasias in children (osteosarcoma, neuroblastoma under one year of age, rhabdomyosarcoma, Wilm's tumor, acute lymphoid leukemia) and in young adults (testis seminoma, teratocarcinoma and embryocarcinoma) [138], while it only contributes a little, if at all, [278, 43, 145, 139] to the cure of adults older than 40 years.

It is precisely at that age, that the incidence of spontaneous tumours in man starts increasing according to an exponential curve (Fig. 1) [164]. In older patients, mortality from cancer increased between 1950 and 1980 (Fig. 2) [138], and the prognosis of many adult tumors,

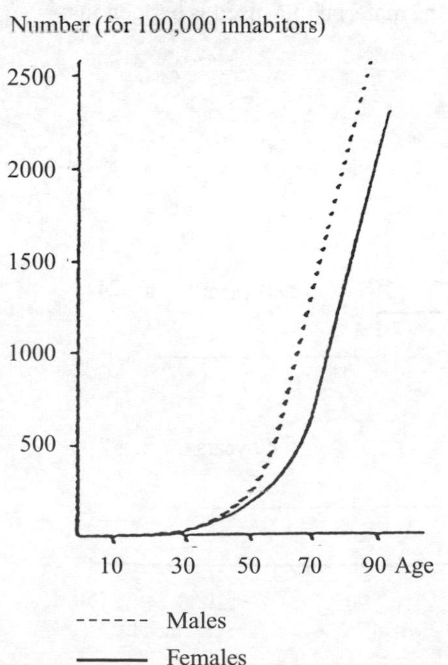

Figure 1. Increase of incidence of cancer with age [164].

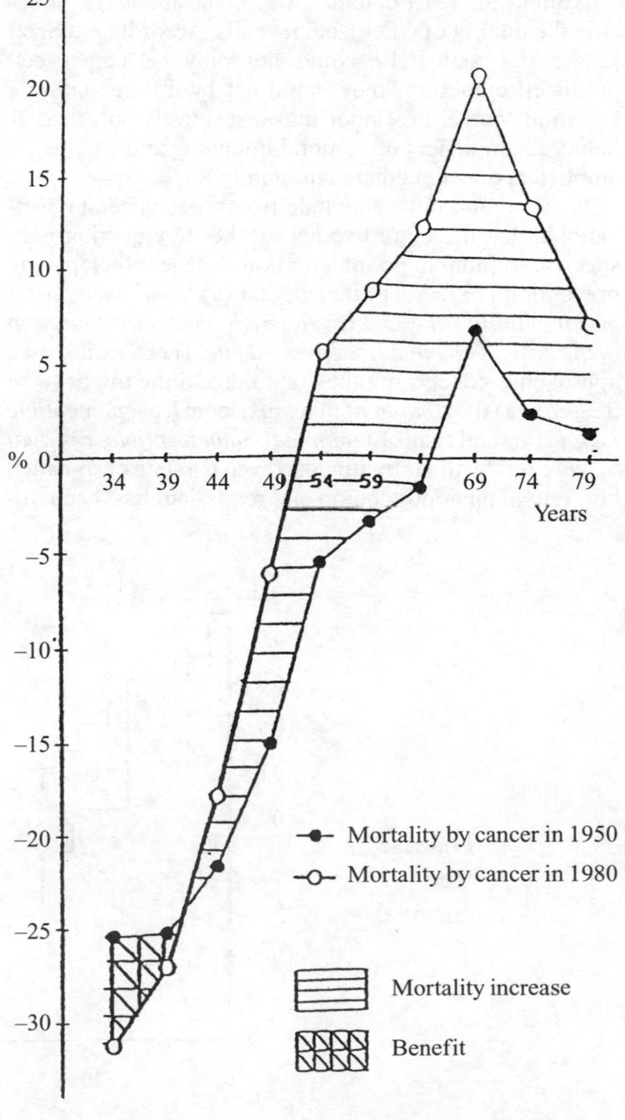

Figure 2. The 75% 'cure' in childhood cancers compared with global increase in age-adjusted mortality [138].

R.K. Oldham (ed.), Principles of Cancer Biotherapy. 3rd ed., 141–178.

such as acute myeloid leukemia, is still generally poor (Fig. 3) [138].

The equivalent age for the occurrence of spontaneous tumors in mice and for their exponential increase of incidence is 16 months [31]. This experimental model shows the probable causal coincidence of occurrence of aging immunodeficiency [31, 36]: the functions of the T-helper cells, of the cytotoxic (killer) T-lymphocytes (CTL), of the natural killer cells (NK) and of B-cell decrease, while that of suppressor cells increases.

These changes are outlined in figure 4 which shows an oversimplified diagram indicating the present day concept of the immune system, cells, molecular factors and their interactions [147]. Figure 5 indicates some ambiguous relationships between inflammatory factors and CD8 T-lymphocyte functions.

Among the least elucidated mechanisms is that inducing the duality of CD4 T-helper cells. According to Scott [254], IL4 and IL12 could not only be helper cell produced cytokines, they could act by differentiating a common 'naive' precursor into respectively so-called T-helper 2, amplifiers of humoral immunity and T-helper 1, amplifiers of cell mediated immunity.

One can and must conclude from these general observations, that there are two approaches to emerging non-specific immunologic intervention in cancer therapy and prevention [137, 221] : the attempt (a) *to enhance a normal immunity state* and (b) *to reach immunorestauration in the case of an immunodepressed one*. There are also two approaches concerning the conditions of the tumor to be treated : (a) the *treatment* of a *bulky* or at least *perceptible neoplasia*, and that of a *minimal, imperceptible, residual disease* left by other treatments (even if a state of so-called but only apparently complete remission has been induced), and which will be the source of local or systemic relapses, (b) the *prevention of tumor development* from a few, even from one cancer cell (as most neoplasias are monoclonal) [164], which has undergone all stages of malignant transformation [4].

From the first immunotherapy trial we published in 1969 in which we used living BCG [156], to the present state of immunopharmacology, there have been several phases of progress: (a) the development of knowledge of the immunological machinery, shown by Figure 4 [147]; (b) the proliferation of non specific exogenous immunomodulators, some being molecularly defined, even synthetized [137, 239]; (c) the extraction, characterization and preparation of an infinite number of natural factors, called *cytokines*, especially *interleukins* [71] when they are produced by leukocytes, and their artificial production in their so-called recombinant forms [263]; (d) the rather disappointing if not negative results as far as tumor curability is concerned, of their application from which so much was expected and prematurely claimed (possibly because the tumors were bulky) [245], which must lead us to ask wonder if they are not less therapeutically active than the exogenous immunomodulators [134], and to reconsider the return to the latter in practical therapy and prevention of cancer.

THE NOTION OF CANCER IMMUNOTHERAPY

It is imperative at this stage to introduce the basic concept and notion of cancer immunotherapy, including its passive type and its *stricto sensu* adoptive form, especially because these two types were the first introduced, and because the material they used is exogenous.

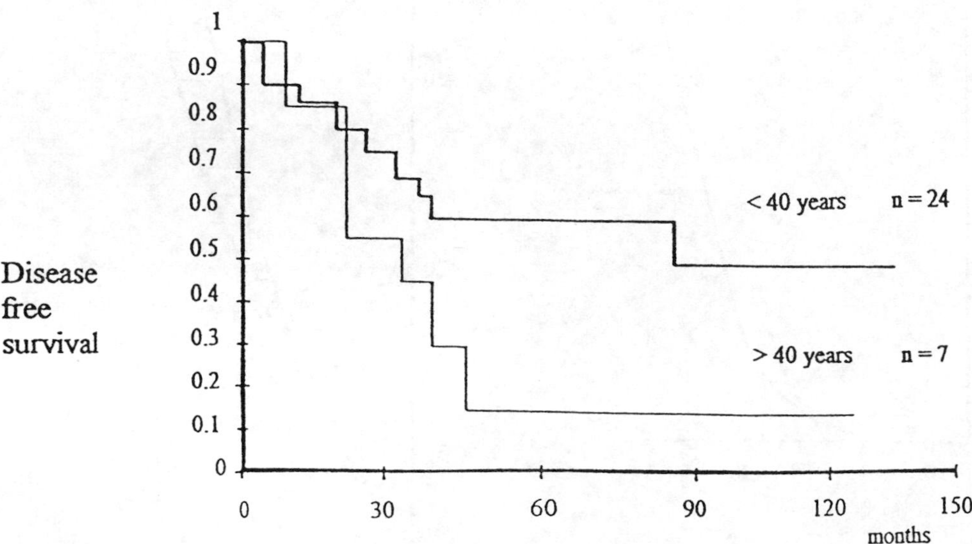

Figure 3. Survival curve in acute myeloid leukemia adult patients: prognosis is better in those under 40 yr of age (among which some are 'curable'), and much poorer in those over 40 yr [138].

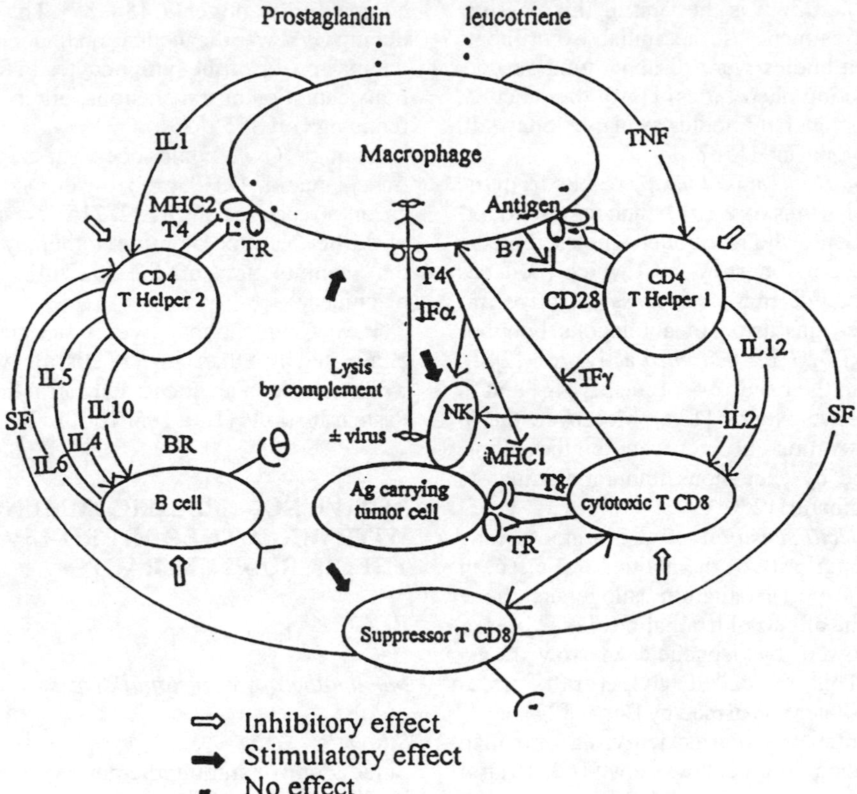

Figure. 4. Oversimplified diagram indicating the present day concept of the immunity system: cells, molecular factors and their interactions [147]. Changes of main functions after 16 months of age in mice [31, 36] are indicated: a decrease, compared to those of young age, of T-helper, of T-killer or cytotoxic cell and of B-lymphocyte functions, and an increase of so called natural killers and the T-suppressor ones. (The black arrows indicate an amplification of the function(s) and the empty one a reduction).
Ag, antigen; BR, B-receptor; CTL, cytotoxic (killer) T lymphocytes; IF, interferon; IL, interleukin; MHC, major histocompatibility complex; NK, natural killers; SF, suppressor factors; TNF, tumor necrosis factor; TR, T-receptor.

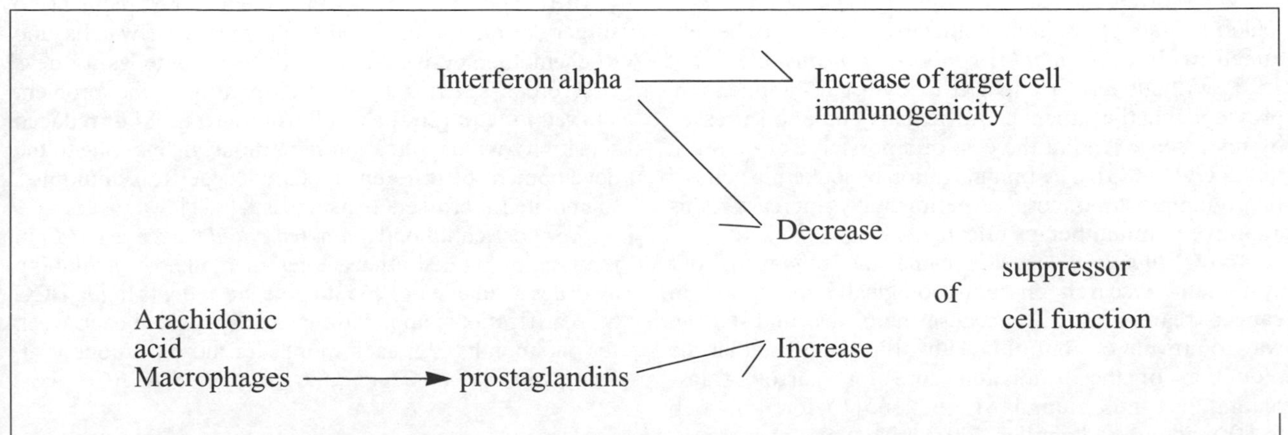

Figure 5. Relationship between inflammation factors and some immunity functions.

Passive immunotherapy was the first of this possible branch of cancer treatment. If the initial experiments using polyclonal antibodies were disappointing (except for their use as targeting oncostatics) [184], the practical interest of the monoclonal antibodies available today still have to be proven and defined [53].

Stricto sensu adoptive immunotherapy results from the reaction of allogeneic (thus *foreign*) lymphocytes, adopted by the cancer patient, who is immunodepressed by the conditioning for the bone marrow graft which produces them. We do not include in *stricto sensu* adoptive immunotherapy, the re-transfusion of autologous lymphocytes after interleukin 2 (IL-2) *in vitro* activation [244], whatever its action in the hands of optimists [244] and in those of more objective experts [134]. Moreover, the *in vitro* lymphocyte activation does not require interleukins, and can be achieved by exogenous immunomodulators such as OK-432 (picibanil) [250].

The notion of *stricto sensu* adoptive immunotherapy resulted from the superiority of the antitumoral effect in leukemic mice, of post-irradiation allogeneic bone marrow graft, over the effects of irradiation alone [163] or of irradiation followed by isogeneic marrow transplantation [159]. This so called GvL (graft versus leukemia effect) was later confirmed by Bortin [27].

Effective on spontaneous murine leukemia, provided that the number of the tumor cells was low [160, 151], it was also effective in our hands, in 1963, on the first human leukemic patient who carried an allogeneic bone marrow graft after a 800 rad total body irradiation [152, 150, 154]. He presented a full chimerism and was free of leukemic cells until he died, two years and a half later, from encephalitis or suicide due to the 'graft versus host disease' (GvH), which he presented as an acute, then a chronic form, illustrating the binding of this reaction to the antileukemic effect, called 'graft versus leukemia' effect [149]. Both the possibility of a full allogeneic graft chimerism, and the reality of its anti-leukemic effects were respectively confirmed at the statistical level in 1975 [271] and 1979 [286] by Thomas and his group.

We showed in man, in 1966, that the 'graft versus leukemia' adoptive immunotherapy could also be obtained with *allogeneic lymphocyte transfusions* [253, 158], without any irradiation or cytostatic application, provided that the patient be sufficiently immunodepressed by his disease, and at the cost of a possibly severe, even lethal GvH [183]. The immunization by leukemic cells of the lymphocyte donors, experimentally increased this adoptive immunotherapy effect [181].

Active immunotherapy became the object of our systematic research on immunological intervention in cancer treatment [137], because there was, in 1969, no way to prevent or control GvH in all patients, neither the reduction of the irradiation dose for marrow transplantation conditioning [161, 162, 165] (before going up to 800 rad, we had applied 400 rad without any success), nor the application of cytostatics which we used after the marrow graft [153], nor that of solubilized histocompatibility antigen(s) [88, 87]. The only method of reducing GvH was the incubation in poor culture medium of the marrow or of the lymphocytes before their respective transplantation or transfusions, but it was simultaneously reducing GvL [155, 55].

Though GvH could occur after syngeneic marrow transplantation [219], probably due to what we considered as 'auto-reactive cells' [222, 218], we chose, as the means of further research on immunotherapy or/and prevention, the manipulation of the patient's own immunologic machinery.

It was evident that living bacteria were more often eliminated by it than cancer cells, and we chose one which was available in an attenuated form: the living BCG from Pasteur Institute [100, 186, 168, 142].

ACTIVE NON SPECIFIC IMMUNOTHERAPY WITH BCG, OTHER MICRO-ORGANISMS AND THEIR CRUDE EXTRACTS

BCG

Immunotherapy of residual disease

Systemic

Since adoptive immunotherapy can only eradicate a tumor if the number of its cells is small [151], the first *experimental study* we conducted consisted in searching if active immunotherapy would obey to this condition, i.e. eradicate the disease if the number of its cells is small enough. We tested experimentally with the L1210 murine leukemia, the effect, according to the grafted cell number, of living BCG injected i.v. after the tumor was established. Figure 6 shows that it could only cure animals if this number was only 10^5 or less [144].

This notion was confirmed on other experimental leukemias [178, 167] and on solid tumors [272] on which BCG was tested. It was experimentally confirmed by several other researchers (see 137).

BCG appeared to be an excellent complement to surgery or radio-therapy when they leave a few cells, and to chemotherapy which always leaves some, as it obeys first order kinetics [259] and confronts the problem showed *in vitro* [266] as well as *in vivo* [208] of reduced sensitivity with application repetitions, mainly due to the development of different types of 'specific', 'multiple', 'cumulated', 'crossed' resistances... [141].

We chose childhood *acute lymphoid leukemia* (*ALL*) in remission obtained after a long chemotherapy including all drugs available in 1965, to give the patients living BCG by scarifications, applications being repeated each week for one month, then each month for more than one year. *Seven out of the 15* children submitted to BCG were*

---

* We eliminate from the present consideration, other patients who were only submitted to active specific immunotherapy.

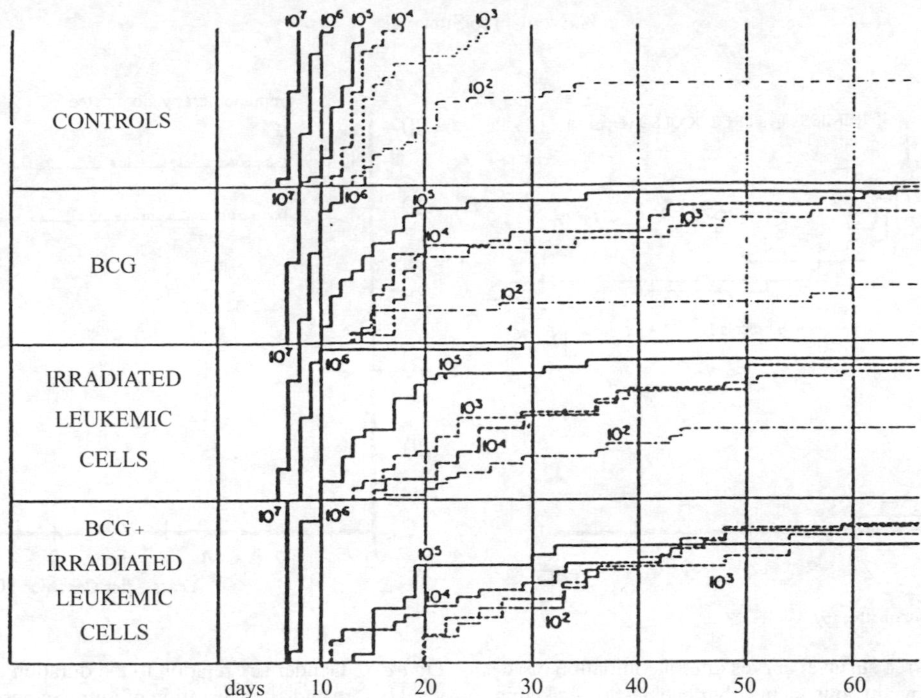

Figure 6. Growth curve population of tumours obtained from mice treated with BCG without or with irradiated cells, the day after transplantation of 10^6 L1210 cells [144].

surviving in normal condition after 12th year [156, 180]; their blood lymphocytes called at that time 'null cells' (to-day considered as NK lymphocytes), had increased in number [108]. These subjects are considered as cured.

We have, since the analysis of this preliminary trial, conducted other studies in which more efficient chemotherapies for ALL were applied. They were adapted as far as their intensity to their predicted prognosis established on age, the cytologic forms and the neoplastic volumes. If the proportion of patients in remission at the end of chemotherapy, varies according to its action, the representation of their survival follows, whatever the length of chemotherapy, a plateau form during the subsequent immunotherapy and after it (Fig. 7), a phenomenon also observed by Sakurai for this disease (Fig. 8) [117]. This makes post-chemotherapy – immunotherapy latest results in contrast to with those of chemotherapy given alone: in this condition, relapses, although rarer and rarer but possibly late, continue to occur, as illustrated (a) by the curves published in 1988 by Steinhorn and Ries for the patients of the 'SEER' areas, United States, and the period 1973-1984 (Fig. 9) [264], and (b) by the proportion reported by Hawkins [92], of those also submitted to chemotherapy only, which, alive at the third year, are still alive after ten years: this proportion was only, in 1989, of 63%.

The three illustrated studies have been chosen as examples, because they were conducted in a period (about ten years ago) where the prognosis was still moderate, which makes the effects of the considered parameters more perceptible.

The enormous randomized trials collected by Terry and Rosenberg [270], did not generally confirm the significance of the superiority of post-chemotherapy BCG over a placebo: we shall discuss later, not only the *common sense significance of statistical significance*, but also the biases such trials suffered from, most being described in the Reizenstein's critical analysis to which 230 such studies were submitted [238]. Their main weakness consisted of neglecting the patient and disease heterogeneities [166], and of *diluting the most important parameters of active immunotherapy action, such as the role of the major histo-compatibility complex (MHC) phenotypes*, as we could show for HLA1 on our BCG immunotherapy cured patients (Table 1) [274], and as Ochiai could observe for HLA2 in his gastric cancer patients (Table 2) [210].

Table 1. HLA1 antigen incidences in our BCG-treated long-term survivors, compared to 591 healthy controls submitted only to chemotherapy [274]

	BCG	Chemotherapy only	
HLA-B17	42.8%	7.3%	P<0.01
HLA-A33	35.7%	1.2%	P<0.01
HLA-B17 or A33	71.4%	8.1%	P<0.001

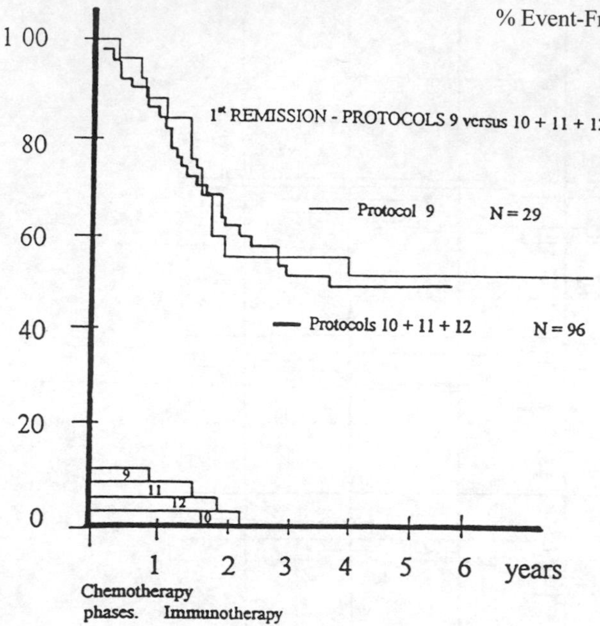

Figure 7. Relapse free survival curves after the initiation of active immunotherapy in our acute lymphoblastic leukemia children, belonging to two groups of protocols which differed as far as the length of pre-BCG chemotherapy (all patients categorised as good and as poor prognosis are included). The various lengths of the 2 types of chemotherapy, short for protocol 9 (1970-1973) and longer but moderate for protocols 10, 11 and 12, are mentioned in the lower left part of the figure.

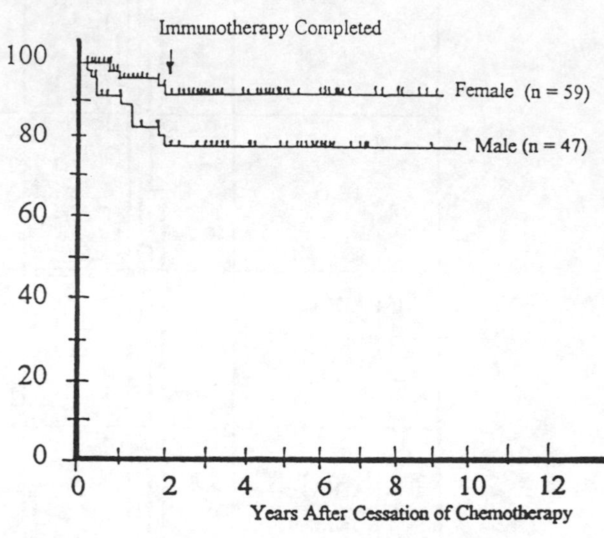

Figure 8. Gender sex relation to the duration of event-free survival before and after cessation of immunotherapy [117].

Table 2. Association of DR4 and survival in 41 gastric cancer patients [210]

	No. of DR4 (+)
No. of patients surviving 3 years p.o.	
23	10(43.5%)
No. of patients who died within 3 years p.o.	
18	3(16.7%)

Chi square test p = 0.0671.
Fisher's exact test p = 0.0955.
p.o., post-operation

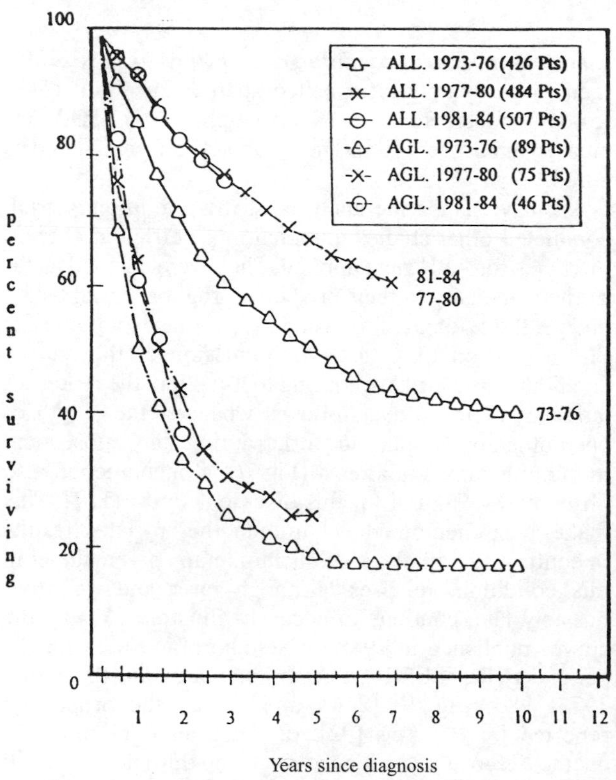

Figure 9. Survival among children with acute lymphoid leukemia only submitted to chemotherapy (white children under 5 and 5-14 yr of age diagnosed with ALL, 9 SEER areas, United States 1973-1984) [264].

Also important is *the cytological type* of the leukemia [180]: the so called microlymphoblastic form of the WHO categorisation [294] (more explicit than the so-called 'FAB' typing 1) [15] seemed to be extremely sensitive to this immunotherapy effect. Patients of the large randomized trials were stratified neither a priori nor a posteriori for any of these factors of the immunotherapy action [270].

Applied to other neoplastic diseases of the lymphoid family, BCG gave, as an adjuvant treatment, a significant

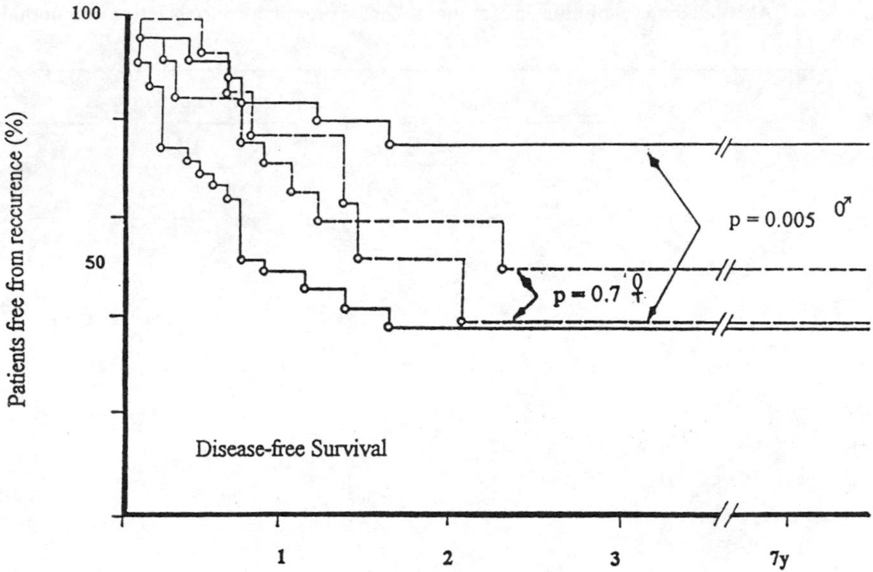

Figure 10. The benefit of BCG immunotherapy in the case of lymphoma is superior in males than in females [96].

effect on *non Hodgkin's lymphoma* (Fig. 10) [96]. The males appear to be more sensitive to BCG effect than the females, which indicates the role of another immunotherapy sensibility parameter, gender. We have found the same advantage of the male sex in a *melanoma* trial [230] which will be considered later.

BCG also produced a transitory benefit to *acute myeloid leukemia* patients, significant at the metanalysis of all trials [282]. Unfortunately, we lack precisions on the fate of the patients, on the immunogenetics and the cytological types of the long survivors. Their knowledge would be more useful than the so-called metanalytic study, whose population is as artificial as those of all randomized trials included in it, as it is the sum of them.

Immunotherapy of perceptible disease

Systemic
The systemic application of BCG in bulky or perceptible neoplasia has always been ineffective [137].

Local
Contrary to the systemic application of BCG, its local injection in the *bladder* for superficial *in situ cancer* has been very effective in all trials [228] conducted after that of Morales [196].

After a 5-year experience with BCG in tumor stage pTis, pTa and pT1 G I-II, Ratliff [234] obtained a lasting remission of 88.5% in 78 patients treated with BCG Pasteur preparation after transurethral injection. A complete remission in patients with carcinoma *in situ* (12 patients) could be induced in 92% of them. Side-effects, which are of limited duration, are tolerable, well treatable and fully reversible. Lamm confirmed this results, which he compared favorably with those of local chemotherapy [123]. *If interferon alpha applied intravesically, induces also remissions of bladder tumors, only BCG induced cures* [109].

A remarkable result was obtained by Zhu [290] with BCG intra-tumoral injection in the case of *rectal cancer*. A brilliant one was obtained against bovine ocular *squamous cell carcinoma* [247].

Immunoprevention

Systemic
A *possible prevention of spontaneous tumors by BCG vaccination against human tuberculosis applied in children*, has been searched. Some but not all retrospective and epidemiologic studies conducted in Europe, the United States and Canada have suggested that this vaccination could have lowered the mortality from acute leukemia in children and from other cancers [111, 98].

Local
BCG finally behaves as the only active *local adjuvant of vaccine preparation against melanoma* [291].

Mechanisms of action

The first control to be achieved in our and other works, was that of the hypothesis according to which BCG could reduce, cure or prevent tumors via an immunological response enhancement [217]. This is shown on Table 3.

Other functions have been shown to be enhanced: BCG activates macrophages in which it induces the process of *lysosomal exocytosis*, which we will describe later, as

Table 3. Correlation between EAkR leukemia evolution and immunological parameters during active immunotherapy with BCG and irradiated tumour cells [217]

Parameters	Experimental groups						
	I	II		III		IV	V
		A	B	A	B		
Tumour size	–	↓	→	↓	→	–	Controls
% TC in peritoneal fluid	–	↓	→	↓	→	–	Controls
% Lymphocytes at day 13 and 18	–	↑	→	↑	→	–	Controls
% Immunoblast-like cells at day 13 and 18	–	↑	→	↑	→	–	Controls
Complement-dependent antibody-mediated cytotoxicity (CDAC)	0	++	++	++	++	+(+)	0
Spleen	+	++	++	++	++	+	(+)
Direct lymphocyte cytotoxicity (DLC)							
Lymph nodes	0	0	0	0	0	0	0
Spleen	(+)	++	(+)	++	(+)	(+)	(+)
Antibody-dependent lymphocyte-mediated cytoxicity (ADLMC)							
Lymph nodes	0	++	0	++	0	0	0

Groups:
I. Normal controls.
II. Mice receiving 10^5 viable tumour cells (T.C.)i.p. on day 0 and weekly i.v. injections of 1 mg BCG.
III. Mice receiving tumour cells i.p. plus weekly injections of BCG i.v. and of 10^7 irradiated tumour cells s.c.
IV. Mice receiving tumour cells i.p. plus weekly injection of irradiated tumour cells s.c.
V. Mice receiving 10^5 tumour cells i.p. on day 0.

Subgroups: IIA and IIIA mice with tumour cell number far below mice from group V.
IIB and IIB mice with tumour cell number not significantly different from group V control mice.

BCG shares it with hyperthermia, an other immunomodifier also influencing macrophages [231, 232].

OTHER MICROORGANISMS: FROM THEIR CRUDE TO MOLECULARLY CHARACTERIZED EXTRACTS

Corynebacterium parvum (*C. parvum*), also called *Propionibacter acnes*, has a half-life of 24 h when given intrapleurally. Its intravenous administration results in hepatic and splenic deposition [110]. Like BCG, it activates macrophages [130]. Some beneficial clinical results have been registered in the case of lung cancer [62].

Pseudomonas aeruginosa is a significant immunomodulator and one of the best tumor necrosis factor (TNF) inducer [63].

From *Corynebacteria* to *Nocardia rubra cell-wall skeleton (CWS)* [118, 211], from *BCG free lipids* [6] to its *water-soluble lipid-free fraction* [102], from the fungal polysaccharide *lentinan* (a beta 1-3 glucan with beta 1-6 branches) [26], to the molecularly defined and purified *muramyl dipeptide and tripeptide* (which are peptidoglycan derivatives) (Fig. 11) [126], there are legions of preparations. The most used is a *protein bound polysaccharide (PSK)*, which has been the object of a comparative randomized trial on patients gastrectomized for a stomach cancer, in which it gave a significant benefit [203] (Fig. 12). The other widely used preparation is a powder of *Streptococus pyogenes* called *picibanil* (OK-432) [275]. This agent has been shown to stimulate the

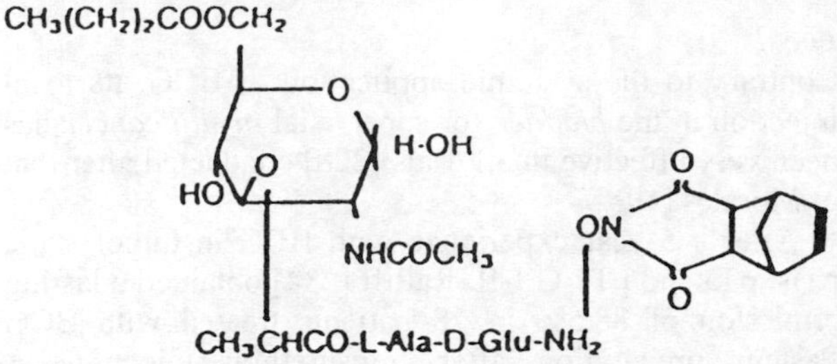

Figure 11. Structure of muramyl dipeptide (6-0-butyryl-*N*-acetylmuramyl-L-alanyl-D-isoglutamine-*N*-hydroxy-5-norbornene-2, 3-dicarboxyimidylester).

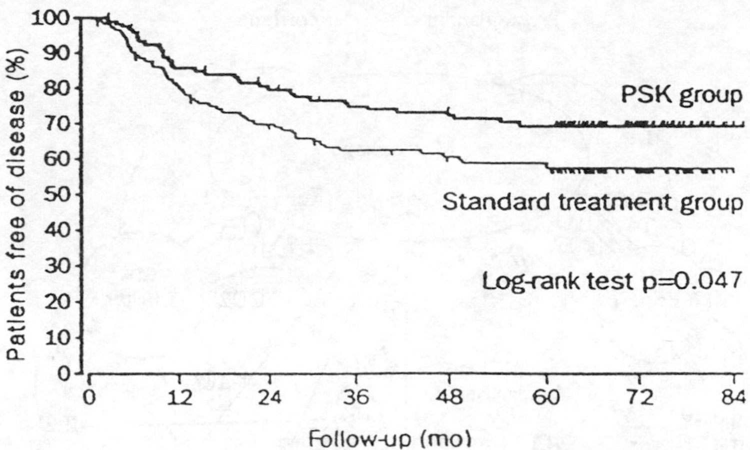

Figure 12. Disease-free survival of gastrectomized patients for stomach cancer, having received as adjuvant treatment, picibanil or a placebo [203].

production of interferons and of interleukin-2 [284, 277], while it reduces suppressor cell effects [276].

The structure of *muramyl dipeptide* is shown in Figure 11. It is reported to replace whole mycobacteria in Freund's complete adjuvant and may cross-react with BCG. The inoculation of muramyl dipeptide into the footpads of BCG-primed mice elicits an increased antibody production against it, as well as delayed hypersensitivity reaction. BCG-primed mice had high helper T-cell activity, and muramyl dipeptide increases the generation of effector T cells. It can cause a regression of mouse tumor metastases and its intralesional injection with an adjuvant can lead to the regression of mouse hepatoma [126].

Molecularly characterized and/or synthetized immuno-modulators and their analogues

A more consistent progress was achieved with extracted or synthetized molecules possessing an immunomodulating power, which are easier to study pharmacologically than microorganisms and their crude extracts.

Bestatin

Bestatin is typical of very instructive exogenous, molecularly defined and available immunomodulators. It is naturally produced by *Actinomycetes olivoreticuli*, from which it was extracted by Hamao Umezawa and his coworkers [280], who noted its capacity to enhance immune responses in experimental tumor therapy [106]. Its molecular structure is represented on Figure 13 [267]. Its basic action mechanism lies in its capacity to inhibit leucine aminopeptidase and aminopeptidase B [129].

We observed [135, 185, 65] that it increases the levels of interleukin 1 and of interleukin 2 production (Fig. 14) in *young mice*. These effects, confirmed by the Umezawa group [258], reveal its action on macrophages and on T-helper 1 cells (Fig. 15).

It also increases antibody production, thus stimulating B cells [135, 185, 65, 227] and the so-called T-helpers 2

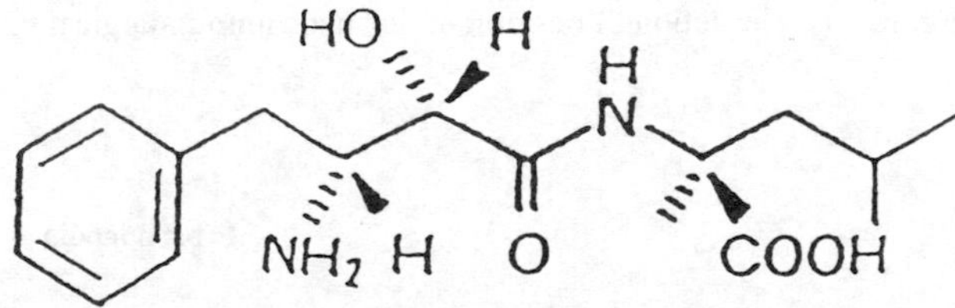

Figure 13. Chemical structure of Bestatin. (±)-N-[(2S. 3R)-3-amino-2-hydroxy-4-phenylbutanoyl] L-leucine (MW: 308.38).

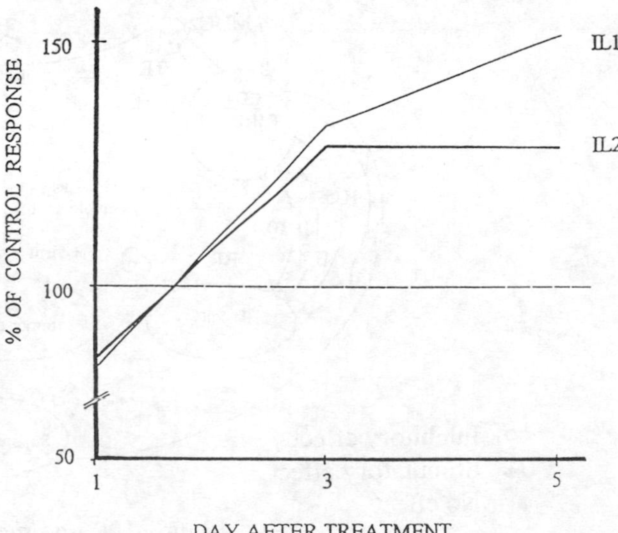

Figure 14. IL1 and IL2 production, stimulated *in vitro* respectively by LPS and Con A, are slightly amplified 3 and 5 days after a 3-day treatment with bestatin.

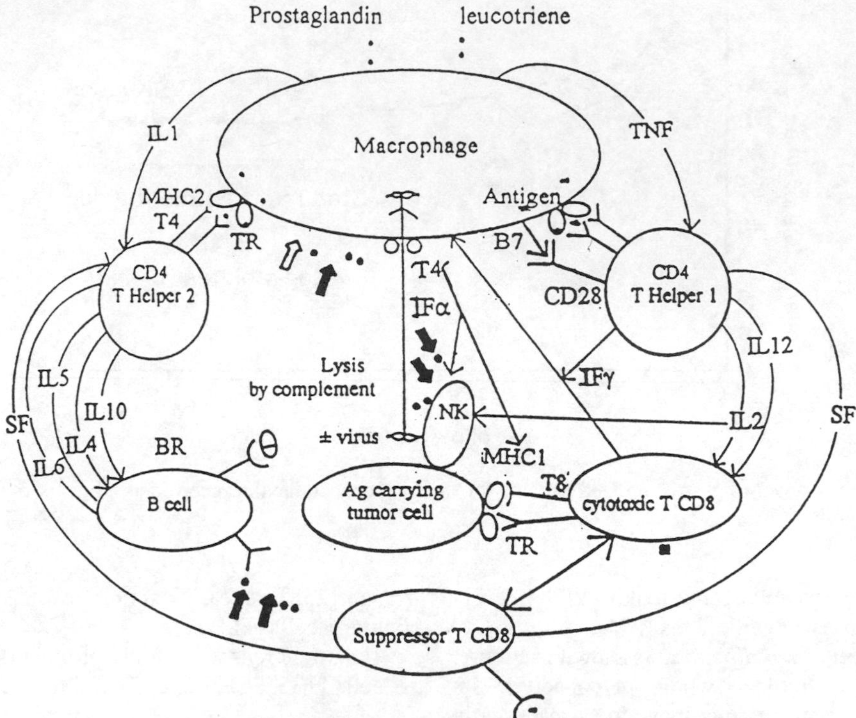

Figure 15. The action of bestatin on the main immunological functions in young mice.

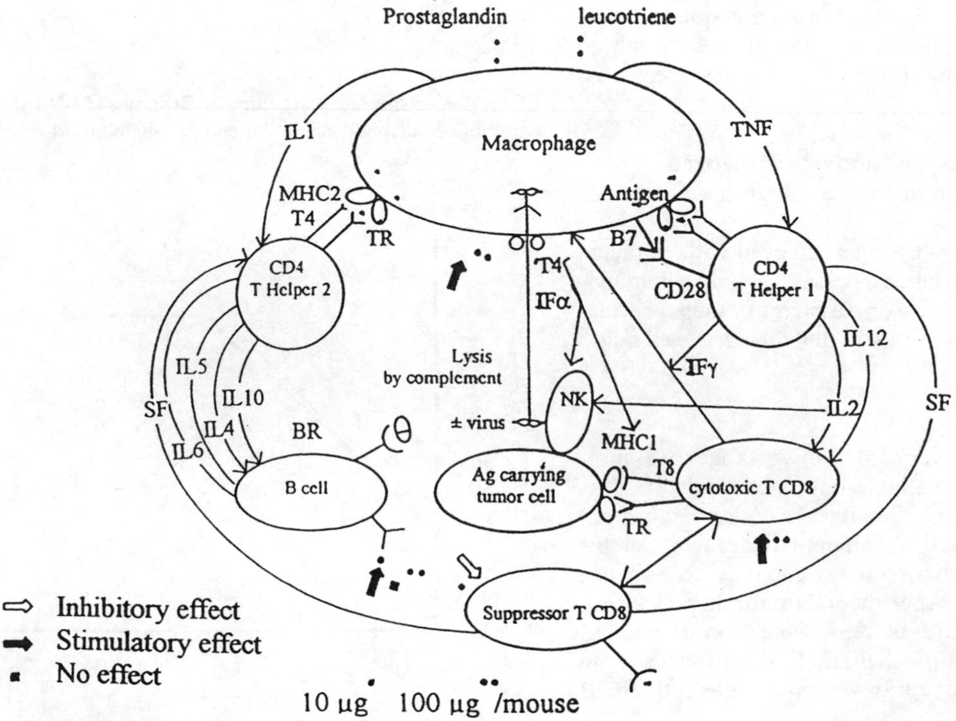

Figure 16. Restoration by bestatin given at the dose of 10 or 100 μg per mouse, of the main immunologic functions of old mice. Ag, antigen; BR, B-receptor; CTL, cytotoxic (killer) T lymphocytes; IF, interferon; IL, interleukin; MHC, major histo-compatibility complex; NK, natural killers; SF, suppressor factors; TNF, tumor necrosis factor; TR, T-receptor.

which are the B cell amplifiers. This is also demonstrated by the increase of interleukin 6 production [69].

It enhances the NK cell action more than that of the T-cytotoxic one which, in young animals, is not significantly increased by bestatin: it behaves as if the increased interleukin 2 excess was only devoted to the natural killers.

We were very impressed when we observed, during the systematic comparison we make in our screening for immunorestorator search [174, 67], the effect in *old mice*. The macrophage functions and the antibody production are increased in old as well as in young animals but, contrary to what is seen in the latter, the NK cell function is not increased by bestatin (Fig. 16) [32]. T-cytotoxicity, contrarily to what is seen in young animals, is enhanced (Fig. 16) [67, 32].

This *restoration of aging T-cell immunodepression* was applied to the *prevention of the risk of spontaneous murine tumors* appearing at the 16th month (Table 4) and exponentially increasing in number later [67, 32] (which happens in man at and after 40 years of age) (Fig. 1) [164].

This notion was brilliantly illustrated *in man* by the analysis of a Japanese phase III trial of adjuvant active immunotherapy of *acute myeloid leukemia*, comparing bestatin to a placebo [225, 226]. Figure 17 shows that, while there was no difference between the survivals of the patients younger that 40, whether they received bestatin or the placebo, there was a great one in older patients: while the survival rate was 10% in controls, it increased in the bestatin group, to 50 %.

Neprina [204] showed a beneficial effect of bestatin used as an adjuvant of chemoradiotherapy of local bladder cancer. *It restored the irradiation impaired immune system* by inhibiting suppressive activity and normalizing T-lymphocyte and natural killer cell actions. Blomgren also showed, in bladder cancer patients immuno-depressed by radiotherapy, that bestatin induced immuno-restoration [20, 21].

We studied the effect of bestatin in the cases of cancer and of the HIV1-AIDS complex in phase 2 trials [185, 173]. We observed a moderate but statistically significant increase of the CD4/CD8 ratio (Fig. 18), the more so that the number prior to treatment was less decreased. The patients were divided in two groups based on their $CD8^+$ T

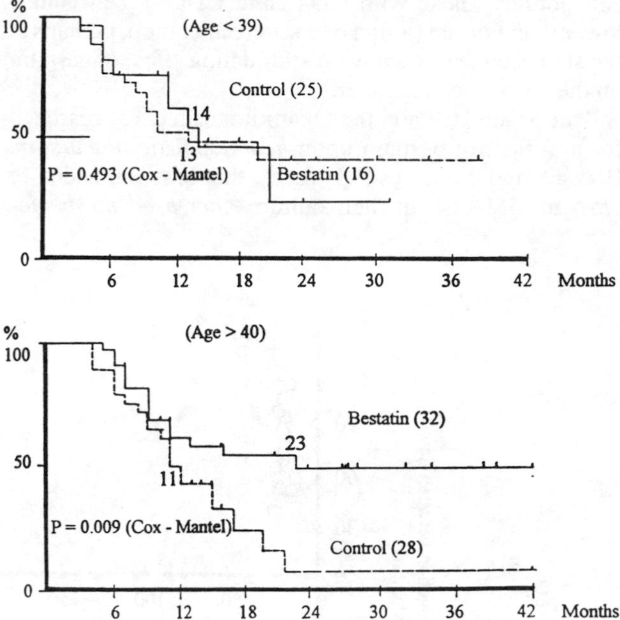

Figure 17. Adjuvant immunotherapy with bestatin did not produce any benefit before 40 years of age, but it increased the survival incidence from 10 to 50% in older patient [225, 226].

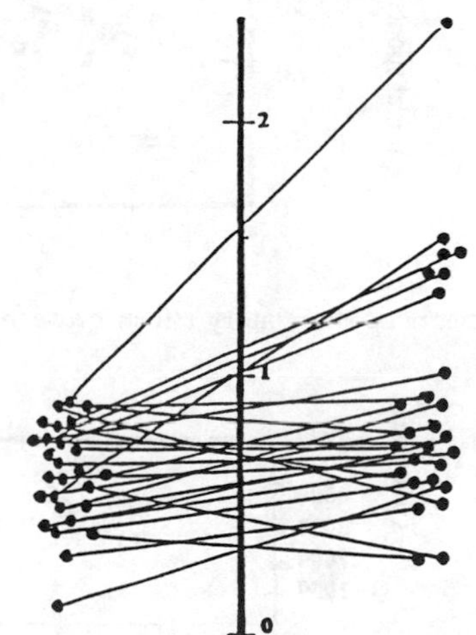

Figure 18. A phase II trial of bestatin in cancer patients and HIV carriers; The effect on decreased CD4/CD8 ratio.

Table 4. Comparison between immunodeficiency and spontaneous tumor incidence between 16 and 28 months. Immunity and tumors in mice of the same age after 12 months of application of bestatin or tuftsin or levamisole.

	Controls			Mice treated with		
	Bestatin exp.	Tuftsin exp.	Levamisole exp.	Bestatin	Tuftsin	Levamisole
				between the 16th and the 28th m		
Killer T-cells				N*	N	N
Cytotoxic macrophages				N	N	N
Tumors (%)	36	27	30	0	5	7

* N : Restored to normal.

cell counts. Those with $CD4^+$ and $CD8^+$ T cell counts lower than normal (a sign of a severe alteration, perhaps at the stem-cell level), show no stimulating effect of bestatin on the $CD4^+$ T cell number.

Our group [19] and the Okamura team [213] searched for an effect of bestatin upon *hematopoietic precursors*. Blazsek and ourselves [19] found that bestatin, added *in vitro* to GM-CSF in their culture, *increased the hemopoietic total cell production* (Fig. 19), *including that of the megakaryocytes* (Fig. 20) [19]. This last enhancement seems in vivo to be partly due to the increase of IL6 by bestatin [69] and, according to Okamura [213], to that of the GM-CSF itself.

Whatever the mechanism, we applied this effect to the treatment of *myelodysplasia* and registered in 6 out of 6 patients, a significant and rapid *increase of the white*

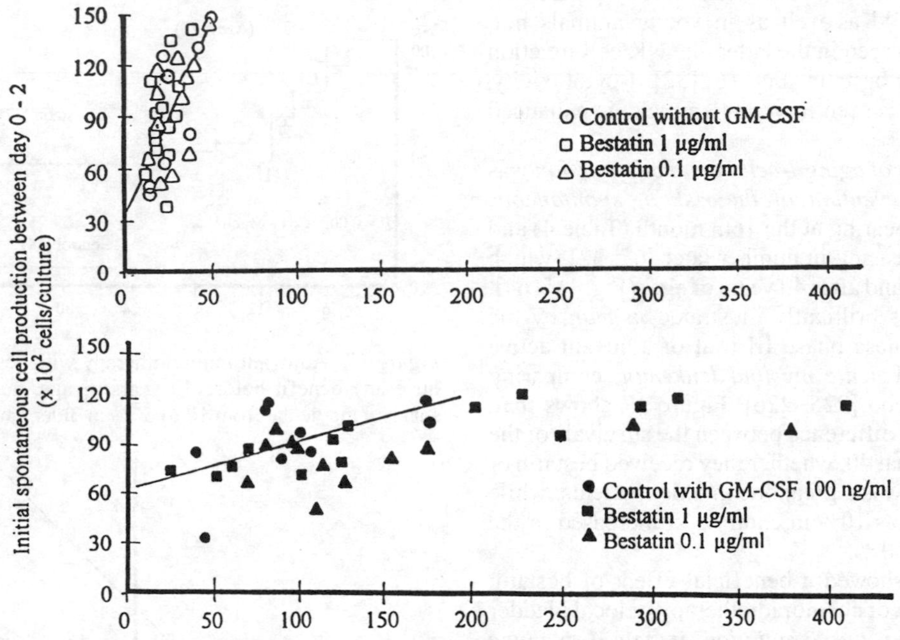

Figure 19. Synergistic stimulatory effects between bestatin and GM-CSF on the hematopoietic cells colony numbers [19].

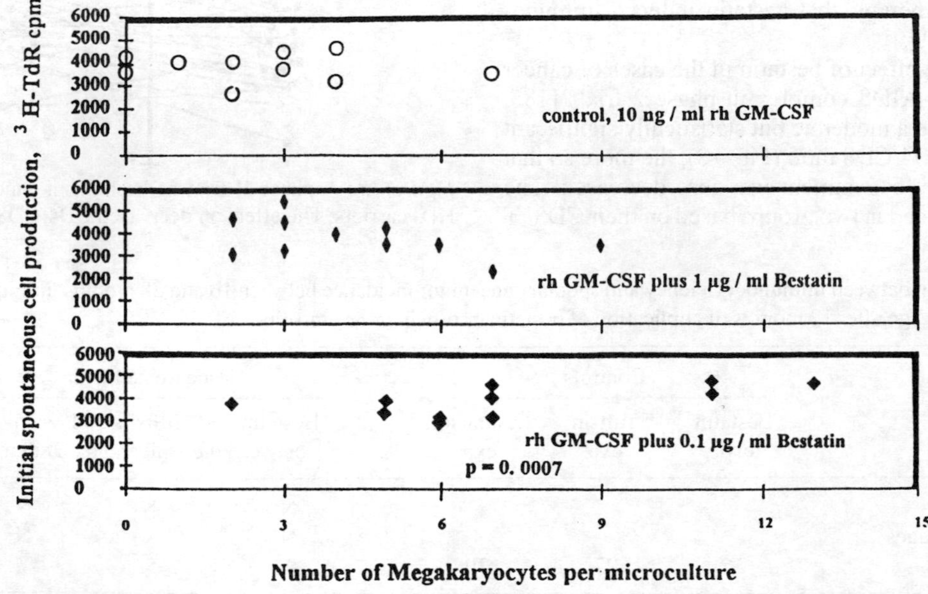

Figure 20. Stimulation of megakaryocytopoiesis by rh GM-CSF and bestatin in organotypic hematon-culture [19].

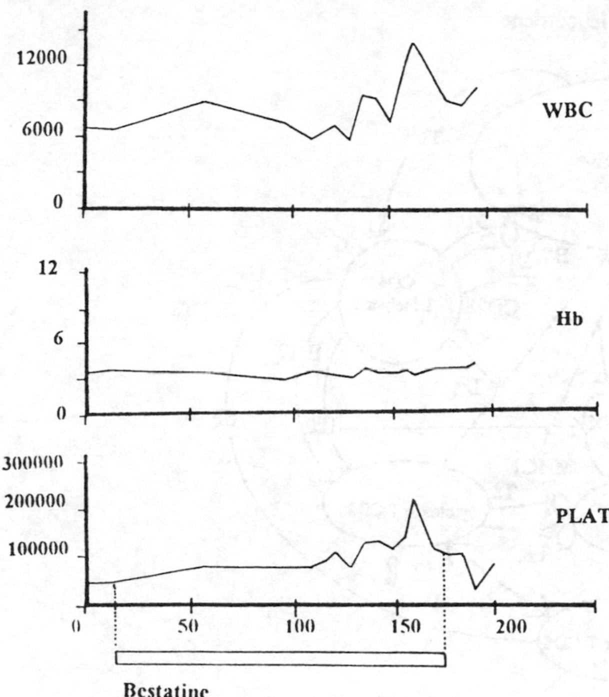

Figure 21. Beneficial effect of bestatin on the thrombocyte number in a 73 years old man suffering from dysmyelopoiesis.

blood cells, including granulocytes, and of platelets: a typical example of the effect obtained is given on Figure 21 [179].

It is interesting to note that natural substances, such as thymic factors [2, 80] and enkephalins [281, 47, 252, 136], known to enhance T-cell production and to be physiologically degradated by amino-peptidases, are structurally protected by bestatin.

Although its exact mechanism *in vivo* is not completely elucidated, it is now well established that it acts as a competitive inhibitor of leucine-aminopeptidase and aminopeptidase B. These enzymes are members of the zinc-binding metalloprotease superfamily, like the aminopeptidase N (or CD13 cell surface antigen) [112, 131], and an important role is attributed to these ecto-enzymes in modulating the physiological level of a number of biological mediators, such as angiotensin and insulin [269].

Not less interesting is the possible protective effect of tuftsin, another naturally produced peptide, resulting from immunoglobulin molecule degradation [140].

Tuftsin and analogues

Tuftsin (TFST) was discovered by Fidalgo and Najjar [60] when they observed the binding of IgG to blood monocytes and neutrophiles [61]. This binding did not stimulate phagocytosis *in vitro*, but one of its Ig peptide sequence did. It is an oligopeptide spontaneously produced by the spleen in two enzymatic steps, the cleavage by an endocarboxy-peptidase at the carboxyterminal arginine, and that by leukokinase at its aminoterminal threonine [201] (Fig. 22). It is also a part of the Fc fragment of the IgA chain [206]. The active tetrapeptide was isolated and sequenced [205, 249, 198]. Its structure is: *Thr-Lys-Pro-Arg*. It was synthetized [207, 82] and called tuftsin.

Interestingly enough, splenectomy affects phagocytosis and the half-life of erythrocytes [197, 202], a disorder corrected by the administration of immunoglobulins. A syndrome called *hyposplenia*, which may be hereditary or acquired, is characterized by eczema, respiratory infections and adenitis [260, 199, 104, 44, 45]. It is related to a point mutation resulting in the replacement of lysin by glutamic acid in tuftsine structure. *This abnormal tetrapeptide is a tuftsine antagonist* [22]. *The tripeptide Lys-Pro-Arg*, resulting from tuftsine enzymatic degradation (including by leucine-aminopeptidase), behaves identically [22].

Tufstin analogs listed on Table 5 were synthetized in the hope that some would be more active than tuftsin: this turned out to be true [66, 133, 119, 200, 95].

Table 5. Tufstin synthetized analogs

(Gly^1)-tuftsin	(For-Met^1)-tuftsin
(Met^1)-tuftsin	Indomethacin-tufstin
Formyl-tuftsin	Indomethacin-(des-Thr^1)-tuftsin

Tuftsin

Residues: 289 290 291 292

NH2--Gln-Val-His-Asn-Ala-Lys-Thr-Lys-Pro-Arg-Glu-Gln-Tyr--COOH

↑ ↑

Points of enzymatic cleavage

Figure 22. Cleavage of tuftsin as a part of the Fc fragment of the heavy chain of IgG.

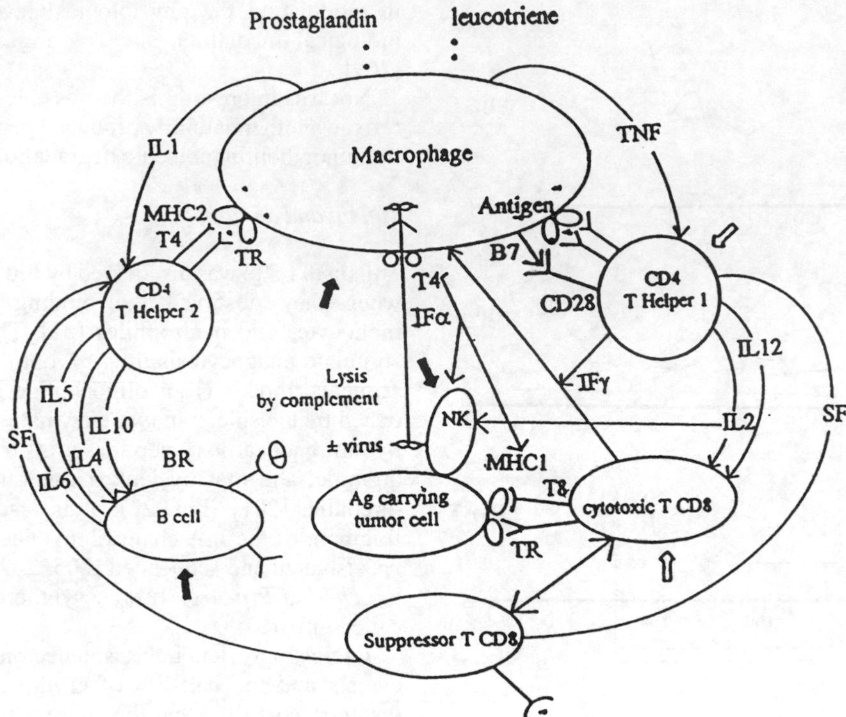

Figure 23. Action of tuftsin on the main immunologic functions in young mice (25 µg).

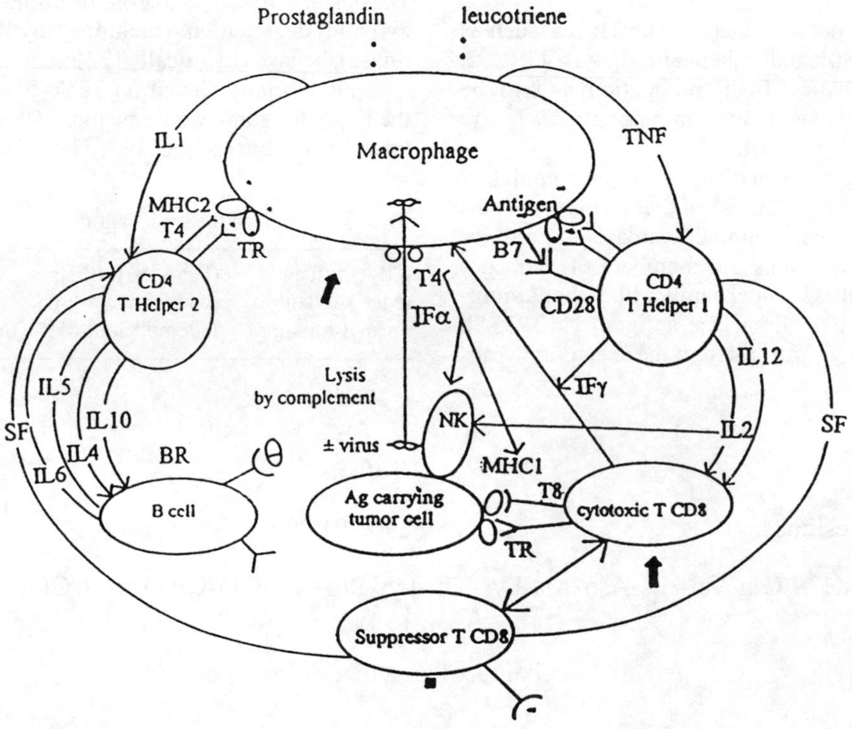

Figure 24. Effect of tuftsin according to dosage on the immunologic functions in old mice (25 µg).

TFST exerts as major pharmacological action, the stimulation of the macrophage functions [64] (a macrophage has 72, 000 TFST receptors [81], which are independent of Fc-receptors). Its endocytosis, when bound to the cells, resembles that of the epidermal growth factor [3]. Phagocytosis is highly stimulated by tuftsin.

Other cells of the immunologic system are also activated [64], as summarized on Figure 23 for *young mice* (less than 16 months old), and a different, restorating effect, is found in *old mice* [35], as for bestatin [32] (Fig. 24).

The spontaneous tumor incidence registered in tuftsin treated mice, is also significantly reduced, compared to controls (Table 4) [35].

The different actions of the analogues slightly differ with each other as far as some parameters [66, 33]. Figures 25 and 26 give the examples of two targets, macrophages and NK cells [66]. They have not been compared as far as the anti-tumoral effect is concerned.

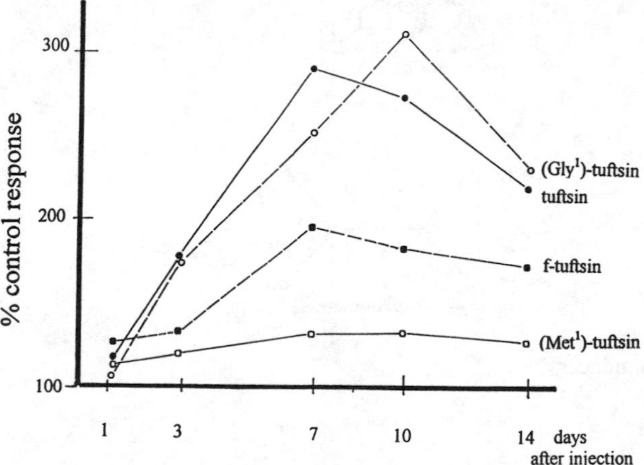

Figure 25. Macrophage chemiluminescence of several tuftsin analogs.

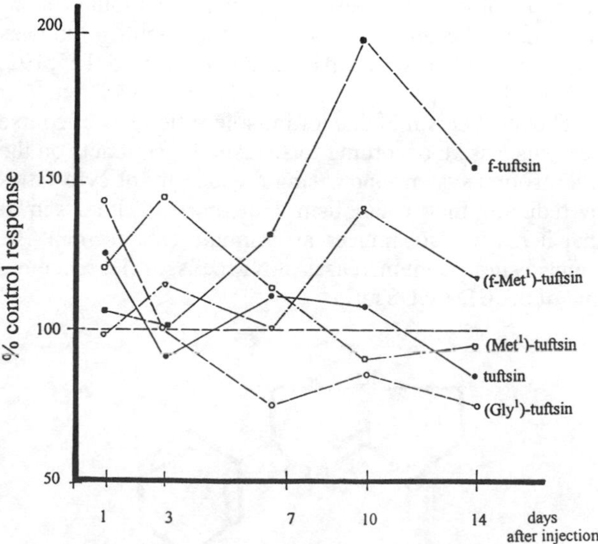

Figure 26. Spleen cell NK activity of several tuftsin analogs.

Unfortunately, the study of tuftsin in man was limited to a phase 1 study, although its results were very encouraging [40]. There was no clinical trial on any of its analogues, only because they were published before being the object of a patent.

TFST mobilizes intra-cellular calcium and modulates cAMP and cGMP levels.

Double stranded polynucleotides

Braun and his coworkers [13] found the same effect on cyclic AMP regulation in lymphocytes of *polyriboinosinic acid-polyribocytidylic acid (polyI-polyC)* (Fig. 27) and of *polyribo-uridylic acid-polyribo-adenilic acid (polyU-polyA)*. It is thus logical to describe here these immunomodulators. The relationship between the effect on c-AMP in lymphocytes and macrophages can possibly be explained by a non specific growth factor effect as we shall consider later [191].

The two quoted polynucleotides are indeed immunostimulators for the production of antibodies. They also stimulate several cellular immunity functions, especially those of the NK cells, and cytokines, particularly interferon [265, 37], increasing its concentration in microgram amounts: they thus were classified as 'interferon inducers'.

This action is not specific as illustrated by Figure 28 which shows the structure of other agents such as 12-0-tetradecanoyl-phorbol-13-acetate and other phorbol

IDP
CDP
POLYNUCLEOTIDE PHOSPHORYLASE
– Ip Ip Ip Ip Ip –
Cp Cp Cp Cp Cp
POLYINOSINIC ACID (POLY I)
POLYCYTIDYLIC ACID (POLY C)
Na Cl
Phos. Buffer
ICIC
ICIC
DOUBLE STRANDED POLY I – POLY C

Figure 27. Synthesis of the polynucleotide polyI-polyC.

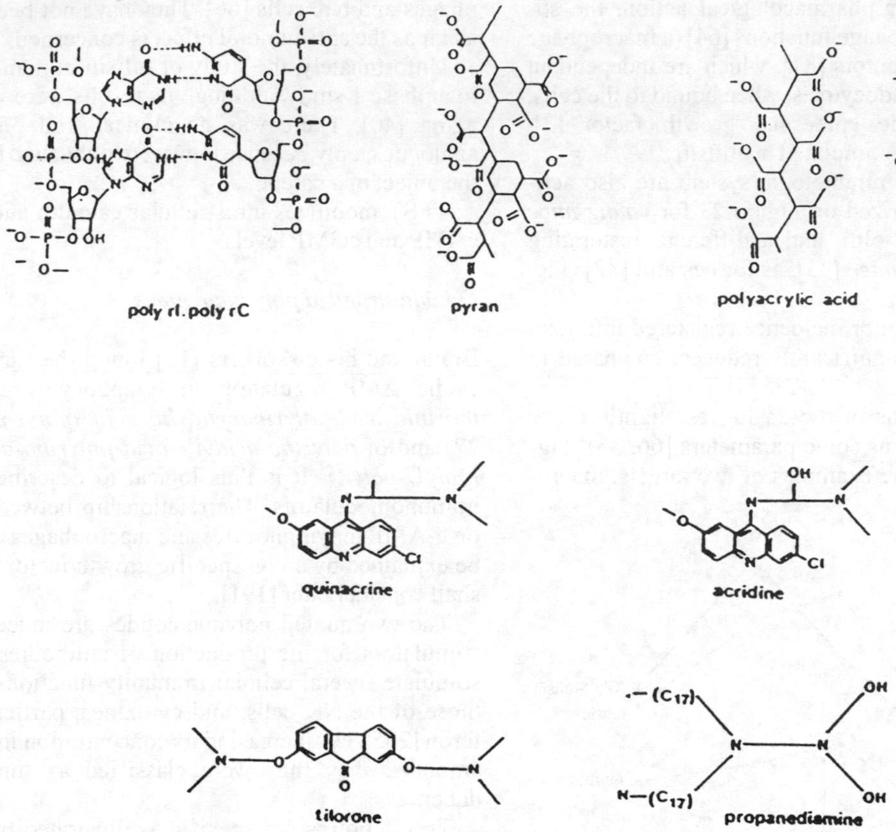

poly rI.poly rC pyran polyacrylic acid coam

quinacrine acridine

tilorone propanediamine

Figure 28. Structural features of other synthetic so called 'interferon inducers'.

esters [116], tirolone, statolon, Newcastle disease virus [77], or its oncolysate [39], and probably those of many others viruses which enhance the production of this cytokine [265]. Most of them stimulate NK cell action [77].

We obtained, with polyI-polyC, a significant effect on the experimental L 1210 leukemia [172] and in a phase 2 trial of human acute lymphoid leukemia [157]. The Lacours [121] obtained, with polyA-polyU an adjuvant effect in a murine breast cancer and the same effect in human patients, which will be described later.

Breast cancers being induced in mice by a virus [9], one can wonder if the action is not due to the induction of interferon antiviral action [265]. In fact, it was shown that it works directly on virus free cells [283].

Levamisole

Levamisole (Fig. 29) is an anthelminthic. It was first considered to inhibit T-suppressor cell activity and to increase interferon induction and lymphokine-induced macrophage phagocytosis [86].

It also restores depressed immunity in aging mice [34, 33] and reduces the incidence of spontaneous tumors (Table 4).

It has given discrete results as adjuvant therapy of acute myeloid leukemia [128] breast cancer [273], and in melanoma [261].

But levamisole has especially attracted interest in the case of colon cancer, especially when combined to 5-fluorouracil because the benefit of their application is as high as unexplained as will be discussed later [5, 125, 192, 132, 115].

The mechanism of this levamisole action has of course been discussed: according to Astashkin [7], it acts on the microsomal system, increasing the activity of cytostatics by reducing their catabolism. Holcombe [97] has shown that it really also induces an immuno-enhancement: he found a significant increases of NK cells, of IL2 receptors and of the CD4/CD8 ratio.

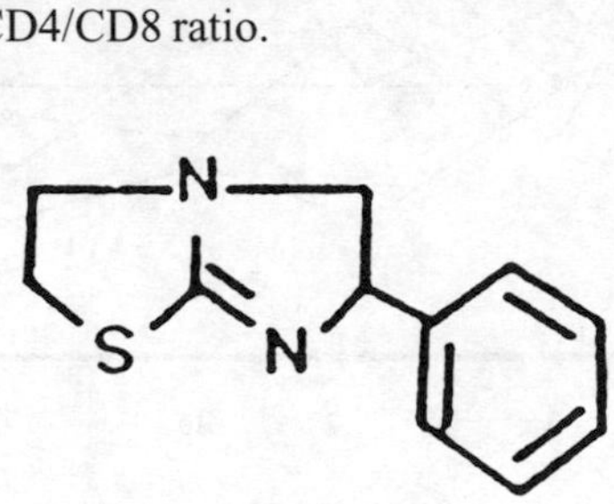

Figure 29. Structure of levamisole.

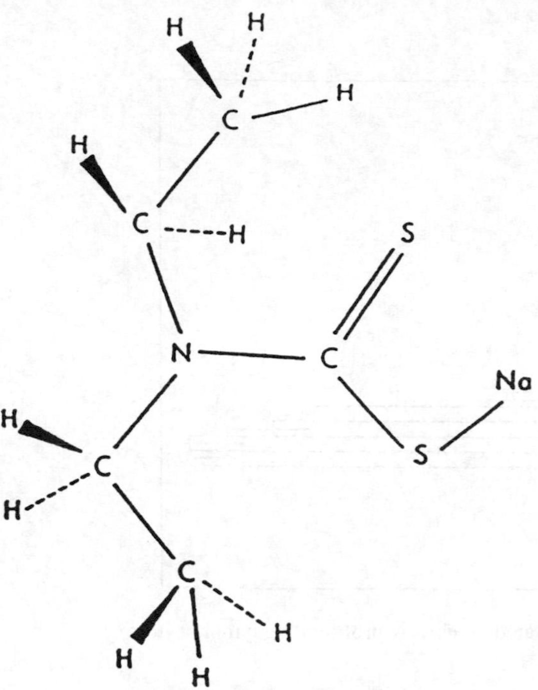

Figure 30. Structure of imuthiol.

Imuthiol

The structure of imuthiol, sodium diethyldithio-carbamate (DTC), is shown in Figure 30. It has been claimed to stimulate both helper and cytotoxic T cells, NK cells, and macrophages in young mice given 0.5 mg/mouse subcutaneously.

Doses of 8-10 mg/kg/week for 6 months improved in man delayed-type hypersensitivity (from 2.5 mm infiltration to 8.2 mm) and the mean T-helper cell number (from 265 to 457/mm^3) in 11 patients with stage 3-5A AIDS [124].

Vitamin A derivatives

Vitamin A (retinol) exerts some immunopotentiation [288]. So does its precursor *beta carotene*, without being as toxic [78]. As vitamin A may, indeed, at its active doses, induce dangerous side effects, the latter agent is more often prescribed than it, as are its retinoic acid isomers, *13-cis retinoic acid and all-trans-retinoic acid.* Both support not only the retinol functions without presenting its toxicity, but complementary effects: the cis suppresses the metaplasia of the smoker bronchi due to tobacco [83], while the all trans-isomer is capable to induce remissions of the *promyelocytic acute leukemia*. This remissions by differentiation of a malignant disease presenting chromosomal abnormalities, were discovered in China by Huang in 1987 [99] and confirmed by Degos [50].

Retinoids act as immunomodulators, especially on thymus cell differentiation [51, 52].

Vitamin D derivatives

While vitamin D deficiency was known to induce reversible myelofibrosis [46], *1-alpha-25-dihydroxy vitamin D_3* was shown to induce monocytic differentiation and bone resorption [10].

Since it binds to some breast cells and may stimulate their growth [68], one must be aware of the ambiguity of its action. This is probably but superficially explained by its relationship with some growth factors: growth factor beta-1 exerts, among them, an antiproliferating effect on murine tumors and hematopoietic progenitor cells [79].

Growth factors being in cooperative or antagonistic relationship with hormones, one is not surprised to learn the role played by 1-alpha-25-dihydroxy vitamin D_3 in modulating circulating hormone levels [91]. Its structure being near to that of steroids, it is not either surprising that it exerts significant, both short-term and long term effects, on bone and calcium metabolism in the case of post-menopausal osteoporosis [72].

Zinc

It is usual in biology to bring together vitamins and so-called metal oligo-elements. Zinc gluconate, the deficiency of which in domestic animals, is known to be responsible for severe infections due to immune deficiency, is a catalyser of lymphocyte proliferation (Fig. 31) [18]. It has significantly increased the CD4/CD8 ratio in a phase 2 trial we conducted in humans (Fig. 32) [175].

Enzymes

We have seen the effect of enzyme inhibitors with bestatin. Different enzymes have been studied as immunomodulators. We shall consider only three types of preparations.

A mixture of *proteolytic enzymes* [38] was proposed to cleave the immune complexes, and as naive as it may appear in first approximation, it reduces their serum level as well as does *plasmapheresis* [209].

Neuraminidase was used to affect cell surface sialic acid [101] of the tumor cells. But it also affects that of lymphocytes and macrophages [256], which probably explains phagocytosis increase [127].

Phospholipase A2 [30] is an *in vivo* immunomodulator affecting most types of cells involved in immunity. Its action illustrates the role of phospholipids of the plasma membrane which are actively involved in the signal transmission via their fatty acid moieties across the membrane in response to external stimuli. The alteration of the arachidonic acid plays a predominant regulatory role. In this metabolic cycle, a fatty acid is usually cleaved from a phospholipid (such as phosphatidylcholine) by phospholipase A2 (Fig. 33) [241].

We had noted on Figure 4, the role on macrophage function of prostanoids and leukotrienes, which also play a role in inducing or multiplying suppressor cells [243].

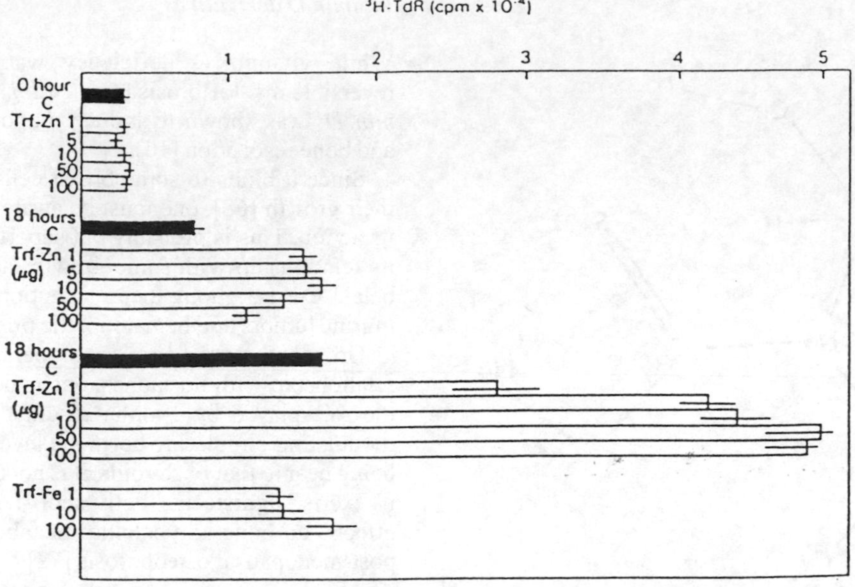

Figure 31. The effects of zinc 2+ or iron-transferrin on resting, preactivated or actively proliferating lymphocytes.

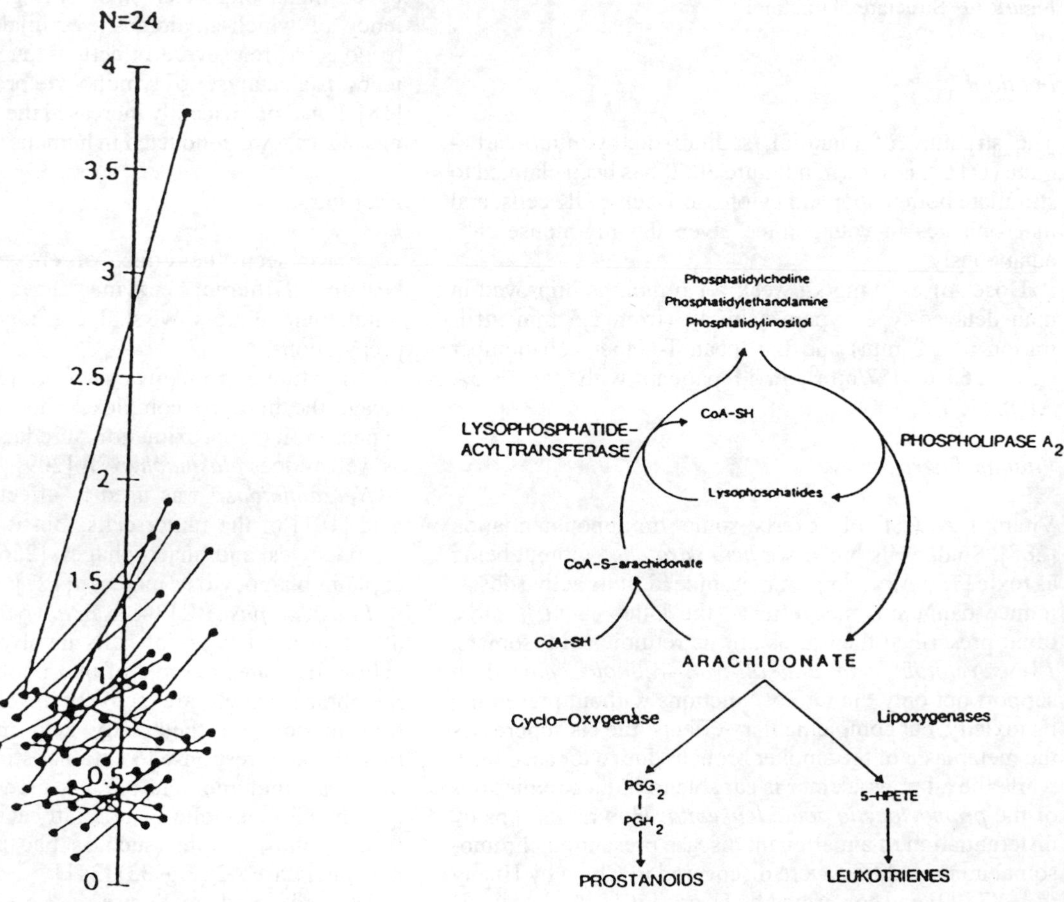

Figure 32. CD4/CD8 ration in the phase II trial of zinc gluconate [175].

Figure 33. The role of phospholipase A2.

Cimetidine and considerations on suppressor cell inhibition

Cimetidine, which decreases the production of prostaglandins and which is a H2 receptor antagonist [107, 57] reduces the suppressor cell function.

A possible side effect, particular to bone marrow transplanted patients which can occur, is myelosuppression [188].

Its action is not specific, while some immunomodulators previously studied, when they reduce the suppressor cell number, do it specifically in relation with the antigen which has initiated the reaction: it is probably the case of most immunomodulators, from BCG [75] to bestatin, what we have seen in man (Fig. 34) [146]. Their high dose, as those of IL2 and of the antigen itself, is one of the common factor inducing suppression (Fig. 35) [56].

Some *oncostatics* and other *cytostatics*, and/or *virostatics* may also induce antigen-specific suppressor cells [224, 223, 11, 29]. This suggests that an antitumor effect may be supported by two actions: a direct one, against neoplastic cells, and an indirect one, against suppressor cells.

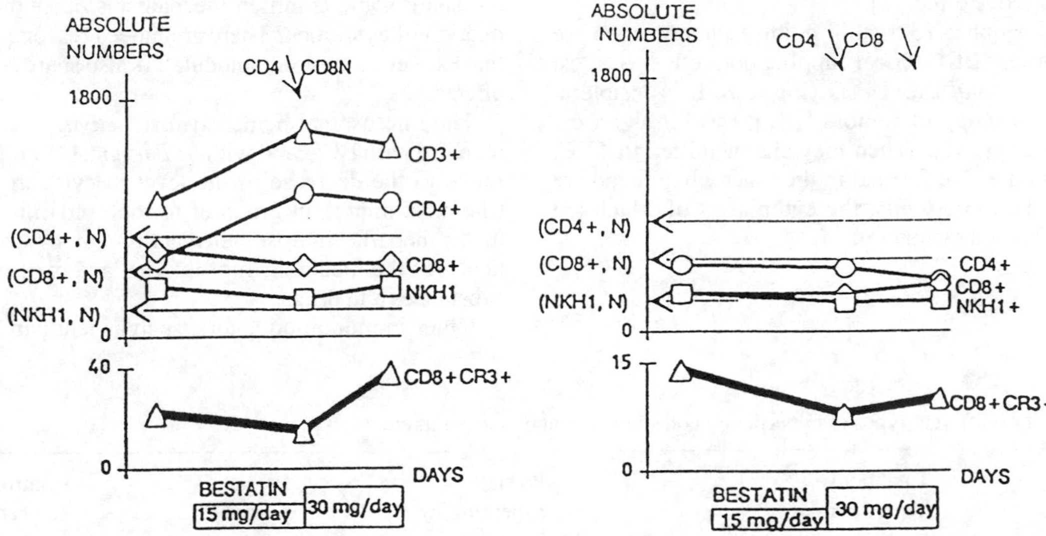

Figure 34. Effect of bestatin according to its dose, and the CD8 lymphocyte number, on immune parameters in man, especially the CD4 and the suppressor cell numbers [146].

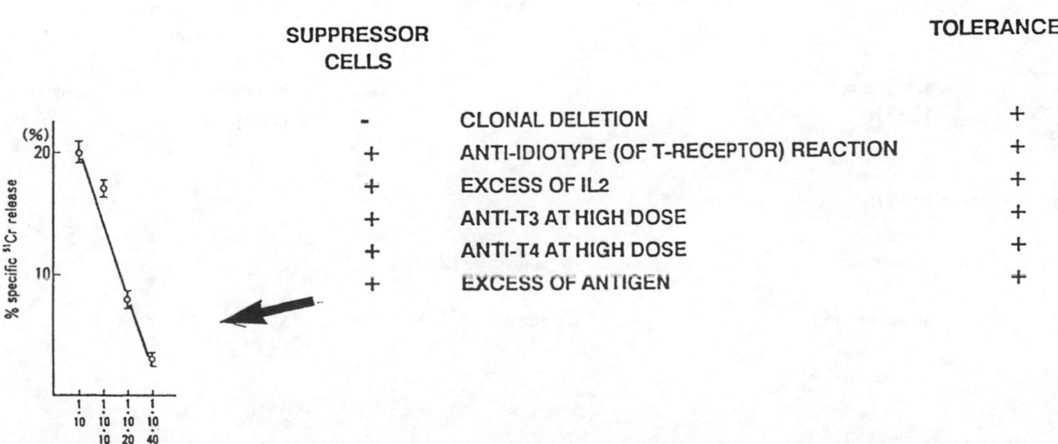

Figure 35. Correlation according to Ebihara [56] between several immunologic parameters or factors and the presence of suppressor cells or tolerance.

Hyperthermia

Total body hyperthermia, contrarily to the effect of most physical elements, ionising radiation [21] and even ultraviolet radiation including those of the sun, which are immunodepressive [49], induces, at a temperature of 40ºC, an immuno-enhancing effect [1, 257, 84]. At 42ºC, it does the contrary [1] (Table 6).

Local hyperthermia, applied at the temperature which may partially destroy tumors (43 to 45ºC) and can prevent metastasis [215], restore general immunity when it is deficient, but induces no significant change when its functions are normal [268]. Very curiously, levamisole, combined with local hyperthermia, is antagonistic to its tumor-destructive effect [8].

We shall emphasize at this point a phenomenon we observed after BCG local application on a Kaposi sarcoma, *lysosomal exocytosis* (Fig. 36). It is visible at electron microscopy of tumors [232], as well as on the peritoneal cells [231]. When they are submitted to 43ºC, lysosomal bodies are formed in the macrophages and are injected to the tumor cells, the cytoplasms of which are affected first, then the nuclei.

Different and/or common mechanism(s) of some action(s) of exogenous immunomodulators

We presented as exogenous immunomodulators, very different types of agents, from BCG to synthetized molecules, and to hyperthermia. They can exert specific effects, as far as the antigen which induces the reaction studied in each experiment is concerned.

Most if not all, from BCG [236] to hyperthermia [231, 232], affect macrophages.

Most can probably, when given at high doses stimulate suppressor cells. They seem, at small doses, to be able to inhibit them in case of immunodepression [148].

A question arises however. Don't some of them if not all, share some common mechanisms other than the induction of cytokines? There are indeed reasons to suggest that exogenous immunomodulators also share some direct effects.

The microsomal heme *oxydase activity* was shown to increase with BCG and with *C. Parvum*, [187]. This could relate to the decrease of the level of cytochrome P-450 (the most important group of ferroporphyrinic enzymes) in the hepatic microsomal reactions of hydroxylations, hence of the metabolism of internal and exogenous such substances and drugs.

Other immunomodulators, such as lentinan [248] and

Table 6. Effect of different types of hyperthermia on some immunologic parameters

	Total body hyperthermia		Prostate hyperthrophy local	Prostate cancer local	Control subjects local
	40ºC	42ºC (1 h)	transrectal hyperthermy at 45ºC [215]		
T cytotoxic lymphocyte proliferation number	stimulation [1]	reduction [1]	stimulation [268]	restoration [268]	no change
CD4 number	stimulation [257]			restoration [268]	no change
CD suppressives	reduction [257]				
CD4/CD8	stimulation		stimulation [268]		
NK	stimulation [1]		stimulation [268]		
IL1	stimulation [84]				
IL2	stimulation [84]				
IF	stimulation [84]				

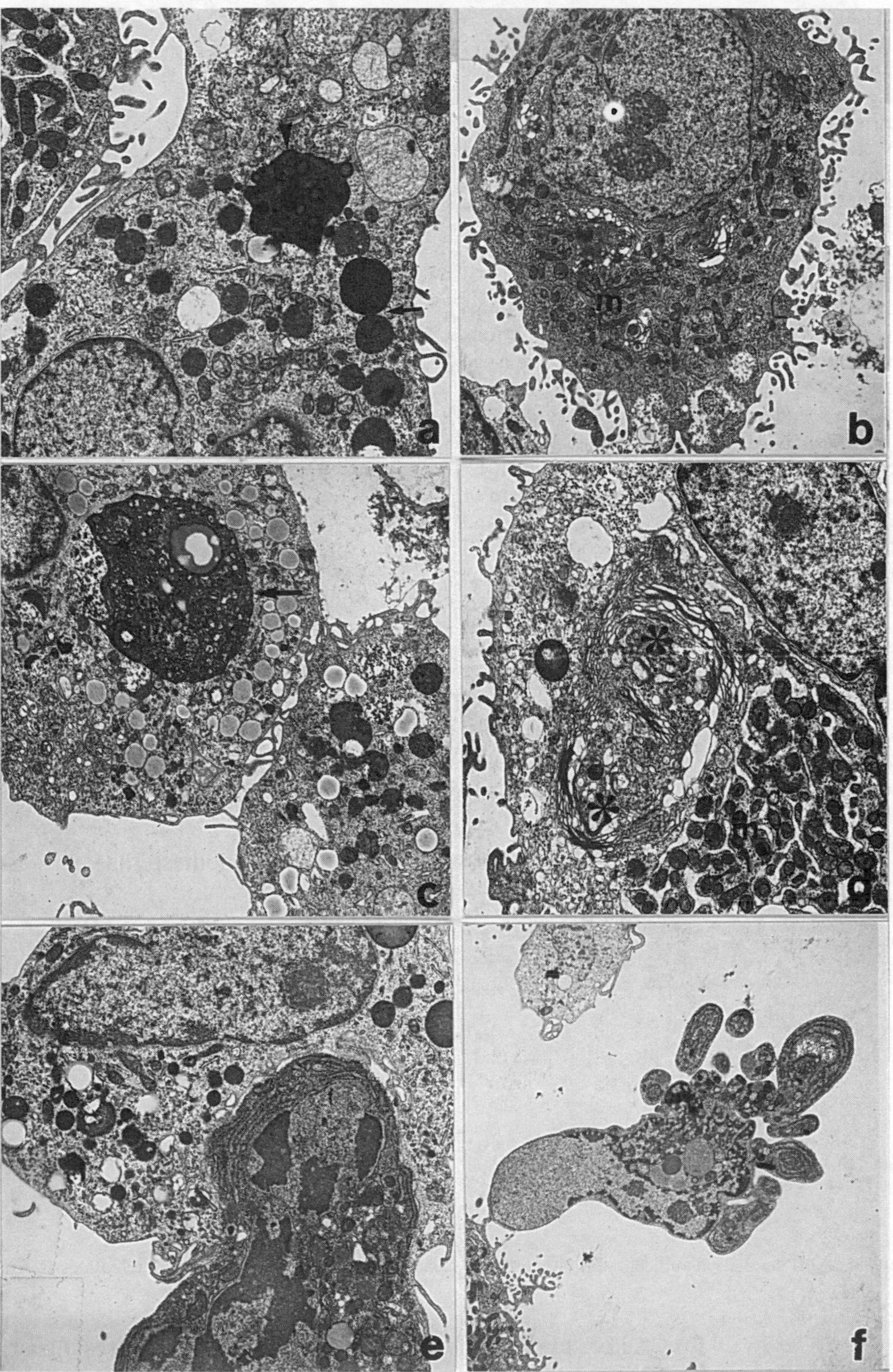

Figure 36. The ultrastructural features of peritoneal macrophages before (a, c, e) and after (d, c, f) hyperthermic treatment; a) macrophage showing accumulation of primary (arrow and secondary (arrow-head) lysosomes (x 12000); b) degranulated macrophage containing numerous mitochondria (m) (x 8000); c) presence of a large phagocytic inclusion (x 9000); d) particular of degranulated macrophage with multiple Golgi complexes (asterisks) in juxtanuclear region and condensed mitochondria (m) (x 12000); e) macrophage in the process of engulfing a cell, probably of neoplastic +derivation (x 10000); f) apoptotic degeneration of a macrophagic cell (x 7000).

lipopeptides [190], as well as *some cytokines, such as interferon* [194] *and interleukin 1* [59] reduce *the level of hepatic microsomal cytochrome P-450*. Nitric oxide seems to be the mediator of this reduction [113].

This decrease of this electron carrier, i.e. of this action of hepatic microsomal hydroxylation by various substances, plays a role by increasing their life span, their concentration and their functions. Muramyl dipeptide activates the macrophages *release of* O_2^- in vitro (Fig. 37), which could be in relation with its effect as local adjuvant, capable of replacing Freund's adjuvant [126].

The search of a *growth factor effect* is the second approach for the discovery of some probable direct actions of exogenous immuno-modulators; it has been discussed for tuftsin and for polynucleotides. These agents *of different structures identically mobilize intra-cellular calcium and modulate cAMP and cGMP level*. Figure 38 describes the situation of cAMP between ATP and AMP, and its main functions; it shows the action mechanism of cAMP modulators which *enhance adenyl-cyclase*, and reminds us that methylxanthines such as theophylline and caffeine, inhibit phosphodiesterase which transforms cAMP into AMP [13/191]. This is one of the complex functions of the so-called growth factors (Fig. 39) [103, 251, 246].

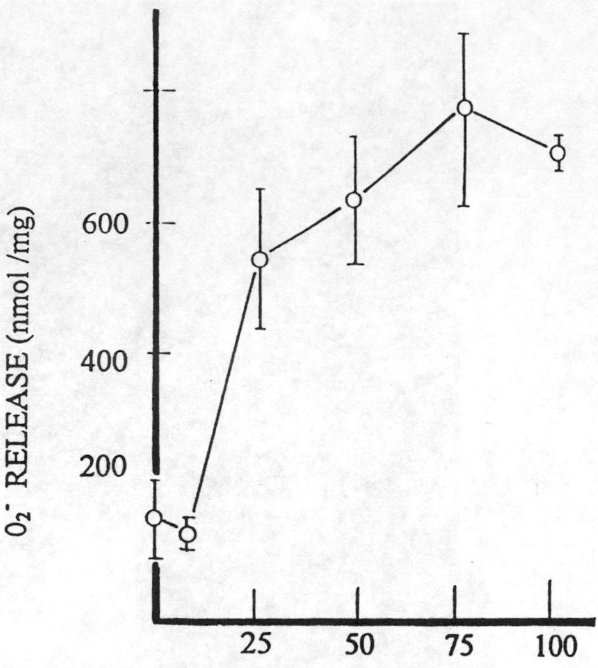

Figure 37. Effect on O_2^- release by mouse macrophages after *in vivo* pretreatment with muramyl dipeptide [126].

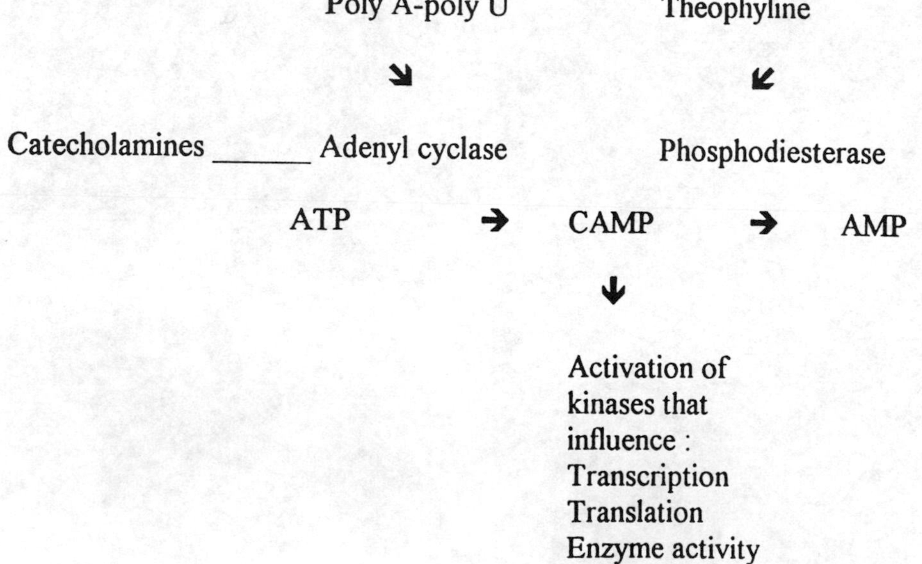

Figure 38. Steps in cAMP formation and degradation, outlining the site of influence of tuftsin, polynucleotides and methylxanthines.

Growth factor + receptor	Activation of protein kinase specific of tyrosinic residues (thus of tyrosinic phosphorylation).
	Activation of phosphatidyl inositol turnover.
	Mobilisation of free calcium and activation of Na^+ and K^+ pumps.

Figure 39. Main mechanisms of growth factor action.

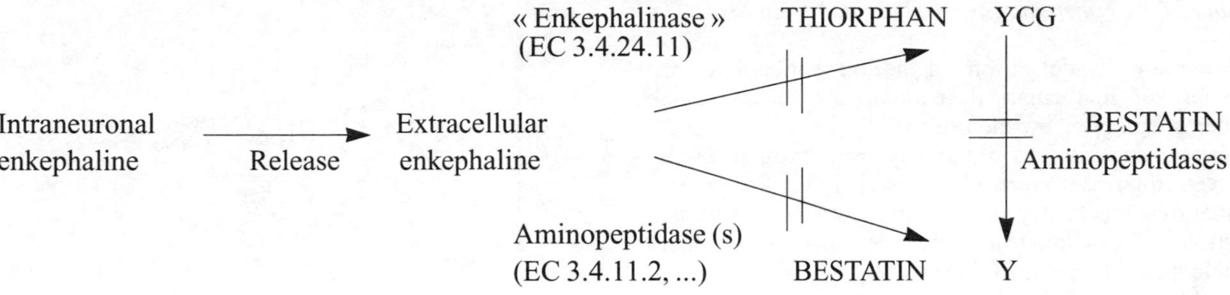

Figure 40. Bestatin inhibits endogenous enkephaline catabolism *via* aminopeptidase inhibition.

The fact that *transforming growth factor beta* [262], behaves as a suppressive agent, especially by inhibiting tumor-specific cytotoxic T-lymphocytes [105], supports this hypothesis. Moore [195] and Sen [255] listed these factors and their relationship with oncogens and antioncogens.

We mentioned the direct or indirect other actions of some agents, studied as immunity immunomodulators, and which may act in other fields of physiology or pathology. Bestatin is an antagonist of the amino-peptidase which destroys enkephalins (Fig. 40), hence its role to enhance this endogenous opioid agent [252, 136], and a possible mechanism of its NK cell enhancement [70].

TOLERANCE OF EXOGENOUS IMMUNOMODULATORS

Side effects of exogenous immunomodulators have rarely been observed, even for living BCG [137]. Their tolerance contrasts with cytokines which are toxic at high doses [93].

However, so called auto-immunity syndromes [42], even immune complexes [85] have not been searched systematically. It should be done in the future. A case of 'multiple inflammatory leucoencephalopathy', associated with levamisole, administered for five weeks at the total dose of 1, 500 mg in a melanoma patient, was described [114].

GENERAL REMARKS AND QUESTIONS

The need to improve the quality of research

The need for respect of a proper terminology

The term 'adoptive immunotherapy' used to describe cellular active immunotherapy [244] is inaccurate.

Following the classical terminology in immunology, we called (a) '*passive immunotherapy or prevention*', the direct or indirect use of antibodies [184, 53]; (b) *active immunotherapy or prevention* [137], the *in vivo* intervention on the own immunological system of the patients, applied either after (for therapy) or before (for prevention) the tumor is established. The *in vitro* manipulation of the patient system components, i.e. its lymphocytes, macrophages, immunoglobins, cytokines.... followed by their own re-infusion(s) belong to active immunotherapy: it is the case of the re-administration of autologous lymphocytes manipulated *in vitro*: calling such intervention 'adoptive' immunotherapy [244] is neither logical nor correct, *as autologous cells, not being foreign, cannot be 'adopted'*. (c) *Strico sensu adoptive immunotherapy* [159, 27, 152, 149] refers to the act realized by *foreign donor bone marrow stem cell grafts* or *lymphocyte transfusions*. The actors of the immunologic reactions directed against normal cells of the recipient and called GvH, and against leukemic cells and called GvL are allogeneic, thus foreign T-lymphocytes, which are indeed adopted.

The terminological relationship between 'immunomodulators' and 'biologic response modifiers' is ambiguous

Some authors have replaced the term 'immunomodulators' by that of 'biological response modifiers' (BRM)?

We have no objection to including the immunomodulators in the BRM, if the practical sense of the latter is correct, including all physiological and pharmacological substances, from hormones to neuromediators, from wine to water, which is not the case. Immunomodulators may indeed have a non immunological action: BCG stimulates hematopoietic cell entry into the cycle [137], and bestatin is the only growth and differentiation factor today available in practice for platelets [19, 179]. But applying GCSF to a patient risking aplasia and death, from a superintensive chemotherapy [182] is not immunotherapy.

The cytokines, the discovery and preparations of which have represented great effort and progress, are so numerous and the object of so many contradictions in their physiologic and pharmacologic roles, that the BRM description and even its concept will soon be chaotic.

The need for a coherent sense of statistical evaluation

Statistics are, by definition, 'a discipline including the ensemble of mathematical methods used to evaluate problems complex by themselves or concerning great numbers of subjects, so that the only results presented will be given in term of probability' [242]. Thus, if the great number of subjects may be a possible characteristic of the question to be studied, it is neither a necessary nor a sufficient characteristic of the answer [287].

Trials concerning moderate or even small numbers of patients may give the exact answer to a question, if there are no biases, for example due to heterogeneity of the subject population, or prematurity of analysis and publication.

According to Reizenstein [238], who submitted 230 clinical trials to a critical analysis, most randomized trials with large numbers of patients, suffer from imperfections and even faults.

More subtle is the critical judgment of some methods used, which affect the results. In 1969, we published, as a 'preliminary communication' in the Lancet [156], the result of a study conducted on a small number of patients, of 'active immunotherapy in acute leukemia patients', in which BCG appeared capable of prolonging the chemotherapy induced remissions of some patients which were, 12 years later, considered as cured. The Medical Research Council Leukaemia Committee and Working Party on Leukaemia in Childhood published in 1971 [293], the result of a large randomized trial which did not confirm the significance of the superiority of BCG as an adjuvant treatment of chemotherapy in acute lymphoid leukemia patients over a placebo.

Figure 41 shows that BCG significantly increased the number of blood lymphocytes, and Figure 42 that the BCG patient curve is different of the placebo one (which indicates a beneficial effect) until the 50th week. At this time, one control happens to be at a level slightly inferior

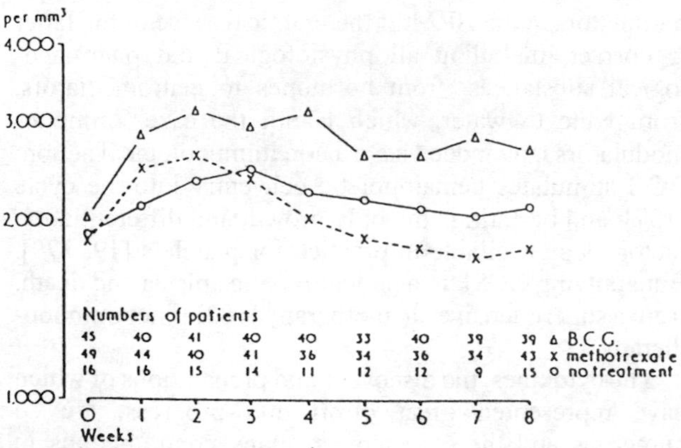

Figure 41. Effect of post-chemotherapy-BCG immunotherapy on absolute blood lymphocyte counts in the concorde. Plotted points are the mean values for all relevant patients whose lymphocyte counts were done at the stated time. (All calculations were done on a logarithmic scale).

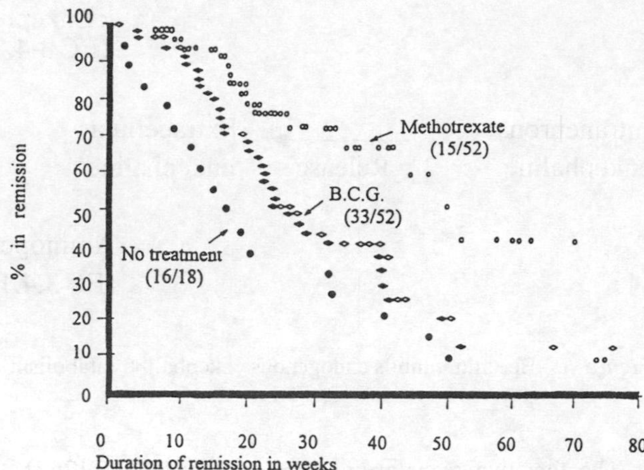

Figure 42. Remission duration after chemotherapy induction, according to randomized adjuvant application of BCG or methotrexate or placebo. The percentages of subjects in remission at the different times were calculated by standard actuarial methods. Each symbol represents one patient. Open symbols are for patients still in their first remission; closed symbols for relapsed patients. Figures in parentheses indicate the numbers relapsed as of March 1st 1971 and total numbers in respective groups [293].

but near that of one BCG patient, while, around the 75th week, two more controls behave so, compared to two BCG patients. One notes that no patient was introduced in the placebo group between the 50th and the 75th weeks, and in the BCG group between the 52th and the 68th weeks.

During this time, all introduced patients were randomized in a methotrexate third branch, which biased the trial, the main if not the only objects being to compare BCG and a placebo. This third branch altered the availability of the patient population. The only data which are valid are the proportions of relapses at the time of publication in the BCG and in the placebo branches, respectively 33/52 and 16/18. And the test of significance used for evaluating BCG should not have masked the abnormal introduction of patients in its branch and in that of the placebo, due to the useless adjunction of a third branch.

The absence of stratification of the patients according to the HLA [274] and to the cytological form [294] parameters is of course another reason for expressing a critical reserve on this trial conclusion.

Another remark about methodology concerns the period of the disease-free-survival on which immunotherapy acts, compared to that on which chemotherapy is effective: the latter affects the cells in divisions, hence reduces the relapse rate in the first part of the curve, that which is rapidly declining, while the first kills the cells in G0 or G1, hence influences the second part of the curve, that of the later relapses. This notion is illustrated by Figure 43, which compares, in the case of breast cancer premenopausal patients, the curves given by two types of chemotherapy, the CMF (cyclophosphamide, methotrexate,

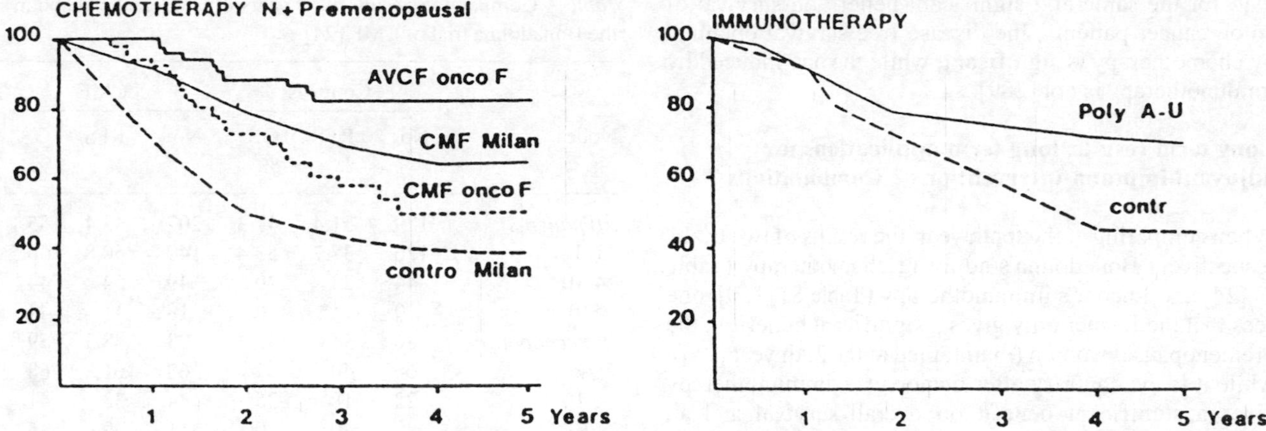

Figure 43. Adjuvant chemotherapy acts on the early part of the disease-free survival exponential curve, and adjuvant active immunotherapy on a later phase.

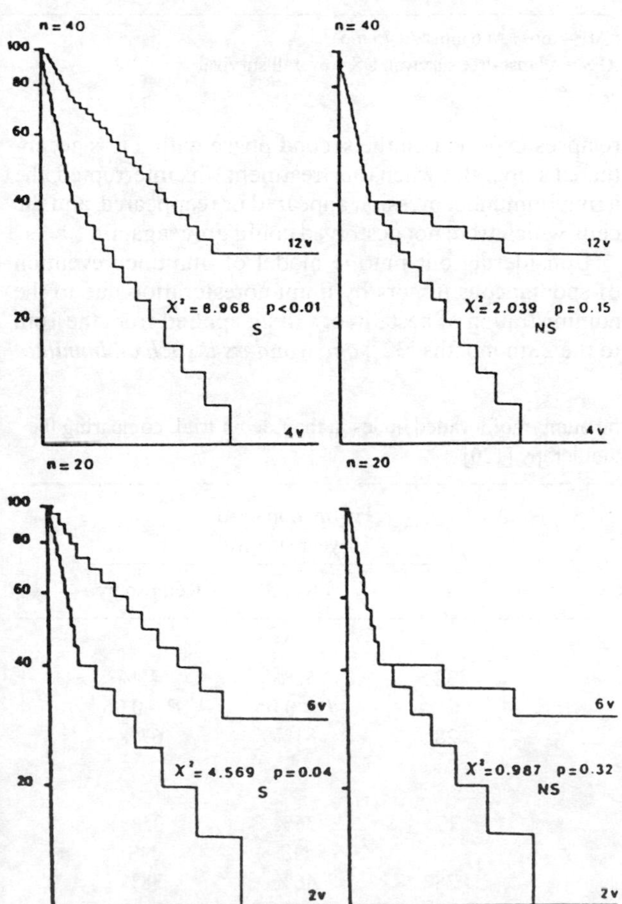

Figure 44. For the same operational benefit, (here 30%), the one given by an adjuvant treatment which works in the initial part of the curve, such as chemotherapy, as see in Figure 43, appears to be significant, while that given by an adjuvant treatment working on the second part, as immunotherapy, appears to be insignificant.

fluorouracil) [23], applied by Bonadonna at Milano, and the AVCF (adriamycine, vincristine, cyclophosphamide, fluorouracil) applied by the OncoFrance group [176], to that given by adjuvant immunotherapy with polyA-polyU [122].

Figure 44 shows that, for the same final benefits, the one obtained by a treatment acting on the beginning of the curve, is significant, while the one obtained by another, acting later, is not [166].

This notion is also illustrated by Figure 45 showing

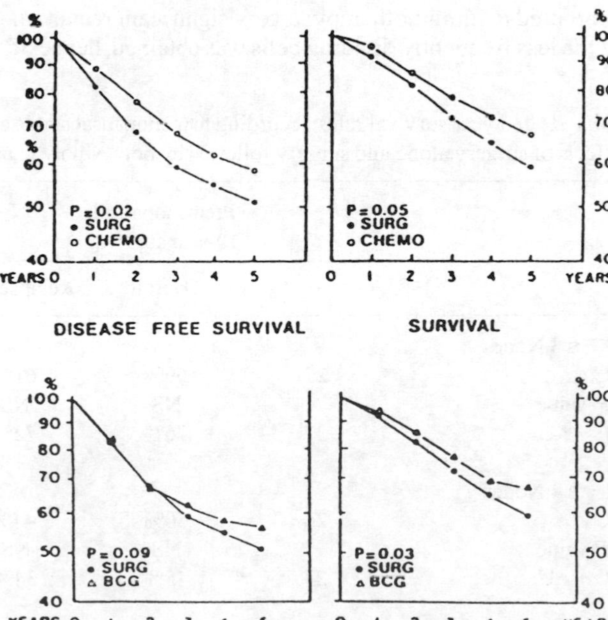

Figure 45. Difference in the significance of disease-free survival increase of colon cancer patients who got, at the fifth year of two trials, the same discrete benefit: it is significant for the trial of chemotherapy, the effect of which affects the first part of the curve, and not significant for the trial of immunotherapy, the effect of which affects the second [289].

that, for the same and significant benefit on survival of colon cancer patients, the disease free survival obtained by chemotherapy is significant, while the one induced by immunotherapy is not [289].

Long term results. long term applications for adjuvant immuno-interventions ? Combinations ?

When comparing at the tenth year, the results of two trials, respectively Bonadonna's adjuvant chemotherapy (Table 7) [24] and Lacour's immunotherapy (Table 8) [120], one sees that the former only gives a significant benefit in the premenopausal women (maintained at the 20th year [25]), while it is the contrary after menopause: immunotherapy gives a significant benefit on overall survival and an almost significant one on relapse-free survival in the patients who had no more than three invaded nodes.

A long term applications of adjuvant immuno-interventions?

These data and considerations must encourage those who are rather disappointed by the last Bonadonna's publication on his result at the 20th years [25], which is of the order of only 10% benefit for overall survival. This fact leads to the conclusion that, by advancing in age, the CMF women of his trial have became immunodepressed, which may have helped the cells having escaped chemotherapy, to grow.

A similar phenomenon occurred in Lacour's patients submitted to immunotherapy: a very significant reduction of the less frequently dividing cells was obtained, hence of relapses expected on the second phase with a less accentuated slope. But when this treatment was interrupted, the aging immunodepression appeared or reappeared, and the cells which were not destroyed could grow again.

Considering our murine model of immunoprevention of spontaneous tumors by immunorestoration due to the administration of bestatin or tuftsin applied from the 16th to the 28th months [32], *one wonders if such an immuno-*

Table 7. Comparative results at 10 years of CMF and placebo in the Bonadonna trial of CMF [24]

	Controls			CMF		
Nodes	No	RFS %	OS %	No	RFS %	OS %
All patients	179	31.4	47.3	207	43.4	55.1
1-3	126	37.7	53.4	140	50.8	60.5
4-10	44	23	40	49	34	44
>10	9	11*	0*	18	11	44
Premenopause	86	31	45	103	48.3	59.0
1-3	60	40	51	68	61	68
4-10	22	18	35	24	33	41
>10	4	0+	0¤	11	9	45
Postmenopause	93	32	50	104	38.2	52.1
1-3	66	35	56	72	42	54
4-10	22	27	45	25	35	46
>10	5	20*	0*	7	14	43

*At 84 mo. +At 6 mo. ¤At 75 mo.
RFS = relapse-free survival. OS = overall survival.

Table 8. Ten year survival rates according to menopausal status and the number of invaded nodes in the Lacour trial, comparing the effects of surgery alone and surgery followed by poly A-poly U immunotherapy [120]

	Premenopausal 10-year survival			Postmenopausal 10-year survival		
	n	Overall	Relapse free	n	Overall	Relapse free
N + ≤ 3 Nodes						
C	27	69%	61%	32	52%	45%
P-value		NS	NS		$P<0.05$	$P=0.06$
C + AU	27	76%	72%	28	81%	67%
N + ≥ 4 Nodes						
C	26	50%	41%	17	35%	35%
P-value		NS	NS		NS	NS
C + AU	27	45%	34%	28	46%	38%
Total N = patients						
C	53	59%	51%	49	52%	45%
P-value		NS	NS		$P=0.07$	NS
C + AU	54	61%	53%	49	66%	54%

° The numbers correspond to 9-year survival rates; no patient has reached a 10-year follow-up in this subset of patients.
NS = Not significant.

intervention should not be applied in humans for a corresponding length of time.

Combinations?

The other suggestion stemming from these data and considerations concerns the use of *combinations of chemotherapy and immuno-therapy*.

Much experimental work has been done on such combinations. It has confirmed what could be expected from the fact that cytostatics for cancer cells are also cytostatics for lymphocytes, hence the success of the sequence chemotherapy-immunotherapy, and the deterioration of the result by the sequence immunotherapy-chemotherapy [171, 170, 169].

The interspersion of cycles of chemotherapy and of immunotherapy may be beneficial, as it may be detrimental. This was the case in a randomized trial on melanoma patients, in which we compared immunotherapy by BCG applied alone, to chemo-immunotherapy: the patients under the combination relapsed before those under immuno-therapy alone (the difference not being significant), and died after relapse significantly earlier (Fig. 46) [230].

But one of the most successful model of adjuvant chemo-immunotherapy is the combination of fluorouracil (5-FU) and of levamisole [193] applied after resection of stage C colon carcinoma. Applying 5-FU (a cycle of 450 mg/m^2/d x 5 followed by weekly injection of 450 mg/m^2 for 48 additional weeks) had not been efficacious in previous trials, and that of levamisole (50 mg 3 times/d for 3 day repeated each 2 weeks for one year), showed no effect in the area where it was applied alone.

The benefit of this combination, marked from the beginning of the treatment, is maintained and amplified at the 8th and 9th years (Fig. 47 and 48). It is of the order of 20% for disease free as well as for global survivals. After correction for the influence of prognostic factors through

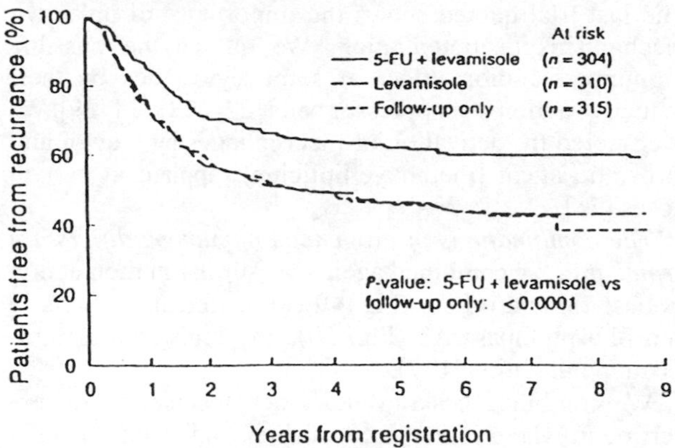

Figure 47. The levamisole-fluorouracil combination for adjuvant therapy trial of colon carcinoma [193]: recurrence-free interval according to treatment arm.
Patients who died without recurrence were censored. 5-Fu = fluorouracil.

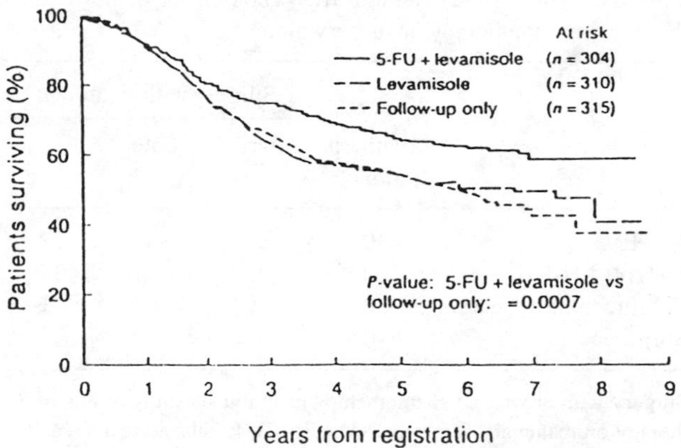

Figure 48. Same trial [193]: survival according to arm.
5-Fu = Fluorouracil

the use of a proportional hazards model, patients receiving FU and levamisole were again found to have a significant survival advantage when compared with patients assigned to observation only; they enjoyed a 33% reduction in mortality rates [193].

This paradoxical results of a significant benefit obtained by combining two agents which appear ineffective when applied alone, has conducted to search for a non immunological effect of levamisole: in fact some of its metabolites enhance the activity of 5-FU [7]. However, recent research by the National Cancer Institute using modern assay technology has confirmed that levamisole does have an immunologic activity, expressed by macrophage stimulation, NK cell and IL-2 receptors increase [97].

Today, the results quoted and all those published, make it possible to draw objectively deducted rules for the numerous possible chemo-immunotherapy combinations.

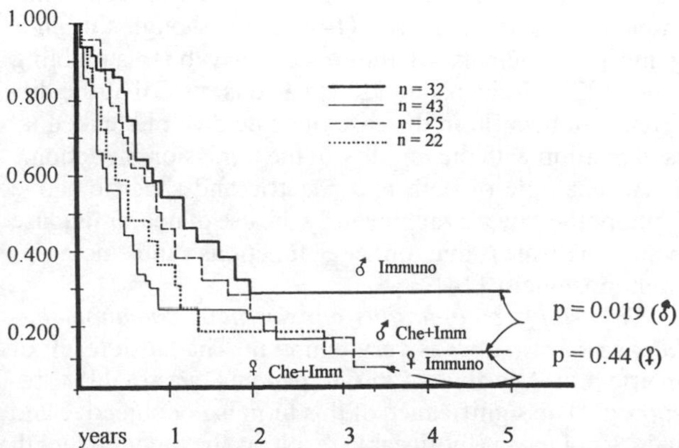

Figure 46. OncoFrance melanoma trial: survival after relapse. The advantage of immunotherapy over immunochemotherapy (to be discussed later) is only significant for males [230].

The last trial quoted shows the importance of unknown mechanisms of potentiation. We quoted the possible immunorestoration effect of some cytostatics by their reductive action on suppressor cells [224, 223, 11, 29]. We even noted the activation of macrophages by a cyto- and virostatic agent (methoxyellipticine), applied at certain doses [73].

The combinations of exogenous immunomodifiers are promising. We combined agents, as similar in their action as bestatin and tuftsin (Fig. 49), or different, as bestatin and phospholipase A2 (Fig. 50), and registered a significant potentiation [177].

We combined bestatin and zinc gluconate in an experiment where the effect of their adjuvant or neo-adjuvant, or double modality, applied in complement of surgical intervention for the treatment of a murine mammary tumor: only the latter modality of immunotherapy gave a significant result (Table 9) [28].

Table 9. Percentages of cured animals carrying the murine mammary (MA 16-C) tumors after chemotherapy, hormonotherapy, immunotherapy or surgery alone

		Surgery with treatment		
	Treatment alone	Early	Late	Early +late
I-OHP	30	50	33	28
D-Trp6-LH-RH	0	33	40	37
Zn gluconate + bestatin	0	0	6	21
Surgery	0			

Surgery with or without chemotherapy or immunotherapy or immunotherapy on mammary carcinoma (MA 16-C). Results are expressed as percentage of lifespan.
I-OHP; oxalatoplatinum

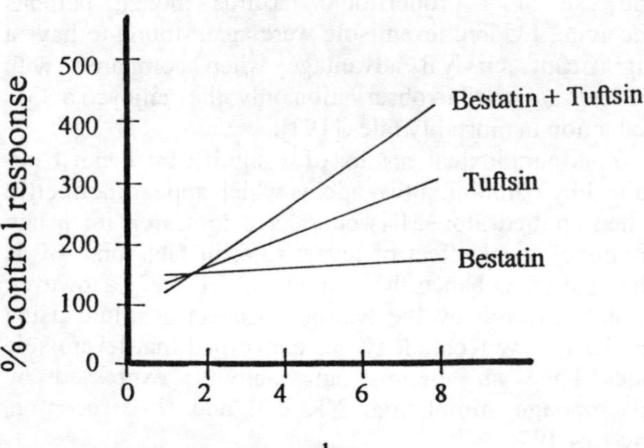

Figure 49. Peritoneal cell chemoluminescence after bestatin (100 μg), tuftsin (25 μg) or their combination.

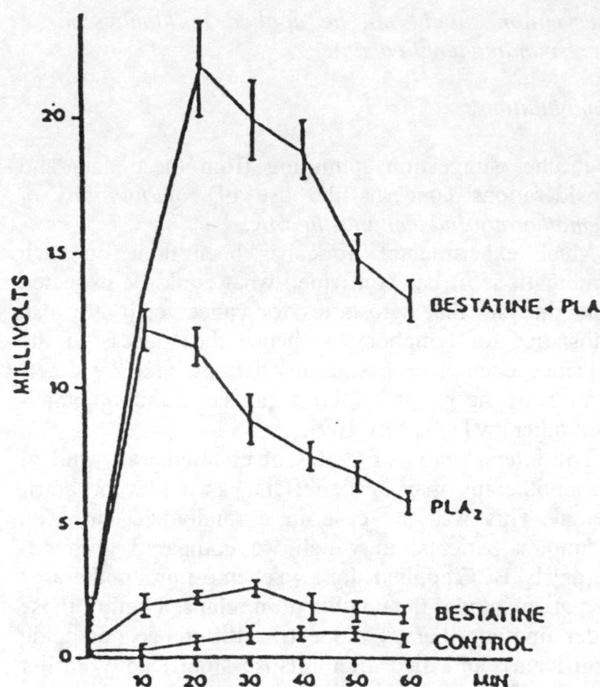

Figure 50. Effects of phospholipase A2 (PLA2) injection on the chemoluminescence response of peritoneal cells from immunostimulated mice. Groups of 10 mice were given, on day-4, bestatin (5 μg/mouse i.p.), with or without i.p. injection of 0.7 units PLA2 per mouse 30 min before cell harvest. Each peritoneal cell suspension was tested individually. The results are expressed as mV/min ± SD.

Besa described improvement of the transformed phase of myelodysplasia, with 13-cis-retinoic acid, alpha-tocopherol and alpha interferon [16]. Hemmi [94] observed the potentiation of all-trans-retinoic acid and of interferon in the differentiation of promyelocytic leukemia cells.

The combination of exogenous immunomodulators with active specific immunotherapy agents has always been successful as we observed it in our first active immunotherapy experiments [144, 216], though the antigenic heterogeneity of tumor cell may be a stumbling block [220]. Reizenstein [237] has observed that the difference in benefit, in the case of acute myeloid leukemia, is in relation with the rapidity of the remission induction.

An example of both non specific and specific active immunotherapy was achieved by the use of neuraminidase which activates macrophage functions and increases immunogenicity [14].

The use of combinations of exogenous immunomodulators and cytokines is very tempting. The latest result of interleukin-2, evaluated in 638 patients, was of 11% 'response'. The significance of this term is not objective and it does not mean a noticeable result, as the medium length was of 4 months [292].

A second evaluation is underway by the FDA which may require another selection of the indications for trials

[292, 48]. Let's not forget that a low level IL2 correlates with a good prognosis in patients with Hodgkin's disease [74], and the role of different interleukins in the genesis of pathologic manifestations is diverse [189, 12].

Even for interferon alpha, some dare ask 'how much of the promise has been accomplished' [283].

Of course, wrong doses and modalities of applications of some cytokines, especially IL2, may have been responsible non only for their possibly high toxicity [90, 58, 214], but also for their inaction.

There may be more to expect from anti-cytokines [54] than from cytokines.

We personally ask ourselves if the time has not come to return (even only temporarily), to exogenous immunomodulators, and conduct correct trials as far as methodology and result interpretation are concerned [134].

We noted the capacity of bestatin and of tuftsin to prevent the occurrence of spontaneous tumors by preventing aging immuno-depression [32]. An epidemiologic study of immunity condition in man after 40 years of age, on one hand, of patients in whom tumors are discovered, on the other hand, would be rewarding. Cases of immunodepression were described [76] in subjects carrying other tumors than the classical neoplasias associated with immunodepression, such as chronic lymphocytic leukemias and Hodgkin's diseases [143].

If the role of immuno-deficiency in oncogenesis has long been debated [137], the high incidence of tumors in subjects immunodepressed for transplantations [229] and in HIV seropositives [17] is evidence of the relationship.

We discussed the role of tumor cells parameters, such as HLA and cytological types, in the effectiveness to active immunotherapy. Herberman [235] confirmed what we have stressed, that its beneficial effect is stronger in immunodepressed patients than in normal ones.

Patients treated for a tumor, especially by radiotherapy [20, 21] and by chemotherapy [137] prescribed as adjuvants, are immunodepressed.

The patients submitted for the same indication to active immuno-therapy, may be immunorestored or immunostimulated for a limited time. Longer application according to the experimental model of immuno-restoration applied in mice between the 16th to the 28th months, should be tempted in man, of course under the control of any risk, especially of auto-immune disease induction [89].

Last question: is it necessary to kill the last cell?

If there is no doubt about the fact that active immunotherapy cures leukemic mice and patients only if they carry a few cells (Figure 51 illustrates the parameters of the tumor volume) [212], it is less certain that, to be cured, the patient's 'last' cell must be killed.

We have observed, several results with long remissions and the plateau form of the relapse free survival curve, in patients the blood of which contained sometimes and transitorily, a few CALLA antigen carrying cells (Fig. 52) [239].

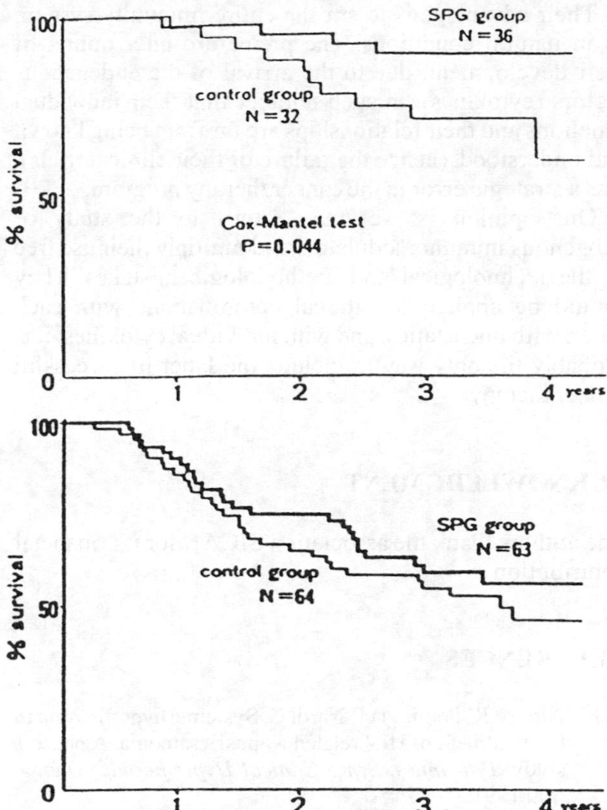

Figure 51. Survival rates in cervical cancer. Top: stage II. Bottom: stage III.

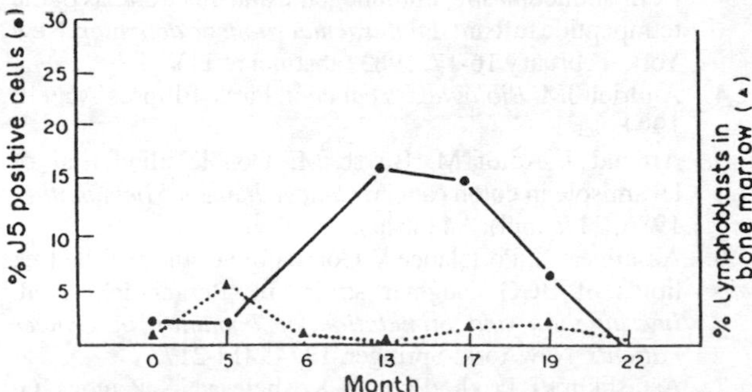

Figure 52. Percentage of CALLA-positive (•) cells and of lymphoblasts (Δ) in the bone marrow of a girl in complete remission 5 years after the treatment of acute lymphatic leukemia. Despite abstention from treatment, there was spontaneous regression and no relapse.

Our final conclusion is that the emergence of cancer immunotherapy and immunorestoration for prevention have been delayed because the first, logical, hence best materials available for them, exogenous immunomodifiers, have not been the object of a correct and sufficient study of their pharmacologic development.

Their advantage is to stir the entire immunity system, as in natural conditions. The premature interruption of their development, due to the arrival of the endogenous factors (cytokines), in such number that their individual functions and their relationships are far from being known and understood, (hence the failure of their clinical trials), was a strategic error in the cancer therapy program.

Our opinion is we must return to the study of exogenous immunomodulators and multiply their use free of the technological and methodologic mistakes. They should be applied in rational combinations with each other, with oncostatics, and with individual cytokines: it is probably the only way to include the latter in successful cancer therapy.

ACKNOWLEDGMENT

The authors thank the association SICAN for its financial contribution.

REFERENCES

1. Alonso K, Pontiggia P, Nardi C. Systemic hyperthermia in the treatment of HIV-related Kaposi's sarcoma. A phase 1 study. *19th Intern Symp Clinical Hyperthermia*, Dubna, Mai 1991.
2. Amoscato AA, Balasubramaniam A, Alexander JW, Babcok GF. Degradation of thymopentin by human lymphocytes: evidence for aminopeptidase activity. *Biochim Biophys Acta* 1988; 955: 164-174.
3. Amoscato AA, Davies PJA, Babcock GF, Nishioka K. Receptor-mediated internalization of tuftsin. In Anon: Conf antineoplastic, immunogenic and other effects of the tetrapeptide tuftsin: *A natural macrophage activator*. New York: February 16-17, 1983 (abstract n° 11).
4. Andrieu JM. *Biologie des cancers*. Paris: Ellipses/Aupelf, 1994.
5. Arnaud J, Adlof M, Buyse M. Double blind trial of levamisole in colon cancer. *Cancer Immunol Immunother* 1986; 23 (suppl): A4 (abstr).
6. Asselinean J, Portelance V. Comparative study of the free lipids of BCG daughter strain. In: Rentchnick P, ed. *Investigation and Stimulation of Immunity in Cancer Patients.* New York: Springer, 1974: 214-217.
7. Astashkin EI, Prikhod'ko AZ, Kosheleva NA, Pautova IG, Nikolaeva IS. Effects of dibasol and levamisole on the microsomal enzyme system. *Farmakologiia I Toksikologiia* 1987; 50: 75-76.
8. Baker D, Sager H, Constable W. The influence of levamisole and hyperthermia on the incidence of metastases from an x-irradiated tumor. *Cancer Invest* 1986; 4: 287-292.
9. Baltimore D. Tumor viruses 1974. *Cold Spring Harbor Symp* 1975; 39: 1187-1200.
10. Bar-Shavit Z, Teitelbaum SL, Reitsma P, Hall A, Pegg LE, Trial J, Kahn, AJ. Induction of monocytic differentiation and bone resorption by 1, 25-dihydroxy vitamin D_3. *Proc Natl Acad Sci* USA 1983; 80: 5907-5911.
11. Bartik MM, Ahn MC, Baumgartel BA, Hendricks RL, Mokyr MB. Presence of an enlarged pool of MOPC-315-specific cytotoxic T lymphocyte precursors in the thymuses of mice that eradicated a large MOPC-315 tumor as a consequence of low-dose melphalan therapy. *Cancer Immunol Immunother* 1990; 32: 43-53.
12. Bataille R, Chappard D, Klein B. The critical role of interleukin-6, interleukin-1B and macrophage colony-stimulating factor in the pathogenesis of bone lesions in multiple myeloma. Int J Clin Lab Res 1992; 21: 283-287.
13. Beers RF, Braun W. *Biological Effects of Polynucleotides.* Heidelberg: Springer, 1971.
14. Bekesi JG, St Artneault G, Holland JF. Increase of leukemia L1210 immunogenicity by *Vibrio cholerae* neuraminidase treatment. *Cancer Res* 1971; 31: 2130-2132.
15. Bennett JM, Catovsky D, Daniel MT, Flandrin G, Galton DA, Gralnick HR, Sultan C. Proposals for the classification of acute leukaemias. *Br J Haematol* 1976; 33: 451-458.
16. Besa EC, Abraham JL, Novell PC. Combination of 13-cis-retinoic acid and alpha-tocopherol for the chronic phase of myelodysplasia. *Third Int Conf Prev Human Cancer* 1988; S4: 13.
17. Biggar RJ, Horm J, Lubin JH, Goedert JJ, Greene MH, Fraumeni Jf, Jr. Cancer trends in a population at risk of acquired immuno-deficiency syndrome. *J Natl Cancer* Inst 1985; 74: 793-797.
18. Blazsek I, Mathé G. Zinc and immunity. *Biomed Pharmacother* 1984; 38: 187-193.
19. Blazsek I, Misset JL, Benavides M, Comisso M, Ribaud P, Mathé G. Hematon, a multicellular functional unit in normal human bone marrow: structural organization, hemopoietic activity and its relationship to myelodysplasia and myeloid leukemias. *Exp Hematol* 1990; 18: 259-265.
20. Blomgren H, Edsmyr F, Esposti PL, Naeslund I. Immunological and hematological monitoring in bladder cancer patients receiving adjuvant bestatin treatment following radiation therapy. A prospective randomized trial. *Biomed Pharmacother* 1984; 38: 143-149.
21. Blomgren H, Edsmyr F, von Stedingk LV, Wasserman J. Bestatin treatment enhances the recovery of radiation induced impairments of the immunological reactivity of the blood lymphocyte population in bladder cancer patients. *Biomed Pharmacother* 1986; 40: 50.
22. Blumenstein M, Layne PP, Najjar VA, Nuclear magnetic resonance studies on the structure of the tetrapeptide tufstin, L-threonyl-L-lysyl-L-propyl-L-arginine, and its pentapeptide analogue, L-threonyl-L-lysyl-L-propyl-L-propyl-L-arginine. *Biochemistry* 1979; 18: 5247-5253.
23. Bonadonna G, Brusamolino E, Valagussa P. Combination chemotherapy as an adjuvant treatment of operable breast cancer. *N Engl J Med* 1976; 294: 405-410.
24. Bonadonna G, Rossi A, Valagussa P. Adjuvant CMF chemotherapy in operable breast cancer: ten years later. *Lancet* 1985; i: 976-977.
25. Bonadonna G, Valagussa P, Moliterni A, Zambetti M, Brambilla C. Adjuvant cyclophosphamide, methotrexate and fluorouracil in node-positive breast cancer. The result at 20 years follow up. *N Engl J Med* 1995; 332: 901-906.
26. Bortin MM, Rimm AA, Saltzstein EC. Cell-mediated immunity in AKR mice treated with lentinan, a fungal polysaccharide. In: Rentchnick P, ed. *Investigation and Stimulation of Immunity in Cancer Patients*. New York: Springer, 1974: 320.
27. Bortin MM, Rimm AA, Salzstein EC. Graft versus leuke-

mia quantitation of adoptive immunotherapy in murine leukemia. *Science* 1973; 179: 811-813.

28. Bourut C, Chenu E, Mathé G. Can neo-adjuvant chemotherapy prevent residual tumors. *J Med Oncol Tumors Pharmacother* 1988; 259-63.
29. Bravo-Cuellar A, Balercia G, Levesque JP, Liu XH, Osculati F. Orbach-Arbouys S. Enhanced activity of peritoneal cells after aclacinomycin injection: effect of pretreatment with superoxide dismutase on aclacinomycin-induced cytological alterations and antitumoral activity. *Cancer Res* 1989; 49: 1578-1586.
30. Bravo-Cuellar A, Homo-Delarche F, Ramos-Zepeda R, Dubouch P, Cabannes J, Orbach-Arbouys S. Increased phagocytic activity of peripheral blood monocytes after intravenous injection of phospholipase A2 to monkeys. *Immunol Letters* 1991; 28: 5-9.
31. Bruley-Rosset M, Florentin I, Kiger N, Schulz J, Davigny M, Mathé G. Age related changes of the immune response and immuno-restoration by stimulating agents. In: Doria G, Eshkol A, eds. *The Immune System: Functions and therapy dysfunction?* New York: Academic Press, 1980: 171-187.
32. Bruley-Rosset M, Florentin I, Kiger N, Schulz J, Mathé G. Restoration of impaired immune functions of aged animals by chronic bestatin treatment. *Immunology* 1979; 38: 75-83.
33. Bruley-Rosset M, Florentin I, Kiger N, Schulz JI, Mathé G. Correction of immunodeficiency in aged mice by levamisole and bestatin administration. *Rec Res Cancer Res* 1980; 75: 139-146.
34. Bruley-Rosset M, Florentin I, Mathé G. Effects of BCG and levamisole on immune response in young adult and aged-immunosuppressed mice. *Cancer Treat Rep* 1978; 62: 1641-1644.
35. Bruley-Rosset M, Hercend T. Immunorestorative capacity of tuftsin after long-term administration to aging mice. *Ann NY Acad Sci* 1983; 419: 242-247.
36. Bruley-Rosset M, Hercend T, Martincz J, Rappaport H, Mathé G. Prevention of spontaneous tumors of aged mice by immuno-pharmacologic manipulation: Study of immune antitumor mechanism. *J Natl Cancer Institute* 1981; 66: 1113-1119.
37. Bruley-Rosset M, Rappaport H. Natural killer cell activity and spontaneous development of lymphoma. Effect of single and multiple injections of interferon into young and aged C57Bl/6 mice. *Int J Cancer* 1983; 31: 381-389.
38. Buschmans E. Personal communication.
39. Cassel WA, Murras DR, Torbin AH, Olkowski ZL, Moore ME. Viral oncolysate in the management of malignant melanoma. I. Preparation of the oncolysate and measurement of immunologic responses. *Cancer* 1977; 40: 672-679.
40. Catane R, Treves AJ, Weiss L. Clinical phase I study of tuftsin. *Proc Am Soc Clin Oncol* 1983; 2: 45 (abstract C-175).
41. Clarysse A, Kenis Y, Mathé G. *Cancer chemotherapy. Its Role in the Treatment Strategy of Hematologic Malignancies and Solid Tumors*. Heidelberg: Springer Verlag, 1976.
42. Cochrane CG, Studies on the localization of circulating antigen-antibody complexes and other macromolecules in vessels. I. Structural studies, *J Exp Red* 1963, 118-489-502
43. Cohen MM, Diamond JM. Medical research. Are we loosing the war on cancer ? *Nature* 1986; 323: 488-489.
44. Constantopoulos A. Congenital tuftsin deficiency. *Ann NY Acad Sci* 1983; 419: 214-219.
45. Constantopoulos A, Najjar VA, Smith JW. Tuftsin deficiency: A new syndrome with defective phagocytosis. *J Pediatr* 1972; 80: 564-572.
46. Cooperberg AA, Singer OP. Reversible myelofibrosis due to vitamine D deficiency rickets. *Can Med Assoc J* 1980; 94: 392.
47. Coquerel A, Dubuc I, Kitabgi P, Costenti J. Potentiation by thiorphan and bestatin of the naloxone-intensive analgesic effects of neurotensin and neuromedin *N. Neurochem Int* 1988; 12: 361.
48. Culliton BJ. FDA panel backs interleukin 2 (news). *Nature* 1992; 355: 287.
49. Deeg HJ, Erickson K, Storb R, Sullivan KM. Photoinactivation of lymphohemopoietic cells: studies in transfusion medicine and bone marrow tranplantation. *Blood Cells* 1992; 18: 151-162.
50. Degos L, Castaigne S, Chomienne C, . Therapeutic trials of acute myeloid leukemia by retinoid acid. In: Waxman S, Ross GB, Takaka F, eds. *Serono Symposia:* Raven Press, 1988: 45.
51. Dennert G. Immunostimulation by retinoic acid. *Ciba Foundation Symposium* 1985; 113: 117-131.
52. Dillehay DL, Cornay WJ, Walia AS, Lamon EW. Effects of retinoids on human thymus-dependent and thymus-independent mitogenesis. *Clinical Immunol Immunopathol* 1989; 50: 100-108.
53. Dillman RO. Antibody therapy. In: Oldham RK, ed. *Principles of Cancer Biotherapy.* New York: Dekker, 1991: 395-432.
54. Dinarello CA. Anti-cytokine strategies. *Eur Cytokine Netw* 1992; 3: 7-17.
55. Doré JF, Diatloff C, Mathé G. Suppression of immunocompetent cells reactivity by incubation at 37ºC. In White cell Transfusions. Paris: *Centre National de la Recherche Scientifique*, 1970: 10.
56. Ebihara T, Koyama S, Fukao K, Osuga T. Lymphokine-activated suppressor (LAS) cells in patients with gastric carcinoma. *Cancer Immunol Immunother* 1989; 28: 218-224.
57. Ershler W, Hacker M. Cimetidine and the immune response. *Clin Immunol Immunopathol* 1982; 26: 10-17.
58. Favalli L, Lanza E, Rozza A, Galimberti M, Villani F. Evaluation of the cardiovascular toxic effect of recombinant interleukin-2 in rats. *Anticancer Res* 1990; 10: 1693-1698.
59. Ferrari L, Jouzeau JY, Gillet P, Herber R, Fener P, Batt AM, Netter P. Interleukin-1 beta differentially represses drug-metabolizing enzymes in arthritic female rats. *J Pharmacol Exper therapeutic* 1993; 264: 1012-1020.
60. Fidalgo BV, Najjar VA. The physiological role of the lymphoid system. III. Leucophilic gamma-globulin and the phagocytic activity of the polymorphonuclear leucocyte. *Proc Natl Acad Sci* USA 1967; 57: 957-964.
61. Fidalgo BV, Najjar VA. The physiological role of the lymphoid system. VI. The stimulatory effect of leucophilic gamma-globulin (leucokinin) on the phagocytic activity of human polymorphonuclear leucocyte. *Biochemistry* 1967; 6: 3385-3392.
62. Fishbein GE. Immunotherapy of lung cancer. *Semin Oncol* 1993; 20: 351-358.
63. Florentin I, Bruley-Rosset M, Davigny M, Mathé G.

Comparison of the effects of BCG and a preparation of heat-killed *Pseudomonas aeruginosa* on the immune response in mice. In: Werner GH, Floch F, eds. *The Pharmacology of Immunoregulation.* New York: Academic Press; 1978: 335.

64. Florentin I, Bruley-Rosset M, Kiger N, Imbach JL, Winternitz F, Mathé G. *In vivo* immunostimulation by tuftsin. *Cancer Immunol Immunother* 1978; 5: 211.
65. Florentin I, Chung V, Davigny M, Mathé G. Immunomodulatory effects of bestatin in immunocompetent mice. In: Mathé G, Umezawa H, eds. Progress in Cancer Chemo-immunotherapy. Tokyo: *Japan Antibiotics Research Association*, 1984: 212.
66. Florentin I, Chung V, Martinez J, Marla J, Le Garrec Y, Mathé G. In vivo immunopharmacological properties of tuftsin (Thr-Lys-Prol-Arg) and some analogues. *Meth Find Exptl Clinic Pharmacol* 1986; 8: 73-80.
67. Florentin I, Kiger N, Bruley-Rosset M, Schulz J, Mathé G. *Effect of seven immunomodulators on different types of immune responses in mice.* In Human Lymphocyte Differentiation. Amsterdam – North Holland: *Biomedical Press*, 1978: 299.
68. Freake HC, Marcocci C, Iwasaki J. 1, 25-dihydroxyvitamin D3 specifically binds to a human breast cancer cell line (T 47D) and stimulates growth. *Biochem Biophys Res Comm* 1981; 101: 1131-1138.
69. Fujisaki T, Otsuka T, Takamatsu Y, Eto T, Harada M, Niho Y. Effects of bestatin hematopoiesis in long-term human bone marrow cultures. *Biomed Pharmacother* 1995; 49: 69-74
70. Gabrilovac J, Martin-Kleiner I, Ikic-Sutlic M, Osmak M. Interaction of leu-enkephalin and alpha interferon in modulation of NK activity of human peripheral blood lymphocytes. *Ann NY Acad Sc* 1992; 650: 140-145.
71. Galazka AR, Weiner J, Barth NM, Oldham RK. Lymphokines and cytokines. In: Oldham RK, ed. *Principles of Cancer Biotherapy.* New York: Dekker, 1991: 327-361.
72. Gallagher JC, Jerpback CM, Jee WS, Johnson KA, Deluca HF, Riggs BL. 1, 25-dihydroxy-vitamin D^3: short- and long-term effects on bone and calcium metabolism in patients with post menopausal osteoporosis. *Proc Natl Acad Sci* USA 1982; 79: 3325-3329.
73. Garcia-Giralt E, Maciera-Coelho A. Methoxy-9-ellipticine. II. Analysis *in vitro* of the mechanism of action. *Rev Europ Etud Clin Biol* 1970; 15: 539-541.
74. Gause A, Roschansky V, Tschiersch A, Smith K, Hasenclever D, Schmits R, Diehl V, Pfreundschuh M. Low serum interleukin-2 receptor levels correlated with a good prognosis in patients with Hodgkin's lymphoma. *Ann Oncology* 1991; 2 suppl 2: 43-47.
75. Geffard M, Orbach-Arbouys S. Enhancement of T-suppressor activity in mice by high doses of BCG. *Cancer Immunol Immunother* 1976; 1: 41-44.
76. Gerosa MA, Olivi A, Rosenblum ML, Semenzato GP, Pezzutto A. Impaired immunocompetence in patients with malignant gliomas: the possible role of Tg-lymphocyte subpopulations. *Neurosurgery* 1982; 10: 571-573.
77. Gidlund M, Orn A, Wigzell H, Senik A, Gresser I. Enhanced NK cell activity in mice injected with interferon and interferon inducers. *Nature* 1978; 273: 759-761.
78. Glover J. The conversion of beta-carotene into vitamin A. *Vitam Horm* 1960; 18: 371.
79. Goey H, Keller JR, Jansen R. Antiproliferative effects of transforming growth factor beta-1 for murine tumors and hematopoietic progenitor cells. *Proc. Ann Meet Am Assoc Cancer Res* 1989; 30: A1295 (abst).
80. Gorvel JP, Vivier I, Naquet P, Brekelmans P, Rigal A, Pierres M. Characterization of the neutral aminopeptidase activity associated to the mouse thymocyte-activating molecule. *J Immunol* 1990; 144: 2899-2907.
81. Gottlieb P, Stabinsky Y, Hazyum E. Tuftsin Receptors. In Anon: *Conf antineoplastic, imunogenic and other effects of the tetrapeptide tuftsin: A natural macrophage activator.* New York, Februrary 16-17, 1983 (abstract n° 9).
82. Gottlieb P, Stabinsky Y, Zakuth V, Spirer Z, Fridkin M. Synthetic pathways to tuftsin and radioimmunoassay. In Anon: *Conf antineoplastic, immunogenic and other effects of the tetrapeptide tuftsin: A natural macrophage activator*. New York, Februrary 16-17, 1983 (abstract n° 2).
83. Gouveia J, Mathé G, Hercend T, Gros F, Lemaigre G, Santelli G, Homasson JP, Gaillard JP, Angebault M, Bonniot JP, Lededente A, Marsac J, Parot R, Pretet S. Degree of bronchial metaplasia in heavy smokers and its regression after treatment with a retinoids. *Lancet* 1982; i: I 710-712.
84. Greeley EH, Helfrich BA, Feuerman LL, Cain CCA, Segre M. Radiant heat-induced hyperthermia in mice: in vivo effects on the immune system. *Int J Hyperthrmia* 1992; 8: 209-220.
85. Haaksenstad AO, Mannik M. The biology of immune complexes. In: Talal N, ed. *Autoimmunity*. New York; Academic Press, 1977.
86. Hadden MJW, Hadden EM. Therapy of secondary T-cell immunodeficiencies with biological substances and drugs. *Med Oncol Tumor Pharmacother* 1989; 6: 11-17.
87. Halle-Pannenko O, Abuaf N, Mathé G. Use of soluble histocompatibility antigen(s) in the control of transplantation reaction: possible dissociation of the roles of H-2 and non H-2 antigens in the prevention of mortality induced by graft-versus-host reactions. *Transpl Proc* 1976; 8: 161-172.
88. Halle-Pannenko O, Martyré M-C, Mathé G. Prevention of graft-versus-host reaction by donor pretreatment with soluble H-2 antigens. *Transplantation* 1971; 2: 414-417.
89. Hang LM, Aguado MT, Dixon FJ, Theofilopoulos AN. Induction of severe autoimmune disease in normal mice by simultaneous action of multiple immunostimulators. *J Exp Med* 1985; 161: 423-428.
90. Harms BA, Rosenfeld DJ, Conhaim RL, Pahl AC, Subramanian R, Storm FK. Pulmonary and systemic fluid filtration after continuous versus bolus interleukin-2 infusion. *Surgery* 1991; 110: 500-507.
91. Haussler MR, Baylink DJ, Hughes MR, Brumbaugh PF, Wergedal JE, Shen FH, Nielsen RL, Counts SJ, Bursac KM, Mc Cain TA. The assay of 1-alpha, 25-dihydroxy vitamin D3: Physiologic and pathologic modulation of circulating hormone levels. *Clin Endocrinol* 1979; 5(supp): 151S-165S.
92. Hawkins MM. Long term survival and cure after childhood cancer. *Arch Dis Child* 1989; 64: 798-807.
93. Hayes TJ. Progress and challenges in the preclinical assessment of cytokines. *Toxicol Letters* 1992; 64-65. spec. n° 291-7.
94. Hemmi H, Breitman TR. Combinations of recombinant human interferons and retinoic acid synergistically induce

differentiation of the human promyelocytic leukemia cell line HL-60. *Blood* 1987; 69: 501-507.

95. Herman ZS, Stachura Z, Opielka L, Siemion IZ, Nawrocka E. Tuftsin and D-Arg^3-tuftsin possess analgesic action. *Experientia* 1981; 37: 76-77.
96. Hoerni B, Durand M, Eghbali H, Hoerni-Simon G, Lagarde C. Adjuvant BCG-therapy of non Hodgkin's malignant lymphomas. In: Salmon SE, Jones SE, eds. *Adjuvant Therapy of Cancer III.* New York: Grune & Stratton, 1981: 99.
97. Holcombe RF, Stewart RM, Betzing KW, Kannan K. Alteration in lymphocyte phenotype associated with administration of adjuvant levamisole and 5-fluorouracil. *Cancer Immunol Immunother* 1994; 38: 394-398.
98. Hoover RN. Bacillus Calmette Guérin vaccination and cancer prevention: A critical review of the human experience. *Cancer Res* 1976; 36: 652-654.
99. Huang ME, Ye YC, Chen SR, Zhao JC, Gu LJ, Cai JR, Zhao L, Xie JX, Shen ZX, Wang ZY. All-trans-retinoic acid with or without low dose cytosine arabinoside in acute promyelocytic leukemia. Report of 6 cases. *Chin Med J* 1987; 100: 949-953.
100. Huchet R, Florentin I, Mathé G. Mechanism of action of BCG as an immunity adjuvant used in cancer active immunotherapy. *Proc Amer Assoc Cancer Res* 1976; 17: 160 (abst).
101. Hughes RC, Sanford BH, Jeanloz RW. Regeneration of the surface glycoproteins of a transplantable mouse tumor cell after treatment with neuraminidase. *Proc Natl Acad Sci USA* 1972; 69: 942-945.
102. Hui IJ. MAAF, a fully water-soluble lipid-free fraction from BCG with adjuvant and antitumor activity. In: Rentchnick P, ed. *Investigation and Stimulation of Immunity in Cancer Patients.* New York: Springer, 1974: 213.
103. Hunter T, Cooper JA. Protein tyrosine kinases. *Ann Rev Biochem* 1985; 54: 897-930.
104. Inada K, Nemeto N, Nishijirna A, Wada S, Hirata M, Yoshida M. A case suspected of tuftsin deficiency. In: Yoshida MA. *Phagocytosis: Its physiology and pathology.* Baltimore: University Park Press, 1979: 158.
105. Inge TH, Hoover SK, Susskind BM, Barrett SK, Bear HD. Inhibition of tumor-specific cytotoxic T-lymphocytic response by transforming growth factor beta. *Cancer Res* 1992; 52: 1386-1392.
106. Ishizuka M, Masuda T, Kanbayashi N, Fukasawa S, Takeuchi T, Aoyagi T, Umezawa H. Effect of bestatin on mouse immune system and experimental murine tumors. *J Antibiot* 1980; 33: 642-652.
107. Jin Z, Kumar A, Cleveland RP, Murray DL, Kaufman DB. Inhibition of suppressor cell function by cimetidine in an murine model. *Clin Immunol Immunopathol* 1986; 38: 350-356.
108. Joseph RR, Belpomme D, Mathé G. Increase in 'null' cells in acute lymphocytic leukaemia in remission on long-term immunotherapy. *Br J Cancer* 1976; 33: 567-570.
109. Kable T, Beer M, Mendoza E, Ikinger U, Link M, Reichert HE, Frangenheim T, Klein E, Fabricius PG. BCG vs interferon alpha for prevention of recurrence of superficial bladder cancer. A prospective randomized study. *Urol Ausg A* 1994; 33: 133.
110. Kaufman M, Marquerson J, Stanley K, Mouritzen C, Hansen H. Distribution of *C parvum* in man. *Cancer Immunol Immunother* 1986; 22: 56-61.
111. Kendrick M, Comstock G. BCG vaccination and cancer in humans. *J Natl Cancer Inst* 1981; 66: 431-437.
112. Kenny AJ, Stephenson SL, Turner AJ. Cell surface peptidase. In: Kenny AJ, Turner AJ, eds. *Mammalian Ectoenzymes*. Amsterdam: Elsevier Science Publishers, 1986: 169.
113. Khatsenko OG, Gross SS, Rifking AB, Vane JR. Nitric oxide is a mediator of the decrease in cytochrome P-450-dependent metabolism caused by immunostimulants. *Proc Natl Acad Sci* USA 1993; 90: 11147-11151.
114. Kimmel DW, Wijdicks EF, Rodriguez M. Multifocal inflammatory leukoencephalopathy associated with levamisole therapy. *Neurology* 1995; 45: 374-376.
115. Kohne-Wompner CH, Schoffski P, Schmoll HJ. Adjuvant therapy for colon adenocarcinoma: current status of clinical investigation. *Ann Oncol* 1994; 5 (suppl 3): 97-104.
116. Kolb J-PB, Senik A, Castagna M. In vitro stimulation of mouse NK cell activity by phorbol esters: a pathway different from interferon-induced activation. *Cellular Immunol* 1981; 65: 258-264.
117. Komada Y, Azuma E, Yamamoto H, Tanaka S, Shimizu K, Kamiya H, Sakurai M, Izawa T. Discontinuing chemo-immunotherapy in childhood acute lymphoblastic leukemia. *Biomed Pharmacother* 1988; 42: 597-603.
118. Konznetzova B, Bizzini B, Cherman JC. Immunostimulating activity of whole cells, cell walls and fractions of anaerobic corynebacteria. In: Rentchnick P, ed. *Investigation and Stimulation of Immunity in Cancer Patients*. New York: Springer, 1974: 275.
119. Kopinska D, Luczak M, Wleklik M, Gomulka S, Kazanowska B. Elongated tufstin analogues: Synthesis and biological investigations. *Ann NY Acad Sci* 1983; 419: 35-43.
120. Lacour J, Lacour F, Ducot B, Spira A, Michelson M, Petit J-Y, Sarrazin D, Contesso G. Polyadenylic-polyuridylic acid as adjuvant in the treatment of operable breast cancer: recent results. *Eur J Surg Oncol* 1988; 14: 311-316.
121. Lacour J, Lacour F, Flamand R. Essai thérapeutique sur le cancer mammaire spontané: chirurgie et ARN synthétique poly A: poly U). *Chir* 1970; 96: 364-368.
122. Lacour J, Lacour F, Spira A, Michelson M, Petit JY, Delage FG, Sarrazin D, Contesso G, Viguier J. Adjuvant treatment with polyadenylic-polyuridylic acid in operable breast cancer. *Lancet* 1980; ii: 161-164.
123. Lamm DL. Optimal BCG treatment of superficial bladder cancer as defined by American trials. *Eur Urol* 1992; 21 suppl.2: 12-16.
124. Lang J, Oberline F, Aleksijevic A, Falkendordt A, Mayer S. Immunomodulator with imuthiol in AIDS. *Cancer Immunol Immunother* 1986; 23 (suppl): A42 (abstr).
125. Laurie JA, Moertel CG, Fleming TR, Wieand HS, Leigh JE, Rubin J. Surgical adjuvant therapy of large-bowel carcinoma: an evaluation of levamisole and the combination of levamisole and fluorouracil. The North Central Cancer Treatment group and the Mayoclinic. *J Clin Oncol* 1989; 7: 1447-1156.
126. Lederer E. From natural products chemistry to immunopharmacology. In Chedid L, Hadden JW, Spreafico F, Dukor P, Willoughby D, eds. *Advances in Immunopharmacology 3.* Proceeding of the Third International Conference on Immuno-pharmacology. Florence, May 6-9, 1985. Pergamon Press, 1986: 3-12.
127. Lee A. Effect of neuraminidase on the phagocytosis of

heterologous red cells by mouse peripheral macrophages. *Proc Soc Exp Biol Med* 1968; 128: 891-894.
128. Lehtinen M. Levamisole in maintenance of acute myeloid leukemia. *Cancer Chemother Pharmacol* 1980, 5 (suppl): 28 (abstract 112).
129. Ley-Hausen G, Gramzow M, Zah RK, Steffen R, Umezawa H, Mueller WE. Immunochemical identification of the cell surface bound leucine aminopeptidase, the target enzyme for the immunostimulant bestatin. *J Antibiot* 1983; 36: 728-734.
130. Lichtenstein A, Berek J. Antitumor effects of pyridine extract from *Propionibacter acnes*. *Cancer Immunol Immunother* 1986; 22: 24-30.
131. Look AT, Ashmun RA, Shapiro LH, Peiper SC. Human myeloid plasma membrane glycoprotein CD13 (gp 150) is identical to aminopeptidase *N. J Clin Invest* 1989; 83: 1299-1307.
132. Lopez M. Adjuvant therapy of colorectal cancer. *Dis Colon Rectum* 1994; 37: S86-S91.
133. Martinez J, Winternitz F. New synthetic and natural tuftsin related compounds and evaluation of their phagocytosis-stimulating activity. *Ann NY Acad Sci* 1983; 419: 23-34.
134. Mathé G. Are recombinant interleukins more or less therapeutically effective than their exogenous inducers? *Biomed Pharmacother* 1994; 48: 413-415.
135. Mathé G. Bestatin, an aminopeptidase inhibitor with a multi-pharmacological function. *Biomed Pharmacother* 1991; 45: 49-54.
136. Mathé G. Beta-endorphin inducers and their catabolism inhibitors in opioid addiction withdrawal. *Biomed Pharmacother* 1993; 47: 299-300.
137. Mathé G. *Cancer Active Immunotherapy, Immunoprophylaxis and Immunorestoration.* New York: Springer, 1976.
138. Mathé G. Cancer 'cures' in children adolescent and young adults, versus general cancer cure failure after 50 years of age. *Biomed Pharmacother* 1988; 42: 227-236.
139. Mathé G. Cancer therapy: it was by persisting that Greeks took troy. *Biomed Pharmacother* 1989; 43: 231-234.
140. Mathé G. Do tuftsin and bestatin constitute a biopharmacological immunoregulatory system? *Cancer Detect Prevent* 1987; suppl 1: 445-455.
141. Mathé G. Don't multiple drug and other cross resistances in cancer therapy compromise (phase 2) efficacy trials? *Biomed Pharmacother* 1993; 47: 361-362.
142. Mathé G. Experience gained in immunotherapy from the immunopharmacology of BCG leading to a second generation of systemic immunity adjuvants. *Comp Immunol Microbiol Infect Disease* 1980; 3: 407-432.
143. Mathé G. Immunity, infection, malignancy and aging: possible immunity restoration and tumor prevention. *Biomed Pharmacother* 1989; 43: 541-543.
144. Mathé G. L'immunothérapie active de la leucémie L1210 appliquée après la greffe tumorale. *Rev Franç Etud Clin Biol* 1968; 13: 301.
145. Mathé G. Oncologists have lost a battle against cancer; biomedicine has not lost the war. *Biomed Pharmacother* 1986; 40: 370-371.
146. Mathé G. Relationship between bestatin dose and the state of the CD8 lymphocyte number of immunologic responses in man. *Biomed Pharmacother*, submitted.
147. Mathé G. SIDA, sceaux, sexe, science. Paris: *La Coutellerie*; 1995.
148. Mathé G. The antigen and exogenous or endogenous immuno-modulator dose and the sens of the reaction. *Biomed Pharmacother* in preparation.
149. Mathé G, Amiel JL. Adoptive immunotherapy of acute leukemia. Experimental and clinical results. *Cancer Res* 1965; 25: 1525.
150. Mathé G, Amiel JL, Schwarzenberg L. Treatment of total body irradiation injury in man. *Ann N Y Acad Sci* 1964; 114: 368-392.
151. Mathé G, Amiel JL, Bernard J. Traitement de souris AkR à l'âge de 6 mois par irradiation totale suivie de transfusion de cellules hématopoïétiques homologues. Incidences respectives de la leucémie et du syndrome secondaire. *Bull Cancer* 1960; 47: 331.
152. Mathé G, Amiel JL, Cattan A, Schneider M. Haematopoietic chimera in man after allogeneic (homologous) bone marrow transplantation. Control of the secondary syndrome. Specific tolerance due to the chimerism. *Br Med J* 1963; 2: 1633.
153. Mathé G, Amiel JL, Niemetz J. Greffe de moelle osseuse après irradiation totale chez des souris leucémiques, suivie de l'administration d'un cytostatique pour réduire la fréquence du syndrome secondaire et ajouter à l'effet antileucémique. *C R Acad Sci* (Paris) 1962; 255: 3602-3605.
154. Mathé G, Amiel JL, Schwarzenberg L, Cattan A, Schneider M, de Vries MJ, Tubiana M, Lalanne C, Binet JL, Papiernik M, Seman G, Matsukura M, Mery AM, Schwarzmann BV, Flaisler A. Successful allogeneic bone marrow transplantation in man. Chimerism, induced specific tolerance and possible antileukemic effects. *Blood* 1965; 25: 179-196.
155. Mathé G, Amiel JL, Schwarzenberg L, Mery AM. A method of reducing the incidence of the secondary syndrome in allogeneic marrow transplantation. *Blood* 1963; 22: 42-52.
156. Mathé G, Amiel JL, Schwarzenberg L, Schneider M, Cattan A, Schlumberger JR, Hayat M, de Vassal F. Active immunotherapy for acute lymphoblastic leukemia. *Lancet* 1969; i: 697-699.
157. Mathé G, Amiel JL, Schwarzenberg L, Schneider M, Hayat M, de Vassal F, Jasmin C, Rosenberg C, Sakouhi M, Choay J. Remission induction with poly IC in patients with acute lymphoblastic leukaemia (preliminary results). *Rev Europ Etudes Clin Biol* 1970; 15: 671-673.
158. Mathé G, Amiel JL, Schwarzenberg L. *Bone marrow transplantation and leukocyte transfusions*. Springfield: Thomas, 1971.
159. Mathé G, Bernard J. Essai de traitement de la leucémie greffée L1210 par l'irradiation X suivie de transfusion de cellules hématopoïétiques normales (isologues ou homologues, lymphoïdes ou myéloïdes, adultes ou embryonnaires). *Rev Franç Etud Clin Biol* 1959; 4: 442.
160. Mathé G, Bernard J. Essai de traitement par l'irradiation X suivie de l'administration de cellules médullaires homologues de souris AkR atteintes de leucémie spontanée très avancée. *Bull Cancer* 1958; 45: 289.
161. Mathé G, Bernard J, Schwarzenberg L, Larrieu MJ, Lalanne C, Dutreix A, Denoix P, Schwarzmann V, Ceoara B. Essai de traitement de sujets atteints de leucémie aigue par irradiation suivie de transfusion de moelle osseuse homologue. *Rev Franç Etud Clin Biol* 1959; 4: 675-704.
162. Mathé G, Bernard J, Schwarzenberg L, Larrieu MJ, Lalanne C, Dutreix A, Amiel JL, Surmont J. Nouveaux

essais de greffe de moelle osseuse homologue après irradiation totale chez des enfants atteints de leucémie aigue en rémission. Le problème du syndrome secondaire chez l'homme. *Rev Hemat* 1960; 15: 115-161.

163. Mathé G, Bernard J, Tran Ba Loc. Effet antileucémique de l'irradiation totale selon la dose d'irradiation et le nombre de cellules tumorales. *Rev Franç Etudes Clin Biol* 1960; 5: 930.

164. Mathé G, Cattan A. Cancérologie. Paris.˙ *Expansion Scientifique Française*. 1976.

165. Mathé G, de Vries MJ, Amiel JL, Cattan A. Les divers aspects du syndrome secondaire compliquant les transfusions de moelle osseuse ou de leucocytes allogéniques chez des sujets atteints d'hémopathies malignes. *Europ J Cancer* 1965; 1: 75.

166. Mathé G, Eriguchi M. Scientific criticisms of the comparison of exponential survival and disease-free survival curves. *Biomed Pharmacother* 1988; 42: 177-186.

167. Mathé G, Halle-Pannenko O, Bourut C. Active immunotherapy of AkR mice spontaneous leukemia. *Rev Eur Etudes Clin Biol Res* 1972; 17: 997-1000.

168. Mathé G, Halle-Pannenko O, Bourut C. BCG in cancer immunotherapy. II. Result obtained with various BCG preparations in a screening study for systemic adjuvants applicable to cancer immunoprophylaxis or immunotherapy. *Natl Cancer Int Monogr* 1973; 39: 107.

169. Mathé G, Halle-Pannenko O, Bourut C. Effectiveness of murine leukemia chemotherapy according to the immune state: Reconsideration of correlation bewteen chemotherapy, tumour cell killing and survival time. *Rec Res Cancer Res.* 1977; 62: 9-12.

170. Mathé G, Halle-Pannenko O, Bourut C. Immune manipulation by BCG administered before or after cyclophosphamide for chemo-immunotherapy of L1210 leukaemia. *Eur J Cancer* 1974; 10: 661-666.

171. Mathé G, Halle-Pannenko O, Bourut C. Interspersion of cyclophosphamide and BCG in the treatment of L1210 leukaemia and Lewis tumour. *Eur. J. Cancer*, 1977; 13: 1095-1098.

172. Mathé G, Hayat M, Sakouhi M, Choay J. L'action immuno-adjuvante du polyIC chez la Souris, et son application au traitement de la leucémie L1210. *C R Acad Sci* 1971; 272: 170-173.

173. Mathé G, Itzhaki M, Orbach-Arbouys S. Bestatin specifically enhances the number of $CD4^+$ T cells in peripheral blood in patients whose $CD8^+$ T cell numbers are also depressed. *Int J Immunotherapy* 1993; 9: 165.

174. Mathé G, Kamel MK, Dezfulian M, Halle-Pannenko O, Bourut C. An experimental screening for 'systemic adjuvant of immunity' applicable to cancer immunotherapy. *Cancer Res* 1973; 33: 1987-1997.

175. Mathé G, Misset JL, Gil-Delgado M, Musset M, Reizenstein P, Canon C. A phase II trial of immunorestoration with zinc gluconate in immunodepressed cancer patients. *Biomed Pharmacother* 1986; 40: 383-385.

176. Mathé G, Misset JL, Plagne R, Belpomme D, Guerrin J, Fumoleau P, Metz R, Delgado M. (OncoFrance Comparative trial project): Superiority of AVCF (adriamycin, vincristine, cyclophosphamide and 5-fluorouracil) as adjuvant chemotherapy for breast cancer. A phase III trial of Association OncoFrance In: Tosiru and Voshida, eds. *Basic Mechanism and Clinical Treatments of Tumor Metastasis*. New York: Academic Press, 1982.

177. Mathé G, Orbach S. Combination of exogenous immunomodulators. *Biomed Pharmacother* 1997 in press.

178. Mathé G, Pouillart P, Lapeyraque F. Active immunotherapy of mouse RC 19 and E female KI leukemias applied after the intravenous transplantation of the tumor cells. *Experientia* 1971; 27: 446-447.

179. Mathé G, Pontiggia P. Several years beneficial effect of bestatin on white cells and platelets numbers in human myelodysplasia. *Biomed Pharmacother* 1995 under press.

180. Mathé G, Pouillart P, Schwarzenberg L, Amiel JL. Attempts at immunotherapy of 100 acute lymphoid leukemia patients. Some factors influencing results. In: *Investigation and Stimulation of Immmunity in Cancer Patients.* Paris & Heidelberg: CNRS & Springer, 1974: 434.

181. Mathé G, Pouillart P, Schwarzenberg L, Schneider M. Transfusions of lymphocytes from non immunized or immunized donors in mice leukaemia therapy. In White cell Transfusions. Paris: *Centre National de la Recherche Scientifique,* 1970: 197-201.

182. Mathé G, Reizenstein P. Intensive cancer chemotherapy and immunotherapy? *Biomed Pharmacother* 1993; 47: 125-126.

183. Mathé G, Schwarzenberg L. The graft versus host reaction after white blood cell transfusions. In White cell Transfusions. Paris: *Centre National de la Recherche Scientifique*, 1970: 101-103.

184. Mathé G, Tran Ba Loc. Effet sur la leucémie L1210 d'une combinaison par diazotation d'A-ménothoptérine et de gamma-globulines de hamsters porteurs de cette leucémie par hétérogreffe. *C R Acad Sci* 1958; 246: 1626-1627.

185. Mathé G, Umezawa H, Misset JL, Brienza S, Canon C, Musset M, Reizenstein P. Immunomodulating properties of bestatin in cancer patients. A phase II trial. *Biomed Pharmacother* 1986; 40: 379-382.

186. Mathé G, Weiner R, Pouillart P. BCG in cancer immunotherapy. I. Experimental and clinical trials of its use in the treatment of leukemia minimum or/and residual disease. *Natl Cancer Int Monogr* 1973; 39: 165.

187. Matsuura MY, Watanabe MH, Fukuda T, Yoshida T, Kuroiwa Y. A sustained increase of microsomal heme oxygenase activity following treatment of rats with Bacillus Calmette-Guérin and Corynebacterium parvum: its possible relation to decrease of cytochrome P-450 content. *J Pharmacobio-Dynamics* 1985; 8: 669-678.

188. Mehta J, Powles RL, Treleaven J, Shields M, Agrawal S, Rege K, Mitchell P, Allard S. Cimetidine-induced myelosuppression after bone marrow transplantation. *Leuk Lymphoma* 1994; 13: 179-181.

189. Michie HR, FRCS(E), Eberlein TJ, Spriggs DR, Manogue KR, Cerami A, Wilmore DW. Interleukin-2 initiates metabolic responses associated with critical illness in humans. *Ann Surg* 1988; 208: 493-503.

190. Migliore-Samour D, Delaforge M, Jaouen M, Mansuy D, Jolles P. In vivo effects of immunostimulating lipopeptides on mouse liver microsomal cytochromes P-450 and on paracetamol-induced toxicity. *Experientia* 1989; 45: 882-886.

191. Moenner M, Barritault D. Les facteurs de croissance et leurs récepteurs. In: Andrieu JM, ed. Biologie des Cancers. Paris: *Ellipses*, 1994: 33-44.

192. Moertel CG, Fleming TR, McDonald JS, Haller DG, Laurie JA, Goodman PJ. Levamisole and fluorouracil for adjuvant therapy of resected colon carcinoma. *N Engl J Med* 1990; 322: 352-358.

193. Moertel CG, Fleming TR, Mcdonald JS, Haller DG, Laurie JA, Tangen CM, Ungerleider JS, Emerson WA, Tormey DC, Glick JH, Veeder MH, Mailliard JA. Fluorouracil plus levamisole as effective adjuvant therapy after resection of stage III colon carcinoma: A final report. *Ann Inter Med* 1995; 122: 321-326.
194. Moochhala SM. Alteration of drug biotransformation by interferon and host defense mechanism. *Annals Acad Med Singapore* 1991; 20: 13-18.
195. Moore MAS. Growth and maturation factors in leukemia. In: Oldham RK, ed. *Principles of Cancer Biotherapy*. New York: Dekker, 1991: 525-583.
196. Morales A, Eidinger D, Bruce AW. Intracavitary bacillus Calmette-Guerin in the treatment of superficial bladder tumors. *J Urol* 1976; 116(2): 180-3.
197. Najjar VA. The clinical and physiological aspects of tuftsin deficiency syndromes exhibiting defective phagocytosis. *Klin Wochensch* 1979; 57: 751-756.
198. Najjar VA, Constantopoulos A. A new phagocytosis-stimulating tetrapeptide hormone, tuftsin, and its role in disease. *J Reticuloendoth Soc* 1972; 12: 197-215.
199. Najjar VA, Konopinska D, Chaudhuri MK, Schmidt DE, Linehan L. Tuftsin, a natural activator of phagocytic functions including tumoricidal activity. *Mol Cell Biochem* 1981; 41: 3-12.
200. Najjar VA, Linehan L, Konopinska D. The antineoplastic effects of tuftsin and tuftsinyltuftsin on B 16/5B melanoma and L 1210 cells. *Ann NY Acad Sci* 1983; 419: 261-267.
201. Najjar VA, Nishioka K. Tuftsin: A physiological phagocytosis-stimulating peptide. *Nature* 1970; 228: 672-673.
202. Najjar VA, Nishioka K, Constantopoulos A, Sato PS. The function and interaction of erythrophilic g-globulin with autologous erythrocytes. In: Rapoport S, Jung M, eds. *VI Int Sym über Struktur und Funktion der Erythrozyten*. Berlin: Akademi-Verlak, 1972: 355-360.
203. Nakazato H, Koike A, Saji S, Ogawa N, Sakamoto J. Efficacy of immuno-chemotherapy as adjuvant treatment after curative resection of gastric cancer. Study group of immunotherapy with PSK for gactric cancer. *Lancet* 1994; 343: 1122-1126.
204. Neprina GS, Panteleeva ES, Vatin OE, Kariakin OB. The immunomodulating action of bestatin in the combined therapy of bladder cancer patients. *Urol Nefrol* (Mosk) 1994; 2: 34-38.
205. Nishioka K, Constantopoulos A, Sato PS, Mitchell WM, Najjar VA. Characteristics and isolation of the phagocytosis-stimulating peptide tuftsin. *Biochem Biophys Acta* 1973; 310: 217-229.
206. Nishioka K, Constantopoulos A, Sato P, Najjar VA. The characteristics, isolation and synthesis of the phagocytosis stimulating peptide tuftsin. *Biochem Biophys Res Commun* 1972; 47: 172-179.
207. Nishioka K, Sato PS, Constantopoulos A, Najjar VA. The chemical synthesis of the phagocytosis tetrapeptide tuftsin (Thr-Lys-Pro-Arg) and its biological properties. *Biochem Biophys Acta* 1973; 310: 230-237.
208. Norton L, Simon R. Tumor size, sensitivity to therapy, and design of treatment schedules. *Cancer Treat Rep* 1977; 61: 1307-1317.
209. Nose Y. After therapeutic plasmapheresis extra-corporeal cellular immunomodulation. *Artif Organs* 1991; 15: 69-73.
210. Ochiai T. Immunotherapy of gastric cancer. In: Mathé G, Reizenstein P, Dicato M, eds. Clinical Trials in Oncology: Ethics, Errors, Methods and Results. Geneva: *Bioscience* Ediprint, 1986: II 87-95.
211. Ohno R, Nakamura H, Kodera MY, Ezaki K, Yokomaku S, Oguma S, Kubota Y, Shibata H, Ogawa N, Masoaka T et al. Randomized controlled study of chemoimmunotherapy of acute myelogenous leukemia (AML) in adults with *Nocardia rubra* cell-wall skeleton and irradiated allogenic AML cells. *Cancer* 1986; 57: 1483-1488.
212. Okamura K, Yajima A. Cervical cancer: chemotherapy and immunotherapy. In: Mathé G, Reizenstein P, Dicato M, eds. Clinical Trials in Oncology: Ethics, Errors, Methods and Results. *Int J Immunother* 1986 II : 101-107.
213. Okamura S, Ompori F, Haga K, Baba H, Kawasaki C, Tanaka T, Suginachi K, Niho Y. Ubenimex stimulates production of colony-stimulating factor from human peripheral mononuclear cells *in vito*. In *Bestatin 16 ICC Proceedings*, Israel, Jerusalem, 1989: (abst)12.
214. Oleksowicz L, Paciucci PA, Zuckerman D, Colorito A, Rand JH, Holland JF. Alterations of platelet function induced by interleukin-2. *J Immmunotherapy* 1991; 10: 363-370.
215. Olkowski ZL, Jedrzejczak WW. Responses of immune system to hyperthermia. *Adv Exp Med Biol* 1990; 267: 507-509.
216. Olsson L, Ebbesen P, Kiger N, Florentin I, Mathé G. The antileukemic effect of systemic nonspecific BCG-immunostimulation versus systemic specific immunostimulation with irradiated isogeneic leukemic cells. *Eur J Cancer* 1978; 14: 355-362.
217. Olsson L, Florentin I, Kiger N, Mathé G. Cellular and humoral immunity to leukemia in BCG-induced growth control growth of a murine leukemia. *J Natl Cancer Inst* 1977; 59: 1297-1306.
218. Olsson L, Kiger N, Mathé G. Autoreactive cells in cancer-active immunotherapy: their cytotoxic potential and genetic restriction. *Transplantation Proceedings* 1980; 12: 167-171.
219. Olsson L, Kiger N, Mathé G. Graft-versus-host disease in recipients of syngeneic bone marrow. Lancet 1980; i: 253.
220. Olsson L, Mathé G. Antigenic heterogeneity of leukemic cells. *Blood Cells* 1981; 7: 281-286.
221. Olsson L, Mathé G. Emerging immunologic approaches to treatment of neoplastic diseases. *Recent Results in Cancer Research*. Vol 80. Berlin – Heidelberg: Springer-Verlag, 1982.
222. Olsson L, Mathé G. Immune reaction with cytotoxic activity to 'self' in natural surveillance of aberrant cells. *Biomed Pharmacother* 1979; 30: 281-282.
223. Orbach-Arbouys S, Andrade-Mena CE, Mathé G. Reversal of immunological tolerance by aclacinomycin through inhibition of suppressor cell activity. *Cell Immunol* 1983; 81: 84-90.
224. Orbach-Arbouys S, Castes M. Augmentation of immune responses after methotrexate administration. *Immunol* 1979; 36: 265-269.
225. Ota K. Efficiency of bestatin for acute nonlymphocytic leukemia. A cooperative bestatin chemoimmunotherapy group study. *Drugs Exp Clin Res* 1984; 10: 643-645.
226. Ota K, Ogawa N. Randomized controlled study of chemoimmunotherapy with bestatin of acute non lymphocytic leukemia in adults. *Biomed Pharmacother* 1990; 44: 93-101.

227. Otsuka T, Okamura S, Ohhara N, Harada M, Hayashi S, Yamaga S, Omori F, Niho Y. Stimulatory effects of bestatin on human B-cell colony formation. *Int J Immunopharmacol* 1988; 10: 587-591.
228. Pagano F, Bassi P, Milani C, Piazza N, Meneghini A, Garbeglio A. BCG in superficial bladder cancer: a review of phase III European trials. *Eur Urol* 1992; 21 suppl.2: 7-11.
229. Penn I, Halgrimson CG, Starzl TE. De novò malignant tumors in organ transplant recipient. *Transpl Proc* 1971; 3: 773-778.
230. Plagne R. Immunotherapy of melanoma. *Int J Immunother* 1986; II: 19-21.
231. Pontiggia P, Barni S, Mathé G, Bertone V, Pontiggia E. Lysosomal exocytosis induced by hyperthermia: a new model of cancer cell death. II. Effects on peritoneal macrophages. *Biomed Pharmacother* 1995; 49: under press.
232. Pontiggia P, Mathé G. A new mode of cancer cell death induced by hyperthermia and non specific (macrophagic) cancer immuno-therapy: lysosomal exocytosis. *Biomed Pharmacother* 1994; 48: 331.
233. Pouillart P, Palangié T, Schwarzenberg L, Mathé G. Effect of BCG on hamopoietic stem cells. *Biomedicine* (Express) 1976; 23: 469-471.
234. Ratliff TL. Role of the immune response in BCG for bladder cancer. *Eur Urol* 1992; 21 suppl.2: 17-21.
235. Reid JW, Cannon GB, Perlin E, Blom J, Connor R, Herberman RB. Immunologically defined prognostic subgroups as predictors of response to BCG immunotherapy. *Rec Res Cancer Res* 1982; 80: 219-226.
236. Reizenstein P, Andersson M, Beran M. Possible mechanisms of immunotherapy action in acute non lymphatic leukemia: macrophage production of colony-stimulating activity. *Rec Res Cancer Res* 1982; 80: 64-69.
237. Reizenstein P, Andersson M, Bjorkholm M, Brenning G, Engstedt L, Gahrton G, Hast R, Holm G, Hornsten P, Killander A, Lantz B, Lindemalm C, Lockner D, Lonnquvist B, Mellstedt H, Palmblad J, Paul C, Simmonsson B, Sjogren AM, Stalfelt A-M, Uden A-M, Wadman B, Oberg G, Osby E. BCG plus leukemic cell therapy in patients with acute nonlymphoblastic leukemia: effect in groups with high and low remission rates. In: Terry W, Rosenberg S, eds. Immunotherapy of Human Cancer. New York; *Excerpta Medica*, 1982: 17-22.
238. Reizenstein P, Delgado M, Gastiaburu J, Lomme L, Ogier C, Pals H, Schellekens J, Whitakker J, Mathé G. Efficacy of an errors in randomized multicenter trials. A review of 230 clinical trials. *Biomed Pharmacother* 1983; 37: 14-24.
239. Reizenstein P, Mathé G. Vriz N, Lomme L. Non specific immunomodulators in oncology and hematology. In: Oldham RK, ed. *Principles of Cancer Biotherapy.* New York: Dekker, 1991: 217-252.
240. Reizenstein P. The monitoring of minimal residual disease in patients with malignant tumor. In: Reizenstein P, Mathé G, Dicato M. eds. *Managing Minimal Malignancy in Man.* Oxford: Pergamon Press, 1988.
241. Resch MK, Goppelt M, Hänsch GM, Körner CF, Martin M, Szamel M. Mechanisms of arachidonic acid turnover implicated in cell activation. In Chedid L, Hadden JW, Spreafico F, Dukor P, Willoughby D, eds. Advances in Immunopharmacology 3. *Proceeding of the Third International Conference on Immuno-pharmacology.* Florence, May 6-9, 1985. Pergamon Press, 1986: 115.
242. Robert P. Le Petit Robert. Paris; *Le Robert,* 1990.
243. Rola-Pleszczynski M. Leukotrienes and the immune system. *J. Lipid Mediat* 1989; 1: 149-159.
244. Rosenberg SA. Adoptive immunotherapy of cancer: accomplishment and prospects. *Cancer Treat Rep* 1984; 68: 233-235.
245. Rosenberg SA. Immunotherapy of patients with advanced cancer using recombinant lymphokines. *Clin Courrier* 1989; 7: 16-20.
246. Rozengurt E. Stimulation of DNA synthesis in quescient cultured cells. Exogenous agents, internal signals and early event. *Curr Top Cell Regal.*1980; 17: 59-88.
247. Rutten VP, Klein WR, Steerenberg PA, De Jong WA, Den Otter W, Ruitenberg EJ. Immunotherapy of bovine ocular squamous cell carcinoma : isolation, culture and characterization of lymphocytes present in the tumor. *Anticancer Res* 1991, 11, 1259-1264.
248. Sasaki K, Sasaki M, Ishikawa M, Takayanagi G. Depression of hepatic microsomal enzyme systems by lentinan in mice. *Japanese J Pharmacol* 1985; 37: 107-115.
249. Sato PS, Constantopoulos A, Nishioka K, Najjar VA. Tuftsin, threonyl-lysyl-prolyl-arginine, the phagocytosis stimulating messenger of the carrier cytophillic gamma-globulin leukokinin. In: Meinhoff J, ed. Chemistry and biology of peptide. Ann Arbor: *Ann Arbor Science Publ,* 1972: 403-408.
250. Satoh K, Kan N, Okino T, Mise K, Yamasaki S, Harada T, Hori T, Ohgaki K, Tobe T. The therapeutic effect of OK-432-combined adoptive immunotherapy against liver metastases from gastric or colorectal cancers. *Biotherapy* 1993; 6: 41-49.
251. Sawyer ST, Krantz SB. Erythropoietin stimulates 45Ca2+ uptake in Friend virus-infected erythroid cells. *J Biol Chem* 1984, 259 p: 2769-2774.
252. Schwartz JC, Cros C. Bestatin and enkephalins. In: Mathé G, Umezawa H, eds. Progress in Cancer Chemo-immunotherapy. Tokyo: *Japan Antibiotics Research Association,* 1984: 243-244.
253. Schwarzenberg L, Mathé G, Schneider M, Amiel JL, Cattan A, Schlumberger JR. Attempted adoptive immunotherapy of acute leukaemia by leucocyte transfusions. *Lancet* 1966; ii: 365-368.
254. Scott Ph. IL-12 initiation cytokine for cell-mediated immunity. *Science* 1993; 260: 496.
255. Sen A, Fareed GC. Oncogens, antioncogens and growth factors. In: Oldham RK, ed. *Principles of Cancer Biotherapy.* New York: Dekker; 1991: 617-635.
256. Sethi KK, Brandis H. Synergistic cytotoxic effect of macrophages and normal mouse serum on neuraminidase-treated murine leukaemia cells. *Eur J Cancer* 1973; 9: 809-819.
257. Shen RN, Lu L, Young P, Shidnia MH, Hornback NB, Boxmeyer HE. Influence of elevated temperature on natural killer cell activity lymphokine-activated killer cell activity and lectin-dependent cytotoxicity of human umbilical cord blood and adult blood cells. *Int J Radiat Oncol Biol Phys* 1994; 29: 921-826.
258. Shibuya K, Hayashi E, Abe F, Takahashi K, Horinishi H, Ishizuka M, Takeuchi T, Umezawa H. Enhancement of interleukin 1 and interleukin 2 released by ubenimex. *J Antibiot* 1987; 40: 363-369.
259. Skipper HE. Kinetic behavior versus response to chemotherapy. *Natl Cancer Int Monogr* 1971; 34: 2-14.

260. Spirer Z, Zakuth V, Orda R, Wiznitzer T. Acquired tuftsin deficiency. In Anon: *Abstracts Conf antineoplastic, imunogenic and other effects of the tetrapeptide tuftsin: A natural macrophage activator.* New York: Februrary 16-17, 1983 (abstract n° 21).
261. Spitler LE, Sagebiel R. A randomized trial of levamisole versus placebo as adjuvant therapy in malignant melanoma. *N Engl J Med* 1980; 303: 11431147.
262. Sporn MB, Robert AB. The transforming growth factor beta: past, present and futur. *Ann NY Acad Sci* 1990; 593: 1-6.
263. Stebbing N. Recombinant DNA-derived organisms as sources of cancer biotherapeutics. In: Oldham RK, ed. *Principles of Cancer Biotherapy.* New York: Dekker; 1991: 73-107.
264. Steinhorn SC, Ries LG. Improved survival among children with acute leukemia in the United States. *Biomed Pharmacother* 1988; 42: 675-681.
265. Stewart WE. *The interferon system.* New York: Springer, 1971.
266. Stout SA, Riley CM, Derendorf H. *In vitro pharmacokinetics and pharmacodynamics of melphalan.* Biennial Conference on Chemo-therapy of Infectious diseases and Malignancies. Munich 26, 1987.
267. Suda H, Takita T, Aoyagi T, Umezawa H. The structure of bestatin. *J Antibiot* 1976; 29: 100-101.
268. Szmigielski S, Sobczynski J, Sokolska G, Stawarz B, Zielinski H, Petrovich Z. Effects of local prostatic hyperthermia on human NK and T cell function. *Int J Hyperthermia* 1991; 7: 869-880.
269. Takahashi SI, Kato H, Sebi T, Takahashi A, Noguchi T, Naito H. Intermediate peptide of insulin degradation in liver and cultures hepatocytes of rats. *Int J Biochem* 1988; 20: 1369-1380.
270. Terry WD, Rosenberg SA, eds. *Immunotherapy of Human Cancer.* Amsterdam: Elsevier North Holland, 1982.
271. Thomas ED, Storb R, Clift RA, Feffer A, Johnson FL, Neiman PE, Lerner KG, Glucksberg H, Buckenr CD. Bone marrow Transplantation. *N Engl J Med* 1975; 292: 832-843.
272. Thompson RB, Alberola V, Mathé G. Evaluation of surgery, chemotherapy and immunotherapy on the Lewis lung tumor. *Rev Eur Etudes Clin Biol* 1972; 17: 900-902.
273. Treurniet-Donker AD, Meischke-de Jongh ML, van Putten WL. Levamisole as adjuvant immunotherapy in breast cancer. *Cancer* 1987; 59: 1590-1593.
274. Tursz T, Hors J, Lipinski M, Amiel JL, Mathé G. HLA phenotypes in long-term survivors treated with BCG immunotherapy for childhood ALL. *N Engl J Med* 1978; 1: 1250.
275. Uchida A, Hoshino T. Effect of immunotherapy with OK-432 in lymphocyte subpopulation and phytomitogen responsiveness i*n vitro*. *Cancer* 1980; 45: 476-483.
276. Uchida A, Hoshino T. Reduction of suppressor cells in cancer patients treated with OK-432 immunotherapy. *Int J Cancer* 1980; 26: 401-404.
277. Uchida A, Micksche M, Hoshino T. Intrapleural administration of OK-432 in cancer patients: augmentation of autologous tumor killing activity of tumor-associated larger granular lymphocytes. *Cancer Immunol Immunother* 1984; 18: 5-12.
278. Ulrich A. *Chemotherapy of Advanced Epithelial Cancer.* Stuttgart: Hippokrates Verlag, 1990.
279. Umezawa H. Small molecular microbial products enhancing immune response. *Antibiot Chemother* 1978; 24: 9-18.
280. Umezawa H, Aoyagi T, Suda H, Hamada M, Takeuchi T. Bestatin, an inhibitor of aminopeptidase B, produced by actinomycetes. *J Antibiot* 1976; 29: 97-99.
281. Van Amsterdam JG, Llorens-Cortes C. Inhibition of enkephalin degradation by phelorphan: effects on striatal (Met^5) enkephalin levels and jump latency in mouse hot plate test. *Eur J Pharm* 1988; 154: 319-324.
282. Vogler WR. Results of randomized trials of immunotherapy for acute leukemia. *Cancer Immunol Immunother* 1981; 9: 15-21.
283. Volz M, Kirkpatrick CH. Interferon 1992: How much of the promise has been realised? *Drugs* 1992; 43: 285-294.
284. Wakasuki M, Kasahara T, Minato N, Hamuro J, Miyata M, Morioka Y. In vitro potentiation of human natural killer cell activity by a streptococcal preparation, OK-432: Interferon and interleukin-2 participation in the stimulation with OK-432. *J Natl Cancer Inst* 1982; 69: 807-812.
285. Webb D, Braun W, Plescia OJ. Antitumor effects of polynucleotides and theophylline. *Cancer Res* 1972; 32: 1814-1819.
286. Weiden PL, Flournoy N, Thomas ED, Prentice R, Fefer A, Buckner CD, Storb R. Antileukemic effect of graft-versus-host disease in human recipients of allogeneic marrow grafts. *New Engl J Med* 1979; 300: 1068-1073.
287. Wider J. Randomizing means, not aims in clinical trial. *Lance*t 1994; 343: 359.
288. Wolf G. Multiple functions of Vitamin A. *Physiol Rev* 1984; 64: 873-937.
289. Wolmark N, Fisher B, Rockette H. Postoperative adjuvant chemotherapy or BCG for colon cancer: Results from NSABP protocol C-01. *J Natl Cancer Inst* 1988; 80: 30-36.
290. Zhu HM. Short-term results of intratumor BCG injection for rectal carcinoma. *Chung Hua Chung Liu Tsa Chih* 1990; 12: 40-42.
291. BCG helps vaccine fight advanced melanoma. *Med Trib* 1993: 12.
292. Interleukin 2 in cancer: select your patients well. *Inpharma* march 28, 1992: 16.
293. Medical Research Council by the Leukaemia Committee and the Working Party on Leukaemia in Childhood: Treatment of acute lymphoblastic leukaemia. Comparison of immunotherapy (BCG), intermittent methotrexate, and no therapy after a five-month intensive cytotoxic regimen (Concord Trial). *Br Med J* 1971; 4: 189-194.
294. WHO. *Neoplastic diseases of haematopoietic and lymphoid tissues*. Genève, 1976.

CANCER VACCINES: TUMOR EPITOPES AND GENE THERAPY

GEORGE C. FAREED and LYNN E. SPITLER
AIDS ReSEARCH ALLIANCE, West Hollywood, California and Jenner Technologies, Inc., Tiburon California

Recent progress in our understanding of the molecular biology of the human immune system and the interplay of soluble growth factors, cytokines and lymphokines, to directly activate immune responses coupled with the molecular characterization of tumor antigens in several human cancers now provide for exciting new treatment approaches for cancer immunotherapy. Many groups are now focusing on overcoming the 'weak tumor-associated' immunity due to insufficient stimulation of helper T lymphocytes through approaches summarized in this chapter.

Cancer cells express novel antigens, which may serve as immunogens capable of eliciting antibody [34, 118] and cellular responses [93, 95] that can mediate tumor destruction directly or indirectly [72, 76]. The efficacy of synthetic tumor components as well as various preparations of suspensions of autologous tumor cells, allogeneic tumor cell lines, or partially purified tumor cell antigens are being investigated in experimental therapy programs [15, 23, 50, 62, 63, 72, 82, 94, 114, 139, 142]. The cellular preparations are generally treated by irradiation, mechanical disruption, or freeze-thaw cycles to render the tumor cells nonviable. They are then used as immunogens, with or without an adjuvant, and administered by various routes (i.e., as intradermal, subcutaneous, intramuscular, or intralymphatic infusions) to immunize cancer patients [115]. These studies have revealed the fairly low toxicity of the immunogens, while providing encouraging clinical responses in advanced cancer patients. The putative tumor antigens present in these undefined immunogen preparations, when distinguishable from normal cellular structures [54, 75, 127, 132, 136], may prove to be the most important components of future cancer vaccines.

Current approaches to the generation of effective antitumor immune responses in patients encompass a wide variety of purified or synthetic, well-defined tumor antigens and a growing list of promising adjuvants (Table 1).

Cancer vaccines are being studied and refined for use in the prophylactic management of several high cancer risk individuals and for adjunctive therapy for solid tissue

Table 1. Approaches to engineered vaccines

Antigens	Adjuvants
• Peptides	• Alumunium Hydroxide (Alum)
• Anti-idiotypic Antibody	• Bacillus Calmette-Guérin (BCG)
• Synthetic Antigen	• Cytokines (IL-2, IL-12, Alpha interferon, GM-CSF)
• Purified Antigen	• Detoxified Endotoxin (DETOX^{TM})
• Heat Shock Protein	• Heat Shock Protein
• Mutant Oncogene	• Immune Stimulating Complexes (ISCOMS)
• Recombinant Vector	• Keyhole Limpet Hemocyanin (KLH)
• Naked DNA	• Lipid molecules
• Gene Transfer	• Liposomes
	• Muramyl dipeptide (MDP) derivatives
	• Monophosphoryl lipid A (MPL)
	• Muamyl tripeptide phosphatidylethanolamine (MTP-PE)
	• Polysaccharides (glucan, lentinan, etc.)
	• Saponin (QS 21)
	• Recombinant Vectors: vaccinia, poxvirus, fowlpox virus
	• Syntex Adjuvant Formulation (SAF-1)
	• T Helper Peptide Epitope

R.K. Oldham (ed.), Principles of Cancer Biotherapy. 3rd ed., 179–191.

tumors (e.g., renal, colon, breast and prostate carcinomas and melanoma). High risk individuals with a genetic susceptibility to cancers are patients with retinoblastoma, neurofibromatosis, xeroderma pigmentosa, familial polyposis coli, and Hodgkin's disease [19]. Chromosomal excess, as in trisomy 21, or chromosomal instability, as in Fanconi's hypoplastic anemia, is associated with an increased incidence of malignancy. Somatic growth disturbances, as seen in hemihypertrophy, may be associated with liver, kidney, or adrenal tumors. Patients with acquired immune deficiency syndrome due to human immune deficiency virus (HIV) infection have significantly increased risks for Kaposi's sarcoma, non-Hodgkin's lymphomas, and rectal carcinoma. Certain large populations, although not having a specific genetic predisposition to cancer, may be at an increased risk owing to their environmental exposure, geographical location, or underlying clinical syndrome (e.g., smokers have a 15- to 50-fold increased risk for lung cancer; fair-skinned individuals living in very sun-exposed countries show greatly increased incidences of malignant melanoma and other skin tumors; patients with ulcerative colitis show a 10- to 30-fold increased risk for gastrointestinal cancer). Prophylactic immunization of these populations could result in enormous social andeconomic benefits if adequate protection against the environmentally provoked malignancy were achieved.

Certain human viral infections are associated with or causative of specific human malignancies: hepatocellular carcinoma (hepatitis B virus, HBV), nasopharyngeal carcinoma and Burkitt's lymphoma (Epstein-Barr virus), cervical carcinoma and possibly certain respiratory tract malignancies (several human papilloma virus strains), and Japanese (human) T cell leukemia (HTLV-I). Where viral etiologies for human malignancies have been established [76, 88, 90, 105, 108], the development of traditional antiviral vaccines has proven to be effective such as that for HBV in hepatocellular cancer prevention. Beyond these, synthetic peptide and recombinant DNA vaccine candidates are close at hand, particularly for HTLV-I (94) and already available for hepatitis B virus [90].

PROTECTIVE ANTICANCER IMMUNE RESPONSES: RELEVANCE OF VACCINE WORK FOR INFECTIOUS DISEASES

The most effective vaccines have been those composed of attenuated strains of infectious agents, such as viruses and other microorganisms, namely, smallpox, yellow fever, poliomyelitis, measles, rubella, and tuberculosis. An attenuated organism may induce a longterm immunity comparable to that generated by a natural infection. The attenuated organisms replicate inefficiently in the host for days or weeks. Therefore, the immunogenic stimulus continues, leading to a 'persisting' antigen effect without the adverse effects of an active infection. During this tume, relevant cytokines are produced and cell activation and/or death takes place, as in a granuloma. This leads to a continuing stimulus of both non-specific and specific response, resulting in long-lived memory cells in this process probably varies depending upon the specific infectious organism.

In order to achieve successful immunization against cancer, a variety of antigen formulations and immunization protocols may have to be tested. The quality and magnitude of immunity produced by these different approaches may ultimately be comparable to those generated by attenuated microbial and viral vaccines. As we shall describe in detail in the discussions that follow, immunotherapy studies with whole cancer cells as immunogens have attempted to mimic attenuation of microorganisms by using radiation or chemical treatments to reduce the viability of the tumor cells, yet permit one or two cell divisions. This may allow a persistent presentation of tumor-associated antigens in their 'natural' forms encountered on tumor cells. These crude, complex antigen preparations generally require the use of immunopotentiating adjuvants [123], such as dead mycobacterial cells in an oil emulsion (Freund's complete adjuvant), muramyl dipeptide, lipopolysaccharide, trehalose dimycolate, or a number of other immunopotentiators, when administered by intradermal or subcutaneous injection.

Unlike a simple foreign infectious agent, cancer cells are highly complex. In addition, most of the antigens in a cancer cell are also present in the normal cellular counterpart. The antigens that will induce an active immune response leading to the regression of a cancer (analogous to the neutralizing antigen of an infectious agent) are thus expected to be rare components of a cancer cell or weakly immunogenic. Considerable refinements of the whole cell preparations will undoubtedly be required. These should be based upon the identification and characterization of critical antigens or antigenic epitopes on cancer cells, which will permit differentiation between soluble and particulate antigens and the production of certain critical components by recombinant DNA technology or peptide synthesis [11, 102, 103]. As previously identified and new natural mediators of growth and differentiation of the immune system (e.g., interleukins, interferons, colony stimulating factors) become available, new classes of adjuvants, capable of converting poor immune responses into strong ones, may be formulated [20]. Results of immunization studies have shown that interleukin-2 [143] administered in reduced dosages subcutaneously is able to enhance the immunogenicity of weak antigens [99, 138]. Active specific immunotherapy combining tumor cell vaccines along with IL-2, GM-CSF, gamma interferon and other lymphokines as adjuvants are under investigation.

IMMUNOLOGIC FUNCTIONS TO BE CONSIDERED FOR AN EFFECTIVE VACCINE

Cancer regression epitopes must be taken up by appropriate antigen-presenting cells, which include macrophages, dendritic cells, reticular cells, Langerhans cells, and eventually B-lymphocytes [3, 92, 141]. The T cell receptor recognizes a processed antigen major histocompatibility complex (MHC) on the B cell surface. The induction of the immune response requires that a helper $CD4^+$ T cell recognize the foreign antigen in the context of a class II MHC molecule on the surface of an antigen presenting cell and cytotoxic $CD8^+$ T cells interact with class I MHC. For most protein antigens, T cells recognize a non-native 'processed' form of the antigen, whereas B cells directly recognize native structures [1, 137]. In contrast to antibodies, which recognize sites all over the surface of globular protein antigens and frequently, although not always, require native tertiary structure, helper T cells appear to recognize only a limited number of antigenic sites and do not seem to recognize structure of higher order than secondary. It has been suggested that amphipathicity (the property of having one hydrophobic face and one hydrophilic face) may be an important property for peptides that can stimulate T cells [17]. These specific immunologic fundamentals must be kept well in mind in the design of any cancer epitope vaccine preparation.

T CELL EPITOPES

An important approach to cancer vaccine design requires identification of tumor-specific epitopes recognized by human T cells and B cells [46, 73, 78]. Recently, T cell epitopes in proteins from a variety of viruses, bacteria and parasites have been characterized. In most experiments, the epitopes were identified by cloning pathogen-specific T cells from a small number of immune donors. While this approach has been a very successful first step in epitope identification, it has a serious disadvantage: unless a large panel of human leukocyte antigen (HLA)-typed immune donors is available, it is difficult to obtain information about HLA-linked responsiveness to the protein or peptide being studied. This information is important, since, in general, a particular T cell epitope is recognized only in association with one, or a few, of the many allelic forms of an MHC-encoded restriction element such as HLA-DR or HLA-A2 [26]. For this reason, non-immune HLA-typed donors may be a useful source of clones and antigen-presenting cells that can be used systematically to assay peptide-MHC associations.

Various antigens have been shown to induce proliferation of T cell from naive donors. With the advent of T cell cloning techniques, several groups have used malaria parasite antigens to select T cell clones from peripheral blood cells of non-exposed donors. The responsiveness of HLA-typed naive donors can be used to study the HLA-associated patterns of responsiveness to synthetic peptides or recombinant proteins. By cloning T cells from naive donors, it was found [120] that responsiveness to a peptide from the *Plasmodium falciparum* circumsporozoite protein was associated with at least seven different HLA-DR alleles. The availability of a bank of T cell clones and APCs derived from HLA-typed donors has another advantage: these cells can be employed in a competition assay to investigate binding of different peptides to HLA restriction elements. Binding is a requirement for responsiveness, although not all peptides that bind to an MHC antigen will induce a response [4, 42]. T helper lymphocytes differentiate into distinct subsets that can be distinguished by their patterns of cytokine secretion. Th1 cells, which secrete IL-2 and INF-gamma among other cytokines, play a key role in generating cell-mediated immunity. Both delayed-type hypersensitivity reactions and cytotoxic T cell (CTL) generation are generated by activation and expansion of Th1 lymphocytes. Th2 lymphocytes secrete IL-4, IL-5, IL-10 and IL-13, cytokines that play a major role in augmenting antibody production by B lymphocytes. Signals which T lymphocytes mujst receiv, in addition to antigen, to proliferate and differentiate into cytoxic effector cells have recently been identified. Costimulators, a class of molecules expressed on the surface of antigen-presenting cells (such as macrophages and denritic cells), serve this function. B7, a costimulatory protein, when expressed on the surface of tumor cells after transfection with the B7 gene, allow poorly immunogenic cells to stimulate a powerful CTL-mediated immune response [25, 130].

Induction of cytotoxic T lymphocytes (CTL) requires not only stimulatory antigen but also cellular interaction among CTL precursor cells, helper T cells and non-T accessory cells [47, 67, 95, 131]. The growth and differentiation of CTL precursors is regulated by soluble factors, of which interleukin-2 (IL-2) is considered to be of prime importance. There are, however, several reports showing that lymphokines other than IL-2 have profound effects on the generation of CTL. These appear to include IL-1, IL-4, IL-5, IL-6, IL-7, IL-12, GM-CSF and gamma interferon [86, 128]. The optimal activation of cytotoxic T lympphocytes requires not only antigenic stimulation but also involves complex cell to cell interactions among diverse types of cells, including helper T cells and macrophages. Signals between these cells are often mediated by soluble factors such as the lymphokines mentioned above.

Despite many lines of evidence for the existence of tumor-associated transplantation antigens (TATA) capable of inducing host-resistance against a tumor [40, 41], establishment of a therapeutic regimen for the complete eradication of tumor cells in a tumor-bearing host by the active induction of anti-tumor protective immunity has not yet been successful. It has been established that although the activation of helper T cells is strictly antigen-specific, their ability to augment T responses is antigen nonspecific, indicating that helper T cells against a given cell surface antigen are capable of assisting T cell responses to other cell surface antigens such as TATA.

Intravesical instillation therapy of bacillus Calmette-Guerin (BCG) is a useful modality for recurrent superficial transitional-cell carcinoma (TCC) of the urinary bladder. The mechanism of BCG effect has not yet been well characterized. BCG was tested *in vitro* for cytokine-mediated antiproliferative activity against T24 and KK47 cells (cell lines established from human TCC of the urinary bladder), and ACHN cells (cell line established from human renal cell carcinoma) using a modified human tumor clonogenic assay. Continuous exposure of cells to BCG at concentrations of more than 5 micrograms/ml in the presence of peripheral blood mononuclear cells (PBMC) consisting of a mixture of 5×10^4 monocytes/dish and 5×10^5 lymphocytes/dish, obtained from healthy donors, significantly inhibited colony formation of T24 and ACHN cells in comparison with growth inhibition in the absence of PBMC ($P > 0.05$). Slightly inhibited colony formation was observed with KK47 cells under the same conditions. At the same time various cytokines were measured in supernatants when BCG and the same conditioned PBMC were co-cultured. Tumor necrosis factor alpha (TNF alpha) and interleukin-1 beta (IL-1 beta) were detected at markedly high levels at 24 h, and interferon gamma (IFN gamma) was detected at 120 h. IL-2 and macrophage-colony-stimulating factor were not detected. Neutralizing anti-TNF alpha monoclonal antibody significantly reduced the anti-proliferative activity of ACHN cells, and anti-IFN gamma antibody reduced that of T24 cells. Thus, cytokines mediated by BCG play an important role in the antitumor activity of BCG and that the sensitivity of bladder cancer cells to the cytokines induced by BCG may differ considerably [77].

ACTIVE SPECIFIC HUMAN IMMUNOTHERAPY STUDIES

One major limitations of these efforts has been the undefined nature of the tumor-cell preparations (generally, intact irradiated cell suspensions or mechanically disrupted lysates). Cells drawn from tissue cultures of autologous tumor cells or continuously passaged tumor-cell lines may undergo significant changes in their antigen-expression profiles during growth in laboratory culture. Membrane proteins may be lost during irradiation of cells, and antigens may be degraded by proteolytic enzymes during the preparation of cell lysates. Different preparations used in previous studies may, therefore, have had variable efficacies even when the same investigating group used similar processes and cell types to prepare the immunogens. Reagents or tests to standardize the preparations for the presence and potency of antigen(s) have not been available. Furthermore, the means of monitoring an individual patient's immune response was not available to adjust the immunization dose and schedule for optimal response.

A systematic search for antibodies against tumor cell-specific components raised in patients undergoing tumor regression may lead to the identification of regression-associated antigens (RAA), immunogens with great potential for cancer prevention as well as active specific immunotherapy of various cancers. Tumor-cell antigens have been identified using antibodies developed in patients immunized by the intralymphatic route with irradiated human tumor cell lines and characterized by significant regression of their tumors [34, 35]. These human tumor cell antigens and antibodies directed against them offer the possibility of novel approaches in the biotherapy of human cancers and are also intriguing candidates for cancer prevention. Sera from immunized patients have been used in sensitive immunoblots [129] to screen extracts of normal and tumor-derived cells, as well as normal and tumor tissue extracts, to identify specific antigens in tumor cells and tissues. These tumor-associated antigens have been further grouped based on their size, ability to react with antibodies from patients experiencing regression of various malignancies, and presence on different human cancer cell types [84].

Results from a number of animal models lend support to the use of tumor cell components in active specific immunization to induce tumor regression [7, 27, 28, 49, 55, 61, 71, 80]. Furthermore, these studies directly demonstrate that preimmunization of animal hosts with tumor cell-derived immunogens can protect against tumor challenge. One of the beststudied systems has been the immunization of cats with FOCMA (feline oncornavirus-associated cell membrane antigen) in order to protect them from subsequent tumor development following challenge with virus [60]. Vaccination of cats using FOCMA-containing lymphoma cells that were heat-inactivated, treated with paraformaldehyde, or disrupted by an alternating freezing and thawing procedure in all cases gave substantial antitumor protection. Neoplasms induced in mice by polycyclic aromatic hydrocarbons, such as 3-methylcholanthrene, express individually distinct tumor-associated transplantation antigens [122]. These antigens are immunogenic in their syngeneic hosts and provide transplantation immunity only against their respective tumors and not against tumors induced by the same or a different carcinogen or against tumors of viral origin. Transplantation immunity in mice can be elicited by prior growth and removal of tumor transplants or by immunization with irradiated tumor cells, tumor-cell membranes, or solubilized antigen preparations. In a murine melanoma model, a purified melanoma-specific glycoprotein antigen with a molecular weight of 65, 000 has been shown to elicit tumor rejection and protection against experimental metastases in immunized mice [49]. Other workers have identified and purified additional tumor rejection antigens from murine tumors [27, 28].

Fusion of BERH-2 rat hepatocellular carcinoma cells with activated B cells produced hybrid cells that lost their tumorigenicity and became immunogenic. Syngeneic rats injected with BERH-2-B hybrid cells became resistant to challenge with parental BERH-2 cells, and rats with established BERH-2 hepatomas were cured by subsequent injection of BERH-2-B cells. Both CD4+ and CD8+ cells were essential for the induction of protective immunity; however, only CD8+ cells were required for the eradication of BERH-2 tumors. The generation of hybrid tumor cells that elicit antitumor immune responses may thus be a useful strategy for cancer immunotherapy [45].

In addition to proteins, certain glycolipids and carbohydrate structures have been shown to possess tumor rejection activity in animals. Tumor-specific glycolipids synthesized in hamster cells virally transformed by SV40 can act as tumor transplantation antigens responsible for specific tumor rejection in syngeneic hosts [10]. A variety of additional carbohydrate structures on animal and human tumors have been detected with monoclonal antibodies. Although most such structures may not be sufficiently immunogenic by themselves, appropriate adjuvants mixed with them may allow their use in vaccines.

A novel animal model system for reticulum cell sarcoma has been elucidated [68] and shown to regress when antibodies specific for host immune T cells were administered. The tumor-specific immune lymphocytes apparently provided growth factors to drive the proliferation of the sarcoma cells. If a similar mechanism exists in human reticulum cell sarcoma or possibly Hodgkin's disease, then either immunization with antigens specific for the T cells or antibody treatment to erradicate the T cell response may have profound therapeutic consequences.

Gene therapy approaches

The local presence of cytokines can drastically alter tumor host immune relations and activate a nonspecific and specific reactions that in some cases leads to induction of anti-tumor responses to otherwise nonimmunogenic tumors. The employment of cytokines in the creation of new antitumor vaccines either via gene therapy or local infiltration is a promising prospect and the subject of much investigation. Analogous effects have been obtained with cytokines inoculated locally and cytokines released from tumor cells engineered to produce them.

Recombinant MUC 1 vaccinia virus has been constructed as a potential vector for immunotherapy of breast cancer. Breast cancer is considered as the major cause of mortality by cancer for women. Although chemotherapy, radiotherapy and surgery have improved the life expectancy of patients bearing tumors, breast cancer is responsible for the death of 42, 000 women per year in USA. In this context, cancer vaccines may add an attractive alternative therapeutic strategy to the current existing treatments. Recombinant vaccinia viruses co-expressing a tumour associated antigen (MUC 1) and an adjuvant cytokine have been constructed, which have potential applications in the active immunotherapy of breast cancer. Indeed, recombinant vaccinia viruses have been extensively used during the past decade to induce a protective response against a whole variety of pathogens, and have proven to be of great value in the elicitation of a cellular immune response leading to the rejection of tumor grafts in mouse models [13].

The local presence of cytokines can drastically alter tumor host immune relations and activate a nonspecific reaction that in some cases leads to induction of specific responses to otherwise nonimmunogenic tumors. The employment of cytokines in the creation of new antitumor vaccines is thus a tempting prospect. Analogous effects have been obtained with cytokines inoculated locally and cytokines released from tumor cells engineered to produce them [38].

In a rational strategy for human prostate cancer gene therapy, efficacy was tested using the Dunning rat prostate carcinoma model. Rats with anaplastic, hormone refractory prostate cancer treated with irradiated prostate cancer cells genetically-engineered to secrete human granulocyte-macrophage colony-stimulating factor (GM-CSF). The results showed longer disease-free survival compared to either untreated control rats or rats receiving prostate cancer cell vaccine mixed with soluble human GM-CSF. A gene modified prostate cancer cell vaccine thus provided effective therapy for anaplastic, hormone refractory prostate cancer in this animal model. An evaluation of the clinical feasibility of gene therapy for human prostate cancer based on these findings was then undertaken. Prostate cancer cells from patients with stage T2 prostate cancer undergoing radical prostatectomy were first transduced with MFG-lacZ, a retroviral vector carrying the beta galactosidase reporter gene. Efficient gene transfer was achieved in each of 16 consecutive cases (median transduction efficiency 35%, range 12 to 65%). Co-transduction with a drug-selectable gene was not required to achieve high yield of genetically-modified cells. Histopathology confirmed malignant origin of these cells and immunofluorescence analysis of cytokeratin 18 expression confirmed prostatic luminal epithelial phenotype in each case tested. Cell yields (2.5×10^8 cells per gram of prostate cancer) were sufficient for potential entry into clinical trials. Autologous human prostate cancer vaccine cells were then transduced with MFG-GM-CSF, and significant human GM-CSF secretion was achieved in each of 10 consecutive cases. Sequential transductions increased GM-CSF secretion in each of 3 cases tested, demonstrating that increased gene dose can be used to escalate desired gene expression in individual patients. These studies show a preclinical basis for proceeding with clinical trials of gene therapy for human prostate cancer [113].

Interleukin-2-secreting mouse fibroblasts transfected with genomic DNA from murine melanoma cells prolong the survival of mice with melanoma. A retrovirus was used to introduce a provirus (pZipNeoSVIL-2) containing the gene for interleukin-2 (IL-2) along with a neor gene (confers resistance to G418) into LM cells, a mouse cell line expressing defined major histocompatibility complex class I antigens (H-2k). After initial selection in growth medium containing G418, IL-2 secretion was confirmed, and the cells were then cotransfected with genomic DNA from B16F1 or B16F10 melanoma cells, along with DNA from a plasmid (pHyg) that confers resistance to hygromycin. After a second round of selection in growth medium containing sufficient quantities of hygromycin to kill 100% of non-transfected cells but without further modification, the unfractionated populations of transfected cells were tested for their immunotherapeutic properties in C57BL/6 mice (H-2b) with established B16 melanomas (H-2b). Animals with melanomas treated with either of the transfected cell populations survived significantly ($P > 0.01$) longer than untreated mice or mice treated with irradiated (5000 rads) B16F1 melanoma cells. The animals also survived longer ($P > 0.05$) than mice with melanoma treated with IL-2-secreting LM cells transfected with genomic DNA from MOPC-315 cells, a nonimmunologically cross-reactive murine tumor. As determined by the capacity of monoclonal antibodies to T-cell subsets to inhibit the anti-melanoma response in a 51Cr release assay, the anti-melanoma immunity in mice immunized with cells transfected with genomic DNA from either B16F1 or B16F10 cells was mediated primarily by Lyt-2.2+ T-cells. These data raise the possibility that a generic, live cell tumor vaccine can be developed that can be modified to provide specificity for the neoplasms of individual patients [74].

The therapeutic effect of a vaccinia colon oncolysate prepared with interleukin-2-gene encoded vaccinia virus was recently studied in a syngeneic CC-36 murine colon hepatic metastasis model. Vaccinia CC-36 murine colon oncolysate (VCO) prepared with interleukin-2-gene encoded recombinant vaccinia virus (IL-2VCO) was used in the treatment of a syngeneic murine colon adenocarcinoma (CC-36) hepatic metastasis to test the beneficial effect of the interleukin-2-gene encoded vaccinia virus over a control recombinant vaccinia virus in producing a vaccinia oncolysate tumor cell vaccine. Results suggest that the IL-2VCO treatment significantly reduced the hepatic tumor burden in comparison with the controls that received either IL-2-gene-encoded recombinant vaccinia virus or a plain recombinant vaccinia virus or vaccinia oncolysate prepared with the plain recombinant virus. The survival of mice treated with IL-2VCO was also improved in comparison with mice treated with other preparations. The induction of a cytolytic T lymphocyte response was examined to elucidate the mechanism of the induction of antitumor responses in IL-2VCO-treated mice. Fresh peripheral blood lymphocytes (PBL) isolated from IL-2VCO-treated mice showed a higher cytolytic activity against CC-36 tumor cell target when compared to PBL from the mice of other treatment groups, suggesting that the IL-2VCO induced an antitumor cytolytic T lymphocyte response. These results suggest that a vaccinia oncolysate, prepared with recombinant vaccinia virus encoding an immunomodulating cytokine gene will enhance antitumor responses in the host [121].

Fibroblasts genetically engineered to secrete interleukin 12 can suppress tumor growth and induce antitumor immunity to a murine melanoma *in vivo*. Interleukin 12 (IL-12), a disulfide-linked heterodimeric cytokine produced primarily by macrophages, is composed of light (p35) and heavy (p40) chains. It binds to a receptor on T-cells and natural killer cells, promoting the induction of primarily a TH1 response *in vitro* and *in vivo*. NIH3T3 cells were stably transfected to express 100-240 units/10^6 cells/48 h of IL-12 using expression plasmids carrying both the murine p35 and p40 genes of murine IL-12. The effects of paracrine secretion of IL-12 on tumor establishment and vaccination models were examined using the poorly immunogenic murine melanoma cell line (BL-6) inC57BL/6 mice. To determine the effects of IL-12 on tumor formation, nonirradiated BL-6 cells were inoculated s.c. into C57BL/6 mice admixed with NIH3T3 cells transfected with both subunits of mIL-12 (3T3-IL-12) or with cells transfected with only the neomycin phosphotransferase gene (3T3-Neo). Compared to mice given injections of BL-6 alone, the day of emergence of detectable tumors was significantly delayed in mice given injections of BL-6 admixed with 3T3-IL-12, but not in mice with BL-6 admixed with 3T3-Neo. Effectiveness in this system was related to the amount of IL-12 expressed by the 3T3-IL-12 and local delivery of IL-12 was found to inhibit tumor growth in a dose dependent manner [124].

Tumor necrosis factor (TNF) produced by genetically engineered tumor cells can lead to very effective tumor rejection; however, experiments conducted to demonstrate systemic protective immunity by TNF-producing tumor cells used as a vaccine have not yet been successful. When observed, tumor suppression does not result from a direct effect of TNF on tumor cells but rather is mediated by the induction of an anti-tumor immune response. It requires a local and continuous presence of TNF at the tumor site. Tumor rejection induced by TNF is dose-dependent and even tumor cell-derived TNF in amounts which cause complete tumor eradication must not be accompanied by toxic side effects. A complex pattern of tumor infiltrating cells has been observed in TNF-producing tumors consisting of macrophages, CD4+ and CD8+ T cells. For tumor suppression, macrophages and CD8+ T cells are needed whereas CD4+ T cells seem to reflect innocent bystander cells. Consistently, TNF is active in T cell deficient mice but in most cases T cells are needed for complete tumor elimination. TNF was active in a number of different tumor models but recent experiments also showed that local TNF failed to induce an anti-tumor response in certain tumor models. Moreover, either depending on the tumor cell line used or on the level of TNF secreted by the tumor, systemic toxicity has been observed, leading to cachexia or wasting of the mice. In one case it has been shown that a TNF gene-transfected tumor showed no tumor growth inhibition *in vivo* but that TNF augmented metastasis of these cells [18].

Transduction of human melanoma cells with interleukin-2 gene reduces tumorigenicity and enhances host antitumor immunity: a nude mouse model. Human melanoma tumor cells were genetically modified *in vitro* by transferring the interleukin-2 (IL-2) gene via a retroviral vector into established or fresh tumor cells. In addition, human melanoma cells were transduced *in vivo* by the direct injection of the IL-2/retroviral vector into melanoma xenografts in nude mice. The gene-modified melanoma cells expressed the IL-2 cytokine gene and secreted biologically active IL-2. Transduction of melanoma cells with the IL-2 gene did not affect the antigenic profile of the cells, but caused a strong abrogation of their tumorigenicity. One million parental cells formed subcutaneous tumors in nude mice. In contrast, various doses of up to 20 x 10^6 IL-2-transduced cells failed to form tumor in the mice Coinjection of IL-2-producing cells with parental cells inhibited tumor formation even when highly tumorigenic doses of parental cells were used. Histochemical analysis of the injection sites of IL-2-modified cells showed an influx of host immune cells, predominantly macrophages, as early as the third day after inoculation. Neutrophils, mast cells, and eosinophils were also seen in the inflammatory exudate. Eventually, transduced cells showed signs of degeneration and necrosis and ultimately died in 4 weeks. Macrophages were seen in parental tumor sites only during the first few days after injection, and then parental tumors exhibited fast, progressive growth. The study suggests that melanoma cells transduced with the IL-2 cytokine gene may provide an effective vaccine for melanoma patients, whereas the in vivo transduction of tumors with cytokine genes is feasible and may represent a novel approach for the immunotherapy of cancer patients [2].

POTENTIAL USE OF PURIFIED OR SYNTHETIC TUMOR ANTIGENS

There is a rapidly growing list of tumor-specific antigens identified by use of murine monoclonal antibodies [39, 85, 87, 101, 109, 110, 116, 119]. The basis for selection of monoclonal antibodies against human tumor markers is not necessarily relevant to tumor regression. In contrast, the selection of human-human hybridomas producing tumor cell-reactive monoclonal antibodies from actively immunized cancer patients or the production of human monoclonal antibodies from fusions with draining lymph node cells for particular malignancies may yield antibodies having specificities associated with tumor regression [9, 48, 58, 65, 66]. Improved recombinant DNA techniques [57] for the rapid cloning and microbial expression of antibody genes from human lymphocytes may contribute to this area in the future.

Perhaps the most intriguing antigenic candidates for cancer epitope vaccine use are those surface antigens identified with monoclonal antibodies exclusively on specific malignant human cells [22, 53, 56, 70, 98]. There is a growing number of these antigens, which have been localized *in vivo* using intravenous infusion of monoclonal antibodies [100, 116]. Precise molecular characterization of these antigens, for example, the melanoma p97 [111] or p250 [109], and the ability to produce pure forms of these antigens or selected epitopes derived from them through genetic engineering techniques offer extremely attractive possibilities for highly specific immunogens. In the case of p97, the entire protein, as well as peptide sequences derived from it, could be used to raise polyclonal and monoclonal antibodies in animals [33]. These antibodies could then be screened for their abilities to elicit antibody-mediated cytotoxicity against human melanoma cells. Those immunogens derived from p97 which stimulate antitumor antibody production might become important components of an anti-melanoma vaccine. Specific gangliosides, GD_2 and GD_3, have been associated with certain human melanomas; and, despite their very limited efficacy as active melanoma immunogens [125], dramatic regression of cutaneous metastatic melanoma was recently described after intralesional injection with a human monoclonal antibody to ganglioside GD_2 [59].

Several antitumor monoclonal antibodies have been reported to have a relatively broad range of carcinoma reactivity. Examples of these are monoclonal antibodies to breast tumor-specific mucin epitopes [43], to gp72, a osteosarcoma and colon carcinoma antigen [29], to L6, a human carcinoma-specific lipid structure [51], and to a *ras* oncogene-associated gp74 antigen [112]. These antigens, or epitopes derived from them, may also be meaningfully evaluated as described above for p97; however, much broader immunization potential may exist, with these potentially offering protection against different human carcinomas. Studies with synthetic peptides containing the breast tumor epitope highly associated with tumor cell mucin are currently underway [89]. As a complement to immunization with the purified anticancer epitopes, anti-idiotypic antibodies mimicking the tumor antigens could be exploited for vaccine use [106]. During the onset of an immune response, auto-antiidiotypic antibody complementary to the antigen combining site of the idiotype plays a major role in determining whether a suppressive or inductive response will take place. Substantial anti-tumor immunity (both humoral and cellular) and evidence of clinical responses have been achieved with antiidiotypic antibody vaccines for melanoma [37] and colorectal carcinoma [52].

There have been several reports of the utility of anti-idiotype antibodies (those expressing an idiotypic determinant that mimics the structure of the antigen for the original antibody) as vaccines for different pathogens. Anti-idiotypic antibodies have also been applied in the treatment of B cell lymphoma, but in many cases success may have been limited on account of spontaneous generation of somatic variants [91]. Several studies have shown anti-idiotypic antibodies to induce protective immunity in animal tumor models [24, 69, 79]. Table 2 lists examples of potential cancer epitope vaccines or target structures currently under investigation.

Table 2. Candidate cancer epitope vaccines

Cancer type/Target class	Target structure	Cancer type (syntheticpeptide)
Breast, ovary, pancreas	Tumor mucins	(yes)
Colon, stomach, bone	gp72	–
Lung, colon, breast, ovary	Ganglioside	–
Melanoma	p200-500, p97	(yes)
Prostate	PSA	(yes)
Colon, stomach, lung, cervix, bladder	gp40/30	(yes)
Oncogenes	ERB B2, Ras, BCR-Abl	breast and other carcinomas, leukeimias, myelomas, sarcomas
Oncofetal proteins	CEA	colon, lung, pancreatic, ovarian, and head and neck
Viral proteins	E6, E7 proteins of HPV	cervical
Carbohydrate moieties	Altered mucins	colon, breast, gastric, pancreas
Novel proteins	MAGE family	melanoma, lung and breast

RECENT FINDINGS IN ANIMAL AND HUMAN CANCER VACCINE STUDIES

Several clinical investigations are now underway to evaluate synthetic tumor immunogens and gene therapy approaches for autologus tumor vaccine enhancement after expression of cytokines such as GM-CSF. The expression of the sialyl-Tn (STn) epitope on cancer cells associated mucins is associated with a poor prognosis in several human cancers suggesting that STn may have functional significance in metastasis. Antibodies against the STn-epitope can inhibit metastasis. A synthetic mimic, NANA alpha (2–>6)GalNAc alpha-O-Crotyl (STn-crotyl), of the natural O-linked epitope on mucins, NANA alpha (2–>6)GalNAc alpha-O-serine (STn-serine) was generated and STn-crotyl was conjugated to the carrier protein KLH through the crotyl linker arm. A vaccine containing STn-KLH plus Detox adjuvant was formulated. The immunogenicity of the vaccine was evaluated in BALB/c mice and in metastatic breast cancer patients. Breast cancer patients immunized 2-8 times with 25 or 100 micrograms of the vaccine developed antibodies which recognized the cancer-associated disaccharide NANA alpha (2–>6)GalNAc. Evidence of a clinical response was noted in several of the immunized breast cancer patients with other patients showing prolonged disease stability [83].

Murine B16 melanoma expresses the ganglioside GM3. GM3 shed from tumor cells is immunosuppressive and promotes tumor growth. Reduction or elimination of the shed GM3 could be therapeutic, and the anti-GM3 antibodies may reduce and clear the shed ganglioside. Mice were challenged with tumor cells, with or without inducing anti-GM3 antibody response. Since gangliosides are poor immunogens and T-cell independent antigens, an adjuvant (monophosphoryl lipid A (MPL), a non-toxic lipid A of Salmonella), directed against B-cells, was employed. MPL was incorporated onto liposomes and into the surface membrane of B16 mouse melanoma cells; both are rich in GM3. C57BL/6J mice immunized with MPL-liposomes or MPL-B16 cells responded with elevated levels of anti-GM3 IgM. Non-immunized mice or mice immunized with B16 cells alone or ganglioside GM3 alone (without MPL) elicited poor anti-GM3 IgM response, confirming the GM3's immunologic crypticity and MPL's immunopotentiating effect. MPL's immunopotentiating effect was improved by coupling it to melanoma cell membranes. C57BL/6J mice were immunized with irradiated B16alone or MPL alone or MPL-conjugated irradiated B16. After three weekly immunizations, each mouse received a challenge dose of viable syngeneic B16. Neither MPL alone nor B16 alone had a significant effect on tumor growth or host survival; however, administration of MPL-conjugated B16 cells significantly prevented tumor growth and prolonged survival. Our results indicate that MPL-incorporated B16 cells augment the anti-GM3 IgM response, which may reverse GM3-induced immunosuppression by eliminating tumor-derived GM3, and restore immunocompetence [107].

Patients with melanoma metastatic to distant sites or at high risk for recurrent melanoma have been treated with a polyvalent melanoma cell vaccine (MCV) in phase II protocols. *In vivo* and *in vitro* cell-mediated responses to MCV were assessed in 163 patients who had undergone surgical resection of stage III melanoma. During the first 4 months of vaccine immunotherapy, 135 patients (83%) responded by developing a positive delayed-type hypersensitivity reaction > or = 6 mm to MCV. In a mixed lymphocyte tumor cell reaction using periphera blood lymphocytes, 35 of 42 patients (83%) showed a recall proliferative response to one or more of the three cell lines of MCV. After 4 months of MCV therapy, 8 of 11 patients had an increased mixed lymphocyte tumor cell reaction to autologous melanoma cells. During the first 4 months of vaccine therapy, 16 of 33 patients developed more than a 50% increase in cytotoxic T-cell activity against one of the cell lines of MCV. Overall survival was significantly prolonged in patients with a positive delayed-type hypersensitivity reaction (P = 0.0054) and/or increased cytotoxic T-cell activity (P = 0.02). These findings suggest that MCV induces specific T-cell responses which are correlated with clinical course and suggested that some of these responses were directed against autologous melanomas [14].

Treatment of metastatic melanoma patients with an autologous vaccine modified by the hapten, dinitrophenyl (DNP), resulted in the induction of clinically evident inflammatory responses in metastatic tumors with infiltration by T lymphocytes. The expression of activation markers on those cells appeared to be characteristic of tissue T cells with the memory phenotype with low expression of IL-2 receptors and functional impairment of tumor infiltrating lymphocytes in situ, which the authors attributed to inhibitory molecules produced by melanoma cells [16].

Colorectal carcinoma represents a highly interesting model for the biological development of a solid tumor, the efficacy or primary and secondary prevention and the development of chemotherapeutic and immunologic strategies for adjuvant and/or neoadjuvant treatment is resectable stages. Adjuvant systemic 5-FU/levamisole is currently the standard adjuvant treatment for stage III colon cancer. 5-FU/folinic acid for 6 months seems to achieve equivalent results. Continuous infusion of 5-FU for 7 days postoperatively via the portal vein achieves also a comparable improvement in disease-free and overall survival. Beyond the long term systemic as well as short time intraportal chemotherapy, adjuvant immunotherapy with either 17-1A murine monoclonal antibody or autologous tumor vaccine achieves quite comparable results like adjuvant chemotherapy. For rectal cancer stage II and III adjuvant 5-FU plus radiation is currently the standard. Immunotherapy with 17-1A antibody also may significantly prolong disease-free and overall survival in rectal cancer [117]. The elucidation of natural killer cell (NK) mechanisms for target cell recognition and new ways to activate NK cells may be part of the optimal cancer vaccine [93, 104].

There is substantial evidence demonstrating tumor heterogeneity and the ability of malignant cells within the same tumor mass to express different surface antigens [5, 96, 133, 134]. Certain tumor regression epitopes also may require the presence of suitable amounts of specific HLA class I or II antigens in order to elicit protective immune responses [7, 31]. Many malignant cells have, in fact, markedly reduced expression of HLA antigens [97, 134]; and recent reports describe the conversion of such nonimmunogenic cells into tumor-protecting cells after the transfer and expression of specific HLA (MHC) determinants [126, 135]. Alternatively, treatment of malignant cells with specific interferons or possibly other biological response modifiers may suffice for recovery of needed HLA and other antigenic determinants [7, 8, 36, 44]. Because of the potential for tumor cell variants to evade the immune surveillance produced by cancer epitope immunogens, it will be a major challenge for both tumor immunologists and biologists to formulate vaccines covering as many as possible of the potential epitopes that can be expressed specifically on any target cancer cell. In addition, the presentation of certain of the critical epitopes in the vaccine may require the use of liposomes or other membrane carriers [30, 123] and specific HLA antigens for appropriate immune recognition [6, 26]. The major advances in molecular characterization, cloning and synthesis of tumor antigens, cytokines, costimulatory molecules and adhesion moleucles now permit clinical trials with much greater likelihood for antitumor immunity-enhancement via vaccination and effective tumor immunotherapy.

REFERENCES

1. Abergel C, Loret E, Claverie, J-M. Conformational analysis of T immunogenic peptides by circular dichroism spectroscopy. *Eur J Immunol* 1989; 19: 1969-1972.
2. Abdel-Wahab Z, Li WP, Osanto S, et al. *Cancer Res* 1994; 54(1): 182-189.
3. Ada GL. Antigen presentation and enhancement of immunity: An introduction. In: Vaccincs 86: New Approaches to Immunization, edited by F. Brown, R. M. Channock, and R. A. Lerner, pp. 105-111. *Cold Spring Harbor Laboratories*, 1986.
4. Adorini L, Appella E, Doria G, Nagy ZA. Mechanisms influencing the immunodominance of T cell determinants. *J Exp Med* 1988; 168: 2091-2104.
5. Aisenber AC, Krontires TG, Mak TW, et al. Rearrangement of the gene for the beta chain of the T-cell receptor in T-cell chronic lymphocytic leukemia and related disorders. *N Engl J Med* 1985; 313: 529-543.
6. Alexander MA, Bennicelli J, Guerry IV, D. Defective antigen presentation by human melanoma cell lines cultured from advanced, but not biologically early, disease. *J Immunol* 1989; 142: 4070-4078.
7. Anderson DJ, Berkowitz RS. γ-Interferon enhances expression of class I MHC antigens in the weakly HLA^+ human choriocarcinoma cell line BeWo, but does not induce MHC expression in the HLA^- choriocarcinoma cell line. *J Immunol* 1985; 135: 2498-2501.
8. Abdel-Wahab Z, Li WP‘ Osanto S, Darrow TL, et al. Transduction of human melanoma cells with interleukin-2 gene reduces tumorigenicity and enhances host antitumor immunity: a nude mouse model. *Cell Immunol* 1994 Nov; 159(1): 26-39.
9. Andreasen RB, Olsson L. Antibody-producing human-human hybridomas III. Derivation and characterization of

two antibodies with specificity for human myeloid cells. *J Immunol* 1986; 137: 1083-1090.
10. Ansel S and Blangy D. *In vivo* induction of tumor-specific immunity by glycolip extracts of SV40-transformed cells. *Int J Cancer* 1984; 34: 555-559.
11. Antonia SJ, Uchida J, Cohen S, Cohen MC. Attachment of tumor cells to endothelial monolayers: detection of surface molecules involved in cell-cell binding. *Clinical Immunology and Immunopathology* 1989; 53: 281-296.
12. Austin EB, Robins RA, Durrant LG, Price MR, et al. Human monoclonal anti-idiotypic antibody to the tumour-associated antibody 791T/36. *Immunology* 1989; 67: 525-530.
13. Balloul JM, Acres RB, Geist M, et al. *Cell Mol Biol* (Noisy-le-grand) 1994; 4) Suppl 1: 49-59.
14. Barth A, Hoon DS, Foshag LJ, et al. *Cancer Res* 1994; 54(13): 3342-3345.
15. Berd D, Maguire HC Jr, Mastrangelo MJ. Induction of cell-mediated immunity to autologous melanoma cells and regression of metastases after treatment with melanoma cell vaccine preceded by cyclophosphamide. *Cancer Res* 1986; 46: 2572-2577.
16. Berd D, Maguire HC Jr, Mastrangelo MJ, Murphy G. *Cancer Immunol Immunother* 1994; 39(3): 141-147.
17. Berzofsky JA. Immunogenicity of antigens recognized by T cells. *J Cell Biochem* 1990; Sup 14B: 50.
18. Blankenstein T. Observations with tumour necrosis factor gene-transfected tumours. *Folia Bioil* (Praha) 1994; 40(1-2): 19-28.
19. Bodmer WF. Genetic susceptibility to cancer. In: *Accomplishments in Cancer Research* 1985, edited by JG Fortner and JE Rhoads, pp. 198-211. Philadelphia, Lippincott, 1986.
20. Bonnefoy J-Y, Denoroy M-C, Guillot O, et al. Activation of normal human B cells through their antigen receptor induces membrane expression of IL-1α and secretion of IL-1β. *J Immunol* 1989; 143: 864-869.
21. Brett SJ, Cease KB, Ouyang CS, Berzofsky JA. Fine specificity of T cell recognition of the same peptide in association with different I-A molecules. *J Immunol* 1989; 143: 771-779.
22. Bruland OS, Fodstad O, Stenwig AE, Pihl A. Expression and characteristics of a novel human osteosarcoma-associated cell surface antigen. *Cancer Res* 1988; 48: 5302-5309.
23. Bystryn JC, Jacobsen S, Harris M, et al. Preparation and characterization of a polyvalent human melanoma antigen vaccine. *J Biol Resp Modif* 1986; 5: 211-224.
24. Chen J-J, Saeki Y, Shi L, Kohler H. Tumor idiotype vaccines: VI. Synergistic anti-tumor effects with combined 'internal image' anti-idiotypes and chemotherapy. *J Immunol* 1989; 143: 1053-1057.
25. Chen L, Ashe S, Brady W, et al. Cell 1991; 71: 1093-1099.
26. Crowley NJ, Slingluff Jr CL, Darrow TL, Seigler HF. Generation of human autologous melanoma-specific cytotoxic T-cells using HLA-A2-matched allogeneic malanomas. *Cancer Res* 1990; 50: 492-498.
27. DuBois GC, Appella E, Law LW. Isolation of a tumor-associated transplantation antigen (TATA) from an SV40 induced sarcoma. Resemblance to the TATA of chemically induced neoplasms. *Int J Cancer* 1984; 34: 561-566.
28. DuBois GC, Law LW, Appella E. Purification and biochemical properties of tumor-associated transplantation antigens from methylcholanthrene-induced murine sarcomas. *Proc Natl Acad Sci* (USA) 1982; 79: 7669-7673.
29. Durrant LG, Byers VS, Scannon PJ, et al. Humoral immune responses to XMMCO-791-RTA immunotoxin in colorectal cancer patients. *Clin exp Immunol* 1989; 75: 258-264.
30. Eggers AE. Use of adult fibroblasts coupled to muramyl dipeptide to induce antitumor immunity. *J Biol Resp Modif* 1988; 7: 229-233.
31. Eisenbach L, Hollander N, Greenfeld L, et al. The differential expression of H2K versus H-2D antigens, distinguishing high-metastatic from low-metastatic clones, is correlated with the immunogenic properties of the tumor cells. *Int J Cancer* 1984; 34: 567-573.
32. Estin CD, Stevenson US, Plowman GD, et al. Recombinant vaccinia virus vaccine against the human melanoma antigen p97 for use in immunotherapy. *Proc Natl Acad Sci* (USA) 1988; 85: 1052-1056.
33. Estin CD, Stevenson U, Kahn M, et al. Transfected mouse melanoma lines that express various levels of melanoma-associated antigen p97. *J Nat Cancer Inst* 1989; 81: 445-448.
34. Fareed GC, Lee J-H, Ghosh-Dastidar P, et al. Human tumor regression-associated antigenic determinants. In: *Human Tumor Antigens and Specific Tumor Therapy,* edited by RS Metzgar and MS Mitchell, pp. 317-334. New York, Alan R Liss Inc., 1989.
35. Fareed GC, Mendiaz E, Sen A, et al. Novel antigenic markers of human tumor regression. *J Biol Resp Modif* 1988; 7: 11-23.
36. Fearon ER, Itaya T, Hunt B, et al. Induction in a murine tumor of immunogenic tumor variants by transfection with a foreign gene. *Cancer Res* 1988; 48: 2975-2980.
37. Ferrone S, Chen G, Yang H, et al. Murine antiidiotypic monoclonal antibodies in melanoma: immunochemical characterization and clinical applications. *J Cell Biochem* Sup 1990; 14B: 55.
38. Forni G, Giovarelli M, Cavallo F, et al. *J Immunother* 1993; 14(4): 253-257.
39. Fradet Y, Cordon-Cardo C, Thomson T, et al. Cell surface antigens of human bladder cancer defined by mouse monoclonal antibodies. *Proc Natl Acad Sci* (USA) 1984; 81: 224-228.
40. Fujiwara H, Yoshioka T, Kosugi A, et al. Mechanisms for recognition of tumor antigens and implementation of anti-tumor function by non-cytolytic type of T cells. *Gann Monograph on Cancer Research* 1988; 34: 71-86.
41. Fujiwara H, Yoshioka T, Shima J, et al. Helper T cell against tumor-associated antigens (TAA): Preferential induction of helper T cell activities involved in anti-TAA cytotoxic and antibody responses. *J Immunol* 1986; 136: 2715-2719.
42. Gelman IM, Hanafusa H. Immune regression of Rous sarcoma virus-induced tumors: correlation with MMC class I expression. *J Cell Biochem Sup* 1990; 14B: 96.
43. Gendler S, Taylor-Papadimitriou J, Duhig T, et al. A highly immunogenic region of a human polymorphic epithelial mucin expressed by carcinomas is made up of tandem repeats. *J Biol Chem* 1988; 263: 12820-12823.
44. Giacomini P, Imberti L, Adriano A, et al. Immunochemical analysis of the modulation of human melanoma-associated antigens by DNA recombinant immune interferon. *J Immunol* 1985; 135: 2887-2894.

45. Guo Y, Wu M, Chen H, et al. *Science* 1994; 263(5146): 518-520.
46. Guttinger M, Certa U, Pink JR, Sinigaglia F. Requirements for screening recombinant DNA libraries for T cell epitope expression. *J Immunol Methods* 1989; 121: 225-230.
47. Hamaoka T, Kosugi A, Shima J, et al. T-T cell interaction for the augmented induction of anti-tumor protective immunity and its application to active immunotherapy in tumor-bearing hosts. *Gann Monograph on Cancer Research* 1988; 34: 81-90.
48. Haspel MV, McCabe RP, Pomato N, et al. Generation of tumor cell reactive human monoclonal antibodies using peripheral blood lymphocytes from actively immunized colorectal carcinoma patients. *Cancer Res* 1985; 45: 3951-3961.
49. Hearing VJ, Gersten DM, Montague PM, et al. Murine melanoma-specific tumor rejection activity elicited by a purified, melanoma-associated antigen. *J Immunol* 1986; 137: 379-384.
50. Heicappell R, Shirrmacher V, von Hoegen P, et al. Prevention of metastatic spread by postoperative immunotherapy with virally modified autologous tumor cells. 1. Parameters for optimal therapeutic effect. *Int J Cancer* 1986; 37: 569-577.
51. Hellstrom I, Beaumier PL, Hellstrom KE. Antitumor effects of L6, an IgG2a antibody that reacts with most human carcinomas. *Proc Natl Acad Sci* (USA) 1986; 83: 7059-7063.
52. Herlyn D. Anti-idiotypes in cancer patients. *J Cell Biochem Supp* 1990; 14B: 56.
53. Herlyn M, Koprowski H. Melanoma antigens: immunological and biological characterization and clinical significance. *Annu Rev Immunol* 1988; 6: 283-308.
54. Heyderman E, Chapman DV, Richardson TC, et al. Human chorionic gonadotropin and human placental lactogen in extragonadal tumors. *Cancer* 1985; 56: 2674-2682.
55. Hostetler LW, Ananthaswamy HN, Kripke ML. Generation of tumor-specific transplantation antigens by UV radiation can occur independently of neoplastic transformation. *J Immuno*l 1986; 137: 2721-2725.
56. Hotta H, Ross AH, Huebner K, et al. Molecular cloning and characterization of an antigen associated with early stages of melanoma tumor progression. *Cancer Res* 1988; 48: 2955-2962.
57. Huse WD, Sastry L, Iverson SA, et al. Generation of a large combinatorial library of the immunoglobulin repertoire in phage lambda. *Science* 1989; 246: 1275-1281.
58. Imam A, Mitchell MS, Modlin RL, et al. Human monoclonal antibodies that distinguish cutaneous malignant melanomas from benign nevi in fixed tissue sections. *J Invest Dermatol* 1986; 86: 145-148.
59. Iric RF, Morton DL. Regression of cutaneous metastatic melanoma by intralesional injection with human monoclonal antibody to ganglioside GD2. *Proc Natl Acad Sci* (USA) 1986; 83: 8694-8698.
60. Jarrett W, Jarrett O, Mackey L, et al. Vaccination against feline leukemia virus using a cell membrane antigen system. *Int J Cancer* 1975; 16: 134-141.
61. Jeglum KA, Mangan C, Wheeler JE. Enhanced antitumor effects with intralymphatic delivery using bacillus Calmette-Guerin in animal models. *Cancer Drug Deliv* 1985; 2: 127-132.
62. Jessup JM, McBride CM, Ames FC, et al. Active specific immunotherapy of Dukes B2 and C colorectal carcinoma: Comparison of two doses of the vaccine. *Cancer Immunol Immunother* 1986; 21: 233-239.
63. Juillard GJF, Boyer PJJ, Yamashiro CH. A phase 1 study of active specific intralymphatic immunotherapy (ASILI). *Cancer* 1978; 41: 2215-2225.
64. Kahn M, Hellstrom I, Estin CD, Hellstrom KE. Monoclonal antiidiotypic antibodies to the p97 human melanoma antigen. *Cancer Res* 1989; 49: 3157-3162.
65. Kan-Mitchell J, Imam S, Kempf RA, et al. Human monoclonal antibodies directed against melanoma tumor-associated antigens. *Cancer Res* 1986; 46: 2490-2496.
66. Kan-Mitchell J, Kempf RA, Imam A, et al. Monoclonal antibodies in the development of active specific immunotherapy for melanoma. In: *Monoclonal Antibodies and Cancer Therapy*, edited by RA Reisfeld and S Sell, pp. 523-536. New York, Alan R. Liss, 1985.
67. Kast WM, Offinger R, Peters PJ, et al. Eradication of adenovirus E1-induced tumors by E1A specific CTL. J *Cell Biochem Sup* 1990; 14B: 97.
68. Katz J, Bonavida B. A spontaneous sarcoma dependent on host tumor-specific immune lymphocytes. *BioEssays* 1989; 11: 243-250.
69. Kennedy RC, Dreesman GR, Butel JS, et al. Suppression of in vivo tumor formation induced by simian virus 40-transformed cells in mice receiving antiidiotypic antibodies. *J Exp Med* 1985; 161: 1432-1441.
70. Kennel SJ, Foote LJ, Falcioni R, et al. Analysis of the tumor-associated antigen TSP-180. *J Biol Chem* 1989; 264: 15515-15521.
71. Key MD, Brandhorst JS, Hanna MG. More of the relevance of animal tumor models: immunogenicity of transplantable leukemias of recent origin in syngeneic strain 2 guinea pigs. *J Biol Resp Modif* 1984; 3: 359-365.
72. Key ME, Hoover HC, Hanna MG. Active specific immunotherapy as an adjunct to the treatment of metastatic solid tumors; present and future prospects. *Adv Immunol Cancer Ther* 1985; 1: 195-219.
73. Kilgus J, Romagnoli P, Guttinger M, et al. Vaccine T-cell epitope selection by a peptide competition assay. *Proc Natl Acad Sci* (USA) 1989; 86: 1629-1633.
74. Kim TS, Cohne EP. *Cancer Res* 1994; 54(10): 2531-2550.
75. Klagsbrun M, Sasse J, Sullivan R, et al. Human tumor cells synthesize an endothelial cell growth factor that is structurally related to basic fibroblast growth factor. *Proc Natl Acad Sci* (USA) 1986; 83: 2448-2452.
76. Klein G, Klein E. Evolution of tumours and the impact of molecular oncology. *Nature* 1985; 315: 190-195.
77. Kurisu H, Matsuyama H, Ohmoto Y, et al. *Cancer Immunol Immunother* 1994; 39(4): 249-253.
78. Lamb JR, Ivanyi J, Rees ADM, et al. Mapping of T cell epitopes using recombinant antigens and synthetic peptides. *EMBO* J 1987; 6: 1245-1249.
79. Lee VK, Harriott TG, Kuchroo VJ, et al. Monoclonal antiidiotypic antibodies related to a murine oncofetal bladder tumor antigen induce specific cell-mediated tumor immunity. *Proc Natl Acad Sci* (USA) 1985; 82: 6286-6290.
80. Liang S, Linnenbach A, Zell T, et al. Murine melanoma cells transformed with a human melanoma-derived gene: an experimental model for active immunotherapy of human melanoma. *J Cell Biochem Sup* 1990; 14B: 98.

81. Linnenbach AJ, Wojcierowski J, Wu S, et al. Sequence investigation of the major gastrointestinal tumor-associated antigen gene family, GA733. *Proc Natl Acad Sci* (USA) 1989; 86: 27-31.
82. Livingston PO, Takeyama H, Pollack MS. Serological responses of melanoma patients to vaccines derived from allogeneic cultured melanoma cells. *Int J Cancer* 1983; 32: 567-575.
83. Longenecker BM, Koganty R, MacLean GD. *Adv Exp Med Biol* 1994; 353: 105-124.
84. Lopez de Castro JA. Purification of human HLA-A and HLA-B class I histocompatibility antigens. *Methods Enzymol* 1984; 108: 582-606.
85. Luner SJ, de Vellis J. Immunoprecipitation of a MR 64, 000 glial tumor-associated antigen by monoclonal antibody 217C. *Cancer Res* 1986; 46: 863-865.
86. Maraskovsky E, Chen W-F, Shortman K. IL-2 and IFN-γ are two necessary lymphokines in the development of cytolytic T cells. *J Immunol* 1989; 143: 1210-1214.
87. McBride OW, Merry D, Givol D. The gene for human p53 cellular tumor antigen is located on chromosome 17, short arm (17p13). *Proc Natl Acad Sci* (USA) 1986; 83: 130-134.
88. McDonnell JM, Mayr AJ, Martin WJ. DNA of human papillomavirus type 16 in dysplastic and malignant lesions of the conjunctiva and cornea. *N Engl J Med* 1989; 320: 1442-1445.
89. McKenzie IFC, Xing P-X, Reynolds K, et al. Design of synthetic peptides for breast cancer. *J Cell Biochem Sup* 1990; 14B: 346.
90. Milich DR, Hughes JL, McLachlan A, et al. Hepatitis B synthetic immunogen comprised of nucleocapsid T-cell sites and an envelope B-cell epitope. *Proc Natl Acad Sci* (USA) 1988; 85: 1610-1614.
91. Miller RA, Maloney DG, Warnke R, et al. Treatment of B-cell lymphoma with monoclonal anti-idiotype antibody. *N Engl J Med* 1982; 306: 517-522.
92. Milstein C. From the structure of antibodies to the diversification of the immune response. *EMBO J* 1985; 4: 1083-1092.
93. Minato N. Natural killer cells: characteristics and their role in anti-tumor resistance. *Gann Monograph on Cancer Research* 1988; 34: 99-123.
94. Moy PM, Golub SH, Calkins E, et al. Effects of intra-lymphatic immunotherapy on natural killer activity in malignant melanoma patients. *J Surg Oncol* 1985; 29: 112-117.
95. Nabholz M, MacDonald RD. Cytolytic T Lymphocytes. *Annu Rev Immunol* 1983; 1: 273-306.
96. Natali PG, Giacomini P, Bigotti A, et al. Heterogeneity in the expression of HLA and tumor-associated antigens by surgically removed and cultured breast carcinoma cells. *Cancer Res* 1983; 43: 660-668.
97. Natali PG, Nicotra MR, Bigotti A, et al. Selective changes in expression of HLA class I polymorphic determinants in human solid tumors. *Proc Natl Acad Sci* (USA) 1989; 86: 6719-6723.
98. Nudelman ED, Mandel U, Levery SB, et al. A deries of disialogangliosides with binary 2→3 sialosyllactosamine structure, defined by monoclonal antibody NUH2, are oncodevelopmentally regulated antigens. *J Biol Chem* 1989; 264: 18719-18725.
99. Nunberg JH, Doyle MV, York SM, York CJ. Interleukin 2 acts as an adjuvant to increase the potency of inactivated rabies virus vaccine. *Proc Natl Acad Sci* (USA) 1989; 86: 4240-4243.
100. Oldham RK, Foon KA, Morgan AC, et al. Monoclonal antibody therapy of malignant melanoma: in vivo localization in cutaneous metastasis after intravenous administration *J Clin Oncol* 1984; 2: 1235-1243.
101. Philben VJ, Jakowatz JG, Beatty BG, et al. The effect of tumor CEA content and tumor size on tissue uptake of indium 111-labeled anti-CEA monoclonal antibody. *Cancer* 1986; 57: 571-576.
102. Plummer JM, Goodwin JJ, Osband ME. Successful in vitro immunization of human peripheral blood monocular cells against prostate specific antigens: an approach for antigen specific adaptive immunotherapy of prostatic cancer. *J Cell Biochem Sup* 1990; 14B: 91.
103. Posnett DN, McGrath H, Tam JP. A novel method for producing anti-peptide antibodies. *J Biol Chem* 1988; 263: 1719-1725.
104. Racz T, Sacks PG, Taylor DL, Schantz SP. Natural killer cell lysis of head and neck cancer. *Arch Otolarngol Head Neck Surg* 1989; 115: 1322-1328.
105. Ralston S, Hoeprich P, Akita R. Identification and synthesis of the epitope for a human monoclonal antibody which can neutralize human T-cell leukemia/lymphotropic virus Type I. *J Biol Chem* 1989; 264: 16343-16346.
106. Raychaudhuri S, Saeki Y, Fuji H, et al. Tumor-specific idiotype vaccines. 1. Generation and characterization of internal image tumor antigen. *J Immunol* 1986; 137: 1743-1749.
107. Reddish M, Ravindranath MH, Brazeau SM, Morton DL. *Experientia* 1994; 50(7): 648-653.
108. Reeves WC, Brinton LA, Garcia M, et al. Human papillomavirus infection and cervical cancer in Latin America. *N Engl J Med* 1989; 320: 1437-1441.
109. Reisfeld RA, Schultz G, Cheresh D A. Approaches for immunotherapy of malignant melanoma with monoclonal antibodies. In: *Monoclonal Antibodies and Cancer Therapy*, edited by RA Reisfeld and S Sell, pp. 173-191. New York, Alan R. Liss, 1985.
110. Rettig WJ, Cordon-Cardo C, Koulos JP, et al. Cell surface antigens of human trophoblast and choriocarcinoma defined by monoclonal antibodies. *Int J Cancer* 1985; 54: 469-475.
111. Rose TM, Plowman GD, Teplow DB, et al. Primary structure of the human melanoma-associated antigen p97 (melanotransferin) deduced from the mRNA sequence. *Proc Natl Acad Sci* (USA) 1986; 83: 1261-1265.
112. Roth JA, Ames RS, Restrepo C, et al. Monoclonal antibody 45-2D9 recognizes a cell surface glycoprotein on a human c-Ha-ras transformed cell line (45-342) and a shared epitope on human tumors. *J Immunol* 1986; 137: 2385.
113. Sanda MG, Ayyagari SR, Jaffee Em, Epstein JI. *J Urol* 1994; 151(3): 622-628.
114. Savage HE, Rossen RD, Hersh EM, et al. Antibody development to viral and allogeneic tumor cell-associated antigens in patients with malignant melanoma and ovarian carcinoma treated with lysates of virus-infected tumor cells. *Cancer Res* 1986; 46: 2127-2133.
115. Schild H, von Hoegen P, Schirrmacher V. Modification of tumor cells by a low dose of Newcastle disease virus. *Cancer Immunol Immunother* 1989; 28: 22-28.
116. Schlom J. Basic principles and applications of monoclonal antibodies in the management of carcinomas: The

Richard and Hinda Rosenthal foundation award lecture. *Cancer Res* 1986; 46: 3225-3238.
117. Schmoll HJ. *Ann Oncol* 1994; 5 Suppl 3: 115-121.
118. Seigler HF, Wallack MK, Vervaert CE, et al. Melanoma patient antibody responses to melanoma tumor-associated antigens defined by murine monoclonal antibodies. *J Biol Response Mod* 1988; 8: 37-52.
119. Sell S. Cancer markers: past, present and future. In: Monoclonal Antibodies and Cancer Therapy, edited by RA Reisfeld and S Sell. New York, Alan R. Liss, 1985.
120. Sinigaglia R, Guttinger M, Kilgus J, et al. A malaria T-cell epitope recognized in association with most mouse and human MHC class II molecules. *Nature* 1988; 336: 778-780.
121. Sivanandham M, Scoggin SD, Tanaka N, Wallack MK. *Cancer Immunol Immunother* 1994; 38()4): 259-264.
122. Srivastava PK, DeLeo AB, and Old LJ. Tumor rejection antigens of chemically induced sarcomas of inbred mice. *Proc Natl Acad Sci* (USA) 1986; 83: 3407-3411.
123. Stewart-Tull DES. Immunopotentiating conjugates. *Vaccine* 1985; 3: 40-44.
124. Tahara H, Zeh JH III, Storkus WJ, et al. *Cancer Res* 1994; 54(1): 182-189.
125. Tai T, Cahan LD, Tsuchida T, et al. Immunogenicity of melanoma-associated gangliosides in cancer patients. *Int J Cancer* 1985; 35: 607-612.
126. Tanaka K, Hayashi H, Hamada C, et al. Expression of major histocompatibility complex class I antigens as a strategy for the potentiation of immune recognition of tumor cells. *Proc Natl Acad Sci* (USA) 1986; 83: 8723-8727.
127. Taniguchi N, Lizuka S, Zhe ZN, et al. Measurements of human serum immunoreactive γ-glutamyl transpeptidase in patients with malignant tumors using enzyme-linked immunosorbent assay. *Cancer Res* 1985; 45: 5835-5839.
128. Tepper RI. Cytokines and strategies for anticancer vaccines. *Contemporary Oncology* 1993; 9: 38-53.
129. Towbin H, Staehelin T, Gordon J. Electrophoretic transfer of proteins from polyacrylamide gels to nitrocellulose sheets: procedure and some applications. *Proc Natl Acad Sci* (USA) 1979; 76: 4350-4354.
130. Townsend SE, Allison JP. *Science* 1993; 259-262.
131. Uede T, Yamari T, Shijubo N, et al. *In vivo* factor(s) responsible for CTL induction. *Gann Monograph on Cancer Research* 1988; 34: 91-106.
132. Ullrich SJ, Robinson EA, Law LW, et al. A mouse tumor-specific transplantation antigen is a heat shock-related protein. *Proc Natl Acad Sci* (USA) 1986; 83: 3121-3125.
133. Urban JL, Kripke ML, Schreiber H. Stepwise immunologic selection of antigenic variants during tumor growth. *J Immunother* 1986; 137: 3036-3041.
134. Waldman TA, Davis MM, Bongiovanni KF, et al. Rearrangements of genes for the antigen receptor on T-cells as markers of lineage and clonality in human lymphoid neoplasms. *N Engl J Med* 1985; 313: 776-783.
135. Wallich R, Bulbuc N, Hammerling GJ, et al. Abrogation of metastatic properties of tumour cells by de novo expression of H-2K antigens following H-2 gene transfection. *Nature* 1985; 315: 301-305.
136. Watt KWK, Lee P-J, Timkulu TM, et al. Human prostate-specific antigen: Structural and functional similarity with serine proteases. *Proc Natl Acad Sci* (USA) 1986; 83: 3166-3170.
137. Watts TH, Gariepy J, Schoolnik GK, et al. T-cell activation by peptide antigen: Effect of peptide sequence and method of antigen presentation. *Proc Natl Acad Sci* (USA) 1985; 82: 5480-5484.
138. Weinberg A, Merigan TC. Recombinant interleukin 2 as an adjuvant for vaccine-induced protection: Immunization of guinea pigs with Herpes Simplex virus subunit vaccines. *J Immunol* 1988; 140: 294-299.
139. Weisenburger TH, Jones PC, Ahn SS, et al. Active specific intralymphatic immunotherapy in metastic malignant melanoma: evidence of clinical response. *J Biol Resp Modif* 1982; 1: 57-66.
140. Wettendorff M, Iliopoulos D, Tempero M, et al. Idiotypic cascades in cancer patients treated with monoclonal antibody CO17-1A. *Proc Natl Acad Sci* (USA) 1989; 86: 3787-3791.
141. Wilson IA, Niman HL, Houghten RA, et al. The structure of an antigenic determinant in a protein. *Cell* 1984; 37: 767-778.
142. Wiseman CL, Rao VS, Kennedy PS, et al. Clinical responses with active specific intralymphatic immunotherapy for cancer-A Phase I-II trial. *West J Med* 1989; 151: 283-288).
143. Yamada G, Hatakeyama M, Fujita T, Taniguchi T. Molecular biology of the interleukin-2 system. *Gann Monograph on Cancer Research* 1988; 34: 167-178.

CHEMICAL INDUCERS OF LYMPHOKINES

RICHARD V. SMALLEY and ROBERT K. OLDHAM
Synertron, Inc., Madison, Wisconsin and
Biological Therapy Institute Foundation, Franklin, Tennessee; and University of Missouri, Columbia, Missouri

Several agents have the capacity to 'artificially' initiate or augment an immunologic response and thereby induce or increase cytokine production. The production of lymphokines (including interferons, alpha, beta, and gamma, interleukin 2, tumor necrosis factor beta), several colony-stimulating factors (including interleukin 3), and the monokines (including tumor necrosis factor alpha and interleukin 1) can all be induced by a variety of chemical and natural substances [62, 64, 65, 76, 100, 105, 109, 110, 147]. The nature of the interrelationship among these cytokines, following induction or following the generation of an immune response, is not completely understood. However, interleukin 2 is required for endogenous interferon-gamma production and also may itself be induced following interleukin 1 release by monocytes. The relationship, if any, of interleukin 3 and other colony-stimulating factors and the tumor necrosis factors to these events is unknown. However, agents such as the tumor promoter phorbol myristate acetate, the calcium ionophore A23 187, and bacterial lipopolysaccharide all have cytokine augmenting capabilities as well as other profound effects on the immune system [62, 76, 100]. Frequently, two or more agents are synergistic in these effects. Whether such agents or their analogs can ever be considered therapeutic remains conjectural.

Originally, these agents were developed as 'interferon inducers.' With the advent of recombinant DNA technology, nearly all effort has been placed on the development of the natural effector molecules themselves. However, it may be that these agents, now recognized as general immune stimulants and cytokine inducers, may still have an independent role as antitumor agents.

A number of agents, both natural and synthetic, capable of inducing interferon production either *in vitro* or *in vivo*, have been identified, either serendipitously or by extensive screening in the search for agents with antiviral activity [40, 91, 132, 143, 144]. Several microorganisms, including viruses, some bacteria (e.g., *Brucella abortus, Corynebacterium parvum*), protozoa, rickettsiae, and mycoplasmas, as well as bacterial products such as endotoxin and certain antibiotics, natural and synthetic nucleic acids, the polycarboxylates, complex carbohydrates, and certain low-molecular-weight amines, including the pyrimidinones, the fluorenones and the lipoidal amines, all have been shown to induce circulating interferon levels. In addition, most of these agents have also been shown to have a profound effect on the immune system. While some have also been evaluated in mice and subhuman primates for their antitumor and/or immunomodulating effects, very few have been tested in humans.

The mechanism(s) by which interferon production is induced by these agents is unknown. Some are capable of inducing interferon either *in vitro* or *in vivo*, but many are active only *in vivo*, suggesting that interactions among cellular populations are necessary in certain circumstances. Generally, the antitumor activity and immunomodulating capabilities of interferon inducers have been correlated with their ability to induce demonstrable levels of circulating interferon. However, some interferon inducers augment biological activity without inducing a detectable circulating interferon level, and others may have biological activity independent of their ability to induce interferon production. These remain of some clinical interest. While the lack of sufficient interferon to do all of the desired preclinical and clinical trials undoubtedly led to much of the original interest in inducers, an immune-modulating capability of their own should be sufficient to foster interest in them currently; most of the development currently is taking place in patients with viral diseases.

POLYNUCLEOTIDES

Following the demonstration that interferon induction by viruses appeared to be correlated with double-stranded RNA (dsRNA), a wide variety of double-stranded polynucleotides were synthesized and evaluated. These agents remain the most efficient agents capable of interferon induction, and many have been shown to have immune augmenting capabilities independent of interferon induction. Double-strandedness, RNA as opposed to DNA, and a molecular weight greater than 100,000 are characteristics associated with interferon induction. Beyond these basic criteria, various substitutions have been made and different length chains, both matched and mismatched, have been synthesized and studied with varying results.

Poly I:C was the initial polynucleotide to be evaluated preclinically, and much of the scientific basis and

R.K. Oldham (ed.), Principles of Cancer Biotherapy. 3rd ed., 192–210.

Table 1. Interferon inducers

	Demonstrable IFN induction		Demonstrable antitumor activity		Oral parenteral	Immune augment
	Animals	Humans	Animals	Humans		
Polynucleotides						
Poly I:C	+	–	+	–	P	+
Poly I:C (LC)	+	+	+	+	P	+
Poly I:C (U12)	+	+	+	+	P	+
Poly A:U	+	+	+	+	P	+
Low-molecular-weight compounds						
Pyrimidinones	+	+	+	+	p o	+
Anthraquinones	+	?	+	?	p o	+
Lipoidal amines	+	+	+	?	p o	+
Acridines	+	+	+	?	p o	+
Miscellaneous	+	?	+	?	p o	+
Carboxylates						
MVE-2	+	–	+	–	P	+
Complex carbohydrates						
Acemannan	+	?	+	?	P/Po	+

rationale for the development of polynucleotides rests on data obtained from these original studies in rodents. However, once it was determined that poly I:C was hydrolyzed in mammalian circulation, it was necessary to develop other polynucleotide molecules for clinical study.

Poly I:C (LC) was the first of the 'second generation' polynucleotides to undergo evaluation. This molecule has been shown to be quite toxic at doses associated with active interferon induction in humans, but some clinical trials have suggested that lower, relatively nontoxic doses may well be immunostimulatory although perhaps not capable of inducing demonstrable circulating interferon levels. Two other polynucleotides, poly I:C (U12) and poly A:U, have undergone preliminary evaluation in humans. Both are relatively nontoxic and have been shown to augment biological responses *in vitro* and to have immune-augmenting and antitumor capabilities *in vivo* in both humans and mice.

Poly I:C

Poly I:C has demonstrable antitumor and immune-augmenting activity in several rodent systems and is the most widely studied interferon inducer in these systems [82]. The antitumor effect of this agent has been greater in the slower-growing as opposed to the rapidly dividing murine tumor (i.e., L1210 leukemia) systems. A modest increase in the median survival of animals treated with poly I:C as compared with nontreatment controls has been demonstrated in Ehrlich ascites, two different reticulum cell sarcomas, and in the carcinosarcoma Walker 256 systems. The mechanism of antitumor action is unknown.

Poly I:C (LC)

Preclinical studies

After extensive studies in rodent models, it was learned that poly I:C was not very efficient at interferon induction in primates because of nucleolytic (hydrolytic) activity present in human and other primate circulation. Various complexes were formed in attempts to counteract this hydrolysis. One such formulation, a complex of poly-L-lysine and carboxymethylcellulose followed by the addition of poly I:C, has been the focus of clinical studies. This material, poly I:C (LC), is relatively resistant to hydrolysis by primate sera and is capable of inducing detectable interferon production in both monkeys and humans [81]. Poly I:C (LC) is moderately toxic when administered intravenously (iv) at doses above 4 mg/m^2, a dose which effectively induces interferon in humans [124, 126]. Lower doses have immune-augmenting capabilities that may be substantial and that induce barely detectable levels of circulating interferon. Poly I:C (LC) induces levels of interferon in rodents that are two to three times greater than poly I:C. In monkeys, a dose of 3-5 mg/kg administered iv induces circulating levels of interferon above 3000 units/ml for up to 10 h postinjection, with measurable levels of over 100 units/ml still present 48 h later. In humans, this level of circulating interferon activity has been associated with significant resistance to virus infections and antitumor activity. Poly I:C (LC) is also a good vaccine adjuvant in primates [82]. Antibody production following vaccination with several relatively weak vaccines such as Venezuelan equine encephalomyelitis, *Hemophilus influenza*, or polysaccharide vaccine oral monovalent influenzal strain has been augmented when the vaccine is administered in association with poly I:C (LC). Augmentation was achieved with doses as low as 10μg/kg, a dose that will not induce detectable levels of interferon in the serum of monkeys. The immunomodulating effects of poly I:C (LC) have been extensively studied in murine systems. Chirigos et al. [23] examined the effects of poly I:C (LC), administered systemically, on macrophage function, natural killer (NK) cell cytotoxicity, delayed hypersensitivity, lymphocyte blastogenesis, and interferon induction. The *in vitro* effect on macrophage function was also compared to *in vivo* stimulation. Poly I:C (LC) induced a 60-90% increase in cytotoxicity. No dose-dependent effects were observed over a wide concentration range (0.05-200 μg/ml). A similar assay, using peritoneal macrophages, was performed following the intraperitoneal (ip) administration of 10 and 100 μg per mouse (roughly comparable to 0.5-5.0 mg/kg). Peritoneal macrophages from treated animals again inhibited tumor cell growth, with the peak effect noted 24 h following administration. There was the suggestion that the 100-μg dose augmented cytotoxicity to a greater degree than did the 10-μg dose, but this was not dramatic. However, augmentation was demonstrable for only 3 days following the 10-μg dose and for 6 days following the 100-μg dose. Both doses also augmented NK cytotoxicity as measured by a 4-h ^{51}Cr release assay. Again, the effect was sustained longer following the 100-μg dose. Interferon induction was greater following the 100-μg dose and was demonstrable as early as 4 h after treatment with peak titers occurring at 8 h. Activity as still demonstrable 48 h posttreatment. *In vitro* stimulation by poly I:C (LC) was also shown to augment the mitogenic response of splenic lymphocytes to the T-cell mitogen phytohemagglutinin (PHA) (concentration range 1-100 μg/ml) and to suppress the response to the B-cell mitogen, lipopolysaccharide. No dose dependency was observed in either case. A dose of 4 and 40 but not 400 μg/mouse also augmented delayed hypersensitivity as measured by footpad thickness, 24 and 48 h following a sheep red blood cell challenge.

Poly I:C (LC) was studied [135-137] in the preclinical screen operated for a few years by the Biological Response Modifiers Program (BRMP) of the U.S. National Cancer Institute (NCI) [39]. Poly I:C (LC) demonstrated greater immune-augmenting capacity in this screen than any other agent tested. It induced macrophage cytotoxicity following *in vitro* stimulation at concentrations between 0.0001 and 0.1 μg/ml (a higher concentration suppressed activity), and *in vivo* (ip) administration of a dose of 0.05 – 0.5 mg/kg (lower and higher doses were ineffective) induced levels of cytotoxicity equal or superior to those of any other agent previously studied. Augmentation of NK cytotoxicity was demonstrated by both *in vivo* administration of 0.5 – 1.0 mg/kg (other doses not evaluated) and *in vitro* (0.001 – 10 μg/ml) stimulation. There was a suggestion of concentration dependency. Poly I:C (LC), administered to mice at a dose of 0.5 mg/kg, was equally effective as an immune modulator by iv, ip, intradermal (id), or subcutaneous (sc) administration, although sc administration induced a more prolonged augmentation. Intravenous administration (1 mg/kg) was shown to be effective in augmenting NK activity in a variety of compartments including circulating, splenic, peritoneal, and pulmonary, and was equally effective on splenic NK cytotoxicity whether administered daily, twice a week, or weekly. Contrary to experience with other inducers, an NK hyporesponsive state was not induced by frequent administration. There was a narrow concentration-dependent (1-5 μg/ml) range capable of augmenting T-cell activity, as measured by the mixed leukocyte reaction, but no effect could be shown on the mixed leukocyte-tumor cell reaction, which measures the induction of specific cytotoxicity. Further, poly I:C (LC) acted as a vaccine adjuvant when administered either iv, ip, or admixed (1.25 mg/kg) with a suboptimally effective tumor cell challenge. Circulating interferon blood levels were induced by either 0.5 or 5.0 mg/kg [156].

Poly I:C (LC) was also shown to have significant antitumor activity in a number of animal models and was reported to increase the median life span in tumor bearers to a degree comparable to poly I:C [82]. In the BRMP preclinical screen, poly I:C (LC) was administered therapeutically to animals both prior (1 day) and subsequent 1-8 days) to iv injection of tumor cells (2.5-5.0 x 10^{-4}), using both the UV 2237 and the B16/BL6 melanoma system. In all circumstances, poly I:C (LC) decreased the number of metastases and induced a number of cures. Effectiveness was demonstrable over a dose range of 0.05 and 2.5 mg/kg with a tendency for the highest dose to be more effective with larger tumor burdens. Schedule dependency was demonstrable. Administration of poly I:C (LC) two or three times weekly was more effective than weekly. In addition, poly I:C (LC) was also effective in a 'spontaneous' metastasis model in which animals were treated 3 days following amputation of a limb bearing an 0.8- to 1.0-cm footpad tumor. All such animals without treatment develop lung metastases within 2-3 weeks, while poly I:C (LC) induced cures in 50%. Again, a larger dose tended to be more effective than a smaller one [136]. These data confirm and extend the earlier reports of Chirigos et al. [23].

In summary, poly I:C (LC) has a significant immunomodulating effect on the four major cellular immune compartments in mice as demonstrated both *in vitro* and *in vivo. In vitro* the effective concentration range may be wide (several logs) for augmentation of NK and macrophage cytotoxicity, but *in vivo* the dose range is narrow. Poly I:C (LC) has significant antitumor effects in several murine tumor models, many designed to demonstrate presumed NK or macrophage antitumor activity. Whether this antitumor activity is due to one or more direct immunomodulatory effects or to a secondary effect from interferon induction has not been ascertained. In an early study of poly I:C, antitumor effect was specifically aborted by anti-interferon antibody, suggesting that the induction of interferon was crucial for antitumor activity [46]. The fact that higher doses and more frequent administration may result in better antitumor activity also suggests that interferon may be the mediator. Additional studies evaluating the mechanism of antitumor action are needed in murine models, as are correlation studies comparing these murine data with human studies, before one can be confident that these models will be predictive of the human situation. The murine studies do indicate, however, that poly I:C (LC) is a potent immune stimulant with antitumor activity.

Clinical studies

Several clinical trials were performed in the 70's with poly I:C (LC) under the sponsorship of Dr. Hilton Levy and the National Institute of Allergy and Infectious Diseases. Two of these were classic dose-escalation phase I studies [69, 77-80] in patients with a variety of malignancies. However, these early studies suggested a dose that has subsequently been determined to be poorly tolerated by the vast majority of patients. Several additional phase I-II studies were performed in patients with neurologic disorders [4, 20, 36, 90], multiple myeloma [32], malignant melanoma [50], and the pediatric tumors, acute leukemia and neuroblastoma [75]. These studies generally used a constant fixed dose administered by a variety of schedules. A later study evaluated the effect of two low but tolerable doses on the immune system [126] in a phase IB immune stimulation study.

Levine and associates treated 25 patients, administering poly I:C (LC) iv over a 60-min period at doses ranging from 0.5 to 27 mg/m^2 [77-80]. Groups of three patients were entered at each dose level and received a single dose followed by a 7-day rest, followed in turn by a daily dose administered for 14 days. Side effects consisted of fever, nausea, serum glutanic/oxaloacetic transaminase (SGOT) elevations of greater than 50%, a transient depression of the white blood cell count (lymphocytes) and platelets, both transient asymptomatic mild hypotension in some and significant symptomatic hypotension to a level of 60/0 in others, arthralgia, and acute renal failure. The latter three effects were noted at doses over 12 mg/m^2. Peak serum levels of interferon of 15 units/ml were induced by doses up to 4 mg/m^2, 200 units/ml by doses up to 8 mg/m^2, and over 2000 units/ml by doses of 12 mg/m^2 and greater. Peak levels occurred 5-8 h after administration and lasted for up to 24 h. The authors reported one minor antitumor response in a patient with acute lymphatic leukemia. No antitumor effect was seen in four other patients with acute leukemia, in six patients with sarcoma, three with lymphoma, four with lung cancer, two with renal-cell carcinoma, or one each with hepatoma, myeloma, prostate cancer, or the carcinoid syndrome. An increase in NK cytotoxicity was noted in several patients in association with a high serum titer of interferon. Some patients eventually became refractory to sustained interferon induction, and NK activity also declined [51].

Krown administered poly I:C (LC) iv over 30 min [69] to 14 patients with malignancy. Five patients initiated therapy at a daily dose of 1 mg/m^2 and underwent a dose escalation (doubling) every four doses. Because of toxicity, this schedule was altered and the subsequent nine patients received escalating doses of 0.01, 0.03, 0.1, and 0.3 mg/m^2 daily for the first 4 days, followed by 3 days of therapy at 1 mg/m^2 followed by 3 days of rest; dose escalations (doubling) to tolerance then occurred every 6 days. The major dose-limiting toxicity was either rigor in six patients (at a dose ranging from 2 to 12 mg/m^2) or hypotension in five patients (over a dose range of 0.3-8 mg/m^2). The mean maximum tolerated dose was 4 mg/m^2 and the maximum individually tolerated dose was 12 mg/m^2. However, effects were unpredictable and dose-limiting toxicity was seen over a wide range of doses in various patients. Fever, beginning within 4-8 h of drug administration and lasting 6-12 h, was associated with significant rigors and occurred in all patients at doses greater than 1 mg/m^2. Some dyspnea and chest pain were occasionally noted at doses greater than 4 mg/m^2. Hypotension occurred in nine patients, usually in association with or just after rigors, and reached symptomatic levels (60/0) in five. Compensatory tachycardia did not occur. Hypotension was generally relieved by vigorous saline infusions. Leukopenia less than 200/mm^3 and thrombocytopenia less than 100, 000/mm^3 each occurred in five patients. The bone marrow was cellular in the three patients with cytopenia in whom it was evaluated. No objective antitumor responses occurred in eight patients with melanoma nor in one each with chronic lymphatic leukemia (CLL), breast carcinoma, myeloma, or head and neck cancer. An antitumor effect with less than 50% tumor reduction was noted in one patient with renal-cell carcinoma and in one patient with CLL.

The Children's Cancer Study Group (CCSG) treated 38 children with chemotherapy-refractory acute leukemia with poly I:C (LC) administered iv over a 60-min period [75]. They also found that an initial dose of 9-12 mg/m^2 was intolerable and therefore switched to an escalating schedule beginning with 3 mg/m^2 followed by a 3-mg/m^2 increase every 2 days as tolerated. A dose of 9 mg/m^2, administered daily, was tolerable in most children. Fever was a major side effect regardless of dose, but tachyphylaxis to this side effect was noted. Hypotension, arthralgia, and central nervous system (CNS) toxicity appeared to be dose related, occurring at a dose of 9 mg/m^2 or higher. Severe hypotension, requiring plasma expanders, occurred in five patients and seizures and/or coma in three patients at these higher doses. No objective tumor responses were noted in this series, although one heavily infiltrated marrow became hypoplastic after treatment. In a subsequent trial in children with neuroblastoma, side effects were similar using the same dose and schedule. No objective responses were noted in the 13 patients in this series.

In a small series of seven patients with multiple myeloma, Durie et al. noted one partial response and three minor responses with poly I:C (LC) administered at a dose of 4 mg/m^2 or less three times weekly (tiw). Side effects were minimal; the drug was well tolerated at this relatively low dose [32].

Poly I:C (LC) was administered to 16 patients with malignant melanoma at a dose of 5 mg/m^2 twice weekly by iv injection. Fever and fatigue were dose-limiting. Interferon was consistently induced in all patients within 8 h of injection. No enhancement of interferon induction was detected on the second day when poly I:C (LC) was given on 2 consecutive days. No objective antitumor responses were noted [50].

Engel et al. [36] administered poly I:C (LC) to 21 patients with a variety of nonmalignant neurologic disorders, administering a dose of 1.4-6.4 mg/m^2 weekly by a 60-min iv infusion. All patients developed fever, nausea, and vomiting, while two patients had an increase in SGOT and three developed thrombocytopenia of less than 100,000/mm^3. Hypotension did not occur, although arthralgia was noted 24 h after each dose in all patients. Champney et al. [20] treated 14 patients with neurologic disorders, including eight with a dose of 6-12 mg/m^2 daily for 5 days and five with a dose of 4-6 mg/m^2 administered weekly. Toxicity consisted of fever in 13 of 14 patients, lymphopenia in 10 of 14, and hypotension in seven of 14 (all of the later occurring at doses of 6 mg/m^2 or greater).

Eighteen patients with multiple sclerosis were treated within weekly intravenous doses of poly I:C (LC) starting with 20 μg/kg (100 ug/kg) is roughly comparable to 4-5 mg/m^2). Thereafter, poly I:C (LC) was administered biweekly or monthly for up to 18 months. Fever was the dose-limiting side effect. Serum levels of alpha-interferon peaked at 8-12 h following the poly I:C (LC) infusion and were comparable to an intravenous dose of 3-6 million units of alpha-interferon. There was no correlation between fever and interferon levels, suggesting that other cytokines might be involved. Of interest, serum levels of interferon were higher in males than in females. A marked elevation of serum cortisol levels 4 h postinfusion was also noted. Stabilization of disease was noted in some [3-5, 90].

In a phase IB study performed subsequently to the above studies, Stevenson et al. administered two doses, 1 and 4 mg/m^2, twice a week for 4 weeks and evaluated the effect on immune function in patients with metastatic cancer [126]. Twenty-five patients with metastatic carcinoma were entered. Toxicities observed at the 1 mg/m^2 dose were mild hypotension, fever, nausea, vomiting, fatigue, and headache. These were all reasonably well tolerated by these patients. The first patient treated at the 4 mg/m^2 dose was taken off study after receiving one dose because of severe hypotension (60/0 mm Hg). The subsequent nine patients treated on this arm of the study received an initial dose of 1 mg/m^2 followed by 4 mg/m^2 twice weekly. No further problems with hypotension were encountered, and toxicities in these patients were similar to those seen at the lower dose. This study was then similar to those seen at the lower dose. This study was then expanded and, in all, a total of 59 patients were monitored for changes in immunological functions. Twenty patients received poly I:C (LC) intramuscularly, twice weekly, 12 receiving 1 mg/m^2 and eight receiving 4 mg/m^2; 17 patients received poly I:C (LC) once weekly by a 1-h iv infusion, nine receiving 1 mg/m^2 and eight receiving 4 mg/m^2 and 22 patients received poly I:C (LC) biw by a 1-h iv infusion, 15 at the lower dose and seven at the higher dose. Natural killer cell activity was elevated slightly at the lower dose and was somewhat depressed at the higher dose administered iv. Monocyte function was elevated in all patients and 2', 5'-oligo A synthetase activity was induced by both doses. Monocyte augmentation and enzyme induction were observed at the lower im dose, despite a lack of detectable circulating interferon. Significant levels of circulating interferon activity were detectable following the 4 mg/m^2 iv dose, and somewhat lower but still detectable levels were demonstrable following the lower iv dose. In contrast, 1 mg/m^2 by intramuscular injection induced no detectable levels of circulating interferon activity. Poly I:C (LC) induced an increase in OKT10 positive cells and a small but consistent trend toward an increase in the ratio of Leu-3/Leu-2 positive cells. The lymphocyte response to concanavalin A was depressed following poly I:C (LC) administration [88, 126].

Droller administered poly I:C (LC) to 11 patients with metastatic renal cell carcinoma. Patients received weekly escalating doses of poly I:C (LC) intravenously starting at 4 mg/m^2 and escalating to 10 mg/m^2 for 4 weeks and then continued at their MTD for an additional 4 weeks. Seven patients completed full course of 8 weeks of treatment. Fever and fatigue were significant side effects. Other side effects included hypotension, myalgia, and lethargy [29]. There were no clinical responses, although two patients had regression of isolated metastases, but in both metastases of other sites progressed. Ewel et al [37] studied the effects of poly I:C (LC) in combination with IL-2 in advanced cancer but no clinical responses were seen.

In summary, clinical toxicity following administration of poly I:C (LC) is significant but is dose related. A dose above 12 mg/m^2 is intolerable, a dose between 6 and 12 mg/m^2 causes some concern, but a dose of 4 mg/m^2 or less is tolerable. Objective antitumor responses (complete, partial, or minor) have been noted in some patients with acute leukemia, myeloma, CLL, and renal-cell carcinoma.

Poly I:C (U12) – Ampligen

In an attempt to improve the therapeutic index, a polymer of poly I:C with mismatched base loopings was synthesized by inserting a uracil approximately every 12 nucleotides in the cytosine chain [13]. Poly I:C (U12) has been directly compared with poly I:C in rabbits and mice and was shown to be less antigenic and less pyrogenic *in vivo* [16, 146]. It will activate 2', 5'-A synthetase and kinase activity in Hela cells and is nearly as active as poly I:C in augmenting NK cytotoxicity *in vitro* [96, 163].

Poly I:C (U12) shows strong antiproliferative activity against human carcinoid tumor cells in a clonogenic assay under conditions in which both natural alpha- and beta-interferon are inactive [16]. Clinical experience in patients with carcinoid tumors remains limited. Four patients with this tumor have received relatively low doses of poly I:C (U12) in a phase I study, but no responses were seen [10].

In vivo murine studies, transplanting human renal cell carcinoma cells into athymic mice, reveal poly I:C (U12) to have a strong antitumor effect under circumstances in which these tumors are largely unaffected by alpha-interferon [16]. In comparative studies in which tumor cell lines were grown in petri dishes and the anti-proliferative effects of natural interferons alpha and beta were compared to the effects of poly I:C and poly I:C (U12), independent sensitivity of these lines to interferons and dsRNA were demonstrated. However, use of an antibody to natural beta-interferon did abort some of the polynucleotide-induced cytotoxicity [60]. Additionally, both synergy and antagonism have been demonstrated between beta-interferon and the dsRNA *in vivo* in human bladder tumor xenograft models, indicating that extensive preclinical testing is needed before combination studies are utilized [16, 59].

Hubbel et al. have shown independent sensitivity in an *in vitro* cytotoxicity assay in which human tumor cell lines were grown with and without interferons alpha, beta, and the two polynucleotides poly I:C and I:C (U12). In cell lines resistant to interferon, polynucleotides induced cytotoxicity and vice versa. However, independence is not complete since antibodies to interferon-beta block some of the cytotoxic effect of polynucleotides [62].

A preliminary clinical report discussed the use of poly I:C (U12) in five patients, each of whom received between 10 and 20 mg twice a week intravenously [10, 15, 127]. An objective antitumor effect was observed in one patient with myeloma whose Bence Jones protein decreased from over 5 g/day to less than 2 g/day. Toxicity was nil. It is stated, although data were not provided, that poly I:C (U12) induced 2', 5'-A synthetase and protein kinase activity.

A more complete phase I trial has been performed in which patients received poly I:C (U12) twice weekly by a 30-min intravenous infusion [128]. Groups of one to six patients were entered at one of eight dose levels: 10, 20, 40, 80, 120, 200, 300 and 500 mg. There were three objective responses (two partial and one complete) observed, all in patients with renal-cell carcinoma. There was said to be correlation between the clonogenic assay and the clinical results in patients with renal cell carcinoma. Approximately 50% of renal cell carcinoma specimens are sensitive to ampligen *in vitro* [129-131]. No toxicity or side effects were noted. Neither the length of treatment nor the degree of biological response modification observed were reported.

Cumulative doses of over 4 g have been well tolerated. The drug has been given by iv infusion in doses of 10-500 mg/infusion twice a week, in some instances for more than a year, without significant side effects. Side effects when seen consist of mild fatigue and/or flu-like symptoms similar to but less severe than alpha-interferon side effects. Antibody formation to poly I:C (U12) in these human trials has not been demonstrated [10].

Poly I:C (U12) has been shown to inhibit replication of variants of the human immunodeficiency virus (HIV) and to synergistically enhance the antiviral activity of zidovudine (AZT) [97, 98]. Following these *in vitro* demonstrations, a clinical trial was performed in which 10 patients with either AIDS-related complex (ARC) or AIDS (acquired immune deficiency syndrome) were treated with 200-250 mg intravenously twice a week. No toxicity was observed. Clinical improvement was reported in the patients with AIDS. Eight of the 10 patients were anergic prior to therapy – all recovered delayed hypersensitivity following treatment; there was an improvement in the T4/T8 ratio in the ARC patients; there was a decrease in the HIV RNA levels in all patients in whom it was present pretherapy; and finally loss of inhibition of the RNAase system, which can degrade macromolecular RNA, was demonstrated [14]. Subsequently, studies by Carter et al. [17] reported stable CD4 cell counts and negative P24 antigen serum levels for two years post treatment.

In summary, poly I:C (U12) appears to be well tolerated when administered twice a week by 30-min iv infusion, in doses up to and including 300 mg. Three objective antitumor responses have been reported, two in patients with renal-cell carcinoma and one in a patient with myeloma, and there is also the suggestion of beneficial activity in patients infected with HIV. Additional studies are ongoing in patients with hepatitis and AIDS.

Poly I:C (L)

A single trial with this synthetic polynucleotide was performed in a small number of patients. Alpha-interferon induction was demonstrated, but the trial was aborted prematurely because of antibody production to I:C (L) in over half of the patients [68].

Polyadenylic Acid – Polyuridylic Acid (Poly A:U)

Preclinical studies

In a review of preclinical studies, Johnson reported that poly A:U has immune-augmenting capabilities similar to other polynucleotides despite the fact that it is a very poor inducer of interferon [61]. Augmentation of murine macrophage activity has been shown with an effect on both antigen processing ability and cytotoxicity following *in vitro* stimulation. The potential role or influence of T helper cells in these processes is undetermined. Although poly A:U is not directly mitogenic, it is readily bound by thymocytes and augments release of lymphokine activity, at least as measured by plaque-forming cell activity. Cell surface markers including surface immunoglobulin and T-cell differentiation expression antigens have been increased. The T-suppressor cell activity may also be increased; timing of adjuvant and antigen presentation is crucial – adjuvant presentation prior to antigen contact induces suppressor activity. The *in vitro* response to antigen stimulation of T cells is enhanced by poly A:U with augmentation in the development of but not activity per se of specific cytotoxic cells. Augmentation of B cell activity has also been noted, but it has not been determined whether this is a result of direct stimulation or an indirect effect mediated by T cells.

In a series of studies evaluating the effect of poly A:U on NK cytotoxicity and on the induction of interferon-induced enzyme activity, Hovanessian et al. have reported that augmentation of NK cytotoxicity and induction of protein kinase and 2', 5'-A synthetase occurred in normal or tumor-bearing rodents [55, 159, 161]. In the spontaneous mammary tumor system of C3H mice, 300 µg/mouse of poly A:U augmented NK cytotoxicity in the splenic cells of tumor bearers when administered either as a single agent or combined with cyclophosphamide; synergy was demonstrable in the latter circumstance [161]. When administered to normal mice intravenously, intramuscularly, or intraperitoneally (but not subcutaneously) in doses of 10 µg or greater, poly A:U augmented splenic NK cytotoxicity. The augmentation of NK cytotoxicity correlated with the induction of 2', 5'-A synthetase activity. The duration of augmentation was directly related to dose; a dose of 10, 100, 300 and 600 µg/mouse all quantitatively augmented NK activity equally, but successively higher doses increased the duration of effect from 2 to 6 days. A dose of 1 µg was ineffective in inducing either NK cytotoxicity or 2', 5'-A activity. All doses, however, including 1 µg, induced a dip or fall in NK activity on day 7. In these experiments, as in experiments with poly I:C (LC), hyporesponsiveness was not noted. NK augmentation was repeatedly induced by weekly administration of poly A:U, and when administered daily for 3 days or on a repetitive basis every 4 days, a boost in 2', 5'-A synthetase activity was invariably seen [159]. In separate experiments, it was demonstrated that a dose of 40 µg/mouse (2 mg/kg) or greater was needed to induce demonstrable levels of circulating interferon activity while a dose fivefold less (8 µg/mouse) induced enzyme activity and augmented NK cytotoxicity [55].

In an interesting series of experiments, nude mice, carrying a xenograft of HeLa cells, were treated with either poly A:U, murine alpha/beta-interferon, or human beta-interferon. Murine interferon stimulated protein kinase and 2', 5'-A synthetase activity in the host cells, human beta-interferon stimulated similar activity in the human xenograft, while poly A:U stimulated enzyme activity and demonstrable interferon production in both murine and human (HeLa) cells [115]. All three approaches inhibited tumor growth, poly A:U to a greater extent than either interferon [53]. Thus, human tumor cells may be induced to produce interferon following poly A:U stimulation with subsequent interferon induction of both protein kinase and 2', 5'-A synthetase activity.

Wiltrout et al. compared the effect of poly A:U, poly I:C (U12), and poly I:C (LC) on NK cytotoxicity and interferon production in a variety of murine lymphocyte compartments. A similar concentration (1-100 µg) of each induced respectively 10, 10-25, and 20-40% cytotoxicity. Thus, all three polynucleotides augment NK cytotoxicity, but at a comparable dose poly A:U does so somewhat less effectively [156].

Poly A:U has been shown to augment T-cell response to soluble and cell-bound antigenic stimuli when added to *in vitro* cultures of both murine and human lymphocytes responsive to allogeneic cells or antigens such as PPD [22, 25, 44, 45, 102, 148]. This augmentation is most effectively demonstrated using suboptimal concentrations of antigen. A bell-shaped dose-response curve was demonstrable, but the optimum concentration of poly A:U depended on the antigen involved and the individual tested and ranged from 25 to 1600 µg/ml. This effect, which may be due to an adherent population of cells [102], influenced the speed and magnitude of the response; once cytotoxicity was demonstrable no additional augmentation occurred.

Talmadge et al. have evaluated poly A:U in the BRMP preclinical screen and have demonstrated substantial immune augmentation of macrophage cytotoxicity, and both NK and T-cell cytotoxicity. In addition, poly A:U has antitumor activity in both experimental and spontaneous metastases models, although somewhat less activity, on a milligram for milligram basis, than poly I:C (LC) [134].

Poly A:U has *in vivo* antitumor activity in at least four rodent systems [7, 71, 72, 161]. A dose of 250 µg/mouse (25 times the minimum immune augmenting dose), administered iv weekly for 6 weeks, reduced the number of subsequent metastases and prolonged life when administered as adjuvant therapy following complete surgical removal of the primary spontaneous mammary tumor of C3H mice [71]. Administered at a dose of 200 µg/hamster every other day for 2 weeks, it also reduced the incidence of early metastases in a highly metastasizing transplantable tumor of hamster [71]. Three doses of 15 µg (the minimum immune-augmenting dose) given iv within 5 days of birth delayed and/or prevented the development of a spontaneous mammary tumor in a significant number of C3H mice [72]. Also using a transplanted C3H mammary tumor, the Lacours demonstrated that cyclophosphamide plus poly A:U, 300 µg/mouse every 2 weeks for four doses, was synergistic. Smaller tumors, fewer animals with tumor, and prolongation of life were all noted in the combined treatment group [161]. In these experiments it was also shown that there was a synergistic effect on splenic NK cytotoxicity of tumor-bearing animals, and activity against YAC-1 cells was substantially greater in the combined treatment (poly A:U plus cyclophosphamide) group that in either the single agent or no-treatment groups [161]. Finally, Borden et al. have demonstrated antitumor activity for both poly I:C and poly A:U using the MBT-2 transplantable bladder cell tumor of mice. In these experiments, poly I:C proved to be more effective than poly A:U on a milligram for milligram basis, but tolerable doses of poly A:U (10 mg/kg, 20 times the minimum immune augmenting dose) were effective in delaying tumor growth following the implantation of 10^5 or 10^6 tumor cells. Interestingly, poly I:C was more effective against a larger than a smaller tumor inoculum, and synergy between cyclophosphamide and poly I:C was also demonstrable [7].

Poly A:U has given mixed results as an antitumor agent in murine models. Long-term therapy (weekly at doses of 1.5-2.0 mg/mouse) had divergent results, enhancing the development of C3H spontaneous mammary tumors and decreasing the incidence of spontaneous AKR leukemia [27, 28]. In the AKR leukemia experiments, a dose-response curve was demonstrated; 1500 mg was substantially more effective than lower doses. The differences between these experiments in which poly A:U enhanced mammary tumor development and those of Lacour et al. in which tumor development was delayed or prevented were (a) dose (substantially larger in these experiments), (b) timing (much later in life in these experiments), and (c) longer duration of therapy.

Singh et al. have shown in rats implanted with tumor that surgery and allogeneic blood transfusions are followed by enhanced growth of tumor metastases. This is thought to be due, at least in part, to an immunosuppressive effect of surgery. They administered poly A:U at a dose of 1.5 mg/week as a single dose weekly for 3 weeks to rats who had been inoculated with LS 175 tumor cells on day 0 and who then underwent either syngeneic or allogeneic blood transfusion alone or in combination with abdominal surgery. Using appropriate controls, it could be shown that the administration of poly A:U in this fashion significantly reduced tumor growth [123].

Thus, poly A:U has been shown to be an immune-augmenting agent at doses below those required to induce demonstrable interferon production. Alpha/beta-interferon is induced by doses of 40 μg/mouse (2 mg/kg), while interferon-induced enzyme activity and NK cytotoxicity are augmented by doses fivefold less. The prophylactic use of poly A:U in this dose range will prevent the spontaneous development of a mammary tumor in some but not all mice. Therapeutic antitumor activity has been demonstrated using doses 20-50 times (1-1.5 logs) greater than the minimum immune-augmenting dose, although dose-response trials have not been performed. Doses in the therapeutic range of 200-500 μg/mouse have been shown to be optimum for inducing continual immune stimulation as defined by enzyme induction and NK augmentation.

Clinical studies

Poly A:U was initially evaluated in humans in an exploratory study of 15 patients with a variety of malignancies [150]. It was administered intravenously, at a dose of 15 mg, over a 5- to 10-min period, twice weekly for at least 3 weeks. Significant toxicity was not seen. Immunologically, the effect on delayed hypersensitivity, as measured by skin testing with Dermatophytin-O, mumps antigen, intermediate-strength tuberculin, streptokinase/streptodornase, and sensitization and challenge with dinitrochlorobenzene, was variable with an equal number converting from negative to positive and vice versa. The lymphocyte-proliferative response to both mitogens and antigens was likewise variable but there was a suggestion of augmentation of the *in vitro* lymphocyte response to soluble antigenic stimulation. These *in vivo* lymphocyte proliferation findings were similar to those previously reported for *in vitro* human lymphocyte studies in which poly A:U increased proliferative responses to certain soluble antigens [23, 55, 115, 148, 156]. Absolute lymphocyte counts as well as levels of T cells measured by E-rosette determinations and B cells measured by surface immunoglobulin determination usually decreased following treatment [150].

In a phase I dose-seeking toxicity study, 13 patients received a single dose of either 90, 180, 300, and 450 mg iv [30]. All patients tolerated administration without side effects. The effect of poly A:U on 2', 5'-A synthetase activity and NK cytotoxicity was evaluated 24 and 48 h after administration. However, some patients had been previously heavily treated with cytotoxic chemotherapy and were not evaluable for laboratory evaluation because of leukopenia or lymphopenia. Of the seven evaluable patients, 2', 5'-A synthetase activity and NK cytotoxicity were augmented in four (not necessarily the same four). There appeared to be no substantial influence of dose on either response. Some evidence of biological effect was seen at every dose, although no circulating interferon activity was demonstrable in any patient.

In a large controlled clinical trial poly A:U improved the overall survival of patients (5-year follow up) with operable breast cancer [73]. Patients with stage 1 or 2 adenocarcinoma of the breast were randomized, following mastectomy, to receive either 30 mg poly AU intravenously weekly for 6 weeks or no further therapy. All patients subsequently determined to have histologic node involvement regardless of randomization also received postoperative radiation therapy. Three-year and 5-year analyses revealed that those in the group receiving poly A:U survived longer than those receiving no adjuvant immunostimulatory therapy. Subset analysis indicated that all of the therapeutic benefit from poly A:U was confined to those patients with one to three nodes involved. The benefits noted here compared favorably on an historical basis to those observed with CMF adjuvant cytotoxic therapy [8]. LaCour et al. subsequently reported that poly A:U administered with postoperative local, regional and pelvic radiotherapy was equivalent to CMF chemotherapy as adjuvant therapy for breast cancer [74].

Patients from this trial were evaluated for the induction of a protein kinase that phosphorylates the alpha chain of fibrinogen and whose activity is induced by interferon and by interferon inducers. Fourteen of 16 patients tested had demonstrable activity of these enzyme systems, demonstrating the induction of biological activity by a dose of 30 mg administered weekly [42, 54-57].

In a subsequent trial comparing poly A:U and CMF as adjuvant therapy following mastectomy, 60 mg of poly A:U administered to patients iv, 8 days postmastectomy, has been shown to selectively (in 50% of patients) augment NK cytotoxicity (using the K562 cell as target) and to induce (in 80%) 2', 5'-A synthetase activity in peripheral blood lymphocytes 24-48 h postadministration [58]. Of those patients with low baseline NK cytotoxic activity, augmentation was demonstrable in 11 of 14, while in those with moderate or high baseline activity, augmentation was demonstrable in only eight of 26 patients. The kinetics varied in that the peak response was demonstrable at 24 h in some patients and 48 h in others.

One other group has reported an inability to augment NK cytotoxicity either *in vivo* or *in vitro* [94]. They used a dose of 30 mg iv in patients with advanced cancer and were unable to augment NK activity with poly A:U but could with poly I:C (LC). The concentrations used *in vitro* are unknown.

A trial sponsored by the World Health Organization designed to evaluate poly A:U as adjuvant therapy in patients with melanoma was performed. Patients with stage II melanoma were randomized to receive either poly A:U or no further therapy following surgical removal of all disease. Patients received poly A:U at 60 mg/week for 6 weeks, starting 10 days after surgery. Over 450 patients were entered. The results of this trial were never published but preliminary analyses were said to show no difference in survival.

Youn et al. began a study in late 1984 that involved 206 patients with gastric adenocarcinoma. None of the patients had been previously treated. All patients underwent an attempt at curative resection followed by a randomization between chemotherapy and chemotherapy plus poly A:U. Chemotherapy consisted of 5-FU and those who were randomized to chemoimmunotherapy received, in addition, poly A:U at 100 mg intravenously weekly for 6 weeks immediately postsurgery with a repeat course of 50 mg intravenously, weekly for 6 weeks, at 6 months after surgery. A preliminary analysis in late 1988 revealed that 80% of the patients receiving chemoimmunotherapy and 60% of the patients receiving chemotherapy were alive. Although there was a trend in favor of chemoimmunotherapy, the survival curves were not statistically significantly different ($p \leq .10$, log rank test). Seventy-four percent of the patients receiving chemoimmunotherapy were disease-free 4 years following surgery whereas only 47% of those receiving chemotherapy were alive and free of disease 4 years later ($p \leq .025$, log rank test) [162]. No further follow-up is available. NK cytotoxicity was augmented in the patient receiving poly A:U [160]. The clinical results of that trial have never been published.

In summary, this synthetic polynucleotide, although a relatively poor inducer of interferon, has shown demonstrable antitumor activity in several murine systems, has been associated with prolongation of survival in one human adjuvant clinical trial (breast) and with prolongation of the duration of response in another, has immune-augmenting effects on the immune systems of rodents and humans, and is nontoxic. Preliminary evidence indicates that the minimum immune-augmenting dose is between 30 and 60 mg in humans, but no data are available to indicate what an optimum dose, as defined by continual augmentation, might be. Murine data would indicate that such a dose is an effective antitumor dose, although the effect of a wide variety of doses has not been explored preclinically. There are a small number of ongoing studies with this agent in Europe in viral diseases including hepatitis, but no further studies have been reported evaluating it in patients with cancer.

LOW-MOLECULAR-WEIGHT COMPOUNDS

Various low-molecular-weight synthetic molecules (MW <30,000) are also capable of inducing alpha/beta- and gamma-interferon in murine systems [91, 133, 144]. Although some have undesirable toxicity, preliminary preclinical evaluation of newly developed analogues indicates reduced toxicity and improved therapeutic activity in experimental animals. Some examples of low-molecular-weight inducers are the pyrimidinones, anthraquinones, lipoidal amines, and acridine compounds. A significant advantage for the low-molecular-weight inducers is the induction of biological activity following oral administration.

Pyrimidinones

The pyrimidinones are halogenated molecules whose ability to induce interferon production is dependent upon their molecular structure [132, 133]. Two compounds that have been extensively studied preclinically are APMP (2-amino-5-bromo-6-methyl-4 pyrimidinone), and AIPP (2-amino-5-iodo-6-pheno-4 pyrimidinone). Each has been evaluated for its capability to induce interferon activity (including the type of interferon produced), to modulate the immune response, and to induce antiviral and antitumor activity [38, 48, 95, 132, 133]. Another agent, ABPP has undergone preliminary clinical evaluation [19, 114, 119].

All three agents were investigated because of their ability to protect mice from a variety of fatal viral infections. AIPP was active at doses fourfold lower than ABPP and about 20 times lower than ABMP. ABMP and ABPP were both effective inducers of serum alpha-interferon production in mice, cats, dogs, and cattle, whereas AIPP was an extremely weak inducer of detectable serum interferon levels in these species. AIPP was likewise ineffective at inducing human tonsillar tissue *in vitro* to produce interferon. Interestingly, independent of their interferon-inducing capability, all three were quite effective in augmenting the immune response in mice, including NK-cell activity *in vivo*, macrophage-mediated cytotoxicity either *in vivo* or *in vitro*, and polyclonal antibody formation in both unimmunized and immunized animals. Each agent also induced colony-formation units in the marrow of mice, but none had mitogenic activity or affected the mitogen response, and all three decreased or inhibited T-cell cytotoxicity *in vitro*.

In animal tumor models, all three agents were moderately effective at prolonging survival of mice challenged with low levels (2 x 10^4) of B16 melanoma cells, and all likewise delayed the onset of pulmonary metastases following iv injection of either a poorly (F1) or a highly (F10) metastatic line of B16 melanoma cells. However, none of them was particularly effective in prolonging survival following the ip injection of 2 x 10^6 B16 cells [132]. A similar tumor-load-dependent moderate antitumor effect has been reported in a dimethylhydrazine-induced weakly immunogenic adenocarcinoma of the colon in rats [34]. ABPP also prolonged survival in a naturally occurring murine fibrosarcoma (poorly immunogenic), the C3H spontaneous mammary carcinoma (moderately immunogenic) and the highly immunogenic MCA fibrosarcoma system in C3H mice, but was ineffective in mice that had received whole-body irradiation [95].

Synergy has been demonstrated in several animal tumor models between cytotoxic chemotherapy and the pyrimidinones [35, 83-85]. Although ABPP has been shown to generate LAK activity in peritoneal exudates, it is not an effective antitumor agent when administered to animals with established methycholanthrene-induced sarcomas. However, when administered 12 h following a dose of cyclophosphamide, synergistic therapeutic effects are obtained. Multiple courses of the combination induced cures in the majority of mice with early but established methylcholathrene-induced tumors. The effect of the combination was greater in the immunogenic than in the nonimmunogenic tumors [35].

Sidky et al. have studied the antitumor effect of the pyrimidinones on the growth of MBT-2. ABPP significantly inhibited tumor growth in a dose-dependent manner and with equal potency whether given intraperitoneally or orally. ABPP was administered every 4 days starting 1 day after tumor-cell inoculation. At 100 mg/kg ABPP had an inhibitory effect comparable to 5000 units of beta-interferon, but each was less inhibitory than 10 mg/kg of poly I:C. Other pyrimidinones, however, were more effective than poly I:C in this system and were capable of inducing cures [121].

The basis for the antitumor effect of ABPP is unknown, but pyrimidinones have been shown to augment NK and macrophage cytotoxicity. This effect can be blocked by anti-asialo monosialoganglioside antibodies, radiation, and anti-interferon treatment [85-87]. When cytotoxicity is blocked, antitumor effect is lost also, suggesting the antitumor effect is indirectly related to interferon induction. However, other experiments using the murine tumor method, have shown partial inhibition of uptake of tritiated thymidine, leucine and uridine with an increase of cells as the G2/M phase by flow cytometry. This effect was inhibited by incubation with anti-interferon antibodies [120].

Some reports have also indicated that ABPP has chemopreventive potential. When given to rats three times per week for 4 weeks, beginning 6 h before the carcinogen 7, 12-dimethylbenzanthracene (DBMA), ABPP reduced the incidence and size of tumors, in direct correlation with the titers of induced interferon activity [21]. Similar experiments performed in female C3H/He mice demonstrated the ability of ABPP and beta interferon, administered separately, to decrease the incidence of FANFT-induced transitional cell carcinoma *in vivo* [9].

ABPP (Bropirimine) was the pyrimidinone selected to undergo evaluation in the clinic. In a phase I study in which a dose of 2-5Gm/m^2 was administered once to patients, only low circulating levels of drug were achieved, resulting in low levels of serum interferon and inconsistent immunoaugmentation [114]. Subsequent trials have used higher doses and multiple administrations and have demonstrated interferon production. In a phase II study in patients with AIDS-related Kaposi's sarcoma, 20 patients received a weekly oral dose of 8 g over 8 weeks. Toxicity was acceptable and was confined to adequately controlled gastrointestinal distress (nausea, vomiting, diarrhea) and fatigue. No objective antitumor responses were observed, but immune augmentation was demonstrable. Interferon induction was noted in nine of 10 patients studied, and the degree of induction was correlated with the plasma levels of drug. Augmentation of the lymphocyte mitogenic response to concanavalin A was also noted [19]. In a second phase II trial, patients with renal-cell carcinoma were treated with escalating doses ranging from 4 to 7 g/day for days, with cycles repeated weekly. Preliminary data from this trial suggest that these higher doses may induce interferon production following several weeks of therapy. In addition, they may augment biological activity including NK cytotoxicity, both lymphocyte and monocyte ADCC, 2', 5'-A synthetase, and some lymphocyte surface antigen expression [119]. Studies in bladder cancer, where some antitumor activity was seen in Phase II studies, continue to expand. A phase I trial of orally administered ABPP has been performed in 34 patients with superficial bladder cancer. Toxicity was minimal at total daily dose of over 5000 mg. Responses, including some complete responses, were seen in about a third of patients and were more frequent in patients with CIS and at higher doses and occurred in patients who had failed prior therapy with BCG [116]. The drug is undergoing further clinical evaluation in patients with superficial bladder cancer with the presumed goal of eventual approval for this indication.

Anthraquinones

One group of anthraquinones, the fluorenones, is exemplified by tilorone (diethylaminoethyl-fluorenone) [1, 63, 70, 92, 101]. Tilorone is an orally active molecule with antiviral activity and a potent ability to induce interferon in rodents. Tilorone had antitumor activity when given to animals bearing the Walker carcinosarcoma 256 or the reticulum cell sarcoma A-RCS [70] but was less effective in these systems than poly I:C. Few studies have been performed evaluating the effect of tilorone on the immune system. Tilorone increased the number of plaque-forming cells in splenic harvests [1], but its effect on the cellular system including NK-cell and macrophage activity is unknown. Tilorone has been administered systemically to three patients, but detailed immunologic studies were not performed [63]. Although it is active orally, interest in this and related compounds has not been extensive.

Lipoidal amines

The first lipoidal amine to be described as an interferon inducer was CP20961 [*N, N*-dioctadecyl-*N', N'*-bis(2-hydroxyethyl)propanediamine [52]. Members of this group of compounds have also been shown to be capable of inducing interferon production and of modulating a variety of both specific and nonspecific immune responses [103]. CP20961 and many of the other lipoidal amines induce circulating alpha/beta-interferon in mice, protect mice against a variety of viral infections, and have activity in a number of transplantable murine tumor models. The peak interferon titers following CP20961 administration occur 8-36 h after a single ip injection [52]. *In vitro*, CP20961 induced detectable levels of interferon in peritoneal cells collected from mice and activated their ability to kill tumor cells *in vitro*. Various other lipoidal amines, including CP28888 and CP46665, have been described [66, 157] that differ in their ability to induce interferon and modulate the immune response. For example, CP28888, an aromatic diamine, was about 3-10 times more potent as an inducer than CP20961, yet differed in its ability to modulate the immune response. Likewise, CP46665 failed to induce detectable levels of interferon and did not have antiviral activity against encephalomyocarditis virus *in vivo*. It, however, does have antitumor activity, apparently mediated through activation of macrophage cytotoxicity. The lipoidal amines have been shown to have antitumor effect *in vivo*; they reduce metastases in a variety of transplantable murine tumor model systems [157].

CP20961 was also the first lipoidal amine used in the clinic. In three separate studies, it was given intranasally to humans with rhinovirus infections [26, 106, 125]. In one study, the agent induced high concentrations of interferon locally and had a positive effect on rhinovirus-infected volunteers, while in other studies, although high levels of interferon were induced intranasally, there was no correlation between drug administration and the course of the rhinovirus infection [26, 125, 149]. Time of administration referable to challenge was significant in that the agent had more effect prophylactically than therapeutically. Negative findings with CP20961 may also have been due to the variable nature of the infection, since rhinovirus infections present variable and arbitrary clinical symptoms which the patients were asked to asses for themselves. One of the other aromatic lipoidal amines, CP28888, which had greater potency in mice, was also evaluated in a human challenge study against rhinovirus infection. No effect was observed with this drug and although interferon was detected in the nasal washes, there was no drug-related effect on the outcome of the virus infections.

The potential utility of this class of compounds would appear to lie in its low toxicity and ability to augment various components of the immune system. There appears to be little interest in pursuing it, however.

Flavone acetic acid

Flavone acetic acid (FAA) has been reported to induce interferon and activate NK cells. There have also been reports of TNF induction with this compound. A variety of clinical studies have been done with no interferon induction or clinical efficacy having been reported [49, 145, 155]. While FAA induced significant plasma TNF levels in mice, this effect was not apparent in human studies. Thus, FAA does not appear to have a significant role in the treatment of human malignancies.

Acridines

19-Carboxymethyl-9-acridanone (CMA), the prototype of this class of compounds, has been shown to be a very potent interferon inducer in mice and hamsters. This agent has produced titers in rodents comparable to titers obtained with the best viral inducers. It is capable of inducing high plasma levels of type 1 interferon when given either intraperitoneally, subcutaneously, intramuscularly, or orally. It is highly soluble and has a low level of toxicity. Likewise, it has provided antiviral protection in mice and hamsters against the Japanese encephalitis virus. A reduction in mortality can be obtained by a single dose of CMA administered intraperitoneally, subcutaneously, or intramuscularly [139, 140]. This compound has not induced interferon production in primates, however [141].

C1246, 738 is an orally active acridine compound that is a modulator of cellular and humoral immunity in mice [24, 33, 151, 152]. In rodents, it is also capable of inducing high levels of circulating interferon, protecting against lethal viral infection, and stimulating both natural killer cell and macrophage cytotoxicity. Additionally, CL246, 738 exhibited significant stimulatory activity on cellular immune responses in normal and tumor-bearing mice; it restored the blastogenic response of lymphocytes from tumor bearing mice, enhanced the development of delayed type hypersensitivity, augmented the cytotoxic T lymphocyte response to syngeneic tumor cells, and potentiated the proliferative response of lymphocytes to alloantigens. When administered in combination with a killer tumor-cell vaccine (L1210), the drug displayed immunoadjuvant activity and protected mice against lethal challenge with live tumor cells. In other studies, CL246, 738 was shown to be capable of inducing tumor-inhibitory macrophages both *in vitro* and *in vivo*.

CL246, 738 has displayed significant adjuvant antitumor activity against P388 leukemia, when used in combination with suboptimal doses of mitoxantrone, and substantial activity when used with noncurative surgery in the treatment of B16 melanoma and Lewis lung carcinoma. Further, the compound appeared to have potential antimetastatic activity against the B16-F10 melanoma. These results warrant the investigation of CL246, 738 as an adjuvant to conventional chemotherapy and surgery in the treatment of cancer.

Three phase I studies have been performed. A multicenter single-dose study in patients with AIDS assessed the safety, tolerance and immunomodulating activity of this agent. Twenty-six patients received a single dose ranging from 1 to 50 mg/kg. Three to four patients were entered per dose level. No dose-limiting toxicities were reported, although nausea, vomiting, and diarrhea were seen in three-quarters of the patients. There was some suggestion that toxicity was more severe at a dose of 30 mg/kg or higher. All of the episodes were mild or moderate in severity and resolved within 24 h. Significant modulation of immunologic activity included an elevation of serum interferon alpha in 11 patients, an increase in NK cell activity in over half the patients (primarily in the lower dose group), and minor changes in lymphocyte subsets numbers.

A second phase I single-dose study was performed in patients with inoperable metastatic colorectal carcinoma. Patients received a single dose ranging from 1 to 20 mg/kg. There were no dose-limiting toxicities seen, but nausea, vomiting, and diarrhea were reported in the majority of patients.

A phase I dose-seeking and immunomodulatory evaluation of CL246739 was initiated at the University of Wisconsin in the summer of 1986 in patients with malignancy. Twenty-three patients received a single oral dose every 28 days. Interpatient dose escalation ranged from 5 to 50 mg/kg orally. An additional five patients were entered at a dose of 50 mg/kg, the maximally tolerated dose, to clarify toxicity at that level. About half of the patients completed three or more cycles of therapy. Gastrointestinal disturbances were the most frequently noted side effects, the majority of patients developing nausea, vomiting, and diarrhea. Two of the patients receiving 50 mg/kg developed severe vomiting. There was no chronic fatigue, malaise, or anorexia noted and no clinically significant changes in pulmonary, renal, hepatic, cardiac, or hematologic function were observed. Interferon induction was not demonstrated, but beta 2 microglobulin levels were shown to be increased significantly by the higher dose levels. Cell-mediated immunity, as determined by a T-cell proliferative assay demonstrated a significant increase in T-cell responsiveness against allogeneic cells. There was no augmentation of T-cell response to nonspecific or specific mitogens, nor was there a significant change in either NK-cell function or 2', 5'-A synthetase activity. Pharmacokinetic studies were performed that suggested a dose-response relationship to blood concentrations at the 30-mg/kg dose and above and a half-life greater than 300 h at all dose levels. No objective clinical responses were observed. Findings in this trial have led to a second trial, which has been initiated and is designed to evaluate the effect of a fractionated dosing regimen with CL246, 738 administered over a 3-day period.

Miscellaneous

R-837 [1-(2-Methylpropyl)-1*H*-imidazo]4, 5-*c*[quinolin-4-amine] is an active interferon inducer in mice, guinea pigs, and primates and *in vitro* in human cells. It is also an effective antiviral agent in guinea pigs and mice. When cultured from 48 h with peripheral blood mononuclear cells from normal individuals it can induce type 1 interferon in a dose-responsive fashion [153]. When administered orally to mice over several days, antitumor efficacy is demonstrable. MC-26 cells (a murine colon carcinoma) were injected subcutaneously and intravenously into mice, followed by R-837 administered by a variety of schedules. Antitumor effects were observed; there was no schedule dependency [122].

POLYCARBOXYLATES

Pyran, a synthetic polycarboxylate that is a copolymer of divinyl ether and maleic anhydride, is a crude material of broad molecular weight distribution initially reported in 1967 to induce the production of interferon [93, 111]. Multiple studies have subsequently demonstrated that these compounds do not stimulate high levels of circulating interferon but activate macrophages and augment NK cytotoxicity and are active antitumor agents in a number of transplantable tumor models with low tumor cell burden [99, 117]. The chief limitation of this series of molecules is that they are not easily cleared and they accumulate in the reticuloendothelial system.

MVE-2

MVE-2 is one of the fractions of pyran with a restricted molecular weight of about 15,000. It was developed for clinical evaluation when structure-activity studies with low-molecular-weight compounds suggested that it might retain both macrophage activation and antitumor activity and be better tolerated. MVE-2 has demonstrable macrophage-activating capabilities and demonstrable antitumor efficacy in various murine systems [2, 11] but must be administered within several days of a tumor transplant to be effective. It had an immunomodulating effect in the BRMP preclinical screen, but less so than other agents [138].

Phase I clinical trials with this agent have demonstrated significant toxicity (proteinuria), marginal monocyte immunomodulating capability, and very little antitumor efficacy in over 150 patients with advanced tumor burdens [41, 112, 113, 154]. Based on its relatively weak ability to induce interferon, its relatively weak immunomodulating and antitumor capability in the preclinical screen, its lack of immunomodulating and antitumor activity in clinical studies, and its toxicity, interest in further evaluation has waned.

COMPLEX CARBOHYDRATES

Various complex carbohydrates have been recognized as immune stimulants for many years. Many of these substances have been components of extracts and fold medicines used worldwide. These complex carbohydrates are usually polymers of glucose (glucans), mannose (mannans), xylose (hemicelluloses), or fructose (levans), or are mixtures of these sugars. The chain length and branching, as well as the bonding between sugars, very within this class of compounds. Perhaps the glucans have been most widely studied as immunostimulatory carbohydrates, but the complex mannans have invoked recent interest. Various mannans have been found in yeast, such as *Candida albicans* and *Coccidioides immitis*, as well as in certain plants, such as the aloe vera plant.

One mannan that has been extensively studied is the beta-(1, 4)-linked acetylated mannan of the aloe vera plant called acemannan. This compound is large and contains complex beta-linked mannoses, with most of the material being in excess of 10,000 molecular weight. Antitumor activity has been seen in selected animal models [107], and this complex carbohydrate also has the ability to increase lymphocyte response to alloantigen, probably through monocyte release of interleukin-1 [158]. While it is still early, it appears that complex carbohydrates can have significant antitumor activity and can be interferon and lymphokine inducers, perhaps on a very broad basis. This area has been recently reviewed [142, 149].

These substances have been nontoxic in preclinical and clinical studies, and Phase II clinical trials in HIV infections, ulcerative colitis, and cancer are underway.

SUMMARY AND CONCLUSIONS

Interferon inducers remain an interesting group of agents, which continue to have potential therapeutic value. Several of these compounds are therapeutically active as antitumor and immune-augmenting agents despite the fact that they do not induce detectable levels of circulating interferon. Additionally, several *in vitro* studies utilizing clonogenic assays and xenogeneic grafts have demonstrated both synergistic and antagonistic activity between the interferons and the interferon inducers. This would appear to be a strong indication that these agents have activity independent of their capacity to induce interferon production. Additional clinical evaluation of their effects on the patient's immune system is warranted. Additionally, the administration of a variety of agents in combination would appear to have the potential for significant therapeutic effect. Exhaustive preclinical studies are indicated for evaluating these interferon inducers, in combination with biologicals and other therapeutic agents, to explore their potential for synergy and to rule out antagonistic effects.

Inducers of other lymphokines are likely to gain more attention in the near future. European and Japanese investigators are reinvestigating older 'nonspecific immunostimulants' for lymphokine induction capacity. Picibanil (OK-432), PPD *Bacillus Calmette-Guerin* (BCG), *Corynebacterium parvum*, endotoxin derivatives, and germanium compounds have each been demonstrated to have the capacity for lymphokine induction. The most commonly induced lymphokines have included gamma-interferon, tumor necrosis factor (alpha and beta), interleukin 1, and interleukin 2 (IL-1, IL-2). It is difficult to analyze these reports, because once one mediator is induced (IL-1) it can cause secondary release of other mediators in the lymphokine system. Thus, many of these substances induce fever, and this may be mediated by IL-1. Its release may subsequently cause the release of IL-2, interferon, and tumor necrosis factor. Generally speaking, the levels of these lymphokines/cytokines in the peripheral blood are quite low, but with repeated injections of the stimulant, steady-state blood levels can be achieved. The administration of a bolus dose of peripheral recombinant lymphokine/cytokine can achieve much higher serum peak levels, but infusion is necessary to maintain a steady state comparable to the levels induced by some of these nonspecific stimulants. Therefore, much of the 'older immunotherapy' may be reexplored as investigators are able to define the mediators released subsequent to immune stimulation (See Chapter 7). Whether these approaches are worthy of further clinical investigation, given their historical lack of activity in experimental trials in humans, is conjectural. For the purpose of combination studies, it may be useful to induce a low level of lymphokine stimulation before or during administration of another modality, such as chemotherapy. Combination studies will undoubtedly be designed to explore the hypothesis that such an approach might be therapeutically useful.

As the mechanisms leading to the release of lymphokines/cytokines are better defined, one might expect to see both chemical and biologic induction of lymphokine/cytokine release utilized in the therapeutic approach to cancer. A major question relates to the mechanism of action of these biologicals. If they work as direct cytoxic/cytostatic substances, and if high serum levels are needed, the administration of recombinant molecules will be necessary. On the other hand, if they work at low serum levels, and if the constant availability of these molecules is important for either the inhibition of neoplastic cell growth or the stimulation or maintenance of an immune response, the strategies of lymphokine/cytokine induction may be rewarding. The availability of recombinant lymphokines/cytokines may make available better biologic mediators for the stimulation and release of secondary messages using variations on the physiologic system of lymphokine/cytokine action.

In this regard, it is important to realize that lymphokines/cytokines may be primarily active as locally released mediators. Evidence has accumulated that these mediators are often active in a localized inflammatory or immune response. Often, they are released at the site of inflammation, infection, and perhaps within the inflammatory infiltrate of cancer. As such, they function as local mediators and, with local release and distribution, may have little systemic toxicity. Our current approaches to administering these materials intravenously and achieving serum levels may be problematical. If unacceptable toxicities are reached at serum levels below which there is adequate delivery to the tumor-cell site such as appears to be the case with TNF, the systemic administration of these substances may not be successful. In these cases, the targeting of lymphokines/cytokines with monoclonal antibodies may be a useful approach in an attempt to make these substances accumulate in inflammatory infiltrates in or around tumor nodules. In addition, one can envision the induction and release of lymphokines/cytokines by inducers in these localized sites if an appropriate inflammatory infiltrate is present. For example, LAK cells are known to release various lymphokines [31, 108]. Infusing IL-2-stimulated lymphocytes systemically or regionally is a cellular strategy of lymphokine/cytokine induction (multiple lymphokine/cytokine therapy) that is beginning to show some therapeutic effect [104]. Thus, a long-term strategy of inducing an appropriate inflammatory infiltrate in the tumor nodules followed by systemic lymphokine induction may be worth further consideration.

REFERENCES

1. Adamson RH. Antitumor activity of tilorone hydrochloride against some rodent tumors: preliminary report. *J Natl Cancer Inst* 1971; 46: 431-434.
2. Bartocci A, Papademetriou V, Chirigos MA. Enhanced macrophage and natural killer cell antitumor activity by various molecular weight maleic anhydride divinyl ethers. *J Immunopharmacol* 1980; 2: 149-158.
3. Bever CT Jr, McFarland HF, McFarlin DE, Levy HB. The kinetics of interferon induction by poly I: C (LC) in humans. *J Interferon Res* 1988; 8: 419-426.
4. Bever CT, Salizar AM, Neely E, et al. Preliminary trials of poly I: C (LC) in chronic progressive multiple sclerosis. *Neurology* 1985; 36: 494-498.
5. Bever CT, McFarlin DE, Levy HB. A comparison of interferon responses to poly I: C (LC) in males and females. *J Interferon Res* 1985; 5: 423-428.
6. Borden EC. Personal communication, 1989.
7. Borden EC, Sidky YA, Groveman DS, Bryan GT. Antitumor effects of polynucleotides for mouse transitional cell carcinoma enhanced by cyclophosphamide. *Cancer Res* 1985; 45: 45-50.
8. Borden EC, Verma AJ, Wolberg WH. Potential role of polyribonucleotides in human neoplastic disease. *J Biol Response Modif* 1985; 4: 676-679.
9. Borden EC, Sidky YA, Erturk E, et al. Protection from carcinogen-induced murine bladder carcinoma by interferons and an oral interferon-inducing pyrimidinone, Bropirimine. *Cancer Research* 1990; 50: 1071-1074.
10. Brodsky I, Strayer DR, Krueger LJ, Carter WA. Clinical studies with ampligen (mismatched double-stranded RNA). *J Biol Response Modif* 1985; 4: 669-675.
11. Carrano RA, Kinoshita FK, Imondi AR, Iuliucci JD. MVE-2: preclinical pharmacology and toxicology. In: Hersh EM, Chirigos MA, Mastrangelo M, eds. *Augmenting agents in cancer therapy.* New York: Raven Press, 1981: 345-372.
12. Carter WA, O'Malley JA, Beeson M, et al. An integrated and cooperative study of the antiviral effects and other biological properties of the polyinosinic-polycytidylic acid duplex and its mismatched analogues. III. Chronic effects and immunological features. *Mol Pharmacol* 1976; 12: 440-53.
13. Carter WA, Pitha P, Marshall LW, et al. Structural requirements of the rIn-rCn complex for induction of human interferon. *J Mol Biol* 1972; 70: 567.
14. Carter WA, Strayer DR, Brodsky I, et al. Clinical, immunological and virological effects of ampligen, a mismatched double-stranded RNA, in patients with AIDS or AIDS-related complex. *Lancet* 1987; 1: 1286-1292.
15. Carter WA, Strayer DR, Gillespie DH, et al. Poly IC with mismatched bases, prospects for cancer therapy. In: Hersh EM, Chirigos M, Mastrangelo M, eds. *Augmenting agents in cancer therapy*. New York: Raven Press, 1982; 177- .
16. Carter WA, Hubbell HR, Krueger LJ, Strayer DR. Comparative studies of ampligen (mismatched double-stranded RNA) and interferons. *J Biol Response Modif* 1985; 4: 613-620.
17. Carter WW, Ventura D, Shapiro DE, et al. Mismatched double-stranded RNA. Ampligen (poly(I): poly (C12U), demonstrates antiviral and immunostimulatory activities in HIV disease. *Int J Immunopharmacol* 1991; 13 Suppl 1: 69-76.
18. Chabot GG, Branellec D, Sassi A, et al. Tumor necrosis factor-alpha plasma levels after flavone acetic acid administration in man and mouse. *Eur J Cancer* 1993; 29A: 729-733.
19. Chachoua A, Hochster H, Green M, et al. Phase II trial of bropirimine (ABPP) in patients with AIDS related Kaposi's sarcoma. *Proc Am Soc Clin Oncol* 1988; 7: 6.
20. Champney KJ, Levine DP, Levy HB, Lerner AM. Modified polyriboinosinci-polyribocytidylic acid complex: sustained interferonemia and its physiological associates in human. *Infect Immun* 1979; 25: 831-837.
21. Chang AY-C, Chuang C, Pandya KJ, Wierenga W. Chemoprevention of 7, 12-dimethylbez(a)anthracene (DMBA)

induced rat mammary tumor by 2-amino-5-bromo-6-phenyl-4(3H)-pyrimidinone (ABPP). *J Biol Resp Modif* 1986; 5: 112-116.

22. Chess L, Levy C, Schmukler M, et al. The effect of synthetic polynucleotides on immunologically induced tritiated thymidine incorporation. *Transplantation* 1972; 14: 748-754.
23. Chirigos MA, Papademetrious V, Bartocci A, et al. Immune response modifying activity in mice of polyinosinic: polycytidylic acid stabilized with poly-L-lysine, in carboxymethylcellulose (poly-ICLC). *Int J Immunopharmacol* 1981; 3: 329-337.
24. Citarella RV, Wallace RE, Damiani MR, et al. Antitumor effects of CL 246, 738, a new immunomodulating agent. *Proc Am Assoc Cancer Res* 1983; 24: 193.
25. Cone RE, Marchalonis JJ. Adjuvant action of poly (A: U) on t-cells during the primary immune response *in vitro*. *Aust J Exp Biol Med Sci* 1972; 50: 69-77.
26. Douglas RG Jr, Betts RF. Effect of induced interferon in experimental rhinovirus infections in volunteers. *Infect Immun* 1974; 9: 506-510.
27. Drake WP, Cimino EF, Mardiney MR Jr, Sutherland JC. Prophylactic therapy of spontaneous leukemia in AKR mice by polyadenylic-polyuridylic acid. J Natl *Cancer Inst* 1974; 52: 941.
28. Drake WP, Pendergrast WJ Jr, Kramer RE, Mardiney MR Jr. Enhancement of spontaneous C3H/HeJ mammary tumorigenesis by long-term polyadenylic-polyuridylic acid therapy. *Cancer Res* 1975; 35: 3051-3053.
29. Droller MJ. Immunotherapy of metastatic renal cell carcinoma with polyinosinic-polycytidylic acid. *J Urol* 1987; 137: 202-206.
30. Ducret JP, Caille P, Sancho Garnier J, et al. A phase I clinical tolerance study of polyadenylic-polyuridylic acid in cancer patients. *J Biol Response Modif* 1985; 4: 129-33.
31. Dupere S, Obiri N, Lackey A, et al. *Patterns of cytokines releases by peripheral blood leukocytes of normal donors and cancer patients during interleukin-2 activation in vitro*. New York: Raven Press, 1990.
32. Durie BGM, Levy HB, Voakes J, et al. Ply (I: C)-LC as an interferon inducer in refractory multiple myeloma. *J Biol Response Modif* 1985; 4: 518-524.
33. Durr FE, Citarella RV, Wallace RE, et al. Biological effects of CL 246, 738, a new immunomodulating agent. In: Spitzky HKH, Karrer K, eds. *Proc 13th Int Congress on Chemotherapy.* Vienna: Verlag H. Egermann, 1983: 287.
34. Eggermont AMM, Marquet RL, deBruin RWF, Jeekel J. Effects of the interferon inducer ABPP on colon cancer in rats; the importance of tumor load and tumor site. *Cancer Immunol Immunother* 1986; 22: 217-220.
35. Eggermont AMM, Sugarbaker PH, Marquet RL, Jeekel J. Synergistic antitumor activity of cyclophosphamide and ABPP in the treatment of established and advanced tumors in murine tumor models. *Cancer Immunol Immunother* 1987; 25: 16-24.
36. Engel WK, Cuneo RA, Levy HB. Polyinosinic-polycytidylic acid treatment of neuropathy. *Lancet* 1978; 1: 503-504.
37. Ewel CH, Urba WJ, Kopp WC, et al. Polyinosinic-polycytidylic acid complexed with poly-L-lysine and carboxymethylcellulose in combination with interleukin 2 in patients with cancer: clinical and immunological effects. *Cancer Res* 1992; 52: 3005-3010.
38. Fast PE, Hatfield CA, Sun EL, Stringfellow DA. Polyclonal B- cell activation and stimulation of specific antibody responses by 5-halo pyrimidinones with antiviral and antineoplastic activity. *J Biol Response Modif* 1982; 1: 199-215.
39. Fidler IJ, Berendt M, Oldham RK. The rationale for and design of a screening procedure for the assessment of biological response modifiers for cancer treatment. *J Biol Response Modif* 1982; 1: 15-26.
40. Field AK, Tytell AA, Lampson GP, Hilleman MR. Inducers of interferon and host resistance, II. Multistranded synthetic polynucleotide complexes. *Proc Natl Acad Sci* USA 1967; 58: 1004-1009.
41. Forbes JT, Luck A, Greco FA. MVE-2: phase I study and evaluation of biological response. *Proc Am Assoc Cancer Res* 1982; 23: 134.
42. Galabru J, Buffet-Janvresse C, Riviere Y, Hovanessian AG. Plasma protein kinase activity enhanced by interferon is found in platelets. *FEBS Lett* 1982; 149: 176-80.
43. Goldin A, Venditti JM. Progress report on the screening program at the Division of Cancer Treatment, National Cancer Institute. *Cancer Treat Rep* 1980; 7: 167-176.
44. Graziano KD, Levy CC, Schmukler M, Mardiney MR Jr. Parameters for effective use of synthetic double-stranded polynucleotides in the amplification of immunologically induced lymphocyte tritiated thymidine incorporation. *Cell Immunol* 1974; 11: 47-56.
45. Graziano KD, Mardiney MR Jr. A synergistic effect of synthetic polynucleotides and mercaptoethanol in amplifying the murine mixed lymphocyte reaction. *Transplantation* 1976; 21: 317-322.
46. Gresser I, Maury C, Bandu-M-T, et al. Role of endogenous interferon in the anti-tumor effect of poly I-C and statolon as demonstrated by the use of anti-mouse interferon serum. *Int J Cance*r 1978; 21: 72-77.
47. Grindlay D, Reynolds T. The aloe vera phenomena: a review of the properties and modern uses of the leaf parenchyma gel. *J Ethopharmacol* 1986; 16: 117-151.
48. Hamilton RD, Wynalda MA, Fitzpatrick FA, et al. Comparison between circulating interferon and drug levels following administration of 2-amino-5-bromo-6-phenyl-4(3*H*)-pyrimidinone (ABPP) to different animal species. *J Interferon Res* 1982; 2: 317-327.
49. Havlin KA, Kuhn JC, Craig JB, et al. Phase I clinical and pharmacokinetic trial of flavone acetic acid. *J Natl Cancer Ins* 1991; 83: 124-128.
50. Hawkins MJ, Levin M, Borden EC. An Eastern Cooperative Oncology Group Phase I-II pilot study of polyriboinosinic-polyribocytidylic acid poly-L-lysine complex in patients with metastatic malignant melanoma. *J Biol Response Modif* 1985; 4: 664-668.
51. Herberman RB, Brunda MJ, Cannon GB, et al. Augmentation of natural killer (NK) cell activity by interferon and interferon inducers. In: Hersh EM, Chirigos MA, Mastrengelo M, eds. *Augmenting agents in cancer therapy*. New York: Raven Press, 1981: 253-265.
52. Hoffman WW, Korst JJ, Niblack JF, Cronin TH. *N, N*-Diaoctadecyl-*N', N'*-bis(2-hydroxyethl) propanediamine: antiviral activity and interferon stimulation in mice. *Antimicrob Agents Chemother* 1973; 3: 498-502.
53. Hovanessian AG. *Personal communication*, 1986.
54. Hovanessian AG, Galabru J, Krust B, et al. Interferon and blood coagulation: phosphorylation of fibrinogen and

other plasma proteins by a platelet kinase activity enhanced by interferon. In: DeMaeyer E, Schellekens H, eds. *The biology of the interferon system*. North Holland, New York: Elsevier Biomedical Press, 1983: 323-328.

55. Hovanessian AG, Riviere Y, Montagnier L, et al. Enhancement of interferon-mediated protein kinase in mouse and human plasma in response to treatment with poly A; poly U. *J Interferon Res* 1982; 2: 209-215.
56. Hovanessian AG, Riviere Y, Robert N, et al. Protein kinase in plasma and tissues of mice with high levels of circulating interferon. *Ann Virol Inst Pasteur* 1981; 132E: 175-188.
57. Hovanessian AG, Rollin P, Riviere Y, et al. Protein kinase in human plasma analogous to that present in control and interferon-treated HeLa cells. *Biochem Biophys Res Commun* 1981; 103: 1372-1377.
58. Hovanessian AG, Youn JK, Buffet-Janvress C, et al. Enhancement of natural killer cell activity and 2-5A synthetase in operable breast cancer patients treated with polyadenylic; polyuridylic acid. *Cancer* 1985; 55: 357-362.
59. Hubbell HR, Kvalnes-Krick K, Carter WA, Strayer DR. Antiproliferative and immunomodulatory actions of beta interferon and double stranded RNA individually and in combination on human bladder tumor xenografts in nude mice. *Cancer Res* 1985; 45: 2481-2486.
60. Hubbell HR, Liu R-S, Maxwell BL. Independent sensitivity of human tumor cell lines to interferon and double-stranded RNA. *Cancer Res* 1984; 44: 3252-3257.
61. Johnson AG. Modulation of the immune system by synthetic polynucleotides. *Springer Semin Immunopathol* 1979; 2: 149-168.
62. Kasahara T, Djeu JY, Dougherty SF, Oppenheim JJ. Capacity of human large granular lymphocytes (LGL) to produce multiple lymphokines: interleukin 2, interferon, and colony stimulating factor. *J Immunol* 1983; 131: 2379-2385.
63. Kaufman HE, Centifanto YM, Ellison ED, Brown DC. Tilorone hydrochloride: human toxicity and interferon stimulation. *Proc Soc Exp Biol Med* 1971; 137: 357-360.
64. Klostergaard J, Goodsel D, Granger GA. Induction and characterization of lymphotoxins from tumor promoter-synergized, lectin-stimulated human lymphocytes *in vitro*. *J Biol Response Modif* 1985; 4: 195-209.
65. Kohase M, Henriksen-DeStefano D, May LT, et al. Induction of B2-interferon by tumor necrosis factor: a homeostatic mechanism in the control of cell proliferation. *Cell* 1986; 45: 659-666.
66. Kraska AR, Hemsworth GR, Hoffman WA, Wolff JS. Antitumor activity of CP-20, 961 and CP-28, 888. *Curr Chemother Infect Dis* 1980; 2: 1605.
67. Krown SE. Interferons and interferon inducers in cancer treatment. *Semin Oncol* 1986; 13: 207-217.
68. Krown SE, Kerr K, Stewart WE II, et al. Phase I trials of poly (I, C) complexes in advanced cancer. *J Biol Response Modif* 1986; 4: 640-649.
69. Krown SE, Kerr D, Stewart WE II, et al. Phase I trial of poly ICLC in patients with advanced cancer. In: Hersh EM, Chirigos MA, Mastrangelo M, eds. *Augmenting agents in cancer therapy.* New York: Raven Press, 1981: 165-176.
70. Krueger RF, Mayer GD. Tilorone Hydrochloride: an orally active antiviral agent. *Science* 1970; 169: 1213-1214.
71. Lacour F, Spira A, Lacour J, Prade M. Polyadenylate-polyuridylic acid in adjunct surgery in the treatment of spontaneous mammary tumors in C3H/He mice and transplantable melanoma in hamster. *Cancer Res* 1972; 32: 648-649.
72. Lacour F, Delage G, Chianale C. Reduced incidence of spontaneous mammary tumors in C3H/He mice after treatment with polyadenylate-polyuridylate. *Science* 1975; 187: 256-257.
73. Lacour J, Lacour F, Spira A, et al. Adjuvant treatment with polyadenylic-polyuridylic acid in operable breast cancer: updated results of a randomized trial. *Br Med* J 1984; 288: 589-592.
74. Lacour J, Laplanche A, Delozier T, et al. Polyadenylic-polyuridylic acid plus locoregional and pelvic radiotherapy versus chemotherapy with CMF as adjuvants in operable breast cancer. *Breast Cancer Res Treat* 1991; 19: 15-21.
75. Lampkin BC, Levine AS, Levy H, et al. Phase II trial of poly (I, C)-LC, an interferon inducer, in the treatment of children with acute leukemia and neuroblastoma: a report from the Children's Cancer Study Group. *J Biol Response Modif* 1985; 4: 531-537.
76. Le J, Lin-J-X, Henriksen-DeStefano D, Vilcek J. Bacterial lipopolysaccharide-induced interferon-gamma production: roles of interleukin 1 and interleukin 2. *J Immunol* 1986; 136: 4525-4530.
77. Levine AS, Durie B, Lampkin B, et al. Poly (ICLC): interferon induction, toxicity, and clinical efficacy in leukemia, lymphoma, solid tumors, myeloma, and laryngeal papillomatosis. In: Hersh EM, Chirigos M, Mastrangelo M, eds. *Augmenting agents in cancer therapy*. New York: Raven Press, 1981: 151-163.
78. Levine AS, Durie B, Lampkin B, et al. Interferon induction, toxicity, and clinical efficacy of poly ICLC in hematologic malignancies and other tumors. In: Terry WD, Rosenberg SA, eds. *Immunotherapy of human cancer*. New York: Elsevier North Holland, 1982: 411-418.
79. Levine AS, Levy HB. Phase I-II trials of poly IC stabilized with poly-L-lysine. *Cancer Treat Rep* 1978; 62: 1907-1913.
80. Levine AS, Sivulich M, Wiernik PH, Levy HB. Initial clinical trials in cancer patients of polyriboinosinic-polyribocytidylic acid stabilized with poly-L-lysine, in carboxymethylcellulose [poly(ICLC)], a highly effective interferon inducer. *Cancer Res* 1979; 39: 1645-1650.
81. Levy HB, Baer G, Baron S, et al. A modified polyriboinosinic-polyribocytidylic acid complex that induced interferon in primates. *J Infect Dis* 1975; 132: 434-439.
82. Levy HB, Stephen ES, Harrington D, et al. Polynucleotides in the treatment of disease. In: Hersh EM, Chirigos MA, Mastrangelo M, eds. *Augmenting agents in cancer therapy*. New York: Raven Press, 1981: 135-150.
83. Li LH, Johnson MA, Moeller RB, Wallace TL. Chemoimmunotherapy of B16 melanoma and P388 leukemia with cyclophosphamide and pyrimidinomes. *Cancer Res* 1984; 44: 2841-2847.
84. Li LH, Wallace TL, DeKoning TF. Effect of pyrimidinone in combination with various types of chemotherapeutic drugs. *Proc Am Assoc Cancer Res* 1986; 27: 380.
85. Li LH, Wallace TL, Richard KA, Tracey DE. Mechanism of antitumor action of pyrimidinones in the treatment of B16 melanoma and P388 leukemia. *Cancer Res* 1985; 45: 532-538.
86. Lotzova E, Savary CA, Kahn A, Stringfellow DA. Stim-

ulation of natural killer cells in two random bred strains of athymic rats by interferon inducing pyrimidinone. *J Immunol* 1984; 132: 2466-2569.

87. Lotzova E, Savary CA, Lowlacht M, Murasko DM. Cytotoxic and morphologic profile of endogenous and pyrimidinone activated murine NK cells. *J Immunol* 1986; 136: 732-740.
88. Maluish AE, Reid JW, Crisp EA, et al. Immunomodulatory effects of poly(I, C)-LC in cancer patients. *J Biol Response Modif* 1985; 4: 656-663.
89. Marquet RL, Eggermont AMM, deBruin RWF, et al. Combined treatment of colon adenocarcinoma in rats with tumor necrosis factor and the interferon inducer ABPP. *J Interferon Res* 1988; 8: 319-324.
90. McFarlin DE, Bever CT, Salazar AM, Levy HB. A preliminary trial of poly(I, C)-LC in multiple sclerosis. *J Biol Response Modif* 1985; 4: 544-548.
91. McIntyre OR. Low molecular weight interferon inducers: overview of potential for cancer therapy. In: Hersh EM, Chirigos MA, Mastrangelo M, eds. *Augmenting agents in cancer therapy*. New York: Raven Press, 1981: 229-237.
92. Megel H, Raychaudhuri A, Gibson JP. Immunological responses with tilorone – update. In: Chirigos MA, ed. *Control of neoplasia by modulation of the immune system*. New York: Raven Press, 1977: 409-420.
93. Merigan TC, Regelson W. Interferon induction in many by a synthetic polyanion of defined composition. *N Engl J Med* 1967; 277: 1283-1287.
94. Mickschė M. *Personal communication*, 1984.
94. Milas L, Hersh EM, Stringfellow DA, Hunter N. Studies on the antitumor activities of pyrimidinone-interferon inducers. I. Effect against artificial and spontaneous lung metastases of murine tumors. *J Natl Cancer Inst* 1982; 68: 139-145.
96. Minks MA, West DK, Benvin S, Baglioni C. Structural requirements of double-stranded RNA for the activation of 2'5' oligo (A) polymerase and protein kinase of interferon-treated HeLa cells. *J Biol Chem* 1979; 254: 10180-10183.
97. Mitchell WM, Montefiori DC, Robinson WE Jr, et al. Mismatched double-stranded RNA (ampligen) reduces concentration of zidovudine (Azidothymidine) required for *in vitro* inhibition of human immunodeficiency virus. *Lancet* 1987; 1: 890-892.
98. Montefiori DC, Mitchell WM. Antiviral activity of mismatched double-stranded RNA against human immunodeficiency virus *in vitro*. *Proc Natl Acad Sci USA* 1987; 84: 2985-2989.
99. Morahan PS, Kaplan AM. Macrophage-mediated tumor resistance. In: Chirigos MA, ed. *Control of neoplasia by modulation of the immune system*. New York: Raven Press, 1977: 449-459.
100. Mohr H, Monner D, Plessing A. Calcium inophore A 23 187 in the presence of phorbol ester PMA: a potent inducer of interleukin 2 and interferon-gamma synthesis by human blood cells. *Immunobiology* 1986; 171: 195-204.
101. Munson AE, Munson JA, Regelson W, Wampler GL. Effect of tilorone hydrochloride and congeners on reticuloendothelial system, tumors, and the immune response. *Cancer Res* 1972; 32: 1397-1403.
102. Narayan PR, Kloehn DB, Sundharadas G. Immune response to alloantigens *in vitro*, amplification of the development of cytotoxic T lymphocytes by lipopolysaccharide and polyadenylic-polyuridylic acid. *J Immunol* 1978; 121: 2502-2508.
103. Niblack JF, Otterness IG, Hemsworth GR, et al. CP-20, 961: a structurally novel, synthetic adjuvant. *J. Reticuloendothel Soc* 1979; 26: 655-666.
104. Oldham RK, Bartal AH, Birch R, et al. Regional adoptive immunotherapy with IL-2 activated cells in patients with metastatic cancer. *ASCO* 1988.
105. Palacios R. Production of lymphokines by circulating human T lymphocytes that express or lack receptors for interleukin 2. *J Immunol* 1984; 132: 1833-1836.
106. Panusarn C, Stanley ED, Dirda V, et al. Prevention of illness from rhinovirus infection by a topical interferon inducer. *N Engl J Med* 1974; 291: 57-61.
107. Peng SY, Norman J, Curting, et al. *Decreased mortality of normal murine sarcoma in mice treated with the immunomodulator, acemannan*, 1990; in press.
108. Pawelec G, Schwuler U, Lenz H, et al. Lymphokine release suppressor cell, generation cell, surface markers, and cytotoxic activity in cancer patients receiving natural interleukin-2. *Biother* 1990; in press.
109. Reem GH, Yeh N-H. Interleukin 2 regulates expression of its receptor and synthesis of gamma interferon by human T lymphocytes. *Science* 1984; 225: 429-430.
110. Reem GH, Yeh N-H. Regulation by interleukin 2 of interleukin 2 receptors and gamma-interferon synthesis by human thymocytes: augmentation of interleukin 2 receptors by interleukin 2. *J Immunol* 1985; 134: 953-958.
111. Regelson W. Prevention and treatment of Friend leukemia virus (FLV) infection by interferon-including synthetic polyanions. *Adv Exp Med Biol* 1967; 1: 315-332.
112. Rinehart JJ, Young DC, Neidhart JA. Evaluation of the immunological and toxicological properties of MVE-2 in phase I trials. *Cancer Res* 1983; 43: 2358-2362.
113. Rios A, Rosenblum M, Powell M, Hersh E. Phase I study of MVE-2 therapy in human cancer. *Cancer Treat Rep* 1983; 67: 239-243.
114. Rios A, Stringfellow DA, Fitzpatrick FA, et al. Phase I study of 2-amino-5-bromo-6-phenyl-4(3*H*)-pyridmidinone (ABPP), an oral interferon inducer, in cancer patients. *J Biol Response Modif* 1986; 5: 330-338.
115. Riviere Y, Yovanessian AG. Direct action of interferon and inducers of interferon on tumor cells in athymic nude mice. *Cancer Res* 1983; 43: 4596-4599.
116. Sarosdy MF, Lamm DL, Williams RD, et al. Phase I trial of oral bropirimine in superficial bladder cancer. *The Journal of Urology* 1992; 147: 31-33.
117. Schultz RM, Chirigos MA, Morh SJ, and Woods WA. Tumoricidal effect *in vitro* of peritoneal macrophages from mice treated with pyran copolymer. In: Chirigos MA, ed. *Control of neoplasia by modulation of the immune system*. New York: Raven Press, 1977: 437-448.
118. Shaw GD, Boll W, Taira H, et al. Structure and expression of cloned murine IFN-alpha genes. *Nucleic Acids Res* 1983; 11: 555-573.
119. Shaw DR, Tilden AB, Kirchler TJ, et al. Demonstration of immune modulation during phase II trials of oral borpirimine. *Proc Am Assoc Clin Res* 1989; 30: 381.
120. Shimizu M, Oh-Hashi F, Tsukagoshi S, et al. *In vitro* and *in vivo* antitumor activity of the interferon inducer bropirimine. *Anti-Cancer Drugs* 1995; 6: 158-162.
121. Sidky YA, Borden EC, Wierenga W, Bryan GT. Inhibitory effects of interferon-inducing pyrimidinones on the growth of transplantable mouse bladder tumors. *Cancer*

Res 1986; 46: 3798-3802.
122. Sidky YA, Weeks CE, Hatcher J, et al. Effects of treatment with the oral interferon inducer, R-837, on the growth of mouse colon carcinoma, MC-26. *Proc Am Assoc Cancer Res* 1990; in press.
123. Singh SK, Marquet RL, Westbroek DL, Jeekel J. Abrogation of the tumor promoting effect of allogeneic blood transfusion by polyadenylic-polyuridylic acid. *Cancer Immunol Immunother* 1987; 25: 242-244.
124. Smalley RV, Stringfellow DA. Interferon inducers for clinical use. In: Finter NB, Oldham RK, eds. *Interferon-in vivo use.* Amsterdam, New York: Elsevier Science Publisher, 1985: 337-358.
125. Stanley ED, Jackson GG, Dirda VA, Rubenis MJ. Effect of a topical interferon inducer on rhinovirus infections in volunteers. *J Infect Dis* 1976; 133: A121-A127.
126. Stevenson HC, Abrams PG, Schoenberger CS, et al. Immunomodulatory effects of poly (I, C)-LC in cancer patients. *J Biol Response Modif* 1985; 4: 650-655.
127. Strayer DR, Carter WA, Brodsky I, et al. Clinical studies with mismatched double-stranded RNA. *Tex Rep Biol Med* 1982; 41: 663-671.
128. Strayer DR, Carter WA, Crilley P, et al. Phase I study of mismatched double-stranded RNA (ampligen). *Proc Am Assoc Cancer Res* 1986; 27: 209.
129. Strayer DR, Watson P, Carter WA, Brodsky I. Antiproliferative effect of mismatched double-stranded RNA on fresh human tumor cells analyzed in a clonogenic assay. *J Interferon Res* 1986; 6: 373-380.
130. Strayer DR, Watson P, Mayberry S, et al. Synergism between natural interferon alpha and a novel mismatched double-stranded RNA produces an antiproliferative effect against fresh human tumor cells. *Proc Am Soc Clin Onc* 1986; 5: 230.
131. Strayer DR, Weisband J, Carter WA, Brodsky I. Antiproliferative effect of natural beta interferon on fresh tumor cells analyzed in a clonogenic assay. *J Interferon Res* 1984; 4: 627-633.
132. Stringfellow DA. Induction of interferon with low molecular weight compounds: fluorenone esters, ethers (tilorone), and pyrimidinones. *Methods Enzymol* 1981; 78: 262-284.
133. Stringfellow DA. 6-Aryl primidinones: interferon inducers-immunomodulators-antiviral and antineoplastic agents. In: Hersh EM, Chirigos MA, Mastrangelo M, eds. *Augmenting agents in cancer therapy*. New York: Raven Press, 1981: 215-228.
134. Talmadge JE. *Personal communication*, 1986.
135. Talmadge JE, Adams J, Phillips H, et al. Immunotherapeutic potential in murine tumor models of polyinosinic-polycytidylic acid and poly-L-lysine solubilized by carboxymethylcellulose. *Cancer Res* 1985; 45: 1066-1072.
136. Talmadge JE, Adams J, Phillips H, et al. Immunomodulatory effects in mice of polyinosinic-polycytidylic acid complexed with poly-L-lysine and carboxymethylcellulose. *Cancer Res* 1985; 45: 1058-1065.
137. Talmadge JE, Hartman D. Optimization of an immunotherapeutic protocol with poly (I, C)-LC. *J Biol Response Modif* 1985; 4: 484-489.
138. Talmadge JE, Maluish AE, Collins M, et al. Immunomodulation and antitumor effects of MVE-2 in mice. *J Biol Response Modif* 1984; 3: 354-652.
139. Taylor JL, Schoenherr CK, Grossberg SE. High yield interferon induction by 10-carboxymethyl-9-acradanone in mice and hamsters. *Antimicrob Agents Chemother* 1980; 18: 20-26.
140. Taylor JL, Schoenherr C, Grossberg SE. Protection against Japanese encephalitis virus in mice and hamster by treatment with carboxymethylacradanone, a potent interferon inducer. *J Infect Dis* 1980; 142: 394-399.
141. Taylor JL, Grossberg SE. Chemical induction of interferon: carboxymethylacradanone and other low molecular weight chemicals. *Tex Rep Biol Med* 1981-1982; 41: 158-163.
142. Tizard IA, Carpenter RH, McAnalley BH, Kemph MC. The biological activities of mannans and related complex carbohydrates. *Mol Biother* 1989; 1: 290-296.
143. Torrence PF, De Clercq E. Inducers and induction of interferon. *Pharmacol Ther A* 1977; 2: 1-88.
144. Torrence PF, De Clercq E. Interferon inducers: general survey and classification. *Methods Enzymol* 1981; 78: 291-299.
145. Triozzi PL, Rinehart JJ, Malspeis L, et al. Immunological effects of flavone acetic acid. *Cancer Res* 1990; 50: 6483-6485.
146. Ts'o POP, Alderfer JL, Levy J, et al. An integrated and comparative study of the antiviral effects and other biological properties of the polyinosinic acid-polycytidylic acid and its mismatched analogues. II. *Mol Pharmacol* 1976; 12: 299-312.
147. Vilcek J, Henriksen-Destefano D, Siegel D, et al. Regulation of IFN-gamma induction in human peripheral blood cells by exogenously and endogenously produced interleukin 2. *J Immunol* 1985; 135: 1851-1856.
148. Wagner J, Cone RE. Adjuvant effect of poly (A: U) upon t-cell mediated *in vitro* cytotoxic allograft responses. *Cell Immunol* 1974; 10: 394.
149. Waldman RH, Ganguly R. Effect of CP-20, 961, an interferon inducer, on upper respiratory tract infections due to rhinovirus type 21 in volunteers. *J Infect Dis* 1978; 138: 531-535.
150. Wanebo HJ, Kemeny M, Pinsky CM, et al. Influence of poly(A)-poly(U) on immune response in cancer patients. *Ann NY Acad Sci* 1976; 277: 288-298.
151. Wang BS, Lumanglas AL, Ruszala-Mallon VM, Durr FE. Induction of tumor-inhibitory macrophages with a novel synthetic immunomodulator, 3, 6-bis (2-piperidinoethoxy) acredine trihydrochloride (CL 246, 738). *J Immunol* 1985; 135: 679-683.
152. Wang BS, Ruszala-Mallon V, Wallace RE, et al. Modulation of the immune response to tumors by a novel synthetic compound, *N*{4-}(4-fluorophenyl)(sulfonyl {phenyl}acetamide (CL 259, 763). *Cancer Immunol Immunother* 1986; 22: 8-14.
153. Weeks CE, Gibson SJ. Alpha interferon induction in human blood cell culture by immunomodulator candidate R-837. *J Interferon Res* 1989; 9(suppl 2): S215.
154. Weiner RS, Carr DJ, Moore M, et al. Clinical and biological phase I study of MVE-2 (pyran copolymer). *Proc Am Soc Clin Oncol* 1984; 3: 49.
155. Weiss RB, Greene RF, Knight RD, et al. Phase I and clinical pharmacology study of intravenous flavone acetic acid (NSC 347512). *Cancer Res* 1988; 48: 5878-5882.
156. Wiltrout RH, Salup RR, Twilley TA, Talmadge JE. Immunomodulation of natural killer activity by polyribonucleotides. *J Biol Response Modif* 1985; 4: 512-517.
157. Wolf JS III, Hemsworth GR, Kraska AR, et al. CP-46,

665-1: a novel lipodal amine with antimetastatic and immunómodulatory properties. *Cancer Immunol Immunother* 1982; 12: 97-103.

158. Womble D, Helderman JH. Enhancement of alloresponsiveness of human lymphocytes by acemannan (Carrisyn^{TM}). *Int J Immunopharmac* 1988; 10: 967-974.
159. Youn JK, Hovanessian AG, Riviere Y, et al. Enhancement of natural killer cell activity and 2-5A synthetase in mice treated with polyadenylic-polyuridylic acid. *Cell Immunol* 1983; 79: 298-308.
160. Youn J, Kim B, Min J, et al. Adjuvant treatment of operable stomach cancer with polyadenylic polyuridylic acid in addition to chemotherapy agents: differential effect on natural killer cell and antibody dependent cellular cytotoxicity. *Int J Immunopharmac* 1987; 9: 313-324.
161. Youn JK, Lacour F, Hue G. Inhibition of C3H/He mouse mammary tumor growth by combined treatment with cyclophosphamide and polyadenylic-polyuridylic acid. *Cancer Res* 1982; 42: 4706-4711.
162. Youn JK. Personal communication, 1989.
163. Zarling JM, Schlais J, Eskra L, et al. Augmentation of human natural killer cell activity by polyinosinic acid-polycytodylic acid and its non-toxic mismatched analogues. *J Immunol* 1980; 124: 1852-1857.

LYMPHOKINES AND CYTOKINES

WALTER LEWKO[1], RICHARD V. SMALLEY[2] and ROBERT K. OLDHAM[3]
[1] *Cancer Therapeutics, Inc., Franklin, Tennessee, Synertron,* [2] *Inc., Madison, Wisconsin, Biological Therapy Institute Foundation,* [3] *Franklin, Tennessee; and University of Missouri, Columbia, Missouri*

The study of lymphokines began in the mid 1960s, after the simultaneous discovery by David (1966) and Bloom and Bennett (1966) that *in vitro* activation of lymphocytes leads to the production of factors that inhibit the migration of macrophages [468]. Subsequently, DuMonde et al. (1969) coined the term *lymphokines* to refer to factors that modulate the growth or mobility of a variety of leukocytes [167]. Hundreds of communication molecules have now been described, which are produced by both lymphocytic and nonlymphocytic cells. Nonlymphocytic cells involved in this process include normal macrophages, fibroblasts, mast cells, and eosinophils. It was therefore proposed by Cohen and co-workers in 1977 that this entire class of mediators be termed *cytokines*, in recognition of the contribution from nonlymphocytic components. It is now recognized that cytokines may function in a wide range of activities, including regulation of immunological and inflammatory processes, which not only regulate normal cell growth and differentiation but also participate in repair mechanisms.

Rapid expansion of this field since 1980 has been brought about by a number of technological developments, including tissue culture techniques, monoclonal antibody generation, separation techniques, such as high-performance liquid chromatography, microsequencing, and finally, genetic engineering with recombinant DNA technology. As scientists began exchanging information, it became apparent that various factors that had been independently described shared certain biological activities. Hence, some of these activities were quite likely attributable to the same molecule. Such was the case with γ-interferon, which has the ability to activate macrophages, a property previously ascribed to macrophage activating factor (MAF). On the other hand, there was the realization that a profusion of named factors could have a broad array of crucial biological effects and that these factors could act on cells in either a synergistic or suppressive fashion.

Recombinant DNA techniques capable of directing biosynthesis of lymphokine proteins in both yeast and bacterial systems have provided the impetus for testing many of these homogeneous lymphokine protein products in preclinical models, and in clinical trials. The first of these to become available was γ-interferon, which, in contrast to the α- and β-interferon antiviral proteins, seemed to have broader cellular effects as a lymphokine. Subsequently, other molecules followed in fairly rapid succession, including interleukin 2 (IL-2), granulocyte-macrophage colony-stimulating factor (GM-CSF), granulocyte colony-stimulating factor (G-CSF), and more recently interleukin 1 (IL-1), tumor necrosis factor (TNF), lymphotoxin (LT), macrophage colony-stimulating factor (M-CSF), and interleukins 3-18. The purity and availability of the products are permitting us to define precisely their individual activities and their possible clinical roles.

There are at least five separate approaches to determining the clinical significance of lymphokines. These include therapeutic, diagnostic or predictive, pathogenetic, pharmacologic activities and biologic standardization.

The therapeutic potential of lymphokines can be demonstrated through a number of procedures that are increasingly recognized: (a) *in vivo* reconstitution of lymphoid cell functions of lymphokine-deficient animals in which lymphokines injected into immunosuppressed animals can stimulate leukocyte function and (b) *in vitro* assays.

In humans, the clinical utility of lymphokines may be demonstrated *in vitro* by measuring lymphokine levels in biologic fluids; measuring lymphokine production by lymphoid cells from patients with various clinical conditions; and reconstituting immunoreactivity *in vitro* by addition of exogenous lymphokines. *In vivo* clinical trials with recombinant lymphokine products or lymphokine-inducing agents will provide the foundation for future therapeutic roles.

The pathogenesis of diseases may be elucidated when lymphokine research applied in a therapeutic setting leads to observations that clearly demonstrate the interactions of certain lymphocyte subpopulations, and the response manifested by the *in vivo* administration of lymphokines, as well as the *in vitro* reaction of these same cells to exogenously administered lymphokines in the laboratory. Examples of this are being seen in the various immunodeficiency states, both primary and secondary, in which interleukin-2 has been shown to rectify certain lymphocyte-deficient conditions in HIV-positive individ-

R.K. Oldham (ed.), Principles of Cancer Biotherapy. 3rd ed., 211–265.

uals. However, in HIV-negative individuals with a secondary immunodeficiency, macrophage dysfunction was felt to be the primary defect, since IL-2 was relatively ineffective in correcting the deficiency. Many more examples of this type of clarification of the pathogenesis of disease will be forthcoming as we enter clinical trials with a number of purified recombinant products.

Interest in the immunopharmacology of lymphokines has further elucidated clinical roles. This is exemplified by observations of lymphokine action in combination or sequence with various well-known immunosuppressive drugs, such as cyclophosphamide and cyclosporin-A. It has been observed that cyclophosphamide can facilitate tumor regression mediated by adoptively transferred immune lymphocytes. Cyclosporin-A is known to suppress IL-2 production by selective action of the drug on T-cells responsive to IL-1. These and many similar observations on the interaction of biologic and pharmacologic agents will greatly expand our arsenal of effective antineoplastic regimens.

Finally, work in the area of biologic standardization has revealed that there is some variability in the recombinant DNA lymphokine preparations with regard to their potency despite estimated potencies of equivalent strength. This was well demonstrated by Thurman et al. [715] in a comparative study of six eukaryotic and six recombinant IL-2 preparations supplied by 12 companies at an estimated potency of 1000 units/ml. The study showed that relative potencies actually ranged from 4600 to 11 ru/ml, with the additional finding that various factors besides IL-2 were contained in the preparations, including γ-interferon, BCGF, CSF, MIF, and MAF, as well as endotoxin.

Hence, as we move into an evaluation of the potential clinical applications of several of these lymphokines, we must bear in mind the need to be primarily observational scientists, prepared to leave behind our prior chemotherapeutic prejudices. Furthermore, we must be willing to evaluate each potential lymphokine *in vivo* and *in vitro* for biologic activity at the effector cell level, as well as the tumor target level in our standard tumor models. The complexity associated with these evaluations will prohibit screening large numbers of these agents, as has been done in the past with cytotoxic agents, since most active lymphokines will have effects in multiple assays and act on multiple target cells. We must be open-minded and flexible in this clinical testing. To apply the simple principle of chemotherapy trials would be a serious error. For example, two inactive chemotherapy drugs given as combination chemotherapy will not be active. By contrast, two lymphokines, inactive as single agents, may work well together as they sequentially activate the immune system. Such has already been observed with TNF and IL-2. As one considers the implications of the handful of substances discussed in greater detail in this chapter, it is apparent that the efforts put forth in the painstaking work of these clinical trials will reap rewards that are many times greater than we have seen in the past with comparable drugs used as anticancer agents.

For this chapter we will use the word *cytokine* to broadly include both lymphokines and cytokines. Cytokines are regulatory proteins, produced and secreted by various cells which control immune response, hematopoiesis, tissue morphogesis and wound repair. Secreted cytokines typically act locally as paracrine or autocrine regulators but endocrine responses over some distance may occur. Cell surface receptors exist for each cytokine which specifically bind the cytokine. Receptor subunits may be shared between different cytokines. Binding the cytokine brings about a series of events, typically involving the phosphorylation of certain tyrosine residues on the receptor itself and other cellular proteins. Kinases are the enzymes which carry out phosphorylation. Receptors may themselves be kinases which activate upon binding the specific ligand. In the case of the cytokine receptors, more often the receptor relies on cytosolic kinases (a group referred to as the Janus kinases, specifically Jak1, Trk and Jak 3) which bind the receptor complex just after it binds the cytokine. As the kinase binds the receptor, its phosphorylation activity increases and an array or cellular proteins are phosphorylated and structurally modified due to the added negative phosphate charge. Structural modifications bring about changes, increases or decreases, in each protein's activity. Among these proteins are the nuclear STAT proteins which control gene expression. When phosphorylated, STAT proteins allow gene activation to occur at specific sites. Therefore, a cytokine binds certain cells because they have specific cell surface receptors. Altered patterns of phosphorylation and changing activities of certain proteins including regulators of gene activity bring about the cell response characteristic of the cytokine.

In this chapter, the major cytokines will be discussed with emphasis on IL-2, IL-4, IL-7, IL-12, IL-15. Regulation of cellular immunity will be emphasized for its role in the elimination of tumor and virus infected cells. Hematopoietic roles will be described only briefly. Unfortunately, all the cytokines can not be adequately covered in detail. The long and heavily studied cytokines interleukin 2, tumor necrosis factor and the colony stimulating factors as well as the interferons are more extensively covered in other chapters.

CYTOKINE RECEPTORS: MANY BELONG TO THE HEMATOPOIETIN RECEPTOR SUPERFAMILY

The receptors for IL-2, IL-3, IL-4, IL-5, IL-6, IL-7, IL-9, G-CSF, GM-CSF and Prolactin are all members of the hematopoietin receptor superfamily. (The interferons have their own family of receptors.) Receptors for these cytokines have been cloned and analyzed molecularly. Amino acid sequence reveals segments in the extracellular domains which are common between the members [334]. Common features include among others four cysteine residues, a Trp-Ser-X-Trp-Ser sequence, and a proline rich motif [547]. Tyrosine kinase activation appears to be a common mechanism for signal transduction by these receptors. The receptors do not necessarily have on board kinase activity. Rather a group of kinases referred to as the Janus kinase (JAK) family appear to be the phosphorylation agents. These are cytosol proteins. There are at least 4 members of the JAK family: JAK 1, JAK 2, JAK 3 and Tyk 2 [128, 301, 341]. A variety of studies show that as the cytokine and receptor come together, affinity for the kinase increase and with binding the JAK becomes active; phosphorylation increases [24]. The receptor itself may be phosphorylated. Cellular proteins are phosphorylated. Among these are the STAT family members, signal transducers and activators of transcription. These proteins regulate gene activity. The binding of a given cytokine may bring about the phosphorylation of one or more of these STAT proteins. Phosphorylation activates STAT proteins, increasing their ability to translocate from the cytoplasm into the nucleus where they bind specific DNA regulatory sequences. Gene activation results. These genes are transcribed resulting in a specific profile of gene products which bring about the cytokine's effects.

Receptors may share subunits which carry out common functions [275, 755]. For example, several receptors (IL-2, IL-4, IL-7, IL-15) share a common gamma subunit which is involved in signal transduction. The multiple receptor roles of this gamma chain show themselves in various forms of combined immunodeficiency disease which appear to be due to mutations in that subunit's gene [380, 627]. Since this receptor subunit is shared between several cytokines, the effects of genetic fault have far reaching and generally debilitating effects on the immune response.

Interleukin 1: general hematopoietic response inducer

Interleukin I was originally described as lymphocyte activating factor for its stimulatory effect on thymus cell response to mitogens by Gery, Gershon and Waksman [226]. It is a 17 kDa protein [150] which is produced by macrophages, dendritic cells, T cells, B cells, NK cells, keratinocytes, fibroblasts, endothelial cells, epithelial cells, neurons, astrocytes, glial cells and eosinophils [195, 407, 770]. There are two types of IL-1, $\propto$ and β [422] which are two distinct gene products. Both types bind a common receptor and have similar effects. Secretion increases in response to TNFα [71, 152] and CAMP is required for the induction of IL-1 by TNF in human monocytes [396]. IL-1 has widespread involvement in hematopoiesis augmenting the activities of several stimulatory factors. It synergizes with IL-2 in LAK generation. IL-1 stimulates T cells, induces IL-2 production, IL-2 receptors and cytokine release [150] and is a chemoattractant for T cells [39, 296, 471]. IL-1, together with IL-12, has a role in the secretion of IFN by NK cells in response to infection [297]. There are two forms of IL-1 designated alpha and beta which share relatively little sequence homology (26%) yet have similar biological activities and receptor binding characteristics. Another protein, IL-1 receptor antagonist binds one of the IL-1 receptors and blocking IL-1 activity at that site [695]. There are two high affinity membrane bound receptors (IL-1RI and IL-1RII) which are distinct proteins from separate genes [99]. The function of the IL-1RII is not certain as it does not appear to signal. A soluble form of the IL-1 RII competes for available IL-1 but does not bind IL-1 receptor antagonist [165, 250]. The soluble receptor is generally believed to behave as a negative regulator although it may as well serve as a repository, increasing the effective half life of the protein. IL-1 appears to mediate several inflammatory diseases. IL-1 receptor antagonist, and soluble IL-1 receptor are being tested clinically as anti-inflammatory agents [153]. Elevated IL-1 levels occur with infection and in patients with rheumatoid arthritis [170]. The major interest in IL-1 for cancer patients is in its hematopoietic activities, to augment colony stimulating factors in restoring the patient's blood cells after chemotherapy or in bone marrow transplant.

Properties that have been clearly identified as attributable to IL-1 include its capacity to act as an endogenous pyrogen [154], to induce fibroblast proliferation [639], to promote bone resorption and cartilage degradation [144], and to induce the release of collagenase, phospholipase A and prostaglandin E_2 from synovial cells [129, 467, 549]. IL-1 stimulated chemotaxis in neutrophils [633]. It is present at elevated levels in inflamed joints. In addition, it induces the secretion of acute phase proteins and various cytokines (notably IL-6 and TNF) during the inflammatory response to injury.

IL-1 can stimulate hematopoiesis (causing proliferation and differentiation of pluripotent stem cells in the bone marrow), particularly in combination with certain colony-stimulating factors (CSFs) [469, 476]. It induces the release of some of these CSFs by bone marrow stromal cells, endothelial cells, and fibroblasts. It also acts as an accessory growth factor for certain T and B lymphocytes [332, 368, 549], partly by stimulating the release of other factors that influence the growth and differentiation of these cells. The proliferation of the T_H2 subset of cells that produce interleukins 4, 5 and 6 is enhanced by IL-1, whereas proliferation of T_H1 cells (producing interleukin 2 and interferon gamma) is independent of IL-1 [367]. IL-1 also has the capacity to stimulate dendritic cells. It acts together with GMCSF to promote the maturation of these important professional antigen presenting cells [269].

Interleukin 1 interacts closely with a number of hormones, notably insulin, in the secretion of corticosteroids by upregulating the release of adrenocorticotrophin from the anterior pituitary [54]. Corticosteroids reduce IL-1 production at the level of transcription [377]; however, they increase the expression of IL-1 receptors on the surface of B lymphocytes, thereby enhancing its effect on antibody production [7].

IL-1 has an angiogenic effect, probably through its

proliferative effects on endothelial cells and vascular smooth muscle [385]. In addition, it stimulates the production of leukocyte adherence molecules and other mediators by endothelial cells. IL-1 has direct stimulatory or inhibitory effects on growth of cancer cells depending on the specific disease [309, 548]. It is one of several cytokines which increase intercellular adhesion molecule-1 (ICAM -1) when tested on human melanoma cells [340] for potential effects on immune recognition. In certain ways molecular response and biological effects of IL-1 resemble TNF [257].

The therapeutic implications of this research into IL-1's biological properties is potentially great, and because of its 'two-edged effect' in inflammation (beneficial and harmful), interest is high in the development of both agonists and antagonists of this cytokine. IL-1 itself is being clinically evaluated in a number of indications, most of which are not in the anticancer area and will not be discussed here in any detail, particularly as they have been well reviewed elsewhere [515]. Most importantly, IL-1's role as an inflammatory mediator and its implication in joint disease have stimulated interest and hope in the value of developing antagonists to this cytokine (both natural and synthetic) as an alternative to steroid therapy.

Of most importance for the oncology area, the recognition of IL-1's role as a stimulator of hematopoiesis has led to its being tested in the clinic both singly and in combination with other CSFs as a means of stimulating bone marrow recovery following cytotoxic chemotherapy and radiotherapy based on elegant animal studies [516, 517]. As it decreases the activity of cytochrome P-450 drug metabolism [227], IL-1 may also provide additional advantage in delaying the catabolism of chemotherapeutic agents. IL-1 may also be useful in the treatment of opportunistic infections in immunosuppressed patients (including those with a possible specific IL-1 deficiency), as it has been shown to enhance the resistance of both normal and neutropenic mice to infection with *Pseudomonas aeruginosa* and *Klebsiella pneumoniae* [745]. Direct intralesional injection of IL-1 into animal tumors has led to regressions; however, no useful effect has been shown on distant metastases, hence the clinical application of this observation is probably very limited [501].

In view of its stimulatory effects on both T and B cells, IL-1 is being tested as a vaccine adjuvant, particularly with poorly immunogenic recombinant viral surface protein coat proteins. Interleukin-1's angiogenic properties together with its proliferative effect on fibroblasts and its effect on neutrophil chemotaxis have provided a strong rationale for current clinical studies in the area of wound healing.

Given the recent emphasis on high-dose chemotherapy with peripheral stem-cell or bone-marrow reconstitution and the availability of the colony-stimulating factors to assist in the reconstitution, the use of IL-1 to protect tissues and enhance antitumor effects has a sound rationale [539]. Studies to exploit these combination effects are envisioned or underway.

IL-1 has been used in a variety of treatment regimens, both as standard phase I single agent trials and in combination with both Interleukin-2 and with chemotherapy agents. While preclinical studies utilizing IL-1 did show some antitumor activity in specific models, IL-1 alone in human trials did not show significant anticancer activities. [587, 679].

The combination of IL-1 with IL-2 was explored in human clinical trials based on preclinical experiments, suggesting IL-1 might protect against some of the capillary leak syndrome which is seen with high-dose IL-2 administration [583]. IL-1 at 0.1 microgram per kilogram per day subcutaneously with IL-2 at 1.5 M units/m^2 per day subcutaneously was utilized in one phase I trial and 0.2 micrograms per kilogram per day IV of IL-1 with 0.1 mg/m^2 per day of IL-2 by continuous intravenous infusion was also tried [733]. Some increases in NK and LAK activity were observed as were minor tumor responses in patients with colon cancer, melanoma and renal cancer. The suggestion of clinical activity in phase I trial has prompted phase II trials which are currently underway.

IL-1 has also been used in combination with chemotherapy because of previously observed antitumor activity in preclinical models [319, 369]. Given the direct antitumor activity along with its ability to activate certain aspects of the immune response and increase hematopoiesis, various investigators have suggested that IL-1 would be ideal when combined with chemotherapy.

In vitro studies demonstrated IL-1's synergistic activity with selected forms of chemotherapy [502, 739]. Phase I clinical trials were initiated to determine the tolerance of IL-1 with chemotherapy agents and hypotension was the main dose limiting side effect observed [118, 663]. An increase in neutrophils and platelets along with enhanced marrow cellularity was noted in these studies [663] and some reduction in toxicity to chemotherapy was suggested in some of these trials [118].

Because of the interesting *in vitro* effects as well as the reasonably well tolerated aspect of phase I clinical trials, further trials are currently underway exploring combinations of Interleukin-1 with Cyclophosphamide [644] and Carboplatinum [392]. Further clinical studies to explore the combination of IL-1 with other biological molecules as well as with chemotherapy are warranted and are currently underway.

Interleukin-2: The key cytokine for activated immune cells

IL-2 activity was originally described by Kawaskura and Lowenstein [329] and Gordon and MacLean [241] in back to back papers in *Nature* as a factor in conditioned medium of mixed lymphocyte cultures which stimulated cell division in lymphocytes [478, 625, 626]. Morgan, Ruscetti and Gallo (1976) later called it T cell growth factor. Since then there has been a large volume of research published on this important cytokine which has been reviewed in previous editions of this book [209] and elsewhere.

In 1983, Tanaguchi and colleagues [701] isolated a human IL-2 complementary DNA clone from a high-producer Jurkat leukemia cell line, and established its nucleotide sequence. In 1984, Rosenberg et al. [606] described the isolation of cDNA clones of the gene for IL-2 from the Jurkat cell line, its expression in *Escherichia coli*, and its biological characteristics. The mature secreted protein contains 133 amino acids (the signal peptide consisting of 20 amino acids), constituting a calculated molecular weight of 15, 420.

Initial studies utilized natural IL-2 (nIL-2) purified from lymphoid cells [202, 455, 603, 772]. Variations in molecular weight are due to variation in the degree of glycosylation of the protein [602], which in turn depends upon its source. In contrast to the naturally occurring cytokine, the amino acid sequence of recombinant IL-2 (rIL-2) preparations available for clinical trials possesses methionine at the N-terminal end. Unlike nIL-2, the recombinant version is not glycosylated. Both of these properties (i.e., methionylation and lack of glycosylation) are a reflection of the fact that rIL-2 is produced in *E. coli*. In addition, depending on the manufacturer, the cysteine at position 125 may be substituted by a serine (Cetus/ Chiron) or an alanine (Ortho-Amgen) in order to prevent inappropriate disulfide bridge formation during production between cysteine 125 and one of the other two cysteine residues present in the native sequence (i.e., at positions 58 and 105). Such inappropriate disulfide bridge formation has been shown to result in a much less active species due to the disruption in the tenting structure of the resulting peptide [75]. Nevertheless, other producers of clinical rIL-2 (Glaxo/Biogen and Roche/ Immunex) have managed to overcome the problem of inappropriate disulfide bridge formation without altering the primary sequence of the peptide. This has the potential but as yet unproven advantage of resulting in a peptide that may be less immunogenic in humans. In fact, antibodies are produced in a significant proportion of patients to rIL-2, but not to nIL-2 [12]. Although some investigators have reported that the anti-rIL-2 antibodies are not clinically significant [12, 560], others [350, 361] have detected neutralizing rIL-2 antibodies that may adversely affect treatment outcome.

As multiple preparations of IL-2, both natural and recombinant, became available, the need arose for a standard preparation to enable comparison of preclinical and clinical results. The natural glycosylated Jurkat IL-2 was selected by the Biological Response Modifiers Program (BRMP) of the National Cancer Institute in 1984 as an 'interim reference reagent' because it had been studied the most and differences between the natural glycosylated and the nonglycosylated recombinant IL-2 had not been established. This standard contained 500 units/ml of IL-2 T-cell growth-promoting activity [621]. In a blinded, preclinical comparison of IL-2 from 12 sources (6 naturals and 6 recombinants), the BRMP demonstrated that significant differences in potency in a variety of different assays, as well as composition and other properties, existed among the various IL-2 preparations [715]. These differences must be considered when interpreting the results of both preclinical and clinical studies.

Finally, after an international collaborative study [220], a lyophilized preparation of the interim BRMP IL-2 reference reagent was established in 1987 as the first international standard for IL-2, containing a defined potency of 100 international units (IU/ampoule), which corresponds with the previous BRMP unitage for the liquid preparation. For a valid comparison of study data, the activity of a particular IL-2 preparation should be related to the activity of the international reference preparation.

There are several features of recombinant IL-2 (rIL-2) that merit attention. No differences exist in biological activity between natural IL-2 (nIL-2) and rIL-2 [164, 606]. Furthermore, human rIL-2 is fully active in the mouse, and on a unit per unit basis has the same capability of producing murine lymphokine-activated killer (LAK) cells as the natural murine IL-2. Therefore, it would seem likely that some of the results of studies using human rIL-2 in mice might be extrapolated to the use of human rIL-2 in humans, providing a rationale for clinical applications of rIL-2 based on murine studies.

Pharmacokinetic studies in humans with both nIL-2 and rIL-2 have revealed similar short elimination half-lives of 1-2h following intravenous injection [256, 398, 399]. In mice, the rapid clearance of IL-2 from the serum has been shown to result from renal rather than hepatic catabolism or receptor binding to T cells [160]. After subcutaneous (sc) and intraperitoneal (ip) administration half-life is prolonged to about 4 h following bolus sc injection, longer for sc infusion using a mini-osmotic pump and from 2 to 20 h for the ip route [256, 353, 519]. Although all three routes of administration can induce *in vivo* T-cell proliferation, murine studies have demonstrated that routes and schedules that prolong serum concentrations of rIL-2 more effectively augment T-cell proliferation [93], and, in the case of the sc infusion, lead to a prolongation of mean survival time in tumor-bearing mice [519]. The covalent binding of polyethylene glycol (PEG) to rIL-2 has prolonged the elimination half-life of rIL-2 to 12 h in humans and has been evaluated for safety and antitumor efficacy [453, 801].

Interleukin-2 is a central cytokine in the activation of the immune system. As important as it is in immune function, IL-2 has emerged clinically as the cytokine most widely used in adoptive immunotherapy for cancer. IL-2 is a 15.5 kDa protein produced mainly by activated T cells. Dendritic epidermal T cells involved in antigen presentation also produce IL-2 [431]. In cultures of peripheral blood lymphocytes (PBL), IL-2 drives the activation of natural killer (NK) cells, cytotoxic T lymphocytes (CTL) and lymphokine activated killer (LAK) cells. When added to cultures of dispersed tumor cells, IL-2 stimulates tumor infiltrating lymphocyte (TIL) expansion and antitumor cytotoxicity [610, 723] with the formation of tumor derived activated T cells (TDAC) [382, 416, 417]. LAK [285, 540, 607, 773] and TIL/TDAC [360, 541, 543, 544, 611] cells are being used to in trials of adoptive immunotherapy to treat patients. IL-2 is the major cytokine currently used in the production of these cells. Interferon, IL-4, IL-7, IL-12, IL-15 and other cytokines are also involved as will be discussed in this chapter. B cell growth and differentiation are also influenced by IL2 acting alone or with other cytokines [315, 503, 676].

The IL-2 receptor

As typical of the other cytokines, cell surface receptors mediate IL-2 response. The IL2 receptor has three component subunits alpha, beta and gamma. The IL-2R gamma subunit functions in signaling. It is shared with several other cytokine receptors and is now referred to as the common gamma subunit (γ c). IL-2 binding affinity may be high, moderate or low. Highest affinity binding, as found in activated T cells, involves all three subunits. Moderate affinity binding characteristic of NK cells utilizes the beta and gamma subunits. IL-2 stimulates cytotoxicity in NK cells [264, 732]. A relatively high concentration of IL-2 is required to bring about this effect, related to the intermediate affinity IL-2R in PBL NK cells [335, 551, 659].

During the immune response to a given antigen, activated T lymphocytes express increasingly higher levels of the IL-2 receptor on their surfaces; thereafter receptor levels decline, the cells go into the resting phase of the cell cycle, and the IL-2 receptor is no longer expressed on the cell surface [664]. Monoclonal antibodies to the IL-2 receptor show promise as clinically useful immunosuppressive agents based on the fact that only activated and non resting T lymphocytes bear the IL-2 receptor, and the results of animal models of allograft rejection [336] are particularly encouraging. Similarly spectacular results are anticipated from the recently engineered IL-2/diphtheria toxin conjugate as another approach to achieving antigen-specific immunosuppression.

IL-2 receptor is expressed on a number of carcinoma cell lines. Certain cell lines incubated with IL-2 grew more slowly [792]. Growth of other receptor positive carcinomas and normal keratinocytes was not affected. In certain cell lines, IL-2 potentiated the growth inhibiting effects of other cytokines, including IFN-γ, TNF-∝ and TGF-β. On the other hand, IL-2 downregulated several seemingly important surface molecules including ICAM-1 (involved in lymphocyte binding) and MHC I (involved in antigen recognition and response) and IL-2 downregulates its own receptor (required for continued IL-2 effect) [792]. Therefore, IL-2 has direct effects on tumor cells which could influence growth directly, alter sensitivity to other cytokines or potentially alter cellular immune response.

Immunologic activities of IL-2

Since the discovery of IL-2 and its T-cell growth-promoting activity [55], extensive research has revealed the complex nature of its immunologic effects, both *in vitro* and *in vivo*.

In vitro, IL-2 enhancement of thymocyte mitogenesis is the best-described activity. Exposure to optimal concentrations of IL-2 for as little as 1 h results in thymidine incorporation at 24 h equal to that seen after continuous exposure to IL-2. The targets for this IL-2 activation are heterogeneous, and include helper, suppressor, and cytotoxic T cells and natural killer (NK) cells [65, 366, 653, 654].

Following the report by Henney et al. [264] that IL-2 could augment the cytotoxic activity of murine NK cells, Domzig et al. [158] showed that IL-2 expresses a rapid, dose-dependent increase in the cytotoxic activity of human NK cells *in vitro*. It has been demonstrated that IL-2 can substantially enhance NK responses as well as alloantigen-specific cytolytic T cell activity *in vivo* in murine models [263], and can reverse cyclophosamide-induced suppression of cytotoxic T-cell responses [449].

Of significance was the report that murine and human peripheral blood lymphocytes (PBL) incubated for 3 days in IL-2 could generate a population of cells that were able to lyse a wide variety of fresh and cultured, autologous and allogeneic, natural killer (NK) resistant tumor cells without antigenic stimulation, that is, in a non-major histocompatibility complex (MHC) restricted manner [254, 619]. These lymphokine-activated killer (LAK) cells were shown to be distinct from both classic cytotoxic T lymphocytes (CTL) and NK cells on the basis of cytotoxic specificity and effector cell phenotype [254, 619].

Subsequent research has revealed that this IL-2-dependent cytotoxic activity, called the LAK phenomenon, is mediated in part by activated cytotoxic T cells, but predominantly by activated NK cells [552, 573, 716, 766].

The availability of an abundant supply of rIL-2 to generate LAK cells *in vitro* led to the adoptive transfer of these cells to mice with pulmonary and hepatic sarcoma metastases [492, 493]. When LAK cells were administered concomitantly with repeated injections of rIL-2, significant antitumor effects were seen.

It was originally suggested that very high doses and prolonged exposures to IL-2 *in vitro* were mandatory to achieve maximal LAK cell production and activation. Studies by Yannelli and Oldham have demonstrated that a 'pulse' of high-dose IL-2 for 1 h at the patient's bedside is sufficient to highly activate LAK cells. Several days of infusional IL-2 for constant exposure to IL-2 was needed to produce the responsive precursor cells in the patient such that maximal activation can occur with a 'pulse' of IL-2 *ex vivo* [285].

Although it appeared that the combination of adoptively transferred LAK cells and rIL-2 was necessary for antitumor efficacy [492, 493] high-dose rIL-2 administered alone could generate LAK cells *in vivo* and also could mediate tumor regression in mice [492, 608]. The *in vivo* induction of LAK activity and antitumor response was dependent on the administered dose of rIL-2.

The intravenous administration of IL-2 rapidly causes a redistribution of circulating lymphocytes. The proportion of LAK precursors and NK cells and the NK activity of the NK cells remaining in the circulation decrease [399]. The prompt disappearance of NK cells from the circulation after the administration of IL-2 is believed to be due to IL-2-induced adherence of NK cells to vascular endothelium [31]. A rebound lymphocytosis occurs within 24-72 h after the discontinuation of IL-2 [399, 670], facilitating adoptive immunotherapy by providing an abundant supply of lymphocytes for *in vitro* activation with rIL-2 and reinfusion *in vivo*.

Mediating its immunoregulatory effects by binding to its receptor, IL-2 can stimulate the proliferation of B cells [240, 461] and can enhance the cytotoxic activity of monocytes in a dose-dependent manner [419].

In addition to augmenting non-MHC-restricted cytotoxicity, IL-2 has been reported to significantly enhance antibody-dependent cellular cytotoxicity (ADCC) mediated by lymphocyte effector cells incubated in rIL-2 [655]. It has been suggested that the cells involved in this ADCC lysis are LAK cells, raising the possibility of using this phenomenon in conjunction with antibodies directed against tumor cell surface antigens [655].

In addition to directly influencing the immune system, IL-2 acts indirectly by inducing the secretion of other lymphokines, which exert a multitude of their own immunological effects. These lymphokines include interferon gamma, tumor necrosis factor alpha, lymphotoxin, and interleukin alpha and beta, and appear to play a very important role in both the antitumor efficacy and the toxicities associated with IL-2 immunotherapy of cancer [172, 224, 268, 358, 458].

IL-2 shows promise in model systems as an adjuvant in tumor vaccines [13, 211, 212, 381]. Cells engineered to produce IL-2 were less tumorigenic than unmodified cells. Animals with regressed tumors were generally immune to subsequent challenge by tumor cells.

The immunopotentiating activities, encouraging *in vitro* results, plus successful therapy of animal tumors in preclinical studies provided the rationale for investigations of IL-2 in patients with advanced malignancy and immunodeficiencies.

CLINICAL TRIALS OF RIL-2 IN PATIENTS WITH CANCER

rIL-2 with and without adoptive immunotherapy

Initial clinical studies were performed in patients with cancer and immunodeficiency syndromes utilizing purified natural human IL-2, administered by a variety of routes and schedules. Doses employed were low, due to the limited quantities of IL-2 available at the time, and ineffective; as one might expect in retrospect, toxicity was minimal [403, 450]. The availability of large quantities of recombinant IL-2 (rIL-2) facilitated the initiation of large-scale clinical trials to establish its safety and efficacy.

Early phase I trials with rIL-2 involved dose escalations by either intravenous (iv) bolus or intravenous infusions of varying duration in a variety of schedules [32, 338, 399, 426]. Kern et al. [338] observed no dose-limiting toxicity at lower doses. Significant dose-related toxicities included chills and fever exceeding 40°C, hypotension, dyspnea, malaise, headache, nausea and vomiting, diarrhea, mild anemia, thrombocytopenia and marked eosinophilia, and occasional rash and pruritus. Fluid retention resulting in weight gain to as much as 10-20% of pretreatment weight was observed after cumulative doses of greater than 0.6 – 1.8 x 10^6 IU/kg. Moderate renal and hepatic toxicity characterized by elevations of creatinine, bilirubin, and liver enzymes were noted [400]. Toxicity-limiting doses appeared to be 6 x 10^6 IU/kg as an iv bolus and 18, 000 IU/kg/h by continuous iv infusion. No significant antitumor activity was demonstrated.

The antitumor efficacy demonstrated in murine models with the adoptive transfer of LAK cells in combination with IL-2 [493] led to human trials of the 'adoptive immunotherapy' technique after it was shown that large numbers of autologous peripheral blood lymphocytes could be obtained, activated *in vitro*, and safely reinfused into humans [41, 437].

Rosenberg et al. were the first to report the results of clinical trials of adoptive immunotherapy using rIL-2 in combination with *in vitro* generated lymphokine-activated killer (LAK) cells [607, 609]. Employing a 16-day treatment cycle, they administered rIL-2 by intravenous bolus, 0.6 x 10^6 IU/kg every 8 h for the first 5 days to induce the rebound lymphocytosis, which was previously observed to occur between 24 and 72 h after discontinuing rIL-2. After 2 days of rest, patients underwent five daily leukaphereses (days 8-12) and their harvested lymphocytes were incubated with rIL-2 to generate LAK cells. On days 12, 13, and 15, patients received LAK cells that had been harvested on days 8 and 9, 10, and 11 and 12, respectively. Concomitantly with the reinfusion of LAK cells, rIL-2 was repeated 0.6 x 10^6 IU/kg every 8 h) on days 12-16. Rosenberg also treated patients with rIL-2 alone, using the same dose and schedule of administration but without leukapheresis and reinfusion of LAK cells.

Of 106 evaluable patients treated with both rIL-2 and LAK cells, eight complete responses and 15 partial responses were observed, suggesting an overall response rate of about 22%. Among 46 evaluable patients treated with rIL-2 alone, one complete response and five partial responses were observed, suggesting an overall response rate of about 13%. Renal-cell carcinoma and malignant melanoma appeared to respond best to this therapy, although the number of patients with other malignancies treated with rIL-2 was relatively small. The median duration of response was 10 months for patients experiencing a complete response, and 6 months in those with partial responses. Despite encouraging efficacy, this high-dose iv bolus therapy with rIL-2 resulted in life-threatening toxicities requiring intensive care treatment. Although these toxicities were similar to those previously reported [400], they were of greater severity, and were often due to an apparent increase in capillary permeability and a decrease in systemic vascular resistance, which resulted in hypotension requiring fluid replacement and vasopressors, and interstitial pulmonary edema often requiring endotracheal intubation. Elevated serum creatinine, azotemia, and oliguria as well as hyperbilirubinemia occurred. Anemia and grade 3 thrombocytopenia required transfusions, and neuropsychiatric effects included somnolence, disorientation, and coma. Transient arrhythmias occurred and four patients experienced myocardial infarction, two of which were fatal. These toxicities were attributed to the rIL-2 because LAK cell infusions were previously shown to involve minimal toxicity [41, 437]. However, at least one group has claimed that the combination of rIL-2 and LAK is more toxic than the sum of the two treatments given separately [85].

In an effort to preserve the efficacy but reduce the toxicity of this treatment, West et al. [773] conducted a variation of Rosenberg's scheme of adoptive immunotherapy by administering the rIL-2 by 24-h continuous infusions rather than intermittently by iv bolus injections. Within-patient dose escalations between 6-42 x 10^6 IU/m^2/day suggested that an optimally safe and effective dose was 18 x 10^6 IU/m^2/day.

With 40 evaluable patients, this group claimed to have achieved a tumor response rate comparable to Rosenberg's with a lower incidence of excessive fluid retention and dyspnea. Tolerance and response to treatment correlated with a good performance status, suggesting that efficacy is best in the setting of minimal disease. West et al. did not compare the administration of rIL-2 plus LAK cells with rIL-2 alone, and they conceded that the contribution of LAK cells to tumor response was uncertain.

In an extension of this protocol to 115 evaluable patients, 58% of whom had malignant melanoma and renal-cell carcinoma, an overall response rate of 13% was reported [145], suggesting that the efficacy rate associated with continuous rIL-2 infusion with LAK cells was similar to that of intermittent bolus administration of rIL-2 with LAK cells. There was a trend suggesting that responding patients were more likely to have neither lung nor liver metastases, and to have a post-IL-2 lymphocytosis of 6000/μl or greater.

In an effort to further develop and confirm the efficacy of Rosenberg's adoptive immunotherapy protocol, the National Cancer Institute established the rIL-2/LAK Extramural Trials Working Group (ETWG) in 1986. Comprising six centers in the United States, the ETWG has continued to enroll patients on the Rosenberg high-dose iv bolus regimen and is also studying the continuous infusion of rIL-2 with LAK. Phase II studies [169, 192] have demonstrated an overall response rate of 16-19% in metastatic melanoma and renal-cell carcinoma with a median response duration of about 10 months, consistent with Rosenberg's initial results. Severe toxicities have continued to remain a problem in studies reported by this group.

Paciucci et al. [556] have reported another continuous infusion protocol employing weekly LAK cell infusions followed by 6 days of rIL-2 at escalating doses for up to 4 weeks, which has produced an antitumor response rate and spectrum of toxicities similar to those of West et al. [773]. The dose best tolerated was 20.4 x 10^6 IU/m^2/day, and response appeared to correlate with the magnitude of rebound lymphocyte counts (>7000/μl) following weekly interruptions of rIL-2 infusions.

Due to the serious toxicities associated with high-dose regimens of IL-2, efforts have been devoted to developing dose and schedule modifications that would hopefully be safer without compromising efficacy. One variation of the Rosenberg regimen involved reducing the intermittent bolus dose of rIL-2 to one-third (0.18 x 10^6 IU/kg) and extending its period of administration to day 19 instead of day 16 [171, 677]. The efficacy of this approach appears comparable to that of Rosenberg et al. [609] and West et al. [773], particularly in renal-cell carcinoma and metastatic melanoma, but with less toxicity.

Due to the complexity, cost, and risk of pathogenic contamination associated with IL-2/LAK adoptive immunotherapy, and the observation that rIL-2 generates LAK cells *in vivo* and can, by itself, mediate an antitumor response [263, 608], research has also been devoted to finding a safe and effective regimen of IL-2 that did not involve leukapheresis and reinfusion of LAK cells.

In phase I/II studies, Thompson et al. [711] investigated the effect of dose and duration of infusion of rIL-2 on toxicity and immunomodulation. They compared two doses (3 x 10^5 vs. 3 x 10^6 IU/m^2/day) administered by three different schedules (either daily 2-h or 24-h infusions or 15-min infusions every 8 h). Although antitumor activity was minimal, toxicity and immunomodulation were found to be dependent on both dose and duration of rIL-2 infusion. The maximum tolerable dose was considered to be 3 x 10^6 IU/m^2/day by continuous 24-h infusions; however, this also produced the greatest *in vivo* immunomodulation.

Sondel et al. have also concentrated their efforts on defining the safest and most effective dose and schedule of rIL-2 alone. Their initial work [260, 620, 668] demonstrated that rIL-2 administered by continuous or bolus intravenous infusion at doses of 1 x 10^6 to 3 x 10^6 IU/m^2/day over 4-7 days causes *in vivo* immune activation with acceptable toxicity, but that the rebound lymphocytosis and augmented cytotoxic lymphocyte function returned to baseline within 7 days after therapy was discontinued.

To determine if repetitive courses of rIL-2 would sustain or enhance immunological activation and result in an improved clinical response, this group administered rIL-2 for four consecutive 4-day cycles, each separated by 72-h rest periods. Twenty-eight patients with recurrent or metastatic renal-cell carcinoma or melanoma were assigned to six different treatment groups to compare two doses of rIL-2 (1×10^6 and 3×10^6 IU/m^2/day), and three different modes of intravenous administration (bolus injection, continuous infusion, and a combination of the two). Since indomethacin has commonly been used to control fever and pain induced by rIL-2, they also examined the effect of indomethacin on therapeutic outcome [670].

The typical dose-related toxicities of rIL-2 occurred in all patients but were not life-threatening and did not require intensive care support. The toxicity of four repetitive cycles of rIL-2 was not significantly different from that of one 4-day cycle. The cumulative nature of toxicity was evident as toxic effects appeared to worsen progressively over each 4-day cycle but resolved rapidly during each 3-day rest period. Indomethacin appeared to increase toxicity by augmenting fluid retention, azotemia, and oliguria, but was not very effective as an analgesic and antipyretic in these patients. Continuous infusion appeared more toxic than intermittent bolus, and the combined regimen was intermediate between the two.

Immunomodulation, particularly NK and LAK cell cytotoxic activities, observed at the end of four cycles of rIL-2 was significantly greater than that after the first cycle, and continuous infusion at the higher dose was more immunostimulatory than bolus administration. Three patients who received the higher dose of rIL-2 by continuous infusion or combined bolus/infusion regimens experienced a transient partial response; however, this did not appear to correlate with the degree of immunomodulation.

In another phase I trial of rIL-2 without LAK cells in patients with melanoma and a variety of urological malignancies, Oliver et al. [546] reported that doses of rIL-2 comparable to those employed by Sondel et al. produced desirable immunomodulation with acceptable toxicity. No complete or partial tumor responses were observed, however.

Less intense regimens involving once-daily iv injections, or once- or twice-weekly 24-h iv infusions are being evaluated for toxicity, immunomodulation, and possible tumor response in an effort to determine an immunomodulating dose and schedule of treatment that can be given safely on an outpatient basis for extended periods of time [14, 116, 218, 236, 588]. Initial results suggest that a tolerable and immunomodulating dose exists between 6 and 18×10^6 IU/m^2/day, but an optimum schedule of administration has yet to be defined. In addition, subcutaneous administration, which provides sustained serum concentrations of IL-2, has been evaluated, but the variable bioavailability and the formation of neutralizing antibodies are possible limitations of this route [350, 361, 560]. These regimens may be more effective as adjuvant therapy in the setting of minimal residual disease or in combination with other therapeutic agents.

Although the efficacy of rIL-2 and rIL-2/LAK has been clearly demonstrated in renal-cell carcinoma and melanoma, some responses have also been noted in Hodgkin's and non-Hodgkin's lymphoma, colorectal carcinoma, lung cancer, and ovarian carcinoma. However, the significance of these results is difficult to interpret due to the small numbers of patients treated with these and other disorders. The role of IL-2 therapy in these and other malignancies, therefore, requires further investigation and caution should be exercised in prematurely rejecting rIL-2 as a treatment modality for tumors in which its efficacy has not been properly evaluated.

The cytotoxicity of LAK cells to solid tumors prompted attempts to define the cytotoxicity of LAK cells to malignant hematological cells.

Oshimi el al. [553] were the first to report that peripheral blood lymphocytes (PBL) isolated from patients with leukemia and lymphoma can be activated and expanded *in vitro* to be cytotoxic to autologous ANLL, ALL, and non-Hodgkin's lymphoma blasts. These LAK effector cells were shown to be both T and NK cells.

The studies of Lotzova et al. [404] demonstrated that the functional defects of NK cells observed in leukemia patients could be corrected by culture of NK cells with IL-2. Importantly, cultured NK cells from both the peripheral blood and bone marrow could lyse fresh autologous leukemic cells.

Additional investigations [4, 5, 187] have supported the results of Oshimi and Lotzova by showing that culture with IL-2 of PBL from both adult and pediatric leukemia patients results in the generation and proliferation of NK and LAK effector cells, which demonstrate significant cytotoxicity toward autologous malignant blasts. The clinical implication of these findings is the possibility of either generating *in vivo* antileukemic NK and LAK cytotoxicity with IL-2 or adoptively transferring LAK effector cells to patients with leukemia.

Clinical studies have commenced in order to determine whether the *in vitro* potential of IL-2 translates into therapeutic benefit in leukemia. Believing that the role of IL-2 in the treatment of leukemia is in the setting of minimal residual disease to prevent relapse and improve survival, Gottlieb et al. [242] have reported that IL-2 can be safely administered to patients who have recently received myelosuppressive chemoradiotherapy to induce disease remission, as long as adequate attention is paid to IL-2 dose, duration of administration, and the management of toxicity. Although the pilot nature of this study precluded the determination of any survival benefit, it did demonstrate the possibility of generating *in vivo* antileukemic effects both by patients' PBL activated *in vivo* by rIL-2 infusion [243] and by cytokines (TNF-alpha and IFN-gamma) released secondary to rIL-2 administration [268].

Is rIL-2/LAK more effective than rIL-2 alone?

Early clinical studies of IL-2 performed at the NCI suggested that IL-2 monotherapy did not have significant antitumor activity [398, 399]. The earliest clinical studies showing efficacy utilized the rIL-2/LAK combination; however, subsequent evaluation showed that rIL-2 monotherapy was indeed also associated with antitumor responses [609]. The reasons for the apparent lack of efficacy in the initial IL-2 monotherapy studies are several and probably include the phase I nature of the studies and hence the implicitly advanced nature of the disease of the enrolled patients, the fact that in these studies patients often received only one or only very few doses of IL-2, and the fact that the initial testing of IL-2 monotherapy was rather rudimentary as the results of animal studies of the IL-2/LAK combination [492, 493] suggested that this combined approach would give much more spectacular results in the clinic than monotherapy with IL-2.

Small trials of either rIL-2 monotherapy or rIL-2/LAK combination therapy have left many investigators with the impression that the combined approach gives a somewhat higher response rate than rIL-2 alone [600]. In terms of toxicity, these small, uncontrolled trials suggest that the rIL-2/LAK combination is more toxic than the sum of the two treatments given separately [85]. However, the small numbers of patients treated in these studies plus substantial patient heterogeneity preclude any scientifically valid conclusion concerning the relative merits of rIL-2 versus rIL-2/LAK being drawn from the results of such trials. It is well recognized that small studies can often give misleading results. For example, the results from two published trials would lead one to conclude that the rIL-2/LAK combination has no activity in malignant melanoma [85] and that high-dose rIL-2 monotherapy has no activity in renal-cell carcinoma [2], conclusions that we know cannot be valid based on the many positive results from other trials. The numbers of patients entered into these studies were 14 and 6, respectively.

It is considered essential to differentiate in a scientifically valid way the relative advantages and disadvantages conferred by *ex vivo* generated LAK cells in terms of toxicity and efficacy, since the requirement for *ex vivo* LAK cell generation adds greatly to the difficulty and expense of rIL-2 therapy, to the extent that its application in most hospitals would probably be precluded if such cellular therapy was found to be essential.

Several randomized studies of rIL-2 monotherapy versus rIL-2 plus LAK have been conducted in an attempt to answer these questions [186, 229, 598, 612]. More recent data in randomized studies has suggested that IL-2 was effective alone as compared with the combination with LAK cells in patients with renal cancer, while in patients with melanoma there was some suggestion that LAK cells improved survival [616]. Studies using Interleukin-2 alone have reported partial or complete tumor regression in 15-25% of patients with malignant melanoma or renal cancer [614-617]. These studies utilized high-dose bolus Interleukin-2 as popularized by Rosenberg and co-workers. These studies and others with bolus IL-2 prompted the Food and Drug Administration to approve IL-2 for metastatic renal cancer in 1992.

Continuous infusion Interleukin-2 has been widely used in the United States and Europe with a variety of different regimens reported. The initial studies were conducted by West and Oldham [773] and follow-up studies were done by a variety of other authors [147-149, 223, 752]. Subcutaneous IL-2 has also been utilized, more widely in Europe than in the United States with response rates in the 10-25% range with much lower toxicity [34, 79].

Comparative studies are still underway to determine the optimal regimen with regard to both toxicity and response rates. It is clear that the lower dose regimens such as subcutaneous and low-dose intravenous (bolus or continuous) are less toxic than the higher doses. In addition, at the same dose level infusions of IL-2 may have lower toxicity than bolus doses when compared on a total dose per 24-h basis. The numbers of patients in these clinical trials have been relatively small and comparative studies with larger numbers of patients are needed.

A major limitation for LAK cell therapy has been the laboratory time and expense associated with cell production. Oldham and Yannelli have developed a method for the bedside, inexpensive activation of LAK cells [285]. Clinical trials are underway today with this new, much simpler method of producing LAK cells [147, 148, 534, 535].

Local therapeutic modalities with rIL-2

Due to rIL-2's short serum half-life and severe toxicities following parenteral administration, investigations have explored alternative methods of administering rIL-2 to potentiate its antitumor activity with less toxicity. Local injection of rIL-2 at the tumor site would theoretically achieve higher concentrations for a longer duration and could potentially result in enhanced activation of tumor-infiltrating lymphocytes without the necessity for high intravenous doses.

Intraperitoneal (ip) administration of rIL-2 or rIL-2 with infusion of LAK cells has been reported for intra-abdominal malignancies, and ip concentrations comparable to those used to activate antitumor effector cells *in vitro* have been achieved and maintained for long durations.

Urba et al. administered one-quarter of Rosenberg's systemic rIL-2 doses ip and observed an extended half-life of 8 h [738]. High ip concentrations of IL-2 maintained LAK activity in the peritoneal cavity throughout treatment periods with reduced systemic toxicity. Although IFN-gamma was detected in peritoneal fluid, the 35% clinical response rate did not correlate with concentrations of either rIL-2 or IFN-gamma or ip effector cell activity. Repeated therapy was precluded by the development of intraperitoneal fibrosis, which was hypothesized to be due to rIL-2 induced release of platelet-derived growth factor.

Although the usual rIL-2-related toxicities appear to be less severe after ip administration, possibly because of low concentrations of IL-2 measurable in serum after ip administration, other investigators have also noted severe peritoneal fibrosis, which they attributed to detectable peritoneal concentrations of TNF-alpha [53, 446]. However, another group has observed a significant antitumor effect in ovarian carcinoma at low doses (6×10^4 to 6×10^5 IU/m^2/day) of rIL-2 administered ip, without peritoneal fibrosis [379].

Pizza et al. [576] were the first to report tumor regression resulting from direct injection of purified natural IL-2 into bladder tumors. Response appeared to be dose-dependent, requiring doses of at least 1200 IU, and no adverse effects were experienced by any patients.

Adoptive immunotherapy of brain tumors has also been investigated [43, 448]. Intralesional infusion of rIL-2 with LAK cells caused increased cerebral edema, which was responsible for most of the adverse neuropsychiatric events experienced by the patients. Systemic toxicities were not observed. Antitumor response was minimal and may partly be attributed to the concomitant administration of corticosteroids to decrease intracranial pressure, since there appeared to be a correlation between steroid use and inhibition of LAK inducibility in PBL. This observation is consistent with the finding that corticosteroids decrease IL-2 receptor expression on PBL [588]. Further studies need to be done to define the antitumor efficacy of rIL-2 given directly into the central nervous system to treat brain tumors.

There have also been reports of significant tumor responses produced by injection of rIL-2 into or around the lymphatic system, with minimal toxicity. These have involved the combination of natural IL-2 (60, 000 IU) and LAK cells injected into the lymphatic vessels of the feet of patients with a variety of advanced metastatic malignancies [577], the perilymphatic injection of very low doses of natural IL-2 (1200 units) to patients with head and neck carcinoma [117], and splenic artery perfusion of 9×10^4 to 2.4×10^5 IU/kg/day of rIL-2 in patients with advanced metastatic malignancy. However, a more recent phase II trial of perilymphatic injection of low-dose rIL-2 [345] has not corroborated the major efficacy previously reported by Cortesina et al. [111] using Jurkat Natural IL-2. In view of the importance of local invasion of head and neck carcinoma to the pathogenesis of this malignancy, together with the encouraging results obtained in trials using both natural [111] and recombinant IL-2 [673], this route of administration warrants further investigation.

Intrapleural instillation of rIL-2 has been reported and produced sustained concentrations of rIL-2 in the pleural effusion without serious toxicity [793]. The disappearance of malignant cells in the effusions and the subsequent disappearance of the effusions occurred in nine of 11 patients 4-10 days after the initiation of therapy, and appeared to correlate with the presence of LAK cells in the effusions of the responders.

In addition, continuous perfusion of the bladder with rIL-2 is being studied and appears to produce desirable local immunomodulation without any adverse effects. However, the optimal dosage of rIL-2 remains to be defined [292].

Interleukin-2 has also been given by inter-arterial, continuous subcutaneous, intramuscular routes as well as by inhalation [293]. Huland and co-workers reported that Interleukin-2 by inhalation was as effective as Interleukin-2 intravenously in the treatment of pulmonary metastasis from metastatic renal cancer, a report that remains to be confirmed by other investigators.

IL-2 and tumor-infiltrating lymphocytes

In an effort to reduce the toxicities associated with high-dose administration of rIL-2 and LAK cells, Rosenberg et al. [610, 722] identified a subpopulation of lymphocytes that infiltrate tumors, appropriately termed tumor-infiltrating lymphocytes (TIL). These TIL demonstrated up to 100 times the antitumor efficacy of LAK cells and were active against LAK-resistant tumors in murine models. Although the adoptively transferred TIL were effective without concomitantly administered rIL-2, addition of low doses of rIL-2 enhanced efficacy with potentially less toxicity. The greatest antitumor effects were demonstrated by prior immunosuppression, with either cyclophosphamide or irradiation, followed by TIL and rIL-2 [610]. These encouraging animal experiments set the stage for subsequent clinical trials.

Initially, it was shown that these long-term cultured tumor-derived T-cells could safely be adoptively transferred to humans, but produced minimal antitumor response [359, 417]. In a phase I pilot study, combination therapy with cyclophosphamide, rIL-2, and TIL has been shown to be safe and feasible, but an optimally effective regimen remains to be determined [723]. More recent clinical trials [360, 611], utilizing different rIL-2 regimens with and without cyclophosphamide in combination with TIL, suggest that this therapy may be superior to rIL-2/LAK or rIL-2 alone.

Studies by Oldham and co-workers using Interleukin-2 by continuous infusion with tumor-derived activated cells (TDAC), cultured T-cell derived from the tumor in a manner similar to TIL, have demonstrated the feasibility of preparing large numbers of T cells for therapy. A major problem with the initial TIL studies as conducted by Rosenberg has been the laborious nature of cell production using a system developed by Oldham and co-workers with cells being grown in multiple tissue culture bags. Our group has abandoned that technique because of the high cost and potential for danger with breaks in sterility to develop and adopt a technique using bioreactors. These small bioreactors are capable of growing large numbers of T-cells at a much lower cost with a safer technique for large-scale clinical trials. While these studies have indicated the feasibility of such an approach and defined the cost with reasonable surety, the response rates remain low and in the same range as seen with Interleukin-2 alone or Interleukin-2 combined with LAK cells or other lymphokines such as Interferon. Further studies in this area are necessary, however, to define the optimal therapeutic modality and its role in cancer therapy, especially since the generation of TIL is complex, costly, and technically impossible in many patients with cancer [536, 543, 669]. Most importantly, dose response studies with activated T cells (TIL/TDAC) have not been done. These studies must be done, even though they will be expensive, to fully explore the effects of T cells in cancer treatment.

IL-2 in combination with other therapeutic agents

The enhancement of antibody-dependent cellular cytotoxicity by rIL-2-activated lymphocytes against tumor targets that had been incubated with tumor-specific antibodies [655] raised the possibility of using rIL-2 and monoclonal antibodies in the immunotherapy of cancer. In murine tumor models, significant antitumor activity has now been demonstrated with various regimens of tumor-specific monoclonal antibodies in combination with rIL-2-activated effector cells, generated either *in vivo* or adoptively transferred [230, 330]. These results provide a rationale for clinical trials of rIL-2 and antitumor monoclonal antibodies, which have now begun [808].

It has been demonstrated that cyclophosphamide has potential in facilitating adoptive immunotherapy of cancer by eliminating tumor-induced suppressor T cells [524] as well as reducing tumor burden. Encouraging results have also been obtained in animal studies [561, 660], which have led to clinical trials of low-dose cyclophosphamide in combination with rIL-2 [117, 350, 387, 464]. Recent animal studies suggest that the sequence of rIL-2 and cyclophosphamide administration is important since maximum therapeutic efficacy was demonstrated only when rIL-2 was administered within 1-4 days after cyclophosphamide [333]. In addition, low-dose (300 mg/m^2) cyclophosphamide appears preferable to higher doses in terms of subsequent induction of LAK cells [173]. As yet, antitumor results seem to suggest that there is no advantage of this approach over that of rIL-2 alone; however, further studies are required to define the optimum combination regimen and to clarify the role of such a combination in the immunotherapy of cancer [538].

Based on the proven, yet limited, efficacy of classical combination chemotherapy in the treatment of cancer, ongoing investigations are exploring the safety and efficacy of various combinations of chemotherapeutic agents with rIL-2 [146, 682, 743].

Perhaps the best rationale for combining chemotherapy and Interleukin-2 is in metastatic melanoma. Interleukin-2 alone or with LAK cells, TIL/TDAC cells or Interferon produces consistent response rates in the range of 10-40% with 1-10% of the patients remaining in durable remissions of greater than two years duration (? cure). Thus, Interleukin-2 based regimens represent the best hope for a sustained complete remission in patients with advanced melanoma. By contrast, chemotherapy using various combinations of three to four drugs can produce objective response rates in 40-50% of the patients with much less durable results. Thus, the rationale for combining a high response rate chemotherapy regimen with a long duration effect from Interleukin-2 has been obvious. Studies of DTIC plus IL-2 have not demonstrated response rates in excess of that seen for IL-2 alone [146, 193, 683]. Cisplatinum with Interleukin-2 or with DTIC and Interferon have also been studied with response rates in the 50% range [601]. Multi-agent chemotherapy using various combinations of Cisplatinum, Vinblastine, DTIC, BCNU and Tamoxifen have produced response rates in the 40-60% range in recent trials [378, 597].

Many of these studies have produced somewhat higher response rates but, as yet, there is no evidence of a prolonged duration of response compared to IL-2 alone. Further studies are necessary combining IL-2 with various chemotherapy agents.

Since cytokines possess overlapping immunomodulating activities, research has also been devoted to combining rIL-2 with other cytokines in an attempt to identify synergistic combinations that might enhance antitumor efficacy in the clinic with decreased toxicity. Preclinical results have revealed significant synergistic antitumor effects produced by combinations of rIL-2 with rTNF-alpha, rIFN-alpha, rIFN-beta, and rIFN-alpha A/D hybrid [80, 303, 441, 442, 535] but not with rIFN-gamma [80, 303]. Phase I clinical trials of some of these combinations have demonstrated that they are generally no more toxic than therapy with the individual agents given alone. They have also been shown to be immunomodulating in these patients [361, 465, 560, 649, 767].

Phase II studies with Interleukin-2 plus Interferon have been conducted by a variety of investigators and is the most studied biotherapy combination to date. Multiple preclinical studies were encouraging with regard to activating immune response with the combination of IL-2 and Interferon, suggesting an effect of Interferon on antigen expression which might be exploited when used in combination with IL-2-activated cytotoxic killing. In addition, the antiproliferative activity of Interferon was a possible mechanism by which the anticancer combination of the two could be enhanced. Multiple clinical studies have now been done using Interferon and Interleukin-2 in combination, with each biologic having been given by a variety of different doses, schedules and route of administration. Rosenberg combined high-dose bolus Interleukin-2 with moderate-dose intravenous Interferon with a complete and partial response rate of approximately 41% in patients with melanoma, renal cancer and a few with other malignancies [613]. Follow-up studies by a variety of investigators using different doses and schedules of the two drugs have not been able to confirm the encouraging results reported by Rosenberg [35, 77, 304, 375, 466, 542, 613, 638, 753].

It is apparent from the large number of phase II trials that have been conducted that the combination of Interleukin-2 and Interferon in these doses, schedules and routes of administration have not shown any significant advantage over Interleukin-2 alone and many investigators are now exploring the sequential use of Interleukin-2 and Interferon as a potentially superior strategy.

Toxicity in perspective

The multisystem toxicities (Table 1) associated with rIL-2 therapy have received much attention and are the subject of several reviews [140, 425, 456]. Phase I studies have shown that toxicity is dose-dependent yet reversible shortly after discontinuation of the IL-2. The most frequent dose-limiting toxicities consist of pyrexia, hypotension, oliguria, pulmonary edema, a vascular leak syndrome, and neurotoxicity. Even if antitumor efficacy is positively correlated to the intensity of rIL-2 dose and schedule employed [69, 608, 712], an understanding of the mechanisms of toxicity may permit interventions that minimize the toxicity without compromising efficacy.

The demonstration that LAK cells could lyse normal cells, despite preferential cytotoxicity of malignant cells [124, 553, 668], indicated a potential mechanism of toxicity. The most important dose-limiting toxicity of IL-2 therapy is the vascular leak syndrome (VLS) [618], which appears to be responsible for other observed toxicities [609].

Table 1. Summary of the cytokine sources and effects related to the growth and treatment of cancer [a]

Cytokine	Cell source	Cells influenced	Effect [b]
IL1	Mono/Macros	Macrophages	Activation, PGE2, nitrogen oxide (w/IFNγ)
	B cells	B cells	Growth/differentiation (w/ IL4, IL6), chemotaxis
	T cells	T cells	Growth (w/IL2), chemotaxis, IL2, IL2R, IFNγ.
	NK	LAK	Induction (w/IL2)
	Dendritic cells	NK cells	IFNγ secretion (w/ IL12), cytotoxicity (w/ IFN), IL2R
	Some tumor cells	Some tumor cells	Growth stimululation/inhibition /no effect
	Fibroblasts	Fibroblasts	Growth, PGE2, collagen metabolism
	Keratinocytes	Keratinocytes	Growth
	Endothelial cells	Endothelial cells	PGE2, PGI.
	Glial cells	Glial cells	Growth
	Eosinophils	Eosinophils	Degranulation
	Neurons	Basophils	Degranulation, histamine release
	Epithelial cells	Neutrophils	Chemotaxis
		Liver	Metabolism, protein production
		Adipose	Lipoprotein lipase, decreased fat catabolism
		Synovial cells	PGE2, collagenase, phospholipase A2
		Melanoma	ICAM
		Vasc smooth muscle	Growth, IFN β
		Dendritic cells	maturation (w/ GM-CSF)
IL2	T cells (activated)	NK	Activation/cytotoxicity
	Dendritic cells	LAK	Activation/cytotoxicity
		T cells	Activation/proliferation/cytotoxocity
		PBL	Prolif/CTL generation
		TIL	Prolif/cytotoxicity
		B cells	Differentiation (w/ IL6, IL12)
		Certain tumors	Growth stimul/inhib/no effect
			ICAM/MHCI decreased
			Potentiates other regulators
		Dendritic cells	Proliferation
		Keratinocytes	Proliferation
IL3	T cells (activated)	Multipotent precursors	Growth
	Thymic epithelium	Megacaryocytes	Platelet production
	Keratinocytes	Erthrocyte precursors	RBC production
	Monocytes	Mast cells	Survival/growth (w/IL4)
	Neurons	Natural cytotoxic cells	Growth/TNF secretion

Table 1. (continued)

Cytokine	Cell source	Cells influenced	Effect [b]
	Eosinophils	NK	Activation/proliferation (w/IL-2)
IL3		T cells	Growth (w/IL2)
IL4	Helper T cells	B cells	Growth/Ig secretion (IgE)
	Mast cells		MHCII expression
	NK cells	Tcells	Growth (+/–/no effect)
	Basophils	Th2 cells	Differentiation
	Eosinophils	Monocytes	Growth
	Dendritic cells	Macrophages	Activation/Ag presentation/HLADR
		Fibroblasts	Growth
		Endothelial cells	Growth, VCAM
		PBL(IL2 primed)	Growth
		NK cells	Proliferation (w/ IL2, IL12), IL5 secretion
		Mast cells	Growth (w/IL3)
		LAK (IL2 primed)	Activation (+/–), IL2R decrease
		Dendritic cells	Activation (w/IL2/IL7/GMCSF)
		Hematopoietic cells	Growth (+/–)
		Certain tumors	Decreased growth
IL5	Helper T cells	Eosinophils	Growth differentiation
	NK cells		Chemotaxis (w/IL8 RANTES)
	Eosinophils	B cells	Growth, Ig secretion (IgA, IgM)
		Mast cells	Growth (w/other factors)
		T cells	Differentiation (w/IL2), IL2R
		LAK cells	Activation (w/IL2)
		NK cells	Activation (w/IL2), IL2R
IL6	Fibroblasts	B lymphocytes	Differentiation, Ig secretion (w/ IL2)
	Macrophages	Tcells	Growth, activation (w/ IL2)
	Epithelial cells	Megacaryocytes	Colony growth, platelets
	Endothelial cells	NK cells	Activation, cytotoxicity
	Eosinophils	Hepatocytes	Stimulation
	Certain tumors	Fibroblasts	Differentiation inhibited
	Astrocytes	Intestine cells	Acute phase proteins
	Keratinocytes	Melanoma	Growth inhibition
		Breast cancer	ICAM 1
		Renal cell ca	Growth
IL7	Stroma, marrow	Precursor B cells	Growth/differentiation
	Stroma, thymus	Precursos T cells	Growth/differentiation
	Keratinocytes	Monocytes/Macroph	Growth/activation
	B cells	NK cells	Activation
	Certain carcinomas/	LAK	Activation
	Leukemia/lymphoma	T cells	Growth/differentiation
		Dendritic cells	Growth/ag presentation
		TIL	Activation/proliferation
		Melanoma	ICAM-1 expression
		Certain leukemias/lymphomas	Growth
IL8	Macrophages	Neutrophils	Chemotaxis
	Endothelial cells	T cells	Chemotaxis
	Neutrophils	Mast cells	Chemotaxis
	Epithelial cells	Macrophages	Chemotaxis
	Fibroblasts	Endothelial cells	Chemotaxis
	Keratinocytes	Eosinophils	Chemotaxis
	Granulocytes	NK cells	Chemotaxis
	Melanoma	Melanoma	Growth/metastasis
IL9	T helper cells	Progenitor cells	Growth (w/ GMCSF, w/IL3)

Table 1. (continued)

Cytokine	Cell source	Cells influenced	Effect [b]
IL9		Erythroid precursors	Growth (w/EPO)
		Fetal thymocytes	Growth (w/IL2)
		T cells (activated)	Growth (w/IL2)
		Mast cells	Growth (w/ IL3,IL4)
		B cells	IgE secretion
IL10	Helper T cells	T helper 1 cells	IFN/growth decreased
	Thymocytes	T cells, CD8	IFN decreased. Chemotaxis increased, growth +/–.
	B cells	NK cells	IFN/cytotoxicity decreased
	Monocytes	Spleen cells	IFN decreased
	Mast cells	Monocytes	GMCSF decreased
	Keratinocytes	Macrophages	IL12 decreased, activity decreased.
	Some tumor cells	Mast cells	Growth (w/ IL3,IL4)
		B cells	Growth /differentiation/ survival/MHC II
IL11	Stroma, marrow	Progenitor cells	Growth/colony fomation
		B cells	Ig increased
		T cells	Cytokines increased
		Fibroblasts	Differentiation to adipocytes decreased
		Liver cells	Acute phase proteins increased
IL12	B cells	NK cells	Growth/cytotoxicity/IFN secretion (w/ IL1)
	Macrophages		IFN increased, IL5 decreased
	Dendritic cells	CD8 T cells	w/IL2 Growth/ IFN/ cytotoxicity increase
	Some B cell tumors	CD4 Th1 cells	IFNγ /IL2/growth increased
		CD4 Th2 cells	IL4/IL10/growth decreased
		PBL	LAK Induction
			CTL growth/cytotoxicity
		Thymus, progenitors	Growth (CD8)
		TIL	Growth/cytotoxicity
IL13	T cells	Monocytes/macroph	Nitric oxide decreased
			CD14 (endotoxin receptor) decreased
			MHC II/ cell adhesion increased
		Neutrophils	IL1 receptor antagonist increased
			CD14 (endotoxin receprtor) decreased
		B cells	Growth /Ig Isotype switching/production (w/other cytokines), MHCII
		T cells	Inhibits chemotaxis
IL14	T cells	B cells	Growth, differentiation, memory
	NK cells		
	Follicular denritic cells		
	B cells		
IL15	Epithelium	CTL	Growth/cytotoxicity
	Stroma, marrow	B cells	Proliferation, IgG, IgM, IgA
	PBMC	NK	Growth/cytotoxicity
	Fibroblasts	LAK	Induction
	Keratinocytes	TIL/TDAC	Growth
SCF	Liver Cells	Progenitor cells	Growth
	Stroma, marrow	Mast cells	Growth
	Fibroblasts	Certain tumors	Growth
	Spleen cells		
	Certain tumor cells		
IFN α	Leukocytes	Macrophages	Nitrogen oxide/ superoxide
	Macrophages		TNFα increased
β	Fibroblasts		IL10 decreased
	Epithelial cells		Cytotoxicity increased

Table 1. (continued)

Cytokine	Cell source	Cells influenced	Effect [b]
IFN γ	T cells (Th1 and CD8)		Fc Receptor increased
	NK cells	Cells in general	P1 Kinase
			2'-5' Oligoadenylate Synthetase
			Mx proteins, MHC I /II
		Macrophages	Activation, H_2O_2
		NK cells	Cytotoxicity increased
		B cells	Altered Ig isotype secretion
			Inhibition of IL4 induced functions
		CD8	T cells With IL2 differentiation and cytotoxicity
		CD4 Th1 cells	Increased Growth/cytokine production
		CD4 Th2 cells	Decreased growth/cytokine production
		Endothelial cells	Decreased growth/angiogenesis
		Tumor cells	Decreased growth/increased differentiation
			Decreased sensitivity to NK cells
TNF	Monocytes/Macroph	TIL	Increased cytotoxicity
	Activated T-cells	LAK	Increased cytotoxicity
	NK cells	Endothelial cells	Toxicity, decreased growth
	Endothelial cells	Macrophages	Nitric Oxide (esp w/ IFNγ)
	Mast cells	Dendritic cells	Growth /differentiation (w/ GMCSF)
		Certain tumors	Increased/decreased growth

[a] This is a partial listing and emphasizes cancer related activities.
[b] Activity increased unless otherwise indicated.

Endothelial cell adherence and lysis by IL-2-activated lymphocytes has been suggested to be the cause of increased capillary permeability that results in the VL [31, 124]. LAK cell cytotoxicity to endothelial cells has been reported to be proportional to the dose of rIL-2, the number of LAK cells present, and the duration of contact, but is not due directly to exposure to rIL-2 alone [124, 356]. The IL-2-induced secretion of TNF, IL-1, and IFN-gamma may play a role by regulating the expression of leukocyte adhesion molecules that enhance the binding of lymphocytes to the endothelium [114, 168]. Recent work has shown, however, that these cytokines inhibit LAK cell-mediated endothelial cell lysis and may actually protect patients from the development of the VLS [457]. Interleukin-2-induced secretion of thromboxane A2 appears to be a direct cause of the pulmonary edema that occurs and has also been proposed to be involved in the development of the VLS [185]. Activation of the complement system has been reported to occur in association with the administration of rIL-2, and this has therefore also been suggested as a contributor to the VLS [710]. The above research illustrates the complexity of IL-2's effects, either directly or indirectly on the vascular endothelium, and this is probably why the exact cause of the VLS is still not clearly understood.

Interleukin-2 administration produces a hemodynamic pattern similar to that of septic shock, with decreased vascular resistance leading to hypotension and oliguria [529]. In animals, the administration of TNF produces physiologic changes similar to those caused by endotoxemia, which can be prevented by prior administration of a neutralizing antibody to TNF [728]. After infusion of endotoxin in humans, elevated serum concentrations of TNF have been shown to be temporally associated with flu-like symptoms consisting of fever, chills, headache, myalgia, and nausea [454], which typically occur during IL-2 therapy. Similar responses occur when rTNF is administered directly to patients with cancer [760]. Work by Mier et al. [458] has demonstrated that rIL-2 is not intrinsically pyrogenic, nor is fever caused by endotoxin contamination of the rIL-2 preparations. It has shown, however, that rIL-2 administration results in increased serum concentrations of TNF-alpha, which could be responsible for the fever and other significant toxicities associated with rIL-2 therapy.

Since the antitumor mechanism of rIL-2 is still not well understood, efforts to reduce toxicity may inadvertently compromise efficacy as well. Although researchers have reported that the NK cell is the predominant LAK effector cell [552, 573, 716, 766], a recent study of murine leukemia has shown that depletion of NK cells reduced the toxicity of IL-2 but did not appear to decrease therapeutic efficacy as measured by survival [568]. Attempts to antagonize the toxic effects of TNF by the use of neutralizing antibodies, although effective in some animal models [728], may negate the synergistic efficacy of therapy observed with the combination of rIL-2 and TNF [441, 442]. It is clear that further elucidation of the mechanisms of toxicity as well as antitumor efficacy is needed in order to optimize cancer therapy with IL-2.

Possible determinants of response

Although complete responses to rIL-2 treatment have been observed in clinical trials, most responses have been only partial and of short duration. There are several proposed explanations why the *in vitro* and preclinical potential of IL-2 has not been realized in clinical cancer therapy.

Investigators have found a positive correlation between tumor response and patient performance status, pretreatment lymphocyte counts, and IL-2-induced rebound lymphocytosis [145, 556, 773]. Since the immunologic effects of IL-2 appear to be the result of a combination of cellular activation, cellular proliferation, and induction of cytokine secretion, the status of the immune system and the effects of previous treatments may influence the capability of the patient to respond.

Tumor bulk has been proposed [145, 171, 192, 556, 773] as a possible limitation of responsiveness, and IL-2 may be most effective in the presence of minimal residual disease after tumor debulking with conventional chemo-radiotherapy and/or surgery, that is, as an adjuvant therapy. However, some murine studies [680] have demonstrated that cytoreduction does not influence outcome of IL-2 therapy.

For both LAK and TIL cells only relatively small numbers of cells over a short duration have been infused. The effects of higher cell doses (dose response studies) and chronic repeated administration need to be explored. Oldham has suggested that repeated, chronic administration of activated cells with moderate doses of IL-2 might produce further tumor responses [536, 537]. With bioreactors, unlimited numbers of cells can be produced for such clinical trials.

The formation of neutralizing antibodies has been reported [350, 361] and may adversely affect the *in vivo* generation of LAK activity [361] and possibly antitumor responses.

In early clinical trials with Jurkat IL-2, Lotze et al. [398] reported the presence of a serum inhibitor of IL-2-induced lymphocyte proliferation *in vivo*. Recent investigators [73, 259] have now demonstrated that rIL-4 is a potent inhibitor of rIL-2-induced proliferation and activation of PBL into LAK effectors. These suppressive influences illustrate the complexity of *in vivo* regulatory mechanisms, which may explain the lack of correlation between *in vitro* LAK activity and clinical efficacy [65].

Although much has been learned about the immune system from the *in vitro* and *in vivo* studies of IL-2, additional research is necessary in order to better understand the immune-mediated mechanism(s) responsible for the observed antitumor efficacy of IL-2 so that its therapeutic use can be optimized.

INTERLEUKIN-3

General stimulator of hematopoietic cells

IL-3 is a 28, 000 mw hematopoietic factor which acts on most early multipotential progenitor cells to stimulate growth. It has remarkable effects on platelet production. Synonyms for this pleiotropic cytokine include histamine producing cell stimulating factor, P cell stimulating factor, CFU stimulating activity, mast cell growth factor, Thy 1 inducing factor, multicolony stimulating factor and hematopoietic growth factor [468]. IL-3 is produced by T cells (especially lectin/antigen stimulated T cells), thymic epithelium, keratinocytes and cell lines of monocytic and neuronal lineage [104, 105, 300, 308] and eosinophils [344]. Effects on early erythroid and megakaryocyte growth are marked and rather distinct to IL-3. IL-3 acts as a growth stimulator and primer for other factors which act subsequently to stimulate differentiation. Therefore, the clinical use IL-3 is being tested in combination with other cytokines such as GM CSF, MCSF and EPO for treatment with chemotherapy and in bone marrow transplant patients.

The domain of IL-3 activity includes pluripotential hematopoietic progenitors, early committed precursors in all of the hematopoietic lineages, and members of the granulocyte, macrophage, and mast-cell lineages through their most mature forms. The only hematopoietic cells that are unresponsive to the trophic effects of IL-3 are those in the distal limbs of the erythroid [308] and megakaryocytic [779] pathways. However, Il-3 is quite effective in stimulating megakaryocyte activity and platelet production. Thus, macrophages, granulocytes, and mast cells are supported from pluripotent precursors through the mature forms. However, there is no unequivocal evidence for a direct effect on cells committed to the T- or B-cell lineages. Interleukin-3 differs distinctly from other hematopoietic growth factors, such as GM-CSF, since recent cDNA cloning of both factors now establishes formally their distinct polypeptide sequences [207, 244].

Furthermore, although IL-3 can mimic the action of other known growth factors on neutrophil and macrophage lineages, no other growth factors identified thus far are capable of supporting growth of pluripotential and early committed cells in the erythroid and megakaryocytic lines.

It appears from murine models that IL-3 may circulate unbound to carrier proteins, and has an approximate molecular weight of 33, 800. Interleukin-3 has a plasma half-life of approximately 40 minutes and is filtered by the glomerulus and degraded in the renal tubules [161]. It seems to be released during immune reactions as the link between the immune and hematopoietic systems in generating hematopoietic effector cells.

Stutman and co-workers described natural cytotoxic (NC) cells [558, 690], which are mast-cell-like morphologically and participate in immune reactions, such as tumor rejection [56, 63, 96, 262, 671] and graft-versus-host diseases [103]. They differ from NK cells in their origin, morphology, and their time to lyse targets. Jadus et al. [313, 314] determined that these cells were IL-3-dependent and IL-2-unresponsive. This suggested further that NC cells may use a TNF/LT-like mediator to produce target cell lyses [311].

IL-3 appears to able to specifically activate macrophages without inducing cytotoxicity [205]. IL-3 also stimulates growth and activity in mast cells [427] and basophils [452].

Recent work using a mouse model suggests tumor cell vaccines engineered to produce IL-3 may stimulate tumor antigen presentation by macrophages [581]. It should be noted IL-3 may be a growth factor for certain tumors of hematopoietic cell lineage [37].

In vivo responses to IL-3 injected intraperitoneally in murine systems in dosages ranging from 6 to 200 mg per injection thrice daily for 6 days have shown dose-related rises in peritoneal macrophages, neutrophils, and eosinophils, with peritoneal macrophages exhibiting greatly increased phagocytic activity. Spleen weight increased 100-fold, and rises in mast cells were observed accompanying a two- to fourfold increase in megakaryocytes and nucleated erythroid cells, as well as 10- to 30-fold rises in progenitor cells. It did not, however, produce a rise in total marrow cell numbers [451]. These results suggest that IL-3 may prove useful therapeutically by increasing resistance to a variety of infections by increasing mature cell numbers of nonhematopoietic tissues.

Early phase clinical trials have clearly shown an increase in platelets in patients with thrombocytopenia. Thus, a major use of IL-3 may be in combination with other CSFs in stimulation of bone marrow productive capacity. See chapters 19 and 20 for more detailed information.

INTERLEUKIN-4

The cytokine for B cell and T helper (Th2) response

Interleukin-4 is a 129 amino acid single chain glycoprotein, 20, 000 mol wt which is secreted by certain activated CD4+ helper T cells [49, 365, 386, 487], by mast cells [68, 74], by NK cells [397], basophils [414], eosinophils [522] and antigen presenting dendritic cells [431]. The gene for IL-4 is located on chromosome 5 and was cloned in 1986.

IL-4 was originally referred to as B cell stimulatory factor-1 for its effect on B cell growth and secretion [178, 287, 567, 586]. IL-4 influences pre-B cells differentiation to IgG secreting plasmacytes [357, 582, 675, 751]. IL-4 stimulates immunoglobulin secretion. It has a particularly important role in IgE production [102, 107, 134, 667, 675] related to allergic inflammation [708]. IL-4 also increases the expression of MHC class II on B cells [520]. IL-4 has a remarkable effect on T cell growth and differentiation [1, 86]. IL-4 stimulated outgrowth of monocytes [709], macrophages [518], and increased macrophage antitumor cell activity [115]. IL-4 also stimulated growth of polymorphonuclear leukocytes [180], fibroblasts [474] and endothelial cells. IL-4, together with IL-3, stimulated proliferation of mast cells [735] and IL-4 stimulated cell surface ICAM-1 [742]. IL-4 enhanced proliferation in activated PBL but had little growth promoting effect on unprimed resting cells. Interestingly, timing of cytokine addition is a factor in response. While IL-4 stimulated cells previously activated with IL-2, IL-4 added to cultures simultaneously inhibited proliferation induced by IL-2 [125, 259, 730].

The receptor for IL-4 is found on hematopoietic cells [563], endothelial cells, fibroblasts [525, 718] and several types of cancer [9, 481, 525, 724, 725]. The IL-4 receptor consists of at least 1 peptide chain, 140 kDa, which has been cloned [61]. The IL-4 receptor has protein kinase activity known to phosphorylate various proteins including the IL-4 receptor itself and a 170 kDa protein which in its phosphorylated form binds and activates phoshatidylinositol-3' kinase [334] producing additional activating signals.

In addition to the cellular receptor, IL-4 R also exists in a soluble form found in body fluids [176, 182]. The soluble receptor is smaller in size but retains the binding character of the membrane bound receptor [484]. The soluble receptor is not simply a shed proteolytic product of the membrane receptor. Rather it arises from a separate message from the same gene by a distinct RNA splicing pathway [46, 484]. Mitogen activation of T lymphocytes stimulated production of both the membrane bound [530, 593] and soluble [97] IL-4 receptors in T cells, B cells and macrophages. IL-4 production appeared to be required for soluble receptor production.

The function of the soluble receptor is not certain. Stimulatory [675] and inhibitory [177, 418, 632] functions have been observed. It has been suggested that soluble receptors compete with bound receptors for ligand, effectively decreasing IL-4 activity [181, 418]. The soluble receptor may also serve as a carrier [184] which may protect the ligand from metabolism and excretion thereby increasing its functional halflife [183]. The off rate of the soluble receptor would allow ligand transfer from the soluble to the membrane receptor. Perhaps the same soluble receptor serves both stimulatory and inhibitory functions acting as a buffer for IL-4 activity.

IL-4 shares certain biological activities in common with IL-13. There is sequence homology between the two proteins. While cloned IL-4 receptor does not bind IL-13, IL-4 and IL-13 receptors share a common subunit which functions in signal transduction [67, 809-811].

A recombinant IL-4 antagonist has been produced with tyrosine 124 substituted by aspartic acid [362]. This ligand binds with high affinity to the IL-4 receptor, competes successfully with native IL-4 for the binding site, and inhibits IL-4 dependent proliferation in a T cell line. Same site substituted with several other amino acids produced a receptor binding ligand with partial agonist activity. These results showed that binding and activity (signal generation) can be uncoupled for the IL-4 receptor [362].

Peripheral blood mononuclear cells stimulated with IL-2 developed LAK cytotoxicity toward Daudi tumor cells. In mice IL-4 could induce LAK in the absence of added IL-2 [494, 568]. When mouse PBLs were induced with IL-2, IL-4 tended to enhance LAK activity [494]. In humans, LAK may be induced by IL-4 in cancer patients pretreated with IL-2 but not in normal unprimed lymphocyte donors [273, 312, 324, 325]. In previously untreated cells, IL-4 added with IL-2 inhibited the induction of LAK by IL-2 [73, 259, 273, 324, 674, 775]. Evidently priming with IL-2, *in vivo* or in culture, was necessary for IL-4 activity. Loss of the IL2R may be the means by which IL4 inhibited LAK [389].

IL4 has complex stimulatory and inhibitory effects on T cell growth [487, 488, 803, 804]. IL-4 enhances activity of cytotoxic T cells in a mixed lymphocyte reaction. The timing of IL-4 was critical; IL-4 present during initiation inhibited cytotoxicity whereas IL-4 added 3 days later stimulated activity [325, 326, 674, 775]. When unstimulated PBL's from normal donors were tested, IL-4 alone had no effect. In cultures activated with anti-CD3, IL-4 stimulated growth. In cultured cells from IL-2 pretreated cancer patients, IL-4 alone stimulated growth in 5/11 cultures and enhanced IL-2 stimulated growth in most cases. It appears IL-4 may have beneficial effects on peripheral blood T cells when added after activation or after IL-2 pretreatment.

There is a similar general pattern of IL-4 effect in tumor infiltrating lymphocyte cultures. Cultures with IL-4 in combination with IL-2, grew T cells from human tumors with specific activity against autologous tumor [325, 326, 382, 737. TIL could not be generated using IL-4 only [326]. For certain non-melanoma tumors (sarcomas and renal), IL-4 together with IL-2 produced better growth and specific antitumor activity in many but not all cases [188, 325]. IL-4 produced some growth benefit early in the cultures of certain TIL of bladder and prostate cancer but there was no evidence of benefit for colon cancer or hepatoma. In some cases, an IL-4 benefit in early culture reversed with time [325]. In another study, Jadus et al [312] found that IL-4 in combination with IL-2 tended to produce more cells with increased antitumor cytotoxicity compared to TIL induced with IL-2 only. We developed an IL-4 dependent T cell line from the node specimen of a lymphoma patient. This tumor cell line had a requirement for IL-4 in addition to IL-2 [382].

Other TIL studies did not show remarkable benefits of IL-4. In one study using melanoma cells, the addition of IL-4 with IL-2 to TIL culture medium promoted growth in a minority of cases (5/24), but decreased growth in most cases (17/24). Likewise, specific lysis was enhanced by IL-4 in a minority of cases but depressed in the majority (13/19) [388]. It may be that IL-4 stimulated those T cells optimally activated by tumor antigen but inhibited those cells which have not been activated [388].

IL-4 influences cells involved in antigen presentation. IL-4 is produced by dendritic epidermal T cells. Together with IL-2, also produced by these cells, and IL-7, produced by keratinocytes [431-433], IL-4 appears to have an autocrine stimulatory effect on the growth of these professional antigen presenting cells [432]. During the activation of B cells, IL-4 induced the expression of class II histocompatibility antigens [520]. IL-4 also activated macrophages and appeared to enhance capacity to present antigen [115, 803, 804].

In bone marrow hematopoietic cells, IL-4 may be stimulatory or inhibitory depending of the cell type and physiologic status [592, 657]. IL-4 blocked certain effects of IL-2. IFN gamma inhibited some of the actions of IL-4. IL-4 stimulated IgE production; this was blocked by IFN.

There are two major subsets of helper T cells (Th1 and Th2) [486, 488, 605] and these helper cells have the remarkable effect of steering immune response toward humoral or cellular pathways. The process involves apoptosis, programmed cell death. Several hormones and cytokines including IL-4 regulate apoptosis. Glucocorticoids are immunosuppressive. They stimulate apoptosis in thymocytes and in mature T cells. IL-4, IL-1 and IL-2 [459, 807] inhibited glucocorticoid induced apoptosis. IL-4 specifically rescued Th2 cells from glucocorticoid induced death; IL-2 specifically rescued Th1 cells. Th1 cells secrete predominantly IL-2 and IFN γ. Th1 cells stimulate cellular immunity. Th2 cells secrete IL-4 and IL-10, and stimulate humoral immunity. Th0 cells are precursors which give rise to Th1 and Th2 cells. IL-4 appears to exert primary control over the pathway of differentiation. Th0 cells secrete IL-2, IL-4 and IFN. *In vitro*, addition of IL-4 depressed IL-2 and IFN production, and favored the formation of IL-4 secreting Th2 cells. Decreased IL-4 levels (by anti IL-4 treatment) favored the formation of TH1 cells [1]. IFN γ has a negative influence on TH2 development. Ability to direct the type response is important since certain antigens are better eliminated by one or the other type immunity. Cellular immune response appears to be advantageous in controlling cancer and oncogenic virus infections.

IL-4 appears to have a direct receptor mediated influence on growth of certain tumor cells. IL-4 inhibits the growth of certain carcinomas of colon, breast, head and neck, melanoma, renal cancer cells and certain hematological malignancies. These effects are IL-4 receptor dependent. Lack of response in cell lines was generally related to lack of high affinity receptors for IL-4. IL-4 had a direct inhibitory efect upon the growth of a myeloblastic leukemia cell line which depended on GCSF for growth [305]. Melanoma and renal carcinoma cell growth were inhibited by IL-4 alone and in combination with interferon-γ or tumor necrosis factor-α [283, 284]. Murine sarcoma, colon adenocarcinoma [584, 719] and human renal cancer cells [283, 284, 525], stomach cancer [9, 480, 481] grew more slowly in IL-4 supplemented medium. IL-4 blocked G1-S progression by down regulating several key cell cycle regulating factors [719].

Normal human fibroblasts and endothelial cell lines do contain receptors for IL-4 but IL-4 did not decrease the growth of normal cells [525]. IL-4 inhibited cultured non-Hodgkins lymphoma cells [131] and leukemia cells [8, 589]. TNF and IL-6 levels were decreased. TNF is a growth factor for these tumor cells. These results suggested that IL-4 may block growth in B cell malignancies by interfering with an autocrine loop. Manabe et al. [420] cultured leukemic cells and normal B cells on bone marrow stroma. IL-4 induced apoptosis in the 16 of 21 leukemia cell lines. This included cells with multi drug resistance. No evidence for T cell, NK or stromal cell mediated killing. Unfortunately, cytotoxicity did extend to the normal cells. It was suggested that IL-4 may be of use in cases of high risk lymphoblastic leukemia which was unresponsive to conventional therapy. IL-4 may be of value in controlling the growth of various cancers apart from its effect on the immune system. IL-4 may have a two phase effect on melanoma. Together IL-4, IL-2 and IFN stimulated CD4+ CTL growth; melanoma target cells treated with IL-4 plus IFN increased the recognition and binding of the T cells [479].

In preclinical animal studies, IL-4 inhibited certain glioma, colon and head and neck cell lines growing as xenografts in athymic nude mice. No remarkable infiltration accompanied depressed growth [724, 725]. An acute lymphoblastic leukemia cell line cultured from a child grew in nude mice. IL-7 increased growth while IL-4, tumor necrosis factor and interferon were each inhibitory [253]. Other cases have been reviewed where IL-4 inhibited acute lymphoblastic leukemia, non-Hodgkins lymphoma and multiple myeloma [8]. Capacity to inhibit tumor growth may be an added therapeutic benefit to the more important immune effects of IL-4. Growth inhibition is in most cases just that; decreased growth rate, growth proceeds but at a slower pace.

As IL-4 has so many important and interrelated functions it is interesting that genetically engineered mice defective for IL-4 production, developed a relatively normal immune profile. Serum IgG1 was very low. In response to nematode infection, the normal rise in serum IgE levels failed to occur. Otherwise B and T cells underwent relatively normal development [364].

Because IL-4 has been demonstrated to inhibit the growth of certain hemopoietic tumor cells *in vitro*, clinical studies with IL-4 were designed to look both at the anti-growth activities of the molecule as well as the immunomodulatory capabilities. In addition to the antiproliferative effect on hemopoietic tumor cell lines, inhibition of growth for melanoma, renal cancer, or breast cancer have also been seen [283, 408, 706, 719, 724].

Phase I clinical trials with IL-4 as a single agent explored doses between 600 and 800 micrograms/m^2 in iv and subcutaneous modes of administration. Fatigue, diarrhea, gastritis and arthralgia were dose-limiting toxicities in addition to the usual side effects of interleukins including fever, fluid retention, nausea, vomiting, diarrhea and fatigue [33, 228, 424]. The possibility of cardiac toxicity has been reported [729].

Phase II trials with malignant melanoma and renal cancer [424] demonstrated one complete response in 49 patients treated. IL-4 was also administered in clinical trials alone or in combination with IL-2 [402]. While considerable toxicities were seen, particularly on the gastrointestinal tract, no antitumor responses were seen in 48 patients given IL-4 alone while 6 responses were noted in 28 patients receiving a combination of IL-4 and IL-2.

Clinical results of IL-4 as a single agent have not been encouraging. Ongoing studies of IL-4 plus IL-2 are underway as are studies using genetically engineered tumor cells which secrete IL-4 in vaccine models.

Vaccines of tumor cells genetically engineered to produce IL-4 have had mixed results. In mice vaccinated with IL-4 engineered tumor cells [237, 707, 798] or IL-4 engineered fibroblast cells mixed with tumor cells [574], animals rejected the IL-4 engineered tumors and subsequent challenges by the parental tumor cells [707, 798]. Cures of established tumors have also been reported [13, 237]. These are interesting results. However, it should be noted there are other studies which show that tumor cells engineered to produce cytokines (IL-4, IL-7, TNF$\propto$, or TNF-γ) were not better inducers of immune response than tumor cells mixed with a conventional adjuvant (*C.parvum*) [278].

INTERLEUKIN-5

Augmentation of eosinophils, B cells, T cells, mast cells and NK

IL-5 is a 12-18 kDa protein also known as B cell growth factor II, eosinophil colony stimulating factor, eosinophil differentiation factor and IgA enhancing factor. It is produced by activated helper T cells [693, 694], eosinophils [72, 139, 166] and stimulated NK cells [815]. In NK cells, IL-5 production is enhanced by IL-4 while IL-10 and IL-12 are inhibitory [759]. IL-5 receptor is composed of an IL-5 specific alpha chain and a beta chain which is shared with the GM CSF receptor [705]. This receptor has a soluble form which is synthesized from mRNA, not just shed from the cell surface [705]. IL-5 stimulates growth and differentiation of eosinophils [631, 790] and activates eosinophil function [395]. It potentiates responses in eosinophils, to IL-8 and RANTES [649]. IL-5 stimulates B cell growth [693, 794, 795] and the production of IgA and IgM [699]. It augments IL-2 induced LAK activity in peripheral blood cells [21] and promotes together with other factors mast cell growth and T cell differentiation [794]. IL-5 enhances IL-2 receptors and responsiveness in NK and T cells [328, 699].

Significant tumor activity in preclinical models has not been reported. No clinical trials with this lymphokine have been done.

INTERLEUKIN-6

IL-6 is a 25000 mw glycoprotein produced by a wide variety of cells including fibroblasts, macrophages, lymphocytes, endothelial cells, eosinophils [258]. IL-6 is produced by mesothelioma cells [641], certain melanomas [406] and other cancer cells. The gene for IL-6 is located on chromosome 7p21. Thrombin, which induces clotting and wound healing, stimulates IL-6 production [672]. IL-6 is in a family of structurally related cytokines which include leukemia inhibitory factor, oncostatin M, ciliary neutrotrophic factor and IL-11. These cytokines share similar helical structures. IL-6 binds to a specific IL-6 receptor alpha subunit [791] which in turn binds and activates a receptor gp 130 subunit [697]. This gp130 subunit is responsible for signaling. This subunit is shared between receptors in this cytokine family [221, 342, 390] and this shared subunit appears responsible for the effects these cytokines have in common. The alpha subunit is responsible for binding specificity.

IL-6 has a major role in the regulation of hematopoiesis and immune response [343]. IL-6, which is also referred to as B cell differentiation factor, stimulates B lymphocyte immunoglobulin production [276, 496, 676, 747]. It is a costimulator of T cell growth and cytokine production [747] and enhances, along with other factors, colony formation and megacaryocyte and platelet production [98, 274]. IL-6 also stimulates natural killer cell activity in peripheral blood lymphocytes [210, 302, 665]. It stimulates human thymocytes and T cells [401, 726]. IL-6 is produced by macrophages and may be a macrophage factor involved in the activation of T cells [495]. In mice treated with IL-6, growth and metastasis of Lewis Lung [321] and B16 melanoma [322] were inhibited.

IL-6 has certain direct effects on non-immune cells and tumor cells. It is a hepatocyte stimulatory factor [349]. Intestinal cells produce acute phase proteins in response to inflammation and injury. IL-6 and other cytokines (IL-1, interferon and tumor necrosis factor) stimulated production of these acute phase proteins. IL-6 is secreted in response to clot formation [672] and appears to have a role in blood vessel formation [489]. IL-6 upregulated the levels of ICAM-1, CD54 and CD40 in certain breast cancer cell lines [298]. It was suggested that IL-6 may be involved in epithelium-stroma signalling in breast tissue. In melanoma, IL-6 often inhibits the early tumor cells but not the growth of the advanced disease [405, 406]. Resistance may develop in IL-6 sensitive cells. In some but not all cases, resistance was associated with loss of the IL-6 receptor α subunit, responsible for specific IL-6 binding [661]. In cultured renal cells, IL-6 was secreted and found to stimulate growth in an autocrine manner [460].

IL-6 appears to have a role in cachexia. In mice, colon adenocarcinoma cells produced elevated serum IL-6 and cachexia; antibodies to IL-6 depressed cachexia. The drug Suramin interfered with the binding of IL-6 to its receptor and reversed cachexia in tumor bearing mice [685, 686].

IL-6 demonstrates tumor growth inhibition *in vivo* in several mouse models [322, 495]. These studies seem to indicate an immunological mechanism for the IL-6 effect with the generation of tumor-specific CTL, but not LAK cells, when mice were treated with IL-6 and experienced shrinkage of pulmonary metastases.

In addition to being active immunologically, IL-6 also alters angiogenesis and inhibits endothelial cell proliferation, another potential mechanism of action [442].

More recently, mRNA coding for IL-6 has been identified in 50% of renal carcinomas and in most renal carcinoma cell lines [354, 700]. IL-6 has stimulated growth *in vitro* for some renal cancer cell lines, so the effects of IL-6 on genitourinary neoplasms may be multifactorial. IL-6 was also found to have a direct autocrine growth effect on certain human multiple myelomas [327].

Clinical trials with IL-6 demonstrated the usual side effects seen with other cytokines in initial phase I trials [764]. Given an increase in platelet cell numbers with Interleukin-6, current trials are focusing on effective doses and schedules for platelet production stimulation but future studies will need to explore both immune function and the antitumor effects in hemopoietic neoplasms as well as selected human solid tumors.

It is interesting and curious that serum IL-6 in melanoma patients is a prognostic factor for poor survival and lack of response to IL-2 therapy [704]. *In vitro* there are studies suggesting IL-6 may be a growth factor for renal cancer cells [460].

For the most part, current interest in IL-6 for the treatment of cancer patients is based on its leukopoietic and thrombopoietic activities in compromised patients [746]. In a phase I study, several toxicities were noted. 120 hr infusion IL-6, 30 ug/day was the maximum tolerated dose; 100 µg/day was also tested. Bilirubin elevations (4) atrial fibrillation (1, 2 at higher dose) hypotension (1) confusion (1, 3 at higher dose). Also noted at high dose, confusion and slurred speech indicating neurotoxicity. In a subsequent phase II trial with renal cell carcinoma patients, using 30 µg/day, 120 hr continuous iv, repeated every 21 day, confirmed the toxicity and showed only modest anticancer benefit. Fourteen patients were studied, There were 2 partial responses, 6 and 8 month durations, 1 minor response, 3 stable and 8 progressive diseases. Toxicities included atrial fibrillation, a/v premature contractions, elevated bilirubin, anemia and a number w/ the usual complaints including some neurotoxicity. Results did not warrant continuation. Good preclinical results and the suggestion of benefit here indicate IL-6 may be of benefit in another format perhaps in combination therapy. Anemia may be due to increased plasma volume. Toxicities were alarming but manageable and reversible. Weiss et al. [768] and Weber et al. [764] also carried out a phase I with IL-6. In vaccination studies, IL-6 engineered mouse mammary tumor cells offered some protection to a subsequent challenge by unmodified tumor cells [13].

INTERLEUKIN-7

IL-7 was first described by Namen et al. [504, 505] as a factor produced by stromal cells in mouse bone marrow which stimulated progenitor cells of B-lymphocytes to multiply and develop. IL-7 is a glycoprotein of 25, 000 molecular weight. In addition to bone marrow stroma [239, 504, 505], IL-7 is also produced by thymus stromal cells [630], keratinocytes [25, 270, 431] and certain carcinomas [320], leukemias [206, 578, 589] and lymphomas [197, 351]. IL-7 is secreted by normal B cells and certain malignant B cell lines [50]. IL-7 is not detected in normal T cells [797].

The IL-7 receptor was found on B cell precursors but not on mature B cells, consistent with its role in the early stages of B cell maturation [120, 121]. The IL-7 receptor is a member of the hematopoietin receptor family. There is a soluble form of the receptor which is not simply shed from the cell surface but is produced by a specific mRNA [238]. The IL-2 R γ chain is a part of the IL-7 receptor. It enhances the binding of IL-7 to the core receptor proteins and participates in signalling [352, 521]. Lack of active γ chain in patients with severe combined immunodeficiency disease (XSCID) results in loss of the IL-7 receptor function. This contributes to poor immune response in these individuals. Three different IL-7 binding affinities have been observed [29, 200, 562]. The physiologic significance of these differing affinities is not certain though the high affinity receptor appears to be responsible for cell division [557]. In human T cells, response to IL-7 depends on the activation state. In resting cells, IL-7 induces certain cellular proteins (CD25 IL2 R) but no proliferation. In activated cells IL-7 is a potent inducer of cell division [247, 483]. T cells contain two distinct IL-7 receptor proteins, separate gene products, p90 present in high concentration in unstimulated cells and p76 which is in activated cells [27]. The p76 receptor protein appears to be the high affinity receptor responsible for IL-7-induced T cell proliferation. Immunosuppressive drugs cyclosporin and FK506 inhibit IL-7 stimulated growth, apparently by interfering with the formation of the P76 receptor [201].

IL-7 has important influences on several different immune cell types. Genetically deficient knockout mice, lacking IL-7 were severely lymphopenic. It appears IL-7 was an absolute requirement for the development of T and B cells [754]. Interestingly, it is unusual for the loss of any one cytokine to cause such impairment. This is probably due to redundancy of cytokine functions, which is not the case for IL-7.

Among its many functions, IL-7 induced proliferation and antitumor activity in human blood monocytes and macrophages [11, 310]. It stimulated lymphokine activated killer cells [410, 634, 684]. While IL-2 induced better melanoma cell kill, IL-7 induced kill with a different pattern of lymphokine release [511, 512] and without TNF secretion and toxicity towards normal cells [635]. It was required for IL-1 and GM-CSF induced outgrowth of mouse thymocytes [265]. IL-7 is a growth/differentiation factor for fetal pre-T cells [23], thymocytes [265, 533, 750, 776] and mature CD4+ and CD8+ T lymphocytes [26, 91, 204, 247, 393, 483, 769]. IL-7 stimulated early thymic cell expansion and differentiation allowing the outgrowth of certain T cell precursors while regulating the generation of TCR αβ cells [579]. It was the only cytokine among 16 factors tested capable of inducing rearrangement of the T cell receptor V(D)J region and expression of the RAG1 and RAG2 genes which are involved in gene rearrangement [490]. This implicated IL-7 in the development of the diversity of the T cell receptor repertoire early in T cell development. IL-7 can stimulate the IL-2 receptor (CD25) in resting T cells [27] and may act alone or with IL-2 to initiate T cell growth. IL-7 stimulated the development of antitumor cytotoxicity in T cells [10, 52, 272, 277, 411], which persisted long-term in culture without frequent antigenic restimulation [411]. It has synergistic effects with IL-2 [736] and with IL-12 [445] on T cell outgrowth and cytotoxicity. IL-2 stimulated antigen induced outgrowth of effector cells from memory CD8+ T cells; IL-7 could replace IL-2 and act independently of it [355]. IL-7 induced the secretion of several cytokines from human peripheral blood T cells including IL-2, IL-4 and IL-6, IFN [28]. In T cell cultures, IL-7 stimulated secretion of IL-3, GM-CSF and IL-4 secretion; unstimulated cells did not respond to IL-7 [156, 157]. IL-7 stimulated peripheral blood T cell growth, cytokine secretion and IL-2 receptors and this effect was not dependent on IL-2 [112]. Therefore, IL-7 shares several activities with IL-2 and while it influences IL-2 response, IL-7 does not necessarily work through IL-2.

IL-7 appears to have a part in antigen presentation to initiate immune response. It is a growth factor for mouse dendritic epidermal T cells [431, 433]. Keratinocytes which surround the dendritic cells in skin produce IL-7 and TNF α [431, 432]. Together these two cytokines stimulated dendritic cell growth. IL-7 increased levels of the costimulatory protein B7 on T cells [797] and also on pre B cells [135]. Increased intracellular adhesion molecule 1 accompanied the change in B7. IFNγ blocked the stimulatory effect of IL-7 on pre B cells. Apoptosis, programmed cell death, resulted [213]. Cytokines interact in a complex manner to regulate response during antigen presentation.

Interleukin-2 is used to activate and grow tumor infiltrating lymphocytes for patient treatment. It appears IL-7 may be beneficial in TIL production. IL-2 generally stimulates good initial growth; tumor cells are killed early in primary culture as TIL cells grow. But antitumor activity is often difficult to maintain over the long periods of time in culture. This is especially the case when tumor cells are not available as a source of antigen to restimulate the T cells. Some investigators have reported difficulty maintaining CD4 helper cells in IL-2 induced cultures. IL-7 treated TIL cultures frequently produced CD4 + cells with better antitumor specificity than those from IL-2 treated cultures [108]. IL-7 alone stimulated the growth of certain renal cancer TIL cultures and enhanced IL-2-induced growth in others [151]. Growth and antitumor activity persisted during long term culture. Antigen restimulation was not required to maintain significant antitumor activity. Others have reported IL-7 may not be beneficial at the initiation of TIL culture but rather IL-7 stimulated growth and cytokine secretion in cultures which were already responding to IL-2 [656].

Mice treated with rhuIL-7 exhibited dose responsive increase in T cells, CD8/CD4 ratio, B cells, macrophages and NK cells. Lung metastases of Renca renal cancer cells were reduced. These results suggested a benefit in treating immunocompromised patients and patients with cancer [351].

In model studies, nude mice with human colon cancer xenografts lived longer when treated with human T cells and rhuIL-7 than when treated with either alone. The antitumor activity appeared due to interferon from CD8+ cells, not cytolysis. Interestingly, injected interferon was not that effective suggesting local continuous release was better than systemic interferon therapy [498].

IL-7 appears to be a good vaccine adjuvant in experimental models. Tumorigenesis was decreased in mice inoculated with IL-7 gene engineered plasmacytoma cells [277], glioma cells [22] and fibrosarcoma cells [439]. The animals which rejected the engineered tumor cells developed immunity to subsequent injections of the parental cells [22, 439]. The pattern of immune cell infiltrate depended on the tumor. T cells responded, CD4 cells in the case of the plasmacytoma [277], CD8 cells in the glioma [22] and fibrosarcoma [439]. Complement receptor rich macrophages, eosinophils and basophils were also remarkable [279, 439].

Aside from its influence of immune cells, IL-7 also has a direct effect on certain tumors which could influence therapy. It was one of several cytokines which upregulated intercellular adhesion molecule-1 (ICAM-1) on human melanoma cells. This protein is involved in immune recognition and anticancer action [340]. On the other hand, there are several reports that IL-7 stimulated cancer growth. IL-7 increased the growth of several leukemia cell lines [253, 428, 477, 532, 559, 727]. Sezary lymphoma cell lines responded to IL-7 and IL-2 with increased and in certain cases synergistic growth [123, 197]. The effect of IL-7 may be autocrine or paracrine. IL-7 mRNA was detected in certain cell lines [197]. In one study, a patient's ALL cells and a derived cell line were growth responsive to IL-7 in culture [253] but did not secrete IL-7. In another study the cells of patients with chronic lymphocytic leukemia contained IL-7 R and produced IL-7 which stimulated growth [206]. Abnormal cytokine secretion by tumor cells may be responsible for immune system abnormalities common in CLL patients [206].

Transgenic mice have been developed which expressed IL-7 in lymphoid tissues [596]. These animals had remarkable skin T cell infiltrates, the result of the powerful influence of IL-7 on lymphocyte development. These transgenic mice also produced T and B cell lymphomas. This model system shows that the IL-7 locus could act as an oncogene.

Given that Interleukin-7 has a stimulatory capacity for cytotoxic T cells, LAK cells, and induces cytokine secretion by lymphoid cells, it would seem to be an interesting compound to use in the cellular therapy of cancer. Preclinical findings suggest that IL-7 gene-modified tumor cells would appear to be useful. This is based on preclinical findings cited above and the possibility of IL-7 gene insertion into activated lymphocytes with the purpose of stimulating stronger or longer-lasting T-cell activity in *ex vivo* generated cells for human trials. Such clinical trials are being considered but no results are yet available.

INTERLEUKIN-8

The chemotactic cytokine

IL-8 is a potent chemotactic and proinflammatory cytokine [436, 491]. It was first described as a chemoattractant for neutrophils [642, 756]. IL-8 is secreted by a variety of cell types and it influences the migration of several important immune regulatory cells. IL-8, a relatively small protein, 8000 mw, is produced by macrophages [642], endothelial cells [231, 585, 643, 688], neutrophils [87, 765] epithelial cells [47, 678], fibroblasts [372], keratinocytes [372, 799], granulocytes [698], mast cells [472] and eosinophils [796]. Certain tumor cells also produce IL-8 including melanoma [636], squamous cell carcinoma [799] colon adenocarcinoma [647]. IL-8 secretion is controlled by various factors such as IL-1 [372, 647], IL-3 [761], IL-5 [648], GM-CSF [440, 761], TNF [372, 687], Vitamin D, [799], lipopolysaccharide [647] and fibrin [585].

There are two different receptors for IL-8, referred to as alpha and beta [282, 374, 485, 499]. Both bind IL-8 with similar high affinities but the two receptors differ in their abilities to bind other members of the chemokine family [374, 639]. There are receptors for IL-8 on neutrophils, T cells, mast cells, dermal macrophages, endothelial cells and keratinocytes [337]. IL-8 has little effect on B cells. It is a chemoattractant for T cells [39] and neutrophils [491]. In dogs injected with human IL-8 the site was infiltrated mainly with neutrophils [713]. Neutrophils respond to IL-8 with the production of superoxide anion, degranulation with the release of hydrolytic enzymes such as elastase, and migration through endothelium of capillaries [40, 84, 291, 572]. IL-8 also induces locomotion in IL-2 activated peripheral blood NK cells [650]. Inasmuch as IL-8 is an attractant to antigen presentation cells such as macrophages and eosinophils [133, 649, 651], IL-8 may have an important role in the initiation of immune response as well as the recruitment of effector cells which carry out the response.

Fibrin is frequently observed in vessels associated with inflammation, trauma and cancer. The addition of fibrin to cultured endothelial cells induced the release of IL-8 [585]. The physical act of blood clotting may stimulate cytokine release and cell migration. Besides IL-8 there are several additional proteins and peptides which are chemotactic to immune cells; macrophage inflammatory protein α (MIP), IL1α, and RANTES (regulated on activation, normal T cell expressed and secreted) to mention a few. These interact to stimulate migration. Interferon γ, while not chemotactic itself, tends to enhance the chemotactic response. Certain cytokines released by T cells inhibit chemotaxis (IL-10, IL-2, IL-13, IL-4). These inhibitors appear to function not in preventing migration but rather they act locally to detain migrating immune cells to effectively gather these cells at the site of inflammation [318].

The release of IL-8 or other chemotactic factors by tumors may have anticancer effects as infiltrating macrophages, granulocytes and lymphocytes accumulate within the tumor. But there is evidence that IL-8 may benefit tumor development and spread. In melanoma, IL-8 has been shown to be an autocrine growth factor [636, 662]. IL-8 stimulated tumor cell movement. Metastasis of melanoma cells in a nude mouse model was correlated with the tumor's capacity to produce IL-8 [662]. Developing tumors require adequate blood supply and may benefit from the angiogenic activity IL-8 has with its ability to stimulate capillary endothelial cell growth and migration [347, 688]. IL-8 may act directly on tumor cells or the tumor may take advantage of IL-8's effects on normal cells to stimulate tumor metastasis and growth.

INTERLEUKIN-9

Costimulation in hematopoietic response

IL-9 is a 32-39 kDa protein which is produced by T helper cells. It was first discovered in the conditioned medium of a HTLV transformed T cell line as a factor which stimulated growth of a human megakaryoblastic leukemia cell line [789]. It is a 144 amino acid protein and it maps to a region of chromosome 5 which contains genes for other cytokines including GM-CSF, IL-3 IL-4 and IL-5. IL-9 is homologous with a mouse factor P40 which stimulates T cells [748]. The receptor for IL-9 has been cloned and characterized [590].

IL-9 has several different functions. It generally acts along with other cytokines as a costimulator. Together with erythropoietin, IL-9 supports erythroid colony (BFU-E) formation [159, 778]. With IL-3 or GM-CSF, IL-9 induced the cloning of hematopoietic progenitor cells [281]. In mice IL-9 with IL-2 stimulated fetal thymocyte proliferation [691]. IL-9 increased growth in activated, but not resting helper T cells and T cell lines [286, 748]. In cultures of mast cells, IL-9 alone enhanced mast cell survival and together with IL-3 and IL-4 stimulated mast cell growth and the secretion of IL-6 [295]. In B cells, IL-9 stimulated the IL-4-induced secretion of IgE [591, 740].

INTERLEUKIN-10

A potent regulator of cell mediated immunity

IL-10 is a 17000 mw protein first characterized in cultures of helper T cells for its ability to inhibit production of interferon by antigen stimulated TH1 cells [189]. IL-10 is now known to be produced by a number of cell types including thymocytes [415], T cells [95, 189], B cells [234, 526], monocytes [142, 143], mast cells [714] and keratinocytes [174].

IL-10 has a number of activities which limit initiation of cellular immunity while enhancing humoral immunity. In some ways IL-10 resembles IL-4. It has several macrophage inhibiting effects and decreased antigen presentation by macrophages to T cells, in particular TH1 [143]. IL-10 inhibited cytokine production by macrophages [143, 191] and macrophage stimulated cytokine production, IL-1, IL-6, TNF by Th1 cells [190]. IL-10 depressed production of peroxide [64] and nitrogen oxide [219] in activated macrophages. Macrophages produce IL-12 which stimulates T cells. IL-10 downregulated IL-12 production and T cell stimulation [363, 497]. In stimulated monocytes, IL-10 and IL-4 depressed the production of macrophage CSF. IL-10 also inhibited dendritic T cell induced production of interferon by TH1, CD4+ and CD8+ T cells [412]. It antagonized NK secretion of INF γ and cytotoxicity induced by IL-12 and TNF ∝ [734]. In mitogen stimulated T cells, IL-10 inhibited cell proliferation and production of IL-2 and IFN-gamma [696] while IL-1 beta was stimulatory. IL-10 depressed the production of IFN by spleen cells. Interestingly, in spleen, IFN was stimulated by IL-4. This is the key difference between IL-4 and IL-10 which otherwise act similarly as they tend to suppress cell mediated immune response.

Not all of IL-10's activities are inhibitory. IL-10 is a growth and differentiation factor for activated B cells [622]. IL-10 stimulated B cell survival and class II MHC expression [234]. Acting together with IL-3 and IL-4, IL-10 stimulated mast cell growth [714]. While IL-10 suppressed the chemotactic response by CD4+ cells to IL-8 [317], it stimulated chemotaxis for CD8+ T cells [317]. In mice, IL-10 stimulated growth and differentiation in T cells [95, 415].

The gene for IL-10 has been cloned [475]. Interestingly, Epstein Barr Virus genes code for an IL-10-like activity called BCRF1. The protein is highly homologous with IL-10 [289, 475, 749]. It appears that at some point in time EBV picked up this gene from a mammalian cell source. Expression in an infected cell would interfere with antiviral immune response. Certain human tumors produce IL-10 [214, 409, 575]. When this is the case, IL-10 may interfere with immune response to the tumor. It appears responsible for tumor cell insensitivity to cytotoxic T cells [409] and has been shown to downregulate HLA class I which is involved in tumor cell recognition by cytotoxic cells [430]. A priori, one might not expect IL-10 be useful in a tumor vaccine preparation. However, interesting results were obtained when mice were vaccinated with mammary adenocarcinoma cells engineered to produce IL-10 [13, 232]. Some mice developed long-term immunity to a subsequent unmodified tumor cell challenge. In this model system, no benefit was obtained using tumor cell vaccines producing IL-6, GM-CSF or TNF-alpha [13]. In another vaccine study IL-10 engineered chinese hamster ovary cells injected into animals failed to form tumors [599]. It was suggested IL-10 may be inhibiting macrophage production of angiogenic factors or tumor growth factors required by the tumor [599].

INTERLEUKIN-11

Progenitor stimulator

Interleukin-11 was discovered as a factor produced by a bone marrow stromal cell line which supported the growth of an IL-6 dependent plasmacytoma cell line [566]. The nucleic acid for this factor was cloned. The monomeric protein is 22, 000 mw and is secreted by stromal fibroblasts.

IL-11 stimulates the growth of hematopoietic progenitor cells [500]. It influences very early stem cells and more committed precursor cells. In some activities IL-11 resembles IL-6. IL-11 receptor contains the gp130 subunit which is also a part of the receptors for IL-6, oncostatin M, ciliary neutortrophic factor and leukocyte inhibitory factor [221, 390]. In mouse cells IL-11 acted synergistically together with IL-3 to stimulate growth of primitive blast colony forming cells [500] as well as megakaryocytes and macrophages. IL-11 stimulated the formation of antibody-producing B cells. T cells are required and appear to be an intermediary in B cell stimulation [566]. It inhibited the differentiation of fibroblast lines into adipocytes as did IL-6 and TNF-alpha [331]. Also IL-11 is among the several cytokines capable of inducing acute phase protein release from hepatic and non hepatic cells [473].

INTERLEUKIN-12

Stimulator of immune responses

During the 1980's it was found that certain B cell lines secreted a factor which acted together with IL-2 to stimulate proliferation, interferon secretion and cytotoxicity in NK cells and T cells [216, 248, 267, 394, 570, 744]. A 70, 000 mw glycoprotein was purified which exhibited these characteristics. It was called natural killer cell stimulatory factor [346] for its remarkable effect on NK cells. Independently, the same agent was isolated from B cells and called cytotoxic lymphocyte maturation factor [681] or T cell stimulating factor [248] for its effect on activated T cells. Now known as IL-12 [255], this cytokine has remarkable effects which extend to several immune cell types with far reaching influences on immune response. IL-12 is secreted mainly by macrophages and B cells [127]. Antigen presenting dendritic cells also produce IL-12 [413]. IL-12 is not secreted by most T cells, bone marrow stroma, or most tumor cells except certain cancers of B cells origin [783].

IL-12 subunits p35 and p40 are coded by two genes on separate chromosomes 3 and 5 respectively [658]. The genes for IL-12 have been cloned [255, 784]. The p35 subunit has homology with certain cytokines, in particular IL-6 and G-CSF [447]. The p40 subunit has homology with the Interleukin-6 receptor extracellular domain [222]. Expression of these two genes does not appear to be coordinately regulated. Curiously, many cells produce the p35 subunit without making p40. But both chains have to be produced and assembled within the cell for secretion to occur [783]. Regulation of secretion appears to be at the level of p40 production [127]. In PBMC cultures, monocytes were the major cell source of secreted IL-12. Monocytes did not produce IL-12 p40 constitutively but expression was induced by bacteria, viruses and parasites [127, 288, 783].

IL-12 receptor has been detected on NK (CD56+) cells and T cells (CD4+ and CD8+) but not B (CD19+) cells [100, 137]. A survey of over 20 established human cell lines of T, B and NK lineage revealed receptor in only 2, both T cells [137, 138]. In PHA stimulated peripheral blood lymphocytes, the receptor bound IL-12 with high affinity Kd = 1-6 x 10-10 M with 1000-9000 sites per cell [100]. Crosslinking studies indicated IL-12 binds directly to a 110, 000 mw protein which is also associated with an 85, 000 mw protein [100]. IL-12 receptor in PBMC is upregulated by PHA or IL-2. Receptor was very low or not detectable in unstimulated cells. With stimulation the receptor was upregulated and the cells became increasingly sensitive to IL-12 [100, 137].

The larger subunit of the IL-12 receptor has been cloned [101]. It is a transmembrane protein, a member of the hematopoietin receptor superfamily, with 516 amino acids in the extracellular domain and 91 amino acids in the cytoplasmic segment. The gene product expressed in COS cells binds IL-12 with a relatively low apparent affinity (5 X 10^{-9} M). An additional subunit appears needed for high affinity binding. The gp 130 protein often associated with cytokine receptors, believed responsible for signal transduction, appears to be a part of the IL-12 receptor complex as well [222].

In cultures, IL-12 increased interferon secretion by peripheral blood lymphocytes [346], T-cells [90] and NK cells [94]. IL-1β appears to be required for IL-12 to induce IFN in NK cells [297]. T cell IFN-γ secretion responded to IL-12 in both CD8+ cytotoxic cells [445] and in CD4+ helper cells [786]. IL-12 induced cytokines regulate NK activity [90], T helper cell development and the induction of cellular immunity. IL-12 also induced IL-2, TNF and GM-CSF production in NK cells [511, 512, 513]. In addition to its NK and T cell stimulating properties, IL-12 acts together with other cytokines to stimulate hematopoiesis [48].

In NK cells, IL-12 increased cell surface adhesion proteins [511, 512, 604], and induced cytotoxicity in human NK cells [94, 604]. It increased secretion of granules containing hydrolytic enzymes and perforin responsible for cell killing [66]. IL-12 is involved in eosinophil regulation and induced growing NK cells to produce IL-5, an eosinophil stimulating cytokine. IL-12 and IL-10 inhibited production of IL-5 [759]. IL-12 also has a role in LAK cell production. PBL cultured 3-5 days in the presence of IL-12 produced LAK cells [217, 511-513]. IL-12 is also a potent inducer of LAK. At least part of the IL-2 effect on LAK appears due to IL-12 for antibodies to IL-12 decreased the response. TNF was costimulatory with IL-12 for LAK induction. Interestingly, IL-4 inhibited IL2 but stimulated IL-12 induction of NK [513].

IL-12 has remarkable effects on the development of T cells. This influence begins early in the thymus where IL-12 stimulates immature progenitor cells to divide increasing the numbers of CD3+ T cells in particular, CD8+ cells [235]. In cultures of peripheral blood T cells, IL-12 quickly stimulated within hours CTL proliferation and cytotoxicity [217, 444]. Increased production of the perforin and hydrolytic enzymes has been observed [215]. In addition to effects on cytotoxicity and proliferation, IL-12 altered the T cell surface [89, 225]. Increased levels of adhesion proteins may influence cell interactions involved in immune recognition, activation and killing. Other cytokines work with IL-12 to stimulate proliferation in T cells; IL-2 and IL-12 together were generally additive [444]. IL-7 acts synergistically with IL-12 on T cells to stimulate both growth and cytotoxicity [445].

In cultured tumor infiltrating lymphocytes activated with anti CD3, IL-12 stimulated growth and autologous tumor cell lysis [20]. The influence of IL-12 was not prevented by antibodies to IL-2. When IL-12 was added to cultures with a low suboptimal dose of IL-2, there was an additive effect on growth and cytotoxicity [20]. These cytokines appear to operate through different mechanisms. But the growth effect of IL-12 alone is transient. Maintenance of growth after 72 hr required further stimulation by IL-2. IL-2 appears to be more potent than IL-12. It remains to be seen whether IL-12 treated TIL cells have added clinical benefit.

IL-12 has a key role in the differentiation of the T helper cell system (Fig 1). Macrophages are a major source of IL-12 and respond to certain infectious organisms with increased IL-12 production. IL-12 has a major influence on interferon secretion. In mice treated with IL-12 there was a remarkable increase in serum IFN γ levels [506, 550]. Many of IL-12's effects appear due at least in part to IFN-γ production [482]. Increased levels of IL-12 stimulate the conversion of precursor helper TH0 cells to TH1 cells. TH1 helper cells produce IL-2, IFN-γ and other cytokines. IFN-γ potentiates further IL-12 production [126]. Th1 cells favor development of cellular immunity over humoral immunity. TH2 helper cells secrete IL-4, IL-10 and other cytokines; these cytokines favor humoral immunity and antibody production. The two helper cell types have antagonistic effects upon one another. IL-4 and IL-10 inhibit IL-12 production by monocytes [734] and by T cells. IL-12 production inhibits TH2 cell proliferation [208]. IL-12 Influences B cell growth and differentiation [316]. IL-12 suppresses the IL-4 induced production of IgE by B cells [339].

In HIV infected individuals, T cells of peripheral blood often fail to grow and produce IL-2 and interferon gamma in response to stimulation. Treatment with IL-12 in culture restored cell growth and cytokine secretion suggesting one of the primary defects in those infected with HIV may be a lack of necessary IL-12 production [94, 106]. Baseline NK activity was very depressed even in asymptomatic patients. When patient PBL's were treated with IL-12, NK cytotoxicity was stimulated to

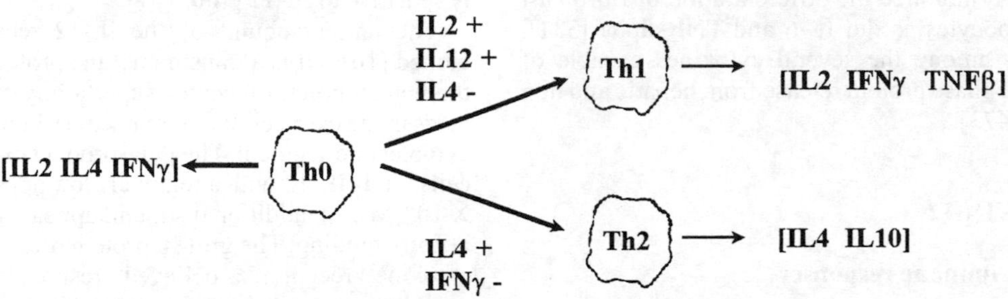

Figure 1. Differentiation of helper T cells. Bracketed cytokines are major secretions of the indicated cell type. TH0 are precursor cells. TH1 cells favor cellular immune response. TH2 cells favor humoral immune response. Additional discussion on regulation is found in the sections on IL10, IL12 and INFγ.

near normal levels [94]. Altered IL-12 activity may be involved in the poor immune response associated with AIDS.

In preclinical studies, mice bearing B16 F10 melanoma, M5076 sarcoma and Renca renal carcinoma benefitted from treatment with IL-12. The antitumor effect did not require NK cells but did depend on T cells, specifically CD8+ T cells [76]. Mice with sarcomas treated with IL-12 showed decreased tumor growth, increased longevity and in some cases complete regressions. Interferon γ was required for the IL-12 effect. The effect appeared to be mediated by CD4+ and CD8+ T cells [506]. IL-12 engineered murine tumor cells may be good anticancer vaccines [802]. IL-12 transfected tumor cells or fibroblasts induced rejection of subsequent tumor implants and inhibited the growth of some established tumors. Simultaneous expression in tumor cell vaccines of IL-12 and B7 costimulatory factor appeared essential for good anticancer response.

The preclinical studies with IL-12 are quite encouraging. This molecule has many similar effects to IL-2 and is more active on a molar basis inducing anticancer responses with less toxicity. For these reasons and others, IL-2 and IL-12 may prove to be effective as combination or sequential biotherapy. Similarly, IL-12 gene insertion may prove an effective strategy for increasing tumor immunogenicity similar to studies underway with IL-2 and IL-4 gene insertion. Finally, the *ex vivo* expansion of T cells with IL-2 might be rendered more specific and more cytolytically effective.

Studies from our laboratories (Oldham and Lewko, personal communication) indicate that IL-12 is effective in activating cytolytic populations of tumor-derived T cells grown *ex vivo* in Interleukin-2. The strategy of IL-2 growth of tumor-derived activated cells with IL-12 stimulation prior to the therapeutic use of these cells seems particularly attractive.

Phase I/II clinical trials are underway.

INTERLEUKIN-13

Anti-inflammatory agent

IL-13 is produced by activated T cells. Two laboratories cloned the gene for IL-13 at about the same time [443, 462]. The recombinant protein has a molecular wt of about 14, 000. Its gene is located on human chromosome 5 in the region of several other cytokines [443]. IL-13 has 30% sequence homology with IL-4 [811]. IL-13 and IL-4 share certain activities [266, 443, 582, 811]. An IL-4 mutant which has higher affinity for the IL-4 receptor, competed for binding with both IL-4 and IL-13 and this mutant IL-4 blocked IgE and B cell proliferation induced by IL-4 or IL-13 [38]. This appears related to a receptor subunit which these cytokines have in common, a subunit which is involved in signaling [809-811].

IL-13 has remarkable anti-inflammatory effects on monocytes and macrophages. It also regulates B-cell growth and function. In monocyte cultures, IL-13 treated cells became more adherent [443]. It enhanced the expression of several surface antigens (CD11b, CD11c, CD23, class II MHC) while it depressed others [443]. IL-13 downregulated the levels of CD14 which is a receptor for endotoxin [785]. CD-14 is involved in monocyte activation and cytokine release [136, 580]. IL-13 decreased several macrophage functions including nitric oxide production by activated cells [160] and the production of several cytokines including TNF-∝ [113]. IL-13 increased neutrophil production of anti-inflammatory factor IL-1ra, an IL-1 antagonist which binds the IL-1 receptor without activating it [141]. In human B cells, IL-13 acted as a costimulator with anti CD40 causing increased proliferation and Ig isotype switching with increased IgE production [582]. In T cells, IL-13 is one of several cytokines (IL-2, IL-4, IL-10) which inhibited chemotaxis induced by IL-8 and Rantes, promoting cell accumulation in the area of an inflammation [318].

INTERLEUKIN-14

B cell growth and memory

IL-14 was originally found in the conditioned media of Burkitt's lymphoma cell lines. It was referred to as high molecular weight B cell growth factor [15, 16]. IL-14 is produced by several cell types including PHA stimulated CD8+, CD4+ (Th1 and Th2), NK T cells, follicular dendritic cells [109, 629] and B cell lymphomas [196]. It is a relatively large glycosylated protein with a molecular wt of 53-65 kDa, depending on carbohydrate content [18]. IL-14 stimulates B cell growth and differentiation [15, 17] but has had no reported activity on T cells. It appears to have a role in B cell memory [17, 528]. Its secretion by B cell malignancies suggests a role IL-4 in the development of these diseases.

INTERLEUKIN-15

IL-15 was first reported by Grabstein et al. [246] as a factor in cultures of monkey kidney epithelium which supported IL-2 dependent growth of a T cell line. The same factor was identified in a human bone marrow stroma line. Independently, Burton et al. [78] discovered a similar activity which was produced by an adult T cell leukemia induced by human T cell lymphotropic virus I. These cells have the IL-2 receptor but with time lose the capacity to produce IL-2. They grow well in culture without cytokine supplementation producing this autocrine growth factor which was called IL-T.

IL-15 is a 14-15 kDa, 114 amino acid protein. The gene for IL-15 has been cloned. The sequence showed this was a distinct cytokine, a member of the helical cytokine family to which IL-2 belongs [246]. Peripheral blood mononuclear cells, epithelial cells and fibroblast lines produce IL-15. It was not detected in activated T cells which do produce IL-2 [246]. It is secreted by placenta, skeletal muscle, and to a lesser extent heart, lung, liver and kidney [246], dermal fibroblasts and keratinocytes [470].

IL-15 competes with IL-2 for its receptor but IL-15 has its own specific receptor and it shares a subunit γc with the IL-2 receptor. This is the same subunit also shared in common with IL-4R, IL-7R and IL-9R. It functions in signal transduction and it is the subunit which is defective in patients with severe combined immunodeficiency disease [42, 233].

IL-15 influences B cells as does IL-2. IL-15 stimulated proliferation and secretion of IgM, IgG, and IgA [30]. It replaced IL-2 in stimulating growth and cytotoxicity in activated cytotoxic T lymphocytes [246] and NK cells [82] and stimulated the growth of an IL-2 dependent CTL cell line [78]. It also induced formation of LAK cells in cultures of peripheral blood lymphocytes [78, 246]. It replaced IL-2, inducing outgrowth of in cultures of tumor derived activated T cells from tumor infiltrating lymphocytes in primary culture [383]. IL-15 also replaced IL-2 for the maintenance of growth of TIL/TDAC cultures which were initially induced with IL-2 and dependent on IL-2 for growth [383]. Whether or not IL-15 will be of therapeutic value over IL-2 in adoptive cellular immunotherapy remains to be seen. IL-15 has many properties in common with IL-2 but there are differences. For one thing, cell growth kinetics appear different; growth of T cells with IL-15 was slower [383]. It may be that the quality of the cytotoxic cells induced by IL-15 alone or together with other locally produced factors such as IL-7 or IL-12 may be different from those of the IL-2 initiated cells. IL-15 may stimulate T cells during the initiation/activation process. Once activated, T cell IL-2 receptor levels rise and IL-2 production by T cells increases for autocrine stimulated growth. Culture conditions which permit T cell outgrowth while maintaining long term antitumor specificity are needed for improved therapy.

Clinical trials for IL-15 are not underway. This molecule is at a level of development slightly behind IL-12 and in many ways the combination of IL-2, 7, 12 and 15 may be particularly desirable in the *ex vivo* production of T cells for therapy. Once the clinical trials with these lymphokines are available as single agents, they can then be used in 'cocktails' *in vivo* or *ex vivo* for T-cell stimulation.

GRANULOCYTE MACROPHAGE COLONY-STIMULATING FACTOR

The set of molecules known as growth and maturation factors includes a large number of quite individual entities. Like many other cytokines, they act through membrane receptors, and, in certain instances, the secretory cell may possess analogous receptors that will permit the growth factor to act upon the generating cell [717].

One of the inherent differences between normal and transformed cells is that transformed cells tend to replicate indefinitely. Certain transforming growth factors produced by RNA tumor viruses that become bound to growth factor receptors on the target cell surface may be capable of inducing a malignant phenotype [132]. Some oncogenes, such as *V-sis* [162, 763] and *V-erb-B* [163], are capable of producing proteins that are homologous to platelet-derived growth factor (PDGF) and epidermal growth factor (EGF). Thus, there is a growing awareness of the relationship that exists between oncogenes, growth factors, and proliferation of tumor cells.

Treatment strategies based upon the development of antibodies to the individual growth factor or its receptors have been explored in several animal models. For example, inhibition of epidermal carcinomas has been observed following treatment with the antibody to the receptor for epidermal growth factor [434]. Furthermore, the inhibition of human small-cell lung cancers by treatment with monoclonal antibodies directed against bombesin autocrine growth factor has been observed [119]. Thus, cell growth factors may very well play an integral role in the understanding and regulation of tumor cell proliferation.

Among the many types of poorly defined hematopoietic growth factors that have been found in the supernatant of certain cell cultures, granulocyte stimulating factor (G-CSF) and granulocyte macrophage colony-stimulating factor (GM-CSF) have made the transition to well-defined entities, now capable of being produced in large quantities by recombinant DNA technology [3, 81]. Both have been approved as drugs and are now widely used as drugs (See Chapters 19 and 20).

In vitro properties of GM-CSF include a demonstrated capability of promoting the survival, growth, and differentiation of granulocytes, macrophages, and in the presence of erythropoietin – erythroid precursors. Like γ-interferon, it can function as a macrophage-activating factor, whereby macrophages are stimulated to cytolysis of certain tumor targets. In addition, neutrophils that have been exposed to GM-CSF show increased cellular chemotaxis. This appears to be due to a rapid increase in the number of cell surface receptors for the *N*-formylated oligopeptides, such as f-Met-Leu-Phe. This increase in receptors corresponds to a period of increased chemotaxis, which is followed by a rapid decrease in the number of receptors over a period of approximately 2 h, at which point there is neutrophil immobilization corresponding to the neutrophil migration-inhibitory factor activity. In addition, during that 2-h period there appears to be a priming of the neutrophil for oxidative metabolism, which almost certainly leads to heightened cytolytic activity.

In vivo responses to GM-CSF have included leukocytosis and reticulocytosis, and rises in the lung content of neutrophils and macrophages, as well as in the liver content of neutrophils, monocytes, and eosinophils. Initial results of testing GM-CSF in monkeys suggest low toxicity and marked efficacy in terms of stimulating myelopoiesis. In addition, the bacterially produced, unglycosylated GM-CSF appears to be as effective as the glycosylated protein produced in mammalian cells by recombinant DNA technology.

The initial half-life of GM-CSF is approximately 7 min, with a slow secondary phase lasting some 89-90 min. Routes of administration, including subcutaneous and intravenous infusion, have appeared equally effective in animal models. Therapeutically, GM-CSF seems capable of reducing naturally occurring or induced cytopenias. In certain parasite-infested models, GM-CSF has demonstrated the ability to promote resolution of the infection.

On the basis of these observations, the place of GM-CSF in the arsenal of biological response modifiers is expected to be in the following areas: (a) prevention and mitigation of chemotherapy- and radiation-induced leukopenia; (b) improvement in host defenses in immunocompromised patients; (c) treatment of infectious and parasitic diseases; (d) induction of antitumor activity *in vivo* both as a direct cytotoxicity [198] and as a result of antibody-dependent cell-mediated cytotoxicity; and (e) facilitation of recovery from autologous and allogeneic transplantation.

Imaginative uses of this biological now include its prechemotherapy usage to boost circulating white cell levels, and to cycle myeloid precursors in a patient's bone marrow prior to undergoing intensive cytoreductive therapy, with discontinuation some 48 h before cytoreductive treatment and reinstitution some 7-10 days after the chemotherapy. The role of cytokines has already significantly affected the current methodology of cytolytic therapy.

Stem cell factor: early progenitor growth without differentiation

SCF was discovered in rat liver cells as a factor responsible for the outgrowth of very early bone marrow progenitor cells [805]. SCF turned out to be the ligand for the receptor encoded by c kit, a proto oncogene [19, 110, 194, 290, 777, 806]. SCF has also been called mast cell growth factor [19] and steel factor. The c-kit receptor protein is a member of the (PDGF/CSF-1 receptor-kinase family [788]. There are two forms of SCF, soluble and membrane bound, produced from alternate splicing of the same pre-mRNA [19, 194, 720, 721]. SCF is produced by several different cell types including bone marrow stroma, fibroblasts, liver and spleen [429, 435]. SCF stimulates growth of early progenitor cells (hematopoietic, lymphoid and myeloid) without inducing differentiation. It will act synergistically with other growth and differentiation factors to stimulate development [122].

SCF and its receptor are produced by several different tumor types [429, 508]. It is not unusual for the same cell to express both the factor and receptor. SCF will usually influence tumor growth by a paracrine mechanism. In this way, for example, the normal fibroblast component of a tumor could serve as the source of SCF for c kit+ carcinoma cells. Tumors which tested positive for c kit and/or SCF included small cell lung carcinoma [271, 628, 652], breast [507], testicular cancer [689], melanoma [509], uterine cervical and ovarian cancer [306]. Interestingly, loss of c-kit expression has been observed with malignant progression in breast cancer [507] and melanoma [508, 509] reminiscent of the loss of estrogen receptor which occurs with progression of estrogen independent growth in breast cancer.

Therapeutic strategies for stem cell factor are similar to those being explored for other growth factors. Any cytokine which has stimulated growth of tumor cells could potentially be inhibited by antibodies to the available cytokine and/or molecular analogs which can fill the receptor and block the cytokine's effect on tumor cell growth. Such strategies are being widely explored for cancer treatment and are further described under Growth and Maturation Factors (Chapter 18).

Interferon: immune modulating, antiviral and cytostatic

Interferon was first described in 1957 as a protein factor secreted in response to viral infection which interfered with subsequent infection by a different virus [307]. This family of proteins was later found to have several antimicrobial and anticancer activities in addition to its antiviral properties. This section will briefly summarize interferon with emphasis on cell mediated antitumor activity. (Please see Chapter 11 for more detailed information.)

The interferon family contains three major proteins: Interferon α, Interferon β (together classified as Type I interferon) and Interferon γ (Type II). Major activities are in the following table.

Table 2. Major functions of the interferon cytokine family members in cellular regulation

Interferon	Major function
α	Antiviral > immune regulation and cytostatic
β	Antiviral > Immune regulation and cytostatic
γ	Immune regulation > cytostatic and antiviral

Type I interferons are secreted in response to viral infection and double stranded RNA [423]. Most mammalian cells are capable of producing type I interferons. Interferons α and β share activities, have considerable homology in amino acid sequence, and share receptors [370]. Interferon β has considerable homology with IL-6 (B cell growth factor). Type I interferons are antiviral and cytostatic. Immune effects are also observed, especially at higher doses.

Interferon γ is distinct in its structure and genetics. It is produced by helper T cells (TH1), cytotoxic-suppressor T cells and NK cells. The IFNγ gene is on chromosome 12 (not 9 as in the case of Type I interferons). It is not induced by viral infection. Rather, it is secreted upon activation of T cells and NK cells with mitogens, phorbol esters or calcium ionophores. Type II interferon functions mainly in the immune regulatory area. IFN γ is less antiviral and cytostatic than the type I interferons.

IFN γ production by T cells is induced by IL-1 and 2 [781], by IL-12 [506, 550] and it is inhibited by IL-10 [189]. Interferon γ contains two identical subunits. It is relatively unstable in acidic pH's and heat. On binding, one IFN γ engages two separate receptor molecules [199]. The receptor for IFN-γ has been cloned [36]. Transfection studies for INF γ receptor proteins show that binding occurred in an otherwise receptor negative cells. As is typically the case, additional cell components were necessary for response. As ligand binds and activates the interferon receptor, the complex then associates with specific cellular kinases (Jak kinases). Interferon γ does not contain on board kinase activity. The cytosolic kinases then phosphorylate and activate specific STAT proteins which then bind and activate transcription at specific gene sites [179].

Mechanisms of interferons' antiviral action depends on the particular virus being eliminated. There are three major pathways of inactivation. 2'5'oligonucleotide synthetase is induced by Interferon types I and II. This enzyme converts ATP to a short polymer which activates an endoribonuclease (RNase L or RNase F) which then cleaves and destroys viral nucleic acid sequences [92, 800]. A second method of inactivating viruses involves interferon induction of P1 Kinase (also called double stranded activatable kinase). P1 Kinase phosphorylates and inactivates elF-2, a protein synthesis initiation factor. Since the P1 kinase is inactive until binding double stranded RNA, the kinase acts specifically to shut down protein synthesis in virus infected cells [595]. Viral and other microbial and parasitic infections may also be controlled by cellular immunity, which is under the influence of interferon. Finally there are the MX proteins, cellular proteins induced by Interferons which inhibit viruses by an uncertain mechanism. MX proteins share homology with GTP binding proteins. It is possible these inhibitors interfere with cell regulation.

Interferons influence several different immune cells with major immune stimulatory effects on macrophages, neutrophils, natural killer cells and T cells [571]. Interferon γ is a very potent inducer of immune effects; α and β interferons are also effective. IFN induces MHC I and MHCII on a variety of cells. MHC is required for correct antigen presentation at the initiation of cellular immune response. Elevated MHC on virus laden and tumor cells enhances cytotoxicity by T cells. IFN γ activates macrophages inducing the enzyme nitric oxide synthetase to metabolize L arginine to produce nitric oxide. Nitrogen oxide has anticancer and antiviral activities. IFN also stimulate macrophages to produce superoxide and tumor necrosis factor [510]. These are cytotoxic and have antitumor activity. They also stimulate increased macrophage cell surface Fc receptor which is involved in tumor cell killing by antibody directed cytotoxicity. IFN also stimulates NK cells in their capacity for non-specific, MHC independent killing of virus infected cells and tumor cells [731]. However it is interesting that tumor cells may be protected from NK cells by pretreatment with interferons, especially interferon γ [771]. The level of protection depends on the cell type; the mechanism is not understood. IFN also influenced immunoglobulin production by B cells [666]. IL-4 stimulated IgG and IgE while interferon depressed these but enhanced IgG2a production.

Interferons have remarkable effects on T cells. We have already discussed T helper cell differentiation, the production of interferon γ and IL-7 by TH1 cells, and the mutual antagonism between these cytokines which favor a cellular immune response vs the humoral immune response of IL-10, IL-5 and IL-4, produced by TH2 cells. IFN also influences growth, differentiation and CTL cytotoxicity [421]. Tumor infiltrating lymphocytes in culture produce several cytokines; interferon γ production correlated with the antitumor activity of TIL treated mice [44]. Interestingly, the correlation was better for IFN secretion than cytotoxicity measured *in vitro*.

IFN has direct growth inhibiting effect on certain cancer cells and normal cells [564]. Sensitive cells contain interferon receptors but the magnitude of antitumor response is not strictly related to the amount of interferon bound per cell. The direct effect tends slow growth rather than cause death. IFN tends to be an antagonist of growth factors. IFN also regulates expression of oncogens such as myc, abl, Ha ras and src in certain tumor cells. Induction of differentiation may accompany or be the reason for growth inhibition. Interferon also blocks angiogenesis, and this is important since the continuous expansion of the vascular system is required to maintain tumor growth.

Preclinical studies show that interferon may be useful as an adjuvant in cancer vaccines. Animals injected with tumor cells engineered to produce interferon γ had reduced tumorigenicity. Animals with regressed tumors were immune to subsequent challenge [212, 762].

All three inferferons are now approved drugs and widely used in the clinic. Clinical studies for the various interferons are described in Chapter 11.

Tumor necrosis factor

Tumor necrosis factor was first described in 1975 as an activity in serum of animals treated first with Bacillus Calmette-Guerin, then with the bacterial toxin lipopolysaccharide. TNF was named for its ability to induce hemorrhagic necrosis in tumors [83, 252]. It was produced by monocytes and macrophages but also by other cell types. Previously, another cytokine was discovered in cultures of T lymphocytes stimulated with antigen [623] or mitogen [249]. This cytokine was called lymphotoxin (LT) after its cell source and its toxic effect on certain types of cells [175, 376, 565, 623]. Later, the gene for LT was cloned from a human lymphoblastoid cell line [251]. LT's structure was related to TNF with about 30% homology in amino acid sequence [6, 569]. LT was then referred to as TNF β. Interestingly, while investigating cachexia and wasting associated with advanced cancer or chronic infection, another factor secreted by macrophages was discovered called cachectin [55, 323]. It was purified from a mouse myeloid cell line and it turned out to be identical with TNF ∝ [55-59].

There are at least two cell surface receptors for TNF α and β [280, 373, 391]. They differ in size (55 and 75 kDa) and molecular properties. Both bind TNF α and TNF β. (A third receptor has been reported in liver which binds TNF ∝ but not TNF β [647]. The P55 and p75 receptors are found in different proportions on different cell types and mediate distinct cellular responses [702]. Neither receptor has kinase activity but activate cytosolic kinases. There is evidence that the two receptors may cooperate by interaction and the passing of the ligand from the larger to the smaller receptor [703]. Soluble tumor necrosis factor receptor found in tissue fluids and culture medium appears to be due to proteolysis [523]. No separate mRNA's have been found for the soluble receptor. There are several cell surface proteins similar in structure to the TNF receptor including FAS (a trigger for apoptosis), CD40 (on B cells) and the receptor for nerve growth factor [45]. Depending on the cell type, TNF induces the expression of a number of proteins including the nuclear regulatory proteins c fos, c jun, cytosolic proteins including nitric oxide synthetase, cell surface markers including several growth factor receptors and adhesion molecules and a number of secreted cytokines (IL-1, TNF itself, IL-6, IL-8, IFN γ, GM-CSF, MCSF, PDGF, NGF) and enzymes including collagenase and plasminogen activator. TNF can inhibit the growth of certain tumors [83, 624, 692], stimulate osteoclast activity, increase fibroblast growth and induce enzyme production in synovial cells [257]. Interestingly, TNF and IL-1, which is also produced by monocytes, share several biological functions [60, 548], even though they are not related molecularly nor do they utilize the same receptors. It appears both cytokines upon binding their receptors activate several cellular protein kinases in common [257].

TNF also inhibits the growth of certain tumor cells directly [692]. The addition of interferon γ often has a synergistic effect on cytotoxicity [203, 780]. However, cells from tumors which were sensitive to TNF in treated animals are not always sensitive to the direct effects of TNF [83]. For many tumors, this cytokine appeared to act systemically to bring about tumor regression. TNF is known to have remarkable inflammatory and toxic effects on vascular endothelium, resulting in vessel disruption and increased blood clotting [514]. Vessels break down or become clogged, shutting off the blood supply to the tumor. TNF also influences the immune system and up-regulates surface antigens involved in recognition. TNF together with IL-2 had synergistic cytotoxic effects in cultured human lymphokine activated killer cells [555], natural killer cells [554] and tumor infiltrating lymphocytes [758]. The addition of TNF with low dose IL-2 produced TIL from long term cultures of ovarian cancer cells with superior tumor cell killing ability [384, 741].

Tumor necrosis factor may be useful as an adjuvant in tumor vaccines. In animal models, tumor cells engineered to produce TNF produced increased immune response [13, 62, 279]. The engineered cells exhibited decreased tumorigenesis and animals with regressed tumors were immune to subsequent tumor challenge. In another approach to vaccination, antigen primed dendritic cells have been used to successfully vaccinate mice against a sarcoma and lung cancer [438]. The dendritic cells were generated from bone marrow cells in culture using GM-CSF and TNF α [88] and then pulsed with specific tumor antigens prior to inoculating the mice [438].

TNF generally inhibits tumor growth, but this is not always the case. TNF appeared to be an autocrine and paracrine growth factor for certain ovarian cancers. TNF induced its own production. IL-1 also stimulated ovarian cancer growth and TNF levels [787]. TNF has also been shown to stimulate lung metastasis in the B16 mouse melanoma model system [531]. Induction of VCAM-1 (Vascular Cell Adhesion Molecule I) by TNF may be responsible for the increase in metastatis [531].

Clinical studies with tumor necrosis factor have been extensive and numerous. Most of the results have indicated that this molecule is not amenable to systemic administration since it's toxicity is quite substantial. TNF can best be visualized as a 'local hormone' such that its effects are best exploited when available at the tumor or inflammatory site for very short-range effects. When injected into the blood, its therapeutic ratio is very low given its high toxicity at serum levels needed to produce any biologic effects at distal sites. Therefore, current strategies with TNF include engineering the TNF gene into tumor cells to increase the vaccination potential of administered cell, insertion of the TNF gene into activated lymphocytes to exploit the TNF activity at the target site, once the lymphocyte has identified tumors by virtue of its receptor for tumor-associated antigens and the regional administration of TNF to limit the systemic effects while exploiting the very active antitumor effects in the tumor bed. These three strategies are now producing a large number of clinical trials which are described in Chapter 22.

ABBREVIATIONS

CFU, colony forming unit; CLL, chronic lymphocytic leukemia; CTL, cytotoxic T lymphocyte; G CSF, EPO; erythropoietin; granulocyte colony stimulating factor; GM CSF, granulocyte macrophage (monocyte) colony stimulating factor; HLA, human leukocyte antigen; ICAM ; intracellular adhesion molecule; IFN, interferon;

Ig, IL-, Interleukin; IL-1ra, Interleukin-1 receptor antagonist; JAK, Janus kinase; LAK, lymphokine activated killer cell; LT, lymphotoxin, TNF β; MHC, major histocompatibility complex; NK; natural killer cell; PBL, peripheral blood lymphocyte; R, receptor; RANTES, regulated on activation, normal T cell expressed and secreted; SCF, stem cell factor; STAT, signal transducers and activators of transcription; TH, helper T cells; TDAC, tumor derived activated T cell; TIL, tumor infiltrating lymphocyte (TDAC and TIL are synonymous); TNF; tumor necrosis factor.

REFERENCES

1. Abehsira-Amar O, Gilbert M, Joliy M, et al. IL-4 plays a dominant role in the differential development of Th0 into Th1 and Th2 cells. *J Immunol* 1992; 148: 3820-9.
2. Abrams J, Rayner A, Wiernik P, Parkinson D. High dose interleukin-2 without lymphokine activated killer cells: inactive in advanced renal cell cancer (meeting abstract). *Proc Annu Meet Am Assoc Cancer Res* 1989; 30: A1507.
3. Adams DO, Hall T, Steplewski Z, et al. Tumor undergoing rejection induced by monoclonal antibodies of the IgG2a isotype contained increased numbers of macrophages activated for a distinctive form of antibody dependent cytostasis. *Proc Natl Acad Sci* (USA) 1984; 81: 3506.
4. Adler A, Albo V, Blatt J, et al. Interleukin-2 induction of lymphokine-activated killer (LAK) activity in the peripheral blood and bone marrow of acute leukemia patients: II. Feasibility of LAK generation in children with active disease and in remission. Blood 1989; 74: 1690.
5. Adler A, Chervenick PA, Whiteside TL, et al. Interleukin 2 induction of lymphokine-activated killer (LAK) activity in the peripheral blood and bone marrow of acute leukemia patients. I. Feasibility of LAK generation in adult patients with active disease and in remission. *Blood* 1988; 71: 709.
6. Aggarwal BB, Henzel WL, Moffat B, et al. Primary structure of human lymphotoxin derived from 1788 lymphoblastoid cell line. *J Biol Chem* 1985; 260: 2334-2344.
7. Akahoski T, Oppenheim JJ, and Matsushima K. Induction of high affinity interleukin 1 receptor on human peripheral blood lymphocytes by glucocorticosteroid hormones. *J Exp Med* 1988; 167: 924-936.
8. Akashi K. Role of interleukin 4 in the negative regulation of leukemia cell growth. *Leukemia and Lymphoma*. 1993; 9: 205-209.
9. Al Jabaari b, Ladyman HM, Larche M, et al. Elevated expression of interleukin 4 receptor in carcinoma. a target for immunotherapy? *British J Cancer* 1989; 59: 910-914.
10. Alderson MR, Sassenfeld HM, Widmer MB. Interleukin 7 enhances cytotoxic T lymphocyte generation and induces lymphokine activated killer cells from peripheral blood. *J Exp Med* 1990; 172: 577-587.
11. Alderson MR, Tough TW, Ziegler SF, Grabstein KW. Interleukin 7 induces cytokine secretion and tumoricidal activity by human peripheral blood monocytes. *J Exp Med* 1991; 173: 923-930.
12. Allegretta M, Atkins MB, Dempsey RA, et al. The development of anti-interleukin-2 antibodies in patients treated with recombinant human interleukin-2 (IL-2). *J Clin Immunol* 1986; 6: 481.
13. Allione A, Consalvo M, Nanni P, et al. Immunizing and curative potential of replicating and nonreplicating murine mammary adenocarcinoma cells engineered with interleukin (IL)-2, IL-4, IL-6, IL-7, IL-10, Tumor Necrosis Factor and gamma-interferon gene or admixed with conventional adjuvants. *Cancer Res* 1994; 54: 6022-6026.
14. Allison MK, Jones SE, McGuffey P. Phase II trial of outpatient interleukin-2 in malignant lymphoma, chronic lymphocytic, leukemia, and selected solid tumors. *J Clin Oncol* 1989; 7: 75-80.
15. Ambrus JL and Fauci AS. Human B cell lymphoma cell line producing B cell growth factor. *J Clin Invest* 1985; 75: 732-730.
16. Ambrus JL, Jurgenson CH, Broom EJ, Fauci AS. Purification to homology of a high molecular weight human B cell growth factor. *J Exp Med* 1985; 162: 1319-1335.
17. Ambrus JL Chesky L, Stephany D, et al. Functional studies examining the subpopulation of human B lymphocytes responding to high molecular weight B cell growth factor. *J Immunol* 1990; 145: 3949-3955.
18. Ambrus JL, Pippin J, Joseph A, et al. Identification of a cDNA for a human high molecular weight B cell growth factor. *Proc Nat Acad Sci USA* 1993; 90: 6330-6334.
19. Anderson DM, Lyman S, Baird A, et al. Molecular cloning of mast cell growth factor, a hematopoietin that is active in both membrane bound and soluble forms. *Cell* 1990; 63: 235-243.
20. Andrews JVR, Schoof DD, Bertagnolli MM, et al. Immunomodulatory effects of Interleukin 12 on human tumor infiltrating lymphocytes. *J Immunotherapy* 1993; 14: 1-10.
21. Aoki T, Kikuchi H, Miyatake S-I, et al. Interleukin 5 enhances interleukin 2 mediated lymphokine activated killer activity. *J Exp Med* 1989; 23: 163-177.
22. Aoki T, Tashiro K, Miyatake S, et al. Expression of murine IL-7 in a murine glioma cell line results in reduced tumorigenicity *in vivo*. *Proc Natl Acad Sci USA* 1992; 89: 3850-3894.
23. Appasamy PM, Kenniston TW, Weng YH, et al. Interleukin 7 induced expression of specific T cell receptor gamma variable region genes in murine fetal liver cultures. *J Exp Med* 1993; 178: 2201-2206.
24. Argetsinger LS, Campbell GS, Yang X, et al. Identification of JAK2 as a growth hormone receptor associated tyrosine kinase. *Cell* 1994; 74: 237-244.
25. Ariizumi K, Meng Y, Bergstresser PR, Takashima A. INF-γ-Dependent IL-7 gene regulation in keratinocytes. *J Immunol* 1995; 154: 6031-6039.
26. Armitage RJ, Namen AE, Sassenfeld HM, Grabstein KH. Regulation of human T cell proliferation by IL-7. *J Immunol* 1989; 144: 938-941.
27. Armitage RJ, Namen AE, Sassenfeld HM, Grabstein KH. Regulation of T cell proliferation by IL-7. *J Immunol* 1990; 144: 938.
28. Armitage RJ, Macduff BM, Ziegler SF Grabstein KH. Multiple cytokine secretion by IL-7 stimulated human T cells. *Cytokine* 1992; 4: 461-469.1992.
29. Armitage RJ, Zeigler SF, Friend DJ, et al. Identification of a novel low affinity receptor for human interleukin-7. *Blood* 1992; 7: 1738.
30. Armitage RJ, MacDuff BM, Eisenman J, et al. IL-15 has stimulatory activity in the induction of B cell proliferation and differentiation. *J Immunol* 1995; 154: 483-490.
31. Aronson FR, Libby P, Brandon EP, et al. IL-2 rapidly

induces natural killer cell adhesion to human endothelial cells. A potential mechanism for endothelial injury. *J Immunol* 1988; 141: 158.

32. Atkins MB, Gould JA, Allegretta M, et al. Phase I evaluation of recombinant interleukin-2 in patients with advanced malignant disease. *J Clin Oncol* 1986; 4: 1380.
33. Atkins MB, Vachino G, Tilg HJ, et al. Phase I evaluation of thrice-daily intravenous bolus interleukin-4 in patients with refractory malignancy. *J Clin Onc* 1992; 10: 1802-1809.
34. Atzpodien J, Korfer A, Evers P, et al. Low-dose subcutaneous recombinant interleukin-2 in advanced human malignancy: A phase II outpatient study. *Mol Biother* 1990; 2: 18-26.
35. Atzpodien J, Korfer A, Franks CR, et al. Home therapy with recombinant interleukin-2 and interferon-α2b in advanced human malignancies. *Lancet* 1990; 335: 1509-1512.
36. Auget M, Dembie Z, Merlin G. Molecular cloning and expression of the human interferon γ receptor. *Cell* 1988; 55: 273-280.
37. Avanzi GC, Brizzi MF, Gianotti J, et al. M-07e human leukemic factor dependent cell line provides a rapid and sensitive bioassay for the human cytokines GM-CSF and IL-3. *J Cell Physiol* 1990; 145: 458-464.
38. Aversa G, Punnonen J, Cocks BG, et al. An interleukin 4 (IL-4) mutant protein inhibits both IL-4 or IL-13 induced human immunoglobulin G4 (IgG4) and IgE synthesis and B cell proliferation: support for a common component shared by IL-4 and IL-13 receptors. *J Exp Med* 1993; 178: 2213.
39. Bacon KB, Westwick J, Camp RDR. Potent and specific inhibition of IL8, IL1α and β induced *in vitro* human lymphocyte migration by calcium channel antagonists. *Biochem Biophys Res Commun* 1989; 165: 349.
40. Baggiolini M, Kernan P. Neutrophil activation: control of shape change exocytosis and respiratory burst. *News Physiol Sci* 1992; 7: 215.
41. Balsari A, Marolda R, Gambacorti-Passerini C, et al. Systemic administration of autologous, alloactivated helper-enriched lymphocytes to patients with metastatic melanoma of the lung. A phase I study. *Cancer Immunol Immunother* 1986; 21: 148.
42. Bamford RN, Grant AJ, Burton JD, et al. The interleukin (IL) 2 beta chain is shared by IL-2 and a cytokine, provisionally designated IL-T that stimulates T cell proliferation and the induction of lymphokine activated killer cells. *Proc Nat Acad Sci USA* 1994; 91: 4940-4944.
43. Barba D, Saris SC, Holder C, et al. Intratumoral LAK cell and interleukin-2 therapy of human gliomas. *J Neurosurg* 1989; 70: 175.
44. Barth RJ, Mule JJ, Speiss PJ, Rosenberg SA. Interferon gamma and tumor necrosis factor have a role in tumor regressions mediated by murine CD8+ tumor infiltrating lymphocytes. *J Exp Med* 1991; 173: 647-658.
45. Bazan JF. Emerging families of cytokines and receptors. *Curr Biol* 1993; 5: 459-462.
46. Beckman MP, Cosman D, Fanslow W, et al. The interleukin 4 receptor: structure function and signal transduction. *Chem Immunol* 1992; 51: 107.
47. Bedard M, Mclure CD, Schiller NL, et al. Release of interleukin 8, interleukin 6, and colony stimulating factors by upper airway epithelial cells: implications for cystic fibrosis. *Am J Respir Cell Mol Biol* 1993; 9: 455.
48. Bellone G, Trinchieri G. Dual stimulatory and inhibitory effect of NK cell stimulatory factor/IL-12 on human hematopoiesis. *J Immunol* 1994; 153: 930-937.
49. Ben-Sasson SZ, Le Gros G, Conrad DH, et al. IL-4 production by T cells from naive donors. *J Immunol* 1990; 145: 1127-1136.
50. Benjamin D, Sharma V, Knobloch TJ, et al. B cell IL7. Human B cell lines constitutively secrete IL-7 and express IL-7 receptors. *J Immunol* 1994; 152: 4749-4757.
51. Berdel WE, Danhauser Riedl S, Steinhauser G, Winton EF. Various human hematopoietic growth factors (interleukin 3, GM CSF, G CSF) stimulate clonal growth of non-hematopoietic tumor cells. *Blood* 1989; 73: 80-83.
52. Bertagnolli M and Herrmann S. IL7 supports the generation of cytotoxic T lymphocytes from thymocytes. *J Immunol* 1990; 145: 1706-1712.
53. Bertoglio S, Melioli G, Baldini E, et al. Intraperitoneal infusion of recombinant interleukin-2 in malignant ascites in patients with gastrointestinal and ovarian cancer. *Acta Med Austriaca* 1989; 16: 81-83.
54. Besedovsky H, del Rey A, Sorkin E, Dinarello CA. Immunoregulatory feedback between interleukin-1 and glucocorticoid hormones. *Science* 1986; 233: 652-654.
55. Beutler B, Mahoney J, Le Trang N, et al. Purification of cachectin, a lipoprotein lipase-suppressing hormone secreted by endotoxin-induced RAW 2264.7 cells. *J Exp Med* 1985; 161: 984.
56. Beutler B, Milsark I, Cerami A. Passive immunization against cachectin/tumor necrosis factor protects mice from lethal effect of endotoxin. *Science* 1985; 229: 869.
57. Beutler B, Greenwald D, Hulmes JD, et al. Identity of tumour necrosis factor and the macrophage secreted factor cachectin. *Nature* 1985; 316: 552-554.
58. Beutler B, ed. *Tumor necrosis factors: the molecules and their emerging role in medicine*. Raven Press New York, 1992 1-590.
59. Beutler B, Tkacenko V, Milasark I, et al. Control of cachechtin (tumor necrosis factor) synthesis: mechanisms of endotoxin resistance. *Science* 1986; 232: 977-979.
60. Beutler BA, Cerami A. Recombinant interleukin 1 suppresses lipoprotein lipase activity in 3T3-L1 cells. *J Immunol* 1985; 135: 3969-3971.
61. Blanchereau J, Briere F, Galizzi JP, et al. Human Interleukin 4. *J Lipid Mediators Cell Signaling* 1994; 9: 43-53.
62. Blankenstein T, Qin Z, Uberla K, et al. Tumor suppression after cell targeted tumor necrosis factor α gene transfer. *J Exp Med* 1991; 173: 1047-1052.
63. Blin N, Stafford DW. Isolation of high molecular weight DNA. *Nucleic Acid Res* 1976; 3: 2303.
64. Bogdan C, Vodovotz Y, Nathan CF. Macrophage inactivation by interleukin 10. *J Exp Med* 1991; 174: 1549.
65. Boldt DH, Mills BJ, Gemlo BT, et al. Laboratory correlates of adoptive immunotherapy with recombinant interleukin-2 and lymphokine-activated killer cells in human. *Cancer Res* 1988; 48: 4409.
66. Bonnema J, Rivlin KA, Ting AT, et al. Cytokine enhanced natural killer cells mediated cytotoxicity. Positive modulatory effects of IL2 and IL12 on stimulus -dependent granule exocytosis. *J Immunol* 1994; 152: 2098-2104.
67. Boulay JL, Paul WE. The interleukin-4 related lymphokines and their binding to hematopoietic receptors. *J Biol Chem* 1992; 267: 20525-20528.
68. Bradding P, Feather IH, Howarth PH, et al. Interleukin 4 is localized and released by human mast cells. *J Exp Med* 1992; 176: 1381.

69. Bradley EC, Louis AC, Paradise CM, et al. Antitumor response in patients with metastatic renal cell carcinoma is dependent upon regimen intensity (meeting abstract). *Proc Am Soc Clin Oncol* 1989; 8: A519.
70. Braun RK, Francini M, Erard F, et al. Human peripheral blood eosinophils produce and release interleukin 8 on stimulation with calcium ionophore. *Eur J Immunol* 1993; 23: 956.
71. Brennan FM, Chantry D, Jackson A, et al. Inhibitory effects of TNF α antibodies on synovial cell interleukin 1 production in rheumatoid arthritis. *Lancet* 1989; 11: 244.
72. Broide DH, Paine MM, Firestein GS. Eosinophils express interleukin 5 and granulocyte macrophage colony stimulating factor mRNA at sites of allergic inflammation in asthmatics. *J Clin Invest* 1992; 90: 1414.
73. Brooks B, Rees RC. Human recombinant IL-4 suppresses the induction of human IL-2 induced lymphokine activated killer (LAK) activity. *Clin Exp Immunol* 1988; 74: 162.
74. Brown MA, Pierce JH, Watson CJ, et al. B cell stimulatory factor-1/Interleukin-4 is expressed by normal and transformed mast cells. *Cell* 1987; 50: 809-818.
75. Browning JL, Mattaliano RJ, Pinchang CE, et al. Disulfide scrambling of interleukin-2: HPLC resolution of the three possible isomers. *Anal Biochem* 1986; 155: 123.
76. Brunda MJ, Luistro L, Warrier RR, et al. Antitumor and antimetastatic activity of interleukin-12 against murine tumors. *J Exp Med* 1993; 178: 1223-30.
77. Bukowski RM, Murthy S, Sergi J, et al. Phase I trial of continuous infusion recombinant interleukin-2 and intermittent recombinant interferon-α_{2a}: clinical effects. *J Biologic Resp Mod* 1990; 9: 538-545.
78. Burton JD, Bamford RM, Peters C, et al. A lymphokine provisionally designated interleukin T and produced by a human adult T cell leukemia line stimulates T cell proliferation and the induction of lymphokine activated killer cells. *Proc Nat Acad Sci USA* 1994; 91: 4935-4939.
79. Butler J, Sleijfer DT, van der Graaf WTA, et al. A progress report on the outpatient treatment of patients with advanced renal cell carcinoma using subcutaneous recombinant interleukin-2. *Semin Oncol* 1993; 20: 16-21.
80. Cameron RB, McIntosh JK, Rosenberg SA. Synergistic antitumor effects of combination immunotherapy with recombinant interleukin-2 and a recombinant hybrid alpha-interferon in the treatment of established murine hepatic metastases. *Cancer Res* 1988; 48: 5810.
81. Cantrell MA, Anderson D, Cerretti DP, et al. Cloning sequence and expression of human granulocyte-macrophage colony stimulating factor. *Proc Natl Acad* (USA) 1985; 82: 6250.
82. Carson WE, Giri JG, Lindenmann MJ, et al. Interleukin (IL) 15 is a novel cytokine that activates human natural killer cells via components of the IL-2 receptor *J Exp Med* 1994; 180: 1395.
83. Carswell EA, Old LJ, Kassel RL, et al. An endotoxin induced serum factor that causes necrosis of tumors *Proc Nat Acad Sci USA* 1975; 25: 3666-3670.
84. Carveth HJ, Bohnsack JF, McIntyre TM, et al. Neutrophil activating factor (NAF) induces polymorphonuclear leukocyte adherence to endothelial cells and to subendothelial matrix proteins. *Biochem Biophys Res Commun* 1989; 162: 387.
85. Cascinelli N, Belli F, Marchini S, et al. A phase II study of the administration of recombinant interleukin 2 plus lymphokine activated killer cells in stage IV melanoma patients. *Tumori* 1989; 75: 233.
86. Casey LS, Lichtman AH, Boothby M. IL-4 induced IL-2 receptor p75 beta chain gene expression and IL-2 dependent proliferation in mouse T lymphocytes. *J Immunol* 1992; 148: 3418-26.
87. Cassatella M, Bazzoni F, Ceska M, et al. IL-8 production by human polymorphonuclear leukocytes: the chemoattractant formylmethionyl leucylphenylalanine induces the pathway . *J Immunol* 1992; 148: 3216.
88. Caux C, Dezutter-Dambuyant D, Schmitt D, Banchereau J. GM-CSF and TNF cooperate in the generation of dendritic Langerhans cells. *Nature* 1992; 360, 258.
89. Cesano A, Visonneau S, Clark SC, Santoli D. Cellular and molecular mechanisms of activation of MHC nonrestricted cytotoxic cells by IL-12. *J Immunol* 1993; 151: 2943.
90. Chan SH, Perussia B, Gupta JW, et al. Induction of interferon γ production by natural killer cell stimulatory factor: characterization of responding cells and synergy with other inducers. *J Exp Med* 1991; 173: 869-879.
91. Chazen GD, Pereira GMB, Le Gross G, et al. Interleukin 7 is a T cell growth factor. *Proc Nat Acad Sci USA* 1989; 86: 5923-5927.
92. Chebath J, Benech P, Hovanessian A, et al. Four different forma of interferon induced 2'-5'oligo(A)synthetase identified by immunoblotting in human cells. *J Biol Chem* 1987; 262: 3852-3857.
93. Cheever MA, Thompson JA, Kern DE, Greenberg PD. Interleukin 2 administration *in vivo*: influence of IL-2 route and timing on T cell growth. *J Immunol* 1985; 134: 3895.
94. Chemini J, Starr S, Frank I. Natural killer cell stimulatory factor (NKSF) increases the cytotoxic activity of NK cells from both healthy donors and HIV-infected patients. *J Exp Med* 1992; 175: 789-788.
95. Chen WF, Zlotnik A. IL10: a novel cytotoxic T cell differentiation factor. *J Immunol* 1991; 147: 528.
96. Chien Y, Gascoigne N, Kavaler J, et al. Somatic recombination in a murine T-cell-receptor gene. *Nature* 1984; 309: 322.
97. Chilton PM, Fernandez-Botran R. Production of soluble IL-4 receptors by murine spleen cells is regulated by activation and IL-4. *J Immunol* 151: 5907-5917.
98. Chiu C-P, Moulds C, Coffman RL, et al. Multiple biological activities are expressed by a mouse interleukin 6 cDNA clone isolated from bone marrow stromal cells. *Proc Nat Acad Sci USA* 1988; 85: 7099-7103.
99. Chizzonite R, Truitt T, Kilian PL, et al. Two high affinity interleukin 1 receptors represent separate gene products. *Proc Nat Acad Sci USA* 1989; 86: 8029.
100. Chizzonite R, Truitt T, Desai BB, et al. IL-12 Receptor. I. Characterization of the receptor on phytohemagglutinin-activated human lymphoblasts. *J Immunol* 1992; 148: 3117-3124.
101. Chua AO, Chizzonite R, Desai BB, et al. Expression cloning of a human IL-12 receptor component. *J Immunol* 1994; 153: 128-136.
102. Claasen JL, Levine AD, Buckley RH. Recombinant human IL-4 induces IgE and IgG synthesis by normal and atopic donor mononuclear cells. *J Immunol* 1991; 144: 123-130.
103. Clamin H. Mast cells, T-cells, and abnormal fibrosis. *Immunol Today* 1985; 6: 192.

104. Clark-Lewis I, Schrader JW. P-cell stimulating factor: biochemical characterization of a new T-cell-derived factor. *J Immunol* 1981; 127: 1941.
105. Clark-Lewis I, Kent SBH, Schrader JW. Purification to apparent homogeneity of a factor stimulating the growth of multiple lineages of hemopoietic cells. *J Biol Chem* 1984; 259: 7488.
106. Clerici M, Lucey DR, Berzofsky JA, et al. Restoration of HIV-mediated immune responses by interleukin 12 *in vitro*. *Science* 1993; 262: 1721-1724.
107. Coffman RL, Bond MW, Carty J, et al. B cell stimulatory factor 1 enhances the IgE response of lipopolysaccharide-activated B cells. *J Immunol* 1986; 136: 4538-4541.
108. Cohen PA, Kim H, Fowler DH, et al. Use of Interleukin-7, Interleukin-2 and Interferon-γ to propagate CD4+ T cells in culture with maintained Antigen Specificity. *J Immunother* 1993; 14: 242-252.
109. Contractor V, Pippin J, Russell J, et al. Identification of cDNA and genomic localization for IL14. *FASEB J* 1994; 8: A506.
110. Copeland NG, Gilgert DJ, Cho BC, et al. Mast cell growth factor maps near the steel locus on mouse chromosome 10 and is deleted in a number of steel alleles. *Cell* 1990; 63: 175-183.
111. Cortesina G, De Stefani A, Gioverelli M, et al. Treatment of recurrent squamous cell carcinoma of the head and neck with low doses of interleukin-2 injected perilymphatically. *Cancer* 1988; 62: 2482.
112. Costello R, Brailly H, Mallet F, et al. Interleukin-7 is a potent costimulus of the adhesion pathway involving CD2 and CD28 molecules. *Immunology* 1993; 80: 451-457.
113. Costino G, Soprana E, Thienes CP, et al. IL13 down regulates CD14 expression and TNFα secretion in normal human monocytes. *J Immunol* 1995; 155: 3145-3151.
114. Cotran RS, Pober JS, Gimbrone MA Jr, et al. Endothelial activation during interleukin 2 immunotherapy. A possible mechanism for the vascular leak syndrome. *J Immunol* 1987; 139: 1883.
115. Crawford R, Finboom D, Ohara J, et al. B cell stimulatory factor 1 (Interleukin 4) activates macrophages for increased tumoricidal activity and expression of Ia antigens. *J Immunol* 1987; 139: 135.
116. Creekmore SP, Harris JE, Ellis TM, et al. A Phase I clinical trial of recombinant interleukin-2 by periodic 24-hour intravenous infusions. *J Clin Oncol* 1989; 7: 276 284.
117. Croghan M, Hersh EM, Taylor C, et al. Phase I-II study of low dose cytoxan and recombinant interleukin 2 (IL-2) for the treatment of disseminated carcinoma (meeting abstract). *Proc Annu Meet Am Soc Clin Oncol* 1989; 8: A699.
118. Crown J, Jakubowski A, Kemeny N, et al. A phase I trial of recombinant human interleukin-1β alone and in combination with myelosuppressive doses of 4-fluorouracil in patients with gastrointestinal cancer. *Blood* 1991; 78: 1420-1427.
119. Cuttitta F, Mulshine J, Moody TW, et al. Bombesin-like peptide can function as autocrine growth factors in human small cell lung cancer. *Nature* 1985; 316: 823.
120. Dadi KH and Roifman CM. Interleukin 7 receptor mediates the activation of phosphatidyl-3 inositol kinase in human B-cell precursors. *Biochem Biophys Res Commun* 1993; 192: 450-64.
121. Dadi KH and Roifman CM. Activation of phosphatidylinositol-3 kinase by ligation of the interleukin 7 receptor on human thymocytes. *J Clin Invest* 1993; 92: 1559-63.
122. Dai CH, Krantz SB, Zsebo KM. Human burst forming units erythroid need direct interaction with stem cell factor for further development *Blood* 1991; 78: 2493-2497.
123. Dalloul A, Laroche L, Bagot M, et al. Interleukin-7 is a growth factor for Sezary lymphoma cells. *J Clin Invest* 1992; 90, 1054-1060.
124. Damle NK, Doyle LV, Bender JR, Bradley EC. Interleukin 2-activated human lymphocytes exhibit enhanced adhesion to normal vascular endothelial cells and cause their lysis. *J Immunol* 1987; 138: 1779.
125. Damle NK, Doyle LV. Distinct regulatory effects of IL-4 and TNF- during CD3-independent initiation human T cell activation. *Lymphokine Res* 1989; 8: 85.
126. D'Andrea A, Aste-Amezaga M, Valiante NM, et al. Interleukin-10 inhibits human lymphocyte INF- production by suppressing natural killer cell stimulatory factor/interleukin 12 synthesis in accessory cells. *J Exp Med* 1993; 178: 1041-1048.
127. D'Andrea A, Rangaraju M, Valiante NM, et al. Production of natural killer cell stimulatory factor (interleukin 12) by peripheral blood mononuclear cells. *J Exp Med* 1992; 176: 1387-1398.
128. Darnell JE, Kerr IM, Stark GR. Jak-STAT pathways and transcriptional activation response to IFNs and other extracellular signalling proteins. *Science* 1994; 264: 1415-1421.
129. Dayer JM, de Rochemonteix B, Burrus B, et al. Human recombinant interleukin 1 stimulates collagenase and prostaglandin E_2 production by synovial cells. *J Clin Invest* 1986; 77: 645-648.
130. Dedhar D. Gaboury L, Galloway P, Evans C. Human granulocyte macrophage colony stimulating factor is a growth factor for a variety of cell types of non-hematopoietic origin. *Proc Nat Acad Sci USA* 1988; 83: 9253-9257.
131. Defrance T, Fluckinger AC, Rossi JF, et al. Antiproliferative effects of Interleukin-4 on freshly isolated non-hodgkin malignant B cell lymphoma cells. *Blood* 1992; 79: 990-996.
132. DeLarco JE, Todaro GJ. Growth factors from murine sarcoma virus-transformed cells. *Proc Natl Acad Sci* (USA) 1978; 75: 4001.
133. Del Pozo V, De Andreas B, Martin E, et al. Eosinophil as antigen presenting cells: activation of T cell clones and T cell hybridoma by eosinophils after antigen processing. *Eur J Immunol* 1992; 22: 1919.
134. Del Prete G, Maggi E, Parronchi P, et al. IL4 is an essential factor for the IgE synthesis induced *in vitro* by human T cell clones and their supernatants. *J Immunol* 1988; 140: 4193-4198.
135. Dennig D, O'Reilly RJ. L7 induces surface expression of B7/BB1 on Pre-B cells and an associated increase in their costimulatory effects on T cell proliferation. *Cellular Immunol* 1994; 153: 227-238.
136. Dentener MA, Bazil V, Von Asmuth EJU, et al. Involvement of CD14 in lipopolysaccharide induced tumor necrosis factor α, IL6, and IL8 release by human monocytes and alveolar macrophages. *J Immunol* 1993; 150: 2885.
137. Desai BB, Quinn PM, Wolitzky AS, et al. IL-12 Receptor II. Distribution and expression of receptor expression. *J Immunol* 1992; 148: 3125-3132.

138. Desai BB, Truit T, Honasoge S, et al. Expression of functional IL-12R on a human IL2-dependent cell line. *J Immunol* 1993; 150: 207A.
139. Desreumauz P, Janin A, Colombel JF, et al. Interleukin 5 messenger RNA expression by eosinophils in the intestinal mucosa of patients with coeliac disease. *J Exp Med* 1992; 175: 293.
140. DeVita VT Jr, Hellman S, Rosenberg SA, eds. In: *Biologic Therapy of Cancer*, Second Edition. Philadelphia, J.B. Lippincott Company, 1995: pp. 235-249.
141. DeWaal Malefyt R, Figdor C, Huijbens R, et al. Effects of IL13 on phenotype, cytokine production and cytotoxic function of human monocytes. *J Immunol* 1993; 151: 6370-6381.
142. DeWaal Malefyt R, Haansen J, et al. IL-10 and viral IL10 strongly reduce antigen specific T cell proliferation by diminishing the antigen presenting capacity of monocytes vial downregulation of class II MHC expression. *J Exp Med* 1991a; 174: 915.
143. De Waal Malefyt R, Abrams J, Bennett B, et al. Interleukin 10 (IL-10) inhibits cytokine synthesis by human monocytes: an autoregulatory role of IL-10 by monocytes. *J Exp Med* 1991b; 174: 1209.
144. Dewhirst FE, Stashenko PP, Mole JE, Tsurumachi T. Purification and partial sequence of human osteoclast activating factor: identity with interleukin-1 beta. *J Immunol* 1985; 135: 2562-2568.
145. Dillman RO, Barth N, Oldham RK, et al. Continuous interleukin-2 and lymphokine-activated killer cells in advanced cancer (meeting abstract). *Proc Annu Meet Am Soc Clin Oncol* 1989; 8: A730.
146. Dillman RO, Oldham RK, Barth NM, et al. Recombinant interleukin-2 and adoptive immunotherapy alternated with dacarbazine therapy in melanoma: A National Biotherapy Study Group Trial. *J Natl Cancer Inst* 1990; 82(16): 1345-1349.
147. Dillman RO, Oldham RK, Tauer KW, et al. Continuous Interleukin-2 and lymphokine activated killer cells for advanced cancer: An NBSG trial. *J Clin Oncol* 1991; 9: 1233-1240.
148. Dillman R, Church C, Oldham RK, et al. Inpatient continuous infusion interleukin-2 in 788 cancer patients: the NBSG experience. *Cancer* 1993; 71: 2358-2370.
149. Dillman RO. The clinical experience with Interleukin-2 in cancer therapy. Cancer Biotherapy 1994; 9(3): 183-210.
150. Dinarello CA. Biology of interleukin 1. *FASEB* J 1988; 2: 108-115.
151. Dinarello CA, Goldin NP, Wolf SM. Demonstration and characterization of two distinct human leukocyte pyrogens. *J Exp Med* 1974; 139: 1369.
152. Dinarello CR, Cannon JG, Wolff SM, et al. Tumor necrosis factor (Cachectin) is an endogenous pyrogen and induces production of interleukin 1. *J Exp Med* 1986; 163: 1433.
153. Dinarello CA. Blocking Interleukin 1 receptors. *Int J Clin Lab Res* 1994; 24: 61-79.
154. Ditonno P, Tso CL, Sakata T, et al. Regulatory effects of interleukin-7 on renal tumor infiltrating lymphocytes. *Urological Res* 1992; 20: 205-210.
155. Doherty TM, Kastelein R, Menon S, et al. Modulation of murine macrophages function by IL-13. J *Immunol* 1993; 151: 7151.
156. Dokter WH, Sierdsema SJ, Esselink MT, et al. IL7 enhances expression of IL-3 and granulocyte-macrophage-CSF mRNA in activated human T cells by post transcriptional mechanisms. *J Immunol* 1993; 150: 2584-90.
157. Dokter WH, Sierdsema SJ, Esselink MT, et al. Interleukin 4 mRNA and protein in activated human T cells are enhanced by Interleukin 7. *Exp Hematology* 1994; 22: 74-79.
158. Domzig W, Stadler BM, Herberman RB. Interleukin 2 dependence of human natural killer (LAK) cell activity. *J Immunol* 1983; 130: 1970.
159. Donohoe RE, Yang YC, Clark SC. Human P40 T cell growth factor (interleukin 9) supports erythroid colony formation. *Blood* 1990; 75: 2271-2275.
160. Donohue JH, Rosenberg SA. The fate of interleukin-2 after *in vivo* administration. *J Immunol* 1983; 130: 2203.
161. Donohue JH, Rosenstein M, Chang AE, et al. The systemic administration of purified interleukin-2 enhances the ability of sensitized murine lymphocyte lines to cure a disseminated syngeneic lymphoma. *J Immunol* 1984; 132: 2123.
162. Doolittle RF, Hunmkapillar MW, Hood LE, et al. Simian sarcoma virus oncogene, Vsis, is derived from the gene encoding a platelet-derived growth factor. *Science* 1983; 221: 275.
163. Downward J, Yarden Y, Mayes E, et al. Close similarity of epidermal growth factor receptor and V-erb B oncogene protein sequences. *Nature* 1984; 307: 521.
164. Doyle MV, Lee MT, Fong S. Comparison of the biological activities of human recombinant interleukin-2(125) and native interleukin-2. *J Biol Response Modif* 1985; 4: 96.
165. Dripps DJ, et al. *J Biol Chem* 1991; 266: 10331.
166. Dubucquoi S, Desreumaux P, Janin A, et al. Interleukin 5 synthesis by eosinophils: association with granules and immunoglobulin -dependent secretion. *J Exp Med* 1994; 179: 703.
167. DuMonde DC, Wolstencraft RA, Panavei GS, et al. *Nature* 1969; 224: 38.
168. Dupere S, Obiri N, Lackey A, et al. Patterns of cytokines released by peripheral blood leukocytes of normal donors and cancer patients during interleukin-2 activation *in vitro*. *J Biol Modif* 1990; 9(2): 140-148.
169. Dutcher JP, Creekmore S, Weiss GR, et al. A Phase II study of interleukin-2 and lymphokine-activated killer cells in patients with metastatic malignant melanoma. *J Clin Oncol* 1989; 7: 477.
170. Eastgate JA, Wood N, DiGiovine FS, et al. Correlation of plasma IL1 levels with disease activity in rheumatoid arthritis. *EMBO* 1991; 10: 4025.
171. Eberlein TJ, Schoof DD, Jung S, et al. A new regimen of interleukin 2 and lymphokine-activated killer cells. *Arch Intern Med* 1988; 148: 2571.
172. Economou JS, McBride WH, Essner R, et al. Tumour necrosis factor production by IL-2-activated macrophages *in vitro* and *in vivo*. *Immunology* 1989; 67: 514.
173. Eiseman J, Melink T, Bell M, et al. Determination of an optimal immunomodulatory dose for cyclophosphamide in combination with interleukin-2 (meeting abstract). *Proc Am Assoc Cancer Res* 1989; 30: A1501.
174. Enk CD, Sredni D, Blauvelt A, Katz SI. Induction of IL-10 gene expression in human keratinocytes by UVB exposure *in vivo* and *in vitro*. *J Immunol* 1995; 154: 4851-4856.
175. Evans CH. Lymphotoxin – An immunologic hormone with anti-carcinogenic and anti-tumor activity. *Cancer Immunol Immunother* 1982; 12: 181.

176. Fanslow WCK, Clifford K, Vandenbos T, et al. A soluble form of the interleukin 4 receptor in biological fluids. *Cytokine* 1990; 2: 398.
177. Fanslow WCK, Clifford K, Park LS, et al. Regulation of alloreactivity *in vivo* by IL-4 and the soluble IL-4 receptor. *J Immunol* 1991; 147: 535.
178. Farrar J, Hilfiker M, Johnson B, et al. Identification of a T-cell derived B-cell growth factor distinct from interleukin-2. *J Exp Med* 1982; 155: 914-923.
179. Farrar MA, Schreiber RD. The molecular biology of interferon γ and its receptor. *Ann Rev Immunol* 1993; 11: 571-611.
180. Favre C, Saeland S, Caux C, et al. Interleukin-4 has growth promoting activity on cord blood cells. *Blood* 1990; 75: 67-73.
181. Fernandez-Botran R. Soluble cytokine receptors and their role in immunoregulation. *FASEB* 1991; 5: 2567.
182. Fernandez-Botran R, Vitetta ES. A soluble high affinity interleukin-4 receptor is present in the biological fluids of mice. *Proc Nat Acad Sci USA* 1990; 87: 4202.
183. Fernandez-Botran R, Vitetta ES. Evidence that soluble interleukin -4 receptors may act as transport proteins. *J Exp Med* 1991; 174: 673.
184. Fernandez-Botran R, Sanders VM, Oliver KG, et al. Evidence that soluble interleukin-4 receptors may act as transport proteins. *J Exp Med* 1991; 174: 673.
185. Ferro TJ, Johnson A, Everitt J, Malik AB. IL-2 induces pulmonary edema and vasoconstriction independent of circulating lymphocytes. *J Immunol* 1989; 142: 1916.
186. Fildes R. Proleukin – the first interleukin to reach the market? *The Clinical Impact of the Interleukins*, London, April 10-11, 1989.
187. Findley HW Jr, Mageed AA, Nasr SA, Ragab AH. Recombinant interleukin-2 activates peripheral blood lymphocytes from children with acute leukemia to kill autologous leukemic cells. *Cancer* 1988; 62: 1928.
188. Finke JH, Rayman P, Hart L, et al. Characterization of tumor infiltrating lymphocyte subsets from human renal cell carcinoma: specific reactivity defined by cytotoxicity interferon γ secretion and proliferation. *J Immunother with Emphasis on Tumor Immunology* 1994; 15: 91-104.
189. Fiorentino DF, Bond MW, Mosmann TR. Two types of mouse T helper IV: TH2 clones secrete a factor that inhibits cytokine production by Th1 clones. *J Exp Med* 1989; 170: 2081-95.
190. Fiorentino DF, Zlotnik A, Viera P, et al. IL-10 acts on the antigen presenting cell to inhibit cytokine production by TH1 cells. *J Immunol* 1991a; 146: 3444-3451.
191. Fiorentino DF, Zlotnik A, Mosmann TR, et al. IL-10 inhibits cytokine production by activated macrophages. *J Immunol* 1991b; 147: 3815.
192. Fisher RI, Coltman CA Jr, Doroshow JH, et al. Metastatic renal cancer treated with interleukin-2 and lymphokine-activated killer cells. *Ann Intern Med* 1988; 108: 518.
193. Flaherty LE, Liu PY, Fletcher WS, et al. Dacarbazine and outpatient interleukin-2 in treatment of metastatic malignant melanoma: Phase II Southwest Oncology Group trial. *J Natl Cancer Inst* 1992; 84: 893-894.
194. Flanagan JG, Chan DC, Leder P. Transmembrane form of the kit growth factor is determined by alternative splicing and is missing in the S1d mutant. *Cell* 1991; 64: 1025-1035.
195. Fontana A, Kristensen F, Dubs R, et al. Production of prostaglandin E and interleukin-1 like factor by cultured astrocytes and CG glioma cells. *J Immunol* 1982; 129: 2413-2419.
196. Ford RJ, Tamayo A, Marker B, Ambrus JL. IL-14 and growth control in human B cell lymphomas. *FASEB J* 1992; 8: A1021.
197. Foss FM, Koc Y, Stetler-Stevenson MA, et al. Costimulation of cutaneous T cell lymphoma cells by Interleukin 7 and interleukin 2: potential autocrine and paracrine effectors in the Sezary syndrome. *J Clin Oncol* 1994; 12: 326-335.
198. Foulke RS, Marshall MH, Trotta PP, von Hoff DD. *In vitro* assessment of the effects of granulocyte monocyte colony stimulating factor on primary human tumors and derived tumor cell lines. *Cancer Res* 1990; 50: 6264-6267.
199. Fountoulakis M, Zulauf M, Lustig A. Stoichiometry of interaction between interferon-γ and its receptor *Eur J Biochem* 1992; 209: 781-787.
200. Foxwell BML, Taylor Fishwick DA, Simon JL, et al. Activation induced changes in expression and structure of the IL7 receptor in human T cells. *Int Immunol* 1992; 4: 277.
201. Foxwell BM, Willcocks JL, Taylor-Fishwick DA, et al. Inhibition of activation induced changed in the structure of the T cell interleukin-7 receptor by cyclosporin A and FK506. *Eur J Immunol* 1993; 23: 85-89.
202. Frank MB, Watson J, Gillis S. Biochemical and biologic characterization of lymphocyte regulatory molecules. VIII. Purification of interleukin-2 from a human T-cell leukemia. *J Immunol* 1981; 127: 2361.
203. Fransen L, Van de Hayden J, Ruysshaert R, et al. Recombinant tumor necrosis factor: its effects and its synergism with interferon γ on a variety of normal and transformed human cell lines. *Eur J Cancer and Clin Oncol* 1986; 22: 419-426.
204. Fraser CC, Thacker JD, Hogge DE, et al. Alterations in lymphopoiesis after hematopoietic reconstitution with IL-7 virus infected bone marrow. *J Immunol* 1993; 151: 2409-2418.
205. Frendl G, Beller DI. Regulation of macrophage activation by IL3. I. IL-3 functions as a macrophage activating factor with unique properties inducing Ia and lymphocyte function associated antigen 1 but not cytotoxicity. *J Immunol* 1990; 144: 3392.
206. Frishman J, Long B, Knospe W, et al. Genes for interleukin 7 are translated in leukemia cell subsets of individuals with chronic lymphocytic leukemia. *J Exp Med* 1993; 177: 955-64.
207. Fung MC, Hapel AJ, Mymer S, et al. Molecular cloning of cDNA for murine interleukin-3. *Nature* 1984; 307: 233.
208. Gajewski TF, Schell SR, Nau G, Fitch FW. Regulation of T cell activation: differences among T cell subsets. *Immunol Rev* 1989; 111: 79-110.
209. Galazaka AR, Weiner J, Barth NM, Oldham RK. Lymphokines and cytokines. In: *Principles of Cancer Biotherapy*, RK Oldham ed. Marcel Dekker Inc., New York, 1991, pp 327-361.
210. Gallagher G, Stimson WH, Findlay J et al. Interleukin 6 enhances the induction of human lymphokine activated killer cells. *Cancer Immunol Immunother* 1990; 31: 49-52.
211. Gansbacher B, Zier K, Daniels B, et al. Interleukin 2 gene transfer into tumor cells abrogates tumorigenicity and induces protective immunity. *Exp Med* 1990a; 172: 1217-1224.

212. Gansbacher B, Bannerji R, Daniels B, et al. Retroviral vector mediated γ-interferon gene transfer into tumor cells generates potent and long lasting antitumor immunity. *Cancer Res* 1990b; 50: 7820-7825.
213. Garvy BA Riley RL. IFN gamma abrogates IL-7 dependent proliferation in per-B cells coinciding with onset of apoptosis. *Immunology* 1994; 81: 381-8.
214. Gastl GA, Abrams JS, Nanus DM, et al. Interleukin 1 production by human carcinoma cell lines and its relationship to interleukin 6 expression. *Int J Cancer* 1993; 55: 96.
215. Gately MK, Desai BB, Wolitky AG, et al. Regulation of human lymphocyte proliferation by a heterodimeric cytokine, IL-12 (Cytotoxic lymphocyte maturation factor). *J Immunol* 1991; 147: 874-882.
216. Gately MK, Wilson DE, Wong HL. Synergy between recombinant Interleukin 2 and interleukin 2 depleted lymphokine containing supernatants in facilitating allogeneic human cytolytic T lymphocyte responses *in vitro*. *J Immunol* 1986; 136: 1274.
217. Gately MK, Wolitzky AG, Quinn PM, Chizzonite R. Regulation of human cytolytic lymphocyte responses by interleukin 12. *Cellular Immunology* 1992; 143: 127-142.
218. Gaynor ER, Ellis TM, Harris J, et al. Adjuvant immunotherapy using intermittent 24 hour infusions of recombinant interleukin-2 in patients with surgically resected colon carcinoma at high risk for recurrence (meeting abstract). *Proc Annu Meet Am Soc Clin Oncol* 1989; 8: A739.
219. Gazzinelli RT, Oswald IP, James SL, Sher A. IL-10 inhibits parasite killing and nitrogen oxide production by IFNγ activated macrophages. *J Immunol* 1992; 148: 1792.
220. Gearing AJH, Thorpe R. The international standard for human interleukin-2. *J Immunol Methods* 1988; 114: 3.
221. Gearing DP, Cameau MR, Friend DJ, et al. The IL-6 signal transducer gp130: an oncostatin M receptor and affinity converter for the LIF receptor. *Science* 1992; 255: 1434.
222. Gearing DP, Cosman D. Homology of the p40 subunit of natural killer cell stimulatory factor (NKSF) with the extracellular domain of the interleukin-6 receptor. *Cell* 1991; 66: 9.
223. Geertsen PF, Hermann GG, von der Maase H, Steven K. Treatment of metastatic renal cell carcinoma by continuous intravenous infusion of recombinant interleukin-2: A single-center phase II study. *J Clin Oncol* 1992; 10: 753-759.
224. Gemlo BT, Palladino MA Jr, Jaffe HS, et al. Circulating cytokines in patients with metastatic cancer treated with recombinant interleukin 2 and lymphokine-activated killer cells. *Cancer Res* 1988; 48: 5864.
225. Germann T, Gately MK, Schoenhaut DS, et al. Interleukin 12/T cell stimulating factor, a cytokine with multiple effects on T helper type 1 (TH1) but not TH2 cells. *E J Immunol* 1993; 23: 1762-1770.
226. Gery I, Gershon RK, Waksman BH. Potentiation of the T-lymphocyte response to mitogens. II. The cellular source of potentiating mediators. *J Exp Med* 1972; 136: 143.
227. Ghezzi P, Saccardo B, Villa P, et al. Role of interleukin-1 in the depression of liver drug metabolism by endotoxin. *Infect Immun* 1986; 54: 837-840.
228. Ghosh AK, Smith K, Prendiville J, et al. A phase-I study of recombinant human interleukin-4 administered by the intravenous and subcutaneous route in patients with advanced cancer – immunological effects. *Eur Cytokine Network* 1993; 4: 205-211.
229. Gilewski TA, Richards JM, Vogelzang NJ, et al. A phase II study of recombinant interleukin-2 with or without lymphokine activated killer cells in patients with metastatic colon carcinoma (meeting abstract). *Proc Annu Meet Am Soc Clin Oncol* 1989; 8: A499a.
230. Gill I, Agah R, Mazumder A. Synergistic antitumor effects of interleukin-2 and the monoclonal antibody Lym-1 *in vitro* and *in vivo* (meeting abstract). *Proc Annu Meet Am Assoc Cancer Res* 1989; 30: A1445.
231. Gimbrone MA, Obin MS, Brock AF, et al. Endothelial interleukin 8. a novel inhibitor of leukocyte endothelial interactions. *Science* 1989; 246: 1601.
232. Giovarelli M, Musiani P, Modesti A, et al. Local release of IL10 by transfected mouse mammary adenocarcinoma cells does not suppress but enhances antitumor reaction and elicits a strong cytotoxic lymphocyte and antibody dependent immune memory. *J Immunol* 1995; 155: 3112-3123.
233. Giri JG, Adhieh M, Eisenman J, et al. Utilization of the beta and gamma chains of the IL2 receptor by the novel cytokine IL-15. *EMBO* J 1994; 13: 2822-2830.
234. Go NF, Castle BE, Barrett R, et al. Interleukin 10 (IL-10) a novel B cell stimulatory factor: unresponsiveness of X chromosome linked immunodeficiency B cells. *J Exp Med* 1990; 172: 1625-1631.
235. Godfrey DI, Gately M, Zlotnik A. Influence of IL-12 on intrathymic T cell development. *J Immunol* 1993; 150: 11A.
236. Goldstein D, Sosman J, Hank J, et al. Repetitive weekly cycles of interleukin-2: Outpatient treatment with a lower dose of IL-2 maintains heightened NK and LAK activity (meeting abstract). *Proc Annu Meet Am Soc Clin Oncol* 1989; 8: A751.
237. Golumbek PT, Lazenby AJ, Levitsky HI, et al. Treatment of established renal caner by tumor cells engineered to secrete interleukin-4. *Science* 1991; 254: 713-716.
238. Goodwin RG, Friend D, Ziegler SF, et al. Cloning of the human and murine interleukin-7 receptors: Demonstration of a soluble form and homology to a new receptor superfamily. *Cell* 1990; 60, 941.
239. Goodwin RG, Lupton GS, Schmierer A, et al. Human interleukin 7: molecular cloning and growth factor activity on human and murine B-lineage cells. *Proc Nat Acad Sci USA* 1989; 86: 302.
240. Gordon J, Guy GR. The molecules controlling B lymphocytes. *Immunol Today* 1987; 8: 339.
241. Gordon J, MacLean LD. A lymphocyte stimulating factor produced in vitro. *Nature* 1965; 208: 795-796.
242. Gottlieb DJ, Brenner MK, Heslop HE, et al. A phase I clinical trial of recombinant interleukin 2 following high dose chemoradiotherapy for haematological malignancy: applicability to the elimination of minimal residual disease. *Br J Cancer* 1989; 60: 610.
243. Gottlieb DJ, Prentice HG, Heslop HE, et al. Effects of recombinant interleukin-2 administration on cytotoxic function following high dose chemo-radiotherapy for haematological malignancy. *Blood* 1989; 74: 2335.
244. Gough NM, Gough J, Metcalf D. Molecular cloning of cDNA encoding a murine hematopoietic growth regulator, granulocyte-macrophage colony stimulating factor. *Nature* 1984; 309: 763.
245. Grabstein K, Eisenman J, Mochizuki D, et al. Purification

to homogeneity of B-cell stimulating factor: a molecule that stimulates proliferation of multiple lymphokine dependent cell lines. *J Exp Med* 1986; 163: 1405-1414.
246. Grabstein K, Eisenman J, Shanebeck K, et al. Cloning of a T cell growth factor that interacts with the B-chain of the interleukin 2 receptor. *Science* 1994; 264: 965-968.
247. Grabstein KH, Namen AE, Shanebeck K, et al. Regulation of human T cell proliferation by IL7. *J Immunol* 1990; 144: 3015-3020.
248. Grabstein KH, Park LS, Morrissey JP, et al. Regulation of T cell proliferation by T cell stimulating factor-1. *J. Immunol* 1987; 139: 1148-1153.
249. Granger GA, Williams TW. Lymphocyte cytotoxicity *in vitro*: Activation and release of a cytotoxic factor. *Nature* 1968; 218: 1253.
250. Granowitz EV, et al. *J Biol Chem* 1991; 266: 14147.
251. Gray PW, Aggarwal BB, Bentor CV, et al. Cloning and expression of cDNA for human lymphotoxin a lymphokine with tumor necrosis activity. *Nature* 1984; 312: 721-724.
252. Green S, Dobrjansky A, Chiasson MA, et al. *Corynebacterium parvum* as the priming agent in the production of tumor necrosis factor in the mouse. *J Natl Cancer Inst* 1977; 59: 1519.
253. Greil J, Gramatzki M, Burger R, et al. The acute lymphoblastic leukemia cell line SEM with t(4; 11) chromosomal rearrangement is biphenotypic and responsive to interleukin-7. *British J Haematology* 1994; 86: 275-283.
254. Grimm EA, Mazumder A, Zhang HZ, Rosenberg SA. Lymphokine activated killer cell phenomenon. *J Exp Med* 1982; 155: 1823.
255. Grubler U, Chua AO, Schoenhaut DS, et al. Coexpression of two distinct genes required to generate secreted bioactive cytotoxic lymphocyte maturation factor. *Proc Nat Acad Sci USA* 1991; 88: 4143-4147.
256. Gustavson LE, Nadeau RW, Oldfield NF. Pharmacokinetics of Teceleukin (recombinant human interleukin-2) after intravenous or subcutaneous administration to patients with cancer. *J Biol Response Modif* 1989; 8: 440.
257. Guy GR, Chua SP, Wong NS, et al. Interleukin 1 and tumor necrosis factor activate common multiple protein kinases in human fibroblasts. *J Biol Chem* 1991; 266: 14343-14352.
258. Hamid Q, Barkans J, Meng Q, et al. Human eosinophils synthesize and secrete Interleukin 6 *in vitro*. *Blood* 1992; 80: 1496.
259. Han X, Itoh K, Balch CM, Pellis JH. Recombinant interluekin-4 (RIL-4) inhibits interleukin 2 induced activation of peripheral blood lymphocytes. *Lymphokine Cytokine Res* 1988; 7: 227-234.
260. Hank JA, Kohler PC, Hillman GW, et al. Interleukin-2 dependent human lymphokine activated killer cells generated *in vivo* during administration of human recombinant IL-2. *Cancer Res* 1988; 48: 1965.
261. Haranaka K, Satomi N, Sakurai A. Antitumor activity of TNF against transplanted murine tumors and heterotransplanted human tumors in nude mice. *Int J Cancer* 1984; 34: 263.
262. Hedrick SM, Cohen D, Nieson E, et al. Isolation of cDNA clones encoding T-cell specific membrane association proteins. *Nature* 1984; 308: 149.
263. Hefeneider S, Conlon P, Henney C, et al. *In vivo* interleukin 2 administration augments the generation of alloreactive cytolytic T-lymphocytes and resident natural killer cells. *J Immunol* 1983; 130: 222.
264. Henney CS, Kuribayashi K, Kern DE, Gillis S. Interleukin-2 augments natural killer cell activity. *Nature* 1981; 291: 335.
265. Herbelin A, Machzvoine F, Schneider E, et al. IL-7 is requisite for IL-1 induced thymocyte proliferation. Involvement of IL-7 in the synergistic effects of granulocyte macrophage colony stimulating factor or tumor necrosis factor with IL-1. *J Immunol* 1992; 148: 99-105.
266. Herbert JM, Savi P, Laplace M-C, et al. IL4 and IL13 exhibit comparable abilities to produce pyrogen induced expression of procoagulant activity in endothelial cells and monocytes. *FEBS Lett* 1993; 328: 268.
267. Hercend T, Meuer SC, Reinherz EL, et al. Generation of a cloned NK cell line from the 'null cell' fraction of human peripheral blood. *J Immunol* 1982; 129: 1299.
268. Heslop HE, Gottlieb DJ, Bianchi ACM, et al. *In vivo* induction of gamma interferon and tumor necrosis factor by interleukin-2 infusion following intensive chemotherapy or autologous marrow transplantation. *Blood* 1989; 74: 1374.
269. Heufler C, Koch F, Schuler G. Granulocyte macrophage colony stimulating factor and interleukin 1 mediate the maturation of murine epidermal Langerhans cells into potent immunostimulatory dendritic cells. *J. Exp Med* 1988; 167: 700.
270. Heufler C, Topar G, Grasseger A, et al. Interleukin 7 is produced by murine and human keratinocytes. *J Exp Med* 1993; 178: 1109-1114.
271. Hibi K, Takahashe T, Sekido Y, et al. Coexpression of the stem cell factor and the c-kit genes in small cell lung cancer. *Oncogene* 1991; 6: 2291-2296.
272. Hickman CJ, Crim JA, Mostowski HS, Siegel JP. Regulation of human cytotoxic T lymphocyte development by interleukin-7. *J Immunol* 1990; 145: 2415-2420.
273. Higuchi CM, Thompson JA, Lindgren CG, et al. Induction of lymphokine-activated killer activity by interleukin 4 in human lymphocytes preactivated by interleukin 2 *in vitro* or *in vivo*. *Cancer Res* 1989; 49: 6487-6492.
274. Hill RJ, Warren MK, Levin J. Stimulation of thrombopoiesis in mice by human recombinant interleukin 6. *J Clin Invest* 1990; 85: 1242.
275. Hirano T, Matsuda T, Nakajima K. Signal transduction through gp130 that is shared among the receptors for the interleukin related cytokine subfamily. *Stem Cells* 1994; 12: 262-277.
276. Hirano T, Yasukawa K, Harada H, et al. Complementary DNA for a novel interleukin (BSF-2) that induces B lymphocytes to produce immunoglobulin *Nature* 1986; 324: 73-76.
277. Hoch H, Dorsch M, Diamantstein T, Blankenstien T. Interleukin 7 induces CD4+ T cell dependent tumor rejection. *J Exp Med* 1991; 174: 1291-1298.
278. Hoch H, Dorsch M, Kunzendorf U, et al. Vaccination with tumor cells genetically engineered to produce different cytokines: effectively not superior to a classical adjuvant. *Cancer Res* 1993; 53: 1-8.
279. Hoch H, Dorsch M, Kunzendorf U, et al. Mechanism of the rejection induced by tumor cell targeted gene transfer of interleukin 2, interleukin 4, interleukin 7 tumor necrosis factor or interferon γ. *Proc Nat Acad Sci USA* 1993; 90: 2774-2778.
280. Hohmann HP, Remy R, Brockhaus M, et al. Two different cell types have different receptors for tumor necrosis factor (TNFα). *J Biol Chem* 1989; 264: 14927-14934.

281. Holbrook ST, Ohls RK, Schibler KR, et al. Effect of interleukin 9 on clonogenic maturation and cell cycle status of fetal and adult hematopoietic progenitors. *Blood* 1991; 77: 2129-2134.
282. Holmes WE, Lee J, Kuang WJ, et al. Structure and functional expression of a human interleukin-8 receptor. *Science* 1991; 253: 1278.
283. Hoon DSB, Banex M, Okun E, et al. Modulation of human melanoma cells by interleukin-4 and in combination with γ-interferon or α-tumor necrosis factor. *Cancer Res* 1991; 51: 2002-2008.
284. Hoon DSB, Edward O, Banez M, et al. Interleukin 4 alone and with γ-interferon or tumor necrosis factor inhibits the growth and modulates cell surface antigens on human renal cell carcinoma. *Cancer Res* 1991; 51: 5687-5693.
285. Horton SA, Oldham RK, Yannelli JR. Generation of human lymphokine-activated killer cells following brief exposure to high dose interleukin-2. *Cancer Res* 1990; 50: 1686-1692.
286. Hossiau FA, Renauld JC, Stevens M, et al. Human T cell lines and clones respond to IL 9. *J Immunol* 1993; 150: 2634-2640.
287. Howard M, Hilfiker M, Johnson B, et al. Identification of a T cell derived B cell growth factor distinct from Interleukin-2. *J Exp Med* 1982; 155: 914-923.
288. Hsieh CS, Macatonia SE, Tripp CS, et al. Development of TH1 CD4+ T cells through IL12 produced by Listerial-induced macrophages. *Science* 1993; 260: 547-9.
289. Hsu D-H, de Waal Malefyt R, Fiorentino DF, et al. Expression of interleukin 10 activity by Epstein Barr virus protein BCRFI. *Science* 1990; 250: 830-832.
290. Huang E, Nocka K, Beier DR, et al. The hematopoietic growth factor KL is encoded at the Sl locus and is the ligand of the c kit receptor the gene product of the W locus. *Cell* 1990; 63: 225-233.
291. Huber AR, Kunkel SL, Todd RF, Weiss SJ. Regulation of transendothelial neutrophil migration by endogenous interleukin-8. *Science* 1991; 254: 99.
292. Huland E, Huland H. Local continuous high dose interleukin 2: a new therapeutic model for the treatment of advanced bladder carcinoma. *Cancer Res* 1989; 49: 5469.
293. Huland E, Huland H, Heinzer H. Interleukin-2 by inhalation: Local therapy for metastatic renal cell carcinoma. *U Urol* 1992; 13\47: 344-348.
294. Hu-Li J, Shevach EM, Mizuguchi J, et al. B cell stimulatory factor-1 (interleukin-4) is a potent costimulant for normal resting T lymphocytes. *J Exp Med* 1987; 165: 157-172.
295. Hultner L, Druez C, Moeller J, et al. Mast cell growth enhancing activity (MEA) is structurally related and functionally identical to the novel mouse T cell growth factor P40/TCGF1II. *Eur J Immunol* 1990; 20: 1413-1416.
296. Hunninghake GW, Glazier MM, Monick MM, Dinarello CR. Interleukin-1 is a chemotactic factor for T lymphocytes. *Am Rev Respir Dis* 1987; 135: 66.
297. Hunter CA, Chizzonite R, Remmington JS. IL-1β is required for IL-12 to induce production of IFNγ by NK cells. *J Immunol* 1995; 155: 4347-4354.
298. Hutchins D, Steel CM. Regulation of ICAM-1 (CD54) expression in human breast cancer cell lines by interleukin 6 and fibroblast derived factors. *Int J Cancer* 1994; 58: 80-84.
299. Ihle JN, Keler J, Oroszlan S, et al. Biological properties of homogenous interleukin-3. *J Immunol* 1983; 131: 282.
300. Ihle JN, Keler J, Oroszlan S et al. Biological properties of interleukin-3. *J Immunol* 1983; 131: 282.
301. Ihle JN, Witthuhn BA, Yamamoto K, et al. Signaling by the cytokine superfamily: JAKs and STATs. *Trends in Biochemical Sciences* 1994; 19: 222-227.
302. Iho S, Shau HY, Golub SH. Characteristics of Interleukin 6 enhanced lymphokine activated killer cell function. *Cell Immunol* 1991; 135: 66-77.
303. Iigo M, Sakurai M, Tamura T, et al. *In vivo* antitumor activity of multiple injections of recombinant interleukin 2, alone and in combination with three different types of recombinant interferon, on various syngeneic murine tumors. *Cancer Res* 1988; 48: 260.
304. Ilson D, Motzer R, Kradin R, et al. A phase-II trial of interleukin-2 and interferon alfa-2a in patients with advanced renal cell carcinoma. *J Clin Oncol* 1992; 10: 1124-1130.
305. Imai Y, Nara N, Tohda S, et al. Antiproliferative and differentiative effects of recombinant interleukin-4 on a G-CSF-stimulating-dependent myeloblastic leukemic cell line. *Blood* 1991; 78: 471-478.
306. Inoue M, Kyo S, Fujita M, et al. Coexpression of the c-kit receptor and the stem cell factor in gynecological tumors *Cancer Res* 1994; 54: 3049-3053.
307. Isaacs A, Lindenman J. Virus interference. *Proc R Soc* 1957; 147: 258-267.
308. Iscove NN. Erythropoietin independent stimulation of early erythropoiesis in adult marrow cultures byconditioned medium of lectin stimulated mouse spleen cells. In: Golde D, Kline MJ, Metcalf D, Fox CF, eds. *Hematopoietic Cell Differentiation. Academic Press, New York* pp37-52.
309. Ito R, Kitadai Y, Kyo E, et al. Interleukin 1 acts as an autocrine growth stimulator for human gastric carcinoma cells. *Cancer Res* 1994; 54: 4102-41206.
310. Jacobsen FW, Veiby OP Jacobsen SE. IL-7 stimulates CSF-induced proliferation of murine bone marrow macrophages and Mac-1+ myeloid progenitors *in vitro*. *J Immunol* 1994; 153: 270-276.
311. Jadus MR, Schmunk G, Djeu JY, Parkman RJ. Morphology and mechanism of interleukin 3 dependent natural cytotoxic cells: tumor necrosis factor as a possible mediator. *Immunol* 1986; 137: 2774- .
312. Jadus MR, Good RW, Crumpacker DB, Yannelli JR. Effects of Interleukin 4 upon human tumoricidal cells obtained from patients bearing solid tumors. *J Leukocyte Biol* 1991; 49: 139-151.
313. Jadus MR, Schmunk G, Djeu JY. Morphology and lytic mechanisms of interleukin 3 dependent natural cytotoxic cells: tumor necrosis factor as their probable mode of action. *J Immunol* 1986; 136: 783.
314. Jadus MR, Parkman R. The selective growth of murine newborn-derived suppressor cells and their probable mode of action. *J Immunol* 1986; 136: 783.
315. Jelinek DF, Splawski JB, Lipsky PE. The roles of IL-2 and IFNγ in human B cell activation, growth and differentiation. Eur *J Immunol* 1986; 16: 925.
316. Jelinek DF and Braten JK. Role of IL-12 in human B lymphocyte proliferation and differentiation. *J Immunol* 1995; 154: 1606.
317. Jinquan T, Larsen CG, Gesser B, et al. Human IL-10 is a chemoattractant for CD8+T lymphocytes and an inhibitor of IL-8-Induced CD4+ T lymphocyte migration. *J Immunol* 1993; 151: 4545-51.

318. Jinquan T, Deleuran B, Gesser B, et al. Regulation of human T lymphocyte chemotaxis *in vitro* by T cell derived cytokines IL-2, IFN-λ, IL-4, IL-10, and IL-13. *J Immunol* 1995; 154: 3742-3752.
319. Johnson CS, Chang MJ, Braunschweiger PG, Furmanski P. Acute hemorrhagic necrosis of tumors induced by interleukin-1α: effects independent of tumor necrosis factor. *J Natl Cancer Inst* 1991; 83: 842-848.
320. Kaashoek JG, Mout JR, Falkenburg JHF, et al. Cytokine production by the bladder carcinoma cell line 5637. *Lymphokine Cytokine Res* 1991; 10: 231.
321. Katz A, Shulaman LM, Revel M, et al. Combined therapy with IL6 and inactivated tumor cell suppressed metastasis in mice bearing 3LL lung carcinomas. *Int J Cancer* 1993; 53: 812-818.
322. Katz A, Schulman LM Porgador A et al. Abrogation of B16 melanoma metastases by long term low dose interleukin 6 therapy. *J Immunother* 1993; 13: 98-109.
323. Kawakami M, Cerami A. A study of endotoxin induced decrease of lipoprotein lipase activity. *J Exp Med* 1981; 154: 631-639.
324. Kawakami Y, Custer M, Rosenberg SA, Lotze M. Interleukin-4 regulates Interleukin-2 induction of lymphokine activated killer activity from human leukocytes. *J Immunol* 1989; 142: 3452.
325. Kawakami Y, Haas, GP, Lotze MT. Expansion of tumor infiltrating lymphocytes from human tumors using the T cell growth factors interleukin-2 and interleukin-4. *J Immunotherapy* 1993; 14; 336-347.
326. Kawakami Y, Rosenberg SA, Lotze MT. Interleukin 4 promotes the growth of tumor infiltrating lymphocytes cytotoxic for human autologous melanoma. *J Exp Med* 1988; 168: 2183-91.
327. Kawano M, Hirano T, Matsuda T et al. Autocrine generation and requirement of BSF-2/IL-6 for human multiple myelomas. *Nature* 1988; 332: 83-85.
328. Kawano M, Matsushima K, Masuda A, et al. A major 50 kDa human B cell growth factor II induces both Tac antigen expression and proliferation by several lymphocytes. *Cell Immunol* 1988; 111: 273-286.
329. Kawasakura S, Lowenstein L. A factor stimulating DNA synthesis derived from the medium of leucocyte cultures. *Nature* 1965; 208: 794-795.
330. Kawase I, Komuta K, Hara H, et al. Combined therapy of mice bearing a lymphokine-activated killer-resistant tumor with recombinant interleukin 2 and an anti-tumor monoclonal antibody capable of inducing antibody-dependent cellular cytotoxicity. *Cancer Res* 1988; 48: 1173.
331. Kawashima I, Ohsumi J, Mita-Honjo K, et al. Molecular cloning of the cDNA encoding adipogenesis inhibitory factor and identity with interleukin 11. *FEBS Lett* 1991; 283: 199-202.
332. Kaye J, Gillis S, Mizel SB, et al. Growth of a cloned helper T cell line induced by a monoclonal antibody specific for the antigen receptor: interleukin 1 is required for the expression of receptors for interleukin 2. *J Immunol* 1984; 133: 1339-1345.
333. Kedar E, Ben-Aziz R, Epstein E, Leshem B. Chemoimmunotherapy of murine tumors using interleukin-2 (IL-2) and cyclophosphamide. IL-2 can facilitate or inhibit tumor growth depending on the sequence of treatment and the tumor type. *Cancer Immunol Immunother* 1989; 29: 74.
334. Keegan AD, Pierce JH. The interleukin-4 receptor: signal transduction by a hematopoietin receptor. *J Leuk Biol* 1994; 5: 272-279.
335. Kehri JH, Dukovich M, Whalen G, et al. Novel interleukin 2 receptor appears to mediate IL2-induced activation of natural killer cells *J Clin Invest* 1988; 81: 779.
336. Kelley VE, Gaulton GN, Hattori M, et al. Anti-interleukin 2 receptor antibody suppresses murine diabetic insulitis and lupus nephritis. *J Immunol* 1988; 140: 59.
337. Kemeny L, Ruzicka T, Dobozy A, Michel G. Role of Interleukin 8 receptor in skin. *International Arch Allergy and Immunology* 1994; 104: 317-322.
338. Kern P, Toy J, Dietrich M. Preliminary clinical observation with recombinant interleukin 2 in patients with AIDS or LAS. *Blut* 1985; 50: 1.
339. Kiniwa M, Gately M, Grubler U, et al. Recombinant interleukin-12 suppresses the synthesis of immunoglobulin E by interleukin-4 stimulated human lymphocytes. *J Clin Invest* 1992; 90: 262-266.
340. Kirnbauer R, Charvat B, Schauer E, et al. Modulation of intracellular adhesion molecule 1 expression on human melanocytes and melanoma cells: evidence for a regulatory role of IL-6, IL-7 TNFβ, and UVB light. *J Invest Dermat* 1992; 98: 320-326.
341. Kirken RA, Rui H, Howard OM, Farrar WL. Involvement of JAK-family tyrosine kinases in hematopoietin receptor signal transduction. *Prog Growth Factor Res* 1994; 5: 195-211.
342. Kishimoto T, Akira S, Taga T. Interleukin 6 and its receptor: a paradigm for cytokines. *Science* 1992; 258: 593-597.
343. Kishimoto T, Hirano T. Molecular regulation of B lymphocyte response. *Ann Rev Immunol* 1988; 6: 485-512.
344. Kita HT, Onishi T, Okubo Y, et al. Granulocyte /macrophage colony stimulating factor and interleukin 3 release from human peripheral blood eosinophils and neutrophils. *J Exp Med* 1991; 174: 745.
345. Klasa RJ, Silver HKB. Phase 1-2 trial of interleukin-2 splenic artery perfusion in advanced malignancy (meeting abstract). *Proc Annu Meet Am Soc Clin Oncol* 1989; 8: A686.
346. Kobayashi M, Fitz L, Ryan M, et al. Identification and purification of natural killer cell stimulatory factor (NKSF), a cytokine with multiple biological effects on human lymphocytes. *J Exp Med* 1989; 170: 827-845.
347. Koch AE, Polverini PK, Kunkel SL, et al. Interleukin 8 as a macrophage derived mediator of angiogenesis. *Science* 1992; 258: 1798-1801.
348. Koettnitz K and Kalthoff FS. Human interleukin 4 receptor signalling requires sequences contained within two cytoplasmic regions. *E J Immunol* 1993; 23: 988-991.
349. Koi A. The role of interleukin 6 as the hepatocyte stimulating factor in the network of inflammatory cytokines. *Ann NY Acad Sci* 1989; 557: 1-8.
350. Kolitz JE, Wong GY, Welte K, et al. Phase I trial of recombinant interleukin-2 and cyclophosphamide: augmentation of cellular immunity and T-cell mitogenic response with long-term administration of rIL-2. *J Biol Response Modif* 1988; 7: 457.
351. Komschlies KL, Back TT, Gregorio TA, et al. Effects of rhIL7 on leukocyte subsets in mice: implications for antitumor activity. *Immunology* 1994; 61: 95-104.
352. Kondo M, Takeshita T, Higuchi M, et al. Functional participation of the IL2 receptor gamma chain in IL-7 receptor complexes. *Science* 1994; 263: 1453-1454.

353. Konrad MW, Bradley EC. The pharmacokinetics of a recombinant IL-2 muteine given by five routes in a number of phase I trials (meeting abstract). *Proc Annu Meet Am Soc Clin Oncol* 1986; 5: A920.
354. Koo AS, Armstrong C, Bochner B, et al. Interleukin-6 and renal cell cancer: production, regulation, and growth effects. *Cancer Immunol Immunother* 1992; 35: 97-105.
355. Kos FJ, Mullbacher A. IL2 independent activity of IL-7 in the generation of secondary antigen-specific cytotoxic T cell responses *in vitro*. *J Immunol* 1993; 150: 387-393.
356. Kotasek D, Vercellotti GM, Ochoa AC, et al. Mechanism of cultured endothelial injury induced by lymphokine-activated killer cells. *Cancer Res* 1988; 48: 5528.
357. Kotowicz K, Callard RE. Human immunoglobulin class and IgG subclass regulation: dual action of interleukin 4. *Eur J Immunol* 1993; 23: 2250.
358. Kovacs EJ, Beckner SK, Longo DL, et al. Cytokine gene expression during the generation of human lymphokine-activated killer cells: early induction of interleukin 1-beta by interleukin 2. *Cancer Res* 1989; 49: 940.
359. Kradin RL, Boyle LA, Preffer FI, et al. Tumor-derived interleukin-2 dependent lymphocytes in adoptive immunotherapy of lung cancer. *Cancer Immunol Immunother* 1987; 24: 76.
360. Kradin RL, Kurnick JT, Lazarus DS, et al. Tumor-infiltrating lymphocytes and interleukin-2 in treatment of advanced cancer. *Lancet* 1989; 1: 577-580.
361. Krigel RL, Padavic-Shaller KA, Rudolph AR, et al. A Phase I study of recombinant interleukin 2 plus recombinant beta-interferon. *Cancer Res* 1988; 48: 3875.
362. Kruse N, Tony HP, Sebald W. Conversion of human interleukin 4 into a high affinity antagonist by a single amino acid replacement. *EMBO Journal* 1992; 11: 3237-3244.
363. Kubin M, Kamoun M, Trinchieri G. Interleukin 12 synergizes with B7/CD28 interaction in inducing efficient proliferation and cytokine production of human T cells. *J Exp Med* 1994; 180: 211-22.
364. Kuhn R, Rajewski K, Muller W. Generation and analysis of Interleukin-4 deficient mice. *Science* 1991; 254: 707-709.
365. Kupper T, Horowitz M, Lee F, et al. Autocrine growth of T cells independent of growth factor for a cloned antigen specific helper T cell. *J Immunol* 1987; 138: 4280.
366. Kuribayshi K, Gillis S, Kern D, et al. Murine NK cell cultures: effects of interleukin-2 and interferon on cell growth and cytotoxic reactivity. *J Immunol* 1981; 126: 2321.
367. Kurt-Jones EA, Beller DI, Mizel SB, Unanui ER. Identification of a membrane-associated interleukin 1. *Proc Natl Acad Sci* (USA) 1985; 82: 1204-1208.
368. Kurt-Jones EA, Hamburg S, Ohara J, et al. Heterogeneity of helper/inducer T lymphocytes. *J Exp Med* 1987; 166: 1774-1787.
369. Lachman LB, Dinarello CA, Llanska ND, Fidler IJ. Natural and recombinant human interleukin-1β is cytotoxic for human melanoma cells. *J Immunol* 1986; 136: 3098-3103.
370. Langer JA, Pestka S. Interferon Receptors. *Immunol Today* 1989; 12: 393-400.
371. Larsen CG, Anderson AO, Oppenheim JJ, Matsushima K. The neutrophil activating protein (NAP-1) is also chemotactic for T lymphocytes. *Science* 1989; 243: 1464.
372. Larsen CG, Anderson AO, Oppenheim JJ, Matsushima K. Production of Interleukin 8 by human dermal fibroblasts and keratinocytes in response to interleukin 1 or tumor necrosis factor. *Immunology* 1989; 68: 31.
373. Le J, Vilcek J. Tumor necrosis factor and interleukin 1: Cytokines with multiple overlapping biological activities. *Lab Invest* 1987; 56: 234-248.
374. Lee J, Horuk R, Rice GC, et al. Characterization of two high affinity human interleukin-8 receptors *J Biol Chem* 1992; 267: 16283.
375. Lee KH, Talpaz M, Rothberg JM, et al. Concomitant administration of recombinant human interleukin-2 and recombinant interferon α-2A in cancer patients: a phase I study. *J Clin Oncol* 1989; 7: 1726-1732.
376. Lee SH, Aggarwal BB, Rinderknecht E, et al. The synergistic antiproliferative effect of gamma-interferon and human lymphotoxin. *J Immunol* 1984; 133: 1083.
377. Lee SW, Tsou AP, Chan H, et al. Glucocorticoids selectively inhibit the transcription of the interleukin 1 beta gene and decrease the stability of interleukin 1 beat mRNA. *Proc Natl Acad Sci* (USA) 1988; 85: 1204-1208.
378. Legha S, Ring S, Bedikian A, et al. Biochemotherapy using interleukin-2 + interferon alpha-2a (IFN) in combination with cisplatin (C), vinblastine (V) and DTIC (D) in patients with metastatic melanoma. *Melanoma Research* 1993; 3: 32.
379. Lembersky B, Baldisseri M, Kunschner A, et al. Phase I-II study of IP low dose interleukin-2 in refractory stage III ovarian cancer (meeting abstract). *Proc Annu Meet Am Soc Clin Oncol* 1989; 8: A636.
380. Leonard WJ, Noguchi M, Russel SM, McBride OW. The molecular basis of severe combined immunodeficiency: the role of the interleukin-2 receptor gamma chain as a common gamma chain, gamma c. *Immunological Reviews* 1994; 138: 61-86.
381. Levitsky JW, Simons H, Vogelstein B, Frost P. Interleukin 2 produced by tumor cell bypasses T helper function in the generation of an antitumor response. *Cell* 1990; 60: 397-403.
382. Lewko WM, Good, RW, Bowman D, et al. Growth of tumor derived activated T cells for the treatment of cancer. *Cancer Biotherapy* 1994; 9(3): 211-224.
383. Lewko WM, Smith TL, Bowman DJ, et al. Interleukin-15 and the growth of tumor derived activated T-cells. *Cancer Biotherapy* 1995; 10: 13-20.
384. Li WY, Lusheng S, Kanbour A, et al. Lymphocytes infiltrating human ovarian tumors: synergy between tumor necrosis factor and interleukin 2 in the generation of CD8+ effectors from tumor infiltrating lymphocytes. *Cancer Res* 1989; 49: 5979.
385. Libby P, Warner SJC, Friedman GB. Interleukin 1: a mitogen for human vascular smooth muscle cells that induces the release of growth-inhibitory prostanoids. *J Clin Invest* 1988; 81: 487-498.
386. Lichtman A, Kurt-Jones E, Abbas A. B cell stimulatory factor 1 and not interleukin 2 is and autocrine growth factor for some helper T lymphocytes. *Proc Nat Acad Sci* 1987; 84: 824.
387. Lindemann A, Hoeffken K, Schmidt RE, et al. A Phase II study of low-dose cyclophosphamide and recombinant human interleukin-2 in metastatic renal cell carcinoma and malignant melanoma. *Cancer Immunol Immunother* 1989; 28: 275.
388. Lindgren CG, Thompson JA, Higuchi CM, Fefer A. Growth and autologous tumor lysis by tumor infiltrating

lymphocytes from metastatic melanoma expanded in interleukin 2 or interleukin 2 plus Interleukin 4. *J. Immunother* 1993; 14: 322-328.

389. Lindqvist C, Ostman AL, Okerblom C, Akerman K. Decreased interleukin-2 beta chain receptor expression by interleukin-4 on LGL: influence on the IL-2 induced cytotoxicity and proliferation. *Cancer Lett* 1992; 64: 43-49.
390. Liu J, Modrell B, Aruffo A, et al. Interaction between oncostatin M and the signal transducer, gp130. *Cytokine* 1994; 6: 272-278.
391. Loetscher H, Pan TC, Lahm HW, et al. Molecular cloning and expression of the human 55kd tumor necrosis factor receptor. *Cell* 1990; 61: 351.
392. Logan TF, Bishop M, Mintun MA, et al. Phase I trial of interleukin-1α and carboplatin in patients with metastatic disease to the lung: effects on tumor blood flow evaluated by positron emission tomography. *Proc ASCO* 1994; 35: 198.
393. Londei M, Verhoef A, Hawrylowicz C, et al. Interleukin 7 is a growth factor for mature human T cells. Eur *J Immunol* 1990; 20: 425-428.
394. London L, Perussiia B, Trinchieri G. Induction and proliferation *in vitro* of resting human natural killer cells: expression of surface activation antigens *J.Immunol* 1985; 134: 718.
395. Lopez AF, Sanderson CJ, Gamble JR, et al. Recombinant human interleukin 5 is a selective activator of human eosinophil function. *J Exp Med* 1988; 167: 219.
396. Lorenz JJ, Furdon PJ, Taylor JD, et al. A cyclic 3'5'-monophosphate signal is required for the induction of IL-1β by TNF-α in human monocytes. *J Immunol* 1995; 155: 836-844.
397. Lorenzen J, Lewis CE, McCracken D, et al. Human tumor associated NK cells secrete increased amounts of interferon-γ and interleukin-4. British *J Cancer* 1991; 64: 457-462.
398. Lotze MT, Frana LW, Sharrow SO, et al. *In vivo* administration of purified human interleukin 2. I. Half-life and immunologic effects of the Jurkat cell linc-derived interleukin 2. *J Immunol* 1985; 134: 157.
399. Lotze MT, Matory YL, Ettinghausen SE, et al. *In vivo* administration of purified human interleukin 2. II. Half life, immunologic effects, and expansion of peripheral lymphoid cells *in vivo* with recombinant interleukin 2. *J Immunol* 1985; 135: 2865-2875.
400. Lotze MT, Matory YL, Rayner AA, et al. Clinical effects and toxicity of interleukin-2 in patients with cancer. *Cancer* 1986; 58: 2764.
401. Lotze M, Jirik F, Kabouridis P, et al. B cell stimulating factor-2/interleukin 6 is a co-stimulant for human thymocytes and T lymphocytes. *J Exp Med* 1988; 167: 1253-1258.
402. Lotze M. Role of IL-4 in the antitumor response. IL-4: Structure and Function (H Spits ed), CRC Press, Boca Raton, *FL* 1992; 111: 274-280.
403. Lotze MT, Robb R, Sharrow SO, et al. Systemic administration of interleukin-2 in humans. *J Biol Response Modif* 1984; 3: 475.
404. Lotzova E, Savary CA, Herberman RB. Induction of NK cell activity against fresh human leukemia in culture with interleukin 2. *J Immunol* 1987; 138: 2718.
405. Lu C, Vickers MF, Kerbel RS. Interleukin 6: a fibroblast derived growth inhibitor of human melanoma cells from early but not advanced stages of tumor progression. *Proc Nat Acad Sci USA* 1992; 89: 9215-9219.
406. Lu C, Kerbel RS. Interleukin 6: undergoes transition from paracrine growth inhibitor to autocrine growth stimulator during human melanoma progression. *J Cell Biol* 1993; 120: 1281-1288.
407. Luger TZ, Stadler BM, Katz SI, et al. Epidermal cell (keratinocyte)-derived thymocyte-activating factor (ETAF). *J Immunol* 1981; 127: 1493-1498.
408. Luo H, Rubio M, Biron G, et al. Antiproliferative effect of interleukin-4 in B chronic lymphocytic leukemia. *Blood* 1991; 10: 418-425.
409. Luscher U, Filgueira L, Juretic A, et al. The pattern of cytokine gene expression in freshly excised human metastatic melanoma suggests a state of reversible anergy of tumor infiltrating lymphocytes. *Int J Cancer* 1994; 57: 612.
410. Lynch DH and Miller RE. Induction of murine lymphokine activated killer cells by recombinant IL-7. *J Immunol* 1990; 145: 198.
411. Lynch DH and Miller RE. Interleukin 7 promotes Long term in vitro growth and antitumor cytotoxic T lymphocytes with immunotherapeutic efficacy *in vivo*. *J Exp Med* 1994; 179: 31-42.
412. Macatonia SE, Doherty TM, Knight SC, O'Garra A. Differential effect of IL-10 on dendritic cell induced T cell proliferation and IFN-gamma production. *J Immunol* 1993; 150: 3755-3765.
413. Macatonia SE, Hosken NA, Litton M, et al. Dendritic cells produce IL-12 and direct the development of Th1 cells form naive CD4+ T cells *J Immunol* 1995; 154: 5071-5079.
414. MacGlashan D Jr, White JM, Huang S, et al. Secretion of IL4 from human basophils. J Immunol 1994; 152: 3006.
415. MacNeil IA, Suda T, Moore KW, et al. IL-10, a novel growth factor for mature and immature T cells. *J Immunol* 1990; 145: 4167.
416. Maleckar JR, Fridell CS, Lewko WM, et al. Tumor derived activated cells: cell culture conditions and characterization. In : Stevenson HC (Ed) *Adoptive cellular immunotherapy of cancer*. Marcel Dekker, Inc. New York. 1989. p159-173.
417. Maleckar JR, Fridell CS, Sferruzza A, et al. Activation and Expansion of tumor derived activated cells (TDAC). J *Nat Cancer Inst* 1989; 1: 1655-1660.
418. Maliszewski CR, Sato TA, VandenBos T, et al. Cytokine Receptors and B cell functions. I. Recombinant soluble receptors specifically inhibit IL-4 and IL-4 induced B cell activities in vitro. *J Immunol* 1990; 144: 3028.
419. Malkovsky M, Loveland B, North M, et al. Recombinant interleukin-2 directly augments the cytotoxicity of human monocytes. *Nature* 1987; 325: 262.
420. Manabe A, Cousan-Smith E, Kumagai M, et al. Interleukin-4 induces programmed cell death (apoptosis) in cases of high risk acute lymphoblastic leukemia. *Blood* 1994; 83: 1731-1737.
421. Maraskovsky E, Chen WF, Shortman K. IL-2 and IFN-γ are two necessary cytokines in the development of cytotoxic T cells. *J Immunol* 1989; 143: 1210-1214.
422. March CJ, Mosley B, Larsen A, et al. Cloning, sequence and expression of two distinct human interleukin-1 complementary DNAs. *Nature* 1985; 315: 641-647.
423. Marcus PI. Interferon induction of viruses: double stranded ribonucleic acid as the common proximal molecules. *Interferons*. 1985; 3: 113-175.

424. Margolin K, Aronson FR, Sznol M, et al. Phase II studies of recombinant human IL-4 in advanced renal cancer and malignant melanoma. *J Immunother* 1994; 15: 147-153.
425. Margolin KA, Rayner AA, Hawkins MJ, et al. Interleukin-2 and lymphokine-activated killer cell therapy of solid tumors: analysis of toxicity and management guidelines. *J Clin Oncol* 1989; 7: 486.
426. Marolda R, Belli F, Prada A, et al. A phase I study of recombinant interleukin-2 in melanoma patients: toxicity and clinical effects. *Tumori* 1987; 73: 575.
427. Marshall JS, and Bienenstock J. The role of mast cells in inflammatory reactions of the airways, skin and intestine. Curr Opin *Immunol* 1990; 6: 853.
428. Matsuda M, Motoji T, Oshimi K, Mizoguchi H. Effects of interleukin 7 on proliferation of hematopoietic malignant cells. *Exp Hematol* 1990; 18: 965-967.
429. Matsuda R, Takahashi T, Nakamura S, et al. Expression of the c-kit protein in human solid tumors and in corresponding fetal and adult normal tissues. *Am J Pathol* 1993; 142: 339-349.
430. Matsuda M, Salazar F, Petersson M, et al. Interleukin 10 pretreatment protects target cells from tumor and allospecific cytotoxic T cells and downregulates HLA class I expression. *J Exp Med* 1994; 180: 2731.
431. Matsue H, Bergstresser PR, Takashima A. Keratinocyte derived IL-7 serves as a growth factor for dendritic epidermal T cells in mice. *J Immunol* 1993; 151: 6012-6019.
432. Matsue H, Cruz PD, Bergstresser PR, Takashima A. Cytokine expression by epidermal subpopulations. *J Invest Dermatol* 1992; 99: 425.
433. Matsue H, Bergstresser PR, Takashima A. Reciprocal cytokine mediated cellular interactions in mouse epidermis: promotion of $\gamma\delta$ T cell growth by IL-7 and TNFα and inhibition of keratinocyte growth by γ interferon. *J Invest Dermatol* 1993b; 101: 543.
434. Masui H, Kawamoto T, Sato JD, et al. Growth inhibition of human tumor cells in athymic nude mice by anti-epidermal growth factor receptor monoclonal antibodies. *Cancer Res* 1984; 44: 1002.
435. Matsui Y, Zsebo KM, Hogan LM. Embryonic expression of hematopoietic growth factor encoded by Sl locus and the ligand for c kit. *Nature* 1990; 343: 667-669.
436. Matsushima K, Oppenheimer JJ. Interleukin 8 and MCAF: Novel inflammatory cytokines inducible by IL-1 and TNF$\propto$. *Cytokine* 1989; 1: 2-13.
437. Mazumder A, Eberlein TJ, Grimm EA, et al. Phase I study of the adoptive immunotherapy of human cancer with lectin activated autologous mononuclear cells. *Cancer* 1984; 53: 896.
438. Mayordoma JI, Zorina T, Storkus WJ, et al. Bone marrow derived dendritic cells pulded with synthetic tumor peptides elicit protective and therapeutic antitumor immunity. *Mature Medicine* 1995; 1: 1297-1302.
439. McBride WH, Thacker JD, Comora S, et al. Genetic modification of a murine fibrosarcoma to produce Interleukin 7 stimulates host cell infiltration and tumor immunity. *Cancer Res* 1992; 52: 3931-3937.
440. McCain RW, Dessypris EN, Christman JW. Granulocyte/macrophage colony stimulating factor stimulates human polymorphonuclear leukocytes to produce interleukin 8 in vitro. *J Respir Cell Mol Biol* 1993; 8: 28.
441. McIntosh JK, Mule JJ, Krosnick JA, Rosenberg SA. Combination cytokine immunotherapy with tumor necrosis factor alpha, interleukin 2 and alpha-interferon and its synergistic antitumor effects in mice. *Cancer Res* 1991; 49: 1408.
442. McIntosh JK, Mule JJ, Merino MJ, Rosenberg SA. Synergistic antitumor effects of immunotherapy with recombinant interleukin-2 and recombinant tumor necrosis factor-alpha. *Cancer Res* 1988; 48: 4011.
443. McKenzie ANJ, Culpepper JA, De Waal Malefyt R, et al. Interleukin 13, a novel T cell derived cytokine that regulates human monocyte and B cell function. *Proc Nat Acad Sci USA* 1993; 90: 3735-3739.
444. Mehrota PT, Wu D, Crim JA, et al. Effects of IL-12 on the generation of cytotoxic activity in human CD8+ T lymphocytes. *J Immunol* 1993; 151: 2444-2452.
445. Mehrota PT, Grant AJG and Siegel JP. Synergistic effects of IL7 and IL12 on Human T cell activation. *J Immunol* 1995; 154: 5093-5102.
446. Melioli G, Sertoli MR, Bruzzone M, et al. A phase I study of recombinant interleukin-2 intraperitoneal infusion in patients with neoplastic ascites: toxic effects and immunologic results. *Am J Clin Oncol* 1991; 14: 231-237.
447. Merberg DM, Wolf SF, Clark SC. Sequence similarity between NKSF and the IL-6/G-CSF family. *Immunol Today* 1992; 14: 77.
448. Merchant RE, Merchant LH, Cook SHS, et al. Intralesional infusion of lymphokine-activated killer cells and recombinant interleukin-2 for the treatment of patients with malignant brain tumor. *Neurosurgery* 1988; 23: 725.
449. Merluzzi VJ, Welte K, Mertelsmann R. Expansion of cyclophosphamide-resistant cytotoxic precursors *in vitro* and *in vivo* by purified human interleukin-2. *J Immunol* 1983; 131: 806.
450. Mertelsmann R, Welte K, Sternberg C, et al. Treatment of immunodeficiency with interleukin-2: initial exploration. *J Biol Response Modif* 1984; 4: 483.
451. Metcalf D. *In vivo* response to recombinant multi-CSF and GM-CSF (abstract). Biological Therapy of Cancer: A 1986 Update, Chapel-Hill, N.C.
452. Metcalf D. Control of granulocytes and macrophages: molecular, cellular and clinical aspects. *Science* 1991; 254: 529.
453. Meyers F, Paradise C, Scudder S, et al. A phase I study including pharmacokinetics of pegylated interleukin 2 in patients with advanced cancer (Meeting Abstract). *Proc Annu Meet Am Soc Clin Oncol* 1989; 8: A274.
454. Michie HR, Manogue KR, Spriggs DR, et al. Detection of circulating tumor necrosis factor after endotoxin administration. *N Engl J Med* 1988; 318: 1481.
455. Mier JW, Gallo RC. Isolation and purification of human T-cell growth factor. *Proc Natl Acad Sci* (USA) 1980; 77: 6134.
456. Mier JW, Aronson FR, Numerof RP, et al. Toxicity of immunotherapy with interleukin-2 and lymphokine-activated killer cells. *Pathol Immunopathol Res* 1988; 7: 459.
457. Mier JW, Brandon EP, Libby P, et al. Activated endothelial cells resist lymphokine-activated killer cell-mediated injury. Possible role of induced cytokines in limiting capillary leak during IL-2 therapy. *J Immunol* 1989; 143: 2407.
458. Mier JW, Vachino G, Van der Meer JWM, et al. Induction of circulating tumor necrosis factor (TNF alpha) as the mechanism for the febrile response to interleukin-2 (IL-2) in cancer patients. *J Clin Immunol* 1988; 8: 426.

459. Migliorati G, Pagilacci C, Moraca R, et al. Interleukins modulate glucocorticoid induced thymocyte apoptosis. *Int J Clin Lab Res* 1992; 21: 300-3.
460. Miki S, Iwano Y, Miki Y, et al. Interleukin 6 functions as an in vitro autocrine growth factor in renal cell carcinoma. *FEBS Lett* 1989; 250: 607-610.
461. Mingari MC, Gerosa F, Carra G, et al. Human interleukin-2 promotes proliferation of activated B cells via surface receptors similar to those of activated T cells. *Nature* 1984; 312: 641.
462. Minty A, Chalon P, Derocq JM, et al. Interleukin 13: A novel human lymphokine regulating inflammatory and immune responses Nature 1993; 362: 248-250.
463. Mitchell LC, Davis LS, Lipsky PE. Promotion of human T lymphocyte proliferation by IL-4. *J. Immunol* 1989; 142: 1548-1557.
464. Mitchell MS, Kempf RA, Harvel W, et al. Low-dose cyclophosphamide and low-dose interleukin-2 for malignant melanoma. Bull NY Acad Med 1989; 65: 128.
465. Mittelman A, Huberman M, Fallon B, et al. Phase I study of recombinant interleukin 2 and recombinant human interferon alpha in patients with melanoma, renal cell carcinoma, colorectal cancer and malignant B-cell disease (meeting abstract). *Proc Annu Meet Am Soc Clin Oncol* 1989; 8: A696.
466. Mittelman A, Puccio C, Ahmed T, et al. A phase II trial of interleukin-2 by continuous infusion and interferon by intramuscular injection in patients with renal cell carcinoma. *Cancer* 1991; 68: 1699-1702.
467. Mizel SB, Dawyer JM, Krane SM, et al. Stimulation of rheumatoid synovial cell collagenase and prostaglandin production by partially purified lymphocyte-activating factor (interleukin-1). *Proc Natl Acad Sci* (USA) 1981; 78: 2474.
468. Mizel SB. The interleukins. FASEB J 1989; 3: 2379-2388.
469. Mochizuki DY, Eisenman JR, Conlon PJ, et al. Interleukin 1 regulates hematopoietic activity, a role previously ascribed to hemopoietin 1. *Proc Natl Acad Sci* (USA) 1987; 84: 5267-5271.
470. Mohamadzadeh M, Takashima A, Dougherty I, et al. Ultraviolet B radiation up regulates the expression of IL-15 in human skin. *J Immunol* 1995; 155: 4492-4496.
471. Moissec P, Yu CL, Ziff M. Lymphocyte chemotactic activity of interleukin 1. *J Immunol* 1984; 133: 2007.
472. Moller A, Lippert U, Lessmann D, et al. Human mast cells produce IL8. *J Immunol* 1993; 151: 3261.
473. Molmenti EP, Ziambaras T, Perlmutter DH. Evidence for an acute phase response in human intestinal epithelial cells. *J Biol Chem* 1993; 268: 12116-14124.
474. Monroe JG, Haldar S, Prystowsky MB, Lammie P. Lymphokine regulation of inflammatory process: IL4 stimulates fibroblast proliferation. *Clin Immunol Immunopathol* 1988, 49: 292.
475. Moore KW, Viera P, Fiorentino DF, et al. Homology of cytokine synthesis inhibitor factor (IL-10) to the Epstein Barr virus gene BCRFI. *Science* 1990; 248: 1230-1234.
476. Moore MAS, Warren DJ. Synergy of interleukin-1 and granulocyte colony-stimulating factor: *in vivo* stimulation of stem-cell recovery and hematopoietic regeneration following 5-fluorouracil treatment of mice. *Proc Natl Acad Sci* (USA) 1987; 84: 7134-7138.
477. Morel F, Delwail V, Brizard A, et al. Effects of sCD23 on proliferation of leukemic cells from a patient with chronic myelogenous leukemia during blast crisis. *Amer J Hematology* 1993; 44: 60-62.
478. Morgan DA, Ruscetti FW, Gallo RC. Selective *in vitro* growth of T-lymphocytes from normal human bone marrows. *Science* 1976; 193: 1007.
479. Morisaki T, Morton DL, Uchiyama A, et al. Characterization and augmentation of CD4+ cytotoxic T cell lines against melanomas. *Cancer Immunol Immunother* 1994; 39: 172-178.
480. Morisaki T, Uchiyama A, Yuzuki D, et al. Interleukin 4 regulates G1 cell cycle progression in gastric carcinoma cells. *Cancer Res* 1994; 54: 1113-8.
481. Morisaki T, Yuzuki D, Lin R, et al. Interleukin 4 receptor expression and growth inhibition of gastric carcinoma cells by interleukin-4. *Cancer Res.* 1992; 52: 6059-6065.
482. Morris SC, Madden KB, Adamovicz JJ, et al. Effects of IL12 on *in vivo* cytokine gene expression and Ig isotype selection. *J Immunol* 1994; 152: 1047-1056.
483. Morrissey PJ, Goodwin RG, Nordan RP, et al. Recombinant interleukin 7, pre-B cell growth factor has costimulatory activity on purified mature T cells. *J Exp Med* 1989; 169: 707-716.
484. Mosley B, Beckman MP, March CJ, et al. The murine interleukin-4 receptor: molecular cloning and characterization of the secreted and membrane bound forms. *Cell* 1989; 59: 355.
485. Moser B, Schumacher C, von Tscharner V, et al. Neutrophil activating peptide 2 and melanoma growth stimulatory activity interact with neutrophil activating peptide 1/interleukin 8 receptors on human neutrophils. *J Biol Chem* 1991; 266: 10667.
486. Mosmann TR. Cytokine secretion patterns and cross regulation of T cell subsets. *Immunol Res* 1991; 10: 183-188.
487. Mosmann T, Bond M, Coffman R, et al. T cell and mast cell lines respond to B cell stimulatory factor 1. *Proc Nat Acad Sci USA* 1986; 83: 1857.
488. Mosmann T, Cherwinski H, Bond M, et al. Two types of murine helper T cell clones. 1. Definition to profiles of lymphokine activities and secreted proteins. *J Immunol* 1986; 136: 2348.
489. Motro B, Itin A, Sachs L, et al. Pattern of interleukin 6 gene expression *in vivo* suggests a role for this cytokine in angiogenesis. *Proc Natl Acad Sci USA* 1990; 87: 3092-3096.
490. Muegge K, Vial MP, Durum SK. Interleukin 7: a cofactor for V(D)J rearrangement of the T cell receptor beta gene. *Science* 1993; 261: 93-5.
491. Mukaida N, Harada A, Yasumoto K et al. Properties of proinflammatory cell type specific leukocyte chemotactic cytokines interleukin 8 (IL8) and monocyte chemotactic and activating factor (MCAF). *Microbiol Immunol* 1992; 36: 773-789.
492. Mule JJ, Shu S, Rosenberg SA. The antitumor efficacy of lymphokine-activated killer cells and recombinant interleukin 2 *in vivo*. *J Immunol* 1985; 135: 646.
493. Mule JJ, Shu S, Schwarz SL, et al. Adoptive immunotherapy of established pulmonary metastases with LAK cells and recombinant interleukin-2. *Science* 1984; 225: 1487.
494. Mule JJ, Smith CA, Rosenberg SA. Interleukin-4 (B cell stimulatory factor) can mediate the induction of lymphokine activated killer cell activity directed against fresh tumor cells. *J Exp Med* 1987; 166: 792-7.
495. Mule JJ, Custer MC, Travis WD, et al. Cellular

mechanisms of the antitumor activity of recombinant IL-6 in mice. *J Immunol* 1992; 148: 2622-2629.
496. Muraguchi A, Hirano T, Tang B, et al. The essential role of B cell stimulatory factor 2 (BSF-2/IL-6) for the terminal differentiation of B cells. *J Exp Med* 1988; 167: 332.
497. Murphy EE, Terres G, Macatonia SE, et al. B7 and interleukin 12 cooperate for proliferation and interferon gamma production by mouse T helper clones that are unresponsive to B7 costimulation. *J Exp Med* 1994; 180: 223-231.
498. Murphy WJ, Back TC, Conlon KC, et al. Antitumor effects of interleukin 7 and adoptive immunotherapy on human colon carcinoma xenografts. *J Clinical Invest* 1993; 92: 1918-1924.
499. Murphy P, Tiffany H. Cloning of complimentary DNA encoding a functional human IL-8 receptor. *Science* 1991; 253: 1280.
500. Musashi M, Yang Y-C, Paul SR, et al. Direct and synergistic effects of interleukin 11 on murine hematopoiesis in culture *Proc Nat Acad Sci USA* 1991; 88: 765-769.
501. Nakamura S, Nakata K, Kashimoti S, et al. Anti-tumor effect of recombinant human interleukin-1 alpha against murine syngeneic tumors. *Jpn J Cancer Res* 1986; 77: 767-773.
502. Nakamura S, Kashimoto S, Kajikawa F, Nakata K. Combination effect on recombinant interleukin 1α with antitumor drugs on syngeneic tumors in mice. *Cancer Res* 1991; 51: 215-221.
503. Nakanishi K, Malek TR, Smith KA, et al. Both interleukin 2 and a second T cell derived factor in EL-4 supernatant have activity as differentiation factors in IgM synthesis. *J Exp Med* 1984; 160: 1605.
504. Namen AE, Schierer AE, March CJ, et al. B cell precursor-growth promoting activity and characterization of a growth factor active on lymphocyte precursors. *J Exp Med* 1988; 167: 988-1002.
505. Namen AS, Lupton S, Hjerrild K, et al. Stimulation of B cell progenitors by cloned murine IL-7. *Nature* 1988; 333: 571.
506. Nastala CL, Edington HD, McKinney TG, et al. Recombinant IL12 administration induced tumor regression in association with IFN-production. *J Immunol* 1994; 153: 1697-1706.
507. Natali PG, Nicotra MR, Sures I, et al. Breast cancer is associated with loss of c-kit oncogene product. *Int J Cancer* 1992a; 52: 713-717.
508. Natali PG, Nicotra MR, Sures I, et al. Expression of c kit receptor in normal and transformed human nonlymphoid tissues. *Cancer Res* 1992b; 52: 6139-6143.
509. Natali PG, Nicotra MR, Winkler AB, et al. Progression of human cutaneous melanoma is associated with loss of expression of c-kit proto oncogene receptor. *Int J Cancer* 1992; 52: 197-201.
510. Nathan CF, Murray HW, Wiebe ME, Rubin BY. Identification of Interferon γ as the lymphokine that activates human macrophage oxidative metabolism and antimicrobial activity. *J Exp Med* 1983; 158: 670.
511. Naume B, Espevik T, Sundan A. Gene expression and secretion of cytokines and cytokine receptors from highly purified CD56+natural killer cells stimulated with interleukin 2 interleukin 7 and interleukin 12. Eur *J Immunol* 1993b; 23: 1831-8.
512. Naume B, Gately M, Espevik T. A comparative study of IL-12 (cytotoxic lymphocyte maturation factor), IL-2, and IL-7 induced effects on immunomagnetically purified CD56+ NK cells. *J Immunol* 1992; 148: 2429-2436.
513. Naume B, Gately MK, Desai BB, et al. Synergistic effects of interleukin 4 and interleukin 12 on NK cell proliferation. *Cytokine* 1993; 5: 38-46.
514. Nawroth P, Handley D, Matsueda G, et al. Tumor necrosis factor/cachechtin-induced intravascular fibrin formation in meth A fibrosarcomas. *J Exp Med* 1988; 168: 637-647.
515. Neta R, Oppenheim JJ. Why should internists be interested in interleukin-1? *Ann Intern Med* 1988; 109: 1-3.
516. Neta R, Oppenheim JJ. Cytokines in therapy of radiation injury. *Blood* 1988; 72: 1093-1095.
517. Neta R, Douches SD, Oppenheim JJ. Interleukin-1 is a radioprotector. *J Immunol* 1986; 136: 2483-2488.
518. Nicholls SE, Heyworth CM, Dexter TM, et al. IL-4 promotes macrophage development by rapidly stimulating lineage restriction of bipotent granulocyte macrophage colony forming cells. *J Immunol* 1995; 155: 845-853.
519. Nishimura T, Uchiyama Y, Yagi H, Hashimoto Y. Administration of slowly released recombinant interleukin 2. *J Immunol Methods* 1986; 91: 21.
520. Noelle R, Krammer P, Ohara J, et al. Increased expression of Ia antigens on resting B cells. A new role for B cell growth factor 1. *Proc Nat Acad Sci USA* 1984; 81: 6149.
521. Noguchi M, Nakamura Y, Russel SM, et al. Interleukin receptor gamma chain a functional component of the interleukin 7 receptor. *Science* 1993; 262: 1877-1880.
522. Nonaka M, Nonaka R, Wooley K, et al. Distinct immunohistochemical localization of IL-4 in human inflamed airway tissues. IL-4 is localized to eosinophils in vivo and is released by peripheral blood eosinophils. *J Immunol* 1995; 155: 3234-3244.
523. Nophar Y, Kemper O, Brakebusch C, et al. Soluble forms of tumor necrosis factor receptors (TNF-R's). The cDNA for the type I TNF-R cloned using amino acid sequence data of its soluble form, encodes both the cell surface and a soluble form of the receptor. *EMBO J* 1990; 9: 3269-3278.
524. North RJ. Cyclophosphamide-facilitated adoptive immunotherapy of an established tumor depends on elimination of tumor-induced suppressor T cells. *J Exp Med* 1982; 55: 1063.
525. Obiri N, Hillman GG, Haas GP, et al. Expression of high affinity interleukin-4 receptors on human renal cell carcinoma cells and inhibition of tumor growth *in vitro* by interleukin-4. *J Clin Investigation* 1993; 91: 88-93.
526. O'Garra A, Chang R, Hatings R, et al. Ly IB (B-1) cells are the main source of B-cell derived IL-10. *Eur J Immunol* 1992; 22: 711.
527. Ogasawa M, Rosenberg S. Enhanced expression of HLA molecules and stimulation of autologous human tumor infiltrating lymphocytes following transduction of melanoma cells with γ interferon genes. *Cancer Res* 1993; 53: 3561-3568.
528. Ogawa N, Itoh M, Gately Y. Abnormal production of B cell growth factor in patients with systemic lupus erythmatosis. *Clin Exp Immunol* 1992; 89: 26-38.
529. Ognibene FP, Rosenberg SA, Lotze M, et al. Interleukin-2 administration causes reversible hemodynamic changes and left ventricular dysfunction similar to those seen in septic shock. *Chest* 1988; 94: 750.
530. Ohara J, Paul WE. Upregulation of the interleukin 4/B cell stimulatory factor receptor expression. *Proc Nat Acad Sci USA* 1988; 85: 8221.

531. Okahara H, Yagita H, Miyake K, Okumura K. Involvement of very late activation antigen 4 (VLA-4) and Vascular Cell Adhesion Molecule 1 (VCAM-1) in tumor necrosis factor α enhancement of experimental metastasis. *Cancer Res* 1994: 54; 3233-3236.
532. Okayashiki K, Miyauchi J, Ohyashiki JH, et al. Interleukin 7 enhances colony growth and induces CD 20 antigen of a Ph+ acute lymphoblastic leukemia cell line. *Leukemia* 1993; 7: 1034-40.
533. Okazaki H, Ito M, Sudo T, et al. IL-7 promotes thymocytes bearing α/β or γ/δ T cell receptors *in vitro*: Synergism with IL-2. *J Immunol* 1989; 143: 2917-2922.
534. Oldham RK. Biological approaches to cancer therapy. *1st Italian/American Symposium on Immunobiologic Aspects in Oncology*, New York City, September 1990.
535. Oldham RK, Blumenschein G, Schwartzberg L, et al. Combination biotherapy utilizing interleukin-2 and alpha-interferon in patients with advanced cancer: An NBSG trial. *Mol Biother* 1992; 4: 4-9.
536. Oldham RK. Cancer cures: by the people, for the people, at what cost? *Mol Biother* 1990; 2(1): 2-3.
537. Oldham RK. Cancer and diabetes: are there similarities? *Mol Biother* 1990; 2(3): 130-131.
538. Oldham RK, Stark J, Barth NM, et al. Continuous infusion interleukin-2 and cyclophosphamide as treatment of advanced cancer: An NBSG trial. *J Natl Cancer Inst* 1990.
539. Oldham RK, Thurman GB. Effects of cytokines on recovery from radiation exposure. In: Rotman M, Rosenthal CJ, eds. *Medical radiology – Diagnostic imaging and radiation oncology. Concomitant continuous infusion chemotherapy and radiation*. Springer-Verlag, New York, 1990.
540. Oldham RK, Dillman RO, Yannelli JR, et al. Continuous infusion interleukin-2 and tumor derived activated cells as treatment of advanced solid tumors: an NBSG trial. *Mol Biother* 1991; 3(2): 68-73.
541. Oldham RK. Therapy with tumor derived activated lymphocytes. In: *Tumor Immunology*. Goldfarb R and Whiteside T, eds. Marcel Dekker, New York, pp. 251-271, 1992.
542. Oldham RK, Blumenschein G, Schwartzberg L, et al. Combination biotherapy utilizing interleukin-2 and alpha-interferon in patients with advanced cancer. an NBSG trial. *Mol Biother* 1992; 4: 4-9.
543. Oldham RK, Lewko W, Good R, et al. Growth of tumor derived activated T-cells for the treatment of cancer. *Cancer Biotherapy* 1994; 9(3): 211-224.
544. Oldham RK, Lewko WM, Good RW, Sharp E. Cancer biotherapy with interferon, interleukin 2 and tumor derived activated cells (TDAC). *In Vivo* 1994; 8: 653-664.
545. Oldham RK and Lewko WM. *Personal Communication*.
546. Oliver RTD, Crosby D, Nouri A, et al. Evaluation of the effect of continuous infusion recombinant interleukin-2 on peripheral blood leucocytes of patients with terminal malignancy. *Br J Cancer* 1989; 60: 934.
547. O'Neal KD, and Yu-Lee L. The proline rich motif (PRM): a novel feature of the cytokine/hematopoietin receptor superfamily. *Lymphokine Cytokine Res.* 1993; 12: 309-312.
548. Onozaki K, Matsushima K, Aggarwal BB, Oppenheim JJ. Human interleukin 1 is a cytocidal factor for several tumor cell lines. *J Immunol* 1985; 135: 3962-3968.
549. Oppenheim JJ, Kovacs EJ, Matsushima K, Durum SK. There is more than one interleukin-1. *Immunol Today* 1986; 7: 45-56.
550. Orange JS, Wolf SF, Biron CR. Effects of IL12 on the response and susceptibility to experimental viral infections. *J Immunol* 1993; 152: 1253.
551. Ortaldo JR, Mason AT, Gerard JP, et al. Effects of natural and recombinant IL2 on regulation of IFN gamma production and natural killer activity: lack of involvement of Tac antigen for these immunoregulatory effects. *J Immunol* 1984; 133: 779.
552. Ortaldo JR, Mason A, Overton R. Lymphokine-activated killer cells. Analysis of the progenitors and effectors. *J Exp Med* 1986; 164: 1193.
553. Oshimi K, Oshimi Y, Akutsu M, et al. Cytotoxicity of interleukin 2-activated lymphocytes for leukemia and lymphoma cells. *Blood* 1986; 68: 938.
554. Ostensen ME, Thiele DL, and Lipsky PE. Tumor necrosis factor enhances cytolytic activity of human natural killer cells. *J Immunol* 1987; 138: 4185.
555. Owen-Schaub LB, Gutterman JU, Grimm EA. Synergy of tumor necrosis factor and interleukin 2 in the activation of human cytotoxic lymphocytes: Effect of tumor necrosis factor and Interleukin 2 in the generation of human lymphokine activated killer cell cytotoxicity. *Cancer Res* 1988; 48: 788-792.
556. Paciucci PA, Holland JF, Glidwell O, et al. Recombinant interleukin-2 by continuous infusion and adoptive transfer of recombinant interleukin-2 activated cells in patients with advanced cancer. *J Clin Oncol* 1989; 1989: 869.
557. Page TH, Willcocks JL, Taylor-Fishwick DA, Foxwell BMJ. Characterization of a novel high affinity human IL-7 receptor. Expression on T cells and association with IL-7 driven proliferation. *J Immunol* 1993; 151: 4753-4763.
558. Paige CJ, Figarella EF, Cuttito M, et al. Natural cytotoxic cells against solid tumors in mice: II. Some characteristics of the effector cells. *J Immunol* 1978; 121: 1827.
559. Pandrau D, Frances V, Martinez Valdez H, et al. Characterization of a t(1; 19) pre-B acute lymphoblastic leukemia (ALL) cell line which proliferates in response to IL-7. *Leukemia* 1993; 7: 635-42.
560. Paolozzi F, Zamkoff K, Doyle M, et al. Phase I trial of recombinant interleukin-2 and recombinant B-interferon in refractory neoplastic diseases. *J Biol Response Modif* 1989; 8: 122.
561. Papa MZ, Yang JC, Vetto JT, et al. Combined effects of chemotherapy and interleukin-2 in the therapy of mice with advanced pulmonary tumors. *Cancer Res* 1988; 48: 122.
562. Park LS, Friend DJ, Schmierer AE, et al. Murine interleukin 7 (IL-7) receptor. Characterization on an IL7 dependent cell line. *J Exp Med* 1990; 171: 1073.
563. Park LS, Friend D, Sassenfeld HM, Urdal DL. Characterization of human B cell stimulatory factor 1 receptor. *J Exp Med* 1987; 166: 476-488.
564. Pauker K, Cantrell K, Henle W. Quantitative studies on viral interference in suspended L cells. III. Effects of interfering viruses and interferon on growth rate of cells. *Virology* 1962; 17: 324-334.
565. Paul NL, Ruddle NH. Lymphotoxin. *Ann Rev Immunol* 1986; 6: 407-438.
566. Paul SR, Bennett F, Calvetti JA, et al. Molecular cloning of a cDNA encoding interleukin 11, a novel stromal cell derived lymphopoietic and hematopoietic cytokine. *Proc Nat Acad Sci USA* 1990; 87: 7512.

567. Paul WE, Ohara J. B-cell stimulatory factor-1/interleukin 4. *Annu Rev Immunol* 1987; 5: 429, 460.
568. Peace DJ, Cheever MA. Toxicity and therapeutic efficacy of high-dose interleukin 2. *In vivo* infusion of antibody to NK-1.1 attenuates toxicity without compromising efficacy against murine leukemia. *J Exp Med* 1989; 169: 161.
569. Pennica D, Nedwin GE, Hayflick JS, et al. Human tumor necrosis factor: precursor structure, expression and homology to lymphotoxin. *Nature* 1984; 312: 724.
570. Perussia B, Ramoni C, Anegon I, et al. Preferential proliferation of natural killer cells among peripheral blood mononuclear cells cocultured with B lymphoblastoid lines. *Nat Immun Cell Growth Regul* 1987; 6: 171.
571. Pestka S, Langer JA, Zoon KC, et al . Interferons and their actions. *Ann Rev Biochem* 1987; 56: 727-777.
572. Peveri P, Walz A, Dewald B, Baggiolini M. A neutrophil activating factor produced by human mononuclear phagocytes. *J Exp Med* 1988; 167: 1547.
573. Phillips JH, Lanier LL. Dissection of the lymphokine-activated killer phenomenon. Relative contribution of peripheral blood natural killer cells and T lymphocytes to cytolysis. *J Exp Med* 1986; 164: 814.
574. Pippin BA, Rosenstein M, Jacob WF, et al. Local IL-4 delivery enhances immune reactivity to murine tumors: Gene therapy in combination with IL2. *Cancer Gene Therapy* 1994; 1: 35-42.
575. Pisa P, Halapi E, Pisa EK, et al. Selective expression of interleukin 10, interferon γ, and granulocyte macrophage colony stimulating factor in ovarian cancer biopsies. *Proc Nat Acad Sci* 1992; 89: 7708.
576. Pizza G, Severini G, Menniti D, et al. Tumour regression after intralesional injection of interleukin 2 in bladder cancer. Preliminary report. *Int J Cancer* 1984; 34: 359.
577. Pizza G, Viza D, De Vinci C, et al. Intralymphatic administration of interleukin-2 in cancer patients: a pilot study. *Lymphokine Res* 1988; 7: 45.
578. Plate JMD, Knospe WH, Harris JE, Gregory SA. Normal and aberrant expression of cytokines in neoplastic cells from lymphocytic leukemias. *Human Immunol* 1993; 36: 249-258.
579. Plum J, De Smedt M, Leclerq G. Exogenous IL-7 promotes the growth of CD33-CD4-CD8-CD44+CD25+/- precursor cells and blocks the differentiation pathway of TCR-alpha beta cells in fetal thymus organ culture. *J Immunol* 1993; 150: 2706-2716.
580. Pugin J, Schurer-Maley C-C, Leturcq D, et al. Lipopolysaccharide activation of human endothelial and epithelial cells is mediated by lipopolysaccharide binding protein and soluble CD14. *Proc Nat Acad Sci USA* 1993; 90: 2744.
581. Pulaski B, Maltby K, Sastri N, et al. IL-3 enhances presentation of exogenous tumor antigen with class I by a rare subpopulation of host macrophages. *Proc AACR* 1995; 36: 474 # 2826.
582. Punnonen J, Aversa G, Cocks BG, et al. Interleukin 13 induces interleukin 4 independent IgG4 and IgE synthesis and CD 23 expression by B cells. *Proc Nat Acad Sci USA* 1993; 90: 3730-3735.
583. Puri R, Travis W, Rosenberg S. Decrease in interleukin-2-induced vascular leakage in the lungs of mice by administration of recombinant interleukin-1 alpha *in vivo*. *Cancer Res* 1989; 49: 969.
584. Puri RK, Ogata M, Leland GM, et al. Expression of high affinity Interleukin 4 receptors on murine sarcoma cells and receptor mediated cytotoxicity of tumor cells to chimeric protein between Interleukin 4 and pseudomonas exotoxin. *Cancer Res* 1991; 51: 3011-3017.
585. Qi J, Kreutzer DL. Fibrin activation of vascular endothelial cells. Induction of IL-8 secretion. *J Immunol* 1995; 155: 867-876.
586. Rabin EM, Ohara J, and Paul WE. B cell stimulatory factor 1 activates resting B cells. *Proc Nat Acad Sci USA* 1985; 82: 2935-2939.
587. Redman BG, Abubakr Y, Chou T, et al. Phase II trial of recombinant interleukin-1β in patients with metastatic renal cell carcinoma. *Proc Am Soc Clin Oncol* 1994; 13: 255.
588. Reed JC, Abidi AH, Alpers JD, et al. Effect of cyclosporin A and dexamethasone on interleukin 2 receptor gene expression. *J Immunol* 1986; 137: 150.
589. Reittie JE, Hoffbrand AV. Interleukin-4 (IL-4) inhibits proliferation and spontaneous cytokine release by chronic lymphocytic leukemia cells. *Leukemia Res* 1994; 18: 55-60.
590. Renauld JC, Druez C, Kermouni A, et al. Expression cloning of murine and human Interleukin 9 receptor DNAs. *Proc Nat Acad Sci USA* 1992; 89: 5690-5694.
591. Renauld JC, Houssiau F, Louahed J, et al. Interleukin 9 Int *Rev Exp Pathol* 1993; 34: 99-109.
592. Rennick D, Yang G, Muler-Sieburg C, et al. Interleukin 4 (B cell stimulatory factor 1) can enhance or antagonize the factor dependent growth of hematopoietic progenitor cells. *Proc Nat Acad Sci USA* 1987; 84: 6889.
593. Renz H, Domenico J, Gelfand EW. IL-4 dependent up-regulation of IL-4 receptor expression in murine T and B cells. *J Immunol* 1991; 146: 3049.
594. Restifo NP, Speis PJ, Karp SE, et al. Non-immunogenic sarcoma transduced with the cDNA for interferon γ elicits CD8+T cells against the wild type tumor: correlation with antigen presentation capability. *J Exp Med* 1992; 175: 1423-1431.
595. Rice A, Kerr I M. Interferon mediated double stranded RNA dependent protein kinase is inhibited in extracts from vaccinia infected cells. *J Virol* 1984; 50: 229-236.
596. Rich BE, Campos-Torres J, Tepper RI, et al. Cutaneous lymphoproliferation and lymphomas in interleukin 7 transgenic mice. *J Exp Med* 1993; 177: 305-316.
597. Richards J, Mehta N, Schroeder L, Dordal A. Sequential chemotherapy/immunotherapy for metastatic melanoma. *Proc Am Soc Clin Oncol* 1992; 11: 1189.
598. Richards JM, Vogelzang NJ, Ramming K, et al. Preliminary results of a randomized trial of recombinant human interleukin-2 given by continuous venous infusion with or without lymphokine activated killer cells (meeting abstract). *Proc Annu Meet Am Soc Clin Oncol* 1988; 7: A618.
599. Richter G, Kruger-Krasagakes S, Hein G, et al. Interleukin 10 transfected into Chinese Hamster Ovary Cells Prevents Tumor Growth and Macrophage Infiltration. *Cancer Res* 1993; 53: 4134-4137.
600. Riddell S, Cheever MA, Greenberg PD. Interleukin-2 in cancer immunotherapy. *ISI Atlas Sci Immunol* 1988; 175.
601. Rixe O, Benhammouda A, Antoine E, et al. Final results of a prospective multicentric study on 91 metastatic malignant melanoma (MMM) patients treated by chemo-immunotherapy (CH-IM) with cisplatin interleukin (IL-2) interferon-α (IFN). *Proc Am Soc Clin Oncol* 1994; 13: 399.

602. Robb RJ, Smith KA. Heterogeneity of human T-cell growth factors due to variable glycosylation. *Mol Immunol* 1981; 18: 1087.
603. Robb RJ. Human T-cell growth factor: purification and interaction with a cellular receptor. *Lymphokine Res* 1982; 1: 37.
604. Robertson MJ, Soiffer RJ, Wolf SF, et al. Response of human natural killer cells to natural killer cell stimulatory factor: Cytolytic activity and proliferation of NK differentially regulated by NKSF. *J Exp Med* 1992; 175: 779-788.
605. Romagnani S. Human TH1 and TH2 subset: Regulation of differentiation and role in protection and immunopathology. *Int Arch Allergy Immunopathology Int Arch Allergy Immunol* 1992; 98: 279-285.
606. Rosenberg SA, Grimm EA, McGrogan M, et al. Biological activity of recombinant human interleukin-2 produced in *Escherichia coli*. *Science* 1984; 223: 1412.
607. Rosenberg SA, Lotze MT, Muul LM, et al. Observations on the systemic administration of autologous lymphokine-activated killer cells and recombinant interleukin-2 to patients with metastatic cancer. *N Engl J Med* 1985; 313: 1485.
608. Rosenberg SA, Mule JJ, Speiss PJ, et al. Regression of established pulmonary metastases and subcutaneous tumor mediated by the systemic administration of high-dose recombinant interleukin 2. *J Exp Med* 1985; 161: 1169.
609. Rosenberg SA, Lotze MT, Muul LM, et al. A progress report on the treatment of 157 patients with advanced cancer using lymphokine-activated killer cells and interleukin-2 or high-dose interleukin-2 alone. *N Engl J Med* 1987; 316: 889.
610. Rosenberg SA, Spiess P, LaFreniere R. A new approach to the adoptive immunotherapy of cancer with tumor-infiltrating lymphocytes. *Science* 1986; 233: 1318.
611. Rosenberg SA, Packard BS, Aebersold PM, et al. Use of tumor-infiltrating lymphocytes and interleukin-2 in the immunotherapy of patients with metastatic melanoma. *N Engl J Med* 1988; 319: 1676.
612. Rosenberg SA. Immunotherapy of patients with advanced cancer using recombinant lymphokines. *Clin Courier* 1989; 7: 16.
613. Rosenberg SA, Lotze MT, Yang JC, et al. Combination therapy with interleukin-2 and alpha-interferon for the treatment of patients with advanced cancer. *J Clin Oncol* 1989; 7: 1863-1874.
614. Rosenberg SA, Lotze MT, Yang JC, et al. Experience with the use of high-dose interleukin-2 in the treatment of 652 cancer patients. *Ann Surg* 1989; 210: 474-485.
615. Rosenberg SA. The immunotherapy and gene therapy of cancer. *J Clin Oncol* 1992; 10: 180-199.
616. Rosenberg SA, Lotze MT, Yang JC, et al. Prospective randomized trial of high-dose interleukin-2 alone or in conjunction with lymphokine-activated killer cells for the treatment of patients with advanced cancer. *J Natl Cancer Inst* 1993; 85: 622-632.
617. Rosenberg SA, Yang JC, Topalian SL, et al. The treatment of 283 consecutive patients with metastatic melanoma or renal cell cancer using high-dose bolus interleukin-2. *JAMA* 1994; 271: 907-913.
618. Rosenstein M, Ettinghausen SE, Rosenberg SA. Extravasation of intravascular fluid mediated by the systemic administration of recombinant interleukin 2. *J Immunol* 1986; 137: 1735.
619. Rosenstein M, Yron I, Kaufmann Y, Rosenberg SA. Lymphocyte-activated killer cells: lysis of fresh syngeneic natural killer-resistant murine tumor cells by lymphocytes cultured in interleukin 2. *Cancer Res* 1984; 44: 1946.
620. Rosenthal NS, Hank JA, Kohler PC, et al. The *in vitro* function of lymphocytes from 25 cancer patients receiving four to seven consecutive days of recombinant IL-2. *J Biol Response Modif* 1988; 7: 123.
621. Rossio JL, Thurman GB, Long C, et al. The BRMP IL-2 Reference Reagent. *Lymphokine Res* 1986; 5(SI): S13.
622. Rousset, F, Garcia E, Peronne C, et al. Interleukin-10 is a potent growth and differentiation factor for activated human B lymphocytes. *Proc Nat Acad Sci USA* 1992; 89: 1890.
623. Ruddle NH, Waksman BH. Cytotoxic effect of lymphocyte-antigen interaction in delayed hypersensitivity. *Science* 1967; 157: 1060-1062.
624. Ruggiero V, Latham K, Baglioni C. Cytostatic and cytotoxic activity of tumor necrosis factor on human cancer cells. *J Immunol* 1987; 138: 2711.
625. Ruscetti FW, Morgan DA, Gallo RG. Selective *in vitro* growth of T-lymphocytes from normal bone marrows. *Science* 1976; 193: 1007-1008.
626. Ruscetti FW, Morgan DA, Gallo RC. Functional and Morphologic Characterization of T cells continuously grown in vitro *J Immunol* 1977; 119: 131-138.
627. Russell SM, Johnson JA, Noguchi M, et al. Interaction of IL-2R and c chains with Jak1 and Jak3: Implications for XSCID and XCID. *Science* 1994; 266: 1042-1044.
628. Rygard K, Nakamura T, Spang-THompsen M. Expression of the protoconcogene cmet and c kit and their ligands, hepatocyte growth factor/scatter factor and stem cell factor in SCLC cell lines and xenografts. *British J Cancer* 1993; 67: 37-46.
629. Sabelko K, Blumenthal D, Ford R, Ambrus J. IL14 producing and responsive cells are found in germinal centers. *FASEB J* 1994; 8: A999.
630. Sakata T, Iwagami S, Tsurata Y, et al. Constitutive expression of interleukin 7 mRNA and production of IL-7 by a cloned murine thymic stromal cell line. *J Leukocyte Biol* 1990; 144: 3015.
631. Sanderson CJ, Campbell HD, Young IG. Molecular and cellular biology of eosinophil differentiation factor (interleukin 5) and its effects on human and mouse B cells. *Immunol Rev* 1988; 109: 29-50.
632. Sato TA, Widmer MB, Finkelman FD, et al. Recombinant soluble murine IL-4 receptor can inhibit of enhance IgE responses in vivo. *J Immunol* 1991; 150: 2717.
633. Sauder DN, Mounessa NL, Katz SI, et al. Chemotactic cytokines: the role of leukocyte pyrogen and epidermal cell thymocyte-activating factor in neutrophil chemotaxis. *J Immunol* 1984; 132: 828.
634. Scala G, Kuang YD, Hall RE, et al. Accessory cell function of human B cells. I. Production of both interleukin-1 like activity and interleukin-1 inhibitory factor by an EBV-transformed B cell line. *J Exp Med* 1984; 159: 1637.
635. Schadendorf D, Bohm M, Moller P, Grunewald T, Czarnetzki BM. Interleukin 7 induces differential lymphokine-activated killer cell activity against human melanoma cell, keratinocytes and endothelial cells. *J Invest Dermatol* 1994; 102: 838-842.
636. Schadendorf D, Moller A, Algermissen B, et al. IL-8 produced by human malignant melanoma cells *in vitro* is

an essential autocrine growth factor. *J Immunol* 1993; 15: 2667-2675.

637. Schendel DJ, Gansbacher B. Tumor specific lysis of Human renal cell carcinomas by tumor infiltrating lymphocytes: Modulation of recognition through retroviral transduction of tumor cells with interleukin 2 complementary DNA and exogenous interferon treatment. *Cancer Res* 1993; 4020-4025.
638. Schiller JH, Hank J, Storer B, et al. A direct comparison of immunological and clinical effects of interleukin-2 with and without interferon-α in humans. *Cancer Res* 1993; 53: 1286-1992.
639. Schmidt JA, Mizel SB, Cohen D, et al. Interleukin-1: a potential regulator of fibroblast proliferation. *J Immunol* 1982; 128: 2177.
640. Schraufstatter IU, Barritt DS, Ma M, et al. Multiple sites on IL-8 responsible for binding to α and β IL-8 receptors. *J Immunol* 1993; 151: 6418-6428.
641. Schmitter D, Lauber B, Fagg B, Stahel RA. Hematopoietic growth factors secreted by seven human pleural mesothelioma cell lines: interleukin 6 production as a common feature. *Int J Cancer* 1992; 51: 296-301.
642. Schroder J, Mrowietz U, Morita E, Christophers E. Purification and partial biochemical characterization of a human monocyte-derived neutrophil activating peptide that lacks interleukin 1 activity. *J Immunol* 1987; 139: 3474.
643. Schroder JM, Christophers E. Secretion of novel and homogeneous neutrophil activating peptides by LPS stimulated human endothelial cells. *J Immunol* 1989; 142: 244.
644. Schuchter L, Neuberg D, Atkins M, et al. A phase I study of interleukin-1 alpha (IL-1) and high dose cyclophosphamide (Cy) in patients with advanced cancer. *Proc Am Soc Clin Oncol* 1994; 13: 133.
645. Schuerer-Maly CC, Eckmann L, Kagoff MF, et al. Colonic epithelial cell lines as a source of interleukin-8: stimulation by inflammatory cytokines and bacterial lipopolysaccharide. *Immunology* 1994; 81: 85-91.
646. Schultz KR, Klarnet JP, Peace DJ, et al. Adoptive transfer of lymphokine-activated killer (LAK) cells augments monoclonal antibody eradication of murine lymphoma without toxicity (meeting abstract). *Proc Annu Meet Am Assoc Cancer Res* 1989; 30: A1441.
647. Schwalb DM, Han H-M, Marino M, et al. Identification of a new receptor subtype for tumor necrosis factor α. *J Biol Chem* 1993; 268: 9949-9954.
648. Schwartzberg L, Tauer K, Birch R, et al. Phase I study of sequential recombinant tumor necrosis factor (rTNF) and recombinant interleukin-2 (rIL-2) in patients with advanced malignancy (meeting abstract). *Proc Annu Meet Am Soc Clin Oncol* 1989; 8: A711.
649. Schweizer RC, Welmers BAC, Raaijmakers JAM, et al. RANTES and Interleukin 8 induced responses in normal human eosinophils: effects of priming with IL5. *Blood* 1994; 83: 3697.
650. Sebok K, Woodside D, al-Aoukaty A. IL-8 induces the locomotion on human IL 2 activated natural killer cells. Involvement of a guanine nucleotide binding protein. *J Immunol* 1993; 150: 1524-1534.
651. Sehmi R, Cromwell O, Wardlaw AJ, et al. Interleukin 8 is a chemoattractant for eosinophils purified from subjects with blood eosinophilia but not from normal healthy subjects. *Clin Exp Allergy* 1993; 23: 1027.
652. Sekido Y, Obata Y, Ueda R, et al. Preferential expression of c-kit protooncogene transcripts in small cell lung cancer. *Cancer Res* 1991; 51: 2416-2419.
653. Shaw J, Caplan B, Paetkau V, et al. Cellular origins of co-stimulator (IL-2) and its activity in cytotoxic T-lymphocyte responses. *J Immunol* 1980; 124: 2231.
654. Shaw J, Monticone V, Paetkau V. Partial purification and molecular characterization of a lymphokine (co-stimulator) required for the mitogenic response of mouse thymocytes *in vitro*. *J Immunol* 1978; 120: 1967.
655. Shiloni E, Eisenthal A, Sachs D, Rosenberg SA. Antibody-dependent cellular cytotoxicity mediated by murine lymphocytes activated in recombinant interleukin 2. *J Immunol* 1987; 138: 1992.
656. Sica D, Rayman P, Edinger M, et al. Interleukin 7 enhances the proliferation and effector function of tumor infiltrating lymphocytes from renal cell carcinoma. *International J Cancer* 1993; 53: 941-947.
657. Sideras P, Palacios R. Bone marrow pre-T and pre-B lymphocyte clones express functional receptors for interleukin (IL)-3 and interleukin 4/BSF-1 and non-functional receptors for IL2. *Eur J Immunol* 1987; 17: 217.
658. Siebruth D, Jabs EW, Warrington JA, et al. Assignment of NKSF/IL-12, a unique cytokine composed of two unrelated subunits to chromosomes 3 and 5. *Genomics* 1992; 14: 59-62.
659. Siegel JP, Sharon M, Smith PL, Leonard WJ. The IL-2 receptor beta chain (p70): role in mediating signals for LAK, NK, and proliferative activities. *Science* 1987; 238: 75.
660. Silagi S, Schaefer AE. Successful immunotherapy of mouse melanoma and sarcoma with recombinant interleukin-2 and cyclophosphamide. *J Biol Response Modif* 1986; 5: 411.
661. Silvani A, Ferrari G, Paonessa G, et al. Down regulation of interleukin 6 receptor alpha chain in interleukin 6 transduced melanoma cells causes selective resistance to interleukin 6 but not to oncostatin M. *Cancer Res* 1995; 55: 2200-2205.
662. Singh RK, Gutman M, Radinsky R, et al. Expression of interleukin 8 correlates with the metastatic potential of human melanoma cells in nude mice. *Cancer Res* 1994; 54: 3232-3247.
663. Smith JW, Urba WJ, Curti BD, et al. The toxic and hematologic effects of interleukin-1 alpha administered in a phase I trial to patients with advanced malignancies. *J Clin Oncol* 1992; 10: 1141-1152.
664. Smith KA. Interleukin-2: Inception, impact and implications. *Science* 1988; 240: 1169-1176.
665. Smyth MJ, Ortaldo JR. Comparison of the effect of IL2 and IL6 on the lytic activity of purified human peripheral blood large granular lymphocytes. *J Immunol* 1991; 146: 1380-1384.
666. Snapper CM, Paul WE. Interferon γ and B cell stimulatory factor I reciprocally regulate Ig isotope production *Science* 1987; 236: 944-947.
667. Snapper CM, Finkelman FD, and Paul WE. Differential regulation of IgG1 and IgE synthesis by interleukin 4. *J Exp Med* 1988; 167: 183.
668. Sondel PM, Hank JA, Kohler PC, et al. Destruction of autologous human lymphocytes by interleukin 2-activated cytotoxic cells. *J Immunol* 1986; 137: 502.
669. Sondel PM, Sosman JA, Hank JA, et al. Tumor-infiltrating lymphocytes and interleukin-2 in melanomas (letter). *N Engl J Med* 1989; 320: 1418.

670. Sosman JA, Kohler PC, Hank JA, et al. Repetitive weekly cycles of interleukin-2. II. Clinical and immunologic effects of dose, schedule, and addition of indomethacin. *J Natl Cancer Inst* 1988; 80: 1451.

671. Southern E. Detection of specific sequences among DNA fragments separated by gel electrophoresis. *J Mol Biol* 1975; 98: 503.

672. Sower LE, Froelich CJ, Carney DH, et al. Thrombin induces IL-6 production in Fibroblasts and Epithelial Cells. *J Immunol* 1995; 155: 895-901.

673. Squadrelli M, Rivoltini F, Gambacorti-Passerini C, et al. *Pilot study of lymphokine activated killer cells and recombinant interleukin-2 in the local treatment of advanced head and neck cancers* (meeting abstract). Sixth NCI/EORTC Symposium on New Drugs in Cancer Therapy, Amsterdam, A192, 1989.

674. Spits H, Yssel H, Paliard X, et al. IL-4 inhibits IL-2 mediated induction of human lymphokine activated killer cells but not the generation of antigen specific cytotoxic T lymphocytes in mixed leukocyte cultures. *J Immunol* 1988; 141: 29-36.

675. Splawski JB, Jelinek DF, Lipsky PE. Immunomodulatory role of IL-4 on the secretion of Ig by human B cells. *J Immunol* 1989; 142: 1569.

676. Splawski JB, McAnally , Lipsky PE. IL2 dependence of the promotion of human B cell differentiation by IL-6 (BSF-2). *J Immunol* 1990; 144: 562.

677. Stahel RA, Sculier JP, Jost LM, et al. Tolerance and effectiveness of recombinant interleukin-2 and lymphokine-activated killer cells in patients with metastatic solid tumors. *Eur J Cancer Clin Oncol* 1989; 25: 965.

678. Standiford T, Kunkel S, Basha M, et al. Interleukin 8 gene expression by a pulmonary epithelial cell line. *J Clin Invest* 1990; 86: 1945.

679. Starnes HF, Hartman G, Torti F, et al. Recombinant human interleukin-1β (IL-1β) has antitumor activity and acceptable toxicity in metastatic malignant melanoma. *Proc Am Soc Clin Oncol* 1991; 10: 292.

680. Steller EP, Ottow RT, Eggermont AMM, et al. Local conditions in the host influence immunotherapy with interleukin-2 and LAK cells. *Cancer Det Prev* 1988; 12: 81.

681. Stern AS, Podlaski FJ, Hulmes JD, et al. Purification to homogeneity and partial characterization of cytotoxic lymphocyte maturation factor from human B-lymphocyte cells. *Proc Nat Acad Sci USA* 1990; 87: 6808-6812.

682. Stoter G, Shiloni E, Gundersen S, et al. Alternating recombinant interleukin-2 and dacarbazine in metastatic melanoma (meeting abstract). *Proc Annu Meet Am Soc Clin Oncol* 1989; 8: A1095.

683. Stoter G, Shiloni E, Aamdal S, et al. Sequential administration of recombinant human interleukin-2 and dacarbazine in metastatic melanoma. A multicentre phase II study. *Eur J Cancer Clin Oncol* 1989; 25: S41-S43.

684. Stotter H, Custer MC, Bolton ES, et al. IL7 induced lymphokine activated killer cell activity and is regulated by IL4. *J Immunol* 1991; 146: 150-155.

685. Strassman G, Jacob CO, Fong M, Bertolini DR. Mechanisms of paraneoplastic syndromes of colon-26: involvement of interleukin 6 in hypercalcemia. *Cytokine* 1993; 5: 463-468.

686. Strassman G. Fong M, Freter CE, et al. Suramin interferes with Interleukin-6 receptor binding *in vitro* and inhibits colon 26 mediated experimental cachexia *in vivo*. *J Clin Invest* 1993; 92: 2152-2159.

687. Strieter R, Kunkel S, Showell H, et al. Endothelial cell gene expression of a neutrophil chemotactic factor by TNF alpha, LPS, and IL-1 Beta. *Science* 1989; 243: 1467.

688. Streiter RM, Kunkel SL, Elner VM, et al. Interleukin-8: a corneal factor that induces neovascularization. *Am J Pathol* 1992; 141: 1279-1284.

689. Strohmeyer T, Peter S, Hartman M, et al. Expression of the hst-1 and c-kit protooncogene in human testicular germ cell tumors. *Cancer Res* 1991; 51: 181-1816.

690. Stutman O, Paige CJ, Figarella EF. Natural cytotoxic cells against solid tumors in mice. I. Strain and age distribution and target cell susceptibility. *J Immunol* 1979; 121: 1819.

691. Suda T, Murray R, Fischer M, et al. Tumor necrosis factor alpha and P40 inducc day 15 murine fetal thymocyte proliferation in combination with IL-2. *J Immunol* 1990; 144: 1783-1787.

692. Sugarman BJ, Aggarwal BB, Hass PE, et al. Recombinant human tumor necrosis factor α: effects on proliferation of normal and transformed cells *in vitro*. *Science* 1985; 230: 943-945.

693. Swain SL, McKenzie DT, Dutton RW, et al. The role of IL-2 and IL-5: characterization of a distinct helper T cell subset that makes IL4 and IL5 (Th2) and requires priming before induction of lymphokine secretion. *Immunol Rev* 1988; 102: 77-106.

694. Swain SL, McKenzie DT, Weinberg AD, Hancock W. Characterization of T helper 1 and 2 cell subsets in normal mice: helper T cells responsible for IL-4 and IL-5 production are present as precursors that require priming before they develop into lymphokine secreting cells. *J Immunol* 1994; 141: 3445.

695. Symons JA, Young PR, Duff GW. *Proc Natl Acad Sci USA* 1995; 92: 1714.

696. Taga K, Tosato G. IL-10 inhibits human T cell proliferation and IL-2 production. *J Immunol* 1992; 148: 1143-1148.

697. Taga T, Hibi M, Yamasaki K, et al. Interleukin 6 triggers the association of its receptor with a possible signal transducer gp130. *Cell* 1989; 58: 573-581.

698. Takahashi GW, Andrews DF, Lilly MB, et al. Effect of granulocyte macrophage colony stimulating factor and interleukin 3 on interleukin 8 production by human neutrophils and monocytes. *Blood* 1993; 81: 357.

699. Takatsu T. Interleukin 5 and its receptor. Prog Growth *Factor Res* 1991; 3: 87.

700. Takenawa J, Kaneko Y, Fukumoto M. Enhanced expression of interleukin-6 in primary human renal cell carcinomas. *J Nat Cancer Inst* 1991; 83: 1668-1672.

701. Tanaguchi T, Matsui H, Fujita T, et al. Structure and expression of a cloned small cDNA for human interleukin-2. *Nature* 1983; 302: 305.

702. Tartaglia LA, Weber RF, Figari IS, et al. The two different receptors for tumor necrosis factor mediate distinct cellular responses. *Proc Nat Acad Sci USA* 1991; 88: 9292.

703. Tartaglia LA, Pennica D, Goeddel DV. Ligand passing: the 75 kDa tumor necrosis factor (TNF) receptor recruits TNF for signalling by the 55-kDa TNF receptor. *J Biol Chem* 1993; 268: 18542-18548.

704. Tartour E, Dorval T, Mosseri V, et al. Serum interleukin 6 and C-reactive protein levels correlate with resistance to IL-2 therapy and poor survival in melanoma patients. *Brit J Cancer* 1994; 69: 911-913.

705. Tavernier J, Devos R, Cornelius S, et al. A human high affinity interleukin-5 receptor (IL-5R) is composed of an IL5 specific alpha chain and a beta chain shared with the receptor for GM-CSF. *Cell* 1991; 66: 1175.
706. Taylor CW, Grogan TM, Salmon SE. Effects of interleukin-4 on the *in vitro* growth of human lymphoid and plasma cell neoplasms. *Blood* 1990; 75: 1114-1118.
707. Tepper RI, Pattengale PK, Leder P. Murine interleukin 4 displays potent antitumor activity *in vivo*. *Cell* 1989; 57: 503-512.
708. Tepper RI, Levinson DA, Stranger BZ, et al. IL-4 induces allergic-like inflammatory disease and alters T cell development in transgenic mice. *Cell* 1991; 62: 457-467.
709. Te Velde AA, Klomp JPG, Yard BA, et al. Modulation of phenotypic and functional properties of human peripheral blood monocytes by IL-4. *J Immunol* 1988; 140: 1548-1554.
710. Thijs LG, Hack CE, Strack van Schijndel RJM, et al. Complement activation and high-dose of interleukin-2 (letter). *Lancet* 1989; ii: 395.
711. Thompson JA, Lee DJ, Lindgren CG, et al. Influence of dose and duration of infusion of interleukin-2 on toxicity and immunomodulation. *J Clin Oncol* 1988; 6: 669.
712. Thompson JA, Peace DJ, Klarnet JP, et al. Eradication of disseminated murine leukemia by treatment with high-dose interleukin 2. *J Immunol* 1986; 137: 3675.
713. Thompsen MK, Larsen CG, Thompsen HK, et al. Recombinant human interleukin 8 is a potent activator of canine neutrophil aggregation migration and leukotriene B4 biosynthesis. *J Invest Dermatol* 1991; 96: 260.
714. Thompson-Snipes LA, Dahr V, Bond MW, et al. Interleukin 10: a novel stimulatory factor for mast cells and their progenitors. *J Exp Med* 1991; 173: 507-510.
715. Thurman GB, Maluish AE, Rossio JL, et al. Comparative evaluation of multiple lymphoid and recombinant human interleukin-2 preparations. *J Biol Response Modif* 1986; 5: 85.
716. Tilden AB, Itoh K, Blach CM. Human lymphokine-activated killer (LAK) cells: identification of two types of effector cells. *J Immunol* 1987; 138: 1068.
717. Todaro GJ. Properties of growth factors produced by sarcoma virus-transformed cells. In: Moore N, ed. *Progress in cancer research and therapy.* Vol. 23: Maturation factors and cancer. Raven Press, New York, 1982: 115-128.
718. Toi M, Harris AL, Bicknell R. Interleukin 4 is a potent mitogen for capillary endothelium. *Biochem Biophys Res Commun* 1991; 174: 1287-1293.
719. Toi M, Bicknel R, Harris AL. Inhibition of colon and breast carcinoma cell growth by interleukin-4. *Cancer Res* 1992; 52: 275-279.
720. Toksoz D, Williams D, Smith KA, et al. Expression of two distinct DNA's of the steel gene (SCF) in deficient murine stromal cell lines. *Exp Hematol* 1992; 20: 138-139.
721. Toksoz D, Zsebo KM, Smith KA, et al. Support of human hematopoiesis in the long term bone marrow cultures by murine stromal cells selectively expressing the membrane bound and secreted forms of the human analog of the steel gene product stem cell factor. *Proc Nat Acad Sci USA* 1992; 89: 7350-7354.
722. Topalian SL, Solomon D, Rosenberg SA. Tumor specific cytolysis by lymphocytes infiltrating human melanomas. *J Immunol* 1989; 142: 3714-3725.
723. Topalian SL, Solomon D, Avis FP, et al. Immunotherapy of patients with advanced cancer using tumor-infiltrating lymphocytes and recombinant interleukin-2: a pilot study. *J Clin Oncol* 1988; 6: 839.
724. Topp MS, Koenigsmann M, Mire-Sluis A, et al. Recombinant human interleukin-4 inhibits growth of some human lung tumor cell lines *in vitro* and *in vivo*. *Blood* 1993; 82: 2837-2844.
725. Topp MS, Papadimitriou CA, Eitelbach F, et al. Recombinant human interleukin 4 has antiproliferative activity on human tumor cell lines derived from epithelial and nonepithelial histologies. *Cancer Res* 1995; 55: 2173-2176.
726. Tosato G, Pike SE. Interferon β2/interleukin-6 is a co-stimulant for human T lymphocytes. *J Immunol* 1988; 141: 1556-62.
727. Touw I, van Agthoven T, van Gurp R, et al. Interleukin 7 is a growth factor of precursor B and T acute lymphoblastic leukemia. *Blood* 1990; 75: 2097-2101.
728. Tracey KJ, Beutler B, Lowry SF, et al. Shock and tissue injury induced by recombinant human cachectin. *Science* 1986; 234: 470.
729. Trehu EG, Isner JM, Mier JW, et al. Possible myocardial toxicity associated with interleukin 4 Therapy. *J Immunotherapy* 1993; 14: 348-351.
730. Treisman J, Higuchi CM, Thompson JA, et al. Enhancement by interleukin 4 of interleukin 2 or antibody induced proliferation of lymphocytes from interleukin 2 treated cancer patients. *Cancer Res* 1990; 50: 1160.
731. Trinchieri G, Santoli D. Antiviral activity induced by culturing lymphocytes with tumor derived or virus transformed cells. Enhancement of natural killer cell activity by interferon and antagonistic inhibition of susceptibility of target cells to lysis. *J Exp Med* 1978; 147: 1314.
732. Trinchieri G, Matsumoto Kobayashi M, et al. Response of peripheral blood resting natural killer cells to interleukin-2. *J Exp Med* 1984; 160: 1147.
733. Triozzi P, Martin E, Kim J, et al. Phase Ib trial of interleukin-1β (IL1β)/interleukin-2 (IL2) in patients with metastatic cancer. *Proc Am Soc Clin Oncol* 1993; 12: 290.
734. Tripp CS, Wolf SF, Unanue ER. Interleukin 12 and tumor necrosis factor ∝ are costimulators of interferon γ production by in severe combined immunodeficiency mice with listeriosis and interleukin 10 is a physiologic antagonist. *Proc Nat Acad Sci USA* 1993; 90: 3725-3729.
735. Tsuji K, Nakahata T, Takagi M et al. Effects of interleukin 3 and interleukin 4 on the development of 'connective tissue type' mast cells: interleukin 3 supports their survival and interleukin 4 triggers and supports their proliferation synergistically with interleukin 3. *Blood* 1990; 75: 421-427.
736. Tsukuda M, Mochimatsu I, Sakumodo M, et al. Synergistic effects of Interleukin 2 and interleukin 7 on the proliferation and autologous tumor cell lysis of tumor associated lymphocytes. *Biotherapy* 1993; 6: 167-174.
737. Tsunoda T, Tanimura H, Yamaue H, et al. The promotive effect of interleukin-4 with interleukin-2 in the proliferation of tumor infiltrating lymphocytes from patients with malignant tumor. *Biotherapy* 1992; 4: 9-15.
738. Urba WJ, Clark JW, Steis RG, et al. Intraperitoneal lymphokine-activated killer cell/interleukin-2 therapy in patients with intra-abdominal cancer: immunologic considerations. *J Natl Cancer Inst* 1989; 81: 602.
739. Usui N, Mimnaugh EG, Sinha BK. A role for the

interleukin 1 receptor in the synergistic antitumor effects of human interleukin 1α and etoposide against human melanoma cells. *Cancer Res* 1991; 51: 769-774.

740. Uyttenhove C, Simpson R, Van Snick J. Functional and structural characterization of P40, a mouse glycoprotein with T cell growth factor activity. *Proc Nat Acad Sci USA.* 1988; 85: 6934-6939.
741. Vaccarello L, Wang YL and Whiteside TL. Sustained outgrowth of auto tumor reactive T lymphocytes from human ovarian carcinomas in the presence of tumor necrosis factor α and interleukin 2. *Human Immunology* 1990; 28: 216-227.
742. Valent P, Bevec D, Mauer D et al. Interleukin 4 promotes expression of mast cell ICAM-1 antigen. *Proc Nat Acad Sci USA* 1991; 88: 3339-3342.
743. Valone FH, Gandara DR, Deisseroth A, et al. Interleukin-2 (IL-2) combined with high-dose cisplatin (HDCP) and 5-fluorouracil (5-FU) in metastatic non-small cell lung (NSCLC) and head and neck cancer (meeting abstract). *Proc Annu Meet Am Soc Clin Oncol* 1989; 8: A755.
744. Van De Griend RJ, Krimpen BA, Ranfeltap CPM and Bolhuis RH. Rapidly expanded natural killer cell clones have strong antitumor cell activity and have surface phenotype of either T, non-T, or null cells. *J Immunol* 1984; 132: 3185.
745. Van der Meer JWM, Barza M, Wolff SM, Dinarello CA. A low dose of recombinant interleukin 1 protects granulocytopenic mice from lethal gram-negative infection. *Proc Natl Acad Sci* (USA) 1988; 85: 1620-1623.
746. Van Gameren MM, Willemse PH, Mulder NH, et al. Effects of recombinant human Interleukin-6 in cancer patients: a phase I-II trial. *Blood* 1994; 84: 1431-1441.
747. Van Snick J. Interleukin 6: an overview. *Ann Rev Immunol* 1990; 8: 253-280.
748. Van Snick J, Goethals A, Renauld J-C, et al. Cloning and characterization of cDNA for a new mouse T cell growth factor (P40) *J Exp Med* 1989; 169: 363-368.
749. Viera P, de Waal Malefyt R, Dang M-N, et al. Isolation and expression of human cytokine synthesis inhibitory factor (CSIF/IL-10) cDNA clones: homology to Epstein Barr virus open reading frame BCRFI. *Proc Nat Acad Sci USA* 1991; 88: 1172-1176.
750. Vissinga CS, Fatur-Saunders DJ and Takei F. Dual role of IL-7 in the growth and differentiation of immature thymocytes. *Experimental Hematology* 1992; 20: 998-1003.
751. Vitetta ES, Ohara J, Myers CD, et al. Serological biochemical and functional identity of B cell stimulatory factor-1 and B cell differentiation factor for IgG1. *J Exp Med* 1985; 162: 1726-1731.
752. Vlasveld LT, Rankin EM, Hekman A, et al. A phase I study of prolonged continuous infusion of low dose recombinant interleukin-2 in melanoma and renal cell cancer. Part I: clinical aspects. *Br J Cancer* 1992; 65: 744-750.
753. Vogelzang NJ, Lipton A, Figlin RA. Subcutaneous interleukin-2 plus interferon alfa-2a in metastatic renal cancer: an outpatient multicenter trial. *J Clin Oncol* 1993; 11: 1809-1816.
754. Von Freeden-Jeffrey U, Viera P, Lucian LA, et al. Lymphopenia in interleukin (IL)-7 gene deleted mice identifies IL-7 and a nonredundant cytokine. *J Exp Med* 1995; 181: 1519-26.
755. Voss SD, Hong R, Sondel PM. Severe Combined Immunodeficiency, Interleukin 2 and the IL-2 receptor: experiments in nature continue to point the way. *Blood* 1194; 83: 626-635.
756. Walz A, Peveri P, Aschauer H, Baggiolini M. Purification and amino acid sequencing of NAF, a novel neutrophil activating factor produced by monocytes. *Biochem Biophys Res Commun* 1987; 149: 755.
757. Wang AM, Creasey AA, Ladner MD, et al. Molecular cloning of the complimentary DNA for human tumor necrosis factor. *Science* 1985; 228: 149.
758. Wang YL, Lusheng S, Kanbaul A, et al. Lymphocytes infiltrating human ovarian tumors: Synergy between tumor necrosis factor α and interleukin 2 in the generation of CD8+ effectors from tumor-infiltrating lymphocytes. *Cancer Res* 1989; 49: 5979-5985.
759. Warren HS, Kinnear BF, Phillips JH, Lanier LL. Production of IL-5 by Human NK cells and regulation of IL-5 secretion by IL-4, IL-10, and IL-12. *J Immunol* 1995; 154: 5144-5152.
760. Warren RS, Starnes HF Jr, Gabrilove JL, et al. The acute metabolic effects of tumor necrosis factor administration in human. *Arch Surg* 1987; 122: 1396.
761. Warringa RAJ, Koenderman L, Kok PTM, et al. Modulation and induction of eosinophil chemotaxis by granulocyte macrophage colony stimulating factor and interleukin 3. *Blood* 1991; 77: 2694.
762. Watanabe Y, Kuribayashi K, Miatake S, et al. Exogenous expression of mouse interferon-γ cDNA in mouse neuroblastoma C1300 cells results in reduced tumorigenicity by augmented antitumor immunity. *Proc Natl Acad Sci USA* 1989; 86: 9456-9460.
763. Waterfield MD, Scarce T, Whittle N, et al. Platelet-derived growth factor is structurally related to the putative transforming protein p28SIS of simian sarcoma virus. *Nature* 1983; 304: 34.
764. Weber J, Yang JC, Topalian SL, et al. Phase I trial of subcutaneous interleukin 6 in patients with advanced cancer. *J Clin Oncol* 1993; 11. 499-506.
765. Wei SJ, Liu JH, Blanchard DK, Djeu JY. Induction of IL8 gene expression in polymorphonuclear leukocytes by recombinant IL-2. *J Immunol* 1994; 142: 244.
766. Weil-Hillman G, Fisch P, Prieve AF, et al. Lymphokine-activated killer activity induced by *in vivo* interleukin 2 therapy: predominant role for lymphocytes with increased expression of CD2 and Leu19 antigens but negative expression of CD16 antigens. *Cancer Res* 1989; 49: 3680.
767. Weiner L, Krigel R, Padavic K, et al. Potentiation of interleukin 2 effects by gamma-interferon in a Phase I clinical trial (meeting abstract). *Proc Annu Meet Am Soc Clin Oncol* 1989; 8: A723.
768. Weiss GR, Margolin KA, Sznol M, et al. Phase II study of the continuous infusion of Interleukin 6 for metastatic renal cell carcinoma. J Immunother 1995; 18: 52-56.
769. Welch PA, Namen AE, Goodwin RG, et al. Human IL-7: a novel T cell growth factor. *J Immunol* 1989; 143(11): 3562-3567.
770. Weller PF, Rand TH, Barrett T, et al. Accessory cell function of eosinophils: HLA DR dependent MHC restricted antigen presentation and interleukin 1α formation. *J Immunol* 1993; 150: 2554.
771. Welsh RM, Karre K, Hansson M, et al. Interferon mediated protection of normal and tumor target cells against lysis by mouse natural killer cells. *J Immunol* 1981; 126: 219-225.

772. Welte K, Chang YW, Mertelsmann R, et al. Purification of human interleukin-2 to apparent homogeneity and its molecular heterogeneity. *J Exp Med* 1982; 156: 435.
773. West WH, Tauer KW, Yannelli JR, et al. Constant infusion recombinant interleukin-2 in adoptive immunotherapy of advanced cancer. *N Engl J Med* 1987; 316: 898.
774. Widmer M. Grabstein K. Regulation of cytolytic T-lymphocyte generation by B cell stimulatory factor 1. *Nature* 1987; 326: 795-798.
775. Widmer M. Acres R, Sassenfeld H, Grabstein K. Regulation of cytolytic cell populations from human peripheral blood by B cell stimulatory factor 1 (interleukin 4). *J Exp Med* 1987; 166: 1447.
776. Widmer MB, Morrissey PJ, Namen AE, et al. Interleukin 7 stimulates the growth of fetal thymic precursors of cytolytic cells: induction of effector function by interleukin 2 and inhibition by interleukin 4. *Int Immunol* 1990; 2: 1055-1061.
777. Williams DE, Eisenman J, Baird A, et al. Identification of a ligand for the c-kit proto-oncogene *Cell* 1990; 63: 167-174.
778. Williams DE, Morrissey PJ, Mochizuki DY, et al. T cell growth factor P40 promotes the proliferation of myeloid cell lines and enhances erythroid burst formation by normal murine bone marrow cells *in vitro*. *Blood* 1990; 76: 906-911.
779. Williams N, Eger RR, Jackson HN, et al. Two factor requirement for murine megakaryocyte colony formation. *J Cell Physiol* 1982; 110: 101.
780. Williamson BD, Carswell EA, Rubin BY, et al. Human tumor necrosis factor produced by human B cell lines. Synergistic cytotoxic interaction with human interferon γ. *Proc Nat Acad Sci USA* 1983; 80: 5397-5401.
781. Wilson AB, Harris JM, Coomb RRA. Interleukin 2 induction of interferon gamma by resting human T cells and large granular lymphocytes: requirement for accessory factors including interleukin-1. *Cellular Immunology* 1988; 113: 130.
782. Witmer-Pack MD, Olivier W, Valinsky J, et al. Granulocyte/macrophage colony stimulating factor is essential for the viability and function of cultured murine epidermal Langerhans cells. *J Exp Med* 1987; 166: 1484.
783. Wolf SF, Sieburth D, Sypek J. Interleukin 12: A key modulator of immune response. *Stem Cells* 1994; 12: 154-168.
784. Wolf SF, Temple PA, Kobayashi M, et al. Cloning of cDNA for natural killer cell stimulatory factor, a heterodimeric cytokine with multiple biologic effects on T and natural killer cells. *J Immunol* 1991; 146: 3074-3081.
785. Wright SD, Ramos RA, Tobias PS, et al. CD14, a receptor for complexes of lipopolysaccharide (LPS) and LPS binding protein. *Science* 1990; 249: 1431.
786. Wu C, Demeure C, Kiniwa M, et al. IL-12 induces production of IFN-γ by neonatal human CD4 T cells. *J Immunol* 1993; 151: 1938-1949.
787. Wu S, Boyer CM, Whittaker RS, et al. Tumor necrosis factor as an autocrine and paracrine growth factor for ovarian cancer: Monokine induction of tumor cell proliferation and tumor necrosis factor alpha production. *Cancer Res* 1993; 53: 1939.
788. Yaden Y, Kuang WS, Yang-Feng T, et al. Human proto-oncogene C kit, a new cell surface receptor tyrosine kinase for an unidentified ligand. *EMBO J* 1987; 6: 3341-3351.
789. Yang YC, Riccaciardi S, Ciarletta A, et al. Expression cloning of a cDNA encoding a novel human hematopoietic growth factor: Human homologue of murine T cell growth factor P40. *Blood* 1989; 74: 1880-1884.
790. Yamagushi Y, Suda T, Suda J, et al. Purified Interleukin 5 supports the terminal differentiation and proliferation of purified eosinophil precursors. *J Exp Med* 1988; 167: 43.
791. Yamasaki K, Taga T, Hirata Y, et al. Cloning and expression of the human interleukin 6 (BSF-2/IFN beta 2) receptor. *Science* 1988; 241: 825-828.
792. Yasamura S, Lin WC, Weidemann E, et al. Expression of interleukin 2 receptors on human carcinoma cell lines and tumor growth inhibition by interleukin-2. *Int J Cancer* 1994; 59: 225-234.
793. Yasumoto K, Miyazaki K, Nagashima A, et al. Induction of lymphokine-activated killer cells by intrapleural instillations of recombinant interleukin-2 in patients with malignant pleurisy due to lung cancer. *Cancer Res* 1987; 47: 2184.
794. Yokota T, Arai N, DeVries et al. Molecular biology of interleukin 4 and interleukin 5 genes and biology of their products that stimulate B cells, T cells and hematopoietic cells. *Immunol Rev* 1988; 102: 137-187.
795. Yokota T, Coffman RL, Hagiwara H, et al. Isolation and characterization of lymphokine cDNA clones encoding mouse and human IgA-enhancing factor eosinophil colony-stimulating activities: relationship to interleukin 5. *Proc Natl Sci* (USA) 1987; 84: 7388-7392.
796. Yousefi S, Hemmann S, Weber M, et al. IL-8 is expressed by human peripheral blood eosinophils. Evidence for increased secretion in asthma. *J Immunol* 1995; 154: 5481-5490.
797. Yssel H, Schneider PV, Lanier LL. Interleukin 7 specifically induces the B7/BB1 antigen on human cord blood and peripheral blood T cells and T cell clones. *Int Immunol* 1993; 5: 753-759.
798. Yu JS, Wei MX, Chjiocca A, et al. Treatment of glioma with engineered interleukin 4 secreting cells. *Cancer Res* 1993; 53: 3125-3128.
799. Zhang JZ, Maruyama K, Iwatsuki K, Kaneko F. Regulatory effects of 1, 25-dihydroxyvitamin D3 and a novel Vitamin D3 analog MC903 on secretion of interleukin 1 alpha (IL-1 alpha) and IL-8 by normal human keratinocytes and a human squamous cell carcinoma cell line (HSC-1). *J Dermatological Sci* 1994; 7: 24-31.
800. Zhou A, Hassel BA, Silverman RH. Expression cloning of 2-5A-dependent RNAase: A uniquely regulated mediator of interferon action. *Cell* 1993; 72: 753-765.
801. Zimmerman RJ, Aukerman SL, Young JD, et al. Schedule dependency of antitumor activity and toxicity of polyethylene glycol-modified IL-2 murine tumors (meeting abstract). *Proc Annu Meet Am Assoc Cancer Res* 1989; 30: A1435.
802. Zitrogel L, Tahara H, Robbins PD, et al. Cancer immunotherapy of established tumors with IL12. Effective delivery by genetically engineered fibroblasts. *J Immunol* 1995; 155: 1393-1403.
803. Zoltnik A, Fisher M, Roehm N, and Zipori D. Evidence for effects of (B cell stimulatory factor 1) on macrophages: enhancement of antigen presenting ability of bone marrow derived macrophages. *J Immunol* 1987; 138: 4275.
804. Zoltnick A, Ransom J, Frank G, et al. Interleukin 4 is a

growth factor for activated thymocytes: possible role in T cell ontogeny. *Proc Nat Acad Sci USA* 1987; 84: 3856.

805. Zsebo KM, Wypych J, McNiece IK, et al. Identification characterization and biological characterization of hematopoietic stem cell factor form Buffalo rat liver conditioned medium. *Cell* 1990; 63: 195-210.
806. Zsebo KM, Williams DA, Geissler EN, et al. Stem cell factor is encoded at the S1 locus of the mouse and is the ligand for the c-kit tyrosine kinase receptor. *Cell* 1990; 63: 312-224.
807. Zubiaga AM, Munoz E, Huber BT. IL-2 and IL-4 selectively rescue Th cell subsets from glucocorticoid induced apoptosis. *J Immunol* 1992; 149: 107-112.
808. Zukiwski AA, Itoh K, Benjamin R, et al. Pilot study of rIL-2 administered with a murine anti-melanoma antibody in patients with metastatic melanoma (meeting abstract). *Proc Annu Meet Am Assoc Cancer Res* 1989; 30: A1448.
809. Zurawski G, de Vries JE. Interleukin 13, an interleukin 4 like cytokine that acts on monocytes and B cells but not T cells. *Immunol Today* 1994; 15: 19-29.
810. Zurawski G, de Vries JE. Interleukin 13 elicits a subset of the activities of its close relative interleukin 4. *Stem Cells* 1994; 12: 169-174.
811. Zurawski SM, Vega F, Huyghe B, Zurawski G. Receptors for interleukin 13 and interleukin 4 are complex and share a novel component that functions in signal transduction. *EMBO* 1993; 12: 3899-3905.

INTERFERONS: THERAPY IN CANCER

RICHARD V. SMALLEY[1], DAVID GOLDSTEIN[2] and ERNEST C. BORDEN[3]
[1] *Synertron, Inc., Madison, Wisconsin,* [2] *Centre for Immunology, Sydney, Australia*
[3] *University of Maryland Cancer Center, Baltimore, Maryland*

> Stimulate the phagocytes. Drugs are a delusion. Find the germ of the disease; prepare from it a suitable antitoxin; inject it three times a day, a quarter of an hour before meals and what is the result? The phagocytes are stimulated; they devour the disease and the patient recovers-unless, of course, he's too far gone.
>
> Sir Ralph Bloomfield Bonnington
> in The Doctors Dilemma
> George Bernard Shaw, 1902

Isaacs and Lindemann, in England, first characterized interferon (IFN) in 1957 and coined the word to signify a protein, elaborated by virus-infected cells, that functions to prevent their infection by a second virus [82]. However, difficulties with chemical isolation and characterization led to great skepticism about the molecule's existence; indeed, 'the scientific community dubbed the discovery "imaginon"' [141].

Time and effort have proven Isaacs and Lindemann right. Interferons are now a well characterized group of proteins. They are a large family of four major immunological types, alpha, beta, gamma, and omega [147]. The alpha and beta interferons were collectively known as the type I interferons while gamma interferon was referred to as type II interferon. There are multiple natural alpha interferon molecules and one natural beta interferon molecule. These type I interferons share a common receptor which is present on nearly all cells in the body. The alpha interferons, originally derived from leucocytes, and beta interferon, originally derived from fibroblasts, are actually secreted by nearly all mammalian cells. Even though they share a common receptor, their activation pathway must differ since the transfection of the human type I receptor gene into murine cells allows alpha but not beta expression [203]. Gamma interferon, on the other hand, is produced by T lymphocytes upon specific antigen recognition. All interferon molecules have antiviral and antiproliferative capacity, and to some extent immunomodulatory activity, although gamma is a stronger immunomodulatory molecule than the type I interferons.

NOMENCLATURE

Alpha interferon is produced following viral stimulation. There are at least fourteen subtypes of alpha interferon, each immunologically related but differing by a number of amino acids [220]. Several nomenclature systems exist for identifying these subtypes. The two commonly used, but unrelated, systems use either lettering A, B, C, D, etc., or numbering 1, 2, 3, etc. to define thc subtypes. A newer proposal, approved by the Nomenclature Committee of the International Society for Interferon Research, has been recently published [147]. A corresponding proposal for nomenclature of the interferon-gene induced proteins is in press.

Three natural alpha interferon pharmaceutical products are currently available for use in patients in various countries in the world. The original Finnish Red Cross partially purified material developed by Cantell and subsequently also produced by others from the buffy coat of peripheral blood is available as Finnferon® in some European countries. A highly purified natural alpha interferon produced by virally stimulated human lymphoma (Namalva) cells has been produced in pharmacologic quantity by Burroughs Wellcome Co (now Glaxo Wellcome) and is known by the trade name Wellferon®. It is marketed in Japan, Canada, Mexico and Europe but not the United States for treatment of hairy cell leukemia (HCL) and some viral disorders. Alferon N® is an aqueous formulation of human alpha interferon proteins with a specific activity of $2x10^8$ IU/mg of protein and is manufactured in the United States by the Purdue Frederick Company. It has been approved in the United States for the intralesional treatment of refractory or recurring external condylomata acuminata in patients over eighteen years of age. These natural alpha interferons contain most, if not all, of the multiple alpha molecules.

In addition to the natural alpha interferon products, there are several pure single alpha molecules obtained by recombinant technology that are available for clinical use. Interferon alpha A (alpha 2) has been pharmacologically produced as recombinant alpha interferon by three companies, Hoffman-LaRoche in Nutley, NJ, Schering Corporation based in Kenilworth, NJ, and Boehringer Ingelheim in Germany. These products are known as

R.K. Oldham (ed.), Principles of Cancer Biotherapy. 3rd ed., 266–283.

Roferon A® (rIFN alfa 2a), Intron A® (rIFN alfa 2b) and Berofor® (rIFN alfa 2c), respectively. The alpha subtype, interferon alpha C (alpha 10) has been produced in pharmacologic quantity in Israel. Roferon A® is manufactured by Roche Laboratories using recombinant DNA technology employing a genetically engineered E coli bacteria containing an interferon alpha 2 gene obtained from a human myeloid leukemia cell line; it has an approximate MW of 19, 000 daltons and a specific activity of 2 x 10^8 IU/mg protein and is approved for use in the United States for the treatment of HCL and AIDS-related Kaposi's sarcoma in patients 18 years of age or older. Intron® A is produced by Schering Corporation and is obtained from the bacterial fermentation of a strain of E coli which bears a genetically engineered plasmid containing an interferon alpha 2 gene from human leukocytes. It has a specific activity of 2 x 10^8 IU/mg protein and is approved in the United States for treatment of patients 18 years of age or older with HCL and for selected patients with condylomata acuminata, AIDS related Kaposi's sarcoma, chronic hepatitis non-A, non-B/C and with chronic hepatitis B.

A recombinant IFN beta, with a single amino acid substitution separating it from the natural beta molecule, was developed by Triton Biosciences, Inc., Berkeley, CA, and is currently manufactured by Berlex and marketed by Chiron Corporation (US) and Schering AG (Germany) under the trade name Betaseron® for treatment of multiple sclerosis. It is obtained by bacterial fermentation of a strain of E coli that bears a genetically engineered plasmid containing the altered gene for human interferon beta. The native gene was obtained from human fibroblasts and altered in a way that substitutes serine for the cysteine residue found in position 17 in the native molecule (interferon $beta_{ser}17$). The recombinant protein is a highly purified molecule with 165 amino acids, a MW of approximately 18, 500 daltons and a specific activity of approximately 32 MU/mg protein; it does not include the carbohydrate side chains found in the native molecule. Betaseron® is approved in the United States for the treatment of ambulatory patients with relapsing-remitting multiple sclerosis. Biogen, Inc has produced a recombinant molecule from the natural beta interferon gene which, since it is produced in eukaryotic cells, is glycosylated. This product, with the trade name Avonex®, has recently been approved in the US for treatment of relapsing forms of multiple sclerosis. Serono also has a beta interferon molecule undergoing clinical trials in Europe and Canada.

Two recombinant gamma interferon molecules have been cloned and clinically developed, one by Genentech, Inc., and one by Biogen, Inc. These will be referred to, respectively, as rIFN gamma (Genentech) with a trade name of Actimmune® and rIFN gamma (Biogen) with a trade name of Immuneron™. Actimmune® is manufactured by bacterial fermentation of a strain of E coli containing the DNA which encodes for the human gamma interferon molecule. It has a specific activity of 30 million units/mg protein, and is approved for clinical use in the United States for reducing the frequency and severity of serious infections associated with chronic granulomatous disease. Immuneron™ is not yet approved for prescription use in the US.

These various products are listed in Table 1. The generic designations will be used throughout this chapter.

Table 1. Interferon nomenclature

IFN	Generic	Trade name
Natural Alpha Interferon		
Cantell IFN	IFN alfa (Le)	Finnferon®
Lymphoblastoid	IFN alfa N1	Wellferon®
Leukocyte Derived	IFN alfa N3	Alferon N®
Recombinant Alpha Interferon		
Alpha A	rIFN alfa 2a	Roferon A®
Alpha A	rIFN alfa 2b	Intron A®
Alpha A	rIFN alfa 2c	Berofor®
Alpha C	rIFN alfa 10	
Recombinant Beta Interferon		
	rIFN beta 1B	Betaseron®
	rIFN beta (Biogen)	Avonex®
Recombinant Gamma Interferon		
	rIFN gamma (Genentech)	Actimmune®
	rIFN gamma (Biogen)	Immuneron™

CLINICAL USE

In the early 1970s, work by Kari Cantell and co-workers led to the production of sufficient quantities of alpha interferon, made from buffy cell layers, to support limited clinical trials in patients with several types of malignancies [37, 189, 190]. This work was expanded in North America by the U.S. National Cancer Institute (NCI) which sponsored trials beginning in 1975 and by the American Cancer Society (ACS) which supported trials beginning in 1978. Despite very limited clinical information, interferon was heralded in the popular press at the time as a significant new drug for the cure of cancer. The early clinical trials with this partially purified natural alpha interferon demonstrated responses in breast cancer, osteosarcoma and lymphoma, comparable to those achievable with chemotherapeutic agents. The wave of enthusiasm and outpouring of venture capital rapidly led to the development of DNA recombinant technology and, following the successful cloning in 1979 by Taniguchi et al. of beta-interferon [196] and the subsequent cloning of the alpha interferon subtypes and gamma interferon, the production of recombinant interferon molecules. Furthermore, the isolation and purification of natural alpha Interferon from Namalva cell cultures led to far greater availability of natural alpha interferon and the number of clinical trials increased dramatically.

The partially purified IFN alfa (Le), used in the early trials sponsored by the NCI and ACS, had a relatively low specific activity and, since it was a supernate, was composed of not only a variety of subtypes of alpha interferon but multiple other cytokines as well. Gutterman et al. [73] and Borden et al. [15], working with patients with breast cancer in the US, and Einhorn et al. [37], working with patients with ovarian carcinoma in Scandinavia, reported response rates of over 20% using this natural alpha interferon product. These results have not been reproduced in these tumors using rIFN alfa 2a or 2b, raising the question of what other active constituent(s) in this interferon preparation may have induced these responses.

B CELL MALIGNANCY

Several B cell malignancies have been shown to be therapeutically sensitive to alpha interferon. Multiple myeloma and non-Hodgkin's lymphoma (NHL) were among the first malignancies to respond in the early trials with the Cantell interferon. Although multiple clinical trials have been performed in patients with both diseases demonstrating activity in these disorders, interferon has not yet been approved in any country for use in these two malignancies. Hairy cell leukemia (HCL) was shown in the early 1980's to be exquisitely sensitive to alpha interferon and this biologic was rapidly approved in most countries for the treatment of this previously untreatable malignancy.

Hairy cell leukemia

Hairy cell leukemia, a B cell malignancy, is a disease with an exquisite sensitivity to alpha interferon and was the first human malignancy to be so identified. Prior to the development of the interferons, no adequate therapy existed for this relatively rare disorder. Splenectomy was the standard approach when treatment was necessary and was useful for controlling pancytopenia for a period of time but had no effect on the leukemic process. Quesada was the first to demonstrate the beneficial effect of alpha interferon in this disease in 1982 [153]. After finding that a dose of 12 MU/m^2 was poorly tolerated, he and his colleagues at the MD Anderson Cancer Center, arbitrarily settled on a regimen of 3 MU (1 MU=10^6 units) administered daily subcutaneously. Several other investigators followed suit and have shown that high response rates are attainable with the potential for a prolonged response duration, even with lower doses. Seventy-five to 80 per cent of patients will obtain major clinical benefit with improvement in hematologic parameters and a decrease in the leukemic (tumor cell) population. Treatment of several months duration is required for maximal benefit and continued treatment is necessary to maintain clinical benefit. Equivalent efficacy has been shown with each of the alpha interferon products and with beta interferon [54, 58, 59, 64, 65, 66, 152, 180, 216, 217, 218]. Gamma interferon is ineffective in this disease [155].

Following Quesada's lead, multiple studies by Golomb et al at the University of Chicago, established an objective anti-leukemic response (CR or PR) rate of 20-25% and an improvement in hematologic parameters in another 60% for an overall major clinical benefit in 80-85% of patients [64-66]. Following cessation of therapy, patients relapsed but remission could be successfully reinduced [64, 154]. The studies by the groups at MD Anderson and the University of Chicago with recombinant alpha interferon led to the approval of alpha interferon in the United States for the treatment of HCL. A significant cost benefit associated with interferon treatment was demonstrated [140] and additional studies with natural alpha interferon demonstrated its superiority over splenectomy, the inadequate standard of therapy prior to the development of alpha interferon [181].

During the mid 1980's, investigators in Innsbruck began to explore the question of dose effect in patients with HCL and determined that a dose as low as 0.5 MU (500, 000 U) was biologically active and immunologically stimulating, as measured by the production of neopterin [53, 80]. They treated a series of patients with either the 'standard' 2 MU/m^2 dose or the low but immunologically stimulating dose of 0.2-0.6 MU/m^2 rIFN alfa 2c daily for 2-3 months followed by less frequent administration [54]. Both doses were effective, but the lower dose was less toxic. The Wellcome HCL study group, using IFN alfa N1, followed this lead and in a prospectively randomized trial compared a low dose, 0.2 MU/m^2, with the standard dose of 2.0 MU/m^2 [180]. The low dose was shown to be as effective as the standard dose in inducing a return to normal of the platelet count (within 36-38 days median) and of the neutrophil count (within 90-130 days median), as well as reducing the need for red cell transfusion support and the incidence of infection. The standard dose, however, was clinically and statistically more effective in its antileukemic effect, i.e., reducing hairy cell infiltration in the marrow. Following six months of therapy, 46% of patients treated with the standard dose had achieved a 50% reduction in infiltration (17% – CR) compared with 25% of patients treated with the low dose (6% – CR) (p=.06 two-tailed Fisher's exact test). Significant drug related toxicity (cardiac, neurologic, neutropenia) occurred in five patients receiving the standard dose and in none receiving the low dose [180].

These studies suggest that a low readily tolerable dose of alpha interferon is biologically and clinically effective but leave open the question of whether or not a less well tolerated higher dose is more efficacious clinically and worth the added financial and side effect cost. The answer, in patients with HCL, is now moot; alpha interferon has been supplanted by cladribine and pentostatin as the treatment of choice, just one decade after it was shown to be the first effective systemic agent for the treatment of this disease.

Multiple myeloma

Interest in the treatment of multiple myeloma with alpha interferon was initially stimulated by the pilot studies of Mellstedt et al. in 1979 and the ACS-supported trial reported in 1980 [115, 136]. Each study demonstrated objective anti-tumor responses in a small number of previously heavily treated patients. A number of phase II trials of both natural and recombinant alpha interferon were subsequently performed and cumulatively suggested that about 20% of patients with multiple myeloma, refractory to cytotoxic chemotherapy, might obtain an objective response to a variety of doses and schedules [21, 27, 29, 30, 129, 130, 151, 213]. Because of these encouraging results in previously treated patients, alpha interferon was compared with cytotoxic chemotherapy in previously untreated patients but chemotherapy proved superior in terms of both response rate and duration of response [4, 103].

Several trials were organized to evaluate the addition of alpha interferon to various combinations of cytotoxic chemotherapy in terms of response induction [28, 102, 131, 132, 137, 168]. The CALGB in the United States evaluated the feasibility of adding a recombinant alpha interferon administered three times a week for the first two weeks of each 28 day cycle to melphalan/prednisone and found the combination tolerable [28]. A large Swedish trial involving over 300 patients evaluated the addition of IFN alfa (Le) administered on days 1-5 and days 22-26 of every four-week cycle to melphalan/prednisone which were given on days 1-4 and demonstrated a benefit in overall response and survival for patients with either IgA or Bence-Jones myeloma but not IgG myeloma [137]. This study was the third in a series of trials performed by this group that demonstrated a clinical benefit from this natural alpha interferon in patients with IgA myeloma. The explanation for benefit only for patients with IgA myeloma in this series of trials is not apparent since other trials have not demonstrated benefit isolated to this specific subset of patients. A substantially smaller trial (33 pts) has also shown no advantage for alpha interferon when added to standard chemotherapy but this trial, even though randomized, evaluated too few patients and cannot be used to rule out added benefit [168]. A multinational group headquartered in Vienna has recently reported on their evaluation of VMCP with or without alpha interferon. Two hundred forty patients were randomized; there was no difference in response rate but fewer patients receiving interferon progressed and the median duration of response was six months longer (12.4 months vs 18.3 months, p<02) for patients receiving alpha interferon [102]. The ECOG has piloted and then prospectively evaluated the addition of alpha interferon to a five drug combination (VBMCP) [131, 132]. There was a trend (six months) towards increased time to progression with rIFN alfa 2 but this was not statistically significant (P=.08).

None of these studies by themselves has yet demonstrated a major clinical advantage with the addition of interferon. However, in this era of meta analyses, Ludwig et al performed a global analysis, including the above mentioned studies (except the ECOG studies) and nine smaller ones, evaluating a total of 1, 518 randomized patients and concluded there was a slight (9.5%) advantage to interferon in terms of response rate [102]. However, any advantage of adding interferon to induction chemotherapy in this disease is too small to be clinically meaningful and is probably not worth the added financial or side effect cost. The Swedish studies leave open to further exploration the persistent intriguing observation of the possible benefits of natural leukocyte alpha interferon in patients with IgA/Bence-Jones myeloma.

Several trials were next established to evaluate the use of alpha interferon as a maintenance agent in patients with myeloma. Following the induction of a response with cytotoxic chemotherapy, various groups randomized patients to receive alpha interferon or no further therapy until the onset of progressive disease [17, 102, 107, 108, 109, 145, 167, 215]. In addition, the Nordic Study Group randomized patients at the start of treatment; those randomized to receive alpha interferon received it continuously [125]. These studies are summarized in Table 2. The US cooperative group trial and the trial in

Table 2. Alpha Interferon maintenance therapy. Multiple myeloma

Author/Reference		# Patients	Duration of response	OS	Dose/ Schedule
Salmon	(167)	193	neg	neg	3 MU tiw
Browman	(17)	177	+	+	2 MU/m^2 tiw
Westin	(215)	120	+	TE	5 MU tiw
Mandelli	(109)	101	+	neg	3 MU/m^2 tiw
Ludwig	(102)	95	+	neg	2 MU tiw
Peest	(145)	71	neg	neg	5 MU tiw
Nordic Group	(125)	583	+	neg	5 MU tiw

TE = Too early.

Germany showed no benefit from interferon therapy. The other five trials have demonstrated either a prolonged time to progression or duration of plateau phase in the interferon maintained group; although two of these were initially reported to have shown benefit on overall survival for patients receiving interferon, a recent update of the Italian study indicates the benefit on survival has been lost [9]. Ludwig et al performed a global analysis for these maintenance studies also and concluded that alpha interferon used as maintenance therapy improves both time to treatment progression (TTP) and overall survival [102].

Very recently, a multi-institutional group in London, England, has been evaluating the effect of maintenance alpha interferon, administered at a dose of 3 MU/m^2 subcutaneous tiw, in a prospectively randomized trial following induction chemotherapy with C-VAMP, then high dose melphalan consolidation with bone marrow transplant rescue, comparing interferon with no maintenance treatment. rIFN alfa 2b has had a beneficial effect on prolonging remission, especially in those patients who achieve a complete remission, and in improving survival, especially in patients with low tumor burden [32].

In summary, alpha interferon is an active agent in myeloma. Current data support its greatest usefulness when used as an agent capable of prolonging remission in patients with low tumor burden; in some of these patients it may also improve survival.

Non-Hodgkin's lymphoma (NHL)

Several clinical trials conducted in the late 1970's with the Cantell interferon suggested efficacy in patients with low and, to a lesser extent, intermediate grade NHL [73, 79, 100, 116]. Single agent trials in the 1980's with the more highly purified recombinant and natural alpha interferons confirmed the efficacy of alpha interferon in patients with NHL [46, 95, 127].

Two single institutions and the CALGB, in three separate trials, combined alpha interferon with an alkylating agent in patients with low grade NHL and demonstrated the combination to be relatively non-toxic and well tolerated. The combination induced a response in 50-75% of patients, more readily in previously untreated individuals [22, 23, 24, 139]. There are currently ongoing randomized trials in patients with low grade NHL evaluating, by direct comparison, the addition of alpha interferon to cytotoxic chemotherapy in the initial treatment of the disease.

The group at MD Anderson, in a single institution non-randomized study, evaluated the use of IFN alfa N1 as maintenance therapy, inducing a response with CHOP plus Bleomycin and then treating patients with IFN alfa N1 until relapse [112]. They concluded, based on historical controls, that alpha interferon prolonged the duration of response but did not improve survival. A prospectively randomized trial, by the EORTC in Europe, has evaluated the use of alpha interferon as maintenance therapy and has also demonstrated a prolongation of response duration [74]. Data are not mature enough to indicate whether survival will be effected. The group at St. Bart's in London, long a leader in evaluating and pursuing new treatments in patients with hematologic malignancy, has conducted a study which randomized patients at two points in the treatment cycle [150]. Slightly over 200 patients were entered on trial. Initially, in this three institution study, patients with low grade lymphoma were randomized between chlorambucil and chlorambucil plus alpha interferon. Patients achieving a response were again randomized between maintenance therapy with alpha interferon and no further treatment. Thus, three of the four subsets received interferon, one in induction, one for maintenance, and the third for both. An interim evaluation reported in 1991, which combined all patients receiving alpha interferon (three groups) and compared them to the single non-interferon group, demonstrated a statistically significant benefit of alpha interferon on duration of response [150]. A final analysis was recently reported following closure of accrual and indicated that only patients achieving a CR (about 25% of patients) benefitted, in terms of length of remission, from interferon maintenance [161]. An intergroup study in the United States (CALGB and ECOG), a larger study with a similar design to the St. Bart study (except for the use of cyclophosphamide instead of chlorambucil), has recently closed to accession. A preliminary analysis evaluating the effect of alpha interferon on the response rate showed no benefit, but longer follow up is necessary before a conclusion can be reached regarding the effect on duration of response and survival [146].

There have been two large prospectively randomized trials performed by cooperative groups in the United States and Europe evaluating the effect of alpha interferon added to four-drug induction cytotoxic chemotherapy [179, 184]. Both trials added alpha interferon to a CHOP-like induction regimen; the Group d'Etude des Lymphomes Folliculaires (GELF) treated only patients with follicular lymphoma but with bulky (>7 cm) disease while the ECOG in the United States studied patients with bulky or symptomatic low grade and intermediate grade NHL. The ECOG used cyclophosphamide, Oncovin®, prednisone and Adriamycin® (COPA) as the chemotherapy regimen, administering alpha interferon for five days (D22-26) of every 28 day cycle for a total of 8-10 months. The GELF used cyclophosphamide, VM 26, prednisone and Adriamycin® monthly for six months and then every two months for an additional twelve months giving alpha interferon three times a week for the entire 18 months. Although the two trials were very similar in design, there were some important differences. Both groups treated patients with bulky, symptomatic disease, all follicular lymphoma in one, and follicular and diffuse in the other while the aggressiveness and length of treatment with both chemotherapy and alpha interferon was different. The GELF demonstrated a better response rate in the group receiving interferon, but had an unusually low response rate in the chemotherapy-only arm. Both studies demonstrated an improved duration of response and time to treatment failure and an improved overall survival. The initial ECOG publication reported an improvement in survival but a subsequent analysis a year later, although demonstrating a consistent 10% increase in survival over a five year period, did not show statistical significance [8]. The GELF has demonstrated a 17% improvement in survival over a three year period which was statistically significant and remains so following an updated analysis in 1995 [26].

In addition to these reported trials, Gams et al. conducted a phase II trial with IFN alfa N1 in previously treated patients with low and intermediate grade lymphoma including diffuse histiocytic lymphoma (DHL), and demonstrated a response in 30-40% of patients in all histologic subsets. This study has been reported only in abstract form but has been fully analyzed. Some patients, more commonly those with DHL, required a change in dose and schedule to 30 MU/m^2 by continuous IV infusion for 10 days in order to obtain a response [49, 50]. It is not clear whether these patients with previously resistant (to alpha interferon therapy) disease responded because of increased dose or continuous schedule. VanderMolen et al. [204], in a study often cited as evidence against a dose response effect of alpha interferon in patients with NHL, randomized patients between 50 MU/m^2 twice a week and 3 MU/m^2 daily and documented seven responses in 20 patients receiving the high intermittent dose and three responses in 19 patients receiving the low daily dose. There was no statistical difference in these response rates. Others have cited this trial as documentation that schedule and dose are immaterial, a conclusion that is not warranted (and was not proposed by the authors) because of the very small numbers of patients. The question of influence of dose and schedule remains unanswered by these two small studies.

Alpha interferon is an active therapeutic agent in patients with NHL, low and intermediate grade, but its role has yet to be clarified. Optimal dose and schedule have yet to be defined and the question of whether higher, less tolerable doses are needed for maximal effect remains unanswered. Additionally, alpha interferon may be most active in patients with lower tumor burdens, i.e. with or following CHOP-like regimens. That daily administration of interferon may be therapeutically superior to intermittent has been suggested and has preclinical support. Assuming a currently planned meta analysis of the effect of alpha interferon in patients with NHL demonstrates efficacy [162], further studies will be needed to define the best dose and schedule and when to use interferon in the treatment of this disease.

Table 3. Randomized IFN/CT studies in NHL

Group/Reference		Chemotherapy	Interferon effect	
			Dur of resp	Survival
		4-Drug		
ECOG	(179,8)	CHOP	+	–
GELF	(184,26)	CVPA	+	+
		3-Drug		
EORTC	(74)	COP	+	TE
		1-Drug		
St. Bart's	(150,161)	C	+	neg
CALGB	(146)	C	neg	neg

TE = Too early.

Chronic myeloid leukemia (CML)

Talpaz et al at MD Anderson have pioneered the use of alpha interferon as treatment for CML [194]. They have conducted a series of uncontrolled trials over the past 13 years which initially demonstrated alpha interferon's ability to control leucocytosis and subsequently demonstrated alpha interferon's unique ability to reduce the size of the Ph^1 positive clone and to induce a clinical and histologic CR. Large multi-institutional randomized trials are now demonstrating the superior benefits of alpha interferon compared to cytotoxic treatment and have established it as the treatment of choice for patients with CML who are not eligible for a bone marrow transplant.

Based upon the demonstration of *in vitro* antiproliferative activity of alpha interferon against CFUs, [12, 122, 133, 156], Talpaz and co-investigators initiated a series of trials in the early 1980's of partially purified alpha interferon in patients with CML and demonstrated not only good hematologic control (which was also achievable with cytotoxic therapy) but also suggested that alpha interferon might decrease the size of the malignant clone, the Ph^1 positive cells in the marrow [192, 194, 195]. Such an effect had met with only limited success using aggressive cytotoxic chemotherapy [182]. They demonstrated that excellent control of leucocytosis, splenomegaly, and clinical symptoms is achievable in over 80% of patients with a complete peripheral blood hematologic response (CHR) in 70%. These results have subsequently been confirmed by Talpaz, et al. and others using the recombinant alpha interferon molecules [6, 123, 138, 191]. Patients most likely to respond are those previously untreated who are first treated with interferon within a year of diagnosis.

Their initial observation that alpha interferon could reduce the size of the malignant clone of cells has now been confirmed; treatment with alpha interferon reduces the number of Ph^1 positive cells in over half of the responding patients with about 20% of patients obtaining a conversion to a cytogenetically normal marrow, confirmed by molecular studies [219]. This is a true pathologic CR. The mechanism by which alpha interferon achieves these results is unknown but the supposition is that alpha interferon has a greater antiproliferative effect against the Ph[1] positive clone than against the normal marrow stem cells and restores a favorable growth advantage to the non-malignant cells. Of unknown significance is the observation that treatment with alpha interferon, as in HCL, causes down regulation of the alpha interferon receptor [10, 163]. There is the suggestion that down regulation occurs to a greater degree in those obtaining a CHR [10].

A prospectively randomized study from Italy first demonstrated alpha interferon's superiority over hydroxyurea [202]. A recently reported, prospectively randomized study by the German CML Study Group has confirmed alpha interferon as the treatment of choice [75, 76]. This study compared the use of IFN alfa 2a, given at a daily dose of up to 9 MU SC, with standard cytotoxic chemotherapy, either busulfan or hydroxyurea. The number of patients with a reduction in the Ph[1] positive clone and the time to progression to accelerated or blast crises were both increased in the interferon group compared to either cytotoxic agent. The overall survival of patients was superior in the group of patients treated with alpha interferon therapy but statistical significance was demonstrable only when interferon was compared to busulfan. This high daily dose was poorly tolerated, however, and 16% of patients had to discontinue alpha interferon therapy. The financial cost of interferon therapy was also substantially higher than for chemotherapy.

These results have been confirmed by a multi-institutional study group in Japan [128]. In this study, newly diagnosed patients with CML in chronic phase were randomized to receive either alpha Interferon or busulfan. Although a complete cytogenetic response occurred in two patients receiving busulfan (not previously noted with this agent), there was a statistically and clinically significant difference in favor of alpha interferon in terms of major cytogenetic response (13 of 80 patients) and in predicted five-year survival rate. Additionally, a UK study using a different approach demonstrated superiority of alpha interferon over no maintenance therapy after induction of a response by either busulfan or hydroxyurea [7].

The question of dose and schedule of alpha interferon and its effect on cytogenetic response has not been directly addressed. A dose of 5 MU/m^2 tiw was shown to be more effective than a dose of 2 MU/m^2 tiw on hematologic response; increasing the higher dose to a daily schedule improved the hematologic response rate still further [6]. Although their studies were uncontrolled, the MD Anderson group has amassed a significant amount of experience and believe that relatively high doses, administered daily, are required for maximum beneficial effect [84]. However, a number of their patients require dose reduction because of lassitude, neurologic problems and/or thrombocytopenia and neutropenia. An uncontrolled, small study has recently been reported from the University of Colorado; the authors came to the conclusion, based on treating 30 patients over a span of three years, that lower doses, given three times a week, are as effective (and less toxic) as a dose of 9-12 MU/day [169]. Because of the small size of the study, this conclusion should be cautiously considered. Until a randomized trial demonstrates otherwise, the higher more frequent dose, although more costly and toxic, appears required for maximum therapeutic benefit, based on the accumulated experience of the MD Anderson group.

Alpha interferon also has clinical utility in patients with other myeloproliferative disorders including essential thrombocytosis and polycythemia rubra vera [61, 72, 94, 178, 193, 198]. Control of the markedly elevated platelet count, decreasing the risk of resultant life-threatening complications can be obtained in nearly all patients with this disorder. The red cell mass, in patients with PRV, can also be reduced leading to symptomatic improvement [178].

Gamma interferon also has demonstrable antiproliferative activity against the CFU in marrow preparations from CML patients. Experience with this molecule is substantially less but clinical and cytogenetic activity have been demonstrated [90]. The CHR rate is less than with alpha interferon; whether this is due to patient selection or other factors is unknown. Cross resistance is not a major factor. Patients refractory to alpha may be sensitive to gamma interferon and vice-versa [90, 177]. As opposed to alpha interferon, down regulation of the gamma receptor has not been observed. Because of the lack of cross resistance and the demonstrable *in vitro* additive (if not synergistic) effect of the combination of gamma and alpha, clinical trials with these two agents might be warranted.

In the space of 10-12 years, alpha interferon has been shown to be the only agent capable of decreasing the malignant clone of cells in patients with CML and has been shown to be superior to chemotherapy in prolonging survival. There have been no studies evaluating in a prospective randomized fashion dose or schedule and

Table 4. IFN vs. CT in CML

Group/ Reference	Comparison	IFN effect on	
		Dur of resp	Survival
Italian Study Group (202)	alpha IFN vs. CT	+	+
German Study Group (75,76)	alpha IFN vs. busulfan alpha IFN vs. HU	+ +	+ neg
Japanese Study Group (128)	alpha IFN vs. busulfan	+	+
UK Study Group (7)	maintenance with α IFN vs. no maintenance	+	+

HU = Hydroxyurea.

until they are performed, the weight of uncontrolled data suggest that alpha interferon should be administered daily in as high a dose as tolerated.

Other lymphomas

Several small phase II studies have been performed in patients with cutaneous T cell lymphoma (CTCL), chronic lymphatic leukemia (CLL), and adult T cell leukemia- lymphoma (ATLL). Alpha interferon has been shown to have an anti-tumor effect in patients with these disorders.

Bunn et al. initially showed that rIFN alfa 2a induced responses in patients with CTCL. Responses were seen in both cutaneous and extracutaneous sites [18, 19]. These encouraging results were followed by a confirmatory report in a small series from Duke and Northwestern [135]. Three complete and 10 partial responses (response rate-59%) were induced and the suggestion of a dose-response relationship was demonstrated. Investigators from Northwestern University then combined rIFN alfa 2a with psoralen plus ultraviolet light irradiation (PUVA) in a Phase I dose escalation trial in which the dose of alpha interferon was escalated from 6 to 30 MU IM tiw [92]. This escalation was based on the steep dose-response relationship observed in the earlier trials. A complete response was obtained in 12 patients (80%). A phase II trial in patients with Sézary syndrome and mycosis fungoides has confirmed this high response rate [91]. No randomized trials have been performed to determine the relative value of the combination.

Several small pilot trials have evaluated the use of alpha interferon in patients with CLL [47, 127, 143, 166, 171]. Alpha interferon appears to have a mild to moderate ability to decrease the population of circulating leukemic cells, especially in patients with early or minimal disease who have not received prior therapy. However, none of these studies strongly suggest a clinically significant benefit from alpha interferon as a single agent.

ATLL has been etiologically associated with infection with HTLV-1, a human retrovirus endemic in southern Japan and the Caribbean basin [148]. All three interferons, alpha, beta, and gamma have been shown to have an occasionally durable anti-tumor effect in a small percentage of patients with the acute form of this disease. Recently, a multi-institutional group studied the two drug combination of rIFN alfa 2b and AZT in 19 patients and induced a major response in 11 patients, including a complete response in 5 [60]. Some of these patients had disease resistant to cytotoxic chemotherapy. Several of the responses were durable.

SOLID TUMORS

Alpha interferon has a demonstrable beneficial effect in patients with some solid tumors; patients with malignant melanoma, renal cell carcinoma, and AIDS related Kaposi's sarcoma have benefitted by treatment with alpha interferon. Alpha interferon has been approved in the US for the treatment of two of these tumors, AIDS-related Kaposi's sarcoma and for high risk patients with malignant melanoma following surgical removal of the primary lesion.

Kaposi's sarcoma

Trials in patients with Kaposi's sarcoma (AIDS) have indicated that about 40% of patients will obtain an anti-tumor response [89]. There has been the suggestion of a dose-response effect, with better results coming with treatment in the range of 20-50 MU/m^2 [34, 70, 158, 207]. Most of these studies indicate benefit is most likely in patients with stage II and III disease, in patients with the absence of a history of opportunistic infection, and in patients with a relatively good lymphocyte (>15, 000/mm^3) and helper lymphocyte (CD_4) count (>400/mm^3). Patients with advanced stage disease and/or poor immune status are less likely to respond [55]. An analysis of 364 patients has suggested prolonged survival for patients with the highest CD4 counts [40]. Studies of interferon in combination with chemotherapy have not shown any benefit over interferon alone [88]. Two studies have evaluated the combination of interferon with AZT and suggest synergy against the HIV virus and possibly also against the tumor, which itself may be virally induced. Prospective randomized trials have not been performed. Unfortunately with the exception of those patients with high CD4 counts, the length of response is only approximately six months and, a significant beneficial effect on survival in the majority of patients remains undefined.

Melanoma

Reported response rates in patients with advanced melanoma vary from 5% to 27%, with an average of about 15%. Some evidence for a dose-response relationship has also been obtained in this disease [31, 87] and an intravenous schedule has allowed higher doses to be used with less associated toxicity [87]. Metastatic malignant melanoma is a difficult malignancy to treat. The response rates for single agent alpha interferon compare favorably with those of single agent cytotoxic agents, but response rates with single cytotoxic agent therapy are low compared to combinations of cytotoxic drugs [111]. Alpha interferon is just beginning to be evaluated in combination with cytotoxic agents [42].

Alpha interferon may have its major impact in patients with high risk of recurrence following removal of the primary lesion. ECOG has recently reported a prospectively randomized study comparing rIFN alfa 2b, administered to patients at high risk for recurrence after surgical removal of the primary lesion, to observation and has shown a demonstrable benefit in terms of time to progression and overall survival [86]. Patients at high risk for recurrence, i.e. with deep penetration or lymph node involvement, received either high dose alpha interferon or no further therapy after surgical removal of a Stage 2 lesion. There was a significant treatment advantage with interferon: the duration of relapse free survival increased from 1.0 years in the untreated group to 1.7 years in patients receiving interferon; the overall survival was 2.8 years in the untreated group to 3.8 years in patients receiving interferon. In node negative patients there was an even greater influence on overall survival. Treatment with interferon was intensive: patients received a dose of 20 MU/m^2 per day IV for one month, followed by a dose of 10 MU/m^2 three times a week subcutaneously for 48 weeks. Treatment at ≥80% of scheduled dose was feasible in the majority of patients through at least the first four months of scheduled treatment.

Renal carcinoma

Alpha interferon has an anti-tumor effect in about 15% of patients with metastatic renal cell carcinoma (RCC) and may be more effective in patients with less bulky disease and when given in higher doses [45, 110, 119, 157, 170, 173, 210]. A large trial comparing the effects of IFN alfa N1 with the combination of IFN alfa N1 and vinblastine revealed no therapeutic advantage to the addition of the chemotherapeutic agent and, interestingly, demonstrated a very high response in a small subset of patients with only pulmonary metastases [121]. An occasional patient with pulmonary metastases and an intact primary renal mass obtained a response in the pulmonary metastases with alpha interferon and could then be converted into a complete response following nephrectomy. A combined surgical-biotherapeutic approach may, therefore, be of significant benefit to some patients, inducing a durable response.

Huber et al., using a previously defined 'optimum biological response modifying' dose of rIFN gamma (Genentech), induced an anti-tumor response in eight of sixteen patients with a relatively low dose of this agent. They demonstrated that a dose of 100 ugm rIFN gamma (Genentech), administered once a week, induced a maximal production of B-2 microglobulin (B2M) and of neopterin, two markers of gamma Interferon's immunostimulatory ability [80]. Patients whose disease was refractory to therapy exhibited significantly lower levels of B2M and neopterin [81].

Interferon to date has not generated significant enough clinical benefit in patients with renal cell carcinoma to support wide usage. Its use in selected patients may be helpful. A recently reported ECOG trial of IFN alfa N-1 as adjuvant therapy following nephrectomy in patients at high risk for recurrence demonstrated no benefit for this agent, even though patients had a low tumor burden [199].

Other solid tumors

Aside from the three solid tumors listed above, there have been trials in many other types of malignancy. There are some encouraging leads. Colon carcinoma is a solid tumor with a low response to therapy. 5-Fluorouracil (5-FU) may induce a relatively brief partial response in 15-20% of patients. rIFN alfa 2a has been shown to enhance the cytotoxic effect of 5-FU *in vitro* and, in pilot clinical trials, the combination induced a partial response in over 60% of patients [5, 211, 212]. However, a prospective randomized trial evaluating the addition of alpha interferon to 5 FU in patients with advanced colorectal cancer has demonstrated no benefit, only added toxicity, from the addition of alpha interferon [78]. Other trials have demonstrated clinical benefit from interferon therapy in patients with carcinoid tumors [118, 126]. Improvement in symptomatology associated with a decrease in 5-hydroxyindoleacetic acid levels has been reported in approximately 50% of patients. Anti-tumor activity has also been demonstrated in patients with squamous cell carcinoma of the cervix when rIFN alfa 2a was combined with 13 cis-retinoic acid. This combination is undergoing further evaluation [97, 98].

MODE OF ACTION

Alpha interferon has an antiproliferative effect, antiviral effect, an immune augmenting effect, and a differentiation effect. Any one or combination of these effects may induce an anti-tumor response. Gamma interferon (Type II IFN) is a more potent immune stimulator of monocyte function and class II HLA activity than are either alpha or beta interferon (Type I IFNs) [206]; however, on a weight basis, the Type I IFNs are 10 times as potent as gamma interferon in their antiviral effect.

Antiproliferative

In vitro studies and murine models have been used to demonstrate the anti-proliferative action of interferons [68, 199]. Decreased tumorigenicity has also been shown in cells pretreated with human interferon [16, 68]. Whether these models are applicable to human tumors *in vivo* remains conjectural. Cell cycle analysis has shown that interferon causes extension of all phases of the cell cycle and prolongation of the overall cell generation time [85, 144, 188]. In some cases, an accumulation of cells in G_0 has been observed, accompanied by a decrease in transition to G_1. This decrease in growth rate may be incompatible with cell life [199].

The critical antiproliferative mechanisms operative at the cellular level have not been elucidated, but it is possible that they may be mediated by the same inhibitors of DNA and RNA synthesis that are found in virus-infected cells. Specifically, induction of 2'5'-oligoadenylate (2, 5 A) synthetase leads to endoribonuclease activation, which in turn inhibits RNA transcription by degrading mRNA linked to dsRNA [159, 172]. In addition, a protein kinase and a phosphodiesterase pathway represent mechanisms of inhibition of protein synthesis which are parallel to, but independent of, 2, 5 A synthetase [172]. Whether these are, in fact, central to antiproliferative as well as antiviral activity remains speculative [197].

Because of its high degree of sensitivity to the Type I interferons, HCL would appear to be an ideal disease in which to determine a mechanism of action for interferon's antitumor effect. Type I interferon receptors are present on hairy cells and are down regulated with therapy [13, 43]. A lack of demonstrable down regulation *in vivo* has been associated with lack of response [14]. Immunologic recovery as manifested by a return of NK activity and normalization of T and B cell counts has been documented [124]; but responses occur without improvement in NK activity [51]. Further, hairy cells were not susceptible to NK cytotoxicity *in vitro* [175]. It has also been shown that alpha interferon, when cultured with peripheral blood mononuclear cells of patients with HCL, gives rise to multi-lineage colonies composed of myeloid and erythroid progenitors – evidence for the existence of circulating hematopoietic stem cells responsive to a differentiation effect of interferon [117]. It has also been shown that the mononuclear cells of HCL are defective in their ability to release tumor necrosis factor (TNF) and that interferon overcomes this – perhaps interferon and TNF then act synergistically as antiproliferative or cytotoxic agents [2, 3]. The low dose – standard dose randomized study with IFN alpha N-1 in patients with HCL supports both of these theories; both doses were comparable in their ability to induce an increase in platelet and neutrophil counts (differentiation) while the standard dose was more effective as an antileukemic (antiproliferative) agent [180]. This is the only prospectively randomized clinical evidence available to support a dose-response effect. Ford et al. and subsequently Pagannelli et al. have shown that HCL proliferation *in vitro* required B cell growth factor (BCGF) and Pagannelli et al. have shown that Type I but not Type II interferon inhibits the effect of BCGF [48, 142]. These observations strongly suggest that interferon's primary anti-tumor effect is an antiproliferative one, at least in this tumor setting.

Antiviral activity

That interferons have antiviral properties is well established and alpha interferon is approved in many countries for the treatment of several forms of viral hepatitis. Whether this effect is the basis for interferon's antitumor effect in tumors possibly related to viral etiologies, such as Kaposi's sarcoma associated with AIDS and ATLL, is unknown. Although other tumors may be of viral origin, most prominently cervical carcinoma, there has not been a major investigative effort mounted in this area and currently the antiviral effect of alpha interferon remains unexploited in the treatment of malignancy.

Immune modulation

Support for immune stimulation as a mechanism of action is found in experiments with animals, in which tumors known to be interferon-resistant *in vitro* have regressed when the animal received systemic treatment with interferon [33, 68]. A variety of immune changes have been described, but the most relevant appear to be the effects on natural killer (NK)-cells and macrophages. *In vitro* work with human lymphocytes shows that interferon increases the cytotoxic potential of NK-cells by recruitment of pre-NK-cells, increasing activity of activated cells, and by augmenting NK-cell-mediated antibody-dependent cell-mediated cytotoxicity [77, 144]. Alpha and beta interferons also appear to cause NK activation at a lower dose and over a shorter time interval than does gamma interferon [200]. In clinical trials, both the dose and route of interferon administration have been shown to effect NK-cell activity significantly. Several trials have suggested that low-dose interferon results in more marked NK-cell activity [35, 36, 39, 93]. This is a confusing issue, however, since others have reported widely differing effects on NK-cell activity, varying from a consistent increase [38, 101, 149] to a consistent decrease [99, 104, 105, 106, 185], in addition to individual variation without discernable pattern [120]. Much of the controversy may be related to the dose of interferon used. Unpublished work from the NCI by Varesio et al. [205] has suggested a bell-shaped curve for both the antiproliferative effect and immune augmentation. These curves do not precisely overlap.

A few clinical studies have examined the long-term immunologic effects of alpha interferon treatment; again, these differ with respect to whether there is an increase [93, 176] or decrease [104, 106] in NK activity. A study by Silver et al. [176] showed that low dose alpha interferon led to an increase in NK activity within 48 hours, which was, however, not sustained despite continued administration. Repeated high-dose interferon gave a more sustained increase of NK activity in the long term, even though it did not lead to the same initial rise as low-dose interferon. However, intravenous administration was used for the high dose, and intramuscular administration for the low dose, and the schedule of therapy was also different (alternate weeks for low-dose versus monthly for high-dose). Both uncontrolled factors, i.e., route of administration and schedule, might have caused the differences noted. An earlier study with lymphoblastoid interferon showed a dose-related decrease in NK activity over a 6-week period, after an initial stimulatory effect; but in that instance the treatment was given three times a week [93]. This suggests that an intermittent schedule may result in different patterns of response.

Since interferon consistently stimulates NK-cells *in vitro*, the inability to reproduce consistent effects of interferon on NK-cell activity in clinical practice suggests a need to explore confounding *in vivo* effects, such as scheduling, dose, or sampling method (peripheral blood versus tumor site). Furthermore, both Type I and Type II interferons have been shown to induce resistance to NK activity *in vitro*. The controversy surrounding NK-cell function after interferon treatment suggests that it may not be a useful immunologic marker.

Macrophages, more consistently than NK-cells, are affected by gamma interferon; indeed, gamma interferon has all the activities of a macrophage-activation factor (MAF) [33, 206]. Gamma interferon acts to increase the number and density of Fc receptors, which in turn are associated with an increase in antigen-presenting function. Enhancements of phagocytosis and also of antiviral activity and cytotoxicity occur [144, 188]. Thus, assays of macrophage/monocyte function may be of more relevance for assessment of gamma interferon action, whereas NK or antiviral activity may be the best choice for alpha or beta interferons. In addition to functional studies, changes in serum molecules, particularly neopterin, tryptophan and beta 2 microglobulin have been found to be very consistent markers of biologic response to interferons. Their relationship to the degree of immune modulation *in vivo* is unclear but recent studies with alpha, beta and gamma interferons have shown the optimal biologic dose to be well below the maximum tolerated dose [52, 63].

The ability to increase cell-surface antigen expression presents another aspect of interferon action that may be important in tumor control. Augmentation has been demonstrated for the expression of Fc receptors on lymphocytes and of Class I and II (Ia) MHC antigens [33, 144, 188] on several other cell types as well. In addition to augmentation of expression, interferon has also been shown to induce HLA expression in a variety of normal cells [165]. In neoplastic cells, interferon has been shown to induce HLA antigen expression and augment tumor-associated antigen (TAA) expression in several cell lines [20, 56, 57, 67]. This work has been expanded and augmentation has been demonstrated *in vitro* in tumor cells obtained from malignant effusions and following the intraperitoneal administration of gamma interferon to patients [62, 71]. The increased expression of TAA occurring concurrently with enhancement of macrophage antigen-presenting function, may improve the endogenous antitumor activity of macrophages.

The actions of interferon in promoting tumor antigen expression suggest another major line of inquiry, namely, the combination of interferon with monoclonal antibody (MoAb) therapy, with or without linkage to a toxin [164]. One of the major stumbling blocks to MoAb therapy has been modulation or poor expression of tumor antigens; if pretreatment with interferon can increase antigen expression, then the effectiveness of subsequent MoAb treatment might be greatly enhanced. However, the risk of similar expression in nontarget areas must be kept in mind, since it is often the level of expression rather than the novel nature of the antigen which characterizes the tumor cell. At least one early trial has demonstrated potential therapeutic effects [214].

An interesting trial has been performed by the group at Stanford University and IDEC Pharmaceutical Corporation in California. These investigators previously reported the use of anti-idiotype antibodies in patients with B cell lymphomas, obtaining a response in 5 of 10 patients including 1 CR [114]. Patients ultimately failed because of the emergence of a dominant clone of antigen (idiotype) negative cells [113]. An animal model was developed to evaluate therapeutic modalities in this setting. Using this model, it was shown that a synergistic effect was obtained with the combination of anti-idiotype antibodies and interferon [11]. rIFN alfa 2a, 12 MU/m^2 SC tiw, was combined with anti-idiotype therapy and administered to twelve patients. Responses were obtained in nine (with 2 CR), not substantially different from the results with anti-idiotype therapy alone. Interferon failed to prevent the emergence of idiotype negative clones. Currently ongoing studies evaluating the combination of alpha interferon and anti CD-20 monoclonal antibody may be clinically more encouraging [69].

Differentiation

Interferons have been shown to have a variety of effects on differentiation. *In vitro* differentiation has been enhanced in mouse myeloid leukemia cells and in erythroblasts of the Friend leukemia system, whereas conversion of mouse 3T3-Li cells into adipocytes and of human monocytes to macrophages has been inhibited [165, 188].

Other evidence supporting an effect on differentiation includes an increased expression of HLA antigens, enhanced excitability of nerve cells, and decreased beating frequency of myocardial cells after interferon treatment [165]. Interestingly, sodium butyrate, a well known differentiating agent, enhances this effect of interferons *in vitro* [165]. An important finding – which may suggest one cellular mechanism for inducing differentiation – is the evidence of decreased c-myc and c-Ha-ras gene expression following interferon treatment, with as much as a 60% decrease in mRNA formation [25]. With 3T3 fibroblasts, this decrease in mRNA has been associated with a reversion to normal cell type. Thus, interferon-induced differentiation appears to be a significant effect and may be part of the antineoplastic action of interferon.

Anti-angiogenesis

Inhibition of experimental angiogenesis by interferons was first demonstrated in a mouse tumor model [174]. This observation was confirmed in infants with life-threatening hemangiomas [41]. Hemangioma regression and significant clinical benefit was demonstrated in more than 80% of seriously effected infants. It is unknown what role, if any, this physiologic effect of alpha interferon plays in inducing anti-tumor activity.

SIDE EFFECTS

While side effects of the Interferons can be debilitating, most appear to be reversible upon cessation of therapy. As one might expect, high doses give rise to more severe manifestations than low doses. The major documented short term side effects are fevers, headache, and myalgia, while fatigue, a long term side effect, can be severe enough to be dose-limiting. Gastrointestinal side effects, in particular, anorexia, nausea, vomiting and/or diarrhea, are neither universal nor severe, but may lead to weight loss, which can be profound with high-dose or prolonged moderate-dose administration. Elevated serum transaminase (but not clinical hepatitis) has also been noted [93, 176, 183]. Hypotension with higher doses of both alpha and gamma interferons can be dose limiting. Both granulocytopenia and thrombocytopenia have occurred, but are rapidly reversible [107, 176] and rarely dose limiting unless the patient has had extensive prior radiation. Margination of leukocytes rather than direct marrow suppression appears responsible.

Central nervous system toxicities, including paresthesias, weakness, somnolence, decreased attention span, short-term memory impairment, confusion, depression, personality change, and even coma at very high doses, have all been seen. EEG abnormalities, including a slowing of the dominant alpha rhythm and diffuse slow waves, have been documented [1, 44, 160, 183].

Exacerbation of coronary artery disease has been reported; although cardiac toxicity may be life-threatening, serious cardiac toxicity due to interferon is unusual. A significant history of coronary artery disease is a relative contraindication for interferon therapy, particularly at high doses. Life-threatening acute pulmonary toxicity, renal failure, and unexplained sudden death have also been noted on rare occasions.

Recently evidence has increased indicating that long term treatment with interferons results in the production of antibodies to interferon. In a study of 51 patients with hairy cell leukemia, neutralizing antibody was detected in 16 patients, six of whom developed some degree of clinical resistance [186]. In a previous review of more than 617 patients who received intramuscular interferon alfa 2a, 25% were reported to have neutralizing antibody [83]. Antibody formation is a significantly less frequent phenomenon in patients treated with either rIFN alfa 2b or IFN alfa N1 [187, 208, 209]. Of the three allelic genes used in the development of recombinant interferon alfa 2, the gene used to produce rIFN alfa 2b is by far the more common allele in North American individuals [96].

SUMMARY

This review of the clinical effects of the interferons indicates that alpha interferon, when used as a single agent, has antitumor effects in a large number of malignancies, perhaps more than any single chemotherapeutic agent. However, like the cytotoxic agents, the interferons will undoubtedly contribute most significantly in combination with cytotoxic drugs, other biologics, or antiviral agents. Clinically, the interferons have proven to be a significant addition to our therapeutic armamentarium and have served well as the prototype for biological therapeutics. Interferon has overcome two misleading labels at opposite ends of the spectrum: of 'imaginon' when most scientists doubted its existence, and more recently that of 'magic bullet', when the public was led to believe it might be the cure-all for cancer. In the context of cancer treatment, interferons are the prototype of the so-called 'fourth arm' of therapy; surgery, radiotherapy, chemotherapy and biotherapy [134]

REFERENCES

1. Adams F, Quesada JR, Gutterman JU. Neuropsychiatric manifestations of human leukocyte interferon therapy in patients with cancer. *J Am Med Assoc* 1984; 252: 938-941.
2. Aderka D, Michalevicz R, Daniel Y, et al. Recombinant interferon alpha-C for advanced hairy cell leukemia. *Cancer* 1988; 61: 2207-2213.
3. Aderka D, Levo Y, Ramot B. Reduced production of tumor necrosis factor (TNF) by mononuclear cells of hairy cell leukemia patients and improvement following leukemia therapy. *Cancer* 1987; 60: 2208-2212.
4. Ahre A, Bjorkholm M, Mellstedt H, et al. Human leukocyte interferon and intermittent high dose melphalan-prednisone administration in the treatment of multiple myeloma. A randomized clinical trial from the myeloma group of central Sweden. *Cancer Treat Rep* 1984; 68: 1331-1338.
5. Ajani J, Rios AH, Ende K, et al. Phase I and II Studies of the combination of recombinant human interferon-alpha and 5-fluorouracil in patients with advanced colorectal carcinoma. *J Biol Resp Modif* 1989; 8: 14-46.
6. Alimena G, Morra E, Lazzarino M, et al. Interferon alpha-2b as therapy for Ph I-positive chronic myelogenous leukemia: A study of 82 patients treated with intermittent or daily administration. *Blood* 1988; 72: 642-647.
7. Allan NC, Richards SM, Shepherd PCA. On behalf of the UK Medical Research Council's Working Parties for Therapeutic Trials in Adult Leukaemia – UK Medical Research Council randomized multicentre trial of interferon alpha N1 for chronic myeloid leukaemia: Improved survival irrespective of cytogenetic response. *Lancet* 1995; 345: 1392-97.
8. Andersen J, Smalley RV. Interferon alfa plus chemotherapy for non-Hodgkin's lymphoma: Five-year follow up. *N Engl J Med* 1993; 329: 1821-1822.
9. Avvisati G, Boccadoro M, Petrucci MT, et al (1993). *Interferon alpha as maintenance treatment in multiple myeloma: The Italian experience (abst), in Program and Abstracts of the IV International Workshop on Multiple Myeloma*, pp 87-88, Rochester, MN.
10. Bartsch HH, Pfizenmaier K, Hanusch A, et al. Sequential therapy with recombinant interferons gamma and alpha in patients with unfavorable prognosis of chronic myelocytic leukemia: clinical responsiveness to recombinant IFN-α

correlates with the degree of receptor down-regulation. *Int J Cancer* 1989; 43: 235-240.

11. Basham TY, Kaminski MS, Ketamura K, et al. Synergistic antitumor effect of interferon and anti-idiotype monoclonal antibody in murine lymphoma. *J Imunnol* 1986; 137: 3019.
12. Bergsagel DE, Haas RH, Messner HA. Interferon alfa-2b in the treatment of chronic granulocytic leukemia. *Invest New Drugs* 1987; 5: 9-17.
13. Billard C, Sigaux F, Castaigne S, et al. Treatment of hairy cell leukemia with recombinant alpha interferon: II. In vivo down-regulation of alpha interferon receptors on tumor cells. *Blood* 1986; 67: 821-826.
14. Billard C, Diez RA, Ferbus D, et al. Lack of in vivo down-regulation of interferon alpha receptors in non-Hodgkin lymphoma cells from patients unresponsive to interferon-alpha therapy. *J Interf Res* 1989; 9(Suppl 2): S202.
15. Borden EC, Holland JF, Dao TL, et al. Leukocyte-derived interferon (alpha) in human breast carcinoma. The American Cancer Society Phase II trial. *Ann Intern Med* 1982; 97: 1-6.
16. Borden E. Interferons, rationale for clinical trials in neoplastic disease. *Ann Intern Med* 1979; 91: 472-479.
17. Browman GP, Bergsagel D, Sicheri D, et al. Randomized trial of interferon maintenance in multiple myeloma: A study of the National Cancer Institute of Canada Clinical Trials Group. *J Clin Onc* 1995; 13: 2354-60.
18. Bunn PA, Foon KA, Ihde DC, et al. Recombinant leukocyte A interferon: An active agent in advanced cutaneous T-cell lymphomas. *Ann Intern Med* 1984; 101: 484-487.
19. Bunn PA Jr, Ihde DC, Foon KA. The role of recombinant interferon alfa-2a in the therapy of cutaneous T-cell lymphomas. *Cancer* 1989; 57: 1689-1695.
20. Carrel S, Schmidt-Kessen A, Giuffre L. Recombinant interferon-gamma can induce the expression of HLA-DR and DC-or DR-negative melanoma cells and enhance the expression of HLA-ABC and tumor-associated antigens. *Eur J Immunol* 1985; 15: 118-123.
21. Case DC Jr, Sonneborn HL, Paul SD, et al. Phase II study of rDNA alpha-2 interferon (Intron A) in patients with multiple myeloma utilizing an escalating induction phase. *Cancer Treat Rep* 1986; 70: 1251-1254.
22. Chisesi T, Capnist G, Vespignani M, et al. Interferon alfa-2b and chlorambucil in the treatment of non-Hodgkin's lymphoma. *Invest New Drugs* 1987; 5: 535-540.
23. Clark RH, Dimitrov NV, Axelson JA. A phase II trial of intermittent leukocyte interferon and high dose chlorambucil in the treatment of non-Hodgkin's lymphoma resistant to conventional therapy. *Am J Clin Oncol* 1989; 12: 75-77.
24. Clark RH, Dimitrov NV, Axelson JA, et al. Leukocyte interferon as a possible biological response modifier in lymphoproliferative disorders resistant to standard therapy. *J Biol Resp Mod* 1984; 3: 613-619.
25. Clemens M. Interferons and oncogenes. *Nature* 1985; 313: 531-532.
26. Coiffier B. Personal Communication, 1995.
27. Cooper MR, Fefer A, Thompson J, et al. Alpha-2-interferon/melphalan/prednisolone in previously untreated patients with multiple myeloma: A Phase I-II trial. *Cancer Treat Rep* 1986; 70: 473-476.
28. Cooper MR. Interferons in the management of multiple myeloma. *Sem Oncol* 1988; 15: 21-25.
29. Costanzi JJ, Pollard RB. The use of interferon in the treatment of multiple myeloma. *Sem Oncol* 1987; 14: 24-28.
30. Costanzi JJ, Cooper MR, Scarffe JH, et al. Phase II study of recombinant alpha 2 interferon in resistant multiple myeloma. *J Clin Oncol* 1985; 3: 654-659.
31. Creagan ET, Ahmann DL, Green SJ, et al. Phase II study of recombinant leukocyte A interferon (RIFN-Alpha-A) in disseminated malignant melanoma. *Cancer* 1984; 54: 2844-2849.
32. Cunningham D, Powles R, Malpas JS, et al. A randomized trial of maintenance therapy with Intron-A following high dose melphalan and ABMT in myeloma [Abstract]. *Proc ASCO* 1993; 12: 364.
33. DeMaeyer-Guignard J, DeMaeyer E. Immunomodulation by interferons: Recent developments. In: *Interferon*, Vol. 6 edited by I. Gresser, pp. 69-86. 1985, New York, Academic Press.
34. Dewit R, Boucher CAB, Veenhof KHN, et al. Clinical and virological effects of high-dose recombinant interferon alpha in disseminated AIDS-related Kaposi's sarcoma. *Lancet* 1988; 2: 1214-1217.
35. Edwards BS, Merritt JA, Fuhlbrigge RL, et al. Low doses of interferon alpha result in more effective clinical natural killer cell activation. *J Clin Invest* 1985; 75: 1908-1913.
36. Edwards BS, Hawkins MJ, and Borden EC. Comparative in vivo and in vitro activation of human NK cells by two recombinant interferons alpha differing in anti-viral activity. *Cancer Res* 1984; 44: 3135-3139.
37. Einhorn N, Cantell K, Einhorn S, et al. Human leukocyte interferon. *Am J Clin Oncol* 1982; 5: 167-172.
38. Einhorn S, Blomgren H, and Strander H. Interferon and spontaneous cytotoxicity in man. *Acta Med Scand* 1978; 204: 477-483.
39. Einhorn S, Ahre A, Blomgren H, et al. Interferon and natural killer activity in multiple myeloma. Lack of correlation between interferon-induced enhancement of natural killer activity and clinical response to human interferon-alpha. *Int J Cancer* 1982; 30: 167-172.
40. Evans LM, Itri LM, Campion M, et al. Alfa interferon 2a in the treatment of AIDS related Kaposi's sarcoma. *J Interf Res* 1989; 9: S207.
41. Ezekowitz RAB, Mulliken JB, Folkman J. Interferon alfa-2a therapy for life-threatening hemangiomas of infancy. *N Eng J Med* 1992; 326: 1456.
42. Falkson CI, Ibrahim J, Kirkwood J, Blum R. A randomized phase III trial of Dacarbazine (DTIC) versus DTIC + interferon alfa 2b (ifn) versus DTIC + Tamoxifen (TMX) versus DTIC + IFN + TMX in metastatic malignant melanoma: An ECOG Trial. *Proc ASCO* 1996; 15: 435.
43. Faltynek CR, Princler GL, Rossio JL, et al. Relationship of the clinical response and binding of recombinant interferon alpha in patients with lymphoproliferative diseases. *Blood* 1986; 67: 1077-1082.
44. Farkilla M, Ilvanainen M, Roine R, et al. Neurotoxic and other side effects of high-dose interferon in amyotrophic lateral sclerosis. *Acta Neurol Scand* 1984; 69: 42-46.
45. Figlin RA, deKernion JB, Maldazys J, Sarna G. Treatment of renal cell carcinoma with alpha (human leukocyte) interferon and vinblastine in combination: A phase I-II trial. *Cancer Treat. Rep* 1985; 69: 263-267.
46. Foon KA, Sherwin SA, Abrams PG, et al. Treatment of advanced non-Hodgkin's lymphoma with recombinant leukocyte A interferon. *N Engl J Med* 1984; 311: 1148-1152.

47. Foon KA, Bottino GC, Abrams PG, et al. Phase II trial of recombinant leukocyte A interferon in patients with advanced chronic lymphocytic leukemia. *Am J Med* 1985; 78: 216.
48. Ford RJ, Kwok D, Quesada J, et al. Production of B cell growth factor(s) by neoplastic B cells from hairy cell leukemia patients. *Blood* 1986; 67: 573-577.
49. Gams R, Gordon D, Guaspari A, et al. Phase II trial of human polyclonal lymphoblastoid interferon in the management of malignant lymphomas. *Proc Am Soc Clin Oncol* 1984; 3: 65 (abstract).
50. Gams R. Personal Communication, 1990.
51. Gastl G, Aulitzky W, Liter E, et al. Alpha interferon induces remission in hairy cell leukemia without enhancement of natural killing. *Blut* 1986; 52: 273-279.
52. Gastl G, Aulitzky W, Tilg H, et al. A biological approach to optimize interferon treatment in hairy cell leukemia. *Immunobiology* 1986; 172: 262-268.
53. Gastl G, Denz H, Abbrederis C, et al. Treatment with low dose human recombinant interferon-alpha-2 ARG induces complete remission in patients with hairy cell leukemia. *Onkologie* 1985; 8: 143-144.
54. Gastl G, Werter M, De Pauw B, et al. Comparison of clinical efficacy and toxicity of conventional and optimum biological response modifying doses of interferon alpha-2C in the treatment of hairy cell leukemia: A retrospective analysis of 39 patients. *Leukemia* 1989; 3: 453-460.
55. Gelmann EP, Preble OT, Steis R, et al. Human lymphoblastoid interferon treatment of Kaposi's sarcoma in the acquired immune deficiency syndrome. *Am J Med* 1985; 78: 737-741.
56. Giacomini P, Imberti L, Aguzzi A, et al. Immunochemical analysis of the modulation of human melanoma-associated antigens by DNA recombinant immune interferon. *J Immunol* 1985; 135: 2887-2894.
57. Giacomini P, Aguzzi A, Pestka S. Modulation by recombinant DNA leukocyte (a) and fibroblast (b) interferons of the expression and shedding of HLA- and tumor-associated antigens by human melanoma cells. *J Immunol* 1984; 133: 1649-1655.
58. Gibson J, Cameron K, Gallagher K, et al. Clinical response of hairy cell leukaemia to interferon-α: results of an Australian study. *Med J of Aust* 1988; 149: 293-296.
59. Gibson J, Gallagher K, Cameron K, et al. Peripheral blood lymphocyte subsets and natural killer cell number and function during α-interferon treatment for hairy cell leukemia. *Aust New Zeal J Med* 1988; 18: 897-898.
60. Gill PS, Harrington W Jr, Kaplan MH, et al. Treatment of adult T-cell leukemia-lymphoma with a combination of interferon alfa and zidovudine. *N Engl J Med* 1995; 332: 1744-1748.
61. Gisslinger H, Ludwig H, Linkesch W, et al. Long-term interferon therapy for thrombocytosis in myeloproliferative diseases. *Lancet* 1989; 1: 634-637.
62. Goldstein D, Guadagni F, Greiner J, et al. Clinical and biological effects of intraperitoneal interferon gamma in a phase 1A/b trial in ovarian carcinoma *J Interf Res* 1989; 9: (2)S115.
63. Goldstein D, Sielaff KM, Storer BE, et al. Human biologic response modification in the absence of serum concentrations: A comparative trial of subcutaneous and intravenous interferon beta ser. *J Natl Cancer Inst* 1989; 81: 1061-1068.
64. Golomb HM, Ratain MJ, Fefer A, et al. Randomized study of the duration of treatment with interferon alfa-2B in patients with hairy cell leukemia. *J Natl Cancer Inst* 1988; 80: 369-373.
65. Golomb HM, Jacobs A, Fefer A, et al. Alpha-2 interferon therapy of hairy cell leukemia: A multi-center study of 64 patients. *J Clin Oncol* 1986; 4: 900-905.
66. Golomb HM, Fefer A, Golde DW. Report of a multi-institutional study of 193 patients with hairy cell leukemia treated with interferon-alfa 2b. *Sem in Oncol* 1988; 15: 7-9.
67. Greiner JW, Hand PH, Naguchi P, et al. Enhanced expression of surface tumor associated antigen on human breast and colon tumor cells after recombinant human leukocyte a-interferon treatment. *Cancer Res* 1984; 44: 3208-3211.
68. Gresser I. How does interferon inhibit tumor growth? In: *Interferon*, Vol. 6, edited by I. Gresser, pp. 93-126. 1985, New York, Academic Press.
69. Grillo-Lopez A. *Personal Communication*, 1996.
70. Groopman J, Gottlieb M, Goodman J, et al. Recombinant alpha-2 interferon therapy for Kaposi's sarcoma associated with the acquired immunodeficiency syndrome. *Ann Intern Med* 1984; 100: 671-676.
71. Guadagni F, Schlom J, Johnston W, et al. Selective Interferon-Induced Enhancement of Tumor-Associated Antigens on a Spectrum of Freshly Isolated Human Adenocarcinoma Cells. *J Natl Cancer Inst* 1989; 81: 502-512.
72. Gugliotta L, Bagnara GP, Catani L, et al. *In vivo* and in vitro inhibitory effect of alpha interferon on megakaryocyte colony growth in essential thrombocythaemia. *Br J Hematol* 1989; 71: 177-181.
73. Gutterman JU, Blumenschein AR, Alexanian R, et al. Leukocyte interferon-induced tumor regression in human metastatic breast cancer, multiple myeloma and malignant lymphoma. *Ann Intern Med* 1980; 93: 399-406.
74. Hagenbeek A, Carde P, Soures R, et al. On behalf of EORTC Lymphoma Cooperative Group. Interferon alfa 2a vs. control as maintenance therapy for low grade non-Hodgkin's lymphoma. *Proc ASCO* 1995; 14: 386.
75. Hehlmann R, Heimpel H, Hasford J, et al. Randomized comparison of interferon alpha with Busulfan and hydroxyurea in chronic myelogenous leukemia. *Blood* 1994; 84: 4064-77.
76. Hehlmann R, Anger B, Messerer D, et al. Randomized study on the treatment of chronic myeloid leukemia (CML) in chronic phase with busulfan versus hydroxyurea versus interferon-alpha. *Blut* 1988; 56: 87-91.
77. Herberman RB, and Ortaldo JR. Natural killer cells: Their role in defenses against disease. *Science* 1981; 214: 24-30.
78. Hill M, Norman A, Cunningham D, et al. Royal Marsden phase III trial of fluorouracil with or without interferon alfa 2b in advanced colorectal cancer. *J Clin Onc* 1995; 13: 1297-1302.
79. Horning SJ, Merigan TL, Krown SE, et al. Human interferon alpha in malignant lymphoma and Hodgkin's disease. *Cancer* 1985; 56: 1305-1310.
80. Huber C, Batchelor JR, Fuchs D, et al. Immune response-associated production of neopterin. *J Exper Med* 1984; 160: 310-316.
81. Huber C, Aulitzky W, Gastl G, et al. Treatment of metastasizing renal cell carcinoma with an 'optimum bio-

logical response modifying' dose of rIFN-gamma. *J Biol Resp Modif* 1989; 8: 335.
82. Isaacs H, Lindemann J. Virus interference 1. The interferon. *Proc R Soc Oncol Biol* 1957; 147: 257-262.
83. Itri LM, Campion M, Dennin RA, et al. Incidence and clinical significance of neutralizing antibodies in patients receiving recombinant interferon alfa 2a by intramuscular injection *Cancer* 1987; 59: 668-674.
84. Kantarjian HM, Smith TL, OBrien S, et al. Prolonged survival in chronic myelogenous leukemia after cytogenetic response to interferon alpha therapy. *Ann Int Med* 1995; 122: 254-61.
85. Kirchner H. Interferons, a group of multiple lymphokines. *Semin Immunopathol* 1984; 7: 347-374.
86. Kirkwood JM, Strawderman MH, Ernstoff MS, et al. Interferon alfa-2b adjuvant therapy of high-risk resected cutaneous melanoma: the Eastern Cooperative Oncology Group Trial EST 1684. *J Clin Oncol* 1996; 14: 7-17.
87. Kirkwood JM, Ernstoff MS, Davis CA, et al. Comparison of intramuscular and intravenous recombinant a-2 interferon in melanoma and other cancers. *Ann Intern Med* 1985; 103: 32-36.
88. Krigel RL, Slywotzky CM, Louiberg M, et al. Treatment of epidemic Kaposi's sarcoma with a combination of interferon-alpha-2b and etoposide. *J Biol Resp Modif* 1988; 7: 359-364.
89. Krown SE. The role for interferon in the therapy of epidemic Kaposi's sarcoma. *Semin Oncol* 1987; 2: 27-33.
90. Kurzrock R, Talpaz M, Kantarjian H, et al. Therapy of chronic myelogenous leukemia with recombinant interferon-alpha. *Blood* 1987; 70: 943-947.
91. Kuzel TM, Roenigk HH, Samuelson E, et al. Effectiveness of interferon alpha 2a combined with phototherapy for mycosis fungoides and the Sézary syndrome. *J Clin Onc* 1995; 13: 257.
92. Kuzel TM, Gilyon K, Springer E, et al. Interferon alfa-2a combined with phototherapy in the treatment of cutaneous T-cell lymphoma. *J Natl Cancer Inst* 1990; 82: 203-207.
93. Laszlo J, Huang AT, Brenkman WD, et al. Phase I study of pharmacological and immunological effects of human lymphoblastoid interferon given to patients with cancer. *Cancer Res* 1983; 43: 4458-4466.
94. Lazzarino M, Vitalle A, Morra E, et al. Interferon alpha-2b as treatment for Philadelphia-negative chronic myeloproliferative disorders with excessive thrombocytosis. *Br J Haematol* 1989; 72: 173-177.
95. Leavitt RD, Ratanatharathorn V, Ozer H, et al. Alfa-2b interferon in the treatment of Hodgkin's Disease and Non-Hodgkin's lymphoma. *Sem Onc* 1987; 14(Suppl 2): 18-23.
96. Liao MJ, Lee N, Dipaola G, et al. Distribution of interferon alpha 2 genes in humans. *J Interferon Res* 1994; 14: 183-185.
97. Lippman SM, Kavanagh JJ, Paredes-Espinoza M, et al. 13 cis-retinoic acid plus interferon alfa 2a: A highly active systemic therapy for squamous cell carcinoma of the cervix. *J Nat Ca Inst* 1992; 84: 241-.
98. Lippman SM, Parkinson DR, Itri LM, et al. 13-cis-retinoic acid plus interferon alfa 2a: Effective combination therapy for advanced squamous cell carcinoma of the cervix. *J Nat Ca Inst* 1992; 84: 235-240.
99. Lotzova E, Savary CA, Gutterman JU, et al. Regulation of natural killer cell cytotoxicity by recombinant leukocyte interferon clone A. *J Biol Resp Modif* 1983; 2: 482-498.
100. Louie AC, Gallagher JG, Sikora K, et al. Followup observations on the effect of human leukocyte interferon in non-Hodgkin's lymphoma. *Blood* 1981; 58: 712-718.
101. Lucero MA, Magdalenat H, Friedman WH, et al. Comparison of effects of leukocyte and fibroblast interferon on immunological parameters in cancer patients. *Eur J Cancer Clin Oncol* 1982; 18: 243-251.
102. Ludwig H, Cohen AM, Polliack A, et al. Interferon-alpha for induction and maintenance in multiple myeloma: Results of two multicenter randomized trials and summary of other studies. *Ann Oncol* 1995; 6: 467-476.
103. Ludwig H, Cortelezzi A, Scheithauer W, et al. Recombinant interferon alfa-2C versus polychemotherapy (VMCP) for treatment of multiple myeloma: a prospective randomized trial. *Eur J Ca Clin Onc* 1986; 22: 1111-1116.
104. Maluish AE, Ortaldo JR, Sherwin SA, et al. Changes in immune function in patients receiving natural leukocyte interferon. *J Biol Resp Modif* 1983; 2: 418-422.
105. Maluish AE, Ortaldo JR, Conlon J, et al. Depression of natural killer cytotoxicity after *in vivo* administration of recombinant leukocyte interferon. *J Immunol* 1983; 131: 503-507.
106. Maluish AE, Leavitt R, Sherwin S, et al. Effects of recombinant interferon-alpha on immune function in cancer patients. *J Biol Resp Modif* 1984; 2: 470-481.
107. Mandelli F, Tribalto M, Cantonetti M, et al. Recombinant interferon alfa-2b (Intron A) as post-induction therapy for responding multiple myeloma patients. M 84 Protocol. *Cancer Treat. Rev* 1988; 15: 43-48.
108. Mandelli F, Avvisati G, Amadori S, et al. Maintenance treatment with alpha 2b recombinant in multiple myeloma patients responding to conventional induction chemotherapy *J Interf Res* 1989; 9: S111.
109. Mandelli F, Avvisati G, Amadori S, et al. Maintenance treatment with recombinant interferon alpha 2b recombinant in multiple myeloma patients responding to conventional induction chemotherapy. *N Engl J Med* 1990; 322: 1430-1434.
110. Marumo K, Murai M, Hagakawa M, et al. Human lymphoblastoid interferon therapy for advanced renal cell carcinoma. *Urology* 1984; 24: 567-571.
111. McClay E, Mastrangelo M, Berd D, et al. Effective combination chemo/hormonal therapy for malignant melanoma: Experience with three consecutive trials. *Int J Cancer* 1992; 50: 553-56.
112. McLaughlin P, Cabanillan F, Hagemeister F, et al. CHOP-Bleo plus interferon for stage IV low-grade lymphoma. *Ann Onc* 1993; 4: 205-211.
113. Meeker T, Lowder J, Cleary ML, et al. Emergence of idiotype variants during treatment of B-cell lymphomas with anti-idiotype antibodies. *N Eng J Med* 1985; 312: 1658.
114. Meeker TC, Lowder J, Maloney DG, et al. A clinical trial of anti-idiotype therapy for B cell malignancy. *Blood* 1985; 65: 1349.
115. Mellstedt H, Ahre A, Bjorkhelm M, et al. Interferon therapy in myelomatosis. *Lancet* 1979; 1: 245-247.
116. Merigan TL, Sikorak K, Breeden JH, et al. Preliminary observations on the effect of human leukocyte interferon in non-Hodgkin's lymphoma. *N Engl J Med* 1978; 299: 1449-1453.
117. Michalevicz R, Revel M. Interferons regulate the *in vitro* differentiation of multilineage lympho-myeloid stem cells in hairy cell leukemia. *Proc Natl Acad Sci USA* 1987; 84: 2307-2311.
118. Moertel CG, Rubin J, Kvols LK. Therapy of metastatic

carcinoid tumor and the malignant carcinoid syndrome with recombinant leukocyte alpha interferon. *J Clin Onc* 1989; 7: 865.

119. Muss HB, Welander C, Caponera M, et al. Interferon and doxorubicin in renal cell carcinoma. *Cancer Treat Rep* 1985; 69: 721-722.
120. Neefe JR, Sullivan JE, Ayoob M, et al. Augmented immunity in cancer patients treated with alpha-interferon. *Cancer Res* 1985; 45: 874-878.
121. Neidhart JA, Anderson SA, Harris JE, et al. Vinblastine Fails to Improve Response of Renal Cancer to Interferon Alfa-n1 (Wellferon); High Response Rate in Patients with Pulmonary Metastases. *J Clin Onc* 1991; 9: 832-837.
122. Neuman HA, Fauser AA. Effect of interferon on pluripotent hemopoietic progenitors (CFU-GEMM) derived from human bone marrow. *Exp Hematol* 1982; 10: 587.
123. Niederle N, Kloke O, May D, et al. Treatment of chronic myelogenous leukemia with recombinant interferon alfa-2b. *Invest New Drugs* 1987; 5: 19-25.
124. Nielsen B, Hokland M, Justesen J, et al. Immunological recovery and dose evaluation in IFN-a treatment of hairy cell leukemia: Analysis of leukocyte differentiation antigens, NK and 2', 5'-oligoadenylate synthetase activity. *Eur J Haematol* 1989; 42: 50-59.
125. Nordic Myeloma Study Group. Interferon-α 2b added to melphalan-prednisone for initial and maintenance therapy in multiple myeloma. *Ann Intern Med* 1996; 124: 212-222.
126. Oberg K, Alm G, Magnusson A, et al. Treatment of malignant carcinoid tumors with recombinant interferon alfa-2b: Development of neutralizing IFN antibodies and possible loss of antitumor activity. *J Nat Ca Inst* 1989; 81: 531-.
127. O'Connell MJ, Colgan JP, Oken MM, et al. Clinical trials of recombinant leukocyte A interferon as initial therapy for favorable histology Non-Hodgkin's lymphomas and chronic lymphocytic leukemia. An Eastern Cooperative Oncology Group Pilot Study. *J Clin Oncol* 1986; 4: 128-136.
128. Ohnishi K, Ohno R, Tomonaga M, et al. A randomized trial comparing interferon-α with busulfan for newly diagnosed chronic myelogenous leukemia in chronic phase. *Blood* 1995; 86: 906-916.
129. Ohno R, Kimura K. Treatment of multiple myeloma with recombinant interferon alfa-2a. *Cancer* 1986; 57: 1685-1688.
130. Oken MM, Kyle RA, Kay NE, et al. A Phase II trial of interferon alpha-2 (rIFN-a2) in the treatment of resistant multiple myeloma (MM). *Proc Am Soc Clin Oncol* 1985; 4: 215 (abstract).
131. Oken MM, Kyle RA, Greipp PR, et al. Alternating cycles of VBMCP with interferon in the treatment of multiple myeloma *Proc Am Soc Clin Oncol* 1988; 7: 225 (abstract).
132. Oken MM, Feong T, Kay NE, et al. The effects of adding interferon (rIFN alfa 2) or high-dose cyclophosphamide to VBMCP to treat multiple myeloma: Results from an ECOG Phase III Trial. *Blood* 1995; 86(suppl 1): 441a.
133. Oladipupo-Williams CK, Svet-Moldavskaya I, Vilcek J. Inhibitory effects of human leukocyte and fibroblast interferons on normal and chronic myelogenous leukemic granulocytic progenitor cells. *Oncology* 1981; 38: 356-360.
134. Oldham RK. Biologicals and biologic response modifiers. The fourth modality of cancer therapy. *Cancer Treat Rep* 1984; 68: 221-232.
135. Olsen EA, Rosen ST, Vollmer RT, et al. Interferon alfa-2a in the treatment of cutaneous T cell lymphoma. *J Am Acad Dermatol* 1989; 20: 395-407.
136. Osserman ET, Sherman WF, Alexanian R, et al. Preliminary results of the American Cancer Society-sponsored trial of human leukocyte interferon in multiple myeloma. *Proc Am Assoc Cancer Res* 1980; 21: 161 (abstract).
137. Österborg A, Björkholm M, Bjöeman M, et al. Natural interferon-alpha in combination with melphalan/prednisone versus melphalan/prednisone in the treatment of multiple myeloma stages II and III. A randomized study from the Myeloma Group of Central Sweden. *Blood* 1993; 81: 1428-34.
138. Ozer H. Biotherapy of chronic myelogenous leukemia with interferon. *Sem Onc* 1988; 15(Suppl 5): 14-20.
139. Ozer H, Anderson JR, Peterson BA, et al. Combination trial of subcutaneous interferon alfa-2b and oral cyclophosphamide in favorable histology, non-Hodgkin's lymphoma. *Invest New Drugs* 1987; 5: 527-523.
140. Ozer H, Golomb HM, Zimmerman H, et al. Cost benefit analysis of interferon alfa 2-b in the treatment of hairy cell leukemia. *J Natl Cancer Inst* 1989; 8: 594-602.
141. Panem S. *The Interferon Crusade*. Washington, D.C., The Brookings Institute, 1985.
142. Pagannelli KA, Evans SS, Hant T, et al. B cell growth factor-induced proliferation of hairy cell lymphocytes and inhibition by Type I interferon *in vitro*. *Blood* 1986; 67: 937-942.
143. Pangalis GA, Griva E. Recombinant alfa-2b-interferon therapy in untreated, stages A and B chronic lymphocytic leukemia. *Cancer* 1988; 61: 869-872.
144. Paulnock DM, and Borden EC. Modulation of immune functions by interferons. In: *Immunity to Cancer*, pp. 545-559. 1985, New York, Academic Press.
145. Peest D, Deicher H, Coldewey R, et al. A comparison of polychemotherapy and melphalan/prednisone for primary remission induction, and interferon-alpha for maintenance treatment, in multiple myeloma. A prospective trial of the German Myeloma Treatment Group. *Eur J Cancer* 1995; 31A: 146-51.
146. Peterson BA, Petroni G, Oken M, Ozer H. Cyclophosphamide vs. Cyclophosphamide plus interferon alfa-2b in follicular low grade lymphomas. A preliminary report of an intergroup trial (CALGB-8691 and EST 7486). *Proc ASCO* 1993; 12: 366.
147. Pitha P. For the Nomenclature Committee of the International Society for Interferon Research. Nomenclature of the human interferon genes. *J Int Res* 1993; 13: 443-444.
148. Poiesz BJ, Ruscetti FW, Gazdar AF, et al. Detection and isolation of type C retrovirus particles from fresh and cultured lymphocytes of a patient with cutaneous T-cell lymphoma. *Proc Natl Acad Sci USA* 1980; 77: 7415-7419.
149. Pope GR, Hadam MR, Eisenburg J, et al. Kinetics of natural cytotoxicity in patients treated with human fibroblast interferon. *Cancer Immunol Immunother* 1981; 11: 1-6.
150. Price CGA, Rohatiner AZS, Steward W, et al. IFN-α 2b in the treatment of follicular lymphoma. Preliminary results of a trial in progress. *Annals Onc* 1991; 2 (suppl) 141-145.
151. Quesada JR, Alexanian R, Hawkins M, et al. Treatment of multiple myeloma with recombinant alpha interferon. *Blood* 1986; 67: 275-278.

152. Quesada JR, Hersh EM, Manning J, et al. Treatment of hairy cell leukemia with recombinant α-interferon. *Blood* 1986; 68: 493-497.
153. Quesada JR, Hersh EM, Rueben J, et al. Alpha interferon for induction of remission in hairy cell leukemia. *N Engl J Med* 1984; 310: 15-18.
154. Quesada JR, Itri L, Gutterman JG. Alpha interferons in hairy cell leukemia (HCL). A five year follow up in 100 patients. *J Interf Res* 1987; 7: 678.
155. Quesada JR, Alexanian R, Kurzrock R, et al. Recombinant interferon gamma in hairy cell leukemia, multiple myeloma, Waldenstrom's macroglobulinemia. *Am J Hematol* 1988; 29: 1-4.
156. Raefsky EL, Platanias LC, Zoumbos NC, et al. Studies of interferon as a regulator of hematopoietic cell proliferation. *J Immunol* 1985; 135: 2507.
157. Ravdin PM, Borden EC, Magers CF, et al. Interferon alfa-N1 and continuous infusion vinblastine for treatment of advanced renal cell carcinoma. *J Biol Resp Mod* 1990; Submitted 1989.
158. Real FX, Oettgen HF, Krown SE. Kaposi's sarcoma and the acquired immunodeficiency syndrome. Treatment with high and low doses of recombinant leukocyte A interferon. *J Clin Oncol* 1986; 4: 544-551.
159. Revel M, Kimch A, Shulman L. Role of interferon-induced enzymes in the antiviral and antimitogenic effects of interferon. *Ann NY Acad Sci* 1980; 350: 459-473.
160. Rohatiner AZS, Prior PF, Burton AC, et al. Central nervous system toxicity of interferon. *Br J Cancer* 1983; 47: 419-422.
161. Rohatiner A, Crowther D, Redford J, et al. The role of interferon in follicular lymphoma. *Proc ASCO* 1996; 15: 418.
162. Rohatiner A. *Personal communication*, 1996.
163. Rosenblum MG, Maxwell BL, Talpaz M, et al. *In vivo* sensitivity and resistance of chronic myelogenous leukemia cells to alpha interferon: Correlation with receptor binding and induction of 2', 5'- oligoadenylate synthetase. *Cancer Res* 1986; 46: 4848-4852.
164. Rosenblum MG, Lamki JL, Murana AJ, et al. Interferon induced changes in pharmacokinetics and tumor uptake of 111In-labelled antimelanoma antibody 96.5 in melanoma patients. *J Natl Cancer Inst* 1988; 80: 160-164.
165. Rossi G. Interferon and cell differentiation. In: *Interferon*, Vol. 6, edited by I. Gresser, pp. 31-68. 1985, New York. Academic Press.
166. Rozman C, Montserrat E, Vinolas N, et al. Recombinant alpha2 interferon in the treatment of B chronic lymphocytic leukemia in early stages. *Blood* 1988; 71: 1295-1298.
167. Salmon SE, Crowley JJ, Grogan TM, et al. Combination chemotherapy, glucocorticosteroids, and interferon alfa in the treatment of multiple myeloma. A Southwest Oncology Group Study. *J Clin Oncol* 1994; 12: 2405-14.
168. Scheithauer W, Cortelezzi A, Fritz E, et al. Combined alpha-2C-interferon/VMCP polychemotherapy versus VMCP as induction therapy in multiple myeloma: A Prospective Randomized Trial. *J Biol Resp Modif* 1989; 8: 109-115.
169. Schofield JR, Robinson WA, Murphy JR, et al. Low doses of interferon-α are as effective as higher doses in inducing remissions and prolonging survival in chronic myeloid leukemia. *Ann Intern Med* 1994; 121: 736-744.
170. Schornagel JH, Verweij J, Ten Bokkel Huinink WV, et al. Phase II Study of recombinant interferon alpha-A and vinblastine in advanced renal cell carcinoma. *J Urol* 1989; 142: 253-254.
171. Schulof RS, Lloyd MJ, Sallings JJ, et al. Recombinant leukocyte A interferon in B-cell chronic lymphocytic leukemia: *In vivo* effects on autologous antitumor immunity. *J Biol Resp Modif* 1985; 4: 310-323.
172. Senn CC. Biochemical pathways in interferon action. *Pharmacol Ther* 1984; 24: 235-257.
173. Sertoli MR, Brunette I, Ardizzoui A, et al. Recombinant alpha-20 interferon plus vinblastine in the treatment of metastatic renal cell carcinoma. *Am J Clin Oncol* 1989; 12: 43-45.
174. Sidky YA, Borden EC. Inhibition of angiogenesis by interferons: Effects on tumor- and lymphocyte-induced vascular responses. *Cancer Res* 1987; 47: 5155.
175. Sigaux F, Castaigne S, Lehn P, et al. Alpha-interferon in hairy cell leukaemia: direct effects on hairy cells or indirect cytotoxicity. *Int J Cancer* 1987; (Suppl)1: 2-8.
176. Silver HKB, Connors JM, Salinas FA. Prospectively randomized toxicity study of high-dose versus low-dose treatment strategies for lymphoblastoid interferon. *Cancer Treat Rep* 1985; 69: 743-750.
177. Silver RT, Coleman M, Benn P, et al. Interferon (rIFN) alfa 2b has activity in treating chronic myeloid leukemia (CML) in rIFN gamma failures. *Proc Amer Soc Clin Onc* 1987; 6: 149 (abstract).
178. Silver RT. Interferon-alpha 2b: A new treatment for polycythemia vera. *Ann Intern Med* 1993; 1091-1092.
179. Smalley RV, Andersen JW, Hawkins, et al. Interferon Alfa Combined with Cytotoxic Chemotherapy for Patients with Non-Hodgkin's Lymphoma – an ECOG Study. *New Eng J Med* 1992; 327: 1336-41.
180. Smalley RV, Anderson SS, Tuttle RL, et al. A randomized comparison of a low dose and a standard dose of alpha interferon (Wellferon[R]) in Hairy Cell Leukemia. *Blood* 1991; 78: 3133-3141.
181. Smalley RV, Connors J, Tuttle RL, et al. Splenectomy vs. Alpha Interferon: A Randomized Study in Patients with Previously Untreated Hairy Cell Leukemia. *Amer J Hematol* 1992; 41: 13-18.
182. Smalley RV, Vogel J, Huguley CM Jr, et al. Chronic granulocytic leukemia: Cytogenetic conversion of the bone marrow with cycle specific chemotherapy. *Blood* 1977; 50: 107-113.
183. Smedley, H.M., Wheeler, T. Toxicity of IFN. In: *Interferon and cancer*, edited by K. Sikora, pp. 203-210. 1983, New York, Plenum.
184. Solal-Celigy P, Lepage E, Brousse N, et al. Recombinant IFN alfa 2b combined with a regimen containing doxorubicin in patients with advanced follicular lymphomas. *N Eng J Med* 1993; 392: 1608-14.
185. Spinna CA, Dahey JL, Durhos-Smith D, et al. Suppression of NK cell cytotoxicity in the peripheral blood of patients receiving interferon therapy. *J Biol Resp Modif* 1983; 2: 458-459.
186. Steis RG, Smith JW, Urba WJ, et al. Resistance to recombinant interferon alfa 2a in hairy cell leukemia associated with neutralizing anti-interferon antibodies *N Engl J Med* 1988; 318: 1409-1413.
187. Steis RG, Urba WJ, Clark JW, et al. Immunogenicity of different types of interferons in the treatment of hairy-cell leukemia. *N Engl J Med* 1988; 319: 1227.
188. Stewart WE, Blanchard DK. Interferons, cytostatic and

immunomodulatory effects. In: *Immunity to Cancer*, pp. 295-307. 1985, New York, Academic Press.

189. Strander H, Cantell K, Inginarison S, et al. Interferon treatment of osteogenic sarcoma: A clinical trial. In: *Conference on Modulation of Host Immune Resistance in the Prevention and Treatment of Induced Neoplasms* 1980; 28: 377-381. Washington, D.C., U.S. Government Printing Office.
190. Strander H, Abramson U, Aparisi T. Adjuvant interferon treatment of human osteosarcoma. *Rec Results Ca Res* 1978; 68: 40.
191. Talpaz M, Kantarjian HM, McCredie K, et al. Hematologic remission and cytogenetic improvement induced by recombinant human interferon alpha A in chronic myelogenous leukemia. *N Eng J Med* 1986; 314: 1065-1069.
192. Talpaz M, Kantarjian HM, McCredie KB, et al. Clinical investigation of human alpha interferon in chronic myelogenous leukemia. *Blood* 1987; 69: 1280-1288.
193. Talpaz M, Kurzrock R, Kantarjian H, et al. Recombinant interferon-alpha therapy of Philadelphia chromosome-negative myeloproliferative disorders with thrombocytosis. *Am J Med* 1989; 86: 554-558.
194. Talpaz M, Trujillo JM, Mittelman WN, et al. Suppression of clonal evolution in two chronic myelogenous leukemia patients treated with leukocyte interferon. *Br J Haematol* 1985; 60: 619-624.
195. Talpaz M, McCredie KB, Mavligit GM, et al. Leukocyte interferon-induced myeloid cytoreduction in chronic myelogenous leukemia. *Blood* 1983; 62: 689-692.
196. Taniguchi T, Ohno S, Fujii-Kuriyama Y, et al. The nucleotide sequence of human fibroblast interferon cDNA. *Gene* 1980; 20: 11-15.
197. Taylor-Papadimitriou J, Ebsworth N, Rozengurt E. Possible mechanisms of interferon-induced growth inhibition. In: *Mediators in Cell Growth and Differentiation*, edited by R.J. Ford, pp. 283-298. 1985, New York, Raven Press.
198. Tichelli A, Gratwohl A, Berger C, et al. Treatment of thrombocytosis in myeloproliferative disorders with interferon alpha-2a. *Blut* 1989; 58: 15-19.
199. Toy J. The interferons. *Clin Exp Immunol* 54: 1-13.
200. Trinchieri G, and Perussia B. Immune interferon: A pleiotropic lymphokine with multiple effects. *Immunol Today* 1985; 6: 131-136.
201. Trump DL, Elson P, Proper TK, et al. Randomized controlled trial of adjuvant therapy with lymphoblastoid interferon in resected high risk renal cell carcinoma. *Proc ASCO* 1996; 15: 253.
202. Tura S, for the Italian Cooperative Study Group on Chronic Myeloid Leukemia. Interferon alfa 2a as compared with conventional chemotherapy for the treatment of chronic myeloid leukemia. *New Engl J Med* 1994; 330: 820-825.
203. Uze G, Lutfalla G, Gresser I. Genetic transfer of a functional human interferon-α receptor into mouse cells: Cloning and expression of its cDNA. *Cell* 1990; 60: 225-234.
204. VanderMolen LA, Steis RG, Duffey PL, et al. Low versus high-dose interferon alpha 2a in relapsed indolent non-Hodgkin's lymphoma. *J Natl Cancer Inst* 1990; 82: 235-238.
205. Varesio L, Blasi E, Thurman G, et al. Recombinant IFN-gamma activates macrophages to become tumoricidal. 1985, Biological Response Modifiers Program, Division of Cancer Treatment, National Cancer Institute, and Preclinical Screening Program. *NCI-FCRF*, Frederick, MD.
206. Vilcek J, Kelke HC, Jumming LE, et al. Structure and function of human interferon gamma. In: *Mediators in Cell Growth and Differentiation*, edited by R.J. Ford, pp. 299-313. 1985, New York, Raven Press.
207. Volberding P, Valero R, Rothman J, et al. Alpha interferon therapy of Kaposi's sarcoma in AIDS. *Ann NY Acad Sci* 1984; 437: 439-447.
208. von Wussow P, Hehlmann R, Hochhaus T, et al. Roferon (rIFN-α2a) is more immunogenic than Intron A (rIFN-α2b) in patients with chronic myelogenous leukemia. *J Interferon Res* 1994; 14: 217-19.
209. von Wussow P, Frund M, Dahle S, et al. Immunogenicity of different types of interferons in the treatment of hairy cell leukemia. *N Engl J Med* 1988; 319: 1226.
210. Vugrin D, Hood L, Laszlo J. A Phase II trial of high-dose human lymphoblastoid alpha interferon in patients with advanced renal carcinoma. *Cancer Treat Rep* 1985; 69: 817-820.
211. Wadler S, Schwartz EL, Goldman M, et al. 5-fluorouracil and recombinant alpha-2a-interferon: An active regimen against advanced colorectal carcinoma. *J Clin Oncol* 1989; 7: 1769-1775.
212. Wadler S, Wiernik PH. Clinical update on the role of fluorouracil and recombinant interferon alfa-2a in the treatment of colorectal carcinoma. *Sem Onc* 1990; 17(Suppl 1): 16-21.
213. Wagstaff J, Loynds P, Scarffe JH. A phase II study of rDNA human alpha 2 interferon in multiple myeloma. *Cancer Treat Rep* 1985; 69: 495-498.
214. Weiner LM, Moldofsky PJ, Gatenby RA, et al. Antibody delivery and effector cell activation in a Phase II trial of recombinant gamma interferon and the murine monoclonal antibody CO-17-1-A in advanced colorectal carcinoma. *Cancer Res* 1988; 49: 1609-1621.
215. Westin J, Rödjer S, Turesson I, et al. Interferon alfa-2b versus no maintenance therapy during the plateau phase in multiple myeloma. A randomized study. *Br J Haematol* 1995; 89: 561-8.
216. Wiernik PH, Schwartz B, Dutcher JP, et al. Successful treatment of hairy cell leukemia with beta ser interferon. *Am J Hematol* 1990; In Press.
217. Worman CP, Catovsky D, Cawley JC, et al. The UK experience withhuman lymphoblastoid interferon in HCL: A report of the first 50 cases. *Leukemia* 1987; 1: 320-322.
218. Worman CP, Nethersell ABW, Bottomley JM, et al. Natural IFN-a therapy in hairy-cell leukaemia (Namalva-Type IFN-Wellferon). *Klin Wochenschr* 1987; 65: 685-687.
219. Yoffe G, Blick M, Kantarjian H, et al. Molecular analysis of interferon-induced suppression of Philadelphia chromosome in patients with chronic myeloid leukemia. *Blood* 1987; 69: 961-963.
220. Zoon KC, Hu R, Nedden DL, et al. Further Studies on the Purification and Partial Characterization of Human Lymphoblastoid Interferon Alphas. In: *The Biology of the Interferon System* 1985, Elsevier Science Publishers, Amsterdam. Stewart WE II, Schellekens H, eds., 1986; p 55-58.

ANTIBODY THERAPY

ROBERT O. DILLMAN
Hoag Cancer Center, Newport Beach, California; and University of California, Irvine, California

The potential of antibody-mediated anticancer therapy has been recognized since the turn of the century when Paul Ehrlich espoused the 'magic bullet' concept [64]. The rationale for this approach is derived from immunological principles which were first recognized in the study of microbiology. Foreign cells, when injected into an animal, induce an immune response characterized by the production of immunoglobulin proteins, called *antibodies*, each of which binds specifically to certain collections of cell surface molecules, termed *antigens*. Chemically such antigens are characterized as glycoproteins, glycolipids, polysaccharides, etc. An antigen found only on cancer cells would be a *tumor-specific antigen*, while one present on some normal tissues, but more prevalent on cancer cells, would be called a *tumor-associated antigen* (TAA).

Antibodies consist of sequences of amino acids that are linked into two heavy chains and two light chains. Each light chain is connected to a heavy chain by a disulfide bridge, and the two heavy chains are connected via disulfide bridges. Chemical separation at these various sites yields portions called Fab, $F(ab')_2$, and Fc (Fig. 1).

Light chains are classified as kappa or lambda based on their composition, and heavy chains as immunoglobulin G (IgG), IgM, IgA, IgD, or IgE, based on their composition. Other differences in heavy chains allow subclass characterization such as IgG1, IgG2A, IgG2B, IgG3, etc. Because of the manner in which various loci for light and heavy chains, located on human chromosomes 2, 14, and 22, can be arranged, there is an almost infinite potential for production of different antibodies with a 'lock-and-key' structural binding capability specific for any given antigen. Antibodies reacting with a specific antigen bind with a variable *affinity*, which is the measure of how tightly multivalent antibody binds to a multivalent antigen. The critical regions associated with binding are located in the 'variable' and more specifically the 'hypervariable' regions of the light and heavy chains of the immunoglobulin molecule.

Conceptually, antibodies directed against a tumor antigen offer potential specificity that is directly related to the degree to which that antigen is found only on tumor cells. At one time it was believed that all cancers were foreign and that tumor-specific antigens would be readily

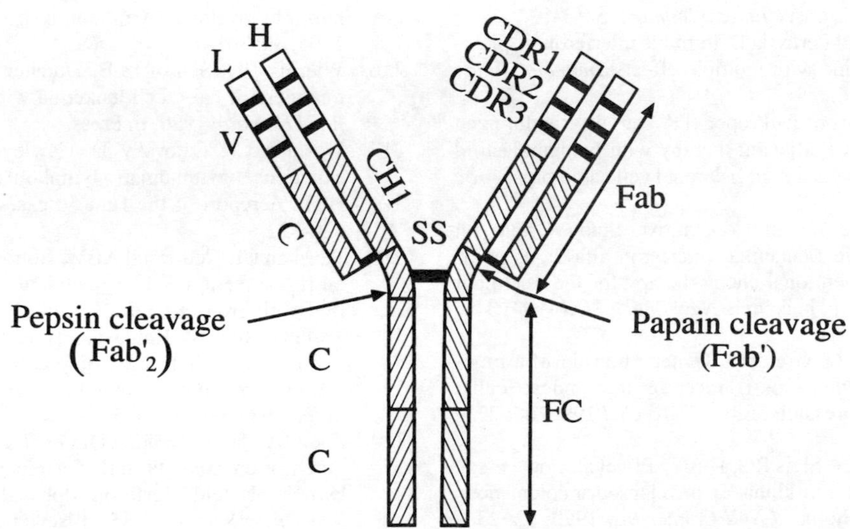

Figure 1. Structure of immunoglobulins and fragments. Two heavy chains are connected by a disulfide bond, and each in turn is connected to a light chain by a disulfide bond.

R.K. Oldham (ed.), Principles of Cancer Biotherapy. 3rd ed., 284–317.

discovered. Unfortunately, this has not been the case and most, if not all, tumor-associated antigens that are relatively tumor specific are found in other tissues as well, but often in very small amounts. Not surprisingly, many tumor-associated antigens are expressed much more heavily during embryonic development. Antibody therapy is theoretically the most tumor specific approach to systemic cancer treatment that has been discovered.

As illustrated in Fig. 2 and Table 1, there are many ways in which antibodies may be used in cancer therapy [48, 59, 182]. In this chapter, we shall review how unconjugated antibodies may be useful in therapy because of their interactions with other elements of the immune system, because of their interactions with specific cell surface molecules or growth factors that are important in the regulation of cell proliferation, or as immunogens to induce antibody antitumor response [57].

In subsequent chapters, the use of conjugated antibodies as carriers of cytotoxic substances including chemotherapy agents, radioisotopes, and natural toxins will be reviewed.

Table 1. Antibodies in cancer therapy

1. ANTIBODIES
   - Cytotoxic
   - Regulatory
   - Immunization
2. IMMUNOCONJUGATES
   - Radiolabeled Antibodies
   - Chemoimmunoconjugates
   - Immunotoxins
   - Immunobiologicals
3. BONE MARROW TRANSPLANTATION
   - Allogeneic
   - Autologous

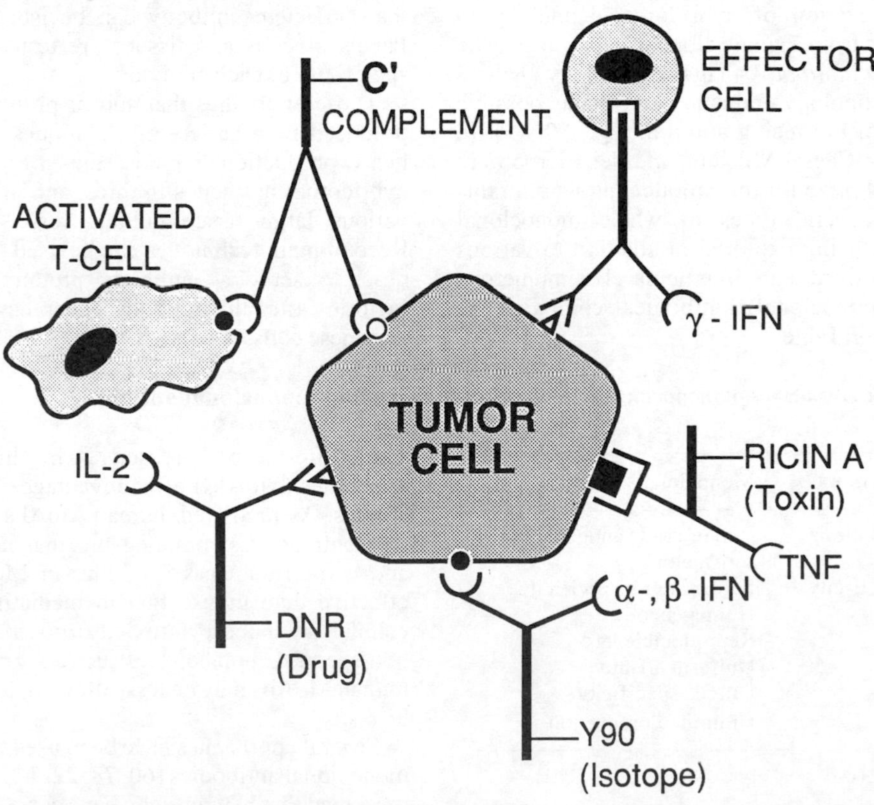

Figure 2. Schematic of potential applications of monoclonal antibodies for cancer therapy. Various antigens, representing the heterogeneity of cancer, are depicted on the tumor cell surface. Bifunctional antibodies are depicted with one Fab directed to a tumor antigen and the other to a biologic response modifier. One antibody has a Fab directed to a CD2 or CD3 receptor on T cells, which results in their activation and enhanced cytotoxicity. The Fc portion of the antibodies are attached to various cytotoxic substances including complement, effector cells (granulocytes, monocytes, killer T cells) of the immune system, and cytotoxic agents such as toxins, radioisotopes, and chemotherapy agents. IFN, interferon; TNF, tumor necrosis factor; IL-2, interleukin-2; DNR, daunorubicin. Ann Intern Med 1989, 111: 592-603. By permission of the American College of Physicians.

ANTIBODY PRODUCTION

Before addressing how antibodies themselves might produce anticancer effects, it is worth considering the issue of mass production of antibodies as potential therapeutic pharmaceuticals. Before 1970, it was virtually impossible to isolate a specific antibody. Rather, collections of antibodies from serum, called antisera, were used. Typically animals were repeatedly immunized with cells or substance of interest, and their sera was collected several weeks later. The specificity of such antisera was enhanced by repeated absorption with tissue that bore antigens other than those specific for a given tumor. Their degree of reactivity was determined by titrations based on serial dilutions. Typically, large animals were immunized in order to yield large volumes of serum. Unfortunately, it was impossible to reproduce a given antiserum exactly. Inasmuch as antibodies were genetically determined for an individual animal, the supply of any given antisera was limited. For these reasons, testing was always limited by quantity and each individual antiserum was of variable purity, consisting of multiple antibodies with various specificities and affinities.

In 1975, George Kohler and Caesar Milstein [132] described the utilization of hybridoma technology to produce antibodies from a single clone of cells – hence the term *monoclonal antibody*. This technology helped launch the biotechnology industry, and made possible mass production of promising antibodies [2, 30, 45]. In 1984, Hans Kohler, Caesar Milstein, and Neils Jerne were awarded the Nobel prize for their pioneering work in this area. There are several types of whole monoclonal antibody products being explored in addition to various Fab'[2], Fab, and linked Fab fragments. The numerous advantages of monoclonal antibodies compared to antisera are shown in Table 2.

Table 2. Comparative advantages of monoclonal antibodies vs. antisera

Antisera (polyclonal)	Monoclonal
Purified antigen to optimize	Cell or crude antigen satisfactory
Absorptions for specificity	Screening for specificity
Heterogeneous	Homogeneous
Variable lots	Reproducible lots
Variable affinities	Uniform affinity
Variable specificities	Unique specificity
Limited quantities	Unlimited production

Mouse/Rat monoclonal antibodies

Monoclonal antibodies directed against human cancer cells were originally derived from mice or other rodents, as illustrated in Fig. 3. The same concept can be applied to other species as well. Briefly, an animal is immunized with tumor cells, tumor cell membranes, or purified tumor-associated antigen.

The animal's immune system initiates an immune response characterized by production of antibodies against the tumor antigens. The antibodies are produced by B lymphocytes, which are found in large quantities in the spleen. The spleen of an immunized animal is removed and minced into a single-cell suspension. These cells are combined with other mouse B cells that have been specifically selected for certain characteristics, including (1) ability to grow in culture as a single clone, (2) inability to produce and secrete immunoglobulin themselves, and (3) inability to grow in the presence or absence of specific medium constituents. In the presence of a cell-fusing substance, such as polyethylene glycol, individual spleen cells with the genetic machinery for making antibody against the tumor fuse with cells from the immortal cell line. By using a process known as limiting dilution, such cells are isolated in wells to maximize the probability that any cell proliferation taking place will have been derived from a single hybridoma, leading to a single clone of cells, that is, a monoclone. The medium in which the cultured cells grow is sampled for secretion of monoclonal antibody. Those clones producing antibody are expanded so that sufficient antibody can be isolated for screening. Panels of cells and tissues are tested to determine the specificity of each antibody.

Those antibodies that appear promising can be mass-produced by a variety of techniques. The techniques of mass production include the *in vivo* expansion of hybridomas as ascites in mice, and *in vitro* expansion in various large tissue culture vessels and bioreactors. Recombinant techniques can be used to allow bacteria or yeast to serve as antibody production and secretory factories after the antibody genes have been introduced into these cells.

Human monoclonal antibodies

There are several reasons why human monoclonal antibodies (MoAbs) offer advantages over those of other species. As predicted, human MoAbs have proven to be substantially less immunogenic, than non-human MoAbs, and certain subclasses of human MoAbs of are more effective than mouse IgG in mediating complement or cellular mediated cytotoxicity *in vitro* [7, 78, 135]. The non-specific uptake, destruction and metabolism of human MoAbs may be less, allowing for prolonged serum levels.

Several approaches have been used for isolating human monoclonal antibodies [60, 78, 222]. In one approach, it is presumed that patients who have cancer have developed at least a limited immune response to their tumor. Lymph nodes are a potential source of B lymphocytes, and regional draining lymph nodes are the first line of immunologic defense against regional tumor. Lymph nodes draining known cancer sites, such as the axillary nodes on the side of a breast cancer, the peribronchial nodes re-

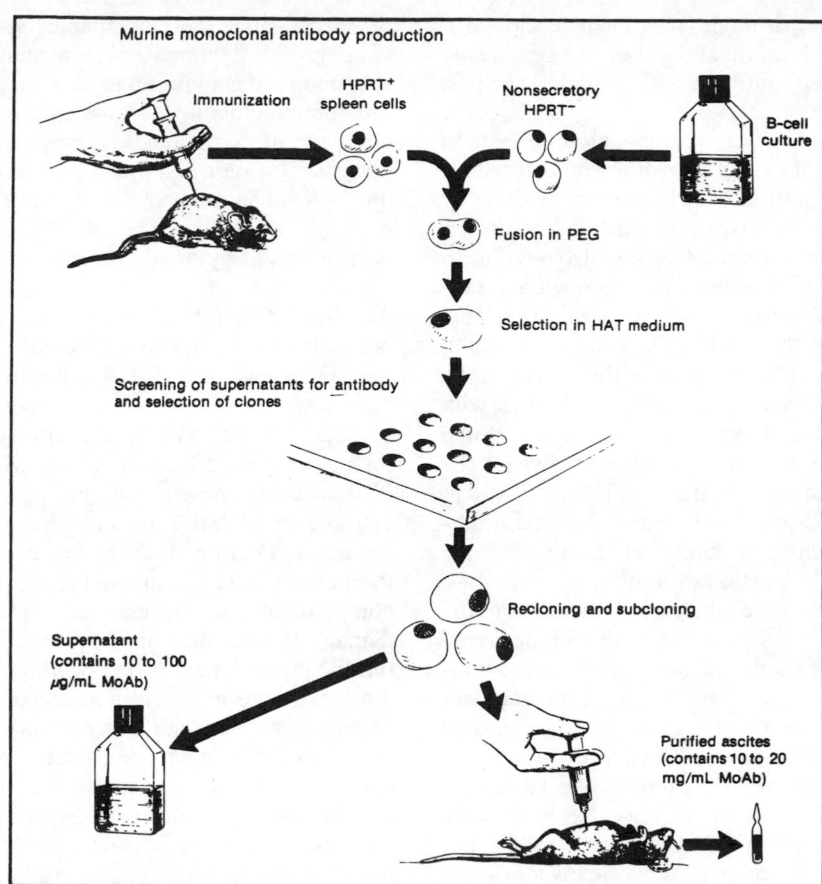

Figure 3. Schema for murine monoclonal antibody production. From Dillman RO, Royston I (1983), Drug Ther 8: 62-74. By permission of Biomedical Information Corporation.

moved at the time of resection of lung cancer, the mesenteric lymph nodes removed with resection of colon cancer, or the inguinal nodes resected following removal of a melanoma on the leg, are all potential sources of B lymphocytes that may have been programmed to make antibodies against the primary cancer. These cells can be fused with other human B cells, selected for similar characteristics as those immortal mouse B-cell lines described above [78]. The resulting human-human hybridoma may produce human monoclonal antibodies [17, 39, 40, 80, 126, 221]. It is also possible to fuse human lymph node B cells with cells from immortal mouse B-cell lines, and still get secretion of human antibody [26, 204, 255], although such hybridomas are often unstable. Other investigators have isolated B lymphocytes from lymph nodes and then infected these cells with Epstein-Barr virus in order to immortalize cells producing human Ig [31, 37, 60, 113].

Another approach to human antibody isolation involves immunization of cancer patients with irradiated autologous cancer cells in order to induce a humoral immune response. Typically irradiated autologous tumor cells are injected into the skin with an immune stimulant such as *Bacillus Calmette-Guerin* (BCG). Immunization is followed 2 to 3 weeks later by the harvesting of peripheral blood B lymphocytes, some of which will be secreting human antitumor antibodies [94]. Using various techniques, investigators have produced human antibodies against breast cancer [26, 127, 204], lung cancer [219], colorectal carcinoma [94], brain tumors [220], stomach cancer [255], and melanoma [75, 113, 119, 226].

Human monoclonals have been more difficult to develop than murine monoclonals because of clonal instability, low secretion rates, and difficulties in mass producing and screening. With improvements in transfection technology and isolation of B-cell growth factors, it should soon be feasible to integrate DNA for human immunoglobulin into cells that can easily produce large quantities of human monoclonal antibodies.

Chimeric/humanized monoclonal antibodies

Because of the difficulties in establishing production of human monoclonal antibodies, and because of the extensive characterization of house MoAbs which react against human TAA, and because of the disadvantages of mouse antibodies, other strategies have been developed to create mouse/human chimeric antibodies and genetically engineered 'humanized' antibodies (Fig. 4) [1, 19, 147, 172, 249].

It is also possible to make bifunctional antibodies in which each antibody arm, or two different antibodies, react with a different antigen [252]. This can be done by chemically linking either two different Fab pairs or $F(ab')_2$ pairs, or two intact antibodies. It is also possible to make quadromas (a hybridoma of two monoclonal antibody-secreting hybridomas), which secrete monoclonal antibodies that react with two different antigenic binding characteristics [39, 231]. One can then select the appropriate quadroma that is producing antibodies with two different antigenic binding characteristics. Such bifunctional antibodies should have high affinity for the target antigens inasmuch as they will lack bivalent binding. It is also possible to class-switch certain antibodies, that is, attach a different Fc portion to the immunoreactive $F(ab')_2$ portion of a given antibody [44, 172]. In the chimeric approach the variable domains of the light and heavy chains of a murine MoAb with desirable specificity, are linked to constant domains of a human immunoglobulin. This is most often done with recombinant techniques in which the mouse genes for the variable domains of amino acids are combined with the human domains for the constant region amino acids. The genes are then inserted into bacteria or yeast for large-scale production. The bacterial preparations are typically not glycosylated while those grown in yeast are glycosylated. It is also possible to isolate the genes specific for the hypervariable amino acid sequences on the light and heavy chains of a desirable murine antibody, and these can then be inserted into the framework of human immunoglobulin to create a 'humanized' monoclonal antibody. This is called 'CDR grafting.' In this instance the only residual mouse amino acid sequences remaining are those which give the antibody its three-dimensional binding specificity. In recent years an increasing number of investigators and companies have developed such chimeric or humanized preparations for superior immunologic activity related to the human Fc portion of the immunoglobulin, and the greatly decreased immunogenicity of such preparations which increases the potential for repeated therapeutic interventions with the monoclonal antibody product [145, 213].

Antibodies as cytotoxic therapy

As outlined in Table 1, there are at least three different rationales for using antibodies alone *in vivo* in approaching cancer treatment. The first two depend on the immune mediated effects of the Fc receptor[161]. The first approach is one in which the antibody mediates an antitumor cytotoxic effects in concert with other components of the host immune system. Complement mediated cytotoxicity (CMC) or complement dependent cytotoxicity (CDC) involves the fixation of complement via the Fc portions of immunoglobulin and activation of the complement protein cascade resulting in membrane damage and cell destruction [73]. In general, most of the murine monoclonal antibodies which have been generated are ineffective in fixing human complement in *in vitro* experiments. As a rule murine IgM antibodies are more likely to fix human complement than other antibody classes. However, IgM immunoglobulins are somewhat more difficult to work with technically because of their size and stickiness. Theoretically their large size could present certain problems in terms of bioavailability and transport into tumor masses, and if administered in large quantities, they might produce hyperviscosity. Certain IgG3 antibodies against disialoganglioside antigens (GD2, GD3) such as those expressed on neuro-ectodermal cells, can also effect CMC [37, 87, 253]. Whether the CMC in these instances is because of the IgG3 subclass, or because of the specific nature of these antigens is unclear. Studies of hemolytic anemia have confirmed that with human antibodies IgM is the most efficient class in

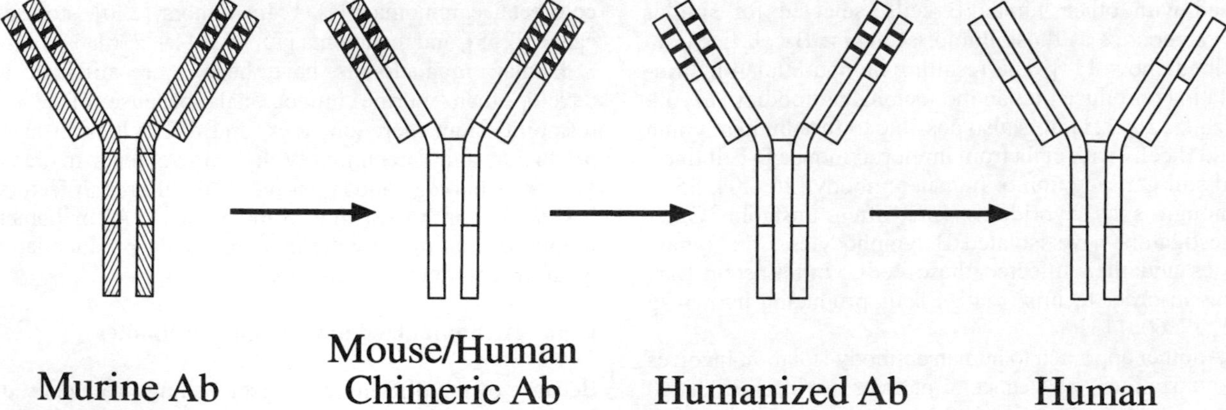

Figure 4. Comparison of mouse, mouse/human chimera, 'humanized,' and human antibodies, illustrating the component of murine amino acid sequences in each.

complement binding followed by IgG1, IgG3, and IgG2. Because complement fixation occurs at the Fc portion of antibody, this approach requires whole intact immunoglobulin rather than antibody subunits.

The second immunological cytotoxic mechanism is that of antibody dependent cell mediated cytotoxicity (ADCC) [97, 98]. Once again, the Fc portion is required for binding of cytolytic cells via their Fc receptors, and correlate with ADCC activity [151]. Many lymphocytes, monocytes, tissue macrophages, and granulocytes have such receptors and can effect tumor cell lysis. Collectively, such cells are referred to as 'effector cells'. Theoretically, antibody can first bind to its cellular target followed by effector cell binding, or alternatively, effector cells may first be linked to antibody, and then be carried to the tumor target. *In vitro*, both methods can produce cytotoxicity and the former approach has produced anti-tumor responses in animal models [101]. *In vivo*, circulating target cells coated with antibody are removed in the liver and spleen, presumably because of Fc receptors on tissue macrophages in these sites. For human antibodies, the ability to bind specifically to macrophages of the reticuloendothelial (RE) system is restricted to IgG1 and IgG3 antibodies and is absent from IgM and other IgG subclasses. There is evidence that mouse monoclonals differ in their subclass binding in humans. Various studies have confirmed that murine IgG2A antibodies, followed by IgG3, are superior to other subclasses in effecting ADCC, apparently because of enhanced Fc receptor binding [103, 111]. In addition, different antibodies of the same subclass and isotype, directed against the same antigen, exhibit different degrees of Fc binding [53]. Murine IgG3 anti-disialoganglioside antibodies have been cytotoxic with human effector cells *in vitro* [35, 98]. Most IgG humanized MoAbs are active [227].

For both ADCC and CMC the *in vivo* anti-tumor effect is dependent on the ability of the host immune system to provide sufficient complement proteins or effector cells to produce cytotoxicity. The use of various biological response modifiers may be useful in augmenting the immune system. To maximize efficiency of effector cell-antibody binding, some investigators have utilized leukopheresis to harvest leukocytes, and then incubated these with antibodies to enrich the antibody-effector cell population. Various lymphokines, such as interleukins-2, -4, and -12 may be useful to enhance the cytotoxic activity of the effector cells. It has been demonstrated that cytotoxicity, either by ADCC or CMC, involves a threshold of antigen binding sites. Lymphokines, such as alpha interferon, may be useful in enhancing target antigen expression [85, 144]. Gamma or immune interferon increases Fc receptors on effector cells and thereby can enhance ADCC [53, 241]. There are good examples from animal models suggesting that various biologicals may be used in combination to maximize an anti-tumor effect. These other biologicals might be used systemically, or targeted specifically by other antibodies.

Regulatory approaches

A second approach to the use of antibodies alone has been termed 'regulatory' to contrast with 'cytotoxic'. It is known that tumor cells have a variety of receptors which are important for growth or proliferative advantages [83]. Table 3 lists a number of such receptors or antigens which may be crucial for tumor cell self renewal, and which have been found in increased quantities in cancer cells and/or other rapidly proliferating cells.

Table 3. Targets for regulatory therapy

CD 20 B-Cell Receptor
Epidermal Growth Factor Receptor (EGF)
Fibronectin
Gastron-Releasing Peptide (GRP)
Her-2Neu Receptor
Idiotypic Immunoglobulin
Interleukin-2 Receptors
Other Oncogene Products or Receptors
Platelet Derived Growth Factor Receptor (PDGF)
Transferrin Receptor

Conceptually, antibodies directed against growth factor receptors may either block or down-regulate the number of receptors available on the cell surface, and thus impair a cell's ability to differentiate and/or divide, ultimately resulting in cell death or apoptosis. Such antigens may also serve as targets for antibodies which can elicit CMC and/or ADCC, or as targets for cytotoxic immunoconjugates. Many receptors internalize after their ligand or an antibody bind to them. Rapid internalization limits the potential for CMC or ADCC, but may be an advantage for the internalization of conjugated cytotoxic chemotherapy agents or toxins.

Probably the most thoroughly studied system for a regulatory approach is the idiotype network which involves anti-idiotype antibodies [76, 115]. A malignant B-cell clone produces cells which express and sometimes secrete a specific antibody with a unique binding ability. The critical molecules in the hypervariable region of the immunoreactive arms of the antibody are the idiotypes which collectively constitute the idiotype of that immunoglobulin and account for its specificity. Under normal conditions memory T cells may signal B cells to produce immunoglobulin via the idiotype when it is expressed on the cell surface. It has also been established that other B cells may produce anti-idiotype antibodies which may be important in negative feedback control of a given B-cell clone which has been activated. How this might relate to B-cell malignancy is depicted simplistically in Fig. 5. A detailed description of the 'network theory' of anti-idiotype regulation is very complex, and beyond the scope of this chapter [77]. In its simplest construct, infusion of an antibody directed against a B-cell lymphoma idiotype might suppress (growth regulate) that clone back to its baseline state. It is also important to note that the idiotype

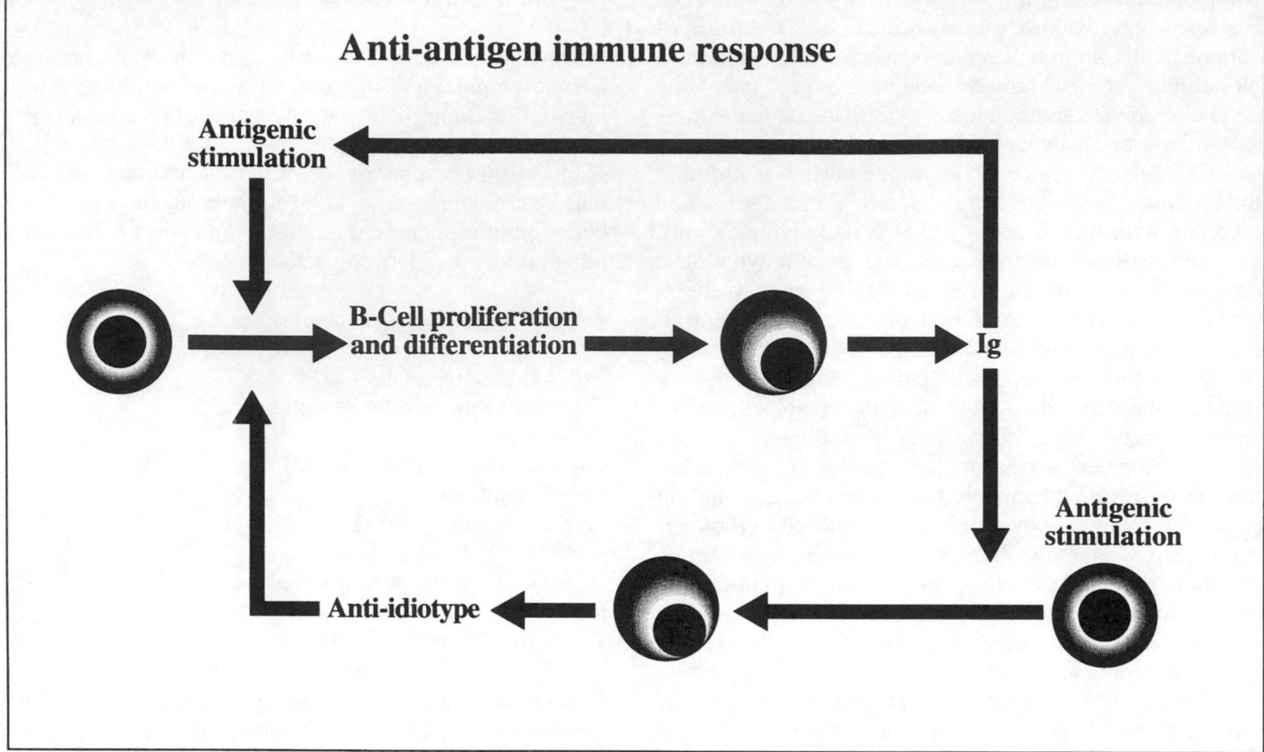

Figure 5. Diagram of anti-idiotype feedback inhibition of B-cell clonal proliferation, based on the specificity of the hypervariable region of the antibodies produced by that clone of cells.

of a given B-cell tumor is the most tumor specific antigen known. The CD20 receptor also appears to be important for signal transduction and proliferation of B lymphocytes. Antibodies which react with CD20 on B lymphocytes, or the receptors for Her-2neu, epidermal growth factor (EGF) receptor, and transferrin receptors are also promising targets for such regulatory approaches [237].

The third application of antibody alone for *in vivo* anti-cancer therapy is actually a method of passive immunization and also is based on idiotype network theory [122, 128]. The idiotype of an immunoglobulin is typically quite immunogenic. Injection of a mouse antibody (AB1) directed against a patient's tumor antigen will lead to production of anti-idiotype antibodies (AB2) directed against the hypervariable determinants of the AB1. Some of these AB2 may present the same three-dimensional antigenic structure as the original tumor antigen. Subsequently, such AB2 anti-idiotype antibodies may induce anti-anti-idiotype antibody (AB3), which because of the 'lock-and-key' structural relationship between antigen and antibody, will have the same binding specificity as the original mouse antibody (AB1), except that it will be a human antibody (AB3) [104, 246]. A more direct approach using this same principle involves simply taking a well-characterized anti-anti-idiotype antibody (AB2) and directly injecting it as an immunogen to try to induce a human AB3 which will react with the tumor antigen. This theoretical approach has been demonstrated in animals and may have application in both cancer and autoimmune diseases [105, 121] Clinical trials are addressing whether this approach can lead to successful production of sufficient antibodies to produce an anti-tumor effect in man (See Chapter 8).

Animal models and antibody therapy

Because of the tremendous number of publications in this area, this section is limited primarily to selected monoclonal antibody animal studies.

The antitumor potential of MoAb therapy has been demonstrated in numerous animal models. Bernstein et al. [3, 11, 12, 13] conducted a series of trials in AKR/J mice with either a transplantable soft tissue leukemia/lymphoma of spontaneous leukemia. Treatment with an IgG2A anti-thy 1.1 murine MoAb was associated with prolonged survival when given one to two hours after subcutaneous inoculation of 10^6 tumor cells, while IgG3 and IgM anti-thy 1.1 were no more effective than placebo. This effect was accomplished even though the MoAb also reacted with normal circulating T cells and normal thymocytes. The therapeutic effects on established transplanted tumor were limited, but the investigators were able to cure animals using a combination of surgical excision of tumor followed by anti-thy 1.1 MoAb with rabbit complement. In AKR/J mice with spontaneous leukemia, anti-thy 1.1 therapy was of no benefit unless it was preceded by cytoreductive cyclophosphamide therapy. All of the antibody isotypes promoted CMC *in vitro*, but only the IgG2A and IgG3 produced effective ADCC. For these reasons, the authors suggested ADCC might be the more important *in vivo* mechanism of antitumor effect. They concluded that IgG2A was superior to IgG3 and that IgM was ineffective in this model, and that curative potential would be best in the adjuvant setting with limited tumor burden. They also noted that IgG2A coated thymocytes were not destroyed *in vivo*, although T lymphocytes were selectively depleted from the spleen and lymph nodes. It took 3.2 mg of IgG2A MoAb to inhibit the growth of 3 x 10^5 SL2 leukemia cells in 83% of mice. Higher cell numbers led to local tumor nodule resistance with antigen positive cells, and the appearance of antigen negative metastases. Extrapolating to man, these experiments suggest that gram quantities of MoAb might be needed for maximum therapeutic effect in human cancer patients, an important point to be addressed later [183].

Other investigators have also used MoAbs against T-cell antigens in animal tumor models. Kirsch and Hammerling used thy 1.2 and LY2.2 in A/thy 1.1 congenic mice inoculated subcutaneously with ASL.1 leukemia or C57BL/6LYT 2.1 congenic mice inoculated with ERLD or ER4 tumors [126]. The MoAb therapy was given intraperitoneally starting 2, 24, or 48 hours after tumor inoculation. In the ALS.1 model, an IgG3 MoAb administered within 24 hours of tumor inoculation prevented tumor development. The IgM antibody was associated with prolonged survival, but did not prevent tumor development. In the LYT 2.1 model, an IgG2A MoAb was associated with prolonged survival in the ERLD tumors, but was associated with a decreased survival in the EL4 model. As in the AKR/J models, this study again pointed out the importance of Ig subclass. In addition, it reminded investigators of the possibility that some MoAbs might stimulate, rather than inhibit, tumor growth [118].

Young and Hakomori [256] treated DBA2 mice with IgM or IgG3 anti-gangliotriosylceramide beginning one day after animals were inoculated with 10^6 cells of mouse lymphoma in the peritoneal cavity. Survival was prolonged when IgG3 was given IP or IV with or without guinea pig complement. Residual tumor cells expressed much less tumor antigen suggesting either selection of antigen depleted cells, or modulation of the antigen as a consequence of exposure to the MoAb. This study again suggested an *in vivo* superiority for IgG over IgM.

Herlyn et al. [102] studied the effects of anti-tumor MoAb in athymic mice bearing human colon carcinoma xenografts. An IgG2A anti-human colorectal carcinoma MoAb, administered IP, was associated with either retardation or complete inhibition of subcutaneous tumor growth. An IgM MoAb to the same antigen produced no effect. These same investigators were also able to retard the development of human melanoma xenografts in athymic mice using an IgG anti-melanoma MoAb [133].

Scheinberg and Strand [202] used a Rauscher leukemia virus induced erythroleukemia in BALB/c mice as a tumor model for testing the effectiveness of MoAb therapy. MoAb 103A was originally prepared against the 70 kilodalton envelope glycoprotein of this virus. Animals were infected with RVB3 virus and subsequently their spleens were removed and analyzed for tumor colony formation. A single 125 mcg dose of MoAb 103A injected within 3 days of virus inoculation caused a 90% reduction in tumor foci compared to controls.

Foon et al. [70] conducted experiments with an IgG1 MoAb which reacts with a chemically induced transplantable hepatocellular carcinoma. This model may be particularly relevant inasmuch as the transplantable tumor metastasized in strain 2 guinea pigs. In addition, these animals are especially susceptible to anaphylactoid reactions. Even though this MoAb failed to mediate ADCC or CMC *in vitro*, IV injections, given shortly after intradermal tumor cell injections, inhibited tumor growth. However, there was little effect on established tumor.

Houghton and Lanier et al. [95, 137] demonstrated the efficiency of anti-idiotype therapy for eliminating the growth of CH1 murine B cell lymphoma using rabbit anti-idiotype serum. Up to 10^3 to 10^4 tumor cells could be eliminated when 100 ul of anti-idiotype serum was given IP within 48 hours of tumor cell inoculation. Anti-tumor effects were preserved even in animals who were genetically C5 deficient, complement depleted by cobra venom factor, or immunosuppressed by splenectomy, thymectomy, sublethal irradiation, or cyclophosphamide chemotherapy. Perek et al. [187] noted antitumor effects with an $F(ab')_2$ anti-idiotype in a lymphoma model suggesting that ADCC and CDC were not required for the response.

Capone et al. [27] obtained tumor regressions in athymic mice bearing established human breast cancers using 100 ug IgG3 or IgG2A anti-breast cancer antibodies injected IP. There was no anti-tumor effect following injection of nonspecific antibody of similar isotype. *In vitro*, both MoAbs were effective in CDC, but not ADCC.

In other animal studies, Masui et al. [158] demonstrated that MoAb against epidermal growth factor inhibited growth of human epidermoid cell line A431 in athymic mice. Trowbridge et al. [234] inhibited growth of human melanoma xenografts in athymic mice using an IgG1 anti-transferrin receptor MoAb which reacts with the transferrin receptor.

Billing and Chatterjee [16] treated nine rhesus monkeys with anti-Ia antibody H-4 to prevent skin graft rejection. Four animals died acutely following IV injection. Lower titers of H-4 were not associated with this complication which was attributed to anaphylaxis.

Stratte et al. [229] studied the effects of anti-human T-cell MoAb anti-leu 1 in one Gibbon ape, 1 rhesus monkey, and 4 chimpanzees whose peripheral blood T cells expressed the same T-cell antigen found on human T cells. Transient decreases in T cells were obtained following slow infusions. All animals developed antimouse antibodies, most of which could be absorbed using immunoglobulin of the same isotype. However, a small amount of the antimouse antibody was reactive with the idiotype (hypervariable region) of the MoAb.

Letvin et al. [141] studied the effects of three different anti-T11 (sheep erythrocyte receptor) MoAbs in rhesus monkeys. Infusions of up to 2 mg/kg over four hours were well tolerated. The IgG2 MoAbs were more effective than an IgG1 in clearing circulating target cells. There were also marked differences among the MoAbs in induction of antigenic modulation.

The following conclusions can be drawn from the heterologous antisera and MoAb therapy studies in animal models. First, MoAb inhibition of tumor cells can occur *in vivo*. Complement fixation is not required for the antitumor effect which seems to vary with the Ig subclass and isotype. Second, antitumor effects on large well established tumors are unimpressive suggesting that passive MoAb therapy may only be effective when given as an adjuvant or in combination with other anti-cancer agents when there is minimal tumor burden. Third, in view of the results with well absorbed heterologous antisera, it seems doubtful that simply combining MoAbs will produce better results than carefully prepared antisera. On the other hand, selection of antibodies to target different antigens to increase the number of antibody molecules binding to a target cell, and to overcome problems of heterogeneity, may still be advantageous [184]. Fourth, there may be a therapeutic advantage for IgG2A and IgG3 subclasses based on various experiments suggesting superior ADCC or CMC with such MoAbs. Finally, passive MoAb therapy has had limited efficacy in situations completely analogous to the human cancer setting, namely spontaneous widely disseminated tumor.

Antisera trials

Although most clinical trials conducted during the past 15 years have utilized monoclonal antibodies, there were numerous clinical studies performed using antisera between 1925 and 1975. These studies with heterologous and isologous antisera and have been reviewed in more detail elsewhere [43, 195, 254]. Such trials were limited by the quantity of purified anti-tumor antisera available, the purity of such preparations, and difficulties producing similar lots of new antibody. Nevertheless, some antitumor effects were noted.

In 1927, Lindstrom [146] treated 10 chronic myelogenous leukemia patients with 15 courses of rabbit antisera. He described therapeutic benefit in five patients, but also noted significant side effects which were attributed to impurities in the preparation. Brittingham and Chaplin [18] treated a CML patient with a series of intramuscular injections of isologous human antisera with minimal benefit. Lazlo et al. [138] reported limited responses in 3 patients with chronic lymphocytic leukemia (CLL) treated with isologous plasma from individuals who had been immunized with lymphocytes. The isoimmune plasma was infused over 30 minutes and produced decreases in circulating lymphocytes, lymph nodes, and spleens in some patients. Fever and chills were the major toxicities noted, and one patient was followed for two years with seven courses of treatment. Herberman et al. [100] treated seven patients with an alloantisera which reacted with histocompatibility antigens. Decreases in circulating lymphocytes were seen, but lasted less than a day and were maximal within an hour of treatment. The patients had decreases in lymph node size. Side effects included fever, chills, nausea, vomiting, and thrombocytopenia. Hamblin et al. [92] treated a CLL patient with sheep anti-CLL idiotype antisera. They observed a drop in circulating leukemia cells associated with fever, hypotension, and bronchospasm.

Anti-thymocyte globulin (ATG) has been used to treat patients with T-cell malignancies. Fisher et al. [69] gave ATG over 6 hours to a patient with Sezary syndrome. Erythroderma resolved, circulating T cells decreased, and lymphadenopathy diminished. Therapy was complicated by hypotension and chills, but prophylaxis with diphenhydramine and steroids seemed to prevent similar side effects during 6 subsequent daily treatments. Inasmuch as this patient had not responded to steroids previously, the results were attributed to ATG. Edelson et al. [62] treated four patients with cutaneous T-cell lymphoma (CTCL) with ATG. They also noted a decrease in circulating T cells, transient antitumor effects, fever, chills, and hypotension. Antihistamines and steroids appeared to prevent side effects with subsequent, repetitive treatments. Wong et al. [251] reported a marked reduction in lymphadenopathy following ATG in a patient with lymphoblastic lymphoma.

Interpretation of these antisera studies was complicated by issues of antibody source, purity and specificity. Certain toxicities were apparent, but it was unclear whether these were due to impurities or to antitumor effects. The antitumor effects themselves could have been induced by such impurities as interferons, interleukins, and tumor necrosis factor. Clinical trials with monoclonal antibodies have confirmed several of these observations, clarified the etiology of various side effects, and defined the promise and problems for using MoAbs alone as anticancer therapy.

Clinical trials of unconjugated monoclonal antibodies in man

The following review covers human clinical trials with unconjugated monoclonal antibodies. Some trials which involved tracer quantities of radiolabeled MoAbs and are also included if in fact patients received large quantities of unmodified antibody. Clinical trials in man with murine monoclonal antibodies began in 1980 in hematopoietic malignancies and subsequently in solid tumors. It should be emphasized that most of the clinical work published to-date has been of a pilot or phase I nature, with mouse monoclonal antibodies, and relatively few patients actually studied. However, in recent years some phase II and III trials have been reported as well as trials of human and humanized antibodies. Modern cancer therapy is dictated by tumor type and, therefore, the remainder of this review is organized by specific malignancy.

Hematopoietic diseases

Summaries of various trials of unconjugated monoclonal antibodies in hematopoietic malignancies are shown in Tables 4-7. The information described is based on publication in the medical literature and cannot be considered all inconclusive because of the volume of unpublished results known only to certain companies who have pursued commercial development of certain antibodies, and the US Food and Drug Administration.

ACUTE LYMPHOCYTIC LEUKEMIA (ALL)

B and pre-B ALL

Murine monoclonal antibody J-5 reacts with the common acute lymphoblastic leukemia antigen CD10 (CALLA). *In vitro* J-5 mediates complement-dependent cytotoxicity in the presence of rabbit complement, but not human complement. Ritz et al. [194] treated 4 acute lymphocytic leukemia (ALL) patients with 1-170 mg infusions of J-5 delivered over 15 minutes to two hours. In those patients with circulating blasts, treatment was followed by a rapid decrease in circulating CALLA$^+$ blasts, but a large number of CALLA-negative lymphoblasts persisted. However, once J-5 was no longer detectable in the serum, the lymphoblasts reexpressed CALLA, consistent with antigenic modulation or cycling of the surface antigen, or down regulation of an antigenic receptor in the presence of the antibody. The transient changes in lymphoblast phenotype noted in these patients were attributed to modulation (internalization) of the CALLA antigen [193]. There was no significant change in degree of bone marrow replacement by lymphoblasts even though J-5 binding was demonstrated. There was no significant toxicity noted in these patients although all 3 patients who had circulating blast cells had temperature elevations in association with therapy.

Dyer et al. [61] treated 5 ALL patients with CAMPATH rat antibodies. CAMPATH reacts with CDw52 antigen which is present on 95% of human peripheral blood B and T lymphocytes, and the antigen is similarly expressed on malignant B and T lymphocytes. Unlike most antibodies used to treat hematopoietic malignancies, CAMPATH does not appear to induce significant antigenic modulation, and is able to lyse lymphocytes in the presence of complement. These patients had prolonged decreases in circulating lymphoblast counts and marrow infiltration by blasts. Repeated treatment was limited because of the human anti-rat antibody (HARA) immune response. For this reason a genetically engineered CAMPATH 1-H was created which retained the 6 rat hypervariable domains in a human IgG1 framework. An early report described significant reductions in circulating blasts in 3 of 7 patients, and complete clearance of blasts in 2 others [130]. Despite these results, and more interesting clinical effects in lymphomas, Burroughs-Wellcome decided to discontinue trials with this agent [63].

T-ALL

Levy and colleagues [142] treated 8 T-cell leukemia patients with two anti-leukemia antibodies which did not induce antigenic modulation, and an anti-CD5 monoclonal antibody later called Leu1 which is associated with antigenic modulation. Patients received from 1 to 92 mg of this antibody alone or in combination 2 or 3 other monoclonal antibodies. Transient reductions in circulating leukemia cell counts were noted with no sustained antitumor effects. In these trials there was no demonstrated advantage associated with giving multiple antibodies, including those which did not induce antigenic modulation.

Table 4. Phase I/II monoclonal antibody trials in acute leukemia

Investigator	MoAB	Ig	Disease	Responders/Treated
Ritz	J-5(CD10)	mIgG1	ALL	0/4
Dyer	CAMPATH	rIgG2b	ALL	3/5
Levy	Leu1(CD5)	mIgG2a	T-ALL	0/8
Waldmann	Anti-TAC(CD25)	mIgG2a	T-ALL	6/19
Ball	Several	mIgM	AML	0/3
Ball	MDX 11(CD15)	mIgM	AML	0/16
Scheinberg	M195(CD33)	mIgG2a	AML	0/10

ALL = acute lymphocytic leukemia.
AML = acute myelocytic leukemia.
m = mouse.
r = rat.

The interleukin-2 receptor is composed of 3 subunits including an alpha chain (p55), a beta chain (p75), and a gamma chain (p65) which combine noncovalently to bind the important lymphokine interleukin-2 [240]. The expression of this receptor is increased in malignant cells of adult T-cell leukemia which is induced by the human T-cell lymphotrophic virus I (HTLV-I) [84, 238]. Waldmann et al. [239] used the anti-TAC (T-activated cells) antibody which is directed against the p55 chain of the interleukin-2 receptor (CD25), in 19 patients with adult T-cell leukemia. Patients received 20, 40, 50, 60, or 100 mg doses over 8 to 445 days with variable total doses ranging from 220 mg over 9 days, 490 mg over 51 days, and 220 mg over 445 days. One patient, who had previously failed aggressive combination chemotherapy had a complete response that lasted for 5 months, and then a partial response which lasted 6 months after retreatment. There were 2 complete and 4 partial responses observed in this trial as well as one mixed response. The duration of remissions ranged from 2 months to 3 years. Another patient had a reduction in peripheral leukemia cells, but had an increase in malignant lymphadenopathy at the same time. These patients were already markedly immunosuppressed, and they may have been further immunosuppressed by this antiactivated T-cell antibody. While on study, one patient developed Kaposi's sarcoma, one Pneumocystis carinii pneumonia, and a third developed Staphylococcal A septicemia. Further evidence of immunosuppression was the fact that only one of the nine patients treated developed antimouse antibodies.

A humanized form of this antibody was developed using genetic engineering techniques; it is called anti-TAC-H and has a human IgG1 constant framework. Thus, this particular antibody is a 'hyperchimeric' in that all components are human except for the hypervariable segments [117]. The murine version of this MoAb was unable to effect ADCC with human effector cells while the humanized antibody is cytolytic in ADCC assays. As expected, this humanized antibody was much less immunogenic in monkeys and in humans with drug resistant graft versus host disease (GVHD). Trials in T-cell leukemia and lymphoma are in progress.

Acute myelocytic leukemia

Ball et al. [5] treated 3 patients with acute myelogenous leukemia (AML) with one or more murine monoclonal antibodies which were relatively specific for AML. The murine monoclonal antibodies used in these studies were all cytotoxic in the presence of rabbit serum as a source of complement, and none induced antigenic modulation *in vitro*. These included 3 IgM, called PMN-81, PMN-29, PM-81, which reacted with glycolipids; the fourth antibody was an IgG2b called AML-2-23 which reacted with a protein antigen. The 3 patients received multiple 8 to 12 hour infusions of 20 to 70 mg of the various antibodies. Treatments were associated with rapid, but transient decreases in circulating blasts and elevations of serum lactic dehydrogenase which suggested that leukemia cells had been destroyed. However, sustained remission of leukemia was not accomplished.

In a subsequent trial, 16 AML patients were treated with a 24-hour continuous infusion of PM81 (also called MDX-11) which reacts with the granulocyte-associated antigen CD15 [6]. Doses from 0.5 to 1.5 mg/kg were given in a dose escalation study. Once again, only transient reductions in circulating blasts were noted, and there did not appear to be an effect on marrow blasts. Circulating CD15 antigen presented a problem in terms of immune complexes. The toxicity observed in this trial: fever, chills, hypotension, tachycardia was the same as the observed with other MoABs which bind to circulating cells. There are plans to perform additional trials with this antibody in AML patients who have been effectively cytoreduced with chemotherapy.

M195 is a murine IgG2a monoclonal antibody which reacts with CD-33 which is found on early myeloid precursors. This receptor is rapidly modulated or down regulated in the presence of M195. Scheinberg et al. [203] injected 10 AML patients were injected with escalating doses of M195 (1, 5, and 10 mg/m^2) up to a total dose of 76 mg. Specific binding to bone marrow cells was demonstrated by tracer radioisotope and by bone marrow biopsy, but rapid antigenic modulation was confirmed *in vivo*. Sustained antitumor effects with unconjugated antibody were not seen. Because of the theoretical limitations of the human antimouse antibody (HAMA) response, a CDR-grafted human IgG1 version of M195 (HuM195) was developed. This construct is able to effect ADCC with human effector cells *in vitro* in contrast to the mouse version. However, antigenic modulation (internalization of antigen/antibody, ligand/receptor) would still be expected to limit ADCC *in vivo*. HuM195 was given as 6 doses administered over 3 weeks with a radiolabelled tracer dose into 13 AML patients, but a decrease in marrow blasts was only noted in one patient. Unconjugated HuM195 is being studied in the setting of minimal tumor burden following cytoreductive chemotherapy.

Chronic lymphocytic leukemia

T101 is a murine IgG2a monoclonal antibody that reacts with the CD5 lymphocyte antigen. This receptor is found on T cells and on the B lymphocytes of chronic lymphocytic leukemia (CLL) and well-differentiated diffuse B-cell lymphoma. This antigen rapidly internalizes after antibody binds to it and was not cytotoxic in *in vitro* assays of CMC or ADCC with human effector cells or human complement. Dillman et al. [46, 49, 50, 52] treated 10 chronic lymphocytic leukemia (CLL) patients with T101. Two patients received 1 to 10 mg over 15 minutes, 2 received weekly doses of 10 mg infused over 2 hours, and 6 received 24-hour infusions of T101 at doses of 10, 50, 100, 150, or 500 mg. Limited unsustained clinical benefit was noted despite confirmation of *in vivo* binding to CLL cells in blood, lymph nodes, and bone marrow. The same T101 antibody was studied by Foon et al. [71, 72] in 13 patients with CLL. Doses of 1, 10, 50, and 100 mg were given and one patient received 140 mg. At all doses there was binding to circulating and bone marrow cells, and a rapid but transient decline in circulating leukemia cell counts. Durable responses were not seen.

Dyer et al. [61] administered the rat CAMPATH antibody to 5 CLL patients. Three had sustained decreases in circulating leukemic cells but only one of the three had resolution of marrow infiltrating by leukemic cells. A sixth CLL patient received a rat/human chimeric IgM CAMPATH antibody and had no response. Burroughs-Wellcome has sponsored clinical trials of CAMPATH 1-H, the human IgG1 construct of this antibody which retains the 6 rat hypervariable domains of the original rat antibody, and clinical responses have been seen in patients who had failed fludarabine chemotherapy. One report claimed responses in 6 of 16 patients who received 30 mg 3 times a week for 16 weeks [114]. However, the response rate observed was considered disappointing; so, the company decided to discontinue the trials [63].

Some patients with chronic lymphocytic leukemia have received infusions of anti-idiotype monoclonal antibodies [33]. These patients are not ideal for anti-idiotype therapy because of the large amounts of free idiotype which are secreted by the leukemia cells. Brief decreases in circulating leukemia cell counts have been seen in these patients following infusion of anti-idiotype antibodies, but sustained antitumor effects have not been noted.

Multiple myeloma

Interleukin-6 (IL-6) is an important growth factor for plasma cells. Klein et al. [129] reported treating a patient with primary plasma cell leukemia whose disease was refractory to chemotherapy. Daily intravenous injections of anti-IL-6 monoclonal antibodies were given. Serial monitoring during the 2 months of treatment was demonstrated a decrease in serum calcium, serum paraprotein, C-reactive protein, and the percentage of cells in S-phase in the bone marrow, but an objective tumor response could not be claimed. There were no major toxicities but decreases in both platelet and white blood cell counts were noted.

Stevenson et al. [228] have developed a mouse/human chimeric antibody to the CD38 antigen which is present on the majority of neoplastic plasma cells. The human IgG1/OKT10 mouse FAB chimeric antibody was able to mediate antibody-dependent cellular cytotoxicity in preclinical trials. Clinical trials with this antibody are in progress.

B-Cell lymphoma

The first report of monoclonal antibody therapy in man involved treatment of a lymphoma patient by Nadler et al. [179]. *In vitro* tests demonstrated cytolysis by complement-mediated cytotoxicity using the patient's serum or animal sources of complement, but AB89 failed to effect antibody-dependent cell-mediated cytotoxicity. On successive days the patient received slow infusions of the monoclonal antibody AB89 at doses of 25, 75, and 150 mg; one month later a 1.5 gm dose was administered. There was a transient decrease in WBC after each treatment, but no significant antitumor effect was noted.

CD20 is a 35 kilodalton antigen with multiple transmembrane domains which does not internalize. It is expressed on normal and malignant B cells. Antibodies binding to surface CD20 can induce a transmembrane signal that can cause a variety of effects including apoptosis. Press et al. [188] treated 4 patients with refractory B-cell lymphoma with monoclonal antibody 1F5 which reacts with CD20. Total treatment was given over 5 to 10 days. Two patients had a 90% reduction in circulating B cells. The total doses delivered were 52 mg in a patient who had progressive disease, 104 mg in a patient who had stable disease, 1, 032 mg in a patient who had a minor response, and 2, 380 mg in a patient who had a partial remission including a 90% reduction in lymph

Table 5. Phase I/II monoclonal antibody trials in chronic lymphocytic leukemia and multiple myeloma

Investigator	MoAB	Ig	Disease	Responders/treated
Dillman	T101(CD5)	mIgG2a	CLL	0/10
Foon	T101(CD5)	mIgG2a	CLL	0/13
Dyer	CAMPATH	rIgG2b	CLL	2/5
Dyer	CAMPATH	chIgM	CLL	0/1
Janson	CAMPATH 1-H	chIg1	CLL	6/16
Klein	Anti-IL-6	–	MM	0/1

CLL = chronic lymphocytic leukemia.
MM = multiple myeloma.
m = mouse.
r = rat.
ch = chimeric.

nodes. Unfortunately, this partial response lasted only 6 weeks.

A mouse/human chimeric version of anti-CD20, called IDEC-C2B8, which contains human IgG1 kappa constant regions and variable murine regions, has been more extensively tested in patients whose had experienced relapse of their indolent B-cell lymphomas. In a phase I trial 15 patients received single doses of 10 to 500 mg per square meter of body surface area [155]. Two partial responses and 4 minor responses were observed. A subsequent phase II trial yielded even more encouraging results [156]. In that trial patients received 375 mg/m2 IV weekly for 4 weeks. There were 3 complete responses and 16 partial responses among 34 evaluable patients for an overall objective response rate of 47%. Most of the responding patients have remained in remission for at least 4-12 months following treatment.

Hekman et al. [96] treated 6 lymphoma patients with a murine IgG2A monoclonal antibody against the B-cell differentiation antigen CD19, a 90 kilodalton glycoprotein on normal and malignant B cells. The CD19 molecule acts as an internalizing receptor which is physically and functionally associated with certain protooncogene phosphokinases. Total doses from 225 to 1, 000 mg were given over 4 hours without major toxicity. One patient was felt to have had a partial remission which lasted 8 months following his first treatment, and then 9 months following a second treatment. Because of the internalization (modulation) of this antigen, immunoconjugate approaches may be preferable for antibodies directed against CD19.

Another group has reported on the treatment of 12 lymphoma patients with 3 different CAMPATH antibodies. As noted earlier, CAMPATH does not appear to induce significant antigenic modulation. There were no significant clinical responses among nine patients who received a rat IgG2b monoclonal antibody [61]. In contrast, although one patient failed to respond to a rat/human IgG1 chimeric version called CAMPATH 1-H, 2 patients with lymphadenopathy, splenomegaly, and bone marrow involvement did respond to that antibody [88]. Doses of 1-20 mg of CAMPATH 1-H induced a complete remission in one patient with lymphoma, and a partial remission in a second patient. Berinstein et al. [10] reported partial responses in 3 of 7 patients who had recurrent indolent lymphoma and received thrice weekly treatment with 30 mg of CAMPATH 1-H. Brown et al. [22] noted one complete responder among 6 lymphoma patients treated with the same dose and schedule. However, as noted in earlier sections, to the surprise of many, the total results from the phase II trials of this agent were not considered encouraging enough for Burroughs/ Wellcome to continue development of the antibody [63].

Table 6. Phase I/II monoclonal antibody trials in B-cell lymphoma

Investigator	MoAB	Ig	Responders/ treated
Nadler	AB89	mIgG	10/1
Press	1F5(CD20)	mIgG2a	1/4
Maloney	IDEC-C2B8(CD20)	chIgG1	21/49
Hekman	(CD19)	mIgG2a	1/6
Dyer	CAMPATH	rIgG2b	0/9
Berinstein	CAMPATH 1-H	chIgG1	3/7
Brown	CAMPATH 1-H	chIgG1	1/6
Hale	CAMPATH 1-H	chIgG1	2/3
Hu	LYM-1	mIgG2a	0/10
Brown	Anti-id	mIgG	9/17
Bertoli	Anti-id	mIgG	0/2
Rankin	Anti-id	mIgG	0/2
Hamblin	Anti-id	chIgG	0/1

m = mouse.
r = rat.
ch = chimeric.

LYM-1 is an IgG2a murine monoclonal antibody that reacts with a polymorphic HLA-Dr antigen on all B cells, but the target antigen is not shed nor does it modulate in the presence of antibody. Ten patients with refractory B cell lymphomas received weekly intravenous infusions of escalating doses of LYM-1 over 4 weeks [109]. There were no significant objective tumor responses observed in this trial.

Despite the enthusiasm for the monoclonal antibody approach with anti-idiotype antibodies, investigation in this area has moved slowly because of the need to develop a specific anti-idiotype antibody for each patient. Subsequent enthusiasm for combinations of anti-idiotype antibodies commonly expressed on B-cell lymphomas dwindled when the frequency of these 'shared' or 'cross reactive' idiotypes was found to be much lower than originally suggested [166, 196]. The largest experience with anti-idiotype antibodies in lymphoma has been reported from Stanford, as initially reported by Meeker et al. [157] and subsequently updated by Brown et al. [20, 21] Seventeen patients received individualized anti-idiotype antibodies at doses ranging from 400 mg to over 9 g. A dramatic, sustained, complete remission was obtained in the first patient treated [162]. He relapsed 7 years later and failed to respond to a second anti-idiotype treatment. In subsequent patients, there have been 8 partial remissions of one to 6 months duration. Favorable responses were associated with increased T-cell infiltration of involved lymph nodes [150]. In some cases, resistance to therapy was shown to result from emergence of idiotype-variant clones [159]. This is not surprising in view of the importance of somatic mutations in the variable region for the versatility of the B-cell immunoglobulin response [38, 139].

The Stanford investigators have combined alpha interferon with anti-idiotype antibodies based on the rationale that alpha interferon might upregulate the idiotype antigen expression, and alpha interferon is known to have antiproliferative effects on follicular B-cell lymphoma cells. Of 12 patients treated in this manner, who received total antibody doses of from 1.7-8 g, there were 2 complete responses and 7 partial responses [21]. Another trial combined chlorambucil with anti-idiotype antibodies and one complete and 7 partial responses were described in 13 patients [154]. One can not conclude that either of these combination therapies is clearly more effective than anti-idiotype antibodies alone because of changes in patient selection and the known efficacy of alpha interferon and chlorambucil themselves, in subsets of patients with follicular lymphoma.

Three other groups have reported on limited trials with anti-idiotype antibodies. Bertoli et al. [14] treated one patient with nodular poorly differentiated lymphoma with 260 mg of IgG3 anti-IgD and another with 870 mg of IgG2a anti-idiotype antibody. There was a transient response in the former and no response in the latter.

Rankin et al. [190] treated 2 lymphoma patients with anti-idiotype antibodies. Escalating doses from 5 to 160 mg were given to total doses of 3.8 and 5.8 g. Minimal antitumor effects were noted. Another report relates an initial experience with a mouse/human chimeric anti-idiotype in a patient with B-cell lymphoma who had no tumor response [93].

Although the theoretical advantages of anti-idiotype antibodies are compelling from an immunologic standpoint, the practical limitations of existing technology, in terms of trying to produce a custom-made anti-idiotype antibody for each patient, render this approach not cost efficient from a commercial development standpoint. For this reason, and because of the encouraging results which have been achieved with antibodies directed to other lymphocyte surface antigens, it is seems likely that this particular approach will remain in the domain of limited research investigation.

T-Cell lymphoma

Although T-cell lymphomas are not very common, there have been a number of trials conducted in these patients because of the early availability of antibodies which reacted with the CD-5 antigen on T lymphocytes. Miller and colleagues [163] reported an early success in a patient with cutaneous T-cell lymphoma (CTCL) who received 17 infusions of 1 to 20 mg of anti-CD5 antibody Leu1 which was administered over a 10-week period. He experienced a partial response which included marked shrinkage of lymph nodes, skin lesions, and a neck mass. There was also a transient decrease in circulating T lymphocytes after each treatment. These same investigators treated 5 additional CTCL patients, and one with a large T-cell lymphoma [165]. Individual patients received 4 to 7 treatments over 2 to 10 weeks at doses of 250 μg to 100 mg infused over 4 to 6 hours for total doses of 13-761 mg. Four patients had brief tumor regressions lasting from 1 to 4 months. Dillman et al. [49] treated 2 patients with multiple 2-hour infusions of the anti-CD5 murine monoclonal antibody T101, and subsequently treated an additional 10 cutaneous T-cell lymphoma patients with T-101 at doses from 10-500 mg, given over 24 hours [52]. With the prolonged infusions, brief antitumor responses lasting from days to weeks were seen in 4 patients. In other trials with T101, Foon et al. [71] administered the antibody to several CTCL patients. Some patients had minimal improvement in skin lesions. Bertram et al. [15] gave T101 to 8 patients with CTCL and to 4 other patients with various T-cell lymphoproliferative disorders. One patient with CTCL had a partial response of his cutaneous lesions that persisted for 3 months. Another patient with convoluted T-cell lymphoma was alleged to have had a complete remission based on a decrease in bone marrow blasts from 6% to 3% which persisted for 2 months following doses of 1-100 mg T101.

Table 7. Passive monoclonal antibody therapy in T-Cell lymphoma

Investigator	MoAB	Ig	Responders/ treated
Miller	Leu1(CD5)	mIgG2a	5/7
Dillman	T101(CD5)	mIgG2a	0/12
Foon	T101(CD5)	mIgG2a	0/12
Bertram	T101(CD5)	mIgG2a	2/12
Knox	Leu3a(CD4)	chIgG	11/7

m = mouse.
ch = chimeric.

Knox and colleagues [131] have treated T-cell lymphoma patients with an anti-CD4 mouse-human chimeric monoclonal antibody. Seven patients received doses of 10, 20, 40, and 80 mg twice a week for 3 consecutive weeks. Circulating cells were coated with antibody but there was no significant change in the number of T cells. Some transient benefit was seen in all patients, but these clinical results were no better than those seen with murine anti-CD5 antibodies.

Solid tumors

Summaries of published trials of monoclonal antibodies in solid tumors are shown in Tables 8-13.

Breast cancer

Ryan et al. [197] treated ten breast cancer patients with three different IgM human anti-breast cancer monoclonal antibodies. These antibodies were selected based on their patterns of tissue reactivity rather than activity with human complement or effector cells. One patient each was treated at dose levels of 1, 2, 4, and 11 mg, and then 3 patients were treated at 20 mg, and 3 other patients received 22 mg in addition to tracer doses of 111-Indium labeled antibody. No tumor regressions were seen in these patients.

L6 is a murine monoclonal antibody which reacts with an antigen which is widely expressed on adenocarcinomas. It is known to mediate complement-dependent cytotoxicity with human complement and antibody-dependent cytotoxicity with human natural killer cells and macrophages. Goodman et al. [81] administered murine anti-L6 antibody to 5 patients with metastatic breast cancer. Patients received daily doses of 5 to 400 mg/m^2 for 7 days, to a total dose of 35 to 2800 mg. One patient who received 400 mg had a complete response. She previously had failed chemotherapy and radiation therapy and her tumor was hormone receptor negative. She had only regional chest wall disease at the time of treatment. The response did not become apparent until about 5 weeks after treatment, and it took about 14 weeks before the complete remission status was obtained. This same antibody was subsequently tested in combination with subcutaneous interleukin-2 in 5 breast cancer patients, one of whom had a transient mixed response. A humanized chimeric form of L6 has also been developed, but no responses were seen in a phase II trial of 21 patients.

Her2-neu, also known as c-erbB-2, is a 185, 000 dalton transmembrane glycoprotein receptor which has partial homology with the receptor for epidermal growth factor (EGF), and has tyrosine kinase activity [201]. HER2-neu is overexpressed in a variety of malignancies, but, so far, most clinical interest has focused on breast cancer. Monoclonal antibody 4D5 is one of the most potent anti-HER2-neu antibodies in terms of cell growth inhibition *in vitro*. The murine 4D5 has been humanized by inserting the complementarity-determining regions (CDRs) of the murine 4D5 into the constant and variable framework of a consensus human IgG1 to produce rHuMAb 4D5 which is more active in ADCC assays than its mouse counterpart [29]. The receptor does not internalize, but is shed into the bloodstream. Two phase I studies in 33 patients with tumors which overexpressed HER2-neu were associated with no tumor responses, but minimal toxicity at single doses of 10-500 mg [8]. However, in a trial of a 250 mg infusion of rHu4D5 followed by weekly rHu4D5 at a dose of 100 mg per treatment, there was one complete response and four partial responses among 44 evaluable patients who previously had received a median of 3 prior chemotherapy regimens [8]. The progression-free interval ranged from 3-17 months. Low grade fever was seen in 15% and was believed to be related to immune complexes formed with shed antigen. At least two additional phase II trials with this agent are planned using the weekly dosing schedule, in addition to a randomized trial with chemotherapy. Other trials of rHu4D5 with cisplatin have been conducted [186].

Colorectal cancer

Numerous clinical studies with antibodies directed against carcinoembryonic antigen (CEA) and other antigens of gastrointestinal mucosa have been reported. Several different IgG1 anti-CEA antibodies at doses from 1 to 80 mg were infused into 30 colorectal cancer patients utilizing single 1- to 2-hour infusions with tracer doses of 111-Indium labeled antibody [54]. In some patients, cross-reactivity with granulocytes led to transient decreases in total white blood count associated with fever and rigors [47]. No tumor regressions were seen. Other trials utilizing anti-CEA antibodies which do not cross-react with granulocytes have been associated with a minimum of side effects, but also were without tumor responses, despite evidence of uptake in tumors [9, 152].

The most intensively studied monoclonal antibody in colorectal cancer is the murine IgG2a monoclonal antibody 17-1A which reacts with most adenocarcinomas and it effects antibody-dependent cell-mediated cytotoxicity with human effector cells *in vitro*. Sears and colleagues [209, 210] reported treating over 60 patients with single intravenous infusions of 15 to 1000 mg. There were no objective regressions solely attributable to antibody during the initial studies, although tumor regressions were associated with monoclonal antibody therapy when used with other treatments in two of the patients. In a phase II trial, one patient with rectal cancer was felt to have had a partial regression of a pelvic recurrence [211].

Other extensive trials with monoclonal antibody 17-1A have been conducted in patients with colorectal carcinoma by Mellstedt and colleagues [74, 160]. Ten patients

Table 8. Passive monoclonal antibody therapy in breast and other cancers

Investigator	MoAB	Ig	Disease	Responders/treated
Ryan	Several	hIgM	Breast	0/10
Goodman	Anti-L6	mIgG2a	Breast	1/5
Baselga	Anti-Her-2neu	hIgG1	Breast	0/33
Baselga	Anti-Her2neu	hIgG1	Breast	5/44

PAP = prostate alkaline phosphatase.
PSA = prostate specific antigen.
h = human.
m = mouse.

received a single 200 to 400 mg dose of 17-1A which was readministered every 4 to 6 weeks. Another 10 patients received the same dose and schedule of antibody but treatment was preceded by the chemotherapy agent, cyclophosphamide, at a dose of 400 mg/m^2 in an effort to possibly decrease the human antimouse response. Fourteen patients received the same dose/schedule of antibody but in this case, antibody was preincubated with autologous peripheral blood mononuclear cells which had been collected from each patient by leukopheresis. Five patients received a total dose of 3.6 g of 17-1A given as 400 mg daily on days 1, 3 and 6, at 3-week intervals for 2 treatment courses. Another 7 patients received 200 to 400 mg every other day up to a total dose of 4.8 to 7.6 g. Six patients received 500 mg 3 days a week, to a total dose of 12 g. Out of this total of 52 patients, there was one complete response and 2 minor responses in the group which received 17-1A preincubated with peripheral blood mononuclear cells. One minor response was also noted among the 10 patients who received 17-1A preceded by cyclophosphamide.

The same 17-1A monoclonal antibody was used administered as one to four 400 mg infusions to treat 25 patients with metastatic colorectal carcinoma by LoBuglio et al. [148]. Eleven patients experienced mild gastrointestinal toxicity during treatment. One of the 25 patients was felt to have achieved a complete remission. Subsequently, this group has treated 8 patients with a chimeric 17-1A monoclonal antibody [149]. Pharmacokinetic studies showed that 17-1A serum levels persisted for longer duration and the human anti-immunoglobulin response was reduced. Despite the IgG4 human subclass heavy chain, which appeared to be optimal in terms of antibody-dependent cell-mediated cytotoxicity, no tumor responses were seen.

Of great significance is the fact that despite the rather disappointing results obtained with murine 17-1A in patients with visible cancer in the phase II setting, an impressive survival advantage has been reported in a randomized trial of adjuvant therapy for patients with Duke's C colon cancer [191]. In this multicenter European trial, 189 patients were randomly assigned to observation alone or postoperative treatment with 500 mg of 17-1A followed by monthly 100 mg infusions for 4 months. There were 4 episodes of anaphylactoid reactions among 371 infusions. After a median follow up of over 5 years, treatment with 17-1A was associated with a 30% reduction in death rate, which is comparable to the reduction in death which has been associated with adjuvant 5-FU regimens. Randomized trials are planned in the United States which will compare 5-FU/levamisole plus placebo to 5-FU/levamisole plus 17-1A.

Table 9. Phase I/II monoclonal antibody trials in colorectal carcinoma

Investigator	MoAB	Ig	Responders/ treated
Dillman	Anti-CEA	mIgG1	0/30
Sears	17-1A	mIgG2a	1/60
Mellstedt	17-1A	mIgG2a	1/52
LoBuglio	17-1A	mIgG2a	1/25
LoBuglio	17-1A	chIgG4	0/8
Herlyn	17-1A id	goIgG	1/30
Khazaeli	chB72.3	chIgG4	0/12
Haisma	16.88	hIgM	0/20

m = mouse.
ch = chimeric.
h = human.
go = goat.

There has been interest in combining 17-1A with gamma interferon because of evidence that the lymphokine-increased Fc receptors on effector cells and also increased expression of the tumor associated antigen. Weiner et al. [243] gave 150 mg of 17-1A on days 2, 3, and 4 in combination with 1.0 x 10^6 IU/m^2 gamma interferon on days 1 to 4, to 19 colorectal cancer patients in an effort to enhance antibody-dependent cell-mediated cytotoxicity, but no antitumor responses were noted. In a second trial in 27 colorectal cancer patients, the same group gave gamma interferon for 4 days followed by 400 mg 17-1A on day 5 [244]. Doses of gamma interferon up to 40 X10^6 U/day were given in this trial. It was found that the low doses of gamma interferon were as effective as the more toxic higher doses in enhancing monocyte cytotoxicity. Objective tumor responses were not seen. The combination of gamma interferon and murine monoclonal antibody 17-1A was also used by Saleh et al. [198] who reported treating 15 patients with metastatic colorectal adenocarcinoma with the combination. Gamma interferon was given days 1 to 15 at a dose of 0.1 mg/m^2 and the 17-1A antibody was infused at a dose of 400 mg on days 5, 7, 9 and 22. No significant objective tumor responses were described.

Herlyn et al. [105] have reported results of an initial effort to induce endogenous human anti-tumor antibodies in patients with colorectal cancer. Earlier clinical trials suggested that 17-1A could induce an anti-idiotype cascade [245]. They gave patients repeated subcutaneous injections of a goat antibody which reacted with the idiotype of antibodies which reacted with the idiotype of monoclonal antibody 17-1A. Thus, the goat antibody had the same structure as the tumor antigen detected by 17-1A. Although the authors demonstrated induction of human antibodies against the target antigen, a significant tumor response was seen in only one of 30 patients so treated.

A 111-Indium conjugate of a mouse antibody called B-72.3 (OncoScint®) was approved for clinical use for radioimmunodetection of cancer in patients with ovarian cancer and colorectal cancer in December 1992, thus earning the distinction of being the first monoclonal antibody pharmaceutical approved for use in cancer patients. Numerous patients received doses of 10 to 40 mg of antibody along with 1 mg doses of radiolabelled antibody [153]. Tumor regressions were not noted in the trials in patients with known colorectal cancer. However, humanized forms of this antibody appeared promising based on *in vitro* assays of ADCC. Khazaeli et al. [123] conducted a trial with a chimeric mouse/human B-72.3 monoclonal antibody with a human IgG4 component. Twelve patients were treated with 3.4 to 6.9 mg of the antibody, with a ^{131}iodine tracer for imaging. Tumor regressions were not seen.

Haisma et al. [87] treated 20 colorectal cancer patients with human IgM monoclonal antibody 16.88, labeled with ^{131}iodine for tumor localization. Patients received an initial 8 mg dose followed one week later by 200, 500, or 1, 000 mg of antibody. Tumor uptake was seen in at least one tumor site in 80% of the patients, but no tumor regressions were reported.

Ziegler et al. [258] treated 5 colorectal cancer patients with the murine L6 antibody in combination with low dose subcutaneous interleukin-2. One patient had a partial response following 7 daily 2-hour infusions, one week of rest, and then 4 days of subcutaneous IL-2.

Lung cancer

Elias et al. [66] treated patients with non-small cell lung cancer with the IgG1 murine monoclonal antibody KS1/4 which detects the same surface antigen as the 17-1A antibody. Five patients received sequential doses of 1, 10, 60, 100, and 1, 000 mg over 2 weeks for a total of 1, 661 mg. Minor upper gastrointestinal toxicity was seen in some patients. No antitumor responses were seen. Goodman et al. [81] infused the L6 murine monoclonal antibodies into 3 patients with non-small cell lung cancer. No tumor responses were seen.

Bombesin-like peptides such as human gastrin-releasing peptide and the peptide bombesin, are sometimes produced by lung cancers. Mulshine et al. [174] infused murine monoclonal antibody 2A11, which reacts with gastrin-releasing peptide, into 12 patients with non-small cell lung cancer. Patients received either 1, 10, or 100 mg/m^2 intravenously 3 times a week for 4 weeks. No tumor regressions were noted. In a phase II trial, 12 patients with small cell carcinoma of the lung were given 2A11 at dose and schedule of 250 mg/m^2 3 times a week for 4 weeks [121]. In this study one patient achieved a complete remission which lasted 5 months. No significant toxicities were observed.

Table 10. Phase I/II monoclonal antibody trials in lung cancer

Investigator	MoAB	Ig	Responders/ treated
Elias	KS1/4	mIgG2a	0/5
Goodman	Anti-L6	mIgG2a	0/3
Mulshine	Anti-GRP	mIgG2a	0/12
Kelly	Anti-GRP	mIG2a	1/12

m = mouse.

Melanoma

Many of the first monoclonal antibodies developed against solid tumors were to melanoma-associated antigens [116]. Several monoclonal antibodies were developed which react with melanotransferrin (p97, p96.5 or gp95 antigen). At the same time, several laboratories generated murine anti-melanoma antibodies which react with the high molecular weight chondroitin sulfated proteoglycan core protein (p240, p280). Other interesting monoclonal antibodies were developed which reacted with the disialoganlioside glycolipids GD2 and GD3 [189, 233].

Halpern and Dillman [54, 91] infused 1 to 50 mg of murine anti-melanoma monoclonal antibodies into melanoma patients as single 2-hour infusions. In most patients, a 1 mg tracer dose of ^{111}Indium radiolabeled monoclonal antibody was given as well. Twenty-four patients received IgG1 monoclonal antibodies directed against the p97 antigen, [89, 224] and another 28 received IgG2A monoclonal antibodies directed against the p240 antigen [91]. No definitive tumor responses were seen in patients with measurable disease. Similar experience has been reported by other investigators utilizing radiolabeled preparations of these same antibodies [125, 176, 177].

Oldham et al. [183] treated 8 patients with murine IgG2A 9.2.27 anti-melanoma antibody which reacts with the P240 antigen. Patients received twice weekly escalating doses of 1, 10, 50, 100, and 200 mg. Tumor biopsies and immunohistochemical staining demonstrated *in vivo* localization in subcutaneous tumors in 6 of 8 patients following doses of 50 mg or greater, but no tumor response were seen.

Goodman et al. [82] treated 4 melanoma patients with a combination of a murine IgG1 anti-P97 and an IgG1 anti-p240. A fifth patient received anti-p97 alone. Escalating antibody doses were administered as 6-hour infusions daily for 10 days to a maximum dose of 50 mg per infusion. No objective tumor regressions were observed.

None of the trials utilizing anti-p97 and anti-p240 murine monoclonal antibodies resulted in objective tumor responses. This may relate to the fact that the antibodies to the p97 and P240 proteoglycan which have been studied do not effect antibody-dependent cell-mediated cytotoxicity or complement-dependent cytotoxicity. More encouraging antitumor effects were described by investigators utilizing murine IgG3 anti-melanoma antibodies directed against the antigens GD3 [108, 236], or GD2 [36]. These antibodies do mediate complement-mediated cytotoxicity and antibody-dependent cell mediated cytotoxicity *in vitro* with human complement and human effector cells. Antibodies directed against these antigens have also been effective in animal tumor models [110].

Twenty-one patients received the anti-GD3 mono-

Table 11. Phase I/II monoclonal antibody trials in melanoma and neuroblastoma

Investigator	MoAB	Ig	Disease	Responders/treated
Halpern	Anti-p97	mIgG1	Melanoma	0/24
Dillman	Anti-p240	mIgG2a	Melanoma	0/28
Oldham	Anti-p240	mIgG2a	Melanoma	0/8
Goodman	Anti-p97/Anti-p240	mIgG2a	Melanoma	0/5
Houghton	R24(GD3)	mIgG3	Melanoma	4/21
Cheung	3F8(GD2)	mIgG3	Melanoma	2/9
Saleh	14G2a(GD2)	mIgG2a	Melanoma	1/12
Murray	14G2a(GD2)	mIgG2a	Melanoma	0/11
Saleh	14G2a(GD2)	chIgG1	Melanoma	0/13
Cheery	3F8(0-D2)	mIgG3	Neuroblastoma	2/8
Murray	14G2a(GD2)	mIgG2a	Neuroblastoma	2/5
Yu	14.18(GD3)	chIgG1	Neuroblastoma	8/17

m = mouse.

clonal antibody R24 intravenously at 1, 10, 30, or 50 mg/m^2 every other day for 2 weeks for total doses of 8, 80, 240, or 400 mg/m [108, 236]. At higher doses all patients developed urticaria and pruritus which typically occurred within 2 to 4 hours following treatment and often appeared around tumor or at sites of previous tumor excision. Antibody uptake in tumor in patients receiving 30 and 50 mg/m^2 was readily demonstrated using biopsies and immunohistochemical analysis. Significant tumor regressions were seen in 2/6, 1/6, 1/6, and 0/3 for each successive dose level. Responses were first noted within 2 weeks of completing treatment, but continued to increase for several months.

The murine IgG3 anti-GD2 antibody called 3F8 was used by Cheung et al. [36] to treat melanoma patients who received 5, 20, 50, or 100 mg/m^2 as 8-hour infusions given daily for 2 to 4 days. The study was closed at the 100 mg/m^2 dose because all patients treated at that dose level developed hypertension. Treatments were associated with focal pain at tumor sites and pain especially over the abdomen, back, and extremities which was felt to perhaps be related to cross-reactivity with neural tissue. Urticaria, fever, nausea, vomiting and sweats were also noted. Inflammatory actions were observed around tumors. Partial responses were reported for 2 of the 9 patients and 2 other patients had a mixed response. Six melanoma patients were given a combination of R24 and 3F8 at doses of only 1-10 mg/m^2; no tumor regressions were seen.

Saleh et al. [199] conducted a phase I trial of a murine anti-GD2 monoclonal antibody called 14G2a (14.18) in 12 patients with melanoma. Single doses from 10 to 120 mg were administered intravenously. This therapy was associated with an abdominal and pelvic pain syndrome, which necessitate narcotic analgesia for control. All 12 patients developed a human anti-mouse antibody (HAMA) response to the murine antibody. One partial response was seen in this small study.

Murray et al. [178] gave murine MoAb 14G2a, an IgG2a switch variant of the IgG3 anti-Gd2 MoAb 14.18, to 11 patients with metastatic melanoma as part of a phase I trial. There were no objective remissions although two patients exhibited mixed responses to the antibody. Generalized pain, fever, rash, paresthesias, weakness, hyponatremia and postural hypotension were the significant toxicities observed. The investigators suggested that 100 mg/m^2 was the maximum tolerated dose of this MoAb.

A chimeric version of the anti-GD2 antibody (ch14.18) with a constant region of human IgG1K has been tested. In a phase I trial in 13 melanoma patient, who received 5 to 100 mg of the MoAb, no tumor responses were seen [200]. As has been seen in other trials of anti-GD2 antibodies in adult patients, the major toxicity associated with this therapy was abdominal/pelvic pain syndrome which necessitated use of intravenous narcotic analgesics.

The R24 anti-GD3 antibody has been given in combination with a variety of different immunostimulatory cytokines in the hopes of enhancing antitumor effects of R24. Caulfield et al. [32] gave R24 with alpha interferon to patients with melanoma. R24 was administered as 5 daily 6-hour infusions in combination with intramuscular interferon alpha 2A. Fifteen patients were treated using dose escalations of the R24. Toxicities were similar to those seen in other trials of R24. No tumor regressions were reported, which was disappointing in view of the apparent activity of R24 and alpha interferon as single agents.

Munn and Cheung [175] had previously demonstrated that interleukin-2 enhanced antibody mediated cellular cytotoxicity by the 3F8 antibody against GD2. Bajorin et al. [4] evaluated the combination of interleukin-2 and mouse monoclonal antibody R24 in 20 patients with metastatic melanoma in a phase I trial IL-2 was given at a dose of 6 x 10^6 IU/m^2 intravenously over 6 hours on days 1 to 5 and 8 to 12, while the anti-GD3 antibody 24 was given on days 8 to 12 at 1, 3, 8, or 12 mg/m^2 per day. Five patients were evaluated at each dose level. The investigators were able to demonstrate some *in vitro* T-cell activation. One patient had a partial response in soft tissue sites lasting 6 months, and 2 other patients had minor responses. Investigators felt that this trial provided further evidence for the lymphocyte activation effects of R24 [246].

In a separate trial, Creekmore et al. [42] gave a higher dose of continuous infusion IL-2 followed by R24. Using the same IL-2 regimen with R24, they previously had seen only one response in 17 patients, while the sequence of the agents yielded 10 responses in 28 patients. However, 5 patients including 2 who died, never received R24 because of IL-2-related toxicity.

R24 has also been given in combination with granulocyte macrophage colony stimulating factor (GM-CSF), macrophage colony stimulating factor (M-CSF), or with tumor necrosis factor (TNF) to melanoma patients. Chachoua et al. [34] gave subcutaneous GM-CSF for 21 days at a dose of 150 μg/m^2/day, and gave R24 by continuous intravenous infusion on days 8 to 15 at doses of 0, 10, or 50 mg/m^2. There were no tumor responses with GM-CSF alone in 5 patients, or the lower R24 dose in 6 patients, but two responses were seen at the 50 mg/m^2 dose in 9 patients. However, 4 of the 9 were unable to complete this single course of therapy because of toxicity. Minasian et al. [168] treated 19 metastatic melanoma patients with a 14-day continuous infusion of recombinant human M-CSF at a dose of 80 μg/kg/day in combination with R24 which was administered daily by intravenous infusion at doses of 1, 3, 10, 0 and 50 μg/m^2/day on days 6 to 10. There were no partial or complete remissions observed, although 3 patients did have a mixed response with regression of some lesions. Minasian et al. [167] conducted a pilot study of R24, and two different doses of TNF. One of the 8 patients treated had a dramatic tumor lysis syndrome in multiple visceral sites of disease.

Mittelman and colleagues have conducted preliminary trials of anti-idiotype antibodies mirroring the gp240 glycoprotein antigen that is common on melanoma cells. In one trial, the MAF11-39 anti-idiotype antibody was injected subcutaneously in 37 patients [169]. Anti-melanoma antibodies were apparently not induced in this study, although one patient had a complete remission of melanoma lesions. In the second trial the MK-23 anti-idiotype antibody was conjugated to keyhole limpet hemocyanin (KLH) and coadministered with BCG (Bacille Calmett-Guerin) in 25 patients [170]. Three partial responses were observed, and 14 of 23 patients developed endogenous human antibodies against gp240.

Neuroblastoma and neuroectodermal tumors

The 3F8 murine anti-GD2 monoclonal antibody was used to treat 8 children with neuroblastoma by Cheung et al. [36]. There were two complete remissions seen, one at a dose of only 5 mg/m^2, and the other at 20 mg/m^2. The abdominal/pelvic pain syndrome seen in patients treated with antibodies directed to this antigen did not appear to be as significant a problem in children as in adults.

Murray et al. [178] gave murine MoAb 14G2a, an IgG2a switch variant of the IgG3 anti-GD2 MoAb 14.18 to 5 patients with neuroblastoma, as part of a phase I trial. Two patients achieved a partial remission. Generalized pain, fever, rash, paresthesias, weakness, hyponatremia and postural hypotension were the significant toxicities observed. Pediatric patients tolerated the agent much better than adults.

Yu and colleagues [257] have treated 17 neuroblastoma patients aged 2 to 8 years with a chimeric ch14.18 antibody using a human IgG1k framework. Granulocyte macrophage colony stimulating factor (GM-CSF) was coadministered in an effort to optimize ADCC *in vivo*. Toxicity was minimal in these children as opposed to the experience in adult patients with melanoma. Significant tumor responses were noted in 8 patients, including 3 complete remissions.

Ovarian cancer

Many monoclonal antibodies which react with breast cancer and some which react with colon cancer also cross-react with epithelial antigens found in ovarian cancer. As noted above, many patients with ovarian cancer have received murine monoclonal antibody B72.3 in conjunction with tracer doses of 111-Indium labelled antibodies. No tumor remissions were reported [153].

Goodman et al. [81] used the L6 murine monoclonal antibody described earlier to treat 9 patients with advanced ovarian cancer. Doses from 5 to 400 mg/m^2 were given daily for 7 days. Decreased levels of the third and fourth components of complement were noted in some patients. There were no objective tumor responses.

Table 12. Passive monoclonal antibody therapy in other carcinomas

Investigator	MoAB	Ig	Disease	Responders/treated
Goodman	Anti-L6	mIgG2a	Ovary	0/9
Kosmos	HMFG1	mIgG2a	Ovary	0/15
Weiner	17-1A	mIgG2a	Pancreas	1/28
Halpern	Anti-PAP	mIgG1	Prostate	0/19
Dillman	Anti-PSA	mIgG1	Prostate	0/4

Kosmos et al. [134] treated 15 ovarian cancer patients with intraperitoneal HMFG1. HMFG1 is a murine IgG1 monoclonal antibody which reacts with epitopes on high molecular weight human milk fat globulin glycoprotein antigen from breast epithelium. It also reacts with 90% of ovarian serous cancers. A dose-dependent *in vitro* T-cell proliferation was observed in 13 of the 15 patients, but no tumor responses were seen.

Pancreatic cancer

Weiner et al. [245] conducted a phase II multicenter trial of the 17-1A murine IgG2a antibody in patients with unresectable pancreatic carcinoma. A dose of 500 mg was given intravenously 3 times a week for 8 weeks, in 28 patients. Because of rapid progression of disease in several patients, only 16 patients received the planned course of 12 g of MoAb. There was one durable partial response.

A trial of gamma interferon plus murine monoclonal antibody 17-1A in pancreatic cancer was carried out by Tempero et al. [231]. Thirty patients with advanced, measurable disease received gamma interferon at a dose of 10^6 U/m^2 daily for 4 days and 150 mg of 17-1A, admixed with autologous leukocytes on days 2, 3 and 4. One patient was felt to have had a complete remission which persisted for 4 months. The median survival for this group of patients was only 5 months. There was no evidence of increased HLA-DR expression on monocytes or lymphocytes following the administration of gamma interferon.

Buchler et al. [23] conducted a prospective randomized trial of adjuvant therapy with the murine IgG1 monoclonal antibody 494/32, which does effect ADCC *in vitro*. The study involved 61 patients, all of whom had undergone a Whipple resection for pancreatic cancer. Patients were randomized to receive either no treatment, or a total of 370 mg of the murine monoclonal antibody over a 10-day period. Analysis after 10 months showed no significant difference in survival between the two treatment groups who had median survivals of 428 days for the treatment group, compared to 386 days for the control group.

Prostate cancer

Halpern and Dillman [54, 90] administered IgG1 murine monoclonal antibodies reactive with prostatic acid phosphatase or prostate specific antigen to 19 patients with metastatic prostate cancer. ^{111}Indium-labeled antibodies showed uptake in some sites of tumor. There were no significant toxicities associated with treatment. Approximately half of the patients developed a human antimouse response. No tumor responses were observed.

Several investigators have conducted radioimmunodetection trials with 111-In CYT-356 from Cytogen, in prostate cancer patients who were about to undergo regional lymph node dissection. Uptake in regional lymph nodes has been confirmed but tumor responses could not be measured in this trial design. Leroy et al. [140] conducted a radioimmunodetection trial in similar patients with ^{123}I-labeled antiprostatic acid phosphatase (PAP) using an F(ab')^2 preparation. Occult disease was imaged, but antitumor effects could not be determined because of the study design.

Stomach cancer

Sears et al. [210] administered the 17-1A murine monoclonal antibody to a small number of patients with gastric carcinoma. Results were similar to those seen in the colorectal cancer trial. The infusions were well tolerated but no objective antitumor responses were observed.

Renal cell carcinoma

While a number of MoAbs have been developed against renal cell carcinoma, few have been extensively tested in clinical trials. Oosterwijk et al. [185] have explored the use of an antibody called G250, originally a murinc IgG2a which was later converted to a mouse/human IgG1 chimeric. Preliminary *in vitro* activity in ADCC assays was considered disappointing.

Monoclonal antibodies as biological response modifiers

Another approach with monoclonal antibodies is to use the antibodies as biological response modifiers, especially to modulate or induce an indirect antitumor action through other components of the immune system. These trials are summarized in Table 13. The best example to date is the OKT3 monoclonal antibody which reacts with the T-cell receptor CD3 [206]. This murine antibody was originally approved for use in patients with kidney transplants as an immunosuppressant to block rejection. Urba et al. [235] treated 36 patients with OKT3 antibody in an effort to activate T cells in the hope of promoting an

Table 13. Clinical trials with anti-CD3 monoclonal antibody

Investigator	MoAB	Ig	Disease	Responders/treated
Richards	anti-CD3 OKT3	mIgG2a	various	1/13
Wiseman	anti-CD3 OKT3	mIgG2a	glioma	3/9
Urba	anti-CD3 OKT3	mIgG2a	various	0/36

antitumor effect. Five patients received a 30 ug dose by intravenous bolus and the other 23 received 3-hour infusions of 1, 10, 30, or 100 ug. An additional 8 patients received the anti-CD3 daily for 14 days by either bolus 3-hour infusion, or 24-hour infusion. The dose-limiting toxicity in this study was headache, accompanied by signs and symptoms of meningeal irritation. Eight of the 16 patients tested exhibited human antimouse antibodies. No tumor responses were observed.

Richards et al. [202] also treated 13 patients with OKT3. Six patients received 50 ug, and 7 received 100 ug. A partial response was described in one patient with metastatic renal cell carcinoma. Again, neurotoxicity was a significant problem and was observed in 11 of the 13 patients after the first treatment. Headache and confusion were noted. In all patients, neurotoxicity was transient and interestingly, did not recur with re-treatment. In both this study and that by Urba et al.[235], a cerebral spinal fluid lymphocytosis was noted in patients who underwent lumbar puncture, and headache was a frequent complaint.

Because of the evidence that OKT3 had stimulated an immune response in the central nervous system, Wiseman et al. [250] initiated a trial with OKT3 in patients with gliomas who had failed conventional therapy and evidence of progressive disease. Patients received 25 to 75 ug of OKT3 over 1-hour, followed a day later by 300 mg per square meter of cyclophosphamide. Three of 9 patients were reported to have had objective tumor regressions, based on brain studies with magnetic resonance imaging. Anticipated side effects included headache, fever, stupor, nausea, emesis, and transient decreases in T-lymphocyte counts, but no severe or life-threatening toxicity.

Several investigators have explored the use of the T-lymphocyte cytokine interleukin-2 in combination with OKT3 because of the potential for synergistic or additive T-cell stimulation. Sosman et al. [225] treated 54 patients with doses of OKT3, ranging between 75 to 600 ug/m^2 followed by high-dose bolus IL-2 therapy. They were unable to significantly enhance the number of circulating T cells expressing the IL-2 receptor, and the tumor response rate was no better than had been observed with IL-2 alone. Buter et al. [24] gave 50 to 400 ug OKT3 with low-dose subcutaneous IL-2. Neurotoxicity was the limiting toxicity at the highest dose. There were no responses among 8 patients, and no enhancement of activated lymphocyte subpopulations was noted.

Weiner and Hillstrom [242] have developed a bispecific antibody which reacts with a murine lymphoma and with murine CD3. Such an approach may soon be tested in man using a bifunctional antibody directed to the CD3 determinant and the human B-cell antigen.

OTHER OBSERVATIONS RELATED TO ANTIBODY THERAPY

In vivo binding to malignant cells

Meticulous screening of immunoglobulin-secreting hybridomas results in selection of monoclonal antibodies which bind to the appropriate target antigen in man. Numerous studies using fluorescein conjugated anti-mouse antibodies have demonstrated that murine monoclonal antibodies readily bind to circulating blood tumor cells in man [5, 15, 46, 52, 165, 179, 216]. Monoclonal antibody binding to solid tumor sites such as lymph nodes, tumor masses, and skin infiltrates has been directly demonstrated using immunofluorescence and immunoperoxidase techniques [52, 108, 183, 218], and indirectly with low doses of monoclonal antibodies conjugated to technetium, indium or iodine, as radioactive tracers [28, 54, 67, 91, 136, 176]. The relative specificity of this uptake was evident by failure to image other lymph node sites, and the successful imaging of nonpalpable nodes which were subsequently proven to contain cancer by surgical excision and histopathology evaluation [171]. In one patient with T-cell lymphoma, a radiolabeled anti-CD5 antibody showed increased uptake in lymph nodes, but injection of radiolabeled anti-melanoma monoclonal antibody of the same subclass was not associated with lymph node uptake [28].

Various studies suggest that uptake in cutaneous tumors is higher than that for solid tumors in other sites or lymph nodes [183]. This in part may relate to cutaneous blood supply. It also may relate to the relatively small size at which cutaneous tumors can be recognized. The apparent differences in uptake may be of particular significance in terms of strategies for treating lymphoproliferative diseases. Some investigators have suggested that direct infusion into the lymphatic system may be superior to intravenous infusions in certain disease settings [232].

Clinical efficacy and mechanisms

The major issue surrounding passive monoclonal antibody therapy is how often is specific *in vivo* binding associated with a significant antitumor response in the absence of prohibitive toxicity. Most studies reported to-date involved mouse antibodies and were of a pilot or phase I design, which would not be definitive tests of monoclonal antibodies as cancer treatment. Nevertheless, it is encouraging that tumor responses following monoclonal antibody therapy have been reported for both hematologic malignancies and solid tumor cancers. Some of the best responses to-date have been described in nodular lymphoma and malignant melanoma, two diseases in which the frequency of spontaneous regressions has led to hypothesis of an existing antitumor immune response. The promising results of adjuvant therapy with murine antibody 17-1A in colorectal cancer has rekindled enthusiasm for exploring the role of antibodies against microscopic residual disease. So far, antitumor effects in man have not been shown to be better when humanized chimeric antibodies are used, despite encouraging *in vitro* results in assays of complement-dependent cytotoxicity and/or antibody-dependent cell-mediated cytotoxicity.

As a general observation, when monoclonal antibodies bind peripheral blood target cells at a sufficient level, the cells are removed in the reticuloendothelial system. Infusions of ^{51}Cr or ^{111}I-labeled autologous tumor cells resulted in marked uptake of the isotope label in the livers and spleens of treated patients [46, 164, 179] Investigators have rarely reported associated decreases in complement levels, although Ritz et al. [194] found deposits of C3 on monoclonal antibody-coated cells in one ALL patient, and complement deposition has been noted in tissues in patients receiving KS1/4 [66] and R24 [236] antibodies. Minor changes in circulating cell viability have been observed following monoclonal antibody binding [179]. These studies suggest that binding of monoclonal antibodies to peripheral blood cells may actually damage the cell membrane and that such cells are then removed in the reticuloendothelial system rather than lysing in the intravascular compartment. The best evidence of cell destruction, rather than sequestration, comes from studies following radiolabeled autologous tumor cells [46, 164, 179], and the finding of an increased lactate dehydrogenase (LDH) associated with decreased AML cells [5].

In those patients in whom tumor regressions have been seen, the mechanism of antibody-mediated tumor regression was not clearly established. Anti-leukemic effects were dependent on the monoclonal antibodies used, the rate and dose of monoclonal antibody infused, the density of antigen expression, and whether there is circulating antigen or antimouse antibodies. Unfortunately, in most instances the anti-leukemic responses are relatively transient. Antibody-coated target cells are removed from the circulating but they are apparently replaced by cells from other organs such as bone marrow, lymph nodes, and possibly spleen, and it appears less likely that they are merely trafficking to other sites and the then re-entering the circulation. The leukemia cell counts usually remain depressed as long as monoclonal antibody levels persist in the circulation, although in many instances the cell count begins to recover in association with entry into the circulation of modulated leukemia cells; which subsequently reexpress the target antigen *in vitro* or *in vivo* once the antibody concentration has dropped to a negligible level. This has definitely been a problem for monoclonal antibodies which reacted with modulating (cycling, internalizing) antigens, but may not be a problem for some monoclonal antibodies, and may be more effective than some other anti-T-cell antibodies because of down regulation of the IL-2 receptor which serves as a growth factor receptor for that tumor.

The explanation for the responses seen in B-cell lymphoma patients treated with anti-idiotype monoclonal antibody has not been elucidated. Investigators have postulated either a direct cytotoxic effect or a regulatory effect via the idiotype network [20, 25, 181, 223]. The most responsive group has been that of nodular poorly differentiated lymphoma (NLPD) or small cleaved follicular center-cell lymphoma. Preliminary analysis suggests that those follicular lymphoma patients who respond have a greater infiltration with T cells prior to therapy [158]. Responses have been more readily achieved in patients with very low levels of circulating idiotype.

The best responses in solid tumors have been achieved with monoclonal antibodies that effect both antibody-dependent cell-mediated cytotoxicity and complement-mediated cytotoxicity. Sequential biopsies in responding melanoma patients who received R24 revealed increasing infiltration with CD3$^+$, CD8$^+$, Ia$^+$ T cells, in the presence of degranulated tissue mast cells [246]. Complement deposition was also noted. Even though responses were seen within 2 weeks of beginning therapy, tumors continued to recede well beyond the treatment period despite the presence of HAMA. These responses may involve a more complex interaction with the host immune system, perhaps triggering a cascade of inflammatory events including activation of T lymphocytes that persist for a long period of time [106]. Unfortunately, most advanced cancer patients do not have tumors that are as easy to analyze sequentially as melanoma. Selection of patients with primarily lymph node or soft tissue disease will facilitate such prospective studies, but will also bias results inasmuch as soft tissue and lymph node metastases tend to be more responsive to any intervention than bone, liver, brain, or other visceral metastases.

We have made observations in two patients which raise questions regarding the possible mechanisms of antitumor affects against microscopic disease [54, 89]. The first patient had undergone a left radical neck dissection for head and neck melanoma. A ^{111}Indium radioimmunodetection study with anti-p97 illuminated 3 apparent lesions in the right neck, although repeated physical examinations and a computerized tomographic scan of the region were negative for tumor. No other lesions or lymph nodes were visualized, but 3 weeks later he developed 3 palpable lymph nodes in the right neck in sites consistent with the scan. A neck resection was recommended but the patient declined the procedure. The neck lesion subsequently resolved and he was known to remain free of disease for over 3 years. A second male patient had had a melanoma resected from his upper back and presented with a known right axillary recurrence. There was uptake of ^{111}Indium anti-p240 in the right axilla but there was also uptake in the left axilla, which was clinically negative. Subsequently, a small left axillary node was found but spontaneously regressed. No other lymphadenopathy was visualized by imaging and no other lymphadenopathy was palpated by examination. Both axillae were explored with confirmation of tumor in the right axilla, but no tumor was found on the left. There are three possible explanations for these intriguing observations of what clearly were antigen specific reactions. First, there may have been a local antitumor effect against microscopic tumor cells. Second, there may have been antibody binding to residual antigen retained in draining regional lymph nodes. Third, there may have been antibody reaction with regional B lymphocytes which were making anti-idiotypic antibody to endogenous anti-p240 or into p97 antibodies.

Dose

There is a dose/response relationship at low monoclonal antibody doses (<10 mg) because of the volume of distribution, nonspecific uptake and metabolism, and the iimportance of number of antibody molecules on cell surfaces for complement, reticuloendothelial, or effector cell-mediated effects. Extrapolation from animal studies and studies of biopsies from patients receiving murine monoclonal antibodies suggests that gram quantities may be needed if tumor saturation is an important issue [183]. Until a larger number of responses is observed, it will be impossible to clearly answer this question. Whether the dose/response relationship holds at higher doses, is unclear. Several investigators have shown that *direct in vivo* tissue binding (as opposed to binding to circulating cells) could only be demonstrated at doses of 30 to 50 mg or higher [49, 52, 108, 183]. Some radiolabeled monoclonal antibody studies have also suggested that more tumors are imaged with doses of 10 mg or greater [86, 90, 91, 177].

Toxicity and side effects

A hierarchy of side effects have been observed during infusion of MoAbs (Table 14) [51, 58]. The toxicities and side effects associated with monoclonal antibody administration may be categorized as allergic or nonallergic in nature. Adverse events have included fever, rigors/chills, sweats, maculopapular erythematous skin rash, urticaria, pruritus, edema, hypotension, headache, nausea, vomiting, diarrhea, fatigue, elevated hepatic transaminases, throat tightness, pain, thrombocytopenia, dyspnea, bronchospasm, anaphylactic shock, and even death. However, adverse events vary greatly depending on the nature of the antibody (mouse or human), the distribution of the target antigen on normal tissues, and whether or not the antibody reacts with circulating cells.

Allergic reactions may be classified as acute or delayed. Because most of the initial monoclonal antibodies were mouse proteins, there was great concern that infusion of these products would be associated with acute anaphylactoid reactions. Fortunately, such complications have been uncommon and have been extremely rare with human or humanized antibodies, such as chimeric antibodies which contain mostly human constant immunoglobulin and only mouse variable region protein or only the idiotypic determinants of a selected mouse antibody. Patients with a known history of allergic reaction to rodents or their byproducts, have typically been excluded from trials of mouse antibodies. Acute allergic reactions have included anaphylactic shock, less severe anaphylactoid reactions such as bronchospasm, dyspnea, and tachycardia, and generalized pruritus and urticaria. The more severe reactions can be successfully managed with epinephrine. The dermatology symptoms may be seen as part of a full anaphylactic reaction with laryngeal edema, hypotension, and bronchospasm, or alone. Pruritus and urticaria alone typically resolve without treatment, but may be responsive to diphenhydramine or epinephrine. Premedication with steroids and/or diphenhydramine does not appreciably effect the frequency of the side effects. Fever, sweats, chills, nausea, and prostration may be a manifestation of a mild acute allergic reaction, but this complex of symptoms is much more commonly associated with a direct antibody/antigen reaction with circulating cells, as discussed below.

Table 14. Summary of side effects and toxicities associated with murine monoclonal antibody infusions

Toxicity	% Patients	% Infusions
Fever	15	12
Transaminasemia	14	9
Rigors/Chills	13	11
Pruritus	12	18
Urticaria	12	6
Diaphoresis	10	10
Nausea	7	3
Vomiting	6	2
Malaise	5	3
Diarrhea	3	2
Hypotension	3	2
Bronchospasm	2	1
Anaphylaxis	<1	<1
Serum Sickness	1	1

For 177 patients with 20 different malignancies receiving 291 infusions of 19 different murine IgG and 3 human IgM monoclonal antibodies.

Because of the anticipated production of human antimouse antibodies (HAMA) in response to murine antibody immunoglobulin exposure, there was concern that delayed reactions such as serum sickness would be a significant problem following infusion of murine monoclonal antibodies. Fortunately, immune complex complications related to HAMA have been uncommon. Classic serum sickness has been seen 2 to 3 weeks following exposure to moderate and high doses of murine antibodies. A typical symptom complex includes fever, malaise, arthralgias/arthritis, myalgias, maculopapular erythematous skin rash, and fatigue. Proteinuria has been rarely observed in these few patients and renal insufficiency extremely rare. Serum sickness can be managed with nonsteroidal, antiinflammatory agents, and corticosteroids in more severe cases.

The most antibody-specific adverse events associated

with infusions of monoclonal antibodies are related to antibody binding to the target antigen. These include direct effects on tumor and nontumor cells which express the antigen, and indirect effects mediated by the secondary release of various cytokines as a result of antibody binding to the target antigen, or formation of immune complexes with circulating soluble antigen. The most predictable symptom complex has been seen in association with monoclonal antibody binding to circulating cells, especially B or T lymphocytes, granulocytes, or leukemia cells. The typical symptom complex includes fever, chills, sweats, prostration, nausea, and sometimes dyspnea and hypotension, which occur within a matter of hours after the antibody is initiated. Studies with radiolabeled cells have shown that once antibody binds to circulating cells, they are removed in the reticuloendothelial system including the lung, liver, and spleen. When large numbers of cells are removed in the lungs, this may be associated with dyspnea and hypotension. For this reason, when it is known that an antibody will react with circulating cells, the initial infusion rate is slow, and high-dose bolus administration is avoided. Many of the symptoms related to the removal of circulating target cells are probably secondary to the release of various cytokines such as various interleukins and interferons. Nearly all patients who have received antilymphocyte and/or antigranulocyte antibodies have experienced such side effects if they had levels of circulating target cells at the time of infusion, and no high titers of endogenous antimouse antibodies to block the effect. The presence of antimouse antibodies actually prevents many of these side effects by altering the pharmacology and bioavailability of the monoclonal antibody which limits binding to the target antigen. Corticosteroids typically will prevent such reactions, but acetaminophen and diphenhydramine have little prophylactic benefit.

Adverse events may also be seen because of direct effects on noncancerous tissue which also expresses the target antigen. This has been especially true for antibodies which cross-react with adenocarcinomas and cells of the gastrointestinal tract. Such antibodies have been associated with a high frequency of diarrhea, nausea and vomiting, abdominal pain, and even large and/or small bowel mucosal damage in some patients. Other antibodies which are known to cross-react with antigens on neural tissue have been associated with specific pain syndromes in some patients. Cross-reactivity with normal tissue antigens is particularly a concern when antibodies are conjugated to cytotoxic substances such as radioisotopes, chemotherapy agents, or natural toxins. The incidence of gastrointestinal toxicity was much greater when a frequently tested adenocarcinoma antibody was given conjugated to a vinca chemotherapy analog, or methotrexate, as compared to administration of the naked antibody. Another adenocarcinoma antibody which cross-reacted with antigens on neural sheaths, produced unacceptable neurotoxicity when conjugated to the A chain of the natural toxin, ricin.

In some instances, monoclonal antibodies are given to patients who are known to have free or soluble circulating antigen. Examples include the circulating idiotype in lymphoma, and carcinoembryonic antigen (CEA), or prostate specific antigen (PSA). Only rarely have symptoms been noted in the presence of the immune complexes formed by the binding of antibody to circulating antigen, probably because of the small size of such complexes since the monoclonal antibody binds to only one determinant on the circulating antigen. For this reason, the presence of circulating antigen is not a contraindication to antibody treatment, although the binding to soluble antigen greatly alters the pharmacokinetics of the antibody. However, acute arthralgias, myalgias, nerve palsies, fever, and skin rashes have occasionally been seen in this setting and attributed to the acute immune complex formation.

One potential adverse event with a cytotoxic antibody preparation is that of tumor lysis syndrome. This has not been described with any of the antibody preparations tested to-date, and therefore prehydration, mannitol, and allopurinol prophylaxis are not routinely administered.

Antibody serum levels and pharmacokinetics

Various enzyme-linked immunosorbent assays (ELISA) and radioimmunoassays (RIA) have been used to measure serum levels of murine monoclonal antibodies during and following infusions. Many have been well standardized and are quantitative [149, 217]. Serum monoclonal antibody levels have been easily detected except during low infusion rates, or in the presence of high levels of circulating antigens, high circulating tumor burden, or in the presence of antimouse antibodies. In the leukemias, monoclonal antibody levels tend to fall rapidly following an infusion because of continuing absorption by circulating cells and entry of additional cells into the circulation. However, with some antibodies, in the presence of antigenic modulation, serum monoclonal antibody levels are sustained for many days to weeks depending on the dose given. Using 24- to 48-hour infusions, peak monoclonal antibody levels of several micrograms have persisted for up to 2 weeks. The significance of serum levels at any time point must be viewed in the light of the variables listed above. In addition to tumor burden, other important variables include circulating antigen, antigenic modulation, and the production of antimouse antibodies. Humanized and chimeric antibodies consistently demonstrate superior pharmacokinetics , such as higher sustained blood levels, compared to their mouse counterparts. This is especially true following repeated administration because of the influence of HAMA on mouse antibody pharmacokinetics.

Free antigen

Many tumor antigens are shed in large quantities, constituting potential blocking factors to monoclonal antibody target cell binding. The immune complexes formed might theoretically produce tissue damage to certain organs, as well. This is a problem for certain antigens that are secreted or shed in large quantities into the circulation, but not for others; although all malignant cells may shed tumor antigens to some extent. Most of the hematopoietic antigens detected by monoclonal antibodies are generally not shed to an extent which interferes with monoclonal antibody detection. However, excess circulating antigen has been a practical problem in the setting of lymphoma. Immediately following treatment, antigen levels decrease precipitously as they complex with antibody, thus allowing the remainder of the monoclonal antibodies to have access to tumor antigen. Thus, the obstacle of circulating antigen can be overcome with higher monoclonal antibody doses. However, immune complex-mediated disease may occasionally be a complication of this approach.

Antigenic modulation/immunoselection

Antigen modulation is actually a dynamic process in which measurement of surface antigen is decreased in the presence of excess antibody. Electron microscopy with autoradiography and ^{125}I-labeled monoclonal antibody studies have shown that modulation is the result of internalization of the antigen and the bound antibody [207, 214]. This is preceded by 'capping' of the antibody-antigen complex, a process during which the complex appears to localize to one region of the cell surface. Monoclonal antibodies directed against many hematopoietic surface antigens and growth factor receptors on solid tumors induce modulation *in vitro* and *in vivo*. Modulation occurs within minutes of exposure to monoclonal antibodies but is reversible once the monoclonal antibody is removed from the system because of the ongoing production or recycling of antigen.

Antigenic modulation must be differentiated from immunoselection which has resulted in the elimination of antigen-positive cells, thereby leaving only cells which express no or only low levels of the target antigen. The conditions for modulation *in vivo* include presence of immunoreactive monoclonal antibodies in the serum, maintenance of a relatively constant cell number, decreased expression of the targeted antigen, and continued expression of another phenotypic marker. In the absence of antibody, the antigen must be re-expressed to prove there is no immunoselection of cells. Modulation consists of antigen expression, antibody binding, antibody-antigen internalization, re-expression, additional binding, etc. This phenomenon has important implications for passive monoclonal antibody therapy because during modulation, there are insufficient quantities of monoclonal antibodies on the cell surface to effect target cell elimination. In terms of circulating cells, there clearly is a threshold of monoclonal antibody-binding that is required before cells are eliminated. In fact, in some cases, cells with a high density of target antigen are rapidly eliminated while cells lower in antigen persist and/or enter the circulation so that total target cell count is relatively unaffected [46, 72, 194]. Modulation, or receptor down regulation, may be desirable for antibodies which act through a regulatory mechanism, perhaps by altering signal transduction. However, rapid internalization greatly limits the therapeutic potential of antibodies which effect complement and/or cell-mediated cytotoxicity but may be helpful where antibodies are conjugated to toxic substances. As a general rule, modulation is much more common for hematopoietic cell antigens than solid tumor antigens.

Human anti-immunoglobulin response (HAMA, HACA, HAHA)

Human antimouse antibodies (HAMA) and other antiglobulin responses to humanized antibodies have been the subject of recent reviews [55, 124]. Because they are foreign proteins, murine monoclonal antibodies were expected to produce HAMA responses in immunocompetent patients. Trials involving repeated exposure to monoclonal antibodies have confirmed that this is a substantial problem, although it is not seen in all patients [56, 208, 215]. Using RIA and ELISA, investigators have detected HAMA in virtually all patients who have received murine monoclonal antibodies except for those with CLL [15, 41, 52, 107, 163]. The fact that HAMA levels have not been detected in CLL probably reflects the immunodeficiency associated with that disorder. It also appears that HAMA is reduced in many B-cell lymphoma patients. Interestingly, in CTCL, many patients who developed HAMA had previously experienced a clinical response to treatment. Once HAMA have been produced, they effectively neutralize most clinical effects of therapy, although targeting of tumor cells can still be demonstrated. It appears that a small percentage of antimouse antibodies react specifically with the idiotype of the mouse protein rather than only with specific murine Ig isotype determinants. Initial efforts to block the antimouse immune response with chemotherapy, radiotherapy, corticosteroids, and cyclosporine, have not been successful. Some investigators have suggested that infusions of high doses of antibody may eliminate the antimouse response, but this has not been substantiated in other studies. One has to follow such patients for a prolonged period of time inasmuch as the mouse antibody excess may block any evidence of antimouse antibodies during the early phase of production. Initial use of high doses is not tolerizing in all patients [55]. Some investigators have suggested that attachment of polyethylene glycol may decrease the immune response [248]. In the presence of HAMA, plasmapheresis and administration of higher doses of antibodies have briefly surmounted the problem.

Immune responses to chimeric (HACA, human antichimeric antibodies) and human (HAHA, human antihuman antibodies) are also readily detected by immunoassays in patients who have received these agents[124].

As predicted, most of the antibodies in HACA are directed to the residual murine determinants. Most of the antibodies in HAHA are directed to allotypic epitopes. However, these preparations are a significant improvement over mouse antibodies because HACA and HAHA tend to appear later and often at lower titers so that repeated intermittent therapy is possible over several months.

A clinical caveat to keep in mind relates to HAMA and to a lesser extent HACA and HAHA. Diagnostic tests with such antibodies may sensitize patients who will then be at risk for later allergic reaction if further antibody doses are given for diagnostic or therapeutic purposes.

Infusion rates/schedules

In the setting of circulating cells that bear the target antigen, rapid infusion rates can be quite toxic. Preparations with microaggregates, pyrogen, or other contaminants are also more of a problem if infused rapidly. Monoclonal antibodies that trigger endogenous immune responses leading to cytokine release and cell activation can also precipitate substantial toxicity if infused rapidly. Most investigators have been satisfied with 2- to 6-hour infusions for delivery of higher doses of antibody, but pure preparations of antibodies which do not react with circulating white blood cells can be given over a few minutes with no untoward effects. Prolonged continuous infusions may be necessary for monoclonal antibodies with regulatory effects in order to keep receptors down-regulated or blocked. This may also be desirable in order to establish a gradient effect in treating solid tumors because of tumor penetration problems. Repeated bolus infusions may be more appropriate for receptors that are rapidly down-regulated when an antibody-dependent cell-mediated cytotoxicity or complement-dependent cytotoxicity mechanism is postulated. Bolus infusions are well tolerated by most patients if the monoclonal antibody preparation is free of aggregates and there is no cross-reactivity with leukocytes. Intermittent bolus infusions may also be preferred if the down-regulated receptor needs to be reexpressed in order for the antibody/antigen (receptor/ligand) to interaction to produce an antitumor effect. Because of HAMA, some investigators have adopted a strategy to deliver the maximum dose of murine monoclonal antibodies within two weeks because HAMA can be detected within 1-week of initiating treatment. If dose is important, rapidly escalating doses over seven to 14 days would be a reasonable approach in exploratory trials in which the toxic effects of various singlc doses are unknown. For human and humanized antibodies, it is reasonable to plan for longer treatment schedules. At present, an insufficient number of responses have been observed to make definitive correlations with dose, infusion rate, or schedule.

Immune complexes

These are formed in the setting of circulating antigen and in the presence of antimouse antibodies. Because monoclonal antibodies have only one determinant, it has been suggested that they are less likely to form large immune complexes. Similarly, the antimouse response may also be relatively limited because of the uniformity of antigenic determinants in the monoclonal antibodies. As noted above, acute and subacute complications associated with immune complexes have been described but are uncommon. This remains a theoretical concern that necessitates appropriate monitoring and observation.

Antibody class and subclass

In lymphoma, anti-idiotype antibodies of various subclasses have produced responses. In melanoma, only murine IgG3 antibodies and humanized anti-CD2 or anti-CD3 antibodies have produced clear-cut responses. The responses seen with murine IgG2A antibodies in T-cell lymphoma have been rather limited. As noted above, it may well be that the mechanism of response is different in these situations. For direct cytotoxic effect, it currently appears that mouse IgG3 and perhaps some IgG2A murine monoclonal antibodies have the potential [227], but the preferred strategy is a humanized form. It may be that some complement-fixing IgM antibodies will be useful, although animal models and limited human studies have not supported this, and size will limit tumor penetration in solid tumors. Human IgG1 antibodies are usually associated with efficient CDC and ADCC [212]. Class and subclass switching of antibodies has enabled us to establish more directly the importance of the Fc receptor as opposed to the nature and density of the target antigen [173].

Antigenic heterogeneity

If a given tumor cell does not express the antigen detected by a given monoclonal antibody, there is no basis for monoclonal antibody-mediated cytolysis or receptor inhibition for that cell. Because of the tremendous heterogeneity in human cancer cell phenotypes [68, 99, 179, 205], it is extremely unlikely that a single monoclonal antibody will be sufficient for antibody-mediated therapy. On the other hand, with our expanded knowledge of tumor cell antigens, it may be possible to employ rationale combinations of monoclonal antibodies to overcome this problem [145]. Ideally, such a combination or 'cocktail' would include monoclonal antibodies in quantities directly related to specific antigen expression on an individual patient's cancer cells rather than fixed proportions being administered to each patient with a given disease [182, 184]. However, just as with chemotherapy, a combination may only be effective if its individual components have some antitumor effects of their own.

Conclusion

The role of monoclonal antibody therapy in cancer treatment is still being defined [59, 143, 184]. The value of passive monoclonal antibody therapy in cancer is still in question despite efforts with humanized chimeric antibodies [57]. It may be that a major limitation of murine monoclonal antibodies relates to the limited types of human antigens recognized by the mouse immune system in addition to problems of HAMA. New technologies such as that of polymerase chain reaction (PCR) [65], offer the hope of vast libraries of human antibodies which may be superior in terms of antigen selection. Human and chimeric antibodies clearly are an immunologic and pharmacologic improvement over most mouse antibodies. There is also the potential for synergistic and additive effects resulting from the use of monoclonal antibodies in combination with other biological response modifiers.

The most encouraging results with murine monoclonal antibodies have been obtained with anti-idiotype and anti-CD20 antibodies in B-cell lymphoma, anti-IL-2 receptor monoclonal antibodies in T-cell acute lymphocytic leukemia, with anti-disialoganglioside antibodies in melanoma and neuroblastoma, and with 17-1A in the adjuvant treatment of colorectal cancer. Initial trials with CAMPATH in B-cell lymphoproliferative disorders were also encouraging, although initial confirmatory trials were disappointing. The best results with anti-idiotype antibody have been achieved in patients with follicular lymphoma, a disease that has as high as a 30% spontaneous regression rate [107], and most of the responses have been of limited durability. In responding patients, this approach has been limited by immunoselection of idiotype variants and the production of antimouse antibodies. In melanoma, the best results have been seen in lung and soft tissue disease. Melanoma has long been considered an immune-responsive tumor, and spontaneous regressions have been noted in that disease as well [230]. Dose response relationships at higher dose levels (>50 mg) have not been established in either the hematologic or solid tumor responses. Except for inhibiting effects via regulatory mechanisms, there appears to be little if any therapeutic future for unconjugated monoclonal antibodies which induce antigenic modulation unless immunization concepts prove to be useful. On the other hand, these may be excellent choices for immunoconjugate therapy. Ongoing studies of unconjugated antibodies used alone continue to focus on these regulatory approaches and on humanized antibodies that are effective in complement-mediated cytotoxicity and antibody-dependent cell-mediated cytotoxicity assays with human complement and human effector cells. The favored clinical trial design for regulatory approval involves the addition of such antibodies to other anticancer therapies, and/or use in the adjuvant setting or other clinical situations of low tumor burden.

ACKNOWLEDGMENTS

This work was supported by the Patty and George Hoag Cancer Center. The author wishes to thank Virginia Battle for her assistance in the preparation of this manuscript.

REFERENCES

1. Adair JR. Engineering antibodies for therapy. *Immunol Rev* 1992; 130: 5-40.
2. Avner BP, Liao SK, Avner B, et al. Therapeutic murine monoclonal antibodies developed for individual cancer patients. *J Biol Response Modif* 1989; 8: 25-36.
3. Badger CC, Bernstein ID. Therapy of murine leukemia with monoclonal antibody against a normal/differentiation antigen. *J Exp Med* 1983; 157: 828-842.
4. Bajorin DF, Chapman PB, Wong G, et al. Phase I evaluation of a combination of monoclonal antibody R24 and interleukin 2 in patients with metastatic melanoma. *Cancer Res* 1990; 50: 7490-7495.
5. Ball ED, Bernier GM, Cornwell III GG, et al. Monoclonal antibodies to myeloid differentiation antigens: In vivo studies of three patients with acute myelogenous leukemia. *Blood* 1983; 62: 1203-1210.
6. Ball ED, Selvaggi K, Hurd D, et al. A phase I clinical trial of serotherapy in patients with acute myeloid leukemia with an IgM monoclonal antibody to CD15. *J Clin Oncol* [in press]
7. Barker E, Mueller BM, Handgretinger R, et al. Effect of a chimeric anti-ganglioside GD2 antibody on cell-mediated lysis of human neuroblastoma cells. *Cancer Res* 1991; 51: 144-149.
8. Baselga J, Tripathy D, Mendelsohn J, et al. Phase II study of recombinant human anti-Her2 monoclonal antibody (rhuMab Her2) in stage IV breast cancer; Her2 shedding dependent pharmacokinetics and antitumor activity. *Proc Am Soc Clin Oncol* 1990; 14: 103.
9. Beatty JD, Duda RB, Williams LE, et al. Preoperative imaging of colorectal carcinoma with 111-In-labeled anticarcinoembryonic antigen monoclonal antibody. *Cancer Res* 1986; 46: 6494-6502.
10. Berinstein NL, Tang SC, Hewitt K. Objective clinical responses in patients with progressive/recurrent low grade lymphoma treated with Campath 11+ monoclonal antibody. *Blood* 84 Suppl 1 1994; 638a.
11. Bernstein ID, Tam MR, Nowinski RC. Mouse leukemia therapy with monoclonal antibodies against a thymus differentiation antigen. *Science* 1980: 207: 68-71.
12. Bernstein ID, Nowinski RC, Tam MR, et al. Monoclonal antibody therapy of mouse leukemia. In: *Monoclonal Antibodies*. Kennett RH, Bechtol TJ, eds. New York: Plenum Press, 1980: 275-291.
13. Bernstein ID, Nowinski RC. Monoclonal antibody treatment of transplanted and spontaneous murine leukemia. In: *Hybridomas in Cancer Diagnosis and Treatment*. Mitchell MS, Oettgen HF, eds. New York: Raven Press, 1982: 97-112.
14. Bertoli LF, Kubagawa H, Mayumi M, et al. Immunotherapy of advanced B cell malignancies with mouse monoclonal antibodies. *Fed Proc* 1984; 43: 1972.
15. Bertram JH, Gill PS, Levine AM, et al. Monoclonal antibody T101 in T-cell malignancies: a clinical, pharmo-

kinetic and immunologic correlation. *Blood* 1986; 68: 752-761.

16. Billing R, Chatterjee S. Prolongation of skin allograft survival in monkeys treated with anti-Ia and anti-blast/ monocyte monoclonal antibodies. *Transplant Proc* 1983; 15: 649-650.
17. Borup-Christensen P, Erb K, Jensenius JC, et al. Human-human hybridomas for the study of antitumor immune response in patients with colorectal cancer. *Int J Cancer* 1986; 37: 683-688.
18. Brittingham TE, Chaplin H. Production of a human anti-leukemic leukocyte serum and its therapeutic trial. *Cancer* 1960; 1: 412-418.
19. Brown BA, Davis GL, Saltzgaber-Muller J, et al. Tumor specific genetically engineered murine/human chimeric monoclonal antibody. *Cancer Res* 1987; 47: 3577-3583.
20. Brown SL, Miller RA, Horning SJ, et al. Treatment of B-cell lymphomas with anti-idiotype antibodies alone and in combination with alpha interferon. *Blood* 1989; 73: 651-661.
21. Brown SL, Miller RA, Levy R. Antiidiotype antibody therapy of B-cell lymphoma. *Semin Oncol* 1989; 16: 199-210.
22. Brown PN, Geisler CH, Nissen NI. Treatment with CAMPATH-1H antibody in patients with relapsed non-Hodgkin lymphoma and chronic lymphocytic leukemia. *Blood* 1994; 84(suppl 1): 653a.
23. Buchler M, Friess H, Schultheiss K-H, et al. A randomized controlled trial of adjuvant immunotherapy (murine monoclonal antibody 494/32) in resectable pancreatic cancer. *Cancer* 1991; 68: 1507-1512.
24. Buter J, Janssen RAJ, Martens A, et al. Phase I/II study of low-dose intravenous OKT3 and subcutaneous inter-leukin-2 in metastatic cancer. *Eur J Cancer* 1993; 29A: 2108-2113.
25. Burdette S, Schwartz RS. Current concepts: Immunology. Idiotypes and idiotypic network. *N Engl J Med* 1987; 317: 219-224.
26. Burnett KG, Masuho Y, Hernandez R et al. Human monoclonal antibodies to breast cancer cells. *In: Monoclonal Antibodies, Diagnostic and Therapeutic Use in Tumor and Transplantation*. Chatterjee SN, ed. PSG Publishing Co., Inc., Littleton, Mass. 1985, pp 47-62.
27. Capone PM, Papsidero LD, Croghan GA, Chu TM. Experimental tumoricidal effects of monoclonal antibody against solid breast tumors. *Proc Natl Acad Sci USA* 1983; 80: 7328-7332.
28. Carrasquillo JA, Bunn PA, Keenan AM, et al. Radioimmunodetection of cutaneous T-cell lymphoma with 111-In-T101 monoclonal antibody. *N Engl J Med* 1986; 315: 673-680.
29. Carter P, Presta L, Gorman C, et al. Humanization of an anti-p185Her2 antibody for human cancer. *Proc Natl Acad Sci* 1992; 89: 4285-4289.
30. Carter PW. Monoclonal antibodies and the biological approach to cancer. *J Biol Response Modif* 1985; 4: 325-339.
31. Casali P, Inghirami G, Nakamura R, et al. Human monoclonals from antigen-specific selection of B-lymphocytes and transformation by EBV. *Science* 1986; 234: 476-478.
32. Caulfield MJ, Barna B, Murthy S, et al. Phase Ia/Ib trial of an anti-GD3 monoclonal antibody (R24) in combination with interferon alpha (rHuIFNa-2a) in patients with malignant melanoma. *J Biol Response Mod* 1990; 9: 319-328.
33. Caulfield MJ, Murthy S, Tubbs RR, et al. Treatment of chronic lymphocytic leukemia with an anti-idiotypic monoclonal antibody. *Cleve Clin J Med* 1989; 56: 182-188.
34. Chachoua A, Oratz R. Liebes L, et al. Phase Ib trial of granulocyte-macrophage colony-stimulating factor combined with murine monoclonal antibody R24 in patients with metastatic melanoma. *J Immunother* 1994; 16: 132-141.
35. Cheresh DA, Honsila CJ, Staffileno LK, et al. Disialoganglioside GD3 on human melanoma serves as a relevant target antigen for monoclonal antibody-mediated tumor cytolysis. *Proc Natl Acad Sci USA* 1985; 82: 5155-5159.
36. Cheung NK V, Lazarus H, Miraldi FD, et al. Ganglioside GD2 specific monoclonal antibody 3F8: A phase I study in patients with neuroblastoma and malignant melanoma. *J Clin Oncol* 1987; 5: 1430-1440.
37. Chiorazzi N, Wasserman RL, Kunkel HG. Use of Epstein-Barr virus-transformed B-cell lines for the generation of immunoglobulin-producing human B-cell hybridomas. *J Exp Med* 1982; 156: 930-935.
38. Cleary ML, Meeker TC, Levy S, et al. Clustering of extensive somatic mutations in the variable region of an immunoglobulin heavy chain gene from a human B cell lymphoma. *Cell* 1986; 44: 97-106.
39. Cole SP, Campling BG, Louwman IH, Kozbor D, Roder JC. A strategy for the production of human monoclonal antibodies reactive with lung tumor cells. *Cancer Res* 1984; 44: 2750-2753.
40. Cote RJ, Morrissey DM, Houghton AN, et al. Generation of human monoclonal antibodies reactive with cellular antigens. *Proc Natl Acad Sci* 1983; 80: 2026-2030.
41. Courtenay-Luck NS, Epenetos AA, Moore R, et al. Development of primary and secondary immune responses to mouse monoclonal antibodies used in the diagnosis and therapy of malignant neoplasms. *Cancer Res* 1986; 46: 6489-6493.
42. Creekmore S, Urba W, Kopp W, et al. Phase IB/II trial of R24 antibody and interleukin-2 in melanoma. *Proc Am Soc Clin Oncol* 1992; 11: 345.
43. Currie GA. Eighty years of immunotherapy: a review of immunobiological methods used in the treatment of cancer. *Int J Cancer* 1972; 26: 141-153.
44. DePinho RA, Feldman LB, Scharff MD. Tailor-made monoclonal antibodies. *Ann Intern Med* 1986; 104: 225-233.
45. Diamond BA, Yelton DE, Scharff MD. Monoclonal antibodies: a new technology for producing serologic reagents. *N Engl J Med* 1981; 304: 1344-1349.
46. Dillman RO, Shawler DL, Sobol RE, et al. Murine monoclonal antibody therapy in two patients with chronic lymphocytic leukemia. *Blood* 1982; 59: 1036-1045.
47. Dillman RO, Beauregard JC, Sobol RE, et al. Lack of radioimmunodetection and complications associated with monoclonal antibody cross-reactivity with an antigen on circulating cells. *Cancer Res* 1984; 44: 2213-2217.
48. Dillman RO. Monoclonal antibodies in the treatment of cancer. *CRC Crit Rev Hematol/Oncol* 1984; 1: 357-386.
49. Dillman RO, Shawler DL, Dillman JB, et al. Therapy of chronic lymphocytic leukemia and cutaneous T-cell lymphoma with T101 monoclonal antibody. *J Clin Oncol* 1984; 2: 881-891.
50. Dillman RO, Beauregard J, Shawler DL, et al. Clinical trial of 24 hour infusions of T101 murine monoclonal

antibody. In: Reisfeld RA, Sell S, eds. Monoclonal antibodies and cancer therapy, UCLA symposia on molecular and cellular biology, new series Alan R. Liss, Inc, New York, NY 1985; 27: 133-146.

51. Dillman RO, Dillman JB, Halpern SE, et al. Toxicities and side effects associated with intravenous infusions of monoclonal antibodies. *J Biol Response* Modif 1986; 5: 73-84.
52. Dillman RO, Beauregard J, Shawler DL, et al. Continuous infusion of T101 monoclonal antibody in chronic lymphocytic leukemia and cutaneous T-cell lymphoma. *J Biol Response Mod* 1986; 5: 394-410.
53. Dillman RO, Johnson DE, Shawler DL. Immune interferon modulation of in vitro murine anti-human T-cell monoclonal antibody mediated cytotoxicity. *J Immunol* 1986; 136: 728-731.
54. Dillman RO, Beauregard J, Ryan KP, et al. Radioimmunodetection of cancer using indium-labeled monoclonal antibodies. International symposium on labeled and unlabeled antibodies in cancer diagnosis and therapy. *NCI Monographs* 1987; 3: 33-36.
55. Dillman RO. The human antimouse and antiglobulin responses to monoclonal antibodies. *Antibody, Immunocon & Radiopharm* 1990; 3: 1-15.
56. Dillman RO, Shawler DL, McCallister TJ, Halpern SE. Human anti-mouse antibody response in cancer patients following single low-dose injections of radiolabeled murine monoclonal antibodies. *Cancer Biother* 1994; 9: 17-28.
57. Dillman RO. Antibodies as cytotoxic therapy. *J Clin Oncol* 1994; 12: 1497-1515.
58. Dillman RO, Beauregard JC, Jamieson M, et al. Toxicities associated with monoclonal antibody infusions in cancer patients. *Molec Biother* 1988; 1: 81-85.
59. Dillman RO. Monoclonal antibodies for treating cancer. *Ann Intern Med* 1989; 111: 592-603.
60. Dorfman NA. The optimal technological approach to the development of human hybridomas. *J Biol Response Modif* 1985; 4: 213-239.
61. Dyer MJS, Hale G, Hayhoe FGJ, et al. Effects of CAMPATH-1 antibodies *in vivo* in patients with lymphoid malignancies: Influence of antibody isotype. *Blood* 1989; 73: 1431-1439.
62. Edelson RL, Raafat J, Berger CL, Grossman M, Troyer C, Hardy M. Anti-thymocyte globulin in the management of cutaneous T-cell lymphoma. *Cancer Treat Rep* 1979; 63: 675-680.
63. Editorial. *Lancet* 1994; 344: 1013.
64. Ehrlich P. Uben den jetzigen stand der Karzinomforschung. In: *The collected papers of Paul Ehrlich*. Vol. II. London: Pergamon Press 1957: 550-557.
65. Eisenberg BI. The polymerase chain reaction. *N Engl J Med* 1990; 322: 178-183.
66. Elias DJ, Hirschowitz L, Kline LE, et al. Phase I clinical comparative study of monoclonal antibody KS1/4 and KS1/4-methotrexate immunoconjugate in patients with non-small cell lung carcinoma. *Cancer Res* 1990; 50: 4154-4159.
67. Epenetos AA, Shepherd J, Britton KE, et al. 123-I radioiodinated antibody imaging of occult ovarian cancer. *Cancer* 1985; 55: 984-987.
68. Fiddler IJ, Hart IR. Biological diversity in metastatic neoplasms: origins and implications. *Science* 1982; 217: 998-1003.
69. Fisher RI, Kobota TT, Mandell GL, et al. Regression of a T-cell lymphoma after administration of anti-thymocyte globulin. *Ann Intern Med* 1978; 88: 799-800.
70. Foon KA, Bernhard MI, Oldham RK. Monoclonal antibody therapy: assessment by animal tumor models. *J Biol Resp Modif* 1982; 1: 277-304.
71. Foon KA, Bunn PA, Schroff RW, et al. Monoclonal antibody therapy of chronic lymphocytic leukemia and cutaneous T-cell lymphoma: preliminary observations. In: Langman RE, Trowbridge IS, Dulbecco R, eds. *Monoclonal antibody and Cancer*. New York: Academic Press 1984; pp39-52.
72. Foon KA, Schroff RW, Bunn PA, et al. Effects of monoclonal antibody therapy in patients with chronic lymphocytic leukemia. *Blood* 1984; 64: 1085-1093.
73. Frank MM. Complement in the pathophysiology of human disease. *N Engl J Med* 1987; 316: 1525-1530.
74. Frodin JE, Harmenberg U, Biberfeld P, et al. Clinical effects of monoclonal antibodies [MAb 17-1A] in patients with metastatic colorectal carcinomas. *Hybridoma* 1988; 7: 309-321.
75. Furukawa K, Yamaguchi H, Oettgen HF, et al. Two human monoclonal antibodies reacting with the major gangliosides of human melanomas and comparison with corresponding mouse monoclonal antibodies. *Cancer Res* 1989; 49: 191-196.
76. Geha RS. Idiotypic-anti-idiotypic interactions in humans. *J Biol Response Modif* 1984; 3: 573-579.
77. Geha RS. Regulation of the immune response by idiotype-anti-idiotype interactions. *N Engl J Med* 1981; 305: 25-28.
78. Glassy MC, Dillman RO. Molecular biotherapy with human monoclonal antibodies. *Molec Biother* 1988; 1: 7-13.
79. Glassy MC, Handley HH, Hagiwara H, et al. UC729-6, a human lymphoblastoid B-cell line useful for generating antibody-secreting human-human hybridomas. *Proc Natl Acad Sci* 1983; 80: 6327-6331.
80. Glassy MC. Immortalization of human lymphocytes from a tumor-involved lymph node. *Cancer Res* 1987; 47: 5181-5188.
81. Goodman GE, Hellstrom I, Brodzinsky L, et al. Phase I trial of murine monoclonal antibody L6 in breast, colon, ovarian, and lung cancer. *J Clin Oncol* 1990; 8: 1083-1092.
82. Goodman GL, Beaumier P, Hellstrom I, et al. Pilot trial of murine monoclonal antibodies in patients with advanced melanoma. *J Clin Oncol* 1985; 3: 340-352.
83. Goustin AS, Leof EB, Shipley GD, et al. Growth factors and cancer. *Cancer Res* 1986; 46: 1015-1029.
84. Greene WC, Leonard WJ, Depper JM, et al. The human interleukin-2 receptor: Normal and abnormal expression in T cells and in leukemias induced by the human T lymphotropic retroviruses. *Ann Intern Med* 1986; 105: 560-572.
85. Greiner JW, Hand PH, Nugochi P, et al. Enhanced expression of surface tumor-associated antigens on human breast and colon tumor cells after recombinant human leukocyte alpha-interferon treatment. *Cancer Res* 1984; 44: 3208-3214.
86. Greiner JW, Guadagni F, Goldstein D, et al. Intraperitoneal administration of interferon-gamma to carcinoma patients enhances expression of tumor-associated glycoprotein-72 and carcinoembryonic antigen on malignant ascites cells. *J Clin Oncol* 1992; 10: 735-746.

87. Haisma HJ, Pinedo HM, Kessel MAP, et al. Human IgM monoclonal antibody 16.88: Pharmacokinetics and immunogenicity in colorectal cancer patients. *J Natl Cancer Inst* 1991; 83: 1813-1819.
88. Hale G, Dyer M, Clark MR, et al. Remission induction in non-Hodgkins lymphoma with reshaped human monoclonal antibody CAMPATH-1H. *Lancet* 1988; 2: 1394-1399.
89. Halpern SE, Dillman RO, Witztum KF, et al. Radioimmunodetection of melanoma utilizing 111-In-96.5 monoclonal antibody: a preliminary report. *Radiology* 1985; 155: 493-499.
90. Halpern SE, Dillman RO. Radioimmunodetection with monoclonal antibodies against prostatic acid phosphatase. In: *Nuclear Medicine in Clinical Oncology*. Winkler C, ed. Springer Verlag, Berlin, Heidelberg 1986; pp 164-170.
91. Halpern SE, Haindl W, Beauregard J, et al. Scintigraphy with In-111-labeled monoclonal antitumor antibodies: Kinetics, biodistribution, and tumor detection. *Radiology* 1988; 168: 529-536.
92. Hamblin TJ, Abdul-Ahad AK, Gordon J, et al. Preliminary experience in treating lymphocytic leukemia with antibody to immunoglobulin idiotypes on the cell surfaces. *Br J Cancer* 1980; 42: 495-502.
93. Hamblin TJ, Cattan AR, Glennie MJ, et al. Initial experience in treating human lymphoma with a chimeric univalent derivative of monoclonal anti-idiotype antibody. *Blood* 1987; 69: 790-797.
94. Haspel MV, McCabe RP, Pomato N, et al. Generation of tumor cell-reactive human monoclonal antibodies using peripheral blood lymphocytes from actively immunized colorectal carcinoma patients. *Cancer Res* 1985; 45: 3951-3961.
95. Haughton G, Lanier LL, Babcock GF, et al. Antigen-induced murine B cell lymphomas. II. Exploitation of the surface idiotype as tumour specific antigen. *J Immunol* 1978; 121: 2358-2362.
96. Hekman A, Honselaar A, Vuist WM, et al. Initial experience with treatment of human B cell lymphoma with anti-CD19 monoclonal antibody. *Cancer Immunol Immunother* 1991; 32: 364-372.
97. Hellstrom I, Garrigues U, Lavie E, et al. Antibody-mediated killing of human tumor cells by attached effector cells. *Cancer Res* 1988; 48: 624-627.
98. Henney CS, Gillis S. Cell-mediated cytotoxicity. In: Paul WE, ed., *Fundamental Immunology*, pp New York, Raven Press, 1984, pp669-684.
99. Heppner GH, Miller BE. Therapeutic implications of tumor heterogeneity. *Semin Onco*l 1989; 16: 91-105.
100. Herberman RB, Orew ME, Rogentine GN, et al. Cytolytic effects of alloantiserum in patients with lymphoproliferative disorders. *Cancer* 1971; 28: 365-371.
101. Heberman RB, Morgan AC, Reisfeld R, et al. Antibody-dependent cellular cytotoxicity (ADCC) against human melanoma by human effector cells in cooperation with mouse monoclonal antibodies. In: *Monoclonal Antibodies and Cancer Therapy*. Reisfeld RA and Sell S, eds. A.R. Liss, Inc., New York. 1985; 27: 193-203.
102. Herlyn DM, Steplewski Z, Herlyn MF, et al. Inhibition of growth of colorectal carcinoma in nude mice by monoclonal antibody. *Cancer Res* 1980; 40: 717-721.
103. Herlyn D, Koprowski H. IgG2A monoclonal antibodies inhibit human tumor growth through interaction with effector cells. *Proc Natl Acad Sci USA* 1982; 79: 4761-4765.
104. Herlyn D, Ross A, Koprowski H. Anti-idiotypic antibodies bear the internal image of a human tumor antigen. *Science* 1986; 232: 100-102.
105. Herlyn D, Wettendorff M, Schmoll E, et al. Anti-idiotype immunization of cancer patients: Modulation of the immune response. *Proc Natl Acad Sch USA* 1987; 84: 8055-8059.
106. Hersey P, Schibeci SD, Townsend P, et al. Potentiation of lymphocyte responses by monoclonal antibodies to the ganglioside GD3. *Cancer Res* 1986; 46: 6083-6090.
107. Hornung SJ, Rosenberg SA. The natural history of initially untreated low grade non-Hodgkin's lymphoma. *N Engl J Med* 1984; 311: 1471-1475.
108. Houghton AN, Mintzer D, Cordon-Cardo C, et al. Mouse monoclonal IgG3 antibody detecting GD3 ganglioside: a phase I trial in patients with malignant melanoma. *Proc Natl Acad Sci USA* 1985; 82: 1242-1246.
109. Hu F, Epstein AL, Naeve GS, et al. A phase Ia clinical trial of LYM-1 monoclonal antibody serotherapy in patients with refractory B cell malignancies. *Hematol Oncol* 1989; 7: 155-166.
110. Iliopoulos D, Ernst C, Steplewski Z, et al. Inhibition of metastases of a human melanoma xenograft by monoclonal antibody to the GD2/GD3 gangliosides. *J Natl Cancer Inst* 1989; 81: 440-444.
111. Imai K, Pellegrino MA, Wilson BS, et al. Higher cytolytic efficiency of an IgG2A than of an IgG1 monoclonal antibody with the same (or spatially close) determinant on a human molecular-weight melanoma-associated antigen. *Cell Immunol* 1982; 72: 239-247.
112. Irie RF, Sze LL, Saxton RE. Human antibody to OFA-1, a tumor antigen produced in vitro by Epstein-Barr virus transformed human B-lymphoid cell lines. *Proc Natl Acad Sci USA* 1982; 79: 5666-5670.
113. Irie RF, Matuski T, Morton DL. Human monoclonal antibody to ganglioside GM2 for melanoma treatment [letter]. *Lancet* 1989; 1: 786-787.
114. Janson D, Hoffman M, Fuchs A, et al. Campath 1-H therapy causes clearing of lymphocytic infiltration of bone marrow in advanced refractory chronic lymphocytic leukemia. *Blood* 84(suppl 10 1994; 526a.
115. Jerne NK. Towards a network theory of the immune system. *Ann Immunol* 1974; 125C: 373.
116. Johnson JP, Riethmuller G. Monoclonal antibodies and melanomas. In: *Handbook of Monoclonal Antibodies, Applications in Biology and Medicine*. Ferrone S and Dierich MP, eds. Noyes pub., Parkridge NJ, 1985; pp347-359.
117. Junghans RP, Waldmann TA, Landolfi NF, et al. Anti-tac-H, a humanized antibody to the interleukin 2 receptor with new features for immunotherapy in malignant and immune disorders. *Cancer Res* 1990; 50: 1495-1502.
118. Kaliss N. Immunological enhancement of tumor homografts in mice: a review. *Cancer Res* 1958; 18: 992-994.
119. Kan-Mitchell J, Iman A, Kempf RA, et al. Human monoclonal antibodies directed against melanoma tumor-associated antigens. *Cancer Res* 1986; 46: 2490-2496.
120. Kelley MJ, Avis I, Linnoila RI, et al. Complete response in a patient with small cell lung cancer treated on a phase II trial using a murine monoclonal antibody (2A11) directed against gastrin-releasing peptide. *Proc Am Soc Clin Oncol* 1993; 12: 339.

121. Kennedy RC, Eichberg JW, Lanford RE, Dreesman GR. Anti-idiotypic antibody vaccine for type B viral hepatitis in chimpanzees. *Science* 1986; 232: 220-223.
122. Kennedy RC, Zhou EM, Lanford RE, et al. Possible role of anti-idiotypic antibodies in the induction of tumor immunity. *J Clin Invest* 1987; 80: 1217-1224.
123. Khazaeli MB, Saleh MN, Liu TP, et al. Pharmacokinetics and immune response of ^{131}I-chimeric mouse/human B72.3 (human γ) monoclonal antibody in humans. *Cancer Res* 1991; 51: 5461-5466.
124. Khazaeli MB, Conry RM, LoBuglio AF. Human immune response to monoclonal antibodies. *J Immunother* 1994; 15: 42-52.
125. Kirkwood JM, Neumann RD, Zoghbi SS, et al. Scintigraphic detection of metastatic melanoma using Indium-111/DTPA conjugated anti-gp240 antibody [ZME018]. *J Clin Oncol* 1987; 5: 1247-1255.
126. Kirch ME, Hammerling U. Immunotherapy of murine leukemias by monoclonal antibody: effect of passively administered antibody on growth of transplanted tumor cells. *J Immunol* 1981; 127: 805-810.
127. Kjeldson TB, Rasmussen BB, Rose C, Zeuthen J. Human-human hybridomas and human monoclonal antibodies obtained by fusion of lymph node lymphocytes from breast cancer patients. *Cancer Res* 1988; 48: 3208-3214.
128. Koprowski H, Herlyn D, Lubeck M, et al. Human anti-idiotype antibodies in cancer patients: is the modulation of the immune response beneficial for the patient? *Proc Natl Acad Sci USA* 1984; 81: 216-219.
129. Klein B, Wijdenes J, Zhang XG, et al. Murine anti-interleukin 6 monoclonal antibody therapy for a patient with plasma cell leukemia. *Blood* 1991; 78: 1198-1204.
130. Kolitz JE, O'Mara KV, Willemze R, et al. Treatment of acute lymphoblastic leukemia with CAMPATH-1H: initial observations. *Blood* 1994; 84 (suppl 1) 301a.
131. Knox SJ, Levy R, Hodgkinson S, et al. Observations on the effect of chimeric anti-CD4 monoclonal antibody in patients with mycosis fungoides. *Blood* 1991; 77: 20-30.
132. Kohler G, Milstein C. Continuous cultures of fused cells secreting antibody of predetermined specificity. *Nature* 1975; 256: 495-597.
133. Koprowski H, Steplewski Z, Herlyn D, et al. Study of antibodies against human melanoma produced by somatic cell hybrids. *Proc Natl Acad Sci USA* 1978; 75: 3405-3409.
134. Kosmos C, Epenetos AE, Colurtenay-Luck NS. Activation of cellular immunity after intracavitary monoclonal antibody therapy of ovarian cancer. *Cancer* 1994; 73: 3000-3010.
135. Larrick JW, Bourla JM. Prospects for therapeutic use of human monoclonal antibodies. *J Biol Response Mod* 1986; 5: 379-393.
136. Larson SM, Brown, JP, Wright PW, et al. Imaging of melanoma with I-131-labeled monoclonal antibodies. *J Nucl Med* 1982; 24: 123-129.
137. Lanier LL, Babcock GF, Raybourne RB, et al. Mechanism of B cell lymphoma immunotherapy with passive xenogeneic anti-idiotype serum. *J Immunol* 1980; 125: 1730-1736.
138. Laszlo J, Buckley CE, Amos DB. Infusion of isologous immune plasma in chronic lymphocytic leukemia. *Blood* 1968; 31: 104-110.
139. Leder P. The genetics of antibody diversity. *Sci Amer* 1980; 243: 102-115.
140. Leroy M. Teillac P, Rain JD, et al. Radioimmunodetection of lymph node invasion in prostatic cancer. *Cancer* 1989; 64: 1-5.
141. Letvin NL, Ritz J, Guida LJ, et al. *In vivo* administration of lymphocyte-specific monoclonal antibodies in nonhuman primates: I. effects of anti-T11 antibodies on the circulating T cell pool. *Blood* 1985; 66: 961-966.
142. Levy R, Miller RA. Biological and clinical indications of lymphocyte hybridomas: tumor therapy with monoclonal antibodies. *Ann Rev Med* 1983; 34: 107-116.
143. Levy R. Will monoclonal antibodies find a place in our therapeutic armamentarium? *J Clin Oncol* 1987; 5: 527-529.
144. Liao S, Kwong PC, Khosravi M, Dent PB. Enhanced expression of melanoma-associated antigens and B2-microglobulin on cultured human melanoma cells by interferon. *J Natl Cancer Inst* 1982; 68: 19-25.
145. Liao SK, Meranda C, Avner BP, et al. Immunohistochemical phenotyping of human solid tumors with monoclonal antibodies in devising biotherapeutic strategies. *Cancer Immunol Immunother* 1989; 28: 77-86.
146. Lindstrom BA. An experimental study of myelotoxic sera. Therapeutic attempts in myeloid leukaemia. *Acta Med Scand Suppl* 1927; 22: 1-169.
147. Liu AY, Robinson RR, Hellstrom AE, et al. Chimeric-mouse-human IgG1 antibody that can mediate lysis of cancer cells. *Proc Natl Acad Sci USA* 1987; 84: 3439-3443.
148. LoBuglio AF, Saleh MN, Lee J, et al. Phase I trial of multiple large doses of murine monoclonal antibody CO17-1A. I Clinic aspects. *J Natl Cancer Inst* 1988; 17: 932-936.
149. LoBuglio AF, Wheeler RH, Trang J, et al. Mouse/human chimeric monoclonal antibody in man: kinetics and immune response. *Proc Natl Acad Sci USA* 1989; 86: 4220-4224.
150. Lowder JN, Meeker TC, Campbell M, et al. Studies on B lymphoid tumors treated with monoclonal anti-idiotype antibodies: Correlation with clinical responses. *Blood* 1987; 69: 199-210.
151. Lubeck MD, Steplewski Z, Baglia F, et al. The interaction of murine IgG subclass proteins with human monocyte Fc receptors. *J Immunol* 1985; 135: 1299-1304.
152. Mach J-P, Chatal J-F, Lumbroso J-D, et al. Tumor localization in patients by radiolabeled monoclonal antibodies against colon carcinoma. *Cancer Res* 1983; 43: 5593-5600.
153. Maguire RT, VanNostrand D. Diagnosis of colorectal and ovarian carcinoma. New York: Marcel Dekker Inc, 1992.
154. Maloney DG, Levy R, Miller RA. Monoclonal anti-idiotype therapy of Ball lymphoma. *Biological Therapy of Cancer Updates* 1992; 6: 1-10.
155. Maloney DG, Liles TM, Czerwinski DK, et al. Phase I clinical trial using escalating single dose infusion of chimeric monoclonal antibody (IDEC C2B8) in patients with recurrent B-cell lymphoma. *Blood* 1994; 84: 2457-2466.
156. Maloney DG, Bodkin D, Grillo-Lopez AJ, et al. IDEC-C2B8: final report on a phase II trial in relapsed non-Hodgkin's lymphoma. *Blood* 1994; 84(suppl 1): 169a.
157. Masui H, Kawamoto T, Sato JD, et al. Growth inhibition of human tumor cells in athymic mice by anti-epidermal growth factor receptor monoclonal antibodies. *Cancer Res* 1984; 44: 1002-1007.

158. Meeker TC, Lowder J, Maloney DG, et al. A clinical trial of anti-idiotype therapy for B cell malignancy. *Blood* 1985; 65: 1349-1372.
159. Meeker T, Lowder J, Cleary ML, et al. Emergence of idiotype variants during treatment of B-cell lymphoma with anti-idiotype antibodies. *Blood* 1985; 65: 1373-1381.
160. Mellstedt H, Frodin J-E, Masucci G, et al. The therapeutic use of monoclonal antibodies in colorectal carcinoma. *Semin Oncol* 1991; 18: 462-477.
161. Metzger H, Kinnet JP. How antibodies work: focus on Fc receptors. *FASEB J* 1988; 2: 311.
162. Miller RA, Maloney DG, Warnke R, et al. Treatment of B-cell lymphoma with monoclonal anti-idiotype antibody. *N Engl J Med* 1981; 306: 517-522.
163. Miller RA, Levy R. Response of cutaneous T cell lymphoma to therapy with hybridoma monoclonal antibody. *Lancet* 1981; 2: 226-230.
164. Miller RA, Maloney DG, McKillop J, Levy R. In vivo effects of murine hybridoma monoclonal antibody in a patient with T-cell leukemia. *Blood* 1981; 58: 78-86.
165. Miller RA, Oseroff AR, Stratte PT, et al. Monoclonal antibody therapeutic trials in seven patients with T-cell lymphoma. *Blood* 1983; 62: 988-995.
166. Miller RA, Hart S, Samoszuk M, et al. Shared idiotypes expressed by human B-cell lymphomas. *N Engl J Med* 1989; 321: 851-857.
167. Minasian LM, Szatrowski TP, Rosenblum M, et al. Hemorrhagic tumor necrosis during a pilot trial of tumor necrosis factor-a and anti-GD3 ganglioside monoclonal antibody in patients with metastatic melanoma. *Blood* 1994; 83: 56-64.
168. Minasian ML, Yao TJ, Steffens TA, et al. A phase I study of anti-GD3 ganglioside monoclonal antibody R24 and recombinant human macrophage-colony stimulating factor inpatients with metastatic melanoma. *Cancer* 1995; 75: 2251-2257.
169. Mittelman A, Chen ZJ, Kageshita T, et al. Active specific immunotherapy in patients with melanoma: A clinical trial with mouse antiidiotypic monoclonal antibodies elicited with synergeneic anti-high-molecular-weight melanoma-associated antigen monoclonal antibodies. *J Clin Invest* 1990; 86: 2136-2144.
170. Mittelman A, Chen ZJ, Yang H, et al. Human high molecular weight melanoma-associated antigen (HMW-MAA) mimicry by mouse anti-idiotypic monoclonal antibody MK2-23: Induction of humoral anti-HMW-MAA immunity and prolongation of survival in patients with stage IV melanoma. *Proc Natl Acad Sci USA* 1992; 89: 466-470.
171. Molodofsky PJ, Sears HF, Mulhearn Jr CB, et al. Detection of metastatic tumor in normal sized retroperitoneal lymph nodes by monoclonal antibody imaging. *N Engl J Med* 1984; 311: 106-107.
172. Morrison SL, Oi T. Genetically engineered antibody molecules. *Adv Immunol* 1989; 44: 65-92.
173. Mujoo K, Kipps TJ, Yang HM, et al. Functional properties and effect on growth suppression of human neuroblastoma tumors by isotype switch variants of monoclonal antiganglioside GD2 antibody 14.18. *Cancer Res* 1989; 49: 2857-2861.
174. Mulshine JL, Avis I, Treston AM, et al. Clinical use of a monoclonal antibody to bombesin-like peptide in patients with lung cancer. *Ann NY Acad Sci* 1988; 547: 360-372.
175. Munn DH, Cheung N-KV. Interleukin-2 enhancement of monoclonal antibody-mediated cellular cytotoxicity against human melanoma. *Cancer Res* 1987; 47: 6600-6605.
176. Murray JL, Rosenblum MG, Sobol RE, et al. Radioimmunoimaging in malignant melanoma with 111-In-labeled monoclonal antibody 96.5. *Cancer Res* 1985; 45: 2376-2381.
177. Murray JL, Rosenblum MG, Lamki K, et al. Clinical parameters related to optimal tumor localization of Indium-111-labeled mouse antimelanoma monoclonal antibody ZME018. *J Nucl Med* 1987; 28: 25-33.
178. Murray JL, Cunningham JE, Brewer H, et al. Phase I trial of murine monoclonal antibody 14G21 administered by prolonged intravenous infusion in patients with neuroectodermal tumor. *J Clin Oncol* 1994; 12: 184-193.
179. Nadler LM, Stashenko P, Hardy R, et al. Serotherapy of a patient with a monoclonal antibody directed against a human lymphoma-associated antigen. *Cancer Res* 1980; 40: 3147-3154.
180. Nicholson GL. Tumor cell instability, diversification, and progression to the metastatic phenotype: From oncogene to oncofetal expression. Cancer Res 1987; 47: 1473-1487.
181. Nisonoff A. Idiotypes: Concepts and applications. *J Immunol* 1991; 147: 2429-2438.
182. Oldham RK. Monoclonal antibodies in cancer therapy. *J Clin Oncol* 1983; 1: 582-590.
183. Oldham RK, Foon KA, Morgan C, et al. Monoclonal antibody therapy of malignant melanoma: *In vivo* localization in cutaneous metastases after intravenous administration. *J Clin Oncol* 1984; 2: 1235-1244.
184. Oldham RK. Monoclonal antibodies: does sufficient selectivity to cancer cells exist for therapeutic application? *J Biol Response Med* 1987; 6: 227-234.
185. Oosterwijk E, Debruyne FMJ, Schalken JA. The use of monoclonal antibody G250 in the therapy of renal-cell carcinoma. *Semin Oncol* 1995; 22: 34-41.
186. Pegram M, Lipton A, Pietras R, et al. Phase II study of intravenous recombinant humanized anti-p185 Her-2 monoclonal antibody plus cisplatin in patients with Her-2 neu overexpressing metastatic breast cancer. *Proc Am Soc Clin Oncol* 1995; 14: 106.
187. Perek Y, Hurwitz E, Burowski D, Haimovich J. Immunotherapy of a murine B-cell tumor with antibodies and $F(ab')_2$ fragments against idiotypic determinants of its cell surface IgM. *J Immunol* 1983; 131: 1600-1603.
188. Press OW, Appelbaum F, Ledbetter JA, et al. Monoclonal antibody 1F5 [anti-CD-20] serotherapy of human B cell lymphomas. *Blood* 1987; 69: 584-591.
189. Pukel CS, Lloyd KO, Travassos LR, et al. GD3, a prominent ganglioside of human melanoma. *J Exp Med* 1982; 155: 1133-1147.
190. Rankin EM, Hekman A, Somers R, et al. Treatment of two patients with B cell lymphoma with monoclonal anti-idiotype antibodies. *Blood* 1985; 65: 1373-1381.
191. Rietmuller G, Schneider-Gadicke E, Schlimok G, et al. Randomized trial of monoclonal antibody for adjuvant therapy of resected Dukes C colorectal carcinoma. *Lancet* 1994; 343: 1177-1183.
192. Richards JM, Vogelzang NJ, Bluestone J.A. Neurotoxicity after treatment with muromonab-CD3. *New Engl J Med* 1990; 323: 487-488.
193. Ritz J, Pesando JM, Notis-McConarty J, et al. Modulation of human acute lymphoblastic leukemia antigen induced

by monoclonal antibody *in vitro*. *J Immunol* 1908; 125: 1506-1514.
194. Ritz J, Pesando JM, Sallan SE, et al. Serotherapy of acute lymphoblastic leukemia with monoclonal antibody. *Blood* 1981; 58: 141-152.
195. Rosenberg SA, Terry WD. Passive immunotherapy of cancer in animals and man. *Adv Cancer Res* 1977; 25: 323-388.
196. Rudders RA, Levin A, Jespersen D, et al. Crossreacting human lymphoma idiotypes. Blood 1992; 80: 1039-1044.
197. Ryan KP, Dillman RO, DeNardo SJ, et al. Breast cancer imaging with In-111 human IgM monoclonal antibodies. *Radiol* 1988; 167: 71-75.
198. Saleh MN, LoBuglio AF, Wheeler RH, et al. A phase II trial of murine monoclonal antibody 17-1A and interferon-gamma: Clinical and immunological data. *Cancer Immunol* 1990; 32: 185-190.
199. Saleh MN, Khazaeli MB, Wheeler RH, et al. Phase I trial of the murine monoclonal anti-GD2 antibody 14G2a in metastatic melanoma. *Cancer Res* 1992; 52: 4342-4347.
200. Saleh MN, Khazaeli MD, Wheeler RH, et al. Phase I trial of the chimeric anti-GD2 monoclonal antibody ch14.18 in patients with malignant melanoma. *Hum Antibod Hybridomas* 1992: 3: 19-23.
201. Schecter AL, Stern DF, Vaidanathan L, et al. The neu oncogene: an erb-B-related gene encoding a 185, 000-Mr tumor antigen. *Nature* 1984; 312: 513-516.
202. Scheinberg DA, Strand M. Leukemic cell targeting and therapy by monoclonal antibody in a mouse model system. *Cancer Res* 1982; 42: 44-49.
203. Scheinberg DA, Lovett D, Divgi CR, et al. A Phase I trial of monoclonal antibody M195 in acute myelogenous leukemia: Specific bone marrow targeting and internalization of radionuclide. *J Clin Onc* 1991; 9: 478-490.
204. Schlom J, Wunderlich D, Teramoto YA. Generation of human monoclonal antibodies reactive with human mammary carcinoma cells. *Proc Natl Acad Sci* 1980; 77: 6841-6845.
205. Schnipper LE. Clinical implications of tumor cell heterogeneity. *N Engl J Med* 1986; 314: 1423-1431.
206. Schoof DD, Selleck CM, Massaro AF, et al. Activation of human tumor-infiltrating lymphocytes by monoclonal antibodies directed to the CD3 complex. *Cancer Res* 1990; 50: 1138-1143.
207. Schroff RW, Farrell MM, Klein RA, et al. T65 antigen modulation in a phase I monoclonal antibody trial with chronic lymphocytic leukemia patients. *J Immunol* 1984; 133: 1641-1648.
208. Schroff RW, Foon KA, Wilburn SB, et al. Human antimurine immunoglobulin responses in patients receiving monoclonal antibody therapy. *Cancer Res* 1985; 45: 879-885.
209. Sears HF, Atkinson B, Mattis J, et al. Phase I clinical trial of monoclonal antibody in treatment of gastrointestinal tumors. *Lancet* 1982; 1: 762-765.
210. Sears HF, Herlyn D, Steplewski Z, et al. Effects of monoclonal antibody immunotherapy on patients with gastrointestinal adenocarcinoma. *J Biol Response Modif* 1984; 3: 136-150.
211. Sears HF, Herlyn D, Steplewski Z, et al. Phase II clinical trial of a murine monoclonal antibody cytotoxic for gastrointestinal adenocarcinoma. *Cancer Res* 1985; 45: 5910-5913.
212. Shakib F, ed. Basic and clinical aspects of IgG subclasses. *New York: Carger*, 1986.
213. Shaw DR, Khazaeli MB, LoBuglio AF. Mouse/human chimeric antibodies to a tumor-associated antigen: biologic activity of the four human IgG subclasses. *J Natl Cancer Inst* 1988; 80: 1553-1559.
214. Shawler DL, Miceli MC, Wormsley SB, et al. Induction of *in vitro* and *in vivo* antigenic modulation by the anti-human T cell monoclonal antibody T101. *Cancer Res* 1984; 44: 5921-5927.
215. Shawler DL, Bartholomew RM, Smith LM, et al. Human immune response to multiple injections of murine monoclonal IgG. *J Immunol* 1985; 135: 1530-1535.
216. Shawler DL, Wormsley SB, Dillman RO, et al. The use of monoclonal antibodies and flow cytometry to detect peripheral blood and bone marrow involvement of a diffuse, poorly differentiated lymphoma. *Int J Immunopharmacol* 1985; 7: 423-432.
217. Shawler DL, McCallister TJ, Sobol RE, et al. Serologic and cellular assays to monitor therapy with murine monoclonal antibodies. *J Clin Lab Anal* 1987; 2: 184-190.
218. Shen JW, Atkinson B, Koprowsky H, et al. Binding of murine immunoglobulin to human tissues after immunotherapy with anti-colorectal carcinoma monoclonal antibody. *Int J Cancer* 1984; 33: 465-468.
219. Sikora K, Wright R. Human monoclonal antibodies to lung cancer antigens. *Br J Cancer* 1981; 43: 696-700.
220. Sikora K, Alderson T, Phillips J, et al. Human hybridomas from malignant gliomas. *Lancet* 1982; 1: 11-14.
221. Sikora K, Alderson T, Ellis J, et al. Human hybridomas from patients with malignant disease. *Br J Cancer* 1983; 47: 135-145.
222. Sikora K. Human monoclonal antibodies. *Brit Med Bull* 1984; 40: 209-212.
223. Sikorska HM. Therapeutic applications of antiidiotype antibodies. *J Biol Respons Modif* 1988; 7: 327-358.
224. Sobol RE, Dillman RO, Smith JD, et al. Phase I evaluation of murine monoclonal anti-melanoma antibody in man: preliminary observations. In: *Hybridomas in Cancer Diagnosis and Treatment*. Mitchell MS, Oettgen HF, eds. New York: Raven Press, 1981; 21: 199-206.
225. Sosman JA, Weiss GR, Margolin KA, et al. Phase IB clinical trial of anti-CD3 followed by high dose bolus interleukin-2 in patients with metastatic melanoma and advanced renal cell carcinoma; clinical and immunologic effects. *J Clin Oncol* 1993; 11: 1496-1505.
226. Starling J, Cote RJ, Marder P, et al. Tissue distribution and cellular location of the antigens recognized by human monoclonal antibodies 16.88 and 28A32. *Cancer Res* 1988; 48: 7273-7278.
227. Steplewski Z, Sun LK, Shearman CW, et al. Biological activity of human-mouse IgG1, IgG2, IgG3, and IgG4 chimeric monoclonal antibodies with antitumor specificity. *Proc Natl Acad Sci USA* 1988; 85: 4852-4856.
228. Stevenson FK, Bell AJ, Cusack R, et al. Preliminary studies for an immunotherapeutic approach to the treatment of human myeloma using chimeric anti-CD38 antibody. *Blood* 1991; 77: 1071-1079.
229. Stratte PT, Miller RA, Amyx HL, et al. In vivo effects of murine monoclonal anti-human T cell antibodies in subhuman primates. *J Biol Respons Modif* 1982; 1: 137-148.
230. Sumner WC, Foraker AG. Spontaneous regression of human melanoma: clinical and experimental studies. *Cancer* 1960; 13: 79-81.

231. Tempero MA, Sivinski C, Steplewski Z, et al. Phase II trial of interferon gamma and monoclonal antibody 17-1A in pancreatic cancer: biologic and clinical effects. *J Clin Oncol* 1990; 8: 2019-2026.
232. Thompson CH, Stacker SA, Salehi N, et al. *Immunoscintigraphy for detection of lymph node metastases from breast cancer*. 1984; 2: 1245-1247.
233. Thurin J, Thurin M, Kimoto Y, et al. Monoclonal antibody-defined correlations in melanoma between levels of GD2 and GD3 antigens and antibody-mediated cytotoxicity. *Cancer Res* 1987; 47: 1229-1233.
234. Trowbridge IS, Domingo DL. Anti-transferrin receptor monoclonal antibody and toxin-antibody conjugates affect growth of human tumour cells. *Nature* 1981; 294: 171-173.
235. Urba WJ, Ewel C, Kopp W, et al. Anti-CD3 monoclonal antibody treatment of patients with CD3-negative tumors: A phase IA/B study. *Cancer Res* 1992; 52: 2394-2401.
236. Vadhan-Raj S, Cordon-Cardo C, Carswell E, et al. Phase I trial of mouse monoclonal antibody against GD3 ganglioside in patients with melanoma: induction of inflammatory responses at tumor sites. *J Clin Oncol* 1988; 6: 1636-1648.
237. Vitetta ES, Uhr JW. Monoclonal antibodies as agonists: an expanded role for their use in cancer therapy. *Cancer Res* 1994; 54: 5301-5309.
238. Waldmann TA. The structure, function, and expression of interleukin-2 receptors on normal and malignant lymphocytes. *Science* 1986; 232: 727-732.
239. Waldmann, TA, Goldman CK, Bongiovanni KF, et al. Therapy of patients with human T-cell lymphotropic virus I-induced adult T-cell leukemia with anti-tac, a monoclonal antibody to the receptor for interleukin-2. *Blood* 1988; 72: 1805-1816.
240. Waldmann TA, Pastan IH, Gansow OA, et al. The multichain interleukin-2 receptor: A target for immunotherapy. *Ann Intern Med* 1992; 116: 148-160.
241. Wallach D, Fellous M, Revel M. Preferential effect of gamma interferon on the synthesis of HLA antigens and their mRNAs in human cells. *Nature* 1982; 299: 833-835.
242. Weiner GJ, Hillstrom JR. Bispecific anti-idiotype/anti-CD3 antibody therapy of murine B cell lymphoma. *J Immunol* 1991; 147: 4035-4044.
243. Weiner LM, Moldofsky PH, Gatenby RA, et al. Antibody delivery and effector cell activation in a phase II trial of recombinant gamma-interferon and the murine monoclonal antibody CO17-1A in advanced colorectal carcinoma. *Cancer Res* 1988; 48: 2568-2573.
244. Weiner LM, Steplewski Z, Koprowski H, et al. Divergent dose-related effects of gamma-interferon therapy on *in vitro* antibody-dependent cellular and nonspecific cytotoxicity by human peripheral blood monocytes. *Cancer Res* 1988; 48: 1042-1046.
245. Weiner LM, Harvey E, Padavic-Shaller K, et al. Phase II multicenter evaluation of prolonged murine monoclonal antibody 17-1A therapy in pancreatic carcinoma. *J Immunother* 1993; 13: 110-116.
246. Welte K, Miller G, Chapman PB, et al. Stimulation of T lymphocyte proliferation by monoclonal antibodies against GD3 ganglioside. *J Immunol* 1987; 139: 1763-1771.
247. Wettendorff M, Hiopoulos D, Tempero M, et al. Idiotypic cascades in cancer patients treated with monoclonal antibody CO17-1A. *Proc Natl Acad Sci USA* 1989; 86: 3787-3791.
248. Wilkinson I, Jackson C-JC, Lang GM, et al. Tolerance induction in mice by conjugates of monoclonal immunoglobulins and monomethoxypolyethylene glycol: transfer of tolerance by T cells and by T cell extracts. *J Immunol* 1987; 139: 326-331.
249. Winter G, Milstein C. Man-made antibodies. *Nature* 1991; 349: 293-299.
250. Wiseman C, Hammock V, Barton L, et al. Clinical responses of primary human CNS tumors to OKT3/cyclophosphamide. *J Immunother* 1994; 16: 245.
251. Wong KK, Sweet DL, Variakoujis D. The treatment of lymphoblastic lymphoma with antithymocyte globulin. *Cancer* 1981; 50: 57-61.
252. Wong JF, Colvin RB. Bi-specific monoclonal antibodies. Selective binding and complement fixation to cells that express two different surface antigens. *J Immunol* 1987; 139: 1369-1374.
253. Woodhouse CS, Morgan AC Jr. Murine monoclonal IgG3 antibodies to human colorectal tumor-associated antigens: production and characterization of antibodies active in both antibody-dependent cellular cytotoxicity and complement-mediated cytolysis. *Cancer Res* 1989; 49: 2766-2772.
254. Wright PW, Hellstrom KE, Hellstrom IE, et al. Serotherapy of malignant disease. *Med Clin North Am* 1976; 60: 607-622.
255. Yoshikawa K, Ueda R, Obata Y, et al. Human monoclonal antibody reactive to stomach cancer produced by mouse-human hybridoma technique. *Jpn J Cancer Res* 1986; 77: 1122-1133.
256. Young WW, Hakomori S. Therapy of mouse lymphoma with monoclonal antibodies to glycolipid: selection of low antigenic variance *in vivo*. *Science* 1981; 211: 487-489.
257. Yu AL, Uttenreuther MM, Kamps A, et al. Combined use of human-mouse chimeric anti-GD2 (ch14.18) in the treatment of refractory neuroblastoma. *Antibody Immunocon Radiopharm* 1995; 8: 61.
258. Ziegler LD, Palazzolo, Cunningham J, et al. Phase I trial of murine monoclonal antibody L6 in combination with subcutaneous interleukin-2 in patients with advanced carcinoma of the breast, colorectum, and lung. *J Clin Oncol* 1992; 10: 1470-1478.

13

IMMUNOTOXINS

LYNN E. SPITLER
Jenner Biotherapies, Inc., San Ramon

Immunotoxins consist of a monoclonal antibody (MoAb) or other targeting agent conjugated to a toxin which has the capability of causing cell death. Although many substances, including chemotherapeutic agents and radionuclides, are toxic to cells, the term 'immunotoxin' has generally been reserved for conjugates in which the toxic moiety is a ribosomal inhibiting protein. These substances act enzymatically to inhibit protein synthesis. Ribosomal inhibiting proteins occur naturally in a variety of bacteria, plants and animals. Many of them are lectins which bind to sugars and agglutinate cells [37, 106]. Examples of ribosomal inhibiting proteins are illustrated in Table 1.

Table 1. Ribosomal inhibiting proteins

Ribosomal inhibiting proteins	Source
Ricin	*Ricinus communis* (Castor bean)
Abrin	*Abrus precatorias*
Gelonin	*Gelonium multiflorum*
Saporin	*Saponaria officinalis*
Pokeweed antiviral protein	*Phytolacca americana*
Diphtheria toxin	*Corynebacterium diphtheriae*
Pseudomonas exotoxin	*Pseudomonas aeruginosa*

Several plant lectins, including the toxins abrin and ricin, are of interest because they are among the most toxic compounds known. Abrin and ricin consist of two peptide subunits known as the A-chain and B-chain (Table 2). The B-chain serves to bind the toxin to the cell membrane via carbohydrate receptors and permit entry of the A-chain into the cell. The A-chain is an enzyme which causes cell death by directly inactivating the 60S ribosomal subunit so that it has a decreased capacity to bind EF-2, thereby inhibiting protein synthesis. Internalization of the A-chain is necessary for the toxic action to occur. To confer specificity on the immunotoxin, it is necessary either to remove the B-chain component or to block its carbohydrate binding sites. The monoclonal antibody then targets the toxin, permitting specific killing of the targeted tissue. The A-chain is such a potent toxin that it has been suggested that one molecule entering the cytosol is sufficient to kill the cell [30].

Table 2. Structure of abrin and ricin

A Chain:	Enzyme which inhibits protein synthesis by binding to ribosomes
B Chain:	Permits internalization of the A chain by binding to carbohydrates (lactose, galactose) on the cell membrane

Some toxins, such as gelonin, saporin, and pokeweed antiviral protein (PAP), consist solely of the A-chain without the B-chain component. Thus, until they are conjugated to a targeting agent, they are relatively non-toxic since they lack the capability to enter the cell.

Diphtheria toxin and pseudomonas exotoxin A each consist of a single polypeptide chain which contains both the binding component and the enzymatic A chain component. Analogous to the situation with the A chain of ricin and abrin, it is thought that a single or a very few molecules of diphtheria toxin A-chain entering the cytosol is sufficient to cause cell death [133]. The use of immunotoxins has been the subject of several recent reviews [7, 18, 53, 58, 92, 98, 99, 119, 120].

PRECLINICAL STUDIES

Extensive preclinical studies *in vitro* and *in vivo* have been reported. A selection of typical studies demonstrating the selectivity and killing capacity of this innovative anticancer approach is presented. Various reviews are cited for a more complete review of the preclinical literature [35].

In vitro

There have been numerous studies documenting the specificity and efficacy of immunotoxins in causing death of the target cell. Gilliland et al. [39] coupled diphtheria toxin A chains to MoAbs against colorectal carcinoma. This conjugate killed 100% of the colorectal carcinoma cells *in vitro*, but did not kill any of the other unrelated malignant and normal cell lines tested. A number of additional *in vitro* studies have demonstrated specific killing

R.K. Oldham (ed.), Principles of Cancer Biotherapy. 3rd ed., 318–337.

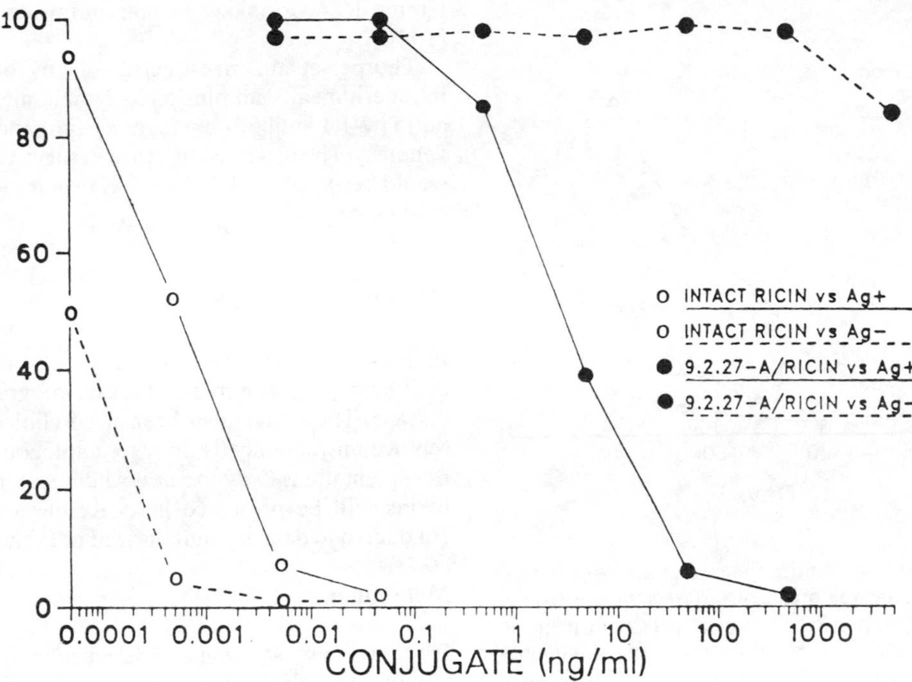

Figure 1. Sensitivity of antigen-positive and -negative human melanoma cells to intact ricin and immunotoxins of 9.2.27 plus ricin A chain.

of cell lines when MoAbs directed toward tumor-associated antigens were coupled to ricin toxin A chain (RTA). Sivan et al. [115] studied an immunotoxin derived from the antimelanoma antibody 9.2.27 which reacts to a high molecular weight proteoglycan associated with melanoma cells. An antigen positive and an antigen negative cell line were shown to have similar sensitivity to intact ricin (Fig. 1). Specific killing of the antigen positive cell line and no toxicity to the antigen negative line was demonstrated when the antimelanoma antibody was conjugated to the purified ricin A chain. They also evaluated a variety of other toxins, using ricin A chain as a standard for comparison. Similar results have been demonstrated for T-leukemia cells [112, 126], guinea pig hepatoma [56], murine B-lymphocytes carrying a specific idiotype [67], human breast carcinoma cells [68], murine T-leukemia cells [11, 134] and acute lymphoblastic leukemia [103]. Similarly, conjugation of antibodies with the A-chains of other plant lectins, such as the A-chain of pokeweed antiviral protein, has also been shown to produce selective cytotoxic effects toward the appropriate cell line [102].

The above referenced studies have involved targeting with antibodies directed towards tumor associated antigens. Another approach involves targeting of the immunotoxin to cell receptors. Thus, immunotoxins have been developed and shown to have specificity for transferrin receptors [44], the IL-2 receptor [96] which is present in large numbers in some leukemias and lymphomas, the epidermal growth factor (EGF) receptors [96], and the IL-6 receptor [96] which is present on some myelomas.

In vivo

In addition to the above *in vitro* studies, immunotoxins consisting of toxins coupled to MoAbs have been shown to have anti-tumor activity *in vivo* in animal studies. The studies most relevant to clinical trials are those in which the immunotoxin is given systemically at some time interval after tumor implantation. The efficacy of an immunotoxin consisting of the D3 antibody to the L10 guinea pig hepatoma conjugated to abrin A chain was investigated [5, 56]. Syngeneic guinea pigs were inoculated with tumor cells intradermally. Seven days later they were divided into groups of five animals each. The control group was given an injection of saline, and the treatment groups were given a single injection of various dosages of immunotoxin. The results showed significant inhibition of tumor growth (Fig. 2). In some animals, regressions persisted and tumors did not reappear, whereas in others, regrowth occurred. In a similar study, tumor growth inhibition was also observed in mice injected with a diphtheria A chain immunotoxin. In other studies, a life prolonging effect was observed following immunotoxin treatment of mice bearing MM46 ascitic tumors [114] and in mice previously injected with murine leukemia L1210/b2L cells [62].

In one study, immunotoxins were shown to be effective therapy of mice bearing a murine B cell tumor after cytoreduction using total lymphoid irradiation and splenectomy [66]. In another study, specific suppression of growth of a murine leukemia by immunotoxins con-

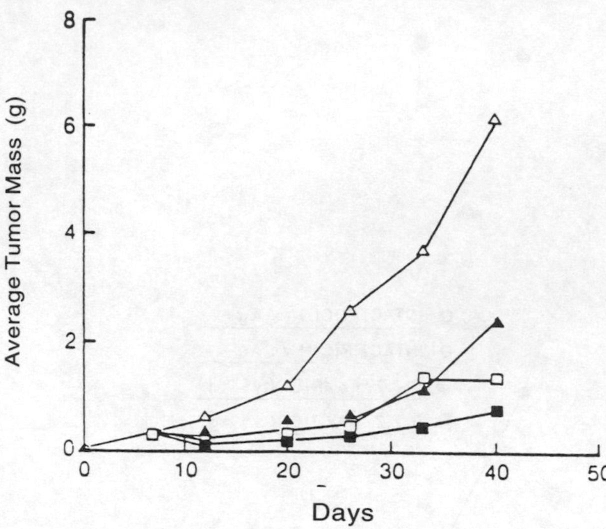

Figure 2. Inhibition by immunoconjugates of growth of primary tumor. L 10 hepatocarcinoma cells (106) were injected i.d. into guinea pigs. Groups of five guinea pigs with palpable tumors received a single treatment of various doses of immunotoxin, (s.c.), saline (△), 60 µg (▲), 120 µg (□), and 240 µg (■).

taining RTA or pokeweed antiviral protein was reported [102].

Thorpe, et al., investigated therapy of mice bearing intraperitoneally administered lymphoma cells using an anti Thy-1.1 antibody conjugated with saporin given intravenously. The observed increase in survival time was what would be expected if 99.999% of the tumor cells had been eradicated [124].

CLINICAL TRIALS

Immunotoxins have been used clinically as biotherapy for malignancy, autoimmune disease, or graft versus host disease. They have also been used clinically *in vitro* to remove unwanted cells prior to autologous bone marrow transplantation. Only the *in vivo* clinical use of immunotoxins will be presented here. Results of clinical trials conducted to date are summarized in Table 3.

Melanoma

By far the largest clinical experience in the use of an immunotoxin in the therapy of malignancy is in the treatment

Table 3. Results of clinical trials of immunotoxin therapy

# Patients	Study design	Result	Ref.
Melanoma			
22	Phase I	Side effects defined, 1CR	122
46	Phase II	3 PR/43 evaluable	123
14	Phase I/II outpatient	Safety in outpatient setting confirmed, 1 PR	Spitler. L. E., and Minor, D., unpublished
12	Phase I, with immunosuppresives	Serum levels of immunotoxin on reinfusion correlated with IgG antibody present at time of reinfusion	78
>50	Phase I, with immunosuppresives	Various immunosuppressive regimens explored, some effective regimens identified	109, 121*
20	Phase I/II with cyclosphomade	4 PR	93*
9	Phase I/II with cyclosporine	Combination therapy well tolerated, No effective immunosuppression	111
13	Phase I single dose escalation	MTD as single infusion found to be 1.25 mg/kg, 1 PR	41, 104
Breast cancer			
5	Phase I continuous infusion	Severe toxic side effects including marked fluid overload and debilitating sensorimotor neuropathy	42
4	Phase I bolus	Toxicity mild. Immunotoxin found to bind to monocytes	131

* Some patients duplicated in these reports.

Table 3. (continued)

# Patients	Study design	Result	Ref.
Colorectal cancer			
17	Phase I	Toxicity similar to other RTA immunotoxins with added observation of proteinuria, regression of smaller hepatic metastases in 2 patients, mixed responses in 5 patients	23
Ongoing	Phase I intralesional	Intralesional injection into hepatic metastasis under CT guidance tolerated	136
Leukemia/Lymphoma			
2	Phase I, anti T cell antibody conjugated to RTA	No toxicity except for slight increase in SG0T in 2nd patient	69
5	Phase I, anti T cell immunotoxin treatment in CLL	No major toxicity. Clinical limited to trainsient fall in WBC	55
14	Phase I, II dose escalation study of XomaZyme H65 in cutaneous T cell lymphoma	MTD was 0.33 mg./Kg/d. Dose limiting toxicity was dyspnea at rest, 4 PR, 6 patients retreated	76
9	Phase I, II study of Xoma Zyme H65 in CLL and lymphoma	2 MR 1 PR	24
41	Phase I, whole(26) or Fab(15) anti CD-22 conjugated to hypoglycosylated RTA using an SMPT linkage	Dose limiting side effects were expressive aphasia, rhabdomyolysis, or pulmonary edema. Responses were seen is 38% of patients given the Fab' construct and 33% given the whole antibody construct	127, 128, 129
24	Phase I dose escalation study of an IL-2-diphtheria toxin conjugate	MTD was 0.1 mg/Kg/d. Dose limiting toxicity was elevation of SGOT. T 1/2 was 4-7 min. Responses were observed in 4 of 24 patients	86
18	Phase I trial of recombinant fusion toxin DAB486Il-2 in patients chemotherapy resistant hematological tumors	Dose limiting toxicity was transient asymptomatic hepatic transaminase elevations	73
23	Phase I study of recombinant fusion toxin DAB486Il-2 in patients with p55 positive cancers	Dose limiting toxicity was renal insufficiency associated with hemolysis; 2 PR	75
25	Phase I, blocked whole ricin conjugated to anti B-4 antibody (anti CD19)	Toxicity consisted of transient grade III elevations of hepatic transaminases; MTD 50 μg/kg/d for 5 days (250 μg total) 1 CR, 2 PR	45, 88, 89
34	Phase I evaluation of blocked whole ricin conjugated to anti B-4 antibody given by 7 day continuous infusion	Major toxicity included grade IV reversible increases in AST and ALT and grade IV decreases in platelet counts; 2 CR, 3 PR	10, 48, 88
13	Phase I evaluation of blocked whole ricin conjugated to anti B-4 antibody given by 7 day continuous infusion, repeated every 14 days	Doses up to 490 μg/kg could be given in a 28 day interval	46

Table 3. (continued)

# Patients	*Study design*	*Result*	*Ref.*
Leukemia/Lymphoma (continued)			
12	Adjuvant therapy with anti-B4-blocked ricin after autologous bone marrow transplantation for patients with B-cell lymphoma	MTD was 40 μg/kg/d for 7 days; dose limiting toxicities were re ersible grade IV thrombocytopenia and elevation of hepatic transaminases; 11 patients remain in CR between 13 and 26 months post ABMT.	46, 47
23	Phase I trial of anti-B4 blocked ricin (B4bR) given as a 28 day continuous infusion, dose escalation	There was lowered toxicity compared to a 7 day schedule and limited or delayed HAMA/HARA allowing higher cumulative dose of B4bR; 2 PR	87
41	Phase II trial of anti-B4 blocked ricin (anti-B4-bR) following autologous bone marrow transplantation; IT given by 7d continuous infusion every 14d.	Toxicities included thrombocytopenia, increases in SGOT/SGPT, capillary leak syndrome, edema, dyspnea, fatigue, myalgias, nausea, HAMA/HARA; 30 patients in CR 6 to 27 months post-ABMT; no relapses occurred in 11 pts in CR at time of ABMT.	49
ongoing	Phase I/II study of RFT5 gamma1 (ab to CD25) conjugated to deglycosylated ricin-A chain in refractory Hodgkin's disease	Too early	31
4	Phase I study of Ber-H2 (ab to CD30) linked to saporin (SO6)	In 3 of the 4 patients there was rapid and substantial reduction in tumour mass of 6-10 weeks duration.	34
18	Phase I trial of anti CD22 IT (IgG-RFB4-SMPT-dgA) given by 8d continuous infusion in pts with >30% CD22+ lymphoma cells	Dose limiting toxicity was vascular leak; 4 PR	108
Ovarian cancer			
23	Phase I, IP administration of antibody OVB3 conjugated to PE	Dose limiting toxicity was encephalopathy progressing to death in 1 patient Abdominal pain and diffuse peritonitis in all patients. Neurologic toxicity thought due to cross-reactivity of antibody with brain tissue	13, 96
Ongoing	Phase I, IP administration of anti ovarian antibody conjugated to PE	Too early	84
12	Phase I, IP administration of anti transferrin receptor ab 454 A12 conjugated to recombinant RTA	At highest dose levels, toxicity similar to other RTA immunotoxins with abdominal pain and peritonitis in addition	13, 14
Ongoing	Pharmacokinetic study of radio labelled ab or immunotoxin following IP administration	Blood levels of 131I rose after administration of antibody whereas they remained low after intraperitoneal immunotoxin administration	22
Small cell lung cancer			
21	Phase I, dose escalation in patients given 7 day continuous infusion of N901-blocked ricin immunotoxin	Toxicity included transient elevation of liver enzymes, thrombocytopenia, hypoalbuminemia, fever, malaise, and capillary leak syndrome; no clinically significant peripheral or central neuropathy. One PR	80, 32, 79

Table 3. (continued)

# Patients	Study design	Result	Ref.
Superficial bladder cancer			
43	Phase I sutdy of TP40, composed of TGF-α fused to modified 40-kDa segment of Pseudomonas exotoxin administered into bladder	Well tolerated; no response in patients with Ta or T1 disease; improvement in 8 of 9 patients with *in situ* disease	40
Graft versus host disease			
1	Phase I, XomaZyme H65	Case report of dramatic response	60
35	Phase I/III, XomaZyme H65	Response in 60% of patients	24
69	Phase III, XomaZyme H65	Response in 57% of patients evaluable	
13	Phase I/II, histoincompatible marrow transplant XomaZyme H65	Significant reduction in Stage II or greater GVHD as compared to historic controls	50, 51
8	Phase I, XomaZyme H65 as pre-emptive therapy of GVHD	Time to recovery of platelets, granulocytes, and lymphocytes enhanced	74
8	Phase I, XomaZyme-CD5 *in vitro* and *in vivo* in patientsundergoing marrow transplant from unrelated donors	Only 2 patients developed GVHD; however there was high morbidity and mortality from virus infections	64
22	Phase I, XomaZyme-CD5 for GVHD prophylaxis in patients undergoing marrow transplant from unrelated donors	Acute GVHD developed in 9 of 15 evaluable patients; 6 of 8 evaluable patients developed chronic GVHD	132
6	Phase I trial of H65-RTA and methylprednisolone for acute GVHD	5 of 6 patients developed Grade III/IV GVHD; 4 died 34 to 78 days post-transplant; H65-RTA was ineffective prophylaxis following allogeneic BMT	65

of melanoma. Over 100 patients have been treated with an immunotoxin consisting of a monoclonal antimelanoma antibody designated XMMME-001 conjugated with ricin A chain. The antibody reacts with a high molecular weight glycoprotein which is associated with the majority of melanomas and has only sparse representation on normal tissues.

A phase I-II trial of the antimelanoma immunotoxin was conducted in 22 patients with metastatic melanoma [122]. The dose of immunotoxin administered ranged from 0.01 mg/kg daily for 5 days to 1 mg/kg daily for 4 days (total dose: 3.2-300 mg). Side effects observed in most patients were a transient fall in serum albumin with an associated fall in serum protein, weight gain, and fluid shifts resulting in edema and mild hypovolemia (Table 4). In addition, patients experienced mild to moderate malaise, fatigue, mylagia, decrease in appetite, and fevers. There was a transient decrease in voltage in electrocardiograms without clinical symptoms, change in serial echocardiograms or elevation of creatine phosphokinase isozyme levels. Symptoms consistent with mild allergic reactions were observed in 3 patients. Except for the

Table 4. Side effects associated with immunotoxin therapy

Immunotoxins made with RTA
- Fall in serum albumin; fluid shifts; weight gain
- Syndrome of malaise, fevers, myalgia
- Decreased voltage on EKG without associated clinical signs/symptoms
- Proteinuria with some, but not all, preparations

Immunotoxins made with PE
- Neurologic changes

Immunotoxins given intraperitoneally
- Side effects associated with the toxic moiety as described above
- Abdominal pain and peritonitis

allergic reactions, the side effects were related to the dose of immunotoxin administered and the side effects, including allergic reactions, were generally transient and reversible. One patient in this phase I study underwent a complete regression of her metastatic melanoma which lasted for over 3 years, even though she had failed to respond to previous quadruple drug chemotherapy.

These encouraging results led to a multicenter cooperative Phase II study to gain additional information about side effects and begin to define efficacy [123]. All patients in this study received a single course of therapy of up to 5 days. Forty-six patients were treated. Side effects were similar to those observed in the Phase I study. In addition, 2 patients experienced serum sickness and 4 patients had a transient fall in platelets to less than 100, 000/cu mm. Of 43 patients evaluable for efficacy, 3 patients had partial responses. These responses are noteworthy in that all patients had previously failed standard chemotherapy and the responses were particularly durable, being still ongoing after 15, 13 and 10 months as of the last follow-up. Additional evidence of biologic activity of the immunotoxin consisting of mixed response or disease stabilization was observed in 9 additional patients.

The transient and mild nature of the observed side effects of the immunotoxin therapy in these studies led to an evaluation of the use of immunotoxins in outpatients. In a study involving 14 patients, it was shown that outpatient administration of the drug was well tolerated, and immunotoxin could be safely administered in an outpatient setting (Spitler, L. E. and Minor, D., unpublished). In that study, 1 patient, who had failed previous chemotherapy, experienced a partial response of 6 months duration.

In the studies described above, therapy was limited to a single course of treatment because there is an immune response to both the murine antibody and ricin A chain components of the immunotoxin (Fig. 3) [109, 122]. In the face of such an immune response, the clearance of immunotoxin is markedly accelerated. The degree of accelerated clearance generally correlates with the strength of the immune response [78]. It is presumed, although it has not been directly shown, that such accelerated clearance of immunotoxin in the face of an immune response would mean that the immunotoxin would not become satisfactorily localized in the tumor.

In view of this, XOMA sponsored a series of pilot clinical trials aimed at evaluating clinical regimens to successfully abrogate the immune response to immunotoxin [109, 121]. To simplify the study and the data analysis, patients received a single infusion of immunotoxin in a dose of 0.4 mg/kg. The immune response was analyzed in serum samples obtained 21 and 28 days after the infusion. Many medical centers collaborated in the conduct of the study. Each center used one or more different immunosuppressive regimens. Results of immune responses in patients receiving immunotoxin in combination with immunosuppressive agents were compared with results obtained in patients receiving immunotoxin alone without immunosuppressive agents. If there was adequate suppression of the immune response and the patient was doing well, immunotoxin was readministered. In some instances, immunotoxin was administered to patients in the face of an immune response if the disease was responding to treatment.

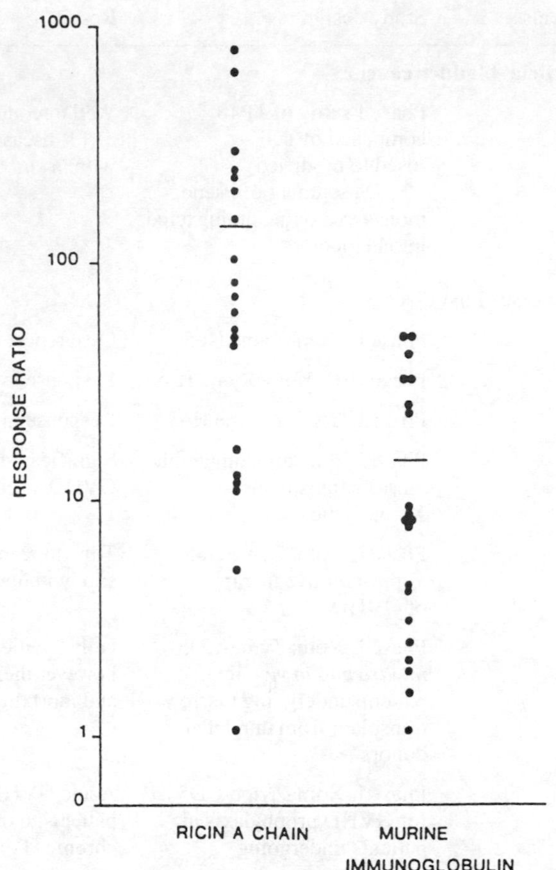

Figure 3. IgG antibody response to immunotoxin components. For each patient, the immune response is expressed as the ratio of the titration end point dilution of the serum sample showing maximum response to the titration end point dilution of the pretreatment serum sample.

Certain regimens were found to be effective in suppressing the immune response to a single infusion of immunotoxins, whereas others were found to be ineffective [121]. Moreover, the efficacy of a particular immunosuppressive agent depended on the dose and timing of administration of that agent. In general, it was found that a more prolonged administration of a lower dose of the immunosuppressive was more effective than a short, high course of therapy. Although certain immunosuppressive regimens were effective in suppressing the immune response to a single infusion of the immunotoxin, there was generally an immune response following repeated infusions. Therefore, in new studies, immunosuppressive regimens identified as most promising have been combined in an effort to more effectively suppress the immune response.

As a part of the evaluation of the effects of immunosuppressive agents on the immune response, there have been reports describing in more detail the results summarized in the above publications. A group of 20 patients were given a dose of immunotoxin of 0.4 mg/kg and 30 minutes later were given cyclophosphamide in a dose of 1,000 mg/m^2 [93]. Four of these patients had partial responses, suggesting the possibility that the addition of cyclophosphamide to the regimen enhanced the efficacy of the immunotoxin. One of these responses lasted over one year.

In another study, 9 patients were given the combination of immunotoxin and cyclosporine A in divided daily doses to achieve serum levels by HPLC of 150-200 ng/ml on days 1-22 [111]. This combination was well tolerated, but effective suppression of the anti-immunoconjugate antibody response was not achieved at the dosage and schedule of administration in this study. Other investigators studying XOMAZYME-Mel evaluated the effects of other immunosuppressive regimens [6, 63]. It was found that patients receiving azathioprine and prednisone combinations had more immunosuppression of the anti-immunoconjugate antibodies than those receiving moderate-dose cyclophosphamide and prednisone, but suppression of the immune response was achieved with high-dose cyclophosphamide alone.

In another trial, dose escalation was evaluated to determine the maximum dose which could be tolerated when the immunotoxin was given once [41]. It was determined that the maximum tolerated dose was 1.25 mg/kg. Moreover, in this study which included 13 evaluable patients, one patient had a complete response lasting for 6 months and two patients had partial responses.

Breast cancer

There have been Phase I evaluations of an antibreast immunotoxin given by two schedules. The antibody used was designated 260F9 which targets an antigen having a molecular weight of 55, 000 expressed by about 50% of human breast carcinomas tested. The toxin is a recombinant ricin A chain which lacks the carbohydrate residue present on ricin A chain isolated from castor beans. In one study, the immunotoxin was given by continuous IV infusion at a dose of 50 μg/kg or 100 μg/1kg/d for 6 to 8 days [42]. Five patients were studied. Severe toxic effects, including marked fluid overload and debilitating sensorimotor neuropathies occurred in most patients. Immunoperoxidase studies suggested that the monoclonal antibody used in the construct of the immunotoxin had cross reactivity with Schwann cells. Targeting of the immunotoxin to these cells may have induced demyelination and the subsequent neuropathy.

In a study conducted simultaneously, four patients were treated with the same immunotoxin given by 1 hour IV injection for 6-8 consecutive days rather than by continuous infusion [131]. Two patients were treated with 10 μg/kg daily and two others with 50 μg/kg daily. Toxicity observed consisted of weight gain, edema, and hypoalbuminemia. This was similar to that observed with the anti-melanoma immunotoxin indicating that it is unrelated to the binding specificity of the antibody and is related to the A chain. Additional investigation revealed that there was detectable binding of the immunotoxin to monocytes at immunotoxin concentrations which were achieved clinically in this trial. The binding appeared to be abrogated by preincubation of the monocytes with human immunoglobulin, suggesting that the binding occurred through the Fc receptor. It was suggested that the binding of the immunotoxin to monocytes might be related to the observed side effects.

Colorectal cancer

A Phase I trial of immunotoxin in 17 patients with colorectal cancer has been completed [23]. The antibody used in generation of the immunotoxin is designated 791T/36 and has specificity for a tumor membrane glycoprotein with a molecular weight of 72,000 associated with colorectal and ovarian carcinoma cells. Side effects were similar to those observed in other clinical trials with the added observation of proteinuria and mental status change not observed in other studies. Mixed responses in which some lesions regressed while others progressed were observed in five patients. Two patients with hepatic metastasis had objective evidence of decreasing size of large metastases and disappearance of smaller lesions.

In another study, the immunotoxin was administered by intralesional injection into hepatic metastasis under CT guidance [136]. For this study, the monoclonal antibody was conjugated to whole ricin in which the binding site of the B chain had been blocked.

Leukemia/Lymphoma

This area has particular potential for successful immunotoxin therapy because the target cells may be more accessable than are the targets for solid tumor therapy. In many cases, the malignant cells are in the circulation. For this reason, leukemia and lymphoma has been the subject of intense interest and a number of clinical trials.

Laurent et al. [69] treated two patients with leukemia with an immunotoxin consisting of an anti-T-cell antibody coupled to ricin A chain. No adverse side effects or toxicity were noted in either patient except for a slight transient increase in serum glutamate-oxaloacetate aminotransferase (SGOT) in the second patient. In the first patient, who received a single dose of 13.5 mg, binding of the immunotoxin to cells *in vivo* was observed and there was a transient decrease in the target cells. This decrease was attributed to the antibody component of the immunotoxin. The blast cell count subsequently increased rapidly and continued to increase until the patient died of septicemia 22 days after the treatment. The second patient was given a dose of 25 mg daily for 3 days combined with chloroquine as an enhancer. *In vivo* binding of the immunotoxin to target cells was demonstrated for a period of 4 hours, commencing 2 hours after the infusion of immunotoxin. In addition, there was a reduction of the leukocytosis attributed to the antibody component. The lowered white cell count remained stable for a period of 2 weeks. The patient died on day 19 of hemorrhage related to the preexisting thrombocytopenia. Rapid clearance of the immunotoxin was noted in these patients.

Another Phase I trial of an anti-T-cell immunotoxin was completed in patients with CLL [55]. Five patients were treated with 6 courses of an anti-CD 5 immunotoxin. Each course consisted of 8 bi-weekly infusions of immunotoxin in a dose of 7 or 14 mg/m^2. There was no major toxicity, and clinical response was limited to a transient fall in WBC. It was observed that the leukemia cells were resistant to killing by the immunotoxin *in vitro*, but became sensitive in the presence of human serum albumin (HSA) conjugated in monensin, suggesting that the therapeutic efficacy might be improved by the addition of HSA-monensin to the regimen.

A Phase I, II dose escalation study of XomaZyme H65 has been completed in patients with cutaneous T-cell lymphoma [76]. Fourteen patients were treated with daily infusions over 10 days of the immunotoxin in doses ranging from 0.2 to 0.5 mg/kg. The maximum tolerated dose (MTD) was determined to be 0.33mg/kg/d for 10 days. Dose limiting toxicity was dyspnea at rest. It was noted that there was an immediate fall in the levels of normal peripheral blood T-cells and a transient decrease in pruritus and erythroderma with clearing of Sezary cells in skin lesions. Partial responses lasting from 3 to 8 months were observed in four of fourteen patients treated. Six patients were retreated without significant difficulty. The development of antibodies against the immunotoxin was associated with a lower peak drug level, but not with enhanced side effects.

A Phase I, II study was initiated in patients with chronic lymphocytic leukemia and lymphoma using XomaZyme H65 [24]. In nine patients treated, there was one partial response and two minimal responses observed.

Ghetie et al. [38] compared immunotoxins specific for the human B cell antigens CD22 and CD19. These immunotoxins consisted of RTA conjugated to an antibody, reactive with CD22 or HD37, an antibody reactive with CD19. Both were shown to be reasonable candidates for *in vivo* therapy in humans. However, the immunotoxin reactive with the CD22 antigen was more potent and reduced protein synthesis more completely. It was therefore suggested that this is the immunotoxin of choice for clinical trials. The antibody reactive with CD22 was conjugated to hypoglycosylated RTA, using a SMPT linkage, which was felt to represent a more stable cross linker [129]. *In vitro* analysis demonstrated that this immunotoxin had an IC50 equal to or greater than that of whole ricin. Toxicity testing in Rhesus monkeys revealed side effects of fall in serum albumin, myalgia, and loss of appetite characteristic of other RTA immunotoxins.

Based on these studies, a clinical trial was completed in patients with hematologic malignancies including refractory B cell leukemia and non-Hodgkins lymphoma [129]. A potent immunotoxin was created consisting of a monoclonal anti-CD22 antibody (RFB4) coupled to deglycosylated ricin A chain. Forty-one patients were treated on a dose escalation schedule; 26 with immunotoxin made from the whole antibody and 15 with an immunotoxin made from the Fab' fragment. Side effects were similar to those observed with other RTA immunotoxins. The MTD for the Fab' construct was 75 mg/m^2 and for the IgG construct it was 36 mg/m^2. Dose limiting toxicity was expressive aphasia, rhabdomyolysis with renal failure, or pulmonary edema. Fewer side effects were noted in patients treated with the whole IgG construct. Response rates at 1 month were 38% for patients treated with the Fab' construct and 33% for patients treated with the whole IgG construct.

A genetically engineered fusion protein was created through the replacement of the diphtheria toxin gene receptor binding domain with the gene for human IL-2. This product, termed DAB_{486}, has been tested in a Phase I dose escalation clinical trial in 24 patients with hematologic malignancy (leukemia or lymphoma) bearing high levels of IL-2 receptors, mainly non-Hodgkins lymphoma and CLL [86]. The MTD was 0.1mg/kg and the dose limiting toxicity was hepatocellular. Clinical responses were noted in 4 of the 24 patients. In another Phase I trial in 18 patients with chemotherapy resistant hematological tumors, the dose limiting toxicity was similarly found to be hepatic transaminase elevations [73]. This led to a further Phase I trial of this recombinant fusion toxin in 23 patients with p55 positive cancers [75]. In this case, the dose limiting toxicity was renal insufficiency associated with hemolysis. There were 2 PRs observed.

An immunotoxin consisting of blocked whole ricin conjugated to the anti-B4 antibody has been developed and extensively evaluated in clinical trials. This antibody reacts with the CD22 antigen on normal and neoplastic B cells and astrocytes. Preclinical studies in cynomolgus monkeys showed minimal to moderate toxicity, primarily hepatic [33], and clinical trials have been initiated [88]. Twenty-five patients were treated with this immunotoxin [45, 89]. The maximum tolerated dose was determined to be 50 μg/kg/d for 5 days. Dose limiting toxicity consisted of transient reversible grade 3 elevation of transaminases, without impaired hepatic synthetic function. In 19 of 22 evaluable patients, there was a loss of B cells. Responses included 1 CR, 2 PR, and transient responses in 8 patients. Therapeutic blood levels were achieved at higher dose levels, but rarely lasted more than four hours. Nine of the patients produced antibody responses to the antibody or ricin components of the immunotoxin.

In view of the short half life of the immunotoxin, a

second trial was conducted in which the immunotoxin was administered by 7-day continuous infusion in a dose escalation study in 34 patients with refractory CD19+ lymphoid malignancy (non T cell ALL, B cell CLL, and non Hodgkins lymphoma, all with multiple relapses) [10, 48, 88]. The MTD was reached at 50 µg/kg/d X 7 days. The dose limiting toxicities included grade IV reversible increases in AST and ALT, and grade IV decreases in platelet counts. Potentially therapeutic serum levels of anti-Br-bR could be sustained for 4 days in patients treated at the MTD. Two CRs and three PRs were observed. In an effort to increase the dose of immunotoxin administered, another Phase I study was done in which the immunotoxin was administered to 13 patients by 7 day continuous infusion and treatment was repeated every 14 days [46]. With this regeman, a dose of up to 490 µg/kg could be given in a 28 day period.

In an effort to achieve better clinical results, the anti-B4-bR immunotoxin was administered by 7-day continuous infusion to 12 patients in complete remission after autologous bone marrow transplantation [47]. The maximum tolerated dose was 40 µg/kg/d for 7 days and potentially therapeutic serum levels could be sustained for 3 to 4 days. Eleven patients remain in CR between 13 and 26 months post ABMT. This led to a Phase I dose escalation trial of B4bR given as a 28 day continuous infusion in 23 patients [87]. There was lowered toxicity compared to the 7 day schedule and limited or delayed immune response to the immunotoxin components allowing a higher cumulative dose of B4bR. Two PRs were noted.

Clinical trials have been initiated in T-cell ALL using an immunotoxin derived from an antibody, termed 4A2, reactive with the CD7 antigen [24]. This is conjugated to RTA with decreased carbohydrate representation, termed RTA 30. Two patients have been treated with a 10-day course of therapy so far.

Ovarian cancer

Metastatic ovarian cancer has attracted special interest of investigators working with clinical trials of immunotoxins. It permits the opportunity for regional administration intraperitoneally. This allows high concentrations of immunotoxin to reach the tumor without the attendant necessity for systemic administration of high doses. An immunotoxin has been prepared utilizing an antibody, OVB3, which reacts uniformly with all ovarian carcinoma cells from all patients. This was conjugated to Pseudomonas exotoxin (PE) to prepare an immunotoxin that kills ovarian cancer cells. A Phase I trial of this immunotoxin, termed OVB3-PE, has been completed [13, 95, 96]. Twenty three patients with refractory ovarian cancer were treated intraperitonally with escalating doses. Doses ranged from 1 µg/kg to 10µg/kg on days 1 and 4. Some patients received 5 µg/kg on days 1, 4, and 7. Dose limiting toxicity was encephalopathy observed at dose levels of 5 µg/kg (x 3) and 10 µg/kg (x 2). Three patients developed encephalopathy with ataxia, aproxia, aphasia, and confusion. One of these patients had focal weakness. In one patient, the encephalopathy progressed to seizures, coma, and death. All patients experienced abdominal pain and diffuse peritonitis. Further study of the antibody demonstrated that it had weak reactivity with the reticular layer of the cerebellum in some examples. It did not demonstrate reactivity with any other brain tissue. It was felt that the neurologic toxicity was likely to be due to crossreactivity of OVB3 to normal human brain tissue, which was not appreciated during preclinical screening. To explain the abdominal pain and peritonitis, the investigators checked the antibody for reactivity to mesothelial cells and none was found. No clinical responses were observed.

In a second Phase I study, this group evaluated the intraperitoneal administration of an immunotoxin in patients with ovarian, mesothelial, renal or gastrointestinal cancer in the peritoneal cavity [13, 14]. The antibody used in the preparation of the immunotoxin was the anti-transferrin receptor antibody 454A12. It was conjugated with recombinant ricin toxin A chain prepared by Cetus Corporation. Twelve patients were treated daily for five days: three at a dose of 5 µg/kg, four at 10 µg/kg and five at 25 µg/kg. At the highest doses, the side effects of hypoalbuminemia, nausea, fever, and peritonitis were observed.

A similar phase I/II clinical trial was initiated in Seattle [83]. In this study, the immunotoxin is derived from antibodies NR-Lu-10 or OVB-3 which react with ovarian and colon cancer. The antibodies are conjugated with PE and the product administered intraperitoneally in patients with ovarian cancer or colon cancer confined to the abdomen. Another trial of intraperitoneal therapy of ovarian cancer involves the use of the anti transferrin receptor antibody 454 A12 conjugated to recombinant RTA (Houston, L., personal communication).

In another study, 131-I-labelled immunotoxin 791T/36-RTA or the monoclonal antibody alone, were administered intraperitoneally to patients with stage III or IV ovarian carcinoma [22]. Following intraperitoneal injection of the antibody, blood levels rose over the first 20-40 hours and then declined whereas blood levels of 131I following intraperitoneal injection of the immunotoxin remained low.

Small cell lung cancer

A Phase I trial was completed with a novel immunotoxin N901-blocked ricin (N901-BR) in patients with small cell lung cancer [80]. This immunotoxin includes a monoclonal antibody which binds to NCAM (CD56) present on small cell lung cancer, cardiac muscle, natural killer cells, and peripheral nerve. The antibody is coupled to blocked ricin, an altered ricin molecule in which the galactose binding sites of the ricin B-chain of the toxin are blocked through the covalent binding of ligands. Twenty patients were treated. The MTD was determined to be 30 µg/kg/d and dose limiting toxicity was capillary leak syndrome. All patients tested developed an immune response to the immunoglobulin. Cardiac function remained normal in 15/16 patients and no patient developed clinically significant peripheral or central neuropathy. There was one partial response.

Graft versus host disease

Acute or chronic graft versus host disease (GVHD) is one of the major potential complications of bone marrow transplantation used in the therapy of leukemia patients. Studies of the use of an anti CD5 antibody-RTA immunotoxin have shown encouraging results regarding the safety and efficacy in therapy of GVHD. An initial case report illustrated dramatic results of this immunotoxin in the treatment of a patient with severe grade III-IV, steroid resistant, acute GVHD [60]. In a larger series of patients, progression of the disease was reversed in 12/25 evaluable patients after the first seven doses of immunotoxin [20]. This study has now been expanded to include 35 patients as a Phase I/II trial and responses have been observed in 60% of patients [24]. A larger, Phase III study has been conducted in 69 patients, with responses in 57% [24]. In another study, an anti-CD3 monoclonal antibody, TI0B9, was used to effect a partial *ex vivo* T cell depletion of histo-incompatible donor marrow in combination with post grafting administration of the anti T cell immunotoxin [51]. Thirteen patients were treated. The results show a significant reduction in Stage II or greater GVHD-(3/13) as compared to historic controls (13/16, $p = 0.001$).

Le Maistre et al. [74] conducted a Phase I study of the anti CD5 immuno-toxin XomaZyme H65 as preemptive therapy of GVHD. Patients undergoing bone marrow transplantation for leukemia, lymphoma, or myelodysplastic syndrome were eligible. Eight patients were treated with the immunotoxin in a dose of 0.1 μg/kg/d. The first group of patients received the immunotoxin on days 7 to 16 post transplant. The second group was treated on days 3 to 16, and the third group was treated on days 0-16. In addition to the toxicity previously noted, it was observed that some patients exhibited proteinuria. It was noted that the time to recovery of counts of platelets, granulocytes, and lymphocytes was enhanced in treated patients. Four patients are alive: two without GVHD, and two with mild GVHD. One patient died of toxic epidermolysis, two of interstitial pneumonitis, and 1 of a pulmonary fungal infection.

There have been 3 additional trials of this immunotoxin as prophylaxis for GVHD in patients undergoing bone marrow transplantation; it was ineffective in all 3 of these studies. In one, only 2 of 8 patients developed GVHD, however there was high morbidity and mortality from virus infections [64]. In another, 6 of 8 evaluable patients developed chronic GVHD [132]. In the third study, the immunotoxin was used in combination with methylprednisone; 5 of 6 patients developed Grade III/IV GVHD [65].

ISSUES RELATED TO IMMUNOTOXIN THERAPY

The results of the clinical trials described above are encouraging and can be used to form the basis for second generation efforts aimed at improving efficacy of the immunotoxins. Issues for consideration in relationship to these second generation efforts are presented in Tables 5 and 6.

Table 5. Issues related to immunotoxin therapy

1. Stability of conjugates *in vivo*
2. Cellular heterogeneity
   - inter tumor
   - intra tumor
   - cell cycle/ploidy
   - antigen expression
3. Access and localization in the tumor
4. Biodistribution
   - binding affinity
   - uptake by the reticuloendothelial system via carbohydrate receptors
   - internalization into cell
   - intracellular distribution
5. Immune response to immunoconjugate
   - murine antibody
   - ribosomal inhibiting protein
6. Potentiators

Stability of conjugates *in vivo*

The most widely used heterobifunctional coupling reagent is N-succinimidyl-3-(2-pyridy-1-dithio) propionate (SPDP). This introduces disulphide bonds between the antibody and RTA. Questions have been raised regarding the stability of these disulphide bonds following *in vivo* administration of the immunotoxin. Blakey et al. [8] have reported that these bonds break down slowly in mice to release free antibody. Others have found that the bonds exhibited adequate stability to permit initiation of clinical trials [77]. Thorpe et al. synthesized a new coupling reagent, 4-succinimidyl-oxy carbonyl-a-methyl-a (2-pyridyldithio) toluene (SMPT), which introduces a disulphide bond which is protected from thiol attack [125]. The immunotoxin produced with this coupling reagent was as effective as one with an unprotected disulphide bond in killing target cells *in vitro* and had a longer blood half-life. It is anticipated that this improved stability of the products *in vivo* will result in improved efficacy.

Cellular heterogeneity

Representation of tumor associated antigens on the cell surface is heterogeneous. This is true for tumors of the same histologic type from different patients (macro-

Table 6. Second generation efforts to improve efficacy of immunotoxin therapy

1. Stability of conjugates *in vivo*
   - Create more stable bonds
2. Cellular heterogeneity
   - Select antibody with broad cross reactivity with tumors of a given histological type
   - Use cocktails of immunoconjugates
   - Combine immunotoxin with interferon
3. Access and localization in the tumor
   - Tumor necrosis factor
   - Vasoactive agents
   - Pre irradiation
   - Continuous infusion
   - Treat smaller tumors (surgical adjuvant therapy)
4. Biodistribution
   - Select antibodies with higher affinity
   - Use site directed conjugation
   - Decrease amount of carbohydrate on the A chain by deglycosylation or use of recombinant A chain
   - Enhance internalization via crosslinking or inclusion of B chain
   - Alter intracellular distribution so that more product enters the cytosol
5. Immune response
   - Agents to suppress immune response
   - Tolerance induction
   - Modify immunoconjugates to make them less immunogenic
   - Plasmaphaphenosis
6. Potentiators
   - Lysosomotropic amines
   - Carboxylic ionophores
   - Calcium channel blockers

heterogeneity) and for different cells from the same tumor from individual patients (microheterogeneity). There is also variation in antigen representation depending on the phase of the cell cycle and cell ploidy.

Antibody selection

There are several possible approaches to address the problem of cellular heterogeneity. One which almost all investigators have used is develop immunotoxin from selected antibodies which have broad cross reactivity with tumors of a given histological type. It is essential that these antibodies be carefully screened not only for reactivity with tumor associated antigens, but also for lack of important reactivity with normal tissues. This screening must be broad and should include *in vitro* screening and *in vivo* distribution studies. Because of the potency of immunotoxins in causing death of cells to which the antibody component binds, significant toxicity could result if there were unrecognized cross reactivity of the antibody with antigens present in normal tissue. This occurred in the trial of the antibreast immunotoxin described above in which the antibody had previously unrecognized reactivity with Schwann cells [42].

Cocktails

Another approach to dealing with cellular heterogeneity is to use cocktails of immunotoxins prepared with antibodies of differing specificity. It has been shown that *in vitro* cytotoxicity of an anti-carcinoembryonic antigen MoAb-RTA immunotoxin is potentiated by a MoAb recognizing a different epitope [21]. This application of cocktails has not been used clinically yet with immunotoxins, but Phase I-II clinical trials have been done using cocktails of antibody-drug immunoconjugates [91, 94].

Interferon

It is recognized that interferons may cause increased representation of certain antigens on the cell surface [15, 43, 82]. In addition, interferons also have direct antigrowth activity for certain tumors. This provides a reasonable basis for considering therapy involving a combination of interferon with immunotoxin. It has been reported that all three interferon types can potentiate monoclonal antibody therapy of lymphomas [3]. It has also been reported that an antibody-drug immunoconjugate demonstrated a synergistic effect with interferon *in vitro* and *in vivo* [81]. Synergistic effects of anti T leukemia immunotoxins and interferon in suppression of the growth of human T leukemia cells transplanted into nude mice has also been demonstrated [113].

Access and localization in tumor

It is clear in the work described above that immunotoxins kill specific target cells *in vitro*. Moreover, clinical efficacy has been most dramatic in therapy of patients with GVHD in which the target cell is readily accessible in the circulation. Perhaps the main reason that immunotoxins have not proved more effective in therapy of solid tumors in patients may be related to limited access of the immunotoxin to the relatively small, poorly vascularized tumor compartment.

It is recognized that less than 1% of radiolabelled antibodies localize in solid tumors. Nonetheless, encouraging evidence of antitumor activity of immunotoxins has been observed in patients. Clinical results obtained to date and information from preclinical data suggest that even a 3-5 fold increase in localization could result in a marked enhancement of the efficacy of these products *in vivo*.

Tumor necrosis factor

Tumor necrosis factor has been reported to have specific effects resulting in enhanced vascular permeability in tumors [12]. In one study, the effects of therapy were evaluated in mice with large, established thymomas.

Thirty percent of the tumors in mice receiving an antibody-drug conjugate and rINF-a partially or completely regressed, while no regressions were observed in animals receiving either product alone [118].

Vasoactive agents

Many vasoactive agents may alter tumor blood flow [57, 59]. While most agents act to decrease blood flow to the tumor, there are a few, such as adrenergic blockers, which act to increase it. It has been reported that administration of B-adrenergic blocking agents were capable of increasing three-fold tumor-to-blood and tumor-to-liver perfusion of 125_I-labelled MoAbs [97, 117]. These B-adrenergic agents, including propranalol, pindolol, and oxyprenolol, were found to increase the antitumor efficacy of antibody drug conjugates. By contrast, prozosin HCL, an a1-adrenergic blocking agent and cyclospasmol, a peripheral vasodilator, did not enhance the tumor perfusion and antitumor efficacy of the immunoconjugate.

Preirradiation

It has long been recognized that radiation causes increased vascular permeability in tumors which may persist for months after completion of the course of radiation. It has been shown that pre-irradiation causes increased localization of monoclonal antibodies in tumors and enhanced efficacy of radiolabelled immunoconjugates in animals [85] and man [72]. It is likely that pre-irradiation would also result in enhanced localization of immunotoxin in the radiated site and that this could result in greater tumor cell killing.

Continuous infusion

In most of the studies conducted to date, the immunotoxin has been given by bolus infusion which results in a peak blood level followed by rapid fall-off of immunotoxin concentration in the blood. Theoretical modelling studies suggest that maintenance of blood levels for more prolonged periods of time would result in enhanced localization of the immunotoxin in the small, poorly vascularized tumor compartment. Thus, administration of the immunotoxin by continuous infusion might result in superior localization and efficacy when compared to bolus infusions.

Surgical adjuvant therapy

Immunotoxins will only kill tumor cells to which the antibody binds, unlike the situation with immunoconjugates made with radionuclides or chemotherapeutic agents which will also kill surrounding tissue. Thus, it is essential that the immunotoxins reach and bind to as many cells as possible in the tumors. As tumors grow larger, they undergo necrosis, and vascular supply is diminished, thereby limiting access to these areas. It has been shown that localization of monoclonal antibodies in tumors is inversely related to tumor size [50, 61]. Surgical adjuvant therapy may be given at a time when all known tumor has been surgically excised, and the histopathology is such that the patient is at high risk for recurrence. In this circumstance, tumor burden is minimal and tumor masses small. Access of the immunotoxin to tumor cells in this setting might well be superior to the circumstance in which one is dealing with a large, poorly vascularized tumor burden.

Biodistribution

Antibody affinity

Antibody affinity is an important determinant of antibody localization. Efforts are underway to create and select antibodies of higher affinity for use in the construct of immunotoxins. Moreover, when the procedures for conjugation of the antibody and toxin is carried out, there may be loss of binding activity because some of the toxin may be adjugated to the binding site. This can be avoided by the use of a site specific conjugation procedure in which the toxin is conjugated to carbohydrate moieties [105]. This results in maintenance of binding activity of the antibody. In addition, this may protect the molecules from uptake via the reticuloendothelial system by interaction with carbohydrate receptors.

Deglycosylation

The ricin A chain contains carbohydrates which react with carbohydrate receptors in the reticuloendothelial system. Immunoconjugates, therefore, have a markedly shorter circulating half life than do the corresponding monoclonal antibodies. This results in less of the product localizing in the tumor. Second generation efforts are aimed at reducing the carbohydrate content of the immunotoxin. One approach to this is to deglycosylate the A chain chemically. Another approach is to use an A chain, such as abrin, which lacks the carbohydrate moieties. Still another approach is to use recombinant A chain created through genetic engineering. This product lacks carbohydrate. Finally, another approach is to separate the naturally occurring molecular weight 33, 000 carbohydrate rich RTA from the 30, 000 RTA which has reduced carbohydrate representation and use only the 30, 000 A chain in production of the immunotoxin. All of these approaches have been tested by various laboratories and all yield immunotoxins with prolonged circulatory half lives.

Internalization

Internalization of the A chain into the cell is essential for killing to occur. It has been reported that crosslinking of immunotoxin molecules on the cell surface through the use of an antimurine immunoglobulin results in greater internalization and enhanced cytotoxicity. Also, it has been suggested that a portion of the B chain can enhance internalization. Thus, in some studies, the immunotoxins have been constructed using whole ricin with the binding site of the B chain blocked. Blocking of the binding site allows specificity of the immunotoxin and also allows enhanced internalization conferred by the B chain. Other studies are aimed at identifying the portion of the B chain responsible for this activity and constructing a molecule with this area present through the use of genetic engineering.

Intracellular distribution

Finally, it is necessary for intracellular distribution of the A chain to the cytosol in order for killing to occur. In one study, it was shown that immunotoxins derived from an anti CD2 and from an anti CD3 antibody showed similar binding to the surface of the target cell, but only the anti CD3 immunotoxin caused cell death [101]. Further study showed that internalization of the A chain was similar, but intracellular distribution was different. Studies to understand the determinants of intracellular distribution are underway, and second generation efforts may involve ways to divert the A chain to the proper compartment.

Immune response

In most of the clinical trials described above, a vigorous immune response to immunotoxin administration has been noted. The exception is in patients with leukemia in whom the immune response may be blunted. In general, in both preclinical and clinical trials, the immune response to the immunotoxin components appears even more vigorous than the response to the corresponding immunoglobin alone. Perhaps this is due to an adjuvant effect of the A chain component. The use of chimeric or human antibodies in the generation of the immunotoxin will not resolve this problem because the response to the A chain will still need to be dealt with.

Agents to suppress immune responses

One approach is to administer the immunotoxin in conjunction with immunosuppressive agents [107]. This was done in the clinical trials described above and has been partially successful. Immunosuppressive agents which have been evaluated include cyclophosphamide, cyclosporine, azathioprenc and prednisone, 6 mercaptopurine, methotrexate, and IV gamma globulin. Further investigation is necessary in order to develop more potent immunosuppressive regimens to prevent an anamnestic response. One concern regarding the use of immunosuppressives is the suggestion that the immune response may be contributing to the efficacy of the immunotoxins and that abrogation of the immune response might diminish this activity. This suggestion has been made because of the observation of delayed and prolonged responses following immunotoxin administration which might be due to the development of an anti-anti-idiotype response.

Tolerance induction

Induction of tolerance to antigens is a well known immunologic phenomenon [29, 116]. Tolerance to specific antigens may be induced by administration of a low dose of the antigen (low zone tolerance) or of a high dose of the antigen (high zone tolerance). Moreover, it has been reported that tolerance could be achieved by administering the antigen with an antibody reactive with L3T4 molecule on T helper cells in mice [4]. Bridges et al. [17] reported that administration of an anti CD4 antibody with immunotoxin in mice delayed the antibody response to the immunotoxin. It has been reported that administration of antigen ricin conjugates *in vitro* causes selective abrogation of antigen-specific human B cell responses [130], but this has not been observed following administration of immunotoxins *in vivo*. Finally, it has been reported that administration of bovine serum albumin (BSA) conjugated to adriamycin to mice caused specific suppression of the immune response to the BSA [16]. In a separate study, others have similarly shown that specific immunosuppression occurs following conjugation of a hapten (ovalbumin) with the chemotherapeutic agent, daunomycin [28]. Similarly, another group reported that the primary immune response to dextran could be selectively and efficiently suppressed or eliminated *in vivo* by the prior administration of a single dose of dextran conjugated to cytosine arabinoside (araC) [1]. It was also reported that administration to mice of a conjugate of the monoclonal antibody 791T/36 with daunomycin resulted in abrogation of the immune response to the antibody [19]. In clinical trials, it was reported that adriamycin immunoconjugates did not result in a diminished immune response [91]. However, the significance of this observation is not clear because the adriamycin was not covalently conjugated to the antibody used in these studies. Results of a second trial suggested that conjugates prepared with mitomycin did result in a lowered immune response to the antibody [94]. All of these represent feasible approaches to dealing with the immune response to the immunotoxin.

Modify immunoconjugates to make them less immunogenic

Modification of antigens by conjugation with polyethylene glycol renders them nonimmunogenic and tolerogenic [2, 26, 70, 71, 110]. Moreover, enzymes so modified retain full enzymatic activity. Studies are underway in a number of laboratories to explore whether modification of monoclonal antibodies or immunoconjugates with polyethylene glycol will render them nonimmunogenic.

Plasmapheresis

Antibodies can be removed from the blood by plasmapheresis with or without the use of a Staphylococcal protein A column. This approach has been used successfully to remove harmful antibodies in a limited number of patients [90]. This procedure could be used to remove antibodies to the immunotoxin components just prior to immunotoxin administration. There is some concern, however, as to whether or not this procedure could remove enough of the antibodies to permit effective treatment. Moreover, such removal of antibodies may stimulate further antibody production with the result that titers might be higher at the time of the next dosing.

Potentiators

A number of substances have been reported to enhance immunotoxin activity *in vitro*. Some of these could be used clinically in an effort to enhance efficacy. Lysosomotropic amines have this activity [25]. Ammonium chloride is the most commonly used *in vitro*, but could not be used *in vivo* in doses sufficient to be effective. Chloroquine is another lysosonotripic amine which also has this activity, and could be used in patients. Monensin is a carboxylic ionophore which strongly increases the rate of protein synthesis inhibition by all immunotoxins tested. Monensin has a low molecular weight and its serum half life would be too short if it were administered unmodified. It has been coupled with human serum albumin to produce a product which retains activity and has a suitable half life [27].

Verapamil has been shown to enhance immunotoxin activity but only at concentrations that are too high for *in vivo* use. Therefore, structural analogues of verapamil have been synthesized and their activity evaluated [100]. Activity was observed, and did not correlate with the calcium-antagonistic activity. One analogue, D792, was found to have greater enhancing potency and less *in vivo* toxicity than verapamil, making it a candidate as a potentiator *in vivo*.

CONCLUSIONS

The preclinical and clinical studies described herein clearly show the potential of immunotoxins for the targeted therapy of cancer (Table 7). A great deal of information has been developed as a result of the Phase I/II clinical trials conducted to date. This information is being used in the development of second generation efforts designed to improve the efficacy of immunotoxins. Targeted therapy of cancer has the potential of being the most important medical advance in this century.

There are many issues to be resolved in order to bring this dream to reality. One major issue is delivery of the immunotoxin to the tumor. Immunotoxins are effective in clearing T-cells from bone marrow *in vitro* for use in transplantation. Use of immunotoxins *in vivo* involves much more complex issues of dose, schedule, route, and delivery (saturation).

Table 7. Summary conclusions from immunotoxin clinical trials

- Immunotoxins can be safely administered and side effects due to the A chain component are transient and well tolerated
- Severe toxicity can result if the monoclonal antibody has unrecognized cross reactivity with normal tissues and targets the toxin inappropriately to an unwanted target
- There is an immune response to both the murine immunoglobulin and toxin components of immunotoxin, except in some patients with leukemia or lymphoma, which precludes repeated courses of treatment
- Second generation efforts aimed at improving the efficacy of immunotoxin therapy are being launched

It is recognized that gram amounts of antibody are necessary in order to achieve saturation of binding sites at the tumor. Because of toxicities, immunotoxins can be administered only in mg amount or, in some cases, µg amounts. Clearly, this does not approach the amount necessary for saturation. But is saturation necessary when dealing with immunotoxins? Presumable it is not, if one believes the reports that one molecule of RTA entering the cytosol is sufficient to kill the cell.

Is the dream of effective targeting limited to an *in vitro* phenomenon, or can it be translated to reality *in vivo*? In this chapter, a number of approaches to enhancing delivery of the immunotoxin to tumors was discussed. The encouraging results in lymphomas, leukemias, and GVHD suggest that it is possible to achieve efficacy following *in vivo* administration of immunotoxin.

Moreover, impressive responses have been observed in rare patients with solid tumors treated with immunotoxins. The reasons for these responses are not understood. Do they relate to antigenic representation on the tumor cells as suggested by the study of Vitetta and Thorpe? Is it related to local factors in the tumors allowing enhanced localization of the immunotoxin in these particular tumors?

Patients and investigators are impatient that advances in this field have not come more rapidly. It is now clear that, like the development of chemotherapy, progress will only be made through the slow process of step by step development, planning each stage on the basis of results to date.

REFERENCES

1. Abu-Hadid MM, Bankert RB, Mayers G L. Antigen-specific drug-targeting used to manipulate an immune response *in vivo*. *Proc Natl Acad Sci USA* 1987; 84: 7232-7236.
2. Abuchowski A, Kazo GM, Verhoest Jr CR, Van Es T, et al. Cancer therapy with chemically modified enzymes. I. Antitumor properties of polyethylene glycol-asparagninase conjugates. *Cancer Biochem Biophys* 1984; 7: 175-186.
3. Basham TY, Palladino MA, Badger CC, et al. Comparison of combinations of interferons with tumor specific and nonspecific monoclonal antibodies as therapy for murine B- and T-cell lymphomas. *Cancer Res* 1988; 48: 4196-4200.
4. Benjamin RJ, Waldmann H. Induction of tolerance by monoclonal antibody therapy. *Nature* 1986; 320: 449-451.
5. Bernhard MT, Foon KA, Oeltmann TN, et al. Guinea pig line 10 hepatocarcinoma model: characterization of monoclonal antibody and *in vivo* effect of unconjugated antibody and antibody conjugated to diphtheria toxin A chain. *Cancer Res* 1983; 43: 4420-4428.
6. Bhardwaj S, Spitler L, Mischak R, et al. Suppression of humoral immune response by oral cyclophosphamide in patients with metastatic melanoma treated with intravenous (I.V.) murine antimelanoma monoclonal antibody ricin-A chain immunotoxin-a Phase I/II study. *Proc Am Soc Clin Oncol* 1988; 7: 167.
7. Blakey DC, Thorpe PE. An overview of therapy with immunotoxins containing ricin or its A-chain. *Ab Immunocon Radiopharm* 1988; 1(1): 1-16.
8. Blakey DC, Watson GJ, Knowles PP, Thorpe PE. Effect of chemical deglycosylation of ricin A chain on the *in vivo* fate and cytotoxic activity of an immunotoxin composed of ricin A chain and anti-Thy 1.1 antibody. *Cancer Res* 1987; 47(4): 947-952.
9. Blakely DC, Wawrzynczak EJ, Wallace PM, Thorpe PE. Antibody toxin conjugates: a perspective. In: *Progress in Allergy; Monoclonal Antibody Therapy*, edited by H Waldmann, 45: 50-90, S. Karger AG, Basel, 1988.
10. Blattler WA. Blocked Ricin: A Potent Effector Molecule for Immunotoxin Therapy. In: *Sixth International Conference on Monoclonal Antibody Immunoconjugates for Cancer*, San Diego, 1991.
11. Blythman HE, Casellas P, Gros O, et al. Immunotoxins: hybrid molecules of monoclonal antibodies and a toxin subunit specifically kill tumor cells. *Nature* 1981; 290: 145-146.
12. Bonavida B, Gifford GE, Kirchner H, and Old LJ, eds. *Tumor Necrosis Factor/Cachectin and Related Cytokines*, Basel, Switzerland, 1988.
13. Bookman MA, FitzGerald D, Frankel A, et al. Intraperitoneal immunotoxin therapy: two clinical studies. In: *Antibody Immunoconjugates, and Radiopharm.*, edited by SE Order, 1990; 3(1): 70.
14. Bookman MA, Godfrey S, Padavic K, et al. Anti-transferrin receptor immunotoxin (IT) therapy: phase I intraperitoneal (*i.p.*) trial. *Proc ASCO* 1990; 9: 187.
15. Borden E C. Augmented tumor-associated antigen expression by interferons. *J Natl Cancer Inst* 1988; 80(3): 148-149.
16. Braslawsky GR, Ligato P, Kaneko T, Greenfield R. Specific immunosuppression of mice by conjugating adriamycin (ADM) to a foreign serum protein. In: *Third International Conference on Monoclonal Antibody Immunoconjugates for Cancer*, p. 162, San Diego, 1988.
17. Bridges SH, Fu-Sheng J, Johnson V, et al. Anti-CD4 modulates the host response to immunotoxin. In: *Fourth International Conference on Monoclonal Antibody Immunoconjugates for Cancer*, edited by I Royston and RD Dillman, p. 154, San Diego, 1989.
18. Byers VS, Baldwin RW. Therapeutic strategies with monoclonal antibodies and immunoconjugates. *Immunology* 1988; 65(3): 329-335.
19. Byers VS, Clegg J, Durrant LG, et al. Abrogation of antibody responses in rats to murine monoclonal antibody 791T/36 by treatment with daunomycin cis-aconityl 791T/36 conjugates. In: *Fourth International Conference on Monoclonal Antibody Immunoconjugates for Cancer*, edited by I Royston and RD Dillman, p. 68, San Diego, 1989.
20. Byers VS, Henslee P, Kernan N, et al. Therapeutic response to a pan T lymphocyte monoclonal antibody-ricin A chain immunotoxin in steroid refractory graft versus host disease (GVHD). *Blood* 1987; 70: 3041.
21. Byers VS, Pawlucyzk I, Berry N, et al. Potentiation of anti-carcinoembryonic antigen immunotoxin cytotoxicity by monoclonal antibodies reacting with co-expressed carcinoembryonic antigen epitopes. *J Immunol* 1988; 140: 4050-4055.
22. Byers VS, Pimm MV, Perkins AC, et al. Biodistribution and biokinetics of intraperitoneally injected immunotoxin 791-RTA and its antibody in recurrent ovarian cancer. *Fourth International Conference on Monoclonal Antibody Immunoconjugates for Cancer*, edited by I Royston and RD Dillman, p. 46, San Diego, 1989.
23. Byers VS, Rodvien R, Grant K, et al. Phase I study of monoclonal antibody-ricin A chain immunotoxin Xoma-Zyme [registered trademark]-791 in patients with metastatic colon cancer. *Cancer Res* 1989; 49: 6153-6160.
24. Byers VS. Therapy of hemotologic manlignancies with anti T-lymphocyte ricin A chain immunotoxins. In: *Fifth International Conference on Monoclonal Antibody Immunoconjugates for Cancer*, edited by I Royston and RD Dillman, p. 13, San Diego, 1990.
25. Casellas P, Bourrie BJP, Gros P, Jansen FK. Kinetics of cytotoxicity induced by immunotoxins: enhancement by lysosomotropic amines and carboxylic ionophores. *J Biol Chem* 1984; 259(15): 9359-9364.
26. Davis FF, Van Es T, Palczuk NC. Non-immunogenic polypeptides. *US Patent No 4*, 296, 097, 1979.
27. Dell'Arciprete L, Colombatt M, Stevanoni G. Potentiation of RTA conjugates by HSA -monensin. *Fourth International Conference on Monoclonal Antibody Immunoconjugates for Cancer*, edited by I Royston and RD Dillman, p. 155, San Diego, 1989.
28. Diener E, Diner UE, Sinha A, et al. Specific immunosuppression by immunotoxins containing daunomycin. *Science* 1986; 231: 148-150.
29. Dresser DW. Tolerance induction as a model for cell differentiation. *Br Med Bull* 1976; 32(2): 147-151.
30. Eiklid K, Olsnes S, Pihl A. Entry of lethal doses of abrin, ricin and modeccin into the cytosol of Hela cells. *Expl Cell Res* 1980; 126: 321-326.
31. Engert A, Gottstein C, Winkler U, et al. Experimental

treatment of human Hodgkin's disease with ricin A-chain immunotoxins. *Leukemia & Lymphoma* 1994; 13(5-6): 441-448.

32. Epstein C, Lynch T, Shefner J, et al. Use of the immunotoxin N901-blocked ricin in patients with small-cell lung cancer. *Int J of Cancer – Supp* 1994; 8: 57-59.
33. Esber HJ, Goad MEP, Zavorskas PA, et al. Preclinical evaluation of an immunoconjugate, blocked ricin and anti-human B-lymphocyte monoclonal antibody, in cynomolgus monkeys. *Fourth International Conference on Monoclonal Antibody Immunoconjugates for Cancer*, edited by I Royston and RD Dillman, p. 150, San Diego, 1989.
34. Falini B, Bolognesi A, Flenghi L, et al. Response of refractory Hodgkin's disease to monoclonal anti-CD30 immunotoxin. *Lancet* 1992; 339(8803): 1195-1196.
35. Foon KA, Bernhard M, Oldham RK. Monoclonal antibody therapy: assessment by animal tumor models. *J Biol Response Modif* 1982; 1: 277-304.
36. Foon KA. Biological response modifiers: the new immunotherapy. *Cancer Res* 1989; 49(7): 1621-1639.
37. Franz H and Ziska P. Affinitins: combining sites containing proteins. In: *Lectins: Biology, Biochemistry, Clinical Biochemistry*, edited by TC Bog-Hansen, Volume 1. Walter de Gruyter, New York, 1981.
38. Ghetie MA, May RD, Till M, et al. Evaluation of ricin A chain-containing immunotoxins directed against CD19 and CD22 antigens on normal and malignant human B-cells as potential reagents for *in vivo* therapy. *Cancer Res* 1988; 48(9): 2610-2617.
39. Gilliland DG, Steplewski Z, Collier RJ, et al. Antibody directed cytotoxic agents: use of monoclonal antibody to direct the action of toxin A chains to colorectal carcinoma cells. *Proc Natl Acad Sci USA* 1980; 77: 4539-4543.
40. Goldberg MR, Heimbrook DC, Russo P, et al. Phase I clinical study of the recombinant oncotoxin TP40 in superficial bladder cancer. *Clin Cancer Res* 1995; 1: 57-61.
41. Gonzalez R, Salem P, Bunn PA, et al. Single-dose murine monoclonal antibody ricin A chain immunotoxin in the treatment of metastatic melanoma: a phase I trial. *Mol Biother* 1991; 3: 192-196.
42. Gould BJ, Borowitz MJ, Groves ES, et al. Phase I study of an anti-breast cancer immunotoxin by continuous infusion: report of a targeted toxic effect not predicted by animal studies. *J Natl Cancer Inst* 1989; 81(10): 775-781.
43. Greiner JW, Fisher PB, Pestka S, Schlom J. Differential effects of recombinant human leukocyte interferons on cell surface antigen expression. *Cancer Res* 1986; 46: 4984-4990.
44. Griffin TW, Pagnini PG, McGrath JJ, et al. *In vitro* cytotoxicity of recombinant ricin A chain-antitransferrin receptor immunotoxin against human adenocarcinomas of the colon and pancreas. *J Biol Resp Modif* 1988; 7(6): 559-567.
45. Grossbard ML, Freedman AS, Ritz J, et al. Serotherapy of B-cell neoplasms with anti-B4-blocked ricin: a phase I trial of daily bolus infusion. *Blood* 1992; 79(3): 576-585.
46. Grossbard ML, Gribben JG, Freedman AS, et al. Immunotherapy with anti-B4-blocked ricin (anti-B4-bR) for B-cell NHL: immunotoxin therapy of minimal residual disease (MRD). *Antibody Immunoconj and Radiopharm* 1992; 5(1): 152.
47. Grossbard ML, Gribben JG, Freedman AS, et al. Adjuvant immunotoxin therapy with anti-b4-blocked ricin after autologous bone marrow transplantation for patients with b-cell non-Hodgkin's lympoma. *Blood* 1993; 81(9): 2263-2271.
48. Grossbard ML, Lambert JM, Goldmacher VS, et al. Anti-B4-blocked ricin: A Phase I trial of 7-day continuous infusion in patients with B-cell neoplasms. *J Clin Oncol* 1993; 11: 726-737.
49. Grossbard ML, O'Day S, Gribben JG, et al. A phase II study of anti-B4-blocked ricin (anti-B4-bR) therapy following autologous bone morrow transplantation (ABMT) for B-cell non-Hodgkin's lymphoma (B-NHL). *Proc ASCO* 1994; 13: 293.
50. Hanna Jr MG, Key ME, Oldham RK. Biology of cancer therapy: some new insights into adjuvant treatment of metastatic solid tumors. *J Biol Response Modif* 1983; 4: 295-309.
51. Henslee PJ, Byers VS, Jennings CD, et al. A new approach to the prevention of graft-versus-host disease using XomaZyme-H65 [registered trademark] following histo-incompatible partialy T-depleted marrow grafts. *Transplant Proc* 1989; 21(1, Part 3): 3004-3007.
52. Henslee PJ, Byers VS, Jennings CD, et al. Reduction of graft versus host disease in Recipients of histoincompatible marrow transplant following administration of XomaZyme [registered trademark]-H65. *Fourth International Conference on Monoclonal Antibody Immunoconjugates for Cancer*, edited by I Royston and RD Dillman, p. 43, San Diego, 1989.
53. Hertler AA, Frankel AE. Immunotoxins: a clinical review of their use in the treatment of malignancies. *J Clin Onc* 1989; in press.
54. Hertler AA, Schlossman DM, Borowitz MJ, et al. An anti-CD5 immunotoxin for chronic lymphocytic leukemia: enhancement of cytotoxicity with human serum albumin-monensin. *Int J Cancer* 1989; 43: 215-219.
55. Hertler AA, Schlossman DM, Borowitz MJ, et al. A phase I study of T101-ricin A chain immunotoxin in refractory chronic lymphocytic leukemia, *J Biol Resp Modif* 1987; 7: 97-113.
56. Hwang KM, Foon KA, Cheung PH, et al. Selective antitumor effect of a potent immunoconjugate composed of the A chain of abrin and monoclonal antibody to a hepatoma associated antigen. *Cancer Res* 1984; 44: 4578-4586.
57. Jain RK, Ward-Hartley K. Tumor blood flow – characterization, modifications, and role in hyperthermia. *IEEE Trans Sonics and Ultrasonics* 1984; SU-31(5): 504-526.
58. Jansen FK, Blythman HE, Carriere D, et al. Immunotoxins: hybrid molecules combining high specificity and potent cytotoxicity. *Immunol Rev* 1982; 62: 185-215.
59. Jirtle R. Chemical modification of tumour blood flow. *Int J Hyperthermia* 1988; 4(4): 355-371.
60. Kernan NA, Byers V, Scannon PJ, et al. Treatment of steroid-resistant acute graft-vs-host disease by *in vivo* administration of an anti-T-cell ricin A chain immunotoxin. *JAMA* 1988; 259(21): 3154-3157.
61. Key ME, Bernhard MI, Hoyer LC, et al. Guinea pig 10 hepatocarcinoma model for monoclonal antibody ser-therapy: *in vivo* localization of a monoclonal antibody in normal and malignant tissues. *J Immunol* 1983; 139: 1451-1457.
62. Kishida K, Masuho Y, Saito M, et al. Ricin A chain conjugated with monoclonal anti-L1210 antibody. *In vitro*

and *in vivo* antitumor activity. *Cancer Immun Immunother* 1983; 16: 93.

63. Khazaeli M, LoBuglio AF, Wheeler R, et al. The effects of immunosuppressive regimens on human immune response to murine monoclonal anti-melanoma antibody-ricin A chain. *Proc Am Assoc Cancer Res* 1988; 29: 418.
64. Koehler M, Hurwitz CA, Krance RA, et al. XomaZyme-CD5 immunotoxin in conjunction with partial T cell depletion for prevention of graft rejection and graft-versus-host disease after bone marrow transplantation from matched unrelated donors. *Bone Marrow Transplantation* 1994; 13(5): 571-575.
65. Krance R, Heslop HE, Mahmoud H, et al. Anti-pan T lymphocyte ricin A chain immunotoxin (H65-RTA) and methylprednisolone for acute GVHD prophylaxis following allogeneic BMT from HLA-identical sibling donors. *Bone Marrow Transplantation* 1993; 11(1): 33-66.
66. Krolick KA, Uhr JW, Slavin S, and Vitetta ES. *In vivo* therapy of a murine B cell tumor (BCL1) using antibody-ricin A chain immunotoxins. *J Exp Med* 1982; 155: 1797-1809.
67. Krolick KA, Villemez C, Isakson P, et al. Selected killing of normal or neoplastic B cells by antibodies coupled to the A chain of ricin. *Proc Natl Acad Sci USA* 1980; 77: 5419.
68. Krolick KA, Yuan D, Vitetta ES. Specific killing of a human breast carcinoma cell line by a monoclonal antibody coupled to the A-chain of ricin Cancer, *Immunol Immunother* 1981; 12: 39-41.
69. Laurent G, Pris J, Farcet J P, et al. Effects of therapy with T101 ricin A-chain immunotoxin in two leukemia patients. *Blood* 1986; 67: 1680-1687.
70. Lee WY, Sehon A. Suppression of reaginic antibodies to drugs employing polyvinyl alcohol as carrier therefor. *US Patent No 4*, 296, 097, 1981.
71. Lee WY, Sehon AH. Suppression of reaginic antibodies. Immunol Rev 1978; 41: 200.
72. Leichner P, Yang N, Wessels B. Dosimetry and treatment planning in radioimmunotherapy. *Int J Radiat Oncol Biol Phys* 1989; in press.
73. LeMaistre CR, Meneghetti C, Rosenblum M, et al. Phase I trial of an interleukin-2 (IL-2) fusion toxin (DAB486 IL-2) in hematologic malignancies expressing the IL-2 receptor. *Blood* 1992; 79: 2547-2554.
74. LeMaistre CF, Meneghetti C, Yau JC, et al. Pre-emptive therapy of graft vs. host disease (GVHD) with a pan-T-cell immunotoxin (IT) is associated with accelerated engraftment. In: *Antibody Immunoconjugates, and Radiopharm*, edited by SE Order, 1990; 3(1): 70.
75. LeMaistre CF, Craig FE, Meneghetti C, et al. Phase I trial of a 90-minute infusion of the fusion toxin DAB486 IL-2 in hematological cancers. *Cancer Research* 1993; 53: 3930-3934.
76. LeMaistre CF; Rosen S, Frankel A, et al. Phase I trial of H65-RTA immunoconjugate in patients with cutaneous T-cell lymphoma.(61) *Blood* 1991; 78(5): 1173-82.
77. Letvin NL, Goldmacher VS, Ritz J, et al. *In vivo* administration of lymphocyte-specific monoclonal antibodies in nonhuman primates: in vivo stability of disulfide-linked immunotoxin conjugates. *J Clin Invest* 1985; 77: 977-984.
78. LoBuglio AF, Khazaeli MB, Lee J, et al. Pharmacokinetics and immune response to Xomazyme-Mel in melanoma patients. *Ab Immunocon Radiopharm* 1988; 1: 305-310.
79. Lynch TJ Jr. Immunotoxin therapy of small-cell lung cancer. N901-blocked ricin for relapsed small-cell lung cancer. *Chest* 1993; 103(4 Suppl): 436S-439S.
80. Lynch TJ, Coral J, Shefner AD, et al. Phase I trial of the novel immunotoxin N901-blocked ricin (N901-BR): demonstration of clinical activity in small cell lung cancer. *Proc of ASCO* 1993; 12, 293.
81. Matsui M, Nakanishi T, Noguchi T, and Ferrone S. Synergistic *in vitro* and *in vivo* anti-tumor effect of daunomycin-anti-96-kDa melanoma-associated antigen monoclonal antibody CL 207 conjugate and recombinant IFN-gamma1. *J Immunol* 1988; 141: 1410-1417.
82. Matsui M, Temponi M, Ferrone S. Characterization of a monoclonal antibody-defined human melanoma-associated antigen susceptible to induction by immune interferon. *J Immunol* 1987; 139: 2088.
83. Morgan AC Jr, Manger R, Pearson JW, et al. Immunoconjugates of Pseudomonas exotoxin A: evaluation in mice, monkeys, and man. *Cancer Detection and Prevention* 1991; 15(2): 137-43.
84. Morgan AC, Siram G, Weiden P, et al. (1989): Pseudomonas exotoxin A immunoconjugates: preclinical and clinical evaluation in mice, monkeys, and man. *Fourth International Conference on Monoclonal Antibody Immunoconjugates for Cancer*, edited by I Royston and RD Dillman, pp. 44-45, San Diego, 1989.
85. Msirikale J, Klein J, Schroeder J, Order S. *Int J Radiat Oncol Biol Phys* 1987; 13: 1839-1844.
86. Murphy J. *Proceedings of the Society of Biological Therapy*, Pittsburgh, 1991.
87. Murray PW, McLaughlin MG, Rosenblum H, et al. Phase I trial of anti-B4 blocked ricin (B4bR) given as a 28 day continuous infusion (CI). *Proceedings of the Society for Biological Therapy* 1994; 48.
88. Nadler L. Anti-B4 blocked ricin immunotoxin therapy for B cell leukemias and lymphomas. *Fourth International Conference on Monoclonal Antibody Immunoconjugates for Cancer*, edited by I Royston and RD Dillman, p. 49, San Diego, 1989.
89. Nadler L. Immunotoxin therapy for B cell malignancies. In: *Fifth International Conference on Monoclonal Antibody Immunoconjugates for Cancer*, edited by I Royston and RD Dillman, p. 13, San Diego, 1990.
90. Nilsson IM, Freiburghaus C, Sundqvist S, Sandberg H. Removal of specific antibodies from whole blood in a continuous extracorporeal system. *Plasma Ther Transfus Technol* 1984; 5: 127-134.
91. Oldham RK, Lewis M, Orr DW, et al. Adriamycin custom-tailored immunoconjugates in the treatment of human malignancies. *Mol Biother* 1988; 1(2): 103-113.
92. Oldham RK. Biological Response Modifiers Program: Subcommittee report. *J Natl Cancer Inst, Monograph* 1983; 63: 235-247.
93. Oratz R, Speyer JL, Wernz JC, et al. Antimelanoma monoclonal antibody-ricin A chain immunoconjugate (XMMME-001-RTA) plus cyclophosphamide in the treatment of metastatic malignant melanoma: results of a phase II trial. *Journal of Biological Response Modifiers* 1990; 9(4): 345-54.
94. Orr D, Oldham R, Lewis M, et al. Phase I trial of mitomycin C immunoconjugates cocktails in human malignancies. *Mol Biother* 1989; 1(4): 229-240.
95. Pai LH, Bookman MA, Ozols RF, et al. Clinical

evaluation of intraperitoneal Pseudomonal exotoxin immunoconjugate OVB3-PE in patients with ovarian cancer. *J Clin Oncol* 1991; 9(12): 2088-2090.

96. Pastan I, FitzGerald D. Novel cytotoxic agents created by the fusion of growth factor and toxin genes. *Fourth International Conference on Monoclonal Antibody Immunoconjugates for Cancer*, edited by I Royston and RD Dillman, pp. 36-37, San Diego, 1989.
97. Pietersz GA, Smyth MJ, Kanellos J, et al. Preclinical and clinical studies with a variety of immunoconjugates. *Ab Immunocon Radiopharm* 1988; 1(1): 79-103.
98. Pimm MV. Drug-monoclonal antibody conjugates for cancer therapy: potentials and limitations. *Crit Rev Ther Drug Carrier Syst* 1988; 5(3): 189-227.
99. Pirker R. Immunotoxins against solid tumors. *J Cancer Res Clin Oncol* 1988; 114(4): 385-93.
100. Pirker R, FitzGerald DJP, Raschack M, et al. Enhancement of the activity of immunotoxins by analogues of verapamil. *Cancer Res* 1989; 49: 4791-4795.
101. Press OW, Vitetta ES, Farr AG, et al. Evaluation of ricin A chain immunotoxins directed against human T cells. *Cellular Immunol* 1986; 102: 10-20.
102. Ramakrishnan S, Houston LL. Prevention of growth of leukemia cells in mice by monoclonal antibodies directed against Thy 1.1 antigen disulfide linked to two ribosomal inhibitors: pokeweed antiviral protein or ricin A chain. *Cancer Res* 1984; 44: 1398.
103. Raso V, Ritz J, Basola M, Schlossman SF. Monoclonal antibody-ricin A chain conjugate selectively cytotoxic for cells bearing the common acute lymphoblastic leukemia antigen. *Cancer Res* 1982; 42: 457.
104. Robinson WA, Adlakha A, Lamb MR, et al. Therapy of metastatic melanoma using single dose murine monoclonal antimelanoma antibody conjugated with ricin A chain (SMMME-001-RTA). *Second International Congress of Melanoma*, Venice, Italy, 1989.
105. Rodwell JD, Alvarez VL, Lee C, et al. Site-specific covalent modification of monoclonal antibodies: *in vitro* and *in vivo* evaluations. *Proc Natl Acad Sci USA* 1986; 83: 2632-2636.
106. Rudiger H. Lectins, an introduction. In: Lectins: Biology, Biochemistry, Clinical Biochemistry, edited by TC Bog-Hansen, Volume 1. Walter de Gruyter, New York, 1981.
107. Santos GW. Immunosuppressive drugs I. *Federation Proceedings* 1967; 26: 907-913.
108. Sausville E, Headlee D, Stetler-Stevenson M, et al. A phase I trial in B-cell lymphoma using anti-CD22 immunotoxin (IT) IgG-RFB4-SMPT-dgA: activity and determinants of toxicity. *Proc ASCO* 1994; 13: 384.
109. Scannon PJ. (1989): Suppression of the human immune response to immunotoxins with drugs. *Fourth International Conference on Monoclonal Antibody Immunoconjugates for Cancer*, edited by I Royston and RD Dillman, p. 63, San Diego, 1989.
110. Sehon AH, Lang GM. The use of nonionic, water soluble polymers for the synthesis of tolerogenic conjugates of antigens. In: *Mediators of Immune Regulation and Immunotherapy*, edited by SK Singhal and TL Delovitch, pp. 190-203, Elsevier Science Publishing Co., Inc., 1986.
111. Selvaggi K, Saria EA, Schwartz R, et al. Phase I/II study of murine monoclonal antibody-ricin A chain (XOMAZYME-Mel) immunoconjugate plus cyclosporine A in patients with metastatic melanoma. *Journal of Immunotherapy* 1993; 13: 201-207.
112. Seon BK. Specific killing of human T leukemia cell by immunotoxins prepared with ricin A chain and monoclonal antihuman T-cell leukemia antibodies. *Cancer Res* 1984; 44: 259.
113. Seon BK, Yokota S, Hara H, Luo Y. Synergistic effects of anti-human leukemia immunotoxins and recombinant a-Interferon in the *in vivo* suppression of tumor growth. *Fourth International Conference on Monoclonal Antibody Immunoconjugates for Cancer*, edited by I Royston and RD Dillman, p. 41, San Diego, 1989.
114. Seto M, Umemoto M, Saito M, et al. Monoclonal anti-MN46 antibody: ricin A chain conjugate; *in vivo* and *in vitro* antitumor activity. *Cancer Res* 1982; 42: 5209.
115. Sivan G, Pearson JW, Bohn W, et al. Immunotoxins to human melanoma associated antigen: comparison of gelonin with ricin and other A-chain conjugates. *Cancer Res* 1987; 47: 3169-3173.
116. Smith RT. Immunological tolerance of nonliving antigens. In: *Advances in Immunology*, edited by WH Taliaferro and JH Humphrey, pp. 67-129. Academic Press, New York, 1961.
117. Smyth MJ, Pietersz GA, McKenzie IFC. Use of vasoactive agents to increase tumor perfusion and the antitumor efficacy of drug-monoclonal antibody conjugates. *JNCI* 1987; 79(6): 1367-1373.
118. Smyth MJ, Pietersz GA, McKenzie IFC. Increased antitumor effedt of immunoconjugates and tumor necrosis factor. *Cancer Res* 1988; 48: 3607-3612.
119. Spitler LE. Clinical Studies: Solid Tumors. In: *Immunotoxins*, edited by Arthur E. Frankel, pp. 491-512. Martinus Nijhoff, Boston, 1988.
120. Spitler LE. Immunotoxins. In *Principles of Cancer Biotherapy*. Edited by Robert K. Oldham, pp.433-456. Marcel Dekker, Inc., New York, 1991.
121. Spitler LE, Mischak R, Scannon P. Therapy of metastatic malignant melanoma using Xomazyme-Mel, a murine monoclonal antimelanoma ricin A chain immunotoxin. *Nuclear Medicine and Biology International Journal of Applied Radiation and Isotopes*, Part B 1989; 16(6): 625-627.
122. Spitler LE, Rio M, del Khentigan A, et al. Therapy of patients with malignant melanoma using a monoclonal antimelanoma antibody-ricin A-chain immunotoxin. *Cancer Res* 1987; 47: 1717-1723.
123. Spitler LE, von Wussow P, Carey RW, et al. Phase II trial of a monoclonal antimelanoma antibody ricin A chain immunotoxin in therapy of malignant melanoma. Second International Conference on Monoclonal Antibody *Immunoconjugates for Cancer*, edited by I Royston and RD Dillman, San Diego, 1987.
124. Thorpe PE, Brown ANF, Bremner JAG, et al. An immunotoxin composed of monoclonal anti-Thy-1.1 antibody and a ribosome inactivating protein from *Saponaria officinalis*: potent antitumor effects *in vitro* and *in vivo*. *J Natl Cancer Inst* 1985; 75: 151-159.
125. Thorpe PE, Wallace PM, Knowles PP, et al. Improved antitumor effects of immunotoxins prepared with deglycosylated ricin A chain and hindered disulfide linkages. *Cancer Res* 1988; 48: 6396-6403.
126. Trowbridge IS, Domingo DL. Anti-transferrin receptor monoclonal antibody and toxin-antibody conjugates affect growth of human tumor cells. *Nature (Lond)* 1981; 294: 171.
127. Vitetta ES. In: *Proceedings of the Society of Biological*

Therapy, Pittsburgh, 1991.

128. Vitetta ES, Stone M, Amlot P, et al. Phase I immunotoxin trial in patients with B-cell lymphoma. *Cancer Research* 1991; 51(15): 4052-8.

129. Vitetta E, Thorpe P. Immunotoxins to treat B cell lymphomas. In: *Fifth International Conference on Monoclonal Antibody Immunoconjugates for Cancer*, edited by I Royston and RD Dillman, p. 13, San Diego, 1990.

130. Volkman DJ, Ahmad A, Fauci AS, Neville Jr DM. Selective abrogation of antigen-specific human B cell responses by antigen-ricin conjugates. *J Exp Med* 1982; 156: 634-639.

131. Weiner LM, O'Dwyer J, Kitson J, et al. Phase I evaluation of an anti-breast carcinoma monoclonal antibody 260F9-recombinant ricin A chain immunoconjugate. *Cancer Res* 1989; 49(14): 4062-4067.

132. Weisdorf D, Filipovich A, McGlave P, et al. Combination graft-versus-host disease prophylaxis using immunotoxin (anti-CD5-RTA [Xomazyme-CD5]) plus methotrexate and cyclosporine or prednisone after unrelated donor marrow transplantation. *Bone Marrow Transplantation* 1993; 12(5): 531-536.

133. Yamaizumi M, Mekada E, Uchida T, Okada Y. One molecule of diphtheria toxin fragment A introduced into a cell can kill the cell. *Cell* 1978; 15: 245-250.

134. Youle RJ, Neville DM Jr. Kinetics of protein synthesis inactivation by ricin A anti-thy 1.1 monoclonal antibody hybrids. *J Biol Chem* 1982; 257: 1598.

135. Yu Y H, Ramakrishnan S, Houston L, et al. Synergistic antitumor activity of immunotoxins reactive with human breast carcinomas. *Fourth International Conference on Monoclonal Antibody Immunoconjugates for Cancer*, edited by I. Royston and R. D. Dillman, p. 40, San Diego, 1989.

136. Zalebert JR, Pielersz G, Toohey B, et al. (1989): Phase I-II study of A ricin monoclonal antibody conjugate in colon cancer. *Fourth International Conference on Monoclonal Antibody Immunoconjugates for Cancer*, edited by I. Royston and R. D. Dillman, p. 47, San Diego, 1989.

DRUG IMMUNOCONJUGATES

ROBERT K. OLDHAM [1] and KENNETH A. FOON [2]

[1] *Biological Therapy Institute Foundation, Franklin, Tennessee; and University of Missouri, Columbia, Missouri*
[2] *Markey Cancer Center, University of Kentucky, Lexington, Kentucky*

Monoclonal antibodies and their immunoconjugates represent the first practical method for the selective treatment of cancer [48]. The three traditional modalities of cancer treatment – surgery, radiotherapy, and chemotherapy – have proven roles in cancer treatment. However, even when applied in optimal fashion, over 50% of patients with cancer still remain incurable [56]. The vast majority of these patients remain incurable because of metastatic disease, which does not respond sufficiently to systemic treatment. Chemotherapy has been the only systemic approach to metastatic cancer. Its limitations, toxicities, and lack of selectivity and efficacy have been repeatedly reviewed. It is apparent from clinical results with systemic treatment that there is a need for more active and more selective approaches to cancer treatment.

Since the original suggestion by Paul Ehrlich that antibodies might be used to treat cancer, investigators have repeatedly – and unsuccessfully – attempted to implement his suggestion. Antibodies have long been known as biological agents with the potential for recognizing tumor tissue as different from the normal tissue of origin. Heteroantisera as selective targeting agents were unsuccessful because of various problems in generation, reproductibility, purification, immunogenecity and clinical use. With the advent of monoclonal antibody technology, a method for the production of unlimited quantities of antibody preparations directed toward one or more antigens and/or antigenic epitopes on the tumor cell membrane became available [16, 17, 54]. While Ehrlich's 'magic bullet' concept has been much discussed, the lack of absolute specificity of any single tumor antigen makes it unlikely that singular and totally specific antigens will be identified for targeting with a single monoclonal antibody preparation (with anti-idiotypic determinants on lymphomas a possible exception). However, there are many indications that quantitative differences in antigens and antigenic patterns exist on cancer cell membranes when compared with the normal counterparts. There are now data indicating that these differences can be exploited in designing selective treatment for patients with cancer [16, 17, 54, 58, 60, 61]. Obviously, current systemic treatment modalities are very nonselective and have considerable toxicity for normal tissues. Depending on how one selects the normal tissue control, drug toxicity may actually be greater to normal tissue than to the cancer. Even in the best of circumstances, considerable toxicity to normal tissue accompanies effective treatment with the currently available drugs. It is now expected that monoclonal antibodies may be used in directing drugs, toxins, biologicals, and isotopes to the tumor cell, and will assist in giving enhanced selectivity to systemic cancer treatment [9-11, 26, 27, 35, 39, 47, 58, 62, 63, 87, 88, 97].

Monoclonal antibody technology now allows for the generation of antibodies or 'cocktails' of antibodies that have some selectivity for cancer tissue as compared with the normal tissue of origin. These antibodies can be tested as unconjugated antibody alone or in conjunction with effector cells. Chapter 12 reviewed these approaches. The 'signal strength' of the antibody may be made more powerful by conjugating antibody to drugs, toxins, biologicals, and radioisotopes. This chapter will focus on the use of drug immunoconjugates for cancer treatment.

THE PROBLEM OF HETEROGENEITY: ANTIBODY-BASED THERAPEUTICS AS A SOLUTION

The problem of tumor-cell heterogeneity (Fig. 1) and the implications for therapy have been reviewed in Chapter 2. Curiously, although tumor-cell heterogeneity has been broadly recognized for more than a decade, clinicians continue to take the simplistic view that treatment need not reflect a specific approach to heterogeneity [78, 94-96]. Thus, treatment is still designed as if there are singular underlying common principles useful in cancer therapy. Single modalities or fixed combinations aimed at eradicating cancer without a strategy designed to approach the problem of tumor-cell heterogeneity still dominate cancer research and treatment [57, 63, 64, 77].

Current data on tumor-cell heterogeneity and the biologic basis of that heterogeneity is covered in Chapter 2 and have been previously reviewed [25]. The basic tenant of these studies is that each primary tumor is composed of a smaller or larger number of clones, each of which has its own genotypic and phenotypic characteristics. Metastasis

R.K. Oldham (ed.), Principles of Cancer Biotherapy. 3rd ed., 338–347.

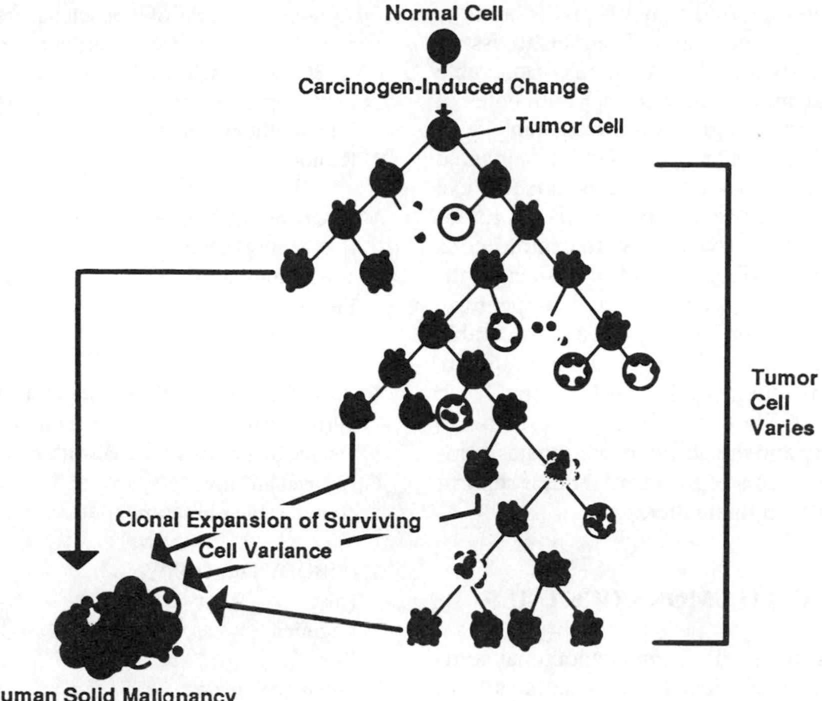

Figure 1. Illustration of tumor cell heterogeneity.

tends to occur from single cells or clumps of cells from within the primary tumor. By virtue of a series of phenotypic analyses, as well as certain kinds of genotypic inferences, these authors and others have demonstrated beyond doubt that heterogeneity is characteristic of both animal and human tumors. Recently, there have been references to the implications of this tumor-cell heterogeneity for treatment, and proposals have been made to approach the problem clinically [55, 56, 77].

There are two types of tumor-cell heterogeneity [69]. There are differences between patients, with heterogeneity being apparent among tumors of the same histological class. This is macroheterogeneity. Tumors such as breast cancer can be very similar by histological examination, and yet lethality can occur in 7 months or 17 years. Clinical observations have made it clear that what is seen under the microscope bears little relationship to the behavior of the cancer in the patient. This sort of 'phenotypic analysis' has led to further investigations, and it is now recognized by most cancer biologists that considerable differences exist among patients with respect to the phenotypic characteristics of the cancer. In addition, there is the problem of heterogeneity within each tumor in each patient; microheterogeneity. Thus, many studies have demonstrated that multiple clones may exist within the primary tumor and that these clones may have different metastatic capabilities, giving rise to heterogeneity even among different deposits in a single patient.

Many still believe that even with heterogeneity between individuals and within each patient's cancer, underlying common features still exist and will allow a general treatment to be developed that might be useful for all cancer, or all of a histological type of cancer. This view supports the 'drug development paradigm, ' wherein drugs are developed as broadly active agents to be tested in different histological types of cancer (see Chapter 3).

Another view is that each cancer and its antigenic phenotype (and behavior) are unique. This view, currently held by a minority of investigators, would suggest the need to individualize treatment for each patient and may even require individual therapeutic manipulations for a single patient over the clinical course of his or her disease based on these differences [61, 64, 67, 69]. Acceptance of this hypothesis would dramatically change cancer treatment and would require a laboratory-clinic interface of a type not often used in cancer therapeutics. With the advent of the 'new biology' using genetically engineered biologicals and monoclonal antibodies, one has diverse mechanisms for the generation of biological responses, which may match the diversity implicit in tumor cell populations. For the first time, there is hope that one can truly approach the heterogeneity of each patient's cancer and the other biologic differences of each patient in a rational manner [37, 56, 61].

RATIONALE FOR IMMUNOCONJUGATES

Most of the early monoclonal antibody clinical trials focused on the use of unconjugated single antibodies (see Chapter 12) in order to determine toxicity, tolerance, the localization of antibody in solid tumor deposits, and the distribution of antibody in normal and neoplastic tissues [19, 29, 50, 51, 73, 74, 81-84]. There is now a considerable body of evidence that murine monoclonal antibodies at doses from 1 mg to several grams are reasonably well tolerated. Although the clinical responses to unconjugated antibody have not been striking, there is unequivocal evidence that antibody does selectively localize in tumor deposits and on individual cancer cells after intravenous injection [58, 81]. Biodistribution studies utilizing antibody conjugated to tracer quantities of isotope have demonstrated excellent tumor imaging, but a considerable amount of the antibody is distributed to the liver, spleen, and other organs of the reticuloendothelial system [1, 12, 13, 36, 43, 45, 94, 98]. The infrequency of response to unconjugated antibody and the ability of conjugates to induce regression of bulky cancer in animal models support the concept of immunoconjugate therapy.

Table 1. Optimization of monoclonal antibody therapy

ANTIBODY SPECIFICITY
Immunoperoxidase
Immunofluorescence
Radiolocalization
ANTIGEN CHARACTERIZATION
Biochemical nature
Topography and density
Epitopes
Heterogeneity
ANTIBODY-ANTIGEN INTERACTION
Turnover of antibody bound to tumor cells
Degree of antibody internalization
Antigen affinity
Antigen levels in serum
ANTIBODY DELIVERY
Dose
Regimen
Route
Pharmacokinetics
Comparison of various cytotoxic agents conjugtated to the same antibody

RATIONALE FOR ANTITUMOR COCKTAILS

There already exists many different monoclonal antibodies to be assessed in clinical trials in patients with solid tumors [16, 17, 61]. A large number of antibodies for lymphoma, melanoma, lung, breast, and colon cancer have been described and characterized. Antibody preparations are available as immunoglobulin M (IgM), IgA, and various subclasses of IgG. A large variety of new monoclonal antibodies, both murine and human, continues to be discovered and developed. Thus, it is apparent that the limitation for the use of monoclonal antibody preparations in treatment will not be due to a shortage of antibody preparations [54].

Although the 'perfect' antibody for use as unconjugated antibody or as a targeting agent has not been identified (and probably never will) for any human cancer, there is a variety of selective antibodies available for clinical investigation. Methods exist to manufacture high-purity (>99%), homogeneous preparations of monoclonal antibodies. Characterization as to antibody isotype, level of purity, degree of contamination by other substances, stability, and other pertinent physical/chemical characteristics is possible. Thus, no insurmountable obstacles exist with respect to testing a wide variety of monoclonal antibodies in patients (Table 1).

Given a wide choice of antibody preparations and the ability to prepare them for the clinic, the next consideration is, how does one select preparations and patients for clinical trials? It seems unlikely that firm rules can be made on the selection of antibody preparations for all solid tumors. Obviously, the distribution of the tumor, its vascularity, its sensitivity to drugs and radiation, and the quantitative expression of antigens on the tumor cell surfaces are all significant factors. Using conjugates of isotopes, drugs, biologicals, and toxins, the issue may be essentially one of biodistribution within the tumor bed and access of the toxic agent to the tumor cell within each tumor nodule. Thus, it is apparent that while certain principles in the use of monoclonal antibody for human solid tumors may be important, each tumor type and, in fact, each individual patient may have to be individually evaluated for the optimal use of a monoclonal antibody preparation [69].

Antibodies whether conjugated or not, presumably must reach the tumor bed to be effective [58]. One general principle has been that smaller antibodies or antibody fragments may more quickly diffuse from the vascular compartment to the tumor bed. Early data from our studies have indicated that the more antibody one infuses into the vascular compartment, the more antibody one delivers to the tumor cell bed [58]. Although access to the tumor bed is clearly quite important, retention within the tumor bed may be equally or more important. The preparations of antibody fragments may diffuse more quickly into the tumor nodule [1], but larger molecules may be retained for a longer time within that same nodule [58]. Therefore, at the level of these elementary principles, there is much to be learned about the use of these antibody preparations in clinical trials, and these clinical trials should not yet be subject to hard and fast rules [54].

On the basis of early assessments of the heterogeneity of malignant melanoma [31], including studies of both melanoma cell lines and fresh biopsies of melanoma nodules, it became obvious that considerable antigenic heterogeneity exists. When the data were analyzed in detail with a panel of antimelanoma monoclonal antibodies, each patient's tumor had its own pattern of reactivity. As an extension of this approach, we have generated antibodies for individual patients, making up to 10 antibodies per patient to analyze heterogeneity [3, 49, 69]. As shown in Figure 2, the flow cytometry patterns for each antibody may differ considerably when tested against the patient's cancer. By additive testing of the individual antibodies, a cocktail of antibodies, consisting of two to five components, can be created to cover all of the cells in the tumor as assessed by flow cytometry and immunoperioxidase staining (Fig. 3).

Our data support the concept that tumor-cell hetero-

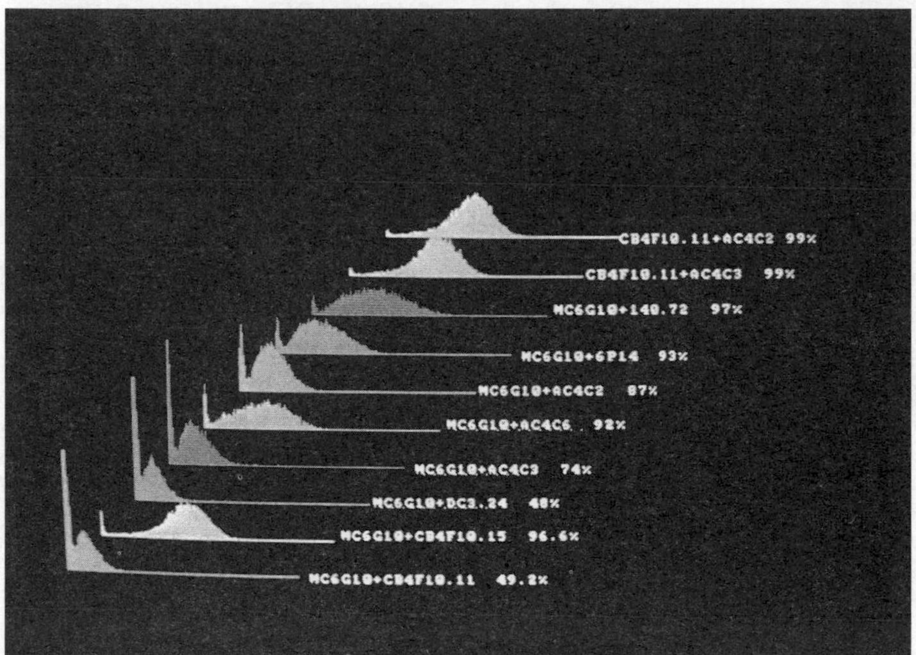

Figure 2. Antibody preparations to a single patient's melanoma as seen on flow cytometry

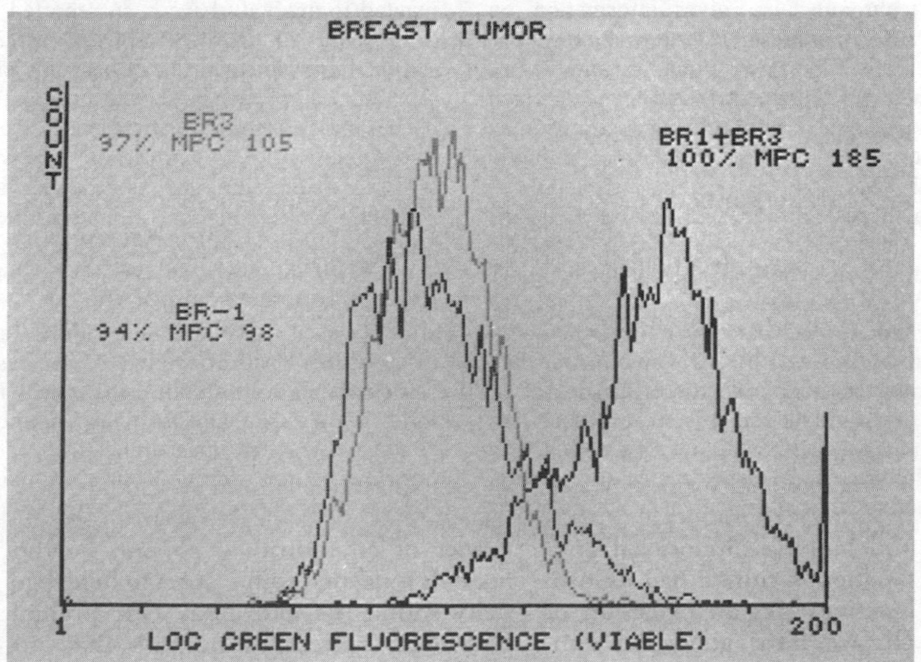

Figure 3. A two-antibody cocktail for melanoma.

geneity will call for the generation of antibodies and/or the use of typing panels to prepare antibody cocktails containing multiple components in an attempt to deliver antibody and its conjugated toxic substance to all the replicating cells in the cancer [69]. This approach should substantially improve the ability to target toxic substances selectively to the cancer of an individual patient. Further analysis is needed with respect to heterogeneity within the individual. Our preliminary data appear to indicate that this microheterogeneity is not striking, and it may be possible to cover it with a sufficiently complex cocktail. However, the possibility of somatic mutation and/or selective pressure in treatment leading to further tumor-cell diversity in patients with metastatic disease is real [21]. In lymphoma, there is evidence to indicate a multiclonality; while it is not completely clear, some of this multiclonality may result from selective pressures induced by treatment with anti-idiotypic antibody [32, 51].

CLINICAL-LABORATORY INTEGRATION FOR DRUG IMMUNOCONJUGATE TRIALS

There are certain important principles in the design and execution of clinical trials using monoclonal antibodies [59, 60, 68]. To learn from these early trials it is necessary to have an active and competent laboratory available for *in vitro* assessments. It is essential to demonstrate that the antibody reaches the tumor nodule. For this, the technique of immunohistology using biopsy specimens subsequent to the infusion of antibody has been quite valuable [37, 58, 81, 82]. The distribution of antibody within the tumor nodule in contrast to surrounding normal tissues can be assessed. This technique also gives information on heterogeneity of antigen expression. *In vitro* overlay with the treatment antibody can assess saturation, and the use of other antibodies can define heterogeneity of antigen expression. Isotope-labeled antibody preparations may also be used to evaluate the biodistribution of antibody [12, 13, 36, 43, 45, 98].

In addition to these techniques using 'fixed' tissue, cytofluorometry can be used to visualize individual cells with respect to antigen distribution, antibody localization, and saturation. When the tumor nodule is disaggregated after *in vivo* treatment, one can determine with great precision the level of antibody localization on individual cells and, by adding exogenous antibody, the degree of saturation on these individual cells [58, 81, 82]. Thus, we have three techniques to assess the delivery of antibody conjugates to the tumor, as well as the degree of saturation of membrane antigens. In addition, actual determinations of heterogeneity within individual tumor biopsies and between patients can easily be made from these studies [69].

The ability to measure antigen and antigen-antibody complexes before and after treatment, and circulating antibody after injection, is critical to an understanding of the pharmacokinetics in these antibody trials [2, 4, 69]. Further, it is important to measure antiglobulin levels initially and after treatment in conducting these clinical trials, since such antiglobulin responses may ultimately be important in the biodistribution, toxicity and efficacy of an infused antibody [18, 58, 79, 80].

CHEMOTHERAPEUTIC DRUG IMMUNOCONJUGATES

The rationale for conjugating antibody to chemotherapeutic drugs is fairly straight-forward. These drugs have been used for many years in clinical studies. The spectrum of activity and the toxicology of these agents are well understood. In addition, there is considerable evidence to support the belief that dose-response curves exist with these drugs in the killing of tumor cells. Their lack of selectivity for cancer and the major problem of normal tissue toxicity is well known. All of these factors constitute a firm basis for attempting antibody delivery to target the chemotherapeutic agent to the tumor site.

Surprisingly, very few clinical studies have been done using antibody-targeted chemotherapy. Perhaps the reason relates to the lower specific activity seen *in vitro* with these conjugates. Compared with immunotoxins, drug conjugates have been less active in preclinical studies, and this finding has discouraged investigators with respect to the possible *in vivo* activity of such preparations [21, 32].

Pre-clinical studies

Preclinical studies using chemotherapeutic agents conjugated to antibody have been reported for a variety of drugs [8, 16, 17, 20, 32, 40, 44, 46, 53, 72, 85, 89]. These studies have indicated that drug conjugates can have *in vitro* and *in vivo* activity. The drugs most often used have been vinca alkaloids, methotrexate, daunorubicin, and doxorubicin. In one study methotrexate was coupled to an IgM monoclonal antibody targeted to a variety of tumors, including mouse teratocarcinoma (7). Deposition of immunoconjugate in viable tumor and lack of binding to antigen negative normal tissue was demonstrated in an *in vivo* animal model. In another study, aminopterin which is a more potent antifolate than methotrexate, was coupled to a monoclonal antibody (75). These investigators demonstrated that administering leucovorin 48-72 hours following a sublethal dose of the aminopterin-antibody conjugate resulted in maintenance of the anti-tumor efficacy of the immunoconjugate and a significant reduction in toxicity. In another report (76), idarubicin, an analogue of daunorubicin, was coupled to a CD19 antibody. A human pre-B-cell acute lymphoblastic leukemia cell line (NALM-6) was implanted into nude mice and this immunoconjugate was demonstrated to have substantial anti-tumor activity, was non-toxic and was stable *in vivo*. They proposed this as an excellent immunoconjugate for clinical trials.

In a different approach (15), investigators studied maytansinoids. These drugs are 100-1,000 times more cytotoxic than common anticancer drugs. These investigators felt that the limitation of drug immunoconjugates is that they act stoichiometrically, requiring much higher intracellular concentrations to achieve the comparable cytotoxicity as compared to a protein toxin where one molecule in the cytoplasm leads to cell death. Maytansine was coupled to a monoclonal antibody via disulfide containing linkers that are cleaved intracellularly to release the drug. They demonstrated antigen specific cytotoxicity of cultured human cells and minimal systemic toxicity in mice with an excellent pharmacokinetic profile. These studies and many others in preclinical models using antibody conjugated to chemotherapeutic agents lend some support to the idea that drug-conjugated antibodies may allow better targeting of chemotherapeutic agents to the tumor site [6, 14, 17, 22, 28, 41, 42, 60, 63, 71, 91, 92, 98].

Novel and recently reported exciting data used a different approach. Src protooncogene family protein tyrosine kinases (PTKs) play a key role in cell function and attempts have been made to develop agents that specifically inhibit Src-family PTKs. In one report (93), a general PTK inhibitor, Genistein, that inhibits all members of the Src PTK family was used to target to cancer cells. Genistein is an isoflavone derived from fermentation broth of *Pseudomonas* spp. It is also a natural occurring tyrosine kinase inhibitor present in soybeans. Genistein inhibits purified Lck kinase from human lymphoid cells at micromolar concentrations. These investigators conjugated Genistein to an anti-CD19 monoclonal antibody. An anti-CD19 antibody was chosen because the CD19 receptor is not shed from cells, it is internalized upon association with antibody and is physically and functionally associated with the Src protooncogene family PTKs including Lck. Human acute lymphoblastic leukemia of the pre-B cell variety was treated in a severe combined immunodeficient mouse model with this immunoconjugate. These investigators demonstrated that the immunoconjugate bound with high affinity to the leukemia cells, inhibited selectively the CD19-associated tyrosine kinases, and triggered rapid apoptotic cell death. Furthermore, at less than one-tenth the maximum tolerated dose, greater than 99.99% of the leukemia cells were killed, which led to 100% long-term event-free survival in these animals.

Clinical trials

Limited trials with drug-labeled monoclonal antibody have been reported. One of the first reports used antibody 791T/36 conjugated to methotrexate [6]. Initial studies with this conjugate demonstrated that methotrexate conjugation did not alter the pharmacokinetics or tumor localization indices for the antibody labeled with ^{131}I [23]. The monoclonal antibody KS1/4 which is expressed on epithelial malignancies and some normal epithelial cells was conjugated to methotrexate (24). Eleven patients with advanced non-small cell carcinoma of the lung were treated up to a maximum tolerated dose of 1750mg/m^2 with a cumulative dose of methotrexate of 40mg/m^2. Toxicities in this study included fever, anorexia, nausea, vomiting, diarrhea, abdominal pain, guaiac positive stools and hypoalbuminemia. Two patients had episodes of aseptic meningitis. One patient had a greater than 50% decrease of two lung nodules. Post-treatment tumor biopsies demonstrated binding of the immunoconjugate to tumor epithelial cells. Some of the gastrointestinal toxicities may also have been secondary to binding of the immunoconjugate to gastrointestinal epithelial cells.

Other studies further support the possibility of clinical trials with drug immunoconjugates [16, 17, 23, 28, 30, 32, 33, 90]. The rationale for such studies has been previously described [59, 64, 66, 68, 69] and the dose-delivery curves for tissue penetration and antigen saturation have been fully described [58, 66, 69, 70]. Issues of antibody specificity, antigen heterogeneity, optimal linkers, drug selection, and specific activity of the immunoconjugate all remain under active investigation.

We have utilized cocktails of antibodies custom tailored to individual patient tumors [64, 67, 69, 70]. These studies have utilized a biopsy of the cancer from each patient and either the generation of new antibodies to that patient's tumor or the use of existing panels of antibodies to type the patient's tumor [3, 49]. From these two methods, cocktails of two to six antibodies were generated and conjugated to doxorubicin [52, 66] or mitomycin-C [70]. The immunoglobulin-to-doxorubicin ratios were in the range of 1: 40 to 1: 60. This level of coupling did not alter the antibody's *in vitro* immunoreactivity, and excellent *in vitro* cytotoxicity was observed on antigen-positive cell lines compared to antigen-negative controls. The spectrum of clinical toxicities was strikingly different for doxorubicin conjugated to antibody as compared with free doxorubicin [66]. More than 1 g of doxorubicin on up to 5 g of antibody was administered over a 3-week period without alopecia or severe bone marrow depression. In several of these patients, antibody delivery was confirmed by biopsy of skin and analysis of cytologically positive pleural fluid. Persistence of antibody conjugates for up to one week posttreatment was noted with doxorubicin doses of 50 mg borne on approximately 300 mg of antibody. These doxorubicin-monoclonal antibody cocktail immunoconjugates were used in 24 patients. Mild toxic reactions were seen in 17/24 (fever, chills, pruritis, and skin rash) after the administration of these drug immunoconjugates. In several patients there was limited antigenic drift among the sequential biopsies within the same patient over time. Five minor responses were seen with these conjugates. Two patients with breast cancer had isolated improvement in skin ulcerations, and three additional patients with other types of cancers had minor responses. None of these responses were sufficient to reach a partial response (50% reduction in mean tumor diameters) by standard oncological criteria.

Toward the end of these studies and at the higher doses of doxorubicin, toxicities were noted in these patients. Urine color turned red, and alopecia with bone marrow suppression was noted. On reexamination of the doxorubicin procured from Adria Laboratories, it was noted that the preparation method for the doxorubicin had changed. A stabilizer (methylparaben) was added to the preparation (RDF-Adriamycin), which likely changed the stability of the doxorubicin immunoconjugates. This change occurred near the end of the study, and the clinical studies were terminated to determine a better method for manufacturing doxorubicin immunoconjugates in light of the changed chemistry [22, 52, 66, 69].

A subsequent study was carried out using mitomycin-C immunoconjugates [70]. Nineteen patients were treated with mitomycin-C conjugated to similar cocktails of monoclonal antibodies. Thrombocytopenia at the 60 mg (mitomycin)dose in this protocol was dose-limiting. The anti-mouse antibody titers were lower in the mitomycin-C compared to the doxorubicin-treated patients [4]. No responses were seen with mitomycin-C immunoconjugates, although several patients had less tumor-related pain after treatment [69].

These studies, while quite preliminary, serve to indicate the potential role in targeting chemotherapeutic agents with monoclonal antibodies. While there are many possible reasons to assume that this approach will not be useful in the clinic, more data concerning the treatment of patients are needed to determine if sufficient quantities of drug can be delivered to the tumor cell to be effective.

The role of drug resistance in cancer treatment is another issue to be considered. The current widely held opinion is that tumor cells, once resistant, cannot easily be treated with the same drug. A variety of approaches using mechanisms to overcome membrane resistance have been suggested. However, antibody-mediated delivery may be another such mechanism, and it is unclear whether doxorubicin-resistant tumor cells will be resistant to doxorubicin conjugates if delivered in appropriate quantities. *In vitro* and animal model data have confirmed sensitivity to doxorubicin conjugate where the cell line was resistant to free drug [17, 20, 22]. These and many other issues will be approachable through the use of drug-antibody conjugates. Other studies comparing drug and toxin conjugates are of interest in regard to the issue of specific activity [21, 23]. While the immunotoxins had a higher specific cytolytic capability *in vitro*, and may be most useful where target cells express low levels of antigens, drug conjugates may be preferable when target cells express a high density of antigens or when large doses of conjugate are needed to penetrate tumors. In these situations higher-specific-activity conjugates (toxins) may be too toxic for clinical use.

CONCLUSIONS

Our studies, as well as many similar studies, clearly indicate the potential for the new selective approach to cancer treatment (Table 2). Selective and effective new anti-cancer approaches are needed in the systemic treatment of human malignancies. Many very toxic molecules are well known to medical science (Table 3). Of key importance is the delivery of these toxic substances to tumor cells in ways that will avoid the undesirable side effects on normal tissues. Given these considerations, it is probably no longer necessary to distinguish between drugs and toxins. Perhaps we should speak of strong and weak drugs (chemicals), in that toxin molecules are simply biological chemicals with a higher degree of toxicity than the chemicals we commonly identify as drugs. This may, however, only partially be the case, since most toxins are complex biologicals and most chemotherapeutic drugs are relatively simple chemicals. Such differences in size and structure may profoundly affect *in vivo* trafficking and immunogenicity.

With the advent of monoclonal antibodies and the pos-

Table 2. Summary of monoclonal antibody (MoAb) serotherapy trials

Murine derived MoAb can be given safely intravenously by prolonged infusion (>1 h) without immediate side effects
Bronchospasm and hypotension have followed rapid infusion and higher doses of monoclonal antibody
Dosages from 1 mg to 5 g have been given safely with careful monitoring
A sustained decline in leukemic cells requires multiple MoAb treatments over several weeks
Skin lesions and lymph nodes can regress following MoAb treatment
There has been no major reduction in the bone-marrow leukemia cells
Antigenic modulation sometimes occurs following MoAb treatment
Free antigen may be detected in the serum following MoAb treatment
Clear evidence of selective localization of infused antibody in solid tumors is available
Antibodies to mouse cells usually develop following MoAb therapy
There is considerable variation with respect to toxicity, bioavailability, and activity related to immunoglobulin class, antigen, and distribution to tumor
Unconjugated antibody appears to have limited anticancer therapeutic value

Table 3. Immunoconjugates with cytotoxic agents

PROTEIN TOXINS AND CYTOTOXINS
Abrin
Ricin
Diphteria
Gelonin
Hematoporphyrin
Purothionine
Pseudomonas exotoxin
Alpha-amanitin
CHEMOTHERAPEUTIC DRUGS
Vindesine
Methotrexate
Daunorubicin
Doxorubicin
Mitomycin-C
Various new drugs with high toxicity profiles
BIOLOGIC AGENTS
Interferon
Tumor necrosis factor
Cobra venom factor

sibility of delivering toxic substances selectively to cancer cells, many toxic chemicals previously rejected as chemotherapeutic agents may now be recognized for use in association with antibody in an immunoconjugate [38, 86]. Pro-drug strategies and methods of *in vivo* activation may add further selectivity [5]. Thus, cancer treatment can now enter a new era, since selective delivery offers the hope of increased specific activity against the cancer with less toxicity to the patient. We are entering an era where costs [55, 65, 69], not technology, will now be the limiting factor in developmental therapeutics.

REFERENCES

1. Andrew AM, Pim MV, Perkins AC, Baldwin RW. Comparative imaging and biodistribution studies with an anti-CEA monoclonal antibody and its F(ab)^2 and Fab fragments in mice with colon carcinoma xenografts. *Eur J Nucl Med* 1986; 12: 168-175.
2. Avner B, Avner BP, Gaydos B, et al. Characterization of a method using viable human target cells as the solid phase in a cell concentration fluorescence immunoassay (CCFIA) for screening of monoclonal antibodies and hybridoma supernatants. *J Immunol Methods* 1988; 113: 123-135.
3. Avner BP, Liao SK, Avner B, et al. Therapeutic murine monoclonal antibodies developed for individual cancer patients. *J Biol Response Modif* 1989; 8(1): 25-36.
4. Avner B, Swindell L, Sharp E, et al. Evaluation and clinical relevance of patient immune responses to intravenous therapy with murine monoclonal antibodies conjugated to adriamycin *Mol Biother* 1991; 3(1): 14-21.
5. Bagshawe KD. Antibody directed enzymes activate prodrugs at tumor site. Order SE, ed. *Antibody Immunoconj. Radiopharm.* 1990; 3(1): 60.
6. Ballantyne KC, Perkins AC, Pimm MV, et al. Localization of monoclonal antibody-drug conjugate 791T/36-methotrexate in colorectal cancer. *STS Abstr* 1986; no. 88.
7. Ballou B, Jaffe R, Persiani S, et al. Tissue localization of methotrexate-monoclonal-IgM immunoconjugates: anti-SSEA-1 and MOPC 104E in mouse teratocarcinomas and normal tissues. *Cancer Immunol Immunother* 1992; 35: 251-256.
8. Belles-Isles M, Page M. *In vitro* activity of daunomycin anti-alpha-fetoprotein conjugate on mouse hepatoma cell. *Cancer (Phila)* 1980; 41: 841-845.
9. Bernhard MT, Foon KA, Oeltmann TN, et al. Guinea pig line 10 hepatocarcinoma model: characterization of monoclonal antibody and *in vivo* efect of unconjugate antibody and antibody conjugated to diptheria toxin A chain. *Cancer Res* 1983; 43: 4420-4428.
10. Berstein ID, Tam MR, Nowinski RC. Mouse leukemia: therapy with monoclonal antibodies against a thumus differentiation antigen. *Science* 1980; 207: 68-70.
11. Blythman HE, Casellas P, Gros O, et al. Immunotoxins: hybrid molecules of monoclonal antibodies and a toxin subunit specifically kill tumor cells. *Nature (Lond)* 1981; 290: 145-146.
12. Carrasquillo JA, Abrams PG, Schroff R, et al. Effect of antibody dose on the imaging and biodistribution of indium-111 9.2.27 anti-melanoma monoclonal antibody. *J Nucl Med* 1988; 29(1): 39-47.
13. Carrasquillo JA, Bunn PA, Kennan AM, et al. Radioimmunodetection of cutaneous T-cell lymphoma with ^{111}In-T101 monoclonal antibody. *N Engl J Med* 1986; 315: 673-680.
14. Chari RJ, Gross JL, Goldmacher VS, et al. Conjugates of monoclonal antibodies and cytotoxic macrolide drugs: potent, target specific antibody-drug conjugates. *Antibody Immunoconj Radiopharm* 1990; 3(1): 64.
15. Chari VJ, Martell BA, Gross JL, et al. Immunoconjugates containing novel maytansinoids: promising anticancer drugs. *Cancer Res* 1992; 52: 127-131.
16. Dillman RO. Monoclonal antibodies in the treatment of cancer. *Crit Rev Hematol Oncol* 1984; 1: 357-386.
17. Dillman RO. Monoclonal antibodies for treating cancer. *Ann Intern Med* 1989; 111: 592-603.
18. Dillman RO. Human antimouse and antiglobulin responses to monoclonal antibodies. *Antibody Immunocon Radiopharm* 1990; 3(1): 1-16.
19. Dillman RO, Shawler DL, Sobol RE. Murine monoclonal antibody therapy in two patients with chronic lymphocytic leukemia. *Blood* 1982; 59: 1036-1046.
20. Dillman RO, Shawler DL, Johnson DE, et al. Preclinical trials with combinations and conjugates of T101 and doxorubicin. *Cancer Res* 1986; 46: 4886-4891.
21. Dillman RO, Johnson DE, Shawler DL. Comparisons of drug and toxin immunoconjugates. *Antibody Immunocon Radiopharm* 1988; 1: 65-77.
22. Dillman RO, Johnson DE, Shawler DL, Koziol JA. Superiority of an acid-labile daunorubicin-monoclonal antibody immunoconjugate compared to free drug. *Cancer Res* 1988; 48: 6097-6102.
23. Embleton MJ. Drug targeting by monoclonal antibodies. *Br J Cancer* 1987; 55: 227-231.
24. Elias DJ, Kline LE, Robbins BA, et al. Monoclonal anti-

body KS1/4-methotrexate immunoconjugate studies in non-small cell lung carcinoma. *Am J Respir Crit Care Med* 150: 1114-1122, 1994.
25. Fidler IJ, Poste G. The cellular heterogeniety of malignant neoplasms: Implications for adjuvant chemotherapy. *Semin Oncol* 1985; 12: 207-221.
26. Fodstad O, Koalheim G, Godal A, et al. Phase I study of the plant protein ricin. *Cancer Res* 44: 862-865.
27. Fodstad O, Oisnes S, Phil A. Inhibitors effect of abrin and ricin on the growth of transplantable murine tumor and of abrin on human cancers in nude mice. *Cancer Res* 1977; 37: 4559-4567.
28. Foon KA, Bernhard MI, Oldham RK. Monoclonal antibody therapy: assessment by animal tumor models. *J Biol Response Modif* 1982; 1: 277-304.
29. Foon KA, Bunn PA, Schroff RW, et al. Monoclonal antibody therapy of chronic lymphocytic leukemia and cutaneous T-cell lymphoma: preliminary observations. In: Boss BD, Langman RE, Trowbridge IS, Dudlbecco R, eds. *Monoclonal antibody and cancer*. New York: Academic Press, 1983: 39-52.
30. Ford CH, Newman CE, Johnson JR, et al. Localization and toxicity study of a vindesine-anti-CEA conjugate in patients with advanced cancer. *Br J Cancer* 1983; 47: 35-42.
31. Krizan Z, Murray JL, Hersh EM, et al. Increased labeling of human melanoma cells *in vitro* using combinations of monoclonal antibodies recognizing separate cell surface antibenic determinants. *Cancer Res* 1985; 45: 4904-4909.
32. Ghose T, Blair AH. Antibody linked cytotoxic agents in the treatment of cancer: current status and future prospects. *J Natl Cancer Inst* 1978; 61: 657-676.
33. Ghose T, Blair AH, Uadia P, et al. Antibodies as carriers of cancer chemotherapeutic agents. *Ann NY Acad Sci* 1985; 446: 213-227.
34. Giardina SL, Schroff RW, Woodhouse CS, et al. Detection of two distinct malignant B-cell clones in a single patient using anti-idiotype monoclonal antibodies and immunoglobulin gene arrangement. *Blood* 1985; 66: 1017-1021.
35. Gilliand DG, Steplewski Z, Collier RJ, et al. Antibody directed cytotoxic agents: use of monoclonal antibody to direct the action of toxin A chains to colorectal carcinoma cells. *Proc Natl Acad Sci USA* 1978; 77: 4539-4543.
36. Goldenberg DM, DeLand FH. History and status of tumor imaging with radiolabled antibodies. *J Biol Response Modif* 1982; 1: 121-136.
37. Goodman GE, Beauimer P, Hellstrom I, et al. Phase I trial of murine monoclonal antibodies in patients with advanced melanoma. *J Clin Oncol* 1984; 3: 340-352.
38. Hinman LM. Calicheamicin immunoconjugates: influence of analog and linker modification on activity *in vivo*. *Antibody Immunocon Radiopharm*. 1990; 3(1): 59.
39. Houston LL, Nowinski R. Cell-specific cytotoxicity expressed by a conjugate of rincin and murine monoclonal antibody directed against Thy. 1.1 antigen. *Cancer Res* 1981; 41: 3913-3917.
40. Hurwitz E, Levy R, Maron, et al. The covalent binding of daunomycin and Adriamycin to antibodies with retention of both drug antibody activities. *Cancer Res* 1975; 3: 1175-1181.
41. Hwang KM, Foon KA, Cheung PH, et al. Selective antitumor effect on L-10 hepato-carcinoma cells of a potent immunoconjugate composed of the A chain fo abrin and monoclonal antibody to a hepatoma-associated antigen. *Cancer Res* 1984; 44: 4578-4586.
42. Hwang KM, Foon KA, Cheung PH, et al. Selective antitumor effect of a potent immunoconjugate composed of the A chain of abrin and monoclonal antibody to a hepatola associate antigen. *Cancer Res* 1984; 44: 4578-4586.
43. Hwang KM, Keenan AM, Frincke J, et al. Dynamic interaction of 111 indium-labeled monoclonal antibodies with surface of solid tumors visualized in vivo by external scintigraphy. *J Nat Cancer Inst* 1986; 76: 849-855.
44. Johnson JR, Ford CMG, Newman E, et al. A vindesine-anti-CEA conjugate cytotoxic for human cancer cell in vitro. *Br J Cancer* 1981; 44: 472-477.
45. Larson SM, Brown JP, Wright PW, et al. Imaging of melanoma with I-labeled monoclonal antibodies. *J Nucl Med* 1983; 24: 123-129.
46. Lee FH, Hwang KM. Antibodies as specific carriers for chemotherapeutic agents. *Cancer Chemother Pharmacol* 1979; 3: 17-25.
47. Levin LV, Griffin TW, Haynes LR, Sedor CJ. Selective cytotoxicity for a colorectal carcinoma cell line by a monoclonal anticarcinoembryonic antigen antibody coupled to the A chain ricin. *J Biol. Response Modif* 1982 1: 149-162.
48. Levy R. Biologicals for cancer treatment: Monoclonal antibodies. *Hosp Pract* 1985; November 15: 67-92.
49. Liao SK, Meranda C, Avner BP, et al. Immunohistochemical phenotyping of human solid tumors with monoclonal antibodies in devising biotherapeutic strategies. *Cancer Immunol Immunother* 1989; 28: 77-86.
50. Miller RA, Levy R. Response of cutaneous T-cell lymphoma to therapy with hybridoma monoclonal antibody. Lancet 1981; 2: 226-230.
51. Miller RA, Maloney DG, Warnke R, et al. Treatment of B-cell lymphoma with monoclonal anti-idiotype antibody. *N Engl J Med* 1982; 306: 517-522.
52. Ogden JR, Leung K, Kundra SA, et al. Immunoconjugates of doxorubicin and murine antihuman breast carcinoma monoclonal antibodies prepared via an n-hydroxysuccinimide active ester intermediate of *cis*-aconityl-doxorubicin: preparation and *in vitro* cytotoxicity. *Mol Biother* 1989; 1(3): 170-174.
53. Ohkawa K, Hibi N, Tsukada Y. Evaluation of a conjugate of purified antibodies against human AFP-dextran-daunorubicin to human AFP-producing yolk sac tumor cell lines. *Cancer Immunol Immunother* 1986; 22: 81-86.
54. Oldham RK. Monoclonal antibodies in cancer therapy. *J Clin Oncol* 1983; 1: 582-590.
55. Oldham RK. Biologicals: new horizons in pharmaceutical development. J Biol Response Modif 1983; 2: 199-206.
56. Oldham RK. Biologicals and biological response modifiers: fourth modality of cancer treatment. *Cancer Treat Rep* 1984; 68: 221-232.
57. Oldham RK. Therapeutic monoclonal antibodies: effects of tumor cell heterogeniety. In: *Present Status of Nontoxic Concepts in Cancer Therapy*, Cancer Treatment Symposium (Germany)' S Karger, 1986.
58. Oldham RK, Foon KA, Morgan AC, et al. Monoclonal antibody therapy of malignant melanoma: *in vivo* localization in cutaneous metastasis after intravenous administration. *J Clin Oncol* 1984; 2: 1235-1242.
59. Oldham RK, Morgan AC, Woodhouse CS, et al. Monoclonal antibodies in the treatment of cancer: preliminary observations and future prospects. *Med Oncol Tumor Pharmocol* 1984p; 1(2): 51-62.

60. Oldham RK. Antibody-drug and antibody toxin conjugates. in: Reif AE, nMitchell MS, eds. *Immunity to cancer*. New York: Academic Press, 1985: 575-586.
61. Oldham RK. Monoclonal antibodies: does sufficient selectivity to cancer cells exist for therapeutic application? *J Biol Response Modif* 1987; 6: 227-234.
62. Oldham RK. Immunoconjugates: drugs and toxins. In: Oldham RK, ed. *Principles of cancer biotherapy*. New York: Raven Press, 1987: 319-335.
63. Oldham RK. Monoclonal antibody therapy. In: Chiao JW, ed. *Biological response modifiers and cancer research*, Vol. 40. New York: Marcel Dekker, 1988: 3-16.
64. Oldham RK, Lewis M, Orr DW, et al. Individually specified drug immunoconjugates in cancer treatment. *Imperial Cancer Research Conference*, England, 1990.
65. Oldham RK. Who pays for new drugs? *Nature* 1988; 332(28): 795.
66. Oldham RK, Lewis M, Orr DW, et al. Adriamycin custom-tailored immunoconjugates in the treatment of human malignancies. *Mol Biother* 1988; 1(2): 103-113.
67. Oldham RK, Lewis M, Orr DW, et al. Individually specified drug immunoconjugates in cancer treatment. In: Ceriani RL, ed. *Breast cancer immunodiagnosis and immunotherapy proceeding*. 1990.
68. Oldham RK. Monoclonal antibodies. In: Nathanson L, ed. Management of advanced melanoma. *Contemporary issues in clinical oncology*. New York: Churchill Livingstone. 1986: 195-207.
69. Oldham RK. Custom tailored drug immunoconjugates in cancer therapy. *Mol Biother* 1991; 3(3): 148-162.
70. Orr DW, Oldham RK, Lewis M, et al. Phase I trial of mitomycin-c immunoconjugate cocktails in human malignancies. *Mol Biother* 1989; 1(4): 229-240.
71. Pavanasasivam G, Pearson JW, Bohn W, et al. Immunotoxins to a human melanoma asociated antigen: comparison of gelonin with ricin and other A-chain conjugates. *Cancer Res* 1987; 47: 3169-3173.
72. Pietersz GA, Smyth MJ, Kanellos J. Preclinical and clinical studies with a variety of immunoconjugates. *Antibody Immunocon Radiopharm* 1988; 1: 79-103.
73. Raso V, Raso J, Basala M, Schlossman S. Monoclonal antibody-ricin A chain conjugate selectivity cytotoxic for cells bearing the common acute lymphoblastic leukemia antigen. *Cancer Res* 1980; 42: 457-464.
74. Ritz J, Schlossman SF. Utilization of monoclonal antibodies in treatment of leukemia and lymphoma. *Blood* 1982; 59: 1-11.
75. Rowland AJ and Pietersz GA. Reduction in the toxicity of aminopterin-monoclonal-antibody conjugates by leucovorin. *Cancer Immunol Immunother* 1994; 39: 135-139.
76. Rowland AJ, Pietersz GA and McKenzie IFC. Preclinical investigation of the antitumour effects of anti-CD19-idarubicin immunoconjugates. *Cancer Immunol Immunother* 1993; 37: 195-202.
77. Schilsky RL. Tumor cell heterogeniety: implications for clinical practice. *Semin Oncol* 1985; 12: 203-206.
78. Schnipper LE. Clinical implications of tumkor cell heterogeniety. *N Engl Med* 1986; 314: 1423-1431.
79. Schroff RW, Farrell MM, Klein RA, et al. T65 antigen modulation in a phase I monoclonal antibody trial with chronic lymphocytic leukemia patients. *J Immunol* 1984; 133: 1641-1648.
80. Schroff RW, Foon KA, Beatty SM, et al. Human anti-murine immunoglobulin responses in patients receiving monoclonal antibody therapy. *Cancer Res* 1985; 45: 879-885.
81. Schroff RW, Morgan AC, Woodhouse CS, et al. Monoclonal antibody therapy in malignant melanoma: factors effecting *in vivo* localization. *J Biol Response Modif* 1987.
82. Schroff RW, Woodhouse CS, Foon KA, et al. Intratumor localization of monoclonal antibody in patients with melanoma treated with antibody to a 250Kd melanoma associated antigen. *JNCI* 1985; 74: 299-306.
83. Sears HF, Herlym D, Steplewski Z, Koprowski H. Effects of monoclonal antibody immunotherapy in patients with gastrointestinal adenocarcinoma. *J Biol Response Modif* 1984; 3: 138-150.
84. Sears HF, Mattis J, Herlyn D, et al. Phase-1 clinical trial of monoclonal antibody in treatment of gastrointestinal tumors. *Lancet* 1982; 1: 762-765.
85. Shawler DL, Johnson DE, Sweet MD, et al. Preclinical trials using an immunoconjugate of T101 and methotrexate in an athymic mouse/human T-cell tumor model. *J Biol Response Modif* 1988; 7: 608-618.
86. Sivam G, Comezoglu FT, Vrudhula VM, et al. Immunoconjugates of a small molecule protein synthesis inhibitor (trichothecene)–an update. *Antibody Immunocon Radiopharm* 1990; 3(1): 63.
87. Sobol RE, Dillman RO, Smith JD. Phase I evaluation of murine monoclonal antimelanoma antibody in man: preliminary observations. In: Mitchell MS, Oettgen HF, eds. *Hybridomas in cancer diagnosis and treatment*. New York: Raven Press, 1981: 199-206.
88. Spitler L. Clin Cancer Lett 1986; 9: 1-2.
89. Stastny JJ and Das Gupta TK. The use of daunomycin-antibody immunoconjugates in managing soft tissue sarcomas: nude mouse xenograft model. *Cancer Res* 53: 5740-5744, 1993.
90. Takahashi T, Yamaguchi T, Noguchi A, et al. Clinical trial of monoclonal antibody-drug conjugate, A7-NCS, for 70 patients with colorectal cancer. *Antibody Immunocon Radiopharm* 1990; 3(1): 60.
91. Thorpe PE, Ross WCJ. The preparation and cytotoxic properties of antibody-toxin conjugated. *Immunol Rev* 1982; 62: 119.
92. Tsukada Y, Hurwitz E, Kashi R, et al. Chemotherapy by intravenous administration of conjugates of daunomycin with monoclonal conventional anti-rat-alpha-fetoprotein antibodies. *Proc Natl Acad Sci USA* 1982; 79: 7896-7899.
93. Uckun FM, Evans WE, Forsyth CJ, et al. Biotherapy of B-cell precursor leukemia by targeting genistein to CD19-associated tyrosine kinases. *Science* 267: 886-891.
94. Vogel C-W, ed. *Immunoconjugates: antibody conjugates in radioimaging and therapy of cancer*. New York; Oxford University Press, 1987.
95. Von Hoff DD. Implications of tumor cell heterogeneity for in vitro drug sensitivity testing. *Semin Oncol* 1985; 12: 327-331.
96. Yarbro JW. Introduction: tumor heterogeniety and the new biology. *Semin Oncol* 1985; 12: 201-202.
97. Youle RJ, Neville DM. Anti-Thy-1.2 monoclonal antibody linked to ricin is a patient cell-type-specific-toxin. *Proc Natl Acad Sci USA* 1980; 77: 5483-5486.
98. Second conference on radioimmunodetection and radioimmunotherapy of cancer. *Suppl Cancer Res* 1990; 50(3): 773s-1059s.

RADIOLABELED MONOCLONAL ANTIBODIES FOR LOCALIZATION AND TREATMENT OF METASTATIC CANCER

HAZEL B. BREITZ[1], PAUL L. WEIDEN[2], ALAN R. FRITZBERG[3], JOHN M. RENO[3] and PAUL G. ABRAMS[3]
[1]*NeoRx-Virginia Mason Clinical Research Unit, Seattle, WA,* [2]*Virginia Mason Medical Center, Seattle, WA,*
[3]*NeoRx Corporation, Seattle, WA*

Current diagnostic imaging procedures are commonly used to view a circumscribed part of the body such as head or thorax. Conventional nuclear medicine imaging procedures such as bone scans may be directed at an organ system, but only recently have single diagnostic imaging procedures become available to search the entire body and all tissues simultaneously for tumor deposits. Antibodies to tumor associated antigens, and ligand-receptor based imaging agents, such as the recently approved somatostatin receptor binding peptide, ^{111}In pentetreotide, offer the opportunity to image tumors directly. Other radiolabeled imaging agents, such as ^{201}thallium, ^{99m}Tc-MIBI and positron emitters such as ^{18}F-fluorodeoxyglucose (FDG) localize in areas of increased cellularity, vascularity or increased metabolism.

External-beam radiation therapy is an essential part of the management of patients with cancer. While current dose fractionation and simulation planning techniques have improved efficacy and reduced toxicity, its general application is in treating local or regional disease. Even when external beam radiation therapy can cure more extensive cancer (e.g., Stage III Hodgkin's disease or metastatic seminoma), the efficacy of standard radiation therapy depends upon the absence of tumor cells outside the radiation ports. Monoclonal antibodies, used as vehicles to target radioactivity directly to tumor cells, offer the promise of overcoming this deficiency in therapy. An appropriate antibody construct could potentially reach and selectively bind to tumor cells anywhere in the body.

In patients with cancer, radioimmunoscintigraphy (RIS) or radioimmunodetection (RAID) is the imaging of radiolabels delivered by antibodies directed against tumor associated antigens. If the antibody is radiolabeled with gamma emitting radionuclides such as ^{99m}Tc, ^{131}I, ^{123}I, or ^{111}In, it may be visualized with a gamma camera which can detect discrete areas of count accumulation. Other diagnostic modalities, such as CT or MRI, may then be directed to suspicious areas to confirm metastatic disease. Several large trials have been conducted establishing the safety of intravenous administration of radiolabeled monoclonal antibodies and they have helped define the clinical utility of RIS in the management of patients with cancer. Of most interest is that, unlike all other diagnostic techniques, successful diagnostic imaging strategies with radiolabeled monoclonal antibodies have direct predictive value in patient selection for radioimmunotherapy including internal radiation dose estimates and treatment outcome.

Radionuclides that emit particulate radiation especially those that deposit energy close to the source, e.g. beta or alpha emitters, have therapeutic potential. Thus, radionuclides such as ^{131}I, ^{186}Re, ^{188}Re, ^{67}Cu, ^{90}Y, ^{211}At, ^{212}Pb, and ^{212}Bi may be linked to antibodies to deliver radiotherapy to tumor cells.

Clearly, the goal in both imaging and therapy applications is to use the specificity of the antibodies to target tumors and avoid normal tissues. This chapter will address the issues of tumor targeting with antibodies, including radionuclide selection (Table 1). Results from clinical trials for detecting and treating cancer will be reviewed.

Table 1. Parameters influencing labeled antibody studies

Antibody	Antigen – Location, cellular density, modulation, circulating density, modulation
	Affinity
	Specificity
	Mass
	Molecular form – Intact, fragments
	Form-murine, chimeric, humanized, human,
Radionuclide	Half-life
	Emissions-type, energy, abundance
	Chemistry
Radiolabel	Specific activity
	Percent protein bound
	Immunoreactivity
	Aggregates
Serum	Pharmacokinetics
	Metabolism
Tumor	Tumor size, vascularity, tumor burden,
Antiglobulins	radiosensitivity

R.K. Oldham (ed.), Principles of Cancer Biotherapy. 3rd ed., 348–368.

CHOICE OF ANTIBODY

Early radiolocalization studies performed with polyclonal antibodies suggested that more homogeneous antibodies were required in order to be clinically useful. Hybridoma technology has permitted careful selection of monoclonal antibodies directed to particular tumors such that antibodies with the highest localization and binding potential and with the lowest cross reactivity may be identified. Reviews of the characteristics of the antibodies that must be considered have been published and will be described briefly [3, 4].

Antigen

Antigen density, location of the antigen, and whether shed or internalized following binding are important in determining tumor localization. Antigen density above 10^5 sites/cell appears to predict for better localization. Whether most of the antigen is expressed on the cell surface or in the stromal matrix surrounding tumor cells must be known. Antibodies to solid tumors can target intracellular antigens or antigens in the mucin pools. In contrast, most lymphoma antigens are found on the cell surfaces. How antigens modulate, internalize and are metabolized once internalized are important issues. Generally, stable cell surface antigens that internalize slowly offer the best target for imaging and therapy with most radionuclides. Circulating antigen, although likely to bind with antibody, does not necessarily interfere with tumor localization [14, 23, 116, 117] .

Specificity

It is typical to initially assess specificity by immunohistochemistry studies on frozen sections of normal and malignant tissues, but localization studies in humans are necessary to determine the ultimate usefulness of a particular antibody. Normal tissue cross-reactivity by immunohistology may not be seen *in vivo* with internal antigens or antigen that is inaccessible to circulating antibodies. Most murine antibodies studied to date have various levels of normal tissue cross-reactivity. When used in RIS applications, quantitative differences in specific binding of antibody to tumor and normal tissues must be sufficient to be able to identify small tumors. In RIT applications, the therapeutic index for tumor and normal tissues must be favorable when compared to untargeted chemotherapy.

Generally, antibodies with less cross-reactivity and those directed to relatively dense and homogeneous cell surface antigens will be the best candidates. Specific localization in tumor sites has been demonstrated using antibody to secreted or intracellular antigens [29] and in some cases to antigens with extensive normal tissue expression. Uptake by human RES cells has been noted with different antibodies or antibody subclasses. Greater localization in the RES of an intact antibody compared with its F(ab')2 fragment has implied that Fc receptors are partially responsible for this interaction [19].

Fc interactions between tumor bound antibody and the immune system can be beneficial in mediating tumor cell destruction via antibody dependent cellular cytotoxicity (ADCC) or complement mediated cytotoxicity (CMC). For example, tumor targeting with radiolabeled antibody L6, an IgG2a antibody which reacts with a membrane bound antigen on human adenocarcinomas, was improved after predosing with cold antibody 24 hours earlier [37]. It was suggested that ADCC and CMC increased tumor permeability and thus improved delivery of subsequent radiolabeled antibody.

Molecular form

Murine monoclonal antibodies may be utilized as the whole antibody, (MW=150, 000 daltons), or fragmented by enzyme digestion to the $F(ab')_2$, (MW=100,000 daltons) and Fab fragments (MW=50, 1000 daltons) or using recombinant DNA technology to generate stabilized Fv fragments(MW 25,000 daltons). The serum half-life of whole murine immunoglobulin in man is approximately 24-30h. The $F(ab')_2$ has an intermediate T½ of approximately 10-12h and may be cleaved to Fab' *in vivo*. Fab or Fab' fragments have a serum T½ of approximately 90 min, and single chain Fv fragments clear from the plasma with an alpha T½ of 0.1 hour and a beta phase clearance of 2.7 hours [48]. Choice of the molecular form depends on an appreciation of the relative rate of tumor uptake and serum clearance. The standard pharmacokinetic 'concentration x time' will influence the antibody accumulation at the tumor. Monovalent Fab and Fv forms may have comparable affinity to whole antibodies but have reduced avidity, and retention at tumor tissue is shorter than with bivalent species.

Choice of antibody form will also be influenced by the choice of radionuclide. For example, faster tumor targeting and blood disappearance are required for the short-lived ^{99m}Tc and ^{123}I than for ^{131}I and ^{111}In. For therapeutic applications the concentration and disappearance time from the serum affect the normal organs as well as the tumor tissue, and normal organ toxicity may be seen as an innocent bystander effect. Animal studies have shown improvements in the ratio of tumor to blood (background) radioactivity when fragments are compared with whole antibodies [48]. While this gain in contrast is useful for radioimaging applications, the loss in fraction of the dose localized (%ID/gm) as well as the loss in time retained at tumor limits the potential for targeted radiotherapy applications for Fab, and especially for Fv constructs. In addition, the major processing organ for Fab and Fv constructs is the kidney and with radionuclide attachment chemistry that results in intracellular retention, the kidney may be a dose limiting organ in radioimmunotherapy.

Affinity

Monoclonal antibodies can be selected with adequate affinities (10^{-8} mol/l or greater) to bind antigen at the tumor site. Higher-affinity antibodies ($\geq 10^{-10}$ mol/l) were suggested to have increased uptake at low doses relative to antigen [143]. Thus, they would then be more likely to complex with circulating antigen, to bind more extensively to low levels of antigen in normal tissues and be more affected by binding site barriers limiting penetration into tumors [149]. However, one controlled human clinical study comparing first generation anti-tumor associated glycoprotein-72 with newer, higher affinity antibody showed no improvement in tumor uptake, nor any alteration in pharmacokinetics nor normal organ distribution [53].

Antibody mass

Localization of some antibodies is influenced by the mass of antibody administered [95, 100, 105, 155]. In patients with melanoma, improved localization and increased rate of tumor detection was noted by Carrasquillo et al using 60 mg ^{111}In 9.2.27 antibody compared with 1 mg of antibody [22], and by Murray et al. with 20 mg ^{111}In ZME-018 antibody compared with 2.5 mg antibody [100]. In patients with colon carcinoma increasing antibody mass of ^{111}In-ZCE025, increased the rate of positive detection of liver lesions by decreasing the relative amount of radiolabeled antibody localizing non-specifically in the liver [105]. However, Miraldi demonstrated that when using 3F8 antibody, only 1 mg was required for 95% accuracy in tumor detection of neuroblastoma [95]. Recently the trend has been to administer the least amount of antibody compatible with a high detection rate for imaging to conserve antibody and to reduce the likelihood of human anti-murine antibody development [91]. Each radiolabeled antibody must be assessed for the lowest antibody dose that is required for successful, effective imaging.

For radioimmunotherapy, the antibody mass dose that will deliver the highest radiation dose to the tumor tissue without toxicity is desirable. The effect of antibody mass on pharmacokinetics and absorbed dose to tumor and normal organs has been studied in several phase I radioimmunotherapy trials in patients with B-cell lymphoma. Press et al studied patients with a trace label of ^{131}I and increasing antibody mass doses to determine the optimal biodistribution for therapy. Increasing the antibody dose of MB-1 to 10 mg/kg improved the tumor to normal organ dose ratio, but with 1F5 and B1 antibodies, biodistribution was unchanged and a favorable distribution could be achieved with 2.5 mg/kg [120]. Kaminski et al administered 10 mg labeled MB-1 either alone or following 135 mg or 685 mg unlabeled antibody and found that the effect on tumor to normal organ absorbed dose ratio was variable [72]. Scheinberg evaluated four dose levels of OKB7, from 0.1 to 40 mg and found that antibody mass dose had little effect on pharmacokinetics [133]. DeNardo et al. showed little difference in pharmacokinetics when administering 5 or 50 mg ^{131}I-Lym-1, although preloading with these doses prolonged clearance and improved distribution. Increasing the antibody dose to 448 mg Lym-1 had no effect on clearance, perhaps suggesting that less than 5 mg Lym-1 saturates the antigenic pool of this antibody [32]. Thus, as for antibody imaging, each antibody must be individually assessed to find the optimal dose of labeled antibody (and of unlabeled antibody) for radioimmunotherapy.

Human anti-murine antibodies (HAMA)

One of the primary concerns in the clinical use of murine monoclonal antibodies has been the development of HAMA. Repeat administration of a murine antibody in the face of existing HAMA can result in the formation of immune complexes with alterations in the normal organ distribution and increased rate of clearance of injected monoclonal antibodies with or without inhibition of the localization of the antibody to tumor cells. Subsequent complex-mediated tissue damage may present as serum sickness or a variant thereof.

Specificity is of primary importance in analyzing an HAMA response and in designing strategies to prevent or minimize it. In most cases, the antiglobulins cross-react with most or all mouse immunoglobulin classes [135]. However, in some cases a component of the HAMA response appears to be specific for the administered antibody (anti-idiotypic). Evidence of anti hapten responses which may occur against the radioisotope chelate have recently been identified [75].

HAMA response rates appear to be dependent upon the disease group being treated, the particular antibody being injected and the antibody form [39, 74]. Patients with chronic lymphocytic leukemia and Hodgkins disease demonstrate decreased HAMA responses after exposure to monoclonal antibodies. Patients with solid tumors have, in general, significant HAMA production, especially in those cases where multiple infusions are given [39, 14].

Several investigators have examined the relative immunogenicity of whole antibody molecules versus fragments [69, 130]. We found that both $F(ab')_2$ and Fab fragments are immunogenic in humans [14] but our data indicates that both types of fragments are less immunogenic than intact antibodies. For example, only a fraction of non-small cell lung cancer patients exposed to NR-LU-10 Fab developed HAMA [47] compared to 100% of patients with a variety of tumor types given intact NR-LU-10 [14]. NR-LU-10 is a murine IgG_{2b} monoclonal antibody that recognizes an epithelial glycoprotein antigen. Sixty one percent of patients with solid tumors given one dose and 86% of patients receiving two doses of the $F(ab')_2$ fragment of NR-CO-02, a murine IgG_1 monoclonal antibody that recognizes the CEA antigen, developed a significant HAMA titer and the mean antibody titer was higher after two doses [14]. Also HAMA responses to a murine $F(ab')_2$ fragment were easier to suppress with Cyclosporin A than were HAMA response to an intact murine antibody [85, 148].

The clinical relevance of HAMA may vary in different clinical circumstances and would be expected to be dependent on HAMA titer. For example, Nabi showed the relative safety of repeated administrations of radiolabeled antibody and the value of antibody imaging in detecting tumor recurrence even in the presence of HAMA [103]. In a multiple dose protocol we reimaged three patients with elevated HAMA levels and found that in one patient with only modestly elevated HAMA titer (80 x baseline), biodistribution was unchanged. In the patients with high HAMA titers (400 and 5000 fold increased) however, there was immediate immune complex formation and localization of activity within the RES with no tumor targeting. A similar alteration in tumor localization was reported with chimeric ^{131}I-B72.3 antibody in patients with elevated anti-antibody levels [94].

Clearly, successful use of radiolabeled antibodies in multi-administration protocols will require neutralizing the impact of HAMA. Consistent elimination of HAMA will most likely require genetically engineered antibody constructs.

CHIMERIC, HUMANIZED AND NOVEL ANTIBODY CONSTRUCTS AND HUMAN ANTIBODIES

In recent years recombinant DNA technology has been applied to monoclonal antibody engineering. The first generation of engineered molecules were human/murine chimeric antibodies produced by substituting the human constant region for the murine constant region, retaining the murine variable portions of the antibody that imparts specificity.

Further genetic engineering of the antibody molecule has produced constructs with only minimal portions of the murine immunoglobulin variable regions. These molecules, known as humanized antibodies, are more than 90% 'human'[68].

Although humanization of monoclonal antibodies and the development of fully human anti-tumor antibodies have so far eliminated the problem of human antiglobulin response[18, 97], it is important to recognize that their use will not eliminate the potential problems associated with an anti-idiotypic response against the unique portions of the engineered monoclonal antibody.

Additional engineering using recombinant DNA technology has produced 'novel antibody constructs'. These include alterations of antibody domains to retain or enhance certain properties, for example, affinity enhancement and addition or elimination of complement fixation activity.

Antibody fragments and single chain antibodies have been produced in bacteria. Fragments from bacteria will dramatically reduce the cost and increase the batch-to-batch homogeneity of the products. Most recently, phage display libraries have produced novel antibody specificities by recombinations of heavy and light regions [65]. Single chain Fv(sFv) molecules of 25 kD have been evaluated in animal studies and found to penetrate into tumors more rapidly but their absolute tumor uptake (%ID/g) and retention is poor due to low avidity. Multivalent dimeric and trimeric molecules, with higher avidities, have shown longer retention at the tumor [73]. The full clinical utility of these new molecules remains to be realized and clinical trials to assess immunogenicity and clinical performance are yet to be reported. Improved complement fixation should enhance effector function and perhaps, specific delivery to target cells.

Choice of radionuclide

The choice of radionuclide with which to label antibodies is governed by several considerations including physical properties such as mode of decay, energy and abundance and half-life; chemical properties affecting protein attachment and *in vivo* handling; and finally production aspects including specific activity, availability at needed scale, and cost. Recognition of the advantages and disadvantages of the available choices is important since different strategies are required to maximize their potential.

Diagnostic

Radionuclides suitable as imaging agents for diagnostic purposes are limited to those with sufficiently high abundance gamma rays, preferably with energies between 100 and 200 keV, for which current gamma cameras are most efficient. Particulate radiation should be minimal to maximize safety. The physical half-life ($T_{1/2}$) must be adequate to permit localization into tumor and background clearance, but not so long as to remain in tissues long after the images are obtained. Properties of radionuclides of primary interest for radiolabeled antibody imaging will be briefly discussed.

Technetium-99m (^{99m}Tc) has been the radionuclide of choice and is used for most nuclear medicine imaging procedures. Its 140-keV gamma-ray energy and high photon flux are ideal for imaging, and current gamma cameras have been optimized for the properties of ^{99m}Tc. The short $T_{1/2}$ of 6 hours and lack of particulate radiation provide a wide margin of safety. ^{99m}Tc is inexpensive, generator produced in high specific activity, and routinely available in all nuclear medicine departments. Its major drawback for antibody labeling is the requirement for rapid kinetics of tumor localization and background clearance because of the short half-life. This is compensated for by the feasibility of using doses of 30 mCi, and by the superior image resolution it provides. Until recently, its complex chemistry hindered efforts to achieve controlled, stable attachment to proteins.

Iodine is easily incorporated into activated aromatic rings such as contained in the tyrosine moiety of proteins by conventional chemistry using several procedures [155]. Iodine-131 (^{131}I), although inexpensive and readily available, has a high gamma-ray energy (364-keV) that degrades images. The relatively long half-life of 8 days and particulate beta emissions limit the total dose that may be administered for imaging studies to 5 mCi. Iodine-123 (^{123}I) has attractive physical qualities for imaging. It has a 159-keV gamma-ray energy and a half-life of 13 hours without particulate radiation, but is very expensive. Radioiodinated proteins are susceptible to radiolabel loss when cell processing occurs. In this instance, enzymatic release of iodine from the tyrosine catabolite occurs.

Indium-111 (^{111}In) has two gamma-ray energies of 173 and 247 keV. The higher energy emission contributes to image degradation, but its $T_{1/2}$ of 67 hours and lack of particulate radiation make ^{111}In a reasonable alternative to ^{99m}Tc and ^{123}I for slower targeting whole antibody forms on the basis of physical characteristics. However, it is moderately expensive, and often requires further purification for antibody labeling.

Therapeutic

The choices of radionuclides for labeling antibodies for therapy are more varied and complex than for the imaging application[145, 150]. It is likely that more than one radionuclide will be suitable. In addition, it has been suggested that therapy radionuclides of different energies and particle types may be more or less suitable in treating different size lesions.

Types of emissions considered are beta particles (electrons with a range of energies), alpha decay (in which helium +2 particles are emitted), and low energy Auger electron emissions which are a byproduct of electron capture decay. While the particulate property of the radiation decay mode determines the therapeutic potential, gamma ray emission often associated with the radiation decay provides the ability to image the biodistribution in vivo, thus indicating tumor localization and non-target uptake and retention. Ideally, gamma radiation should be of low abundance such that contribution to non-target organ irradiation is minimized.

Beta particle decay

A wide range of beta emitter energies of emission and half life are available for radioimmunotherapy. Howell [63], Humm [64] and Wheldon [152] have considered the application of beta emitters with respect to emission energy and penetration, number of cell traversals and size of tumor targets. Beta emitters have the unique advantage of exerting their cytotoxicity by a crossfire effect as only occasional beta particles result in lethal DNA double strand breaks. When sufficient concentration of emissions occur in a tissue volume, the probability of lethal hits increases, predominantly from sources bound to other cells. This crossfire killing property obviates the need for targeting every cancer cell in contrast to antibody targeted delivery of drug or toxin conjugates. This crossfire effect is efficient for tumor masses larger in diameter than the average beta path length. If the clinical target consists of micrometastases as in the adjuvant setting, clusters of cells may range from several thousand (0.1mm) to 10^5 cells (1mm). Low energy emitters such as ^{33}P, ^{121}Sn, ^{177}Lu, or ^{199}Au would have their energy most efficiently absorbed in these size tumors. Medium energy range emitters including ^{47}Sc, ^{67}Cu, ^{131}I, ^{153}Sm and ^{186}Re result in variable fractions absorbed depending on energy range. In larger tumors, high energy beta emitters are efficiently absorbed and ^{32}P, ^{188}Re, or ^{90}Y are more suitable. Comparisons have been made by Humm [64] resulting in estimates of 54% absorption of particles for ^{131}I (0.61 MeV maximum) in a 1 mm cluster while the high energy ^{90}Y (2.3 MeV maximum) results in only 10% beta absorption. Further analysis by Wheldon and coworkers suggest that moderate or lower energy emitters should be used for clusters of up to 10^7 cells while an emitter such as ^{90}Y should be used for tumors of 10^8 cells or greater [152].

Dose rate is another factor modifying therapeutic efficacy, particularly for beta emitters. External beam radiation is given at a much higher rate than internally administered radionuclides. In radioimmunotherapy, radiation is delivered in the range of 10 to 30 rad/hr and continuously decreasing because of decay. Generally, effectiveness of cell killing goes down as the dose rate lowers because more time is available for repair of sub-lethal damage [45]. Considering the dose rate effect, some have suggested that 20 to 30% more rads are needed to sterilize tumors compared to fractionated external beam treatment [38, 46]. Review of radioimmunotherapy in animal xenografts by Wessels, however, suggests dose effects from radioimmunotherapy are comparable to external beam [151]. An inverse effect resulting in enhancement of low dose rate effects has been observed in which cells accumulate in the radiosensitive G_2 stage of the cell cycle which may contribute to efficacy of the low dose rate radiation of radioimmunotherapy. The dose rate factor, while complex, is one that may be important and must be kept in consideration.

Alpha particle decay

With the large He particle emitted, alpha decay results in high linear energy transfer (LET) or energy delivery over a distance of only several cell diameters. This results in the advantages of high potency and lack of oxygen dependence with correspondingly no shoulder on the cell survival curve. The short path length, however, results in the need for much more homogeneous targeting for complete tumor cell kill. Alpha emitters that have been studied for antibody mediated tumor targeting include ^{212}Bi ($t_{1/2}$ 1.06 hr) and ^{211}At ($t_{1/2}$ 7.2 hr). As these are short lived radionuclides, applications have been mainly in leukemia and lymphoma models. Macklis and co-workers[90] determined aspects of ^{212}Bi labeled antibody in lymphoma. Only 27 cell-bound ^{212}Bi atoms and 4 alpha-particle tracks ('hits') of ^{212}Bi were required for a log of target cell killing. The limitation for homogeneous targeting of alpha emitters is greater with solid tumors which are often poorly vascularized and may be access limited by high interstitial pressure due to poor lymphatic drainage [67]. Toxicity to normal tissue can be high due to the potency of alpha radiation and lack of repair potential of double-stranded DNA lesions. However, antibody pretargeting in which a non-radiolabeled antibody is administered first allowing time and dose to achieve greater homogeneity, would enable subsequent injection of the alpha emitter on a rapidly penetrating small molecule to quickly access tumor cells potentially overcoming both short half life and homogeneity issues in the treatment of solid tumors.

Auger-low energy electron emissions

Decay by electron capture results in emission of electrons at a range from a few to several hundred keV. While these are weak energies, occurrence in the proximity of nuclear DNA causes high cellular lethality. Several studies using ^{125}I, ^{123}I, and ^{77}Br on nuclear targeting forms such as halogenated pyrimidines have shown a steep dose response curve with no shoulder [5]. With an internalizing antibody and a mechanism for intracellular translocation to the region of the nucleus, radiotherapy with these emitters can be as selective as the antibody. A significant limitation, however, is that homogeneous tumor cell targeting is required in addition to the nucleus targeting mechanism.

Radionuclide half life

Half life considerations include time for targeting and retention at tumor in order to deliver a tumor dose commensurate with radionuclide dose fraction delivered to tumor. With whole antibodies, maximum tumor uptake requires 24 to 48 hours, but tumor retention can be for several days [15, 48]. Thus, with conventionally radiolabeled antibodies, i.e. injected with radionuclide attached, the half life must be long enough for tumor uptake as well as tumor irradiation during time of useful tumor to non-tumor ratios for normal tissues. As examples, ^{131}I (8 day $t_{1/2}$), ^{186}Re (3.7 day $t_{1/2}$) and ^{90}Y (2.7 day $t_{1/2}$) are suitable for whole antibody pharmacokinetics. When delivered via the pretargeting approach (see section on pretargeting), tumor delivery is essentially immediate and the more important consideration is matching radionuclide half life with time of tumor retention.

The combination of radionuclide physical properties with antibody forms and their pharmacokinetics has been evaluated with respect to optimal radiation delivery potential [154]. Several moderate to high energy beta emitters and ^{211}At as an alpha emitter were modeled as if targeted via whole IgG, $F(ab')_2$ or Fab forms. Combination of physical properties and pharmacokinetics as well as non-target organ uptake and retention data generated on these antibody forms in mice suggested ^{90}Y, ^{153}Sm and ^{186}Re to be the most promising for radioimmunotherapy when used to treat relatively large tumors.

Antibody radiolabeling for imaging

Iodine

The earlier studies of radiolocalization with monoclonal antibodies used ^{125}I or ^{131}I as the radionuclide due to availability and ease of incorporation into tyrosyl residues on antibody as mentioned previously. The release of radioiodine as iodide following cellular processing has for some antibodies compromised tumor retention and resulted in thyroid and stomach uptake. Partial blockage of uptake results from Lugol's solution, but with high therapy doses, concern for toxicity to these organs exists. The release of radioiodine as iodide can be avoided by attachment of the iodide on non-activated phenyl rings using reagents such as *p*-iodophenyl [153].

^{111}Indium

^{111}In has favorable imaging properties and a half-life long enough for use with whole antibody forms and much effort has gone into applications for it with radioimmunoimaging. Indium chemistry is characterized by +3 valence metal chelation and polyamino acids have been utilized as bifunctional chelates. The diethylenetriaminepentaacetic acid (DTPA) chelate used initially was unstable and the released ^{111}In bound to transferrin and thus accumulated in the reticuloendothelial system. For details regarding structural modifications for optimization of stability and minimization of normal organ uptake and retention, reviews are available [49, 54, 62, 112]. In the case of ^{111}In-B72.3, the product Oncoscint™, the polyamino acid chelating agent DTPA was conjugated to the antibody via a glycyltyrosyllysyl (GYK) linker using carbohydrate groups[127]. This allowed the bifunctional chelating group to be located remotely from the antibody binding sites and avoid loss of immunoreactivity of the antibody. Animal studies appeared promising, but in clinical trials problems with detection of hepatic lesions were seen (see discussion elsewhere in the chapter). Other work involved increasing stability by chelate modification. Improvements have been demonstrated in animal model studies as a result of controlled conjugation chemistry as well as optimal numbers of donor atoms and spatial arrangements. Results in patients, however, have been disappointing in that radioactivity uptake and retention in liver has continued to generally be a problem. The most promising results have been seen with benzyl-DTPA derivatives developed by Brandt and Johnson [13] and evaluated in patients by Divgi et al. [40]. They reported 52% visualization of hepatic lesions compared to previous studies in which liver metastases were often 'cold spots' or indistinguishable from normal liver uptake on scans.

Tc-99m

Technetium is available as pertechnetate, +7 oxidation level, and forms stable chelates at various lower oxidation levels depending on a combination of reducing agents and donor atoms. For details on applications to antibody labeling, reviews are available [48, 49, 52, 60]. As appropriate donor atoms are available in proteins for +5 oxidation level chelation of technetium, several groups have optimized binding of ^{99m}Tc to endogenous protein donor atoms, primarily involving sulfhydryl groups [137]. In order to increase stability of binding, bifunctional chelates have been used by several groups. Extensive application of N, S amide thiolate chelating agents with antibody fragments has been developed by Fritzberg et al. [52].

Antibody radiolabeling for therapeutic radionuclides

Yttrium-90

Yttrium-90, (^{90}Y) has high energy beta emission (Emax 2.27 MeV) and has been the object of much effort for radiotherapy via antibody targeting. Although it is a +3 metal and has similar chelation chemistry to indium and iron, yttrium is generally less stably held. Once released, a significant fraction of ^{90}Y is taken up by bone resulting in radiation of bone marrow cells. Dose limiting bone marrow toxicity at relatively low administered radioactivity levels of 15 to 25 mCi has been observed [61, 110]. Also, the accumulation of ^{90}Y in the liver may lead to hepatic toxicity as the second organ of dose limiting toxicity. Gansow and coworkers have synthesized and tested a number of acyclic and cyclic amino acids as bifunctional chelates [54]. Although improvement was seen via the benzyl DTPA analogs, only the cyclic DOTA appeared stable relative to release of ^{90}Y to bone [20].

Rhenium-186/188

The radioisotopes of rhenium, ^{186}Re (E beta 1.07 MeV) and ^{188}Re (E beta 2.12 MeV), have desirable physical properties for radiotherapy and have been investigated for use in radioimmunotherapy. Rhenium is in the same group as technetium on the periodic table. The structures of chelates of technetium and rhenium are virtually identical, but rhenium is harder to reduce from available perrhenate (+7) to lower oxidation level rhenium than is technetium for chelation. In addition, rhenium has slower kinetics of chelation. Both rhenium beta-emitting isotopes can be linked to antibody with the N, S amide thiolate chelate systems as described for ^{99m}Tc [50].

Additional parameters in analyzing radionuclide-antibody studies

In addition to the antibody and the radionuclide, the radiolabeled antibody reagent itself must be evaluated (Table 1).

Knowledge of the specific activity and the percentage of protein-bound counts is critical in interpreting the biodistribution of the radioactivity. High-performance liquid chromatography (HPLC) can separate forms on the basis of hydrodynamic radius which is proportional to molecular weight (gel filtration)and charge (ion exchange), for analysis of the different molecular weights of the radioactive components in the preparation. Thin layer chromatography is used to assess the percentage of protein bound counts. Serum should be monitored for antibody and radioactivity independently. Stable labels will show a serum disappearance parallel to the antibody. Analysis of the labeled material for immunoreactivity to the antigen should be performed and compared to an established standard. Immunoreactivity should be assessed following radiolabeling and based on radioactivity, and not protein, as done in calorimetric developed ELISAs. The only species measured in vivo is the radiolabeled form and when high specific activity radioactivity is used, it is possible that non immunoreactive species are preferentially labeled. Competition experiments with unlabeled antibody can provide an indication of relative affinities.

Parameters affecting the bioavailability of the labeled antibody for the tumor site should be measured following injection. Uptake in tumor depends on the serum concentration over time. Thus, it is important to measure blood disappearance curves, urine excretion, whole-body retention, presence of circulating antigen. Unlabeled antibody may be able to block antigenic sites on normal tissue which interfere with localization at the tumor.

Characteristics of the tumor and its location must considered. Background activity in the areas of particular interest should be low, such that the antibody localization can be distinguished from normal metabolites and cross-reactive sites. The vascularity and size of the tumor will determine the ability of the antibody to penetrate fully into the tumor lesions. For imaging, this is less important than for therapy where localization throughout the tumor is desirable. For therapy, the tumor burden and the radiosensitivity must also be considered.

Biopsies of tumor and other organs should be obtained in animal studies to determine the percent of the injected dose per gram tissue that localized. In patients, when biopsies of tumor are not possible, one must usually be satisfied with quantitative estimation of tumor activity from region of interest (ROI) analysis using the gamma camera images. Counts detected by the gamma camera are compared to a calibration standard for the camera to assess the radioactivity within a particular region of interest, organ or tumor. Time activity curves from selected regions can be used to estimate radiation absorbed dose, knowing the physical characteristics of the radionuclide [15]. These estimates of radiation absorbed dose from therapeutic radiolabeled antibodies can be useful to assess the safety of the radioimmunoconjugate. Although myelosuppression is always the first sign of radiation toxicity in dose escalation studies, and can be easily monitored, prior treatment with myelotoxic chemotherapeutic agents makes correlation of toxicity with estimates of radiation absorbed dose complicated. Thus, one must consider the baseline function, prior therapy as well as the absorbed dose estimates when attempting to predict effects of therapy on normal organs. As yet, data on radiation absorbed dose to tumor is insufficient to correlate with tumor response rates. Continued work in this area is desirable so that tracer studies would be able to accurately predict radiation absorbed dose, which will be valuable in selecting patients for treatment and in treatment planning.

Pretargeting techniques

Conventionally radiolabeled antibodies remain in the blood pool for long periods of time exposing the normal organs, especially the radiosensitive bone marrow, to radiation. This limits the dose that can be safely administered and ultimately limits the efficacy of the approach. Antibodies, being relatively large molecules also do not penetrate the tumor tissue rapidly or to a great extent. An alternative approach is to administer the antibody and the therapeutic radioisotope separately. Of course, some means of bringing them together at the tumor needs to be devised. This is a very attractive approach since the targeting specificity of the antibody is retained, but the whole body radiation dose is substantially decreased if the radioisotope administered as a small molecule rapidly clears the body. Goodwin et al pioneered the use of bifunctional antibodies by pre-localizing an unlabeled antihapten antibody in tumors and then administering a labeled hapten that is cleared from the blood stream rapidly [57].

Another approach utilizing pretargeting takes advantage of the ultra-high affinity avidin-biotin system ($Kd=10^{-15}M$). Amplification of tumor dose is also a possibility with this technique as each avidin has four biotin binding sites[113]. Avidin-biotin is widely used in *in vitro* applications but was first translated into *in vivo* localizing strategies by Goodwin, Meares and McCall[57]. Antibody pretargeting has potential for both imaging and therapy applications. Both avidin and its bacterial counterpart streptavidin have been used in pretargeting applications. Two and three step pretargeting approaches have been described with the antibody carrying either the avidin /streptavidin or biotin [113, 114]. The potential of this approach for therapy applications is particularly great and will be discussed below.

Radioimmunoscintigraphy (RIS)

The first human use of radiolabeled monoclonal antibodies was reported in 1981 by Mach et al. [89] who successfully imaged tumors using ^{131}I-labeled antibodies to CEA. The RIS literature has been reviewed in detail by Larson [80, 81], Kramer [77], Carasquillo [21] and reviews of RIS in melanoma [40], colorectal [104], lung [16] and ovarian and prostate [107] cancer have been published. Radioimmunoscintigraphic studies in a variety of carcinomas using ^{131}I, ^{123}I, ^{111}In, and ^{99m}Tc labeled antibodies and antibody fragments have been carried out [1, 2, 12, 19, 23, 27, 30, 40, 41, 42, 47, 55, 69, 78, 80, 86, 91, 95, 97, 99, 103, 104, 105, 116, 119, 129, 138, 139, 144]. The advantages and disadvantages of the different radionuclides have been discussed above. When sensitivity of detection was compared in the same patient with an ^{111}In and ^{131}I-labeled antibody to CEA, the ^{111}In-labeled antibody detected more of the known lesions than ^{131}I-labeled antibody and showed the lesions with greater certainty [45]. *In vitro*, ^{111}In is found to be retained longer within the cells than ^{131}I, probably due to retention of catabolic products within the lysosomes[92, 106]. Improved sensitivity of ^{99m}Tc compared with ^{111}In labeled to the same antibody, 225.28S was demonstrated by Siccardi [139]. Some of the important findings from the clinical trials and the role of RIS will be discussed.

Melanoma

Larson et al. performed the first systematic human studies of ^{131}I-labeled monoclonal antibodies in patients with melanoma. The unpredictability of the spread of melanoma makes a whole body imaging study particularly valuable for staging patients prior to surgery. Using Fab fragments, they reported approximately 60% of known sites detectable by RIS with more than 90% of the patients having at least one site detected [22, 80].

Salk et al. reported the results of the first formal phase III multicenter trial of a radiolabeled monoclonal antibody for imaging tumors [131]. The Fab fragment of NR-ML-05, an antibody directed at a 250-kD melanoma-associated antigen, was labeled with the ^{99m}Tc-N_2S_2 bifunctional chelate. There was no significant RES localization, although biliary and renal excretion were visualized. Unlabeled whole NR-ML-05 was preinjected to block nontumor, cross-reactive antigen. Important observations from this study included the safety of the procedure. Allergic reactions were observed in only 2% of the patients, all of whom had histories of atopy. HAMA responses, however, were high (over 80%). This study showed that antibody imaging detected an equal number, but a noncongruent set of lesions compared to conventional diagnostic imaging techniques. This observation appeared to be unrelated to antigen distribution, and more related to site and size of the tumor. In a small, but definite, subset of patients the detection of lesions by antibody imaging made a difference in patient care despite the prior evaluation of the patient with standard techniques. The study concluded that as a single test that can evaluate all anatomic regions simultaneously, RIS is highly accurate (97%) for establishing a patient's stage of disease.

Lung cancer

Imaging studies of patients with lung cancer reached a similar conclusion. As a single, noninvasive test, RIS is rapid and accurate for staging patients [12, 78]. Although the sensitivity is approximately 90% for primary tumors, the specificity is not high enough to be useful for diagnosis.

A phase III trial using the ^{99m}Tc N_2S_2 preformed chelate conjugated to the Fab fragment of NR-LU-10, a pancarcinoma antibody, was carried out in patients with previously untreated, newly diagnosed SCLC. The positive predictive value of antibody imaging for establishing a diagnosis of extensive disease was over 95%. (Fig. 1)

Antibody imaging alone was shown to be almost as accurate as a large standard battery of conventional tests (chest x-ray, CT-abdomen, bone scan, CT-head) in distinguishing limited and extensive disease SCLC.

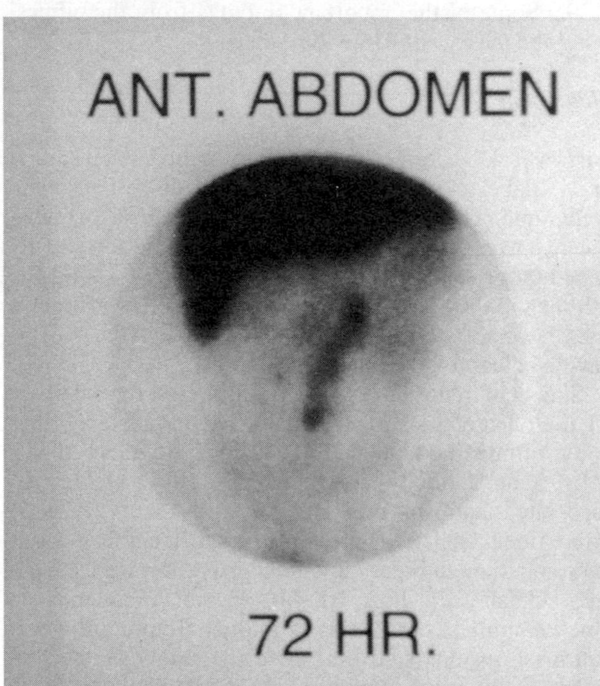

Figure 1. A 75 year old female patient with small cell lung cancer 18 hours following ^{99m}Tc NR-LU-10. She was known to have right supraclavicular lymphadenopathy and a right pleural based mass from a chest CT scan. A bone scan was negative. The posterior chest antibody images demonstrated activity in the known sites of disease, and additionally, right hilar and mediastinal nodes were identified. These were confirmed on CT. The multiple skeletal abnormalities were confirmed to be marrow lesions by MRI and a positive bone marrow aspirate.

Single photon emission tomography (SPECT) imaging markedly improved the detection of pulmonary and mediastinal metastases. Bone marrow metastases were also occasionally detected by the imaging procedure. Second injections of the antibody agent were administered without evidence of altered pharmacokinetics, biodistribution, or toxicity in over 40 patients.*

Colorectal carcinoma

^{111}In-CYT-103 or Oncoscint CR/OV-In, (CYTOGEN Corp., Princeton, NJ) was approved by the US FDA in 1992 as the first diagnostic radioimmunoconjugate for evaluation of recurrent colorectal and ovarian carcinoma. This was based on its accuracy, efficacy, clinical utility and safety. The imaging performance of Oncoscint is similar to that of other immunoconjugates for colorectal carcinoma and will be described. CYT-103 consists of 1 mg of intact monoclonal antibody B72.3 conjugated with the site specific linker chelator GYK-DTPA and is radiolabeled with 5 mCi ^{111}In [127] B72.3 is a murine IgG1 that recognizes a mucin-like high molecular weight protein, referred to as tumor-associated glycoprotein TAG-72, and is expressed in several epithelial derived malignancies. Oncoscint CR/OV was studied in 155 patients with surgically confirmed colorectal carcinoma, 82 with primary disease and 73 with recurrent disease [27, 91]. RIS was carried out at 72-120 hours. The overall sensitivity per patient was approximately 70% and specificity was 77% with an overall accuracy of 70%. For recurrent disease, sensitivity (64%) and specificity (71%) were lower. The overall tumor detection rates for RIS and CT scan were similar (60%) but in only 49% of patients were the CT and antibody scan both positive. The different performances of the two diagnostic modalities depended to some extent on the location of the lesions. In the extrahepatic abdomen and pelvis, the antibody scan was more sensitive than the CT scan: 66% in the abdomen and 74% in the pelvis, compared with 57% and 34% respectively. However, in the liver, CT was more sensitive: 84% vs 41%. This is because localization of ^{111}In in normal liver tissue masks uptake in hepatic metastases. In colorectal cancer patients with carcinomatosis, a situation in which other diagnostic tests are of limited value, the antibody scan was positive in 70% of patients. In 12% of patients, occult disease was identified by RIS.

Patient management was altered in a subset of patients by results of the antibody scan. RIS was useful in defining the presence and extent of disease, in detection of occult lesions, in confirming that suspected disease was localized and therefore resectable, and in clarifying equivocal findings on other diagnostic tests. RIS accurately localized regional or distant metastases more often when compared to standard workup. Of all patients studied,

* This product has now been approved as Verluma for the detection of extensive stage disease in patients with biopsy-confirmed, previously untreated small cell lung cancer.

3.5% had mild or moderate transient adverse events. HAMA developed in 39% of patients within 8 weeks and subsequently decreased in approximately half the patients.

Ovarian cancer

Surwit reported results in a trial of 103 patients with ovarian cancer who received intact antibody, CYT-103 (Oncoscint)[144]. Of 71 patients with ovarian carcinoma, tumor was detected in 48 patients (68%) with RIS, compared with 44% from CT imaging. In 20 of these 71 patients, occult disease was detected. The antibody detected 62 of 105 lesions (59%), Figure 2.

However, false positive localizations occurred in 17 patients, mainly due to nonspecific localization in benign ovarian tumors and in areas of inflammation. The sensitivity was higher in patients with primary disease than those with recurrent disease or those with a negative workup scheduled for second look surgery. Sensitivity also increased with lesion size as lesions ≥ 2 cm were more likely to be detected. In 17 patients with otherwise negative pre-surgical workups, the antibody-based imaging study detected disease in 6 patients. Carcinomatosis was detected in 71% of 38 patients by antibody scan but in only 45% by CT scan. Tumor lesions were correctly identified by both CT and antibody scan in 29 of 70 patients. The antibody images detected lesions in an additional 19 patients with negative CT scans and CT detected lesions in an additional 2 patients. The antibody image aided the presurgical evaluation in 27% of patients, by detecting occult disease, (n=9), or by confirming findings initially identified by other diagnostic tests (n=12). Thus again in this disease, RIS and the CT scan provide complementary information. However, because of low specificity of the antibody, the antibody imaging is not useful in distinguishing primary disease from benign disease. Also, a negative study should not be used to defer otherwise planned surgical exploration.

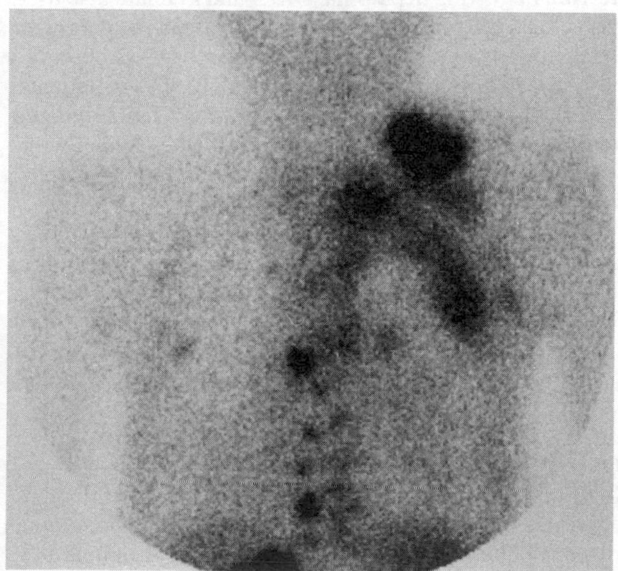

Figure 2. A 44 year old patient with ovarian cancer who had a mildly elevated CA-125 and negative abdominal CT scan. On the anterior abdominal image ^{111}In CYT-103 showed radiactivity in para-aortic lymph nodes which were confirmed at surgery to be the site of recurrent disease. Normal liver shows high radioactivity, typical of ^{111}In-labeled antibody studies.(Image courtesy of Dr. R.Maguire, CYTOGEN Corp; reprinted with permission from Marcel Dekker, inc).

The role of RIS in the management of cancer has been defined by these clinical trials. Total body scans using RIS can be used to stage disease. It can be used as an initial metastatic survey to direct physicians to efficient follow-on workup of the patient. RIS may have a role in the pre-operative workup of patients with a diagnosis of cancer as well as in their post-operative management. By detecting disease outside those regions routinely assessed by conventional techniques, RIS can improve the identification of patients with truly disseminated disease. Thus, results of local therapies (surgery and external beam radiation) may be improved by excluding patients upstaged by antibody imaging. However, the negative predictive value is not generally sufficiently high (i.e., 15-20% false negatives) for imaging to be used as a final determinant for the absence of metastatic disease.

The limitations of RIS are due to the low absolute tumor uptake of radioconjugate and also a low tumor to background ratio from the high level of long circulating conjugate in the blood. Biodistribution of the radioimmunoconjugate catabolites and cross-reactivity of antibodies to normal tissues antigens may interfere with tumor detection. The physical limitations on resolution imposed by gamma camera imaging technology also limit the detectability of lesions. Lesions larger than 2 cm can be generally visualized by planar imaging. Smaller lesions may require tomographic (SPECT) imaging to be visualized [119, 138]. As with all diagnostic techniques, the role of RIS will vary with different tumor types.

Pretargeting techniques

Clinical trials using bifunctional antibodies (BFA) have been reported by Stickney [142] with specificity for CEA as well as ^{111}In-labeled hapten, and by Le Doussal [84] also using an anti-CEA construct but with specificity for radiolabeled bivalent hapten. These bifunctional antibody systems demonstrated successful tumor imaging and reduced RES uptake compared to identical studies with ^{111}In-DTPA radiolabeled anti-CEA antibody. Hepatic metastases were detected as 'hot' spots rather than the 'cold' spots previously described and a high percentage of known lesions were identified. The BFA required 96 h to obtain optimal biodistribution before the radiolabeled hapten. Imaging was performed 72 h later for a total of 1 week from initial injection until results were obtained [142].

In a clinical pretargeting study using the avidin-biotin approach, Kalofonos reported that tumor detection with ^{111}In labeled biotin was improved by the prior administration of Mab-streptavidin conjugate 3 days earlier [70].

Paganelli reported an overall 88% sensitivity and 94% specificity with a 'three step' pretargeting approach using biotinylated antibody, avidin and finally ^{111}In-labeled biotin. Imaging studies were performed within 0.5 to 2 hours following administration of the radiolabeled biotin. A variety of tumors and antibodies were studied using this technique. The procedure was safe and well tolerated and the higher tumor to background activity ratios relative to conventional RIS gave improved sensitivity [113]. Mordorati conducted a cross-over study in patients with uveal melanoma comparing conventional RIS, using ^{99m}Tc, with three step pretargeting in the same patients a week later [96]. Conventional RIS yielded a diagnostic sensitivity of 71% whereas the three step pretargeting procedure showed a 100% diagnostic sensitivity. Dramatically reduced background activity was noted through the use of pretargeting, emphasizing the advantage of using a rapidly localizing and rapidly clearing low molecular weight radioligand.

Gamma detection probes

External scanning is also limited by the attenuation of the gamma rays from the overlying tissues. Small hand held gamma detection probes have been developed which can provide useful complementary information intraoperatively as to the presence and exact location of small lesions. The RIGS^R system localizes ^{125}I-labeled antibodies and is helpful to the surgeon in identifying tumor free margins in the surgical bed and has also identified previously unknown lesions[6]. Other detector probes which detect imageable gamma photons, ^{111}In and ^{99m}Tc are being evaluated in conjunction with pre-operative RIS [76, 97].

Radioimmunotherapy (RIT)

Beierwaltes' successful treatment of metastatic melanoma in a single patient with ^{131}I-labeled polyclonal antibody raised to the patient's own tumor was the first indication that RIT might be feasible [11].

Cheung et al achieved complete regressions of 0.45-2 cm^3 human neuroblastoma nude mouse xenografts by administering 0.5-1 mCi ^{131}I-labeled anti-G_{D2} monoclonal antibody [24]. The critical determinant of response was the radiation dose delivered to tumor, with complete responses achieved only with greater than 4200 rads. We have demonstrated [9] antibody-specific regressions and occasional cures of palpable small cell lung cancer xenografts in nude mice using ^{186}Re-labeled NR-LU-10 when the delivered dose to the tumor was 2800 rads. Recently, we have achieved reproducible cures of larger lung, colon and breast cancer xenografts using our pretargeting strategy [8].

Trends observed in small animals often translate into human studies, but dosing and timing may not be strictly comparable. A 1-cm (1 gm) tumor constitutes 5% of the total mass of the mouse; in a human it is approximately 0.0014%. The rapid metabolic rate and short circulation time of small animals exaggerate the pharmacokinetics of antibodies. Thus, any attempt to compare different agents in animals must be done recognizing the limitations of the model.

There is now emerging an increasing body of RIT clinical trials using radiolabeled antibodies. The pioneers in the human trials in this field are Order et al. who reported initial trials of ^{131}I and ^{90}Y-labeled antiferritin polyclonal antibodies [109, 110]. They showed that ^{131}I-labeled antiferritin polyclonal antiserum could produce regressions of bulky hepatomas [109]. Four of 24 patients had partial responses (PR) and one had complete response (CR). Single doses as high as 150 mCi were given with acceptable hematologic toxicity. Subsequent studies combined cytotoxic agents (5-FU and adriamycin) and external beam radiation with lower doses (50 mCi in divided doses) of antibody-labeled radiation and achieved a response rate of 48% (7% CR; 41% PR). They found monoclonal antiferritin inferior to polyclonal antisera, and ^{90}Y-labeled anti-ferritin to be superior to ^{131}I-anti-ferritin in treating hepatoma. Order and Lenhard also used polyclonal anti-ferritin antibodies to treat patients with Hodgkin's disease [87]. Symptomatic relief was observed in 77% and objective tumor regression in 40% of patients.

The majority of the clinical trials have utilized radiolabeled murine monoclonal antibodies alone, without other concomitant therapy, and ^{131}I, ^{90}Y or ^{186}Re as the radiolabel.

The most impressive results of RIT to date have been achieved in lymphoma, a relatively radiosensitive tumor. Press et al have reviewed results reported by various investigators using non-myeloablative dose of radioactivity and antibodies directed against a variety of lymphoid differentiation antigens, including HLA class II variant molecules, idiotypic immunoglobulin, the CD 5, 20, 21, 22 and 37 antigens, and the IL2 receptor [121]. Overall, 58 of 141 evaluable patients (41%) with hematologic malignancies treated with radiolabeled antibodies achieved objective partial or complete remissions with response durations of 2-15+ months. Myelosuppression, particularly thrombocytopenia was the major toxicity observed [120].

Several of these trials in patients with hematological malignancies deserve additional comment. In one of the first trials, Rosen and co-workers [128] treated a small series of patients with cutaneous T-cell lymphoma with up to 150 mCi of ^{131}I T101 antibody. Dramatic regressions were observed in skin and lymph nodes. Duration of response, however, was short, lasting 2-3 months at best.

Thrombocytopenia was the major toxicity. A second 100 mCi dose administered at 7 days resulted in severe bone marrow suppression.

DeNardo et al. [31, 32] treated 45 patients with B-cell malignancies with ^{131}I-labeled Lym-1. Lym-1 is an IgG2a antibody which reacts with a membrane antigen. Patients received 30-60 mCi ^{131}I-labeled Lym-1 antibody every 2-6 weeks to a total dose of 300-750 mCi, or 40 to 100 mCi/m^2 every 4 weeks. Acute toxicity (e.g., fever, rash) was mild and transient. Repeat doses of 80 mCi/m^2 could be administered with minimal toxicity limited to thrombocytopenia. Responses were observed in 30 of 45 patients, and 95% of patients who received more than 200 mCi of ^{131}I Lym-1 responded.

Kaminski et al. recently reported use of relative low-dose ^{131}I-labeled anti-CD20 (B1) antibody to treat patients with non-Hodgkin's lymphoma. Six of nine patients achieved either complete or partial responses at doses that produced negligible toxicity [72]. However, since three patients had objective responses to tracer infusions before they received radioimmunotherapeutic doses, other antitumor mechanisms may be working in concert in this form of treatment.

Press et al. have explored the use of myeloablative doses of ^{131}I labeled monoclonal antibody with autologous bone marrow support in patients with B cell lymphomas who had failed conventional chemotherapy [120]. In these studies, patients were selected for treatment after tracer studies determined the absorbed dose to tumor to be greater than that to normal organs. Thus 64% of patients screened were eligible for therapeutic doses of radiolabeled antibody. Patients were treated with marrow ablative doses of ^{131}I radiolabeled monoclonal antibody and achieved complete responses in 16 and partial responses in 2 of 19 patients with B-cell lymphoma. Mean response duration is in excess of 19 months. Patients received 234 – 777 mCi ^{131}I labeled MB-1 (anti CD37, IgG1 antibody) or 1F5 or B1 (anti-CD20, IgG2a antibodies). At absorbed doses above 2725 rad to lungs, patients experienced cardiopulmonary toxicity. Results have been most successful with radiolabeled anti-CD20 antibody probably due to the cytotoxicity of this IgG2a antibody in addition to the targeted radiation effect. A phase II study has repeated these results in obtaining responses in 15 of 19 patients [122].

One additional potential therapeutic role for radiolabeled monoclonal antibodies is to augment marrow irradiation prior to marrow transplants in patients with acute leukemia or other malignancies limited to the marrow cavity. Two groups of investigators demonstrated that ^{131}I-labeled monoclonal antibody reactive with the CD33 antigen could be used to treat patients with acute myeloid leukemia [7, 136]. Both groups delivered radiotherapy with relative specificity to the marrow in some, but not all, patients. Success appeared limited by low CD33 expression on target cells and by internalization of the antibody antigen complex leading to deiodination and release of ^{131}I. In a subsequent trial, Mathews et al. sought to overcome some of these problems by using BC8 antibody, a murine anti-CD45 antibody, which does not internalize but is reactive with 85-90% of cases of acute leukemia, and 70% of nucleated cells in normal marrow but not with cells outside the lymphoid or hematopoietic lineages. A recent phase I dose escalation trial demonstrated that ^{131}I-labeled anti-CD45 antibody could deliver 2-4x more radiation to the marrow and spleen than to normal organs, resulting in 20 Gy more radiation to the marrow without excessive toxicity [93].

Several radionuclides have been evaluated which appear to have superior properties to ^{131}I for therapy. Order reported responses following up to 30 mCi ^{90}Y antiferritin antibodies in patients with both Hodgkin's disease and hepatocellular carcinoma in conjunction with chemotherapy [110]. A response rate of 62% was reported recently in 27 patients with advanced Hodgkin's disease with ^{90}Y antiferritin [98]. Marrow toxicity at 30 mCi limited further dose escalation, although multiple infusions were administered in some patients. Bierman reported that 30 mCi ^{90}Y-polyclonal antiferritin combined with high-dose chemotherapy in patients with Hodgkins disease undergoing bone marrow transplantation did not cause any additional adverse effects. The marrow irradiation from the ^{90}Y did not cause increased toxicity nor did it interfere with re-engraftment [10]. Although no definite improvement in outcome could be attributed to the RIT, the lack of additional toxicities with the additional low dose rate irradiation suggests that further similar studies in patients with better performance status are warranted.

Clinical trials have also been initiated with ^{67}Cu. As with other metals, slower clearance from the tumor was noted compared with ^{131}I-labeled antibodies. However, radiation absorbed dose to liver may be a problem with this radionuclide because of localization in normal liver [33].

Radioimmunotherapy trials using monoclonal antibodies in patients with solid tumors began with Larson et al. [80] who performed the first phase I RIT study of a labeled monoclonal antibody fragment in patients with melanoma. Despite good localization of ^{131}I-labeled anti-97.5Fab with estimated doses of 3800-8500 rad to tumor, the antitumor effects were few and modest, one PR was obtained. The bone marrow was the first critical organ of toxicity as has been the case in all subsequent dose escalation RIT trials.

We have studied ^{186}Re-labeled monoclonal antibodies using the preformed chelate, MAG2-GABA in a series of Phase I trials in patients with solid tumors [14, 17, 66, 147]. Our results will be described to illustrate the challenges associated with RIT and the approaches to overcome them. The radioisotope-antibody conjugate is stable, and single doses of up to 300 mCi ^{186}Re/m^2 have been administered with toxicity limited to bone marrow. Murine, chimeric, and more recently, human antibodies labeled with ^{186}Re have been administered. Regional administration, concurrent immunosuppression, dose fractionation and autologous marrow and stem cell harvesting have been studied in an attempt to increase the therapeutic ratio and improve response rates [14, 17, 18, 66, 147].

Rhenium and technetium (Tc) have similar chemical properties and thus both can be conjugated to antibodies using the preformed chelate approach as discussed earlier. Our general approach has been to use the ^{99m}Tc labeled antibody Fab fragment as a tumor imaging agent. If the imaging study showed positive localization, the ^{186}Re-labeled antibody was then administered for therapy. Using the 3.7 day half-life and the imaging photon of ^{186}Re, we could confirm that the antibody-conjugate localized in tumor tissue and follow biodistribution in the normal organs.

^{186}Re-labeled NR-LU-10, a pancarcinoma antibody, was studied initially in fifteen patients with carcinoma of the GI tract, lung, ovary or kidney [14]. Patients were treated with the ^{186}Re immunoconjugate within 2 weeks of a ^{99m}Tc imaging study using the NR-LU-10 Fab fragment. Forty mg NR-LU-10 antibody was labeled with escalating doses of ^{186}Re, from 25 to 120 mCi/m^2. The ^{99m}Tc study was shown to be an accurate predictor of tumor localization of the ^{186}Re immunoconjugate. Severe but reversible myelosuppression was observed at the 120 mCi/m^2, but the absorbed dose to tumor was insufficient for tumor response.

Another study used the F(ab')$_2$ fragment of an anti-CEA variant murine monoclonal antibody designated NR-CO-02. The same antibody fragment was used for both ^{99m}Tc imaging and ^{186}Re therapy. In addition to using the imaging study to select the patients for therapy, we investigated whether predicting absorbed dose from the ^{99m}Tc study could allow us to determine the optimal ^{186}Re activity to be administered for radioimmunotherapy. Thirty-one patients with colorectal, lung or gastric cancer received ^{186}Re-labeled NR-CO-02 F(ab')$_2$. The dose levels studied ranged from 25 to 200 mCi/m^2 ^{186}Re. Pharmacokinetics and images with ^{99m}Tc and ^{186}Re were similar, and on average the predicted dosimetry compared favorably with the actual dosimetry to normal organs. Dosimetry projections were not sufficiently accurate for treatment planning for individual patients [15]. The maximum tolerated dose (MTD) was 125 mCi/m^2 in patients who were heavily pre-treated with radiation or chemotherapy more intensive than antimetabolites (e.g. 5-FU). The MTD was not reached at 200 mCi/m^2 in patients with limited prior therapy, although toxicity was seen in some patients.

We also administered ^{186}Re NR-CO-02 F(ab')$_2$ by hepatic artery catheter to 5 patients with liver metastases, but were unable to determine any advantage in tumor dosimetry from intra-arterial infusion. However, one patient with colon carcinoma achieved a partial response (PR) on two occasions following an intra-arterial dose of 83 and 89 mCi/m^2 respectively of ^{186}Re NR-CO-02 F(ab')$_2$.

Responses of solid tumors to RIT in other trials have also been infrequent in contrast to the lymphoma studies reviewed above. In patients with neuroblastoma, Lashford reported a complete remission(CR) in one of 5 patients [83] and Cheung reported a PR and prolonged stabilization of disease following doses of over 500 mCi ^{131}I-labeled 3F8, an antibody which is specific to GD ganglioside [25]. These patients received autologous bone marrow transplantation to overcome marrow toxicity.

Our initial trials demonstrated some of the challenges associated with current radioimmunotherapy, namely, significant HAMA formation and marrow toxicity prior to responses being achieved (Table 2).

Since single dose therapy is unlikely to produce significant responses in treating non-lymphatic solid tumors, we attempted to reduce HAMA formation to allow for multi-dose trials.

A chimeric derivative of the murine NR-LU-10, called NR-LU-13 was studied in 9 patients [147]. Although HAMA still occurred in 75% of patients following NR-LU-13 (compared with 100% following NR-LU-10), the human anti-chimeric antibody (HACA) titers were typically 10-1000 times lower than after administration of intact murine antibody. HACA responses after administration of other chimeric antibodies have been variable. Weak responses were observed following chimeric 17-1A antibody [88] and after chimeric L6 administration [56]. A higher incidence of HACA, however, has been found following chimeric B72.3 antibody although again this was lower than HAMA after murine B72.3 [94].

Table 2. Problems facing RIT and possible solutions

Problems	Potential solutions
Human-antibodies (HAMA)	• Chimeric antibodies • Humanized genetically engineered antibodies • Human antibodies • Immunosuppressive therapy
Marrow toxicity	• Marrow preservation: 1. Autologous marrow or peripheral blood progenitor cell rescue 2. Colony stimulating factors 3. Marrow protective agents 4. Dose fractionation • Decrease circulating radioactivity by 1. Clearing agent *in vivo* a Anti-antibodies b. Avidin/biotin system 2. Extracorporeal immuno-adsorption column
Inadequate tumor irradiation	• Increase antigenic expression e.g. α interferon, cytokines • Regional administration • Pretargeted approach, e.g., antibody/SA followed by isotope/biotin

Immunosuppression has been used in an attempt to reduce the immune response to monoclonal antibodies. Lederman et al. administered Cyclosporin A to suppress the development of HAMA in studies involving radiolabeled anti-CEA murine monoclonal antibodies with modest success [85]. In our studies, none of three patients given 15 mg/kg Cyclosporin A daily from 2 days prior until 14 days after administration of the murine $F(ab')_2$ fragment of NR-CO-02 developed HAMA. Eighty percent of patients who received Cyclosporin A 9-15 mg/kg daily and the intact murine NR-LU-10 developed HAMA, but the mean titer was lower than in those who had not received immunosuppression. Thus, although either chimeric antibodies or Cyclosporin A could reduce the development of HAMA, neither appeared to eradicate HAMA enough to permit repetitive radioimmunoconjugate administration to patients.

Therefore, we turned to human monoclonal antibodies and have studied two human antibodies labeled with ^{186}Re. Fourteen patients received up to three infusions of 100 mg ^{186}Re-16.88, a human IgM antibody, and eight patients have received single doses of 10 or 100 mg 88BV59, a human IgG antibody [18]. Clearance of these human radioimmunoconjugates was more rapid than expected [146]: 70% of the IgM antibody associated ^{186}Re, and 30% of the IgG associated ^{186}Re was excreted within 24 hours. There was no evidence of human anti-human antibody formation. However, tumor targeting was suboptimal indicating that these particular immunoconjugates were likely to be of limited usefulness for intravenous radioimmunotherapy, but establishing that repetitive doses of human monoclonal antibodies can be administered without evidence of alloimmunization.

The second major challenge facing RIT is marrow toxicity (Table 2). Approaches to reduce marrow toxicity include autologous marrow or peripheral blood progenitor cell harvest with reinfusion when the total body radioactivity is at low levels. For example, we continued dose escalation of ^{186}Re-NR-LU-10 to 300 mCi/m^2, utilizing autologous marrow or stem cell rescue, and have not observed a second organ of toxicity. Two of three patients with ovarian cancer treated in this way have achieved a PR (Fig. 3).

Recently, responses in patients with breast cancer and who received ^{90}Y-labeled BrE-3 antibody and peripheral blood stem cells were reported [140].

Other approaches to reduce marrow toxicity include administration of hematopoietic growth factors [34], dose fractionation [32, 134], or removal of non-targeted (but radiolabeled) antibody by a clearing agent [59]. Such a clearing agent could either be administered intravenously or be extracorporeal, i.e., part of an immunoabsorption column [36]. Candidate clearing agents include anti-antibodies directed at the Fc portion of the immunoconjugate or the avidin/biotin system with one component linked to the immunoconjugate and the other to the clearing agent [59].

DeNardo et al. have employed some of these approaches and have reported responses in patients with advanced breast cancer with multiple doses of ^{131}I-labeled chimeric antibody, L6 [35]. Some patients received G-CSF 7-20 days following infusion while others underwent immunophoresis using a goat anti-mouse antibody to reduce the non-bound circulating antibody. Four of 9 patients who were able to receive more than one dose achieved a PR [124].

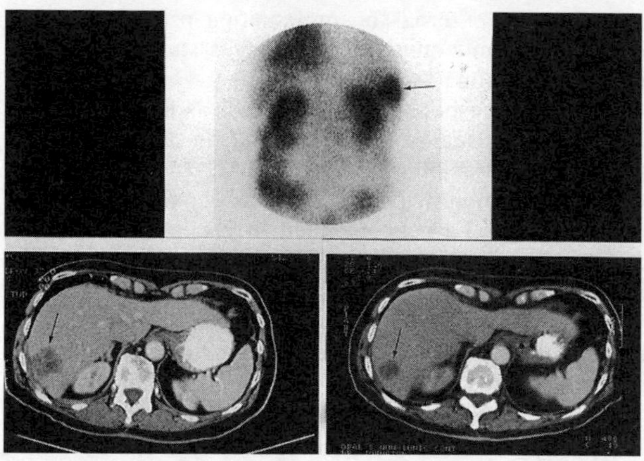

Figure 3. A 69 year old patient with ovarian cancer who achieved a partial response following radioimmunotherapy with 382 mCi ^{186}Re NR-LU-10. The posterior abdomen antibody image demonstrates uptake in a 3.8 cm hepatic metastasis. CT scans before treatment and 6 weeks later show a reduction in size of this metastasis. Additionally, para-aortic and inguinal lymphadenopathy showed a similar decrease in size.

An important reason for the poor results with systemic therapy using radioimmunoconjugates is the low uptake of antibody in tumors. Usually less than 0.01% per gram of the injected activity accumulates in tumor. Explanations for this low accumulation include restricted antigen expression on tumor cells, the small fraction of the cardiac output which reaches the tumor, and poor vascular permeability because of vascular spasm and high interstitial pressure. Decreased lymphatic drainage results in a high pressure gradient compromising transport towards the center. Thus, RIT may be most effective for small tumors which are more vascular, or manipulations to improve tumor blood flow may be worthwhile. Drugs to increase permeability have been studied in animals. Studies have also been performed to increase permeability by external beam radiation prior to administering immunoconjugate, but results vary with tumor type and location [71].

Biological response modifiers such as IL-2 and alpha interferon appear to be successful in increasing the antigenic expression of CEA and TAG-72 and increases targeting in tumors [101, 124] and, in fact, increased response rates have been noted in patients with breast cancer receiving alpha interferon in conjunction with ^{131}I-labeled CC49 RIT [102].

Regional administration of the immunoconjugates for RIT has met with some success because direct tumor cell exposure results in improved binding [26, 44, 66, 83].

Clinical trials with intraperitoneal injections of ^{131}I-, ^{90}Y- and ^{186}Re-labeled antibodies have been undertaken [61, 66, 126, 141]. Encouraging tumor responses were observed in patients with Stage III ovarian carcinoma who had tumor nodules less than 2 cm in diameter. [61, 66, 141]. Stewart reported 5/21 PR following ^{131}I antibodies [141]. Hird reported anti-tumor activity following ^{90}Y-HFMG but marrow toxicity limited the administered dose to <30 mCi, even with the addition of intravenous EDTA to chelate the unbound ^{90}Y [61]. Following intraperitoneal ^{186}Re-labeled NR-LU-10, 5 of 12 patients with minimal ovarian cancer achieved a PR. The MTD following intraperitoneal infusion, 150 mCi/m^2, was higher than following intravenous infusion, because of the reduced blood radioactivity accounting for less marrow exposure [17].

Riva reported results in patients with peritoneal gastrointestinal carcinomatosis who received 100 mCi ^{131}I-FO23C5 via the intraperitoneal and intravenous route. Therapy was administered in conjunction with Cyclosporin A every 3 months with up to 4 injections. Three complete and six partial responses were observed in 34 patients. Seventeen patients received alfa-interferon to increase the expression of CEA, this increased the response rate to 59% compared with 29% without alfa-interferon [126].

Pizer used intra-thecal ^{131}I-tumor specific antibodies for leptomeningeal recurrences of medulloblastoma, and reported 4/11 PR [118]. Riva administered ^{131}I-labeled antibody directly into malignant gliomas and achieved a 40% response rate [125].

We attempted to reduce toxicity by fractionating IP ^{186}Re NR-LU-10 dose. and administering a second dose of intraperitoneal ^{186}Re-NR-LU-10 7 days after the first dose [132]. At the highest dose level of 90 mCi/m^2 twice, i.e., 180 mCi/m^2, there was severe marrow toxicity in one of 3 patients. In contrast, similar toxicity was seen in 2 of 3 patients in the single dose study at only 150 mCi/m^2 [66]

Pretargeting

We are presently developing a pretargeted approach to therapy to reduce marrow toxicity. The step-wise delivery scheme involves as a first step, administration of non-radiolabeled, long-circulating antibody-streptavidin conjugate. After adequate time for the antibody to localize to tumor, a clearing agent is given to remove nonlocalized circulating antibody to the liver where it undergoes metabolism. Finally, a ^{90}Y chelate-biotin conjugate is administered, which localizes quickly to the tumor-antibody-avidin complex. The preclinical performance of our pretargeting system has been detailed by Axworthy and coworkers, who reported 80-100% cures of subcutaneous small cell, breast and colon carcinoma xenografts (250 mm^3) at ^{90}Y doses of up to 800μCi/mouse) with negligible hematologic toxicity [8].

Preliminary clinical data indicate that we have substantially improved the tumor to marrow absorbed dose ratios with acceptable radiation dose to other normal organs. The significant reduction in marrow toxicity we have observed using the pretargeting approach has also been noted by Paganelli and coworkers who administered total doses of 150 mCi ^{90}Y -DOTA-biotin, about 6 – 10 x the MTD by the conventional approach. Negligible hematologic toxicity and no acute or delayed side effects were seen [115]. Anti-tumor effects in patients with advanced bulky colon and ovarian cancers have been observed in our own studies.

Future investigations

The clinical trials have defined the value of RIS in the management of cancer patients, particularly in staging disease with a single diagnostic study. The use of antibody fragments in RIS has enabled the imaging to be performed earlier with adequate tumor to background ratios. The development of non-immunogenic radioimmunoconjugates for imaging will increase the acceptance of this imaging modality. Improvements in gamma camera technology has enabled smaller lesions to be visualized and increasing availability of these systems, with shorter imaging times for SPECT, will add to the efficiency of these studies. Although PET scanning provides improved resolution over gamma camera imaging, and has been evaluated for RIS, the high cost and limited facilities make PET imaging unlikely to become widely available in the foreseeable future.

The theoretical appeal of targeted therapy using radiolabeled antibodies and the tumor regressions observed in pre-clinical studies and in patients with B-cell lymphoma and leukemia have encouraged investigators to pursue solutions to the problems associated with RIT. Phase I trials in patients with solid tumors and phase II trials in patients with lymphoma are ongoing. Tumor regressions in some lymphoma studies have been consistent, and often complete and of long duration. Disappointing results in patients with solid tumors may be due, in part, to the selection of advanced stage patients who have failed prior treatments and have bulky disease.

Progress has been made in reducing the problems of HAMA formation and in decreasing marrow toxicity. Some chimeric antibodies showed comparable results to the murine antibodies although others resulted in poorer biodistribution characteristics. Chimeric antibodies have shown some reduction of the anti-antibody response. Clinical trials with human, humanized and genetically engineered antibodies have begun and the initial clinical study reports on some of the these antibodies indicate no appearance of HAMA allowing repeat dosing.

By radiolabeling the antibody directly, marrow toxicity has limited the amount of radioactivity that can be administered to less than that required to cause significant responses in most situations. Injected doses up to 600 mCi ^{186}Re and 770 mCi ^{131}I have been administered but marrow rescue was necessary at these high dose levels. The use of growth factors in conjunction with peripheral blood progenitor cell harvest has substantially decreased the toxicity of RIT allowing some tumors to receive lethal doses of radiation at tolerable doses to the patient. Either alternatively, or additionally, hematopoietic growth factors and radioprotectors may increase the dose intensity of RIT that can be safely administered to patients. Increasing the tumor to marrow exposure ratio through the use of antibody pretargeting should allow higher total activity to be administered, for the tumor to receive more radiation absorbed dose while marrow function is preserved and for earlier administration of growth factors due to much more rapid clearance of the radioactivity.

The inadequate delivery of radiation to tumor has been the major problem compromising RIT. Increasing the fraction of the radioimmunoconjugate that localizes in the target tumor tissue has been difficult. Regional approaches, such as intraperitoneal administration have increased the response rate. Attempts to increase fractional tumor uptake by upregulating antigen expression using alpha interferon and IL-2 or by increasing tumor blood flow using concurrent external beam radiation have been successful in some studies.

One current dilemma is the proper positioning of RIT and the design of future clinical trials. Should it be used as adjuvant therapy in patients with primary disease? Alternately, should RIT only be used in recurrent disease therapy trials until it proves to offer significant and consistent responses? Wessels has proposed that an additional 1500-2000 rads be delivered by RIT as a boost to external beam XRT [151]. Such an increment could have a dramatic effect on local control after XRT of lung or rectal cancer, for example. Pre-clinical studies with external beam therapy and RIT of liver metastases suggest that toxicities are additive. Thus, RIT with a radioimmunoconjugate that does not localize in normal liver tissue may be beneficial to treat hepatic metastases with additional radiation while sparing the normal liver tissue. Clinical studies with external beam therapy in conjunction with RIT in head and neck cancer are underway [43].

The technologies exist to link appropriate radionuclides to antibody, to redesign the carriers and to make multiple dosing possible. These improved carriers may be able to deliver an increased radiation dose to tumors and induce regressions. The future of radioimmunotherapy in patients with solid tumors appears to lie with one of the pretargeting approaches. The promise of pretargeting is to deliver tumoricidal doses without toxicities associated with current treatments. Recent results suggest that a sufficient commitment of resources may be the major requirement to fulfil that promise.

REFERENCES

1. Abrams P, Fer M, Faubion C, et al. A new procedure for staging small cell lung cancer (SCLC): gamma camera imaging using a technetium-99m labeled monoclonal antibody Fab. *Am Soc Clin Oncol* 1990; 9: A895.
2. Abrams PG, Morgan AC, Schroff RW, et al. Localization and biodistribution studies of a monoclonal antibody in patients with melanoma. In: Reisfeld, Sell, eds. *Monoclonal antibodies and cancer therapy*. New York: Alan R. Liss, 1985: 233-236.
3. Abrams P, Oldham R. Monoclonal antibody therapy of solid tumors. In: Foon KA, Morgan AC Jr, eds. *Monoclonal antibody therapy of human cancer*. Boston: Martinus Nijhoff, 1985: 103-120.
4. Abrams PG, Rossio JR, Stevenson HC, Foon KA. Optimal strategies for developing human monoclonal antibodies. *Methods Enzymol* 1986; 121: 107-119.
5. Adelstein SJ, Kassis AI. Radiobiologic implications of the microscopic distribution of energy from radionuclides. *Nucl Med Biol* 1987; 14: 165-169.
6. Arnold MW, Schneebaum S, Berens A, Mojzisik C, Hinkle G, Martin EW Jr. Radioimmunoguided surgery challenges traditinal decision making in patients with primary colorectal cancer. *Surgery* 1992; 112: 624-630.
7. Appelbaum FR, Matthews DC, Eary JF, et al. Use of radiolabeled anti-CD33 antibody to augment marrow irradiation prior to marrow transplantation for acute myelogenous leukemia. *Transplantation* 1992; 54: 829-833.
8. Axworthy DB, Fritzberg AR, Hylarides MD, et al. Preclinical evaluation of an anti-tumor monocloncal/streptavidin conjugate for pretargeted ^{90}Y radioimmunotherapy in a mouse xenograft model. *J Immunother* 1994; 16(2): 158.
9. Beaumier PL, Vanderheyden J-L, Venkatesan P, et al. Concurrent ^{186}Re radioimmunotherapy and chemotherapy of experimental small cell lung carcinoma. *Antibody, Immunoconjugates and Radiopharmaceuticals* 1991; 4(4): 735-744.
10. Bierman PJ, Vose JM, Leichner PK et al. Yttrium-90-labeled antiferritin followed by high-dose chemotherapy and autologous bone marrow transplantation for poor prognostic Hodgkin's disease. *J Clin Oncol* 1993; 11: 698-703
11. Bierwaltes WH. Radioimmunotherapy of cancer: Historical perspectives and prospects for the future. Text of talk delivered at the NATO Conference on Radiolabeled monoclonal antibody and external scintigraphy. *Science* 1979; 206: 844-847.
12. Biggi A, Gianfranco B, Ferrigno D et al. Detection of suspected primary lung cancer by scintigraphy with Indium-111-anti-carcinoembryonic antigen monoclonal antibodies (type F023C5). *J Nucl Med* 1991; 32(11): 2064-2068.

13. Brandt KD, Johnson DK: Structure-function relationships in indium-111 radioimmunoconjugates. *Bioconjugate Chem* 1992; 3: 118-125.
14. Breitz HB, Weiden PL, Vanderheyden J-L, et al. Clinical experience with Re-186-labeled monoclonal antibodies for radioimmunotherapy: Results of phase I trials. *J Nucl Med* 1992; 33: 1099-1112.
15. Breitz HB, Fisher DR, Weiden PL, et al. Dosimetry of Rhenium-186-labeled monoclonal antibodies: Methods, predictions from technetium-99m-labeled antibodies and results of phase I trials. *J Nucl Med* 1993; 34 (6): 908-917.
16. Breitz HB, Sullivan K, Nelp WB. Imaging lung cancer with radiolabeled antibodies. *Seminars in Nuclear Medicine* 1993; 23(2): 127-132.
17. Breitz HB, Durham JS, Fisher DR, et al. Pharmacokinetics and normal organ dosimetry following intraperitoneal rhenium-186-labeled monoclonal antibody. *J Nucl Med* 1995; 36(5): 754-761.
18. Breitz HB, Seiler C, Weiden P, et al. Re-186 16.88 IgM and 88BV69 IgG human antibody studies to assess potential for radioimmunotherapy. *J Nucl Med* 1994; 34(5): 100P.
19. Buraggi G, Turrin A, Bombardiere E, et al. Immunoscintigraphy of colorectal carcinoma with $F(ab')_2$ fragments of anti-CEA monoclonal antibody. *Cancer Detect Prev* 1987; 10: 335-345.
20. Camera L, Kinuya S, Garmestani K, et al. Comparative biodistribution of indium- and yttrium-labeled B3 monoclonal antibody conjugated to either 2-(p-SCN-Bz)-6-methyl-DTPA (1B4M-DTPA) or 2-(p-SCN-Bz) -1, 4, 7, 10-tetraazacyclododecane tetraacetic acid (2B-DOTA). *Eur J Nucl Med* 1994; 21: 640-646.
21. Carrasquillo JA, Krohn KA, Beaumier P, et al. Diagnosis and treatment for solid tumors with radiolabeled antibodies and immune fragments. *Cancer Treatment Report* 1984; 68: 317-328.
22. Carrasquillo JA, Abrams PG, Schroff RW, Reynolds JC, et al. Effect of ^{111}In-9.2.27 monoclonal antibody dose on the imaging of metastatic melanoma. *J Nucl Med* 1987; 26: 67.
23. Carrasquillo JA, Sugarbaker P, Colcher D, et al. Radioimmunoscintigraphy of colon cancer with iodine-131-labeled B72.3 monoclonal antibody. *J Nucl Med* 1988; 29: 1022-1030.
24. Cheung N-K., Landmeier B, et al. Complete tumor ablation with ^{131}I-labeled disialoganglioside GD2-specific monoclonal antibody against human neuroblastoma xenografted in nude mice. *JNCI* 1986; 77: 739-745.
25. Cheung N-K, Munn D, Kushner BH, Usmani N, Yeh SD. Targeted radiotherapy and immunotherapy of human neuroblastoma with GD2 specific monoclonal antibodies. *Int J Rad Appl Instrum (B)* 1989; 16: 111-120.
26. Colcher D, Esteban J, Carrasquillo JA, et al. Complementation of intracavitary and intravenous administration of a monoclonal antibody (B72.3) in patients with carcinoma. *Cancer Research* 1987; 47: 4218-4224.
27. Collier BD, Abdel-Nabi H, Doerr RJ, et al. Immunoscintigraphy performed with In-111-labeled CYT-103 in the management of colorectal cancer: comparison with CT. *Radiol* 1992; 185(1): 179-186.
28. Czucman MS, Nabi HA, Meredith RM, et al. Radioimmunotherapy of B-cell lymphomas with iodine-131-labeled LL2 monoclonal antibody. *J Immunother* 1994; 16(2): 160 (abs)
29. De Jager R, Abdel-Nabi H, Serafini A, Pecking A, Klein J, Hanna MG. Current status of cancer immunodetection with radiolabeled human monoclonal antibodies. *Semin Nucl Med* 1993; 23(2) 165-179..
30. Delaloye B, Bischof-Delaloye A, Buchegger F, et al. Detection of colorectal carcinoma by emission-computerized tomography after injection of ^{123}I-labeled Fab or $F(ab')_2$ fragments from monoclonal anti-carcinoembryonic antigen antibodies. *J Clin Invest* 1986; 77: 301-311.
31. DeNardo S, DeNardo G, O'Grady LF. Chronic lymphocytic leukemia and non-Hodgkins' lymphoma. *Front Radiat Ther Oncol* 1989; 24: 18
32. DeNardo GL, DeNardo SJ, O'Grady LF, Levy NB, Adams GP, Mills SL. Fractionated radioimmunotherapy of B-cell malignancies with 131-Lym-1. *Cancer Res* 1990; 50: 1014s – 1016s.
33. DeNardo GL, DeNardo SJ, Meares CF et al. Pharmacokinetics of copper-67 conjugated Lym-1, a potential therapeutic radioimmunoconjugate in mice and in patients with lymphoma. *Antibod Immunoconjug and Radiopharm* 1991; 4: 777-785.
34. DeNardo GL, DeNardo SJ, Kukis D et al. Strategies for enhancement of radioimmunotherapy. *NuclMed Biol* 1991; 18: 633-640..
35. DeNardo SJ, O'Grady LF, Warhoe KA, Kroger LA, Hellstrom I, Hellstrom KE, Maddock SW, et al. Radioimmunotherapy in patients with metastatic breast cancer. *J Nucl Med* 1992; 33(5): 862Abstr
36. DeNardo GL, Maddock SW, Sgouros G, Scheibe PO, DeNardo SJ. Immunoadsorption: An enhancement strategy for radioimmunotherapy. *J Nucl Med* 1993; 6: 1020-1027.
37. DeNardo SJ, Mirick GR, Kroger LA et al. The Biologic window for chimeric L6 radioimmunotherapy. *Cancer suppl* 1994; 73: 1023-1032.
38. Dillehay LE, Williams JR. Radiobiology of dose-rate patterns achievable in radioimmunoglobulin therapy. In: *The Present and Future Role of Monoclonal Antibodies in the Management of Cancer*. Front Radiat Ther Oncol. Vaeth JM, Meyer JL, Eds. Karger, Basel, 1990; 24: 96-103.
39. Dillman RO. Human antimouse and antiglobulin responses to monoclonal antibodies. Antibody, Immunoconjugates, and Radiopharmaceuticals 1990; 3(1): 1-15.
40. Divgi CR, Larson SM. Radiolabeled monoclonal antibodies in the diagnosis and treatment of malignant melanoma. *Seminars in Nucl Med* 1989; 19(4): 252-261.
41. Divgi CR, McDermott K, Griffin TW, et al. Lesion-by-lesion comparison of computerized tomography and indium-111-labeled monoclonal antibody C110 radioimmunoscintigraphy in colorectal carcinoma: A multicenter trial. *J Nucl Med* 1993; 34: 1656-1661.
42. Epenetos AA, Mather S, Granowska M, et al. Targeting of iodine-123-labeled tumor-associated monoclonal antibodies to ovarian, breast and gastrointestinal tumors. *Lancet* 1982; II: 999-1004.
43. Epenetos AA. Combined radiolabeled antibodies and radiotherapy for the treatment of head and neck cancer. *J Immunother* 1994; 16(2): 163 (abs).
44. Epenetos AA, Snook D, Durbin H et al Limitations of radiolabeled monoclonal antibodies for localization of human neoplasms. *Cancer Research* 1986; 46: 3183-3191.

45. Fairweather DS, Bradwell AR, Dykes PW, Vaughan AT, Watson-James SF, Chandler S. Improved tumor localization using indium-111 labelled antibodies. *British Med J* 1983; 287: 167-170. .
46. Fowler JF. Radiobiological aspects of low dose rates in radioimmunotherapy. *Br J Radiat Oncol Biol Phys* 1990: 18: 1261-1269.
47. Friedman S, Sullivan K, Salk D, et al. Staging non-small cell carcinoma of the lung using Technetium-99m-labeled monoclonal antibodies. *Hematology/Oncology Clinics of North America* 1990; 4(6): 1069-1078.
48. Fritzberg AR, Beaumier PL, Bottino BJ, Reno JR. Approaches to improved antibody- and peptide-mediated targeting for imaging and therapy of cancer. *J Controlled Release* 1994; 28: 167-173.
49. Fritzberg AR, Wilbur DS. Radiolabeled antibodies for targeted diagnostics. In: *Targeted Delivery of Imaging Agents*. Ed. V. Torchilin, CRC Press, Boca Raton, in press.
50. Fritzberg AR, Vanderheyden J-L, Morgan AC, Schroff RW, Abrams PG. Rhenium-186/-188 labeled antibodies for radioimmunotherapy. In: *Technetium and Rhenium in Chemistry and Nuclear Medicine*. Cortina Intl., Verona, pp615 – 621, 1990.
51. Fritzberg AR, Berninger RW, Hadley SW, Wester DW. Approaches to radiolabeling of antibodies for diagnosis and therapy of cancer. *Pharm Res* 1988; 5: 325-334.
52. Fritzberg AR, Abrams PG, Beaumier PL, et al. Specific and stable labeling of antibodies with technetium-99m with a diamide dithiolate chelating agent. *Proc Natl Acad Sci* 1988; 85: 4025-4029
53. Gallinger S, Reilly RM, Kirsh JC et al. Comparative dual label study of first and second generation antitumor-associated glycoprotein-72 monoclonal antibodies in colorectal cancer patients. *Cancer Research* 1993; 53: 271-278.
54. Gansow OA. Newer approaches to the radiolabeling of monoclonal antibodies by use of metal chelates. *Nucl Med Biol* 1991; 18: 369-381.
55. Goldenberg DM, Kim EE, DeLand FH, et al. Clinical radioimmunodetection of cancer with radioactive antibodies to human chorionic gonadotropin. *Science* 1980; 208: 1284-1286.
56. Goodman GE, Hellstrom I, Yelton DE, et al. Phase I trial of chimeric (human-mouse) monoclonal antibody L6 in patients with non-small cell lung, colon, and breast cancer. *Cancer Immunol Immunother* 1993: 36: 267-273.
57. Goodwin DA, Meares CF, McCall MJ, et al. Pretargeted immunoscintigraphy of murine tumors with indium-111-labeled bifunctional haptens. *J Nucl Med* 1988; 29: 266-334
58. Goodwin DA, Meares CF, Watanabe N et al. Pharmacokinetics of pretargeted monoclonal antibody 2D12.5 and ^{90}Y-Janus-2(p-nitrobenzyl)-1, 4, 7, 10-tetraazacyclododecanetetraacetic acid(DOTA) in BALB/c mice with KHJJ mouse adenocarcinoma: A model for radioimmunotherapy. *Cancer Res* 1994; 54: 5937-5946.
59. Goodwin DA. Tumor pretargeting: Almost the bottom line. *J Nucl Med* 1995; 36(5) 876-879.
60. Griffiths GL, Goldenberg DM, Jones AL, Hansen HJ. Radiolabeling of monoclonal antibodies and fragments with technetium and rhenium. *Bioconj Chem* 1992; 3: 91-99.
61. Hird V, Stewart JSW, Snook D, et al. Intraperitoneally administered ^{90}Y-labeled monoclonal antibodies as a third line of treatment in ovarian cancer, a phase 1-2 trial: problems encountered and possible solutions. *Br J Cancer* 1990; 10: 48-51.
62. Hnatowich DJ. Recent developments in the radiolabeling of antibodies with iodine, indium, and technetium. *Sem Nucl Med* 1990; 20: 80-91,
63. Howell RW, Dandamudi V, Rao, Sastry KSR. Macroscopic dosimtry for radioimmunotherapy: Nonuniform activity distributions in solid tumors. *Med Phys* 1989; 16: 66-74.
64. Humm JL. Dosimetric aspects of radiolabeled antibodies for tumor therapy. *J Nucl Med* 1986; 27: 10-1497.
65. Huse WD, Sastry L, Iverson SA, et al. Generation of a large combinatorial library of the immunoglobulin repertoire in phage. *Science* 1989; 246: 1275-1281.
66. Jacobs AJ, Fer M, Su F-M, et al. A phase I trial of a rhenium-186-labeled monoclonal antibody administered intraperitoneally in ovarian carcinoma: Toxicity and clinical response. *Obstet Gynecol* 1993; 82: 586-593.
67. Jain RK. Determinants of tumor blood flow: a review. *Cancer Res* 1988; 48: 2641-2658.
68. James K. Human monoclonal antibodies and engineered antibodies in the management of cancer. *Semin Cancer Biol* 1990; 1: 243-253.
69. Kalofonos HP, Sivolapenko GB, Courtney-Luck NS, et al. Antibody guided targeting of non-small cell lung cancer using ^{111}In-labeled HMFG1 F(ab')2 fragments. *Cancer Res* 1988; 48: 1977-1984.
70. Kalofonos HP, Rusckowski M, Siebecker DA, et al. Imaging of tumor in patients with In-111-labeled biotin and streptavidin-conjugated antibodies: preliminary communication. *J Nucl Med* 1990; 31: 1791-1796
71. Kalofonos HP, Rowlinson G, Epenetos AA. Enhancement of antibody uptake in human colon xenografts following irradiation. *Can Res* 1990; 50: 159-163..
72. Kaminski MS, Zasadny KR, Francis IR, et al. Radioimmunotherapy of B-cell lymnphoma with [^{131}I]anti-BI (anti-CD20) antibody. *N Engl J Med* 1993; 329(7): 459-465.
73. King DJ, Turner A, Farnsworth APH., et al. Improved tumor targeting with chemically cross-linked recombinant antibody fragments. *Cancer Research* 1994; 54: 6176-6185.
74. Klein JL, Leichner PK, Callahan KM, Laphar KA, Order SE. Effects of anti-antibodies on radiolabeled antibody therapy. *Antibody Immunocon Radiopharm* 1988; 1: 55-64.
75. Kosmas C, Maraveyas A, Gooden CS, Snook D, Epenetos A. Anti-chelate antibodies after intraperitoneal yttrium-90-labeled antibody immunoconjugates for ovarian cancer therapy. *J Nucl Med* 1995; 36(5): 746-753.
76. Krag DN, Haseman MK, Ford P, et al. Gamma probe location of ^{111}Indium-labeled B72.3: An extension of immunoscintigraphy. *Journ Surg Oncol* 1992; 51: 226-230.
77. Kramer EL, Larson SM. Tumor targeting with radiolabeled anti-body for diagnosis and therapy. *Immunology and Allergy Clinics of North America* 1991; 11(2): 301-339.
78. Krishnamurthy S, Morris JF, Antonovic R, Ahmed A, Galey WT, Duncan C, Krishnamurthy GT. Evaluation of primary lung cancer with Indium 111 anti-carcinoembryonic antigen (Type ZCE-025) monoclonal antibody scintigraphy. *Cancer* 1990; 65: 458-465.

79. Langmuir VK. Radioimmunotherapy: Clinical results and dosimetric considerations. *Nucl Med Biol* 1992; 19: 213-225.
80. Larson SM, Brown JP, Wright BW, et al. Imaging of melanoma with I-131-labeled antibodies. *J Nucl Med* 1983; 127: 539-546.
81. Larson SM, Carrasquillo JA, Krohn KA, Brown JP, et al. Localization of ^{131}I-labeled p97 specific Fab fragments in human melanomas as a basis for radiotherapy. *J Clin Invest* 1983; 72: 2101-2114.
82. Larson SM. Radioimmunology: Imaging and therapy. *Cancer Suppl* 1991; 67: 1253-1260.
83. Lashford LS, Davies AG, Richardson RB, et al. A pilot study of 131I monoclonal antibodies in the therapy of leptomeningeal tumors. *Cancer* 1988; 61: 857-868.
84. Le Doussal J-M, Martin M, Gautherot E, Delaage M, Barbet J. *In vitro* and *in vivo* targeting of radiolabeled monovalent and divalent haptens with dual specificity monoclonal antibody conjugates: Enhanced divalent hapten affinity for cell-bound antibody conjugate. *J Nucl Med* 1989; 30: 1358-1366.
85. Ledermann JA, Begent RHJ., Massof C, Kelly AMB, Adam T, Bagshawe KD. A phase-I study of repeated therapy with radiolabed antibody to carcinoembryonic antigen using intermittent or continuous administration of cyclosporin A to suppress the immune response. *Int J Cancer* 1991; 47: 659-664.
86. Leitha T, Walter R, Schlick W, Dudczak R. ^{99m}Tc-Anti-CEA radioimmunoscintigraphy of lung adenocarcinoma. *Chest* 1991; 99: 14-19.
87. Lenhard RE, Order SE, Spunberg JJ, et al. Isotopic immunoglobulin: A new systemic therapy for advanced Hodgkin's disease. *J Clin Oncol* 1985; 3: 1296.
88. LoBuglio AF, Wheeler RH, Trang J, et al. Mouse/human chimeric antibody in man: Kinetics and immune response. *Proc Natl Acad Sci USA* 1989; 86: 4220-4224.
89. Mach JP, Bucheggar F, Forni M, et al. Use of radiolabeled monocolnoal anti-CEA antibodies for detection of human carcinomas by external photoscanning and tomoscintigraphy. *Immunol Today* 1981; 2: 239-249.
90. Macklis RM, Lin JY, Beresford B, Atcher RW, Hines JJ, Humm JL. Cellular kinetics, dosimetry, and radiobiology of a-particle radioimmunotherapy: Induction of apoptosis. *Radiat Res* 1992; 130: 220-226.
91. Maguire RT, Schmelter RF, Pascucci VL et al. Immunoscintigraphy of colorectal adenocarcinoma: Results with site specific radiolabeled B72.3 (^{111}In-CYT-103). *Antibod Immunoconj Radiopharm* 1989; 2: 257-269.
92. Mattes, MJ, Griffiths, GL, Diril, H, et al. Processing of antibody-radioisotope conjugates after binding to the surface of tumor cells. *Cancer* 1994; 73: 787-793.
93. Matthews DC, Appelbaum FR, Eary et al. Development of a marrow transplant regimen for acute leukemia using targeted hematopoeitic irradiation delivered by ^{131}.I-labeled anti-CD45 antibody, combined with cyclophosphamide and total body irradiation. *Blood* 1995; 85(4): 1122-1131.
94. Meredith RM, Khazaeli MB, Plott WE, et al. Phase I trial of iodine-131-chimeric B72.3 in metastatic colorectal cancer. *J Nucl Med* 1992; 33: 23-29.
95. Miraldi FD, Nelson AD, Kraly C, et al. Diagnostic imaging of human neuroblastoma with radiolabeled antibody. *Radiology* 1986; 161: 413-418.
96. Modorati G, Brancato R, Paganelli G, Magnani P, Pavoni R, Fazio F. Immunoscintigraphy with three step monoclonal pretargeting technique in diagnosis of uveal melanoma: preliminary results. *Br J Ophthalmol* 1994; 78(1): 19-23.
97. Moffat FL, Vargas-Cuba RD, Serafini AN et al. Preoperative scintigraphy and operative probe scintimetry of colorectal carcinoma using technetium-99m-88BV59. *J Nucl Med* 1995 36: 738-745.
98. Morton JD, Quadri SM, TYang XZ et al. Treatment of refractory end stage Hodgkin's disease with Yttrium-90 polyclonal antiferritin antibodies. *J Immunother* 1994; 16(2): 160.
99. Murray JL, Rosenblum MG, Sobol RE, Bartholomew RM, et al. Radioimmunoimaging in malignant melanoma with ^{111}In-labeled monoclonal antibody 96.5. *Cancer Res* 1985; 45: 2376-2381.
100. Murray JL, Rosenblum MG, Lamki L, et al. Clinical parameters related to optimal tumor localization of indium-111-labeled mouse antimelanoma monoclonal antibody ZME-018. *J Nucl Med* 1987; 28: 25-33.
101. Murray JL, Zukiwski AA, Mujoo K et al. Recombinant alpha-interferon enhances tumor targeting of an anti melanoma monoclonal antibody in vivo. *J Biol Response Mod* 1990; 4: 556-563.
102. Murray JL, Macey DJ, Grant EJ, et al. Phase II trial of ^{131}I-CC49 Mab plus alpha interferon (rIFN$\propto$) in breast cancer. *J Immunother* 1994; 16(2): 162 (abs).
103. Nabi HA, Doerr RJ, Chan H-W, Balu D, Schmelter RF, Maguire RT. In-111-labeled monoclonal antibody immunoscintigraphy in colorectal carcinoma: safety, sensitivity, and preliminary clinical results. *Radiology* 1990; 175: 163-171.
104. Nabi HA, Doerr RJ. Radiolabeled monoclonal antibody imaging (immunoscintigraphy) of colorectal cancers: current status and future perspectives. *Amer Journ Surg* 1992; 163: 448-456.
105. Nabi HA, Schwartz AN, Higano CS, et al. Colorectal carcinoma: Detection with indium-111 anticarcinoembryonic-antigen monoclonal antibody ZCE-025. *Radiology* 1987; 164: 617-621.
106. Naruki Y, Carrasquillo JA, Reynolds JC, et al. Differential cellular metabolism of In-111, Y-90, and I-125 radiolabeled T101 anti-CD5 monoclonal antibody. *Int J Rad Appl Instrum Br* 1990; 17: 201-207.
107. Neal CE, Swenson LC, Fanning JC, Texter JH. Monoclonal antibodies in ovarian and prostate cancer. *Seminars in Nucl Med* 1993; 23(2): 114-126.
108. Oldham RK, Foon KA, Morgan AC, et al. Monoclonal antibody therapy of malignant melanoma: *In vivo* localization in cutaneous metastases after intravenous administration. *J Clin Oncol* 1984; 2: 1235.
109. Order SE, Klein JL, Leichner PK, et al. Advances in iodine-131 labeled antiferritin immunoglobulin cancer therapy. *Cancer Biol* 1982; 34: 264-267.
110. Order SE, Klein JL, Leichner PK. Radiation therapy of hepatoma with I-131 and Y-90 labeled antiferritin antibodies. *Int. Conf. Monoclonal Antibody Immunoconjugates for Cancer* 1986; 1: 27-28.
111. Order SE, Vriesendorp HM, Klein JL, et al. A phase I study of ^{90}yttrium antiferritin: dose escalation and tumor dose. *Antibody Immunoconjug Radiopharm* 1988; 1(2): 163-168.
112. Otsuka FL, Welch MJ. Methods to label monoclonal antibodies for use in tumor imaging. *Nucl Med Biol* 1987; 14:

243-249

113. Paganelli G, Malcovati M, Fazio F. Monoclonal antibody pretargetting techniques for tumour localization: the avidin-biotin system. *Nucl Med Communications* 1991; 12: 211-234..
114. Paganelli G, Belloni C, Magnani P, et al. Two-step tumor targetting in ovarian cancer patients using biotinylated monoclonal antibodies and radioactive streptavidin. *Eur J Nucl Med* 1992; 19: 322-329.
115. Paganelli G, Magnani P, Meares C, et al. Antibody guided therapy of CEA positive tumors using biotinylated monoclonal antiodies, avidin, and ^{90}Y -DOTA-biotin: initial evaluation. *J Nucl Med* 1993; 34(5): 94P.
116. Patt YZ, Lamki LM, Shanken J, et al. Imaging with indium 111-labeled anticarcinoembryonic antigen monoclonal antibody ZCE-025 of recurrent colorectal or carcinoembryonic antigen-producing cancer in patients with rising serum carcinoembryonic antigen levels and occult metastases. *J Clin Oncol* 1990; 8: 1246-1254
117. Pimm M. Circulating antigen: Bad or good for immunoscintigraphy. *Nuc Med Biol* 1995; 22: 137-145..
118. Pizer BL, Papanastassiou V, Mosely R , Tzanis S, Hancock JP, Kemshcad JT, Coakham HB. Meningeal leukemia and medullablastoma: preliminary expeience with intrathecal radioimmunotherapy. *Antib Immunoconj Radiopharm* 1991; 4(4): 753-761.
119. Podoloff DA, Patt YZ, Curley SA, Kim EE, Bhadkamkar VA, Smith RE. Imaging of colorectal carcinoma with technetium-99m radiolabeled Fab' fragments. *Seminars in Nucl Med* 1993; 23(2): 89-98
120. Press OW, Eary JF, Appelbaum FR, et al. Radiolabeled-antibody therapy of B-cell lymphoma with autologous bone marrow support. *N Engl J Med* 1993; 329(17): 1219-1224.
121. Press OW, Eary JF, Appelbaum FR, Bernstein ID. Radiolabeled antibody therapy of lymphomas. In: DeVita VT, Hellman S, Rosenberg SA, eds. *Biologic Therapy of Cancer* 1994; 4(4): 1-13
122. Press OW, Eary JF, Martin PJ, et al. Preliminary results of a phase II trial of iodine-131-labeled anti-CD20 (B1) antibody therapy with bone marrow rescue for patients with relapsed B cell lymphomas. *J Immunother* 1994; 16(2): 160 (abs).
123. Rao DV, Howell RW. Time-dose-fractionation in radio immunotherapy: Implications for selecting radionuclides. *J Nucl Med* 1993; 34: 1801-1810.
124. Richman CM, DeNardo SJ, O'Grady LF, Valk PE, DeNardo GL. Radioimmunotherapy for breast cancer using escalating fractionated doses of I-131 chimeric (Ch) L6. *J Immunother* 1994; 16(2): 161 (abs).
125. Riva P, Arista A, Sturiale, C., Franceschi, G., et al. Direct intratumor radioimmunotherapy of malignant gliomas: clinical experiences in recurrent or primary tumours. *J Immunother* 1994; 16(2): 163 (abs)
126. Riva P, Tison G, Franchesci N, Casi M , Moscatelli G. Successful treatment of metastatic gastrointestinal cancer by means of radioimmunotherapy. *J Nucl Med* 1992; 33(5): 863 Abst.
127. Rodwell JD, Alvarez VL, Lee C, et al. Site-specific covalent modification of monoclonal antibodies: *In vitro* and *in vivo* evaluations. *Proc Natl Acad Sci USA* 1986; 83: 2632-2636.
128. Rosen ST, Zimmer AM, Goldman-Leiken et al. Radioimmunodetection and radioimmunotherapy of cutaneous T-cell lymphomas using an ^{131}I-labeled T101 monoclonal antibody: anIllinios Cancer Council study. *J Clin Oncol* 1987; (5): 562.. Blood 1986; 68: 241a (abstr).
129. Rusch V, Macapinlac H, Heelan R, et al. NR-LU-10 Monoclonal Antibody Scanning: A Helpful New Adjunct to CT in Evaluating Non-Small Cell Lung Cancer. *J Thorac Cardiovasc Surg* 1993; 106: 200-204
130. Sahakara H, Reynolds JC, Carasquillo JA et al. In vitro complex formation and biodistribution of mouse antitumor monoclonal antibody in cancer patients. *J Nucl Med.* 1989; 30: 1311-1317.
131. Salk D and the Multicenter Study Group. Technetium-labeled monoclonal antibodies for imaging metastatic melanoma: Results of a multicenter clinical study. *Semin Oncol* 1988; 15: 608-618.
132. Salk D, Lesley T, Wiseman G, et al. A phase I trial of a fractionated dose intraperitoneal administration of Rhenium-186 monoclonal antibodies in ovarian cancer. *Antib Immunoconj Radiopharm* 1992; 4: 359 Abst.
133. Scheinberg DA, Straus DJ, Yeh SD, etc. A phase I toxicity, pharmacology, and dosimetry trial of monoclonal antibody OKB7 in patients with non-hodgkin's lymphoma: Effects of tumor burden and antigen expression. *Journal of Clinical Oncology* 1990; 8(5): 792-803
134. Schlom J, Molinolo A, Simpson JF et al. Advantages of dose fractionation in monoclonal antibody-targeted radioimmunotherapy. *J Natl Cancer Inst* 1990; 82: 763-771.
135. Schroff RW, Foon KA, Beatty SM, Oldham RK, Morgan AC. Human anti-murine immunoglobulin responses in patients receiving monoclonal antibody therapy. *Cancer Res* 1985; 45: 879-885.
136. Schwartz MA, Lovett DR, Redner A, et al. Dose-escalation trial of M195 labeled with iodine 131 for cytoreduction and marrow ablation in relapsed or refractory myeloid leukemias. *Journal of Clinical Oncology* 1993; 11(2): 294-303.
137. Schwartz SW, Connett JM, Anderson CJ, Rocque PA, Philpott GW, Guo LW, Welch MJ. Evaluation of a direct method for technetium labeling of intact and $F(ab')_2$ 1A3, an anticolorectal monoclonal antibody. *Nucl Med Biol* 1994; 21: 619-626.
138. Serafini AN, Kotler J, Feun L, et al. Technetium-99m-labeled monoclonal antibodies in the detection of metastatic melanoma. *J Clin Nucl Med* 1989; 14: 580-587.
139. Siccardi AG, Buraggi GL, Callegaro L, et al. Multicenter study of immunoscintigraphy with radiolabeled monoclonal antibodies in patients with melanoma. *Cancer Res* 1986; 46: 4817-4822.
140. Stemmer SM, Johnson R, Kasliwal R, et al. High dose ^{90}Y Mx-DTPA-BrE-3 and autologous hematopoietic stem cell support (AHSCS) for the treatment of advanced breast cancer. *J Immunother* 1994; 16(2): 161 (abs).
141. Stewart JSW, Hird V, Snook D, et al. Intraperitoneal radioimmunotherapy for ovarian cancer: Pharmacokinetics, toxicity, and efficacy of I-131 labeled monclonal antibodies. *Int J Radiation Oncology Biol Phys* 1989; 16: 405-413.
142. Stickney DR, Slater JB, Kirk GA, et al. Bifunctional antibody: ZCE/CHA ^{111}Indium BLEDTA-IV clinical imaging in colorectal carcinoma. *Ant Immun Radiopharm* 1989; 2: 1-13.
143. Sung C, Shockley TR, Morrison PF, Dvorak HF, Yarmush

ML, Dedrick RL. Predicted and observed effects of antibody affinity and antigen density on monoclonal antibody uptake in solid tumors. *Cancer Research* 1992; 52: 377-384.

144. Surwit EA, Childers JM, Krag DN, Katterhagen G, Gallion H, Waggoner S, Mann WJ Jr. Clinical assessment of ^{111}In-CYT-103 immunoscintigraphy in ovarian cancer. *Gynecologic Oncology* 1993; 48: 285-292.
145. Volkert WA, Goeckeler WF, Ehrhardt GJ, Ketring AR. Therapeutic radionuclides: Production and decay property considerations. *J Nucl Med* 1991; 32: 174-185.
146. Waldmann TA, Strober W. Metabolism of immunoglobulin. *Prog Allergy* 1969; 13: 1-10.
147. Weiden PL, Breitz HB, Seiler CA, et al. Rhenium-186-labeled chimeric antibody NR-LU-13: pharmacokinetics, biodistribution and immunogenicity relative to murine analog NR-LU-10. *J Nucl Med* 1993; 34: 2111-2119.
148. Weiden PL, Wolf SB, Breitz HB, et al. Human anti-mouse antibody suppression with Cyclosporin A. *Cancer* 1994; 73(3): 1093-1097
149. Weinstein JN, Eger RR, Covell DG, et al. The pharmacology of monoclonal antibodies. *Ann NY Acad Sci* 1987; 507: 199-210.
150. Wessels BW, Rogers RD. Radionuclide selection and model absorbed dose calculations for radiolabeled tumor associated antibodies. *Med Phys* 1984; 11: 638-645.
151. Wessels BW. Current status of animal radioimmunotherapy. *Cancer Res* 1990; 50: 970s-973s.
152. Wheldon TE, O'Donoghue JA, Bartett A, Michalowski AS. The curability of tumours of differing size by targeted radiotherapy using ^{131}I or ^{90}Y. *Radiotherapy Oncol* 1991; 21: 91-99.
153. Wilbur DS. Radiohalogenation of proteins: an overview of radionuclides, labeling methods and reagents for conjugate labeling. *Bioconjugate Chem* 1992; 3: 433-470.
154. Yorke ED, Beaumier PL, Wessels BW, Fritzberg AR, Morgan AC Jr. Optimal antibody-radionuclide combinations for clinical radioimmunotherapy: A predictive model based on mouse pharmacokinetics. *Nucl Med Biol* 1991; 18: 827-835
155. Zalutsky MR. Radiohalogenation of antibodies: Chemical aspects. In: *Radiolabeled Monoclonal Antibodies for Imaging and Therapy*. Srivastava SC, Ed., Plenum Press, New York, 1988.

16

STEM CELL/BONE MARROW TRANSPLANTATION AS BIOTHERAPY

ROBERT K. OLDHAM

Biological Therapy Institute Foundation, Franklin, Tennessee; and University of Missouri, Columbia, Missouri

AUTOLOGOUS BONE MARROW TRANSPLANTATION

It is clear that bone marrow transplantation has become a major technique in the treatment of metastatic cancer. The use of autologous bone marrow transplantation has allowed for much higher doses of chemotherapy to be given in an attempt to eliminate all of the cancer cells from the patient with the sacrifice of normal bone marrow function in the process. Autologous, cryopreserved bone marrow or peripheral blood stem cells (PBSC) can be reinfused to reconstitute stem cells and bone marrow function. This process is still dose limited by damage to the gastrointestinal tract, liver, lung, heart and other critical organs [20, 36]. Considerable progress has been made using this technique to allow dose escalation with chemotherapeutic agents. Escalation of doses to the level causing damage to secondary target organs is the current limitation of this technique.

The problems of graft versus host disease (GVHD) limits the use of allogeneic bone marrow transplantation (ALBMT), although matching techniques and immunosuppression have improved the results for allogeneic grafts. By contrast, autologous bone marrow transplantation (ABMT) is a technique that does not involve significant GVHD and allows for significant drug dose escalation. Unfortunately, residual tumor cells can exist in autologous bone marrow. Techniques must be developed to effectively eliminate all replicating tumor cells from these specimens such that the cancer is not reinitiated in the patient after cure by high dose therapy.

Considerable progress has been made in leukemias and lymphomas, and there is an ongoing and increasing effort with BMT in solid tumors [53, 65, 78].

Histocompatible donors can be selected leading to successful allogeneic transplants [53, 76]. The perfect transplant only occurs with identical twins (available in less than 1 in 300 transplants), but matching of donors at the HLA-A, -B, -C, and -D loci and selecting for those individuals with negative mixed lymphocyte cultures have improved the results of ALBMT. Engraftment of a stable chimeric state can be demonstrated [74], but GVHD (acute and chronic) results in the recognition of recipient tissues by transplanted donor T lymphocytes and occurs in more than 50% of ALBMT patients. More than half of these individuals will have a fatal outcome [29, 41, 75]. A variety of techniques have been used to attempt to eliminate T cells from these marrow grafts. These have included monoclonal antibodies [57, 63], monoclonal antibody with complement [6, 27, 34, 35, 45, 50, 58, 67, 73, 86], immunotoxins [19, 46, 59, 81], and physical methods [5, 30, 56] to eliminate T cells from the donor graft. Allogeneic BMT is covered later in this chapter, but various techniques to eliminate T cells have been reviewed in a recent book by Gross et al. [31]. Many of the techniques to deplete the T cells for ALBMT are similar to techniques being used to eliminate residual tumor cells in ABMT. Therefore, a review of this literature is critical to the reader who wants to understand all the current techniques available for elimination of subsets of cells from bone marrow prior to transplantation.

ABMT is the most popular current method of bone marrow reconstitution and offers the advantage of avoiding GVHD. Bone marrow cells in numbers (1-5 x 10^{10}) sufficient to reconstitute the individual's marrow function, through the stem-cell transplant, can easily be obtained by multiple punctures of the bone with marrow aspiration and then storage of the separated cells in liquid nitrogen. These cells can be thawed and reinfused after high-dose chemotherapy with consistent reconstitution of the bone marrow. In fact, bone marrows can now be separated and divided in such a way as to prepare one to three grafts from a single bone marrow donor.

More recent application of this reconstituting technique has involved the use of PBSC harvests through leukapheresis. This technique allows for stem cells to be harvested by high volume leukapheresis and represents a selection method for stem cells that avoids many of the problems of tumor cell infiltration in the bone marrow. Although peripheral blood may contain circulating tumor cells, the evidence thus far indicates that considerable positive selection of stem cells can be effected by a peripheral blood harvest. This may obviate purging of bone marrow or at least make the purging process easier by virtue of having fewer tumor cells in the stem-cell preparations. The techniques for removing tumor cells from autologous marrow are numerous and have been extensively discussed elsewhere [42, 55, 61, 80, 84]. This area has been extensively reviewed by multiple authors. Perhaps the two best recent reviews

R.K. Oldham (ed.), Principles of Cancer Biotherapy. 3rd ed., 369–375.

can be found in the work of McIntyre [47] and Gross et al. [31].

THE PREPARATION OF BONE MARROW FOR TRANSPLANTATION IN ABMT

Marrow manipulation must be carried out to preserve the pluripotent hematopoietic stem cell in sufficient numbers to insure engraftment. All of the procedures discussed in this chapter to eliminate tumor cells must be done in such a way to preserve adequate stem-cell activity. Clonogenic assays can be used to determine the number and function of stem cells by assaying these preparations for granulocyte/macrophage colony forming cells (GM-CFC), burst forming unit-erythroid (BFU-E), and granulocyte, erythroid, macrophage, and megakaryocyte colony-forming cells (GEMM-CFC). Long-term bone marrow cultures may also be used with the Dexter culture system to measure cell renewal in these systems. These techniques have been recently reviewed [2, 18, 22, 26, 48]. Recently, simple flow cytometry assessment of CD-34 lymphocyte numbers has been used to predict stem cell numbers. While these assays are useful to measure progenitor proliferation and differentiation, the critical test is marrow engraftment in the patient treated by the ABMT technique.

ABMT hematopoietic recovery is usually seen in the 20- to 40-day period after bone marrow infusion. White blood cell recovery generally precedes platelet recovery; and delayed engraftment can lead to fatal complications. These patients are often isolated from potential surrounding infectious risk and must be carefully monitored for viral, bacterial, and fungal infections during the course of ABMT. Once the white count recovers to the level of 500 granulocytes/mm^3 and the platelet count exceeds 30,000/mm^3, the risk of infection and bleeding markedly decreases. ABMT impairs immune function but much less so than ALBMT. Immune recovery may take months, and in some patients immune competence is never really fully reconstituted [21, 43, 60, 89].

To prepare marrow aspirates for transplantation, some positive selection of the appropriate reconstituting cells by physical means is commonly done. This may include the simple task of cryopreservation, which eliminates a large number of red blood cells, but may also include separation procedures to obtain mononuclear cells from the marrow [7, 17, 37]. Isopyknic centrifugation of Ficoll-Hypaque gradients, isopyknic sedimentation on discontinuous Percoll gradients, and the use of centrifugation in blood-cell separators without a gradient are all techniques that have been used to separate mononuclear cells containing the stem-cell fraction [7, 17, 23, 37]. These techniques have eliminated the problems of clumping and cell lysis, yield high numbers of progenitor stem cells, and routinely give marrow engraftment in patients. The technique of removal, manipulation, and preparation for ABMT and the more recent technique, peripheral stem-cell isolation by leukapheresis in an outpatient setting, are rapidly gaining wide clinical acceptance. These techniques are now available and being utilized broadly in the clinical practice of oncology, such that ABMT has become a major treatment technique in patients with previously refractory solid tumors [3, 8, 24, 25, 40, 68, 71, 77].

TECHNIQUES TO ELIMINATE SPECIFIC SUBPOPULATIONS OF CELLS (TUMOR CELLS AND LYMPHOCYTES) FROM MARROW SPECIMENS

There has been a huge number of specific techniques utilized to attempt to eliminate either tumor cells and/or T cells from bone marrow. Elimination of the former is essential in ABMT, and elimination of the latter is desirable in allogeneic BMT. Some of these techniques depend on a biological agent and thus represent a form of *ex vivo* biotherapy, and others utilize chemotherapy, radiotherapy, or physical techniques to effect marrow purging. Each of these techniques will be reviewed with an emphasis on biotherapeutic techniques for bone marrow purging.

Ex vivo purging with chemotherapy

Various agents have been utilized to exploit the differential toxicity for a specific chemotherapy drug on tumor cells in contrast to the activity on the marrow stem cells. Preclinical studies have demonstrated the effect of corticosteroids [38], VP-16 and Verapamil [9], 4-hydroperoxycyclophosphamide (4-HC) and platinum [54], 1-β-D-arabinofuranosylcytosine (Ara-C) and deoxycytidine [28], VP-16 and corticosteroids [72], and alkyl lysophospholipids (ALP) [85]. These studies indicate that each of these approaches can eliminate tumor cells and/or T cells (glucocorticoids) from marrows to be reinfused. Most of these studies have not progressed to significant clinical studies, but such trials are planned.

Mafosfamide [62] and 4-HC, both relatives of cyclophosphamide, have been utilized in clinical studies to eliminate residual tumor cells. These cyclophosphamide derivatives, as well as other chemotherapy agents, appear to be promising in the elimination of residual tumor cells from these marrow grafts [31].

Biophysical and physical approaches

A variety of biophysical methods, including photoradiation [32], laser photoradiation [33], and isotope-mediated purging [44] have been used to purge marrow of unwanted tumor cells. These studies, sometimes with chemotherapy purging, have primarily been used in preclinical studies, but now investigators are posed to begin clinical studies with these biophysical approaches.

Physical separation methods such as elutriation [52] can be used to positively select bone marrow stem cells for

ABMT, and this technique can be used as a negative selection technique against tumor cells in ABMT and T cells in ALBMT. Clinical studies of this technique are underway and appear promising. Cell separators can be utilized for the separation of mononuclear cells for marrow [1] or peripheral blood stem cells [87] for transplantation. Various other physical approaches have been used, but the most promising and straightforward approaches involve machines that can carry out such processing in an automated format.

Biotherapeutic approaches

A variety of biotherapeutic approaches have been used to treat bone marrow prior to reinfusion. Lymphokine activated killer (LAK) cells induced by interleukin 2 [16] have been used to purge bone marrow of residual tumor cells with interesting preclinical results. Antibody alone and antibody plus complement have been used by a variety of investigators for the elimination of residual tumor cells. The Campath series of antibodies may have the dual use of purging lymphoma or leukemia cells from the marrow and may also be useful in the *in vivo* elimination of residual tumor cells after ABMT. More than 520 patients have been treated in various European transplant centers in an approach to deplete T cells and lessen GVHD in allogeneic BMT [14]. These results certainly demonstrate the usefulness of this approach in eliminating T cells. The application of this technique to ABMT for purging malignant lymphocytes carrying the antigens recognized by the Campath antibodies is the next logical step. In multiple myeloma, antibody plus complement [79] can eliminate residual myeloma cells from the marrow. Antibody plus complement has been used in preclinical and clinical studies [49] to purge myelocytic leukemia cells from marrow prior to ABMT. An interesting study of an antibody conjugated to Adriamycin, where the antibody also fixed complement, has been reported, but the preclinical activities demonstrated insufficient selectivity for clinical application [88].

In addition to antibody alone and antibody-fixing complement, there has been a series of studies using antibody conjugated to toxins, usually ricin, to prepare immunotoxins that can be used in bone marrow purging. These immunotoxins have been used in ABMT for T-cell acute lymphoblastic leukemia [82] and to eliminate T cells to decrease GVHD in ALBMT. These ricin immunotoxins have been utilized in clinical studies with positive preliminary results. Studies are only now beginning with immunotoxins in marrow purging of solid tumors, but the early studies in neuroblastoma [11] and breast cancer [70] are encouraging.

Combination techniques

Investigators are pursuing combination techniques with antibody tied to magnetic spheres (biotherapy plus physical separation) to eliminate residual marrow tumor cells. These studies are very well reviewed by Gross et al. [31] and will not be covered in detail here. Suffice it to say that various physical techniques are being developed where bone marrow is being purged by the dispersion of magnetic beads coated with antibody. These antibody-coated beads attach to tumor cells and can be extracted from bone marrow by passing the preparation over a magnet. By pulling out the residual tumor cells, one can prepare a bone marrow free of residual tumor cells for reinfusion. These studies certainly appear interesting, and further preclinical studies and early clinical applications are being pursued [31].

Stem-cell selection

There is now increasing evidence that biological techniques to select stem cells by positive methods will result in enhanced marrow preparations for ABMT. Antibody to CD-34 can be used to select stem cells from bone marrow or peripheral blood [4, 13]. This technique has mainly been applied to bone marrow, but with the development of PBSC collection techniques [87], the same positive stem-cell selection process could be applied to peripheral blood. High speed clinical cell sorters and antibody-based positive selection systems are both used in clinical trials as methods to select and purify peripheral blood stem cells for ABMT.

A technique with far-reaching implications has recently been developed to culture stem cells continuously *in vitro* [15, 51]. This approach may allow for the repeated infusion of autologous bone marrow stem cells free of any residual tumor cells and without the presence of any immunologically active T cells. The potential for the broad application of culture stem cells is obvious, even to the point of cryopreserving such stem cells for each interested individual, while living and healthy, in anticipation of their use later in life in the presence of disease. Preserving cord blood or fetal tissues for use later in life as stem cells is also being explored. Such techniques, while interesting, bring up the whole question of how far technology should take us in anticipating disease and dealing with the potential for developing specific diseases. There are various social, political, and economic consequences of techniques that may predict or be useful in the treatment of future diseases. In fact, the whole area of genetic therapy is now coming forth as a potential major form of biotherapy. Not only can stem cells be grown *in vitro* for eventual use in reconstituting bone marrow, gene therapy with electroporation and other techniques can be used to insert specific genes in normal or defective human cells [39]. Very primitive stem cells may carry few transplantation antigens and after long-term culture may be useful broadly in reconstituting stem cells. It is clear that biotherapy and gene therapy will lead to tremendous advances and opportunities but also bring forth major considerations of 'who pays for clinical research' and 'who should have access to these new techniques'. (See Chapter 3.)

ALLOGENEIC BONE MARROW TRANSPLANTATION

Allogeneic BMT has been successful in treating certain lymphoid and hemopoietic neoplasms. Initially, the total body irradiation plus high dose chemotherapy followed by ALBMT was felt to work primarily through the cytoreductive effects of the chemoradiotherapy. Innovative suggestions by Professor Georges Mathé as early as 1965 and follow-up evidence reviewed by George Santos in 1972 suggested that there was an anti-tumor effect independent of the chemoradiotherapy from ALBMT. This has more recently been clarified as a form of graft-versus-tumor (GVT) effect similar to the concept of GVHD as has been well understood in allogeneic bone marrow transplantation since the early days of this technique [64]. GVHD has been well characterized for many years. It is known to have an acute and more chronic variety, primarily manifest by a clinical syndrome of skin rash, liver and gastrointestinal dysfunction as well as a variety of autoimmune type effects [64]. A variety of strategies, primarily total body irradiation and/or systemic chemotherapy has been used to reduce the number of T cells from the graft responsible for GVHD. These strategies have been more or less effective, usually requiring lifelong treatment of patients who have experienced allogeneic GVHD.

Of particular interest has been the concept of autologous GVHD which was initially quite a controversial theory. This concept was recently reviewed by Santos [66]. The autoreactive cells found in autologous GVHD can cause damage to a variety of organs, most of which are less severe than that seen in allogeneic BMT. Histocompatibility differences cannot explain this phenomenon since these autologous transplants cannot have histocompatibility differences. Therefore, immune disregulation is felt to play the major role in autologous GVHD. Treatment is usually not necessary since the syndrome is normally benign and symptomatic care is usually sufficient for patients with manifestations of autologous GVHD.

GRAFT-VERSUS-TUMOR EFFECTS

Early evidence that bone marrow cells of allogeneic BMT producing a graft-versus-leukemia effect has prompted the more general idea of graft-versus-tumor (GVT) effect of both ALBMT and ABMT. Most studies found a correlation between GVH and reduced relapse rate for patients with leukemia treated by ALBMT. Similar observations have been seen, though less striking, in ABMT. Santos [66] has summarized the evidence that GVT might be utilized as a therapeutic tool, noting the presence of autoreactive T cells related to Ia antigens in many of these syndromes and also noting that Ia antigens are expressed on leukemias and lymphomas with perhaps similar antigens being present on certain solid tumors. The potential for identifying these cells and using them after *ex vivo* application continues to intrigue investigators in this area. Whether these cells may be purely T cells or be some form of LAK or NK cell is currently under investigation. The ability to grow large numbers of activated T cells opens the possibility of utilizing cells identified by transplantation techniques as useful for their GVT activities.

Recent evidence has provided further credence to the concept that the immune system is active in treating leukemia post allogeneic BMT. This information has come from studies in patients with chronic myelogenous leukemia and includes the following factors.

1. Marrow grafts that have been T-cell depleted have a higher rate of leukemic relapse and less GVHD.
2. An inverse relationship has been seen in HLA identical BMT between the occurrence of GVHD and leukemia relapse.
3. The GVT effect arises from a reduction in leukemic recurrences post allogeneic BMT compared to homozygous twin transplants.
4. Relapsed allogeneic BMT CML patients can be reinduced into complete remission simply by infusing donor leukocytes [83].
5. Summarizing eight reports similar to that of van Rhee [83], a total of 66 patients with relapsed chronic plase CML have received allogeneic peripheral blood mononuclear cells with or without inferferon with complete responses (cytogenic and molecular) of approximately 75%.

CONCLUSION

ABMT and ALBMT offer major opportunities in cancer biotherapy. With ABMT the major question relates to the sensitivity of cancer to a dose escalation strategy of chemotherapy and radiotherapy. If these modalities can eliminate cancer from the patient at doses between the marrow lethal dose and the maximum tolerated dose to the next organ system (gut, liver, lung, heart, etc.), then the technique of ABMT with high-dose therapy may be broadly applicable and curative in certain solid tumors. This technique will always have major, inherent toxicity because of the toxicities of the therapeutic agents. However, short-term toxicity and even some risk of long-term effects would be tolerated by patients with lethal diseases if complete remissions and prolonged remission duration can be engendered. On the other hand, if the dose-response curve for human solid tumors is insufficiently steep to allow for the induction of complete response and improved survival with these techniques, then the broader application of this approach may not be warranted, given the significant toxicities involved.

Recent results, summarized above, using allogeneic peripheral blood mononuclear cells are particularly encouraging, with clear GVT effects now being seen in CML and other leukemias/lymphomas, confirming the earlier, more intuitive observations of Mathé and Santos [64].

Biotherapeutic approaches toward the elimination of residual tumor cells appear to be the most promising with regard to ABMT. Similar approaches to eliminate T cells from allogeneic bone marrow may broaden its application. The two most promising techniques appear to rest in the use of antibody to negatively or positively select appropriate cell populations in marrow transplantation and the use of physical separation methods, such as leukapheresis, to positively select for replicating stem cells. Most specifically, the technique of peripheral blood leukapheresis to select for stem cells, perhaps with their eventual long-term culture for repetitive use, does appear to be a highly promising technique to provide stem-cell reconstitution in patients lethally damaged by high-dose chemotherapy and radiotherapy. These studies are at an early stage but they are rapidly evolving, with the technique of ABMT being already widespread in the clinical practice of oncology [8]. The recent availability of colony-stimulating factors (see Chapters 19 and 20) provides a further mechanism for the manipulation of stem-cell numbers and activity. The outpatient use of autologous bone marrow transplantation through leukapheresis to select the stem cells and the use of colony-stimulating factors to support stem cell growth *in vitro* and *in vivo* appear to be promising approaches in the treatment of advanced solid tumors [10, 12, 69].

REFERENCES

1. Areman EM, Cullis H, Sacher RA, et al. Automated isolation of mononuclear cells using the Fenwall CS3000 blood cell separator. In: *Bone marrow purging and processing*. New York: Wiley-Liss, 1990: 379-385.
2. Ash RC, Detrick RA, Zanjani ED. Studies of human pluripotential hemopoietic stem cells (CFU-GEMM) *in vitro*. *Blood* 1981; 58: 309-316.
3. Beelen DW, Ouabeck K. Graeven U, et al. Acute toxicity and first clinical results of intensive postinduction therapy using a modified busulfan and cyclophosphamide regimen with autologous bone marrow rescue in first remission of acute myeloid leukemia. *Blood* 1989; 74: 1507-1516.
4. Berensen RJ, Bensinger WI, Hill R, et al. Stem cell selection: clinical experience. In: *Bone marrow purging and processing*. New York: Wiley-Liss, 1990: 403-413.
5. Berensen RJ, Levitt LJ, Levy R, et al. Cellular immunoabsorption using monoclonal antibodies. Selective removal of T cells from peripheral blood and bone marrow. *Transplantation* 1984; 38: 136-142.
6. Blazar BR, Quinones RR, Heinitz KJ, et al. Comparison of three techniques for the ex vivo elimination of T cells from human bone marrow. *Exp Hematol* 1985; 13: 123-128.
7. Bodger MP, Hann IM, Maclean RF, et al. Enrichment of pluripotent hemopoietic progenitor cells from human bone marrow. *Blood* 1984; 64: 774-779.
8. Brandwine JM, Callum J, Rubinger M, et al. An Evaluation of outpatient bone marrow harvesting. *J Clin Oncol* 1989; 7: 648-650.
9. Cairo MS, Toy C, Sender L, et al. Combination chemotherapy and Verapamil to purge drug resistant leukemia cells from human bone marrow. In: *Bone marrow purging and processing*. New York: Wiley-Liss, 1990: 47-55.
10. Caron PC, Scheinberg DA. Therapy of acute chronic leukemias using immunologic agents. *Cancer Investigation* 1996; (in press)
11. Cassano WF, Zaytoun AM. Specific killing of neuroblastoma cells *in vitro* by immunotoxins. In: *Bone marrow purging and processing*. New York: Wiley-Liss, 1990: 217-223.
12. Chao NJ, Schriber JR, Grimes K, et al. Granulocyte colony-stimulating factor "mobilized" peripheral blood progenitor cells accelerate granulocyte and platelet recovery after high dose chemotherapy. *Blood* 1993; 81: 2031-2035.
13. Civin CI, Strauss LC, Fackler MJ, et al. Positive stem cell selection: basic science. In: *Bone marrow purging and processing*. New York: Wiley-Liss, 1990: 387-402.
14. Cobbold SP, Hale G, Clark MR, et al. Purging in auto- and allografts: CAMPATH monoclonal antibodies which use human complement and other natural effector mechanisms. In: *Bone marrow purging and processing*. New York: Wiley-Liss, 1990: 139-154.
15. Coutinho LH, Testa NG, Chang J, et al. The use of cultured bone marrow cells in autologous transplantation. In: *Bone marrow purging and processing*. New York: Wiley-Liss, 1990: 415-433.
16. Cramer DV, Long GS. Lymphokine-activated killer (LAK) cell purging of bone marrow. In: *Bone marrow purging and processing*. New York: Wiley-Liss, 1990: 125-137.
17. Ellis WM, Georgiou GM, Roberton DM, et al. The use of discontinuous Percoll gradients to separate populations of cells from human bone marrow and peripheral blood. *J Immunol Methods* 1984; 66: 9-16.
18. Fauser AD, Messner HA. Identification of megakaryocytes, macrophages, and eosinophils in colonies of human bone marrow containing neutrophilic granulocytes and erythroblasts. *Blood* 1979; 53: 1023-1027.
19. Filipovich AH, Vallera DA, Youle RJ, et al. *Ex-vivo* treatment of donor bone marrow with anti-T-cell immunotoxins for prevention of graft-versus-host disease. *Lancet* 1984; 1: 469-472.
20. Frei E III, Canellos GP. Dose: a critical factor in cancer chemotherapy. *Am J Med* 1980; 69: 585-594.
21. Friedrich W, Goldmann SF, Vetter U, et al. Immunoreconstitution in severe combined immunodeficiency after transplantation of HAL-hapolidentical, T-cell-depleted bone marrow. *Lancet* 1984; 1: 761-764.
22. Gartner S, Kaplan H. Long-term culture of human bone marrow cells. *Proc Natl Acad Sci USA* 1980; 77: 4756-4759.
23. Georgiou GM, Roberton DM, Ellis WM, et al. Enrichment from human bone marrow using a discontinuous Percoll gradient and soybean agglutinin in comparison with Ficoll-paque. *Clin Exp Immunol* 1983; 53: 491-496.
24. Gianni AM, Siena S, Bregni M, et al. Granulocyte-macrophage colony-stimulating factor to harvest circulating haemopoietic stem cells for autotransplantation. *Lancet* 1989; ii: 580-585.
25. Goodnough LT, Rudnick S, Price TH, et al. Increased preoperative collection of autologous blood with

recombinant human erythropoietin therapy. *N Engl J Med* 1989; 321: 1163-1168.

26. Gordon MY, Goldman JM, Gordon-Smith EC. 4-Hydroperoxycyclophosphamide inhibits proliferation by human granulocyte-macrophage colony-forming cells. (GM-CFC) but spares more primitive progenitor cells. *Leukemia Res* 1985; 9: 1017-1021.
27. Granger S, Janossy G, Francis G, et al. Elimination of T-lymphocytes from human bone marrow with monoclonal T-antibodies and cytolytic complement. *Br J Haematol* 1982; 50: 367-374.
28. Grant S, Howe C, Kuczynski T. Selective eradication of leukemic (L-CFU) versus normal (CFU-GM) myeloid progenitors in suspension culture utilizing a prolonged exposure in 1-β-D-arabinofuranosylcytosine (Ara-C) and deoxycytidine (dCyd). In: *Bone marrow purging and processing*. New York: Wiley-Liss, 1990: 69-77.
29. Grebe SC, Streilein JW. Graft-versus-host reactions: a review. *Adv Immunol* 1976; 22: 119-221.
30. Greenberg PL, Baker S, Link M, et al. Immunologic selection of hemopoietic precursor cells utilizing antibody-mediated plate binding ('panning'). *Blood* 1985; 65: 190-197.
31. Gross S, Gee AP, Worthington-White DA. Transporting bone marrow for *in vitro* purging before autologous reinfusion. In: *Bone marrow purging and processing*. New York: Wiley-Liss, 1990: 541-549.
32. Gulati S, Atzpodien J, Lemoli RM, et al. Photoradiation methods for purging autologous bone marrow grafts. In: *Bone marrow purging and processing*. New York: Wiley-Liss, 1990: 87-102.
33. Gulliya KS, Batagllino M, Matthews JL. Breast cancer and laser photoradiation therapy: an *in vitro* model for autologous bone marrow purging. In: *Bone marrow purging and processing*. New York: Wiley-Liss, 1990: 103-107.
34. Hale G, Bright S, Chumbley G, et al. Removal of T cells from bone marrow for transplantation: a monoclonal antilymphocyte antibody that fixes human complement. *Blood* 1983; 62: 873-882.
35. Herve P, Racadot E, Flesch M, et al. Prevention of graft-versus-host disease. Elimination of T-lymphocytes from bone marrow cells by complement-dependent cytolysis with a combination of pan-T monoclonal antibodies (letter). *Presse Med* 1984; 13(14): 886-887.
36. Herzig GP. Autologous marrow transplantation for cancer therapy. In: McCullough J, Sandler SG, eds. *Advances in immunobiology, blood cell antigens, and bone marrow transplantation*. New York: Alan R. Liss, 1984: 319-335.
37. Ho WG, Champlin RE, Feig SA, et al. Transplantation of ABH incompatible bone marrow: gravity sedimentation of donor marrow. *Br J Haematol* 1984; 57: 155-162.
38. Kapoor N, Tutschka PJ, Copelan EA. Bone marrow purging with glucocorticoids. In: *Bone marrow purging and processing*. New York: Wiley-Liss, 1990: 39-46.
39. Keating A, Toneguzzo F. Gene transfer by electroporation: a model for gene therapy. In: *Bone marrow purging and processing*. New York: Wiley-Liss, 1990: 491-498.
40. Kessinger A, Armitage JO, Smith DM, et al. High-dose therapy and autologous peripheral blood stem cell transplantation for patients with lymphoma. Blood 1989; 74: 1260-1265.
41. Korngold R, Sprent J. Lethal GVHD across minor histocompatibility barriers: nature of the effector cells and role of the H-2 complex. *Immunol Rev* 1983; 71: 5-29.
42. Krolick KA, Uhr JW, Vitetta ES. Selective killing of leukaemia cells by antibody-toxin conjugates: implications for autologous bone marrow transplantation. *Nature* 1982; 295: 604-605.
43. Lum LC, Seugneuret MC, Storb RF, et al. In vitro regulation of immunoglobulin synthesis after marrow transplantation. I. T-cell and B-cell deficiencies in patients with and without chronic graft-versus-host disease. *Blood* 1981; 58: 431-439.
44. Macklis RM. Radioisotope-mediated purging in bone marrow transplantation. In: *Bone marrow purging and processing*. New York: Wiley-Liss, 1990: 109-123.
45. Martin PJ, Hansen JA. Quantitative assays for detection of residual T cells of T-depleted human marrow. *Blood* 1985; 65: 1134-1140.
46. Martin PJ, Hansen JA, Vitetta ES. A ricin A chain-containing immunotoxin that kills human T lymphocytes *in vitro*. *Blood* 1985; 66: 908-912.
47. McIntyre EA. The use of monoclonal antibodies for purging autologous bone marrow in the lymphoid malignancies. *Clin Haematol* 1986; 15: 249-267.
48. Metcalf D. Detection and analysis of human granulocyte-monocyte precursors using semi-solid cultures. *Clin Haemotol* 1979; 8: 263-285.
49. Mills LE, Ball ED, Howell AL, et al. Efficacy of bone marrow purging in AML using monoclonal antibodies and complement. In: *Bone marrow purging and processing*. New York: Wiley-Liss, 1990: 165-170.
50. Mitsuyasu RT, Chaplin RE, Ho WG, et al. Prospective randomized controlled trial of *ex vivo* treatment of donor bone marrow with monoclonal anti-T cell antibody and complement for prevention of graft-versus-host disease: a preliminary report. *Transplant Proc* 1985; 17: 482-485.
51. Naughton BA, Jacob L, Naughton GK. A three dimensional culture system for the growth of hematopoietic cells. In: *Bone marrow purging and processing.* New York: Wiley-Liss, 1990; 435-445.
52. Noga SJ, Wagner JE, Rowley SD, et al. Using elutriation to engineer bone marrow allografts. In: *Bone marrow purging and processing.* New York: Wiley-Liss, 1990: 345-361.
53. O'Reilly RJ. Allogeneic bone marrow transplantation: current status and future directions. *Blood* 1983; 62: 941-964.
54. Peters RH, Brandon CS, Lobelia AA, et al. Combinations of 4-dydroperoxycyclophosphamide (4-HC) and cisplatin for bone marrow purging in autologous marrow transplantation: an update. In: *Bone marrow purging and processing*. New York: Wiley-Liss, 1990: 57-68.
55. Poynton CH, Reading CL. Monoclonal antibodies: the possibilities for cancer therapy. *Exp Biol* 1984; 43: 13-33.
56. Poynton CH, Reading CL, Dicke KA. In: Dicke KA, Spitzer G, Zander AR, eds. *Autologous bone marrow transplantation*. edited by K.A. Houston: University of Texas M.D. Anderson Hospital and Tumor Institute, 1985: 433-437.
57. Prentice HG, Blacklock HA, Janossy G, et al. Use of anti-T-cell monoclonal antibody OKT3 to prevent acute graft-versus-host disease in allogeneic bone marrow transplantation for acute leukaemia. *Lancet* 1982; 1: 700-703.
58. Prentice HG, Blacklock HA, Janossy G, et al. Depletion of T lymphocytes in donor marrow prevents significant graft-versus-host disease in matched allogeneic leukae-

mic marrow transplant recipients. *Lancet* 1984; 1: 472-476.

59. Quinones RR, Youle RJ, Kersey JH. Anti-T cell monoclonal antibodies conjugated in ricin as potential reagents for human GVHD prophylaxis: effect on the generation of cytotoxic T cells in both peripheral blood and bone marrow. *J Immunol* 1984; 132: 678-683.
60. Rappeport JM, Dunn MG, Parkman R. T lymphocytes in the peripheral blood of bone marrow transplant recipients. *Transplantation* 1983; 36: 674-680.
61. Raso V, Ritz J, Busala M, et al. Monoclonal antibody-ricin A chain conjugate selectively cytotoxic for cells bearing the common acute lymphoblastic leukemia antigen. *Cancer Res* 1982; 42: 457-464.
62. Rizzoli V, Mangoni L. Pharmaceutical-mediated purging with mafosfamide in acute and chronic myeloid leukemias. In: *Bone marrow purging and processing.* New York: Wiley-Liss, 1990: 21-38.
63. Rodt H, Kolb JH, Netzel B, et al. Effect of anti-T-cell globulin on GVHD in leukemic patients treated with BMT. *Transplant Proc* 1981; 13: 257-261.
64. Santos GW. History of bone marrow transplantation. *Clin Haematol* 1983; 12: 611-639.
65. Santos GW. Bone marrow transplantation in leukemia. Current status. *Cancer* 1984; 54: 2732-2740.
66. Santos GW. Syngeneic or autologous graft-versus-host disease. *Int J Cell Cloning* 1989; 7: 92-99.
67. Sharp TG, Sachs DH, Fauci AS, et al. T cell depletion of human bone marrow using monoclonal antibody and complement-mediated lysis. *Transplantation* 1983; 35: 112-120.
68. Sheridan WP, Wolf M, Lusk J, et al. Granulocyte colony-stimulating factor and neutrophil recovery after high-dose chemotherapy and autologous bone marrow transplantation. *Lancet* 1989; ii: 891-895.
69. Sheridan WP, Begley GC, Juttner CA, et al. Effect of peripheral-blood progenitor cells mobilized by filgrastim (G-CSF) on platelet recovery after high dose chemotherapy. *Lancet* 1992; 339: 640-644.
70. Shpall EJ, Anderson IC, Bast RC Jr, et al. Immunopharmacologic purging of breast cancer from bone marrow for autologous bone marrow transplantation. In: *Bone marrow purging and processing*. New York: Wiley-Liss, 1990: 321-336.
71. Siena S, Bregni M, Brando B, et al. Circulation of CD34+ hematopoietic stem cells in the peripheral blood of high-dose cyclophosphamide-treated patients: enhancement by intravenous recombinant human granulocyte-macrophage colony-stimulating factor. *Blood* 1989; 74: 1905-1914.
72. Skala JP, Rogers PCJ, Chan K-W, et al. Effect of methylprednisolone and VP-16 on acute lymphocytic leukemia cells. In: *Bone marrow purging and processing*. New York: Wiley-Liss, 1990: 79-86.
73. Slavin S, Waldmann H, Or R, et al. Prevention of graft-versus-host disease in allogeneic bone marrow transplantation for leukemia by T cell depletion *in vitro* prior to transplantation. *Transplant Proc* 1985; 17: 465-467.
74. Sparkes MC, Crist ML, Sparkes RS, et al. Gene markers in human bone marrow transplantation. *Vox Sang* 1977; 33: 202-205.
75. Sullivan KM, Shulman HM, Storb R, et al. Chronic graft-versus-host disease in 52 patients: adverse natural course and successful treatment with combination immunosuppression. *Blood* 1981; 57: 267-276.
76. Sullivan KM, Storb R. Allogeneic marrow transplantation. *Cancer Invest* 1984; 2: 27-38.
77. Takaue Y, Watanabe T, Kawano Y, et al. Isolation and storage of peripheral blood hematopoietic stem cells for autotransplantation into children with cancer. *Blood* 1989; 74: 1245-1251.
78. Thomas ED. Karnofsky Memorial Lecture. Marrow transplantation for malignant diseases. *J Clin Oncol* 1983; 1: 517-531.
79. Tong AW, Dalton WS, Tsuruo T, et al. Elimination of chemoresistant myeloma clonogenic cells from human bone marrow by monoclonal antibody and complement. In: *Bone marrow purging and processing.* New York: Wiley-Liss, 1990: 15-164.
80. Treleaven JG, Kemshead JT. Removal of tumour cells from bone marrow: an evaluation of the available techniques. *Hematol Oncol* 1985; 3: 65-75.
81. Vallera DA, Quinones RR, Azemove SM, et al. Monoclonal antibody-toxin conjugates reactive against human T lymphocytes. A comparison of antibody linked to intact ricin toxin with antibody linked to ricin A chain. *Transplantation.* 1984; 37: 387-392.
82. Vallera DA. Uckun FM. Bone marrow purging with immunotoxins for treatment of T-cell acute lymphoblastic leukemia (T-ALL). In: *Bone marrow purging and processing*. New York: Wiley-Liss, 1990: 191-205.
83. van Rhee F, Lyn F, Cullous JO, et al. Relapse of chronic myeloid leukemia after allogeneic bone marrow transplant: the case for giving donor leukocyte transfusions before the onset of hematological relapse. *Blood* 1994; 83: 3377-3383.
84. Vitetta ES, Uhr JW. The potential use of immunotoxins in transplantation, cancer therapy, and immunoregulation. *Transplantation* 1984; 37: 535-538.
85. Vogler WR, Olson AC, Berdel WE, et al. Purging leukemia remission marrows with alkyl-lysophospholipids, preclinical and clinical results. In: *Bone marrow purging and processing*. New York: Wiley-Liss, 1990: 1-20.
86. Waldmann H, Polliak A, Hale G, et al. Elimination of graft-versus-host disease by *in vitro* depletion of alloreactive lymphocytes with a monoclonal rat anti-human lymphocyte antibody (CAMPATH-1). *Lancet* 1984; 2: 483-486.
87. Williams SF, Bitran JD, Richards JM, et al. Peripheral blood-derived stem cell collections for use in autologous transplantation after high dose chemotherapy: an alternative approach. In: *Bone marrow purging and processing*. New York: Wiley-Liss, 1990: 461-469.
88. Winter JN, Bass B, Bringman T, Nedwin G. Preclinical evaluation of immunoconjugates consisting of doxorubicin linked to complement-fixing monoclonal antibody DLC-48 for bone marrow purging of B-cell lymphomas. In: *Bone marrow purging and processing.* New York: Wiley-Liss, 1990: 171-183.
89. Witherspoon R, Lum LG, Storb R. Immunologic reconstitution after human marrow grafting. *Semin Hematol* 1984; 21: 2-10.

UPDATE ON THE LABORATORY ASPECTS OF THE CELLULAR IMMUNOTHERAPY OF HUMAN CANCER

JOHN R. YANNELLI
University of Kentucky, School of Medicine, Markey Cancer Center, Lexington, Kentucky

INTRODUCTION

There has been tremendous progress made in the field of cellular immunotherapy over the last six years since the publication of the second edition of *Principles of Cancer Biotherapy*. In our chapter in that Edition, we focused on the nonspecific arm of the cellular immune response (LAK cells, macrophages) and how it could be utilized clinically to cure metastatic cancer [103]. We discussed rapidly developing large scale cell culture technologies used to generate LAK cells and macrophages. Our emphasis was on the generation of the cells in such a way that they could be routinely infused into cancer patients. At the time, we could only hint at what has occurred between 1991 and 1996 in terms of basic lymphocyte biology and cellular immunotherapy. These advances have dramatically affected our most recent approaches to immunotherapy. While we introduced the potential of the specific arm of the immune system in fighting cancer, we could only speculate on the impact tumor infiltrating lymphocytes (TIL) would make in the immunotherapy of tumors. In addition, the various specificities of TIL have allowed the identification of lymphocyte defined tumor antigens on melanoma tumor cells. These discoveries have been of immense value toward expanding and improving our approach to immunotherapies. It is not unreasonable to plan for the day when all manipulations of the immune system will be accomplished *in vivo* through the use of specific vaccines.

The work to be described in this updated chapter of *Principles* will center on CD3+ lymphocytes which bear the αβ form of the T cell receptor. We will not further review LAK cells or macrophages but the reader is encouraged to examine recent references detailing both clinical and laboratory issues regarding their use [53, 71, 72]. It is not to say that these cell types do not contribute to the immune response against cancer and that their function cannot be utilized, however, so much focus is currently on tumor specific T cells that I feel this topic should be reviewed in more detail. Thus, this chapter will show how specific T cells derived from melanoma tumors can be expanded from different anatomic sites, characterized for functional reactivity, and utilized in cellular immunotherapy protocols. In addition, we will introduce some of the recently discovered CTL defined antigens on melanoma tumor cells and discuss how they might be utilized in future vaccine therapies. In light of the large amount of research that has been done over the past ten years, it is hoped that the reader will view the immune response against cancer as a whole (nonspecific and specific) and try to piece together all aspects of it in the fight against cancer. The ultimate goal for everyone is to develop novel and successful ways of fighting an individuals metastatic disease. The reader should appreciate where the field is going and the author suggests that it is time to apply the wealth of information gathered in melanoma to other tumor histologies (lung cancer, breast cancer, colon cancer, renal cell cancer, prostate cancer etc.).

TUMOR INFILTRATING LYMPHOCYTES (TIL)

In addition to tumor cells, solid tumors contain a variable complement of host cells including fibroblasts, endothelial cells, macrophages, dendritic cells and lymphocytes. Early murine studies showed that lymphocytes contained in tumors, termed tumor infiltrating lymphocytes or TIL [73], could be expanded to large numbers *in vitro* in the presence of IL-2. When reinfused into tumor bearing mice, TIL were shown to be efficacious against a variety of solid tumors [84]. TIL have also been derived and expanded from human solid tumors including: multiple histologies [14, 28, 48, 49, 50, 55, 74, 89, 90, 104]; melanoma [1, 3, 25, 30, 31, 35, 36, 37, 38, 59, 61, 75, 76, 79, 80, 92, 105]; renal cell cancer [5, 6, 18, 19, 20, 47, 58, 77, 78, 85]; breast cancer [4, 40, 41, 52, 81, 96]; colon cancer [32, 87, 98, 111]; non renal urologic cancer [27] ; pancreatic adenocarcinoma [41]; head and neck cancer [29]; brain tumors 57, 101]; lung cancer 56, 112, 113]; and ovarian cancer [2, 22, 33, 34, 63]. TIL have also been isolated from blood borne malignancy such as lymphoma [39, 54, 82, 83] and most recently in our lab from B-CLL (Yannelli et al., unpublished observation). When TIL are expanded *in vitro* in the presence of natural or recombinant Interleukin-2 (IL-2), the cellular events which occur are proliferation and in some cases, activation to a tumoricidal state. Because of this activated tumoricidal state, TIL have been used in

R.K. Oldham (ed.), Principles of Cancer Biotherapy. 3rd ed., 376–386.

clinical trials for the treatment of patients with metastatic disease [72].

Growth of TIL from human solid tumors

The growth of TIL for human clinical trials has been accomplished by three techniques including: 1) growth of TIL from single cell suspensions using conventional cell culture vessels [1, 75, 89, 104], growth of TIL from small pieces of tumor (tumor chunks) using conventional cell culture vessels [49, 55, 72]and growth of TIL from single cell suspensions using hollow fiber bioreactor technology [22, 46, 50]. In all cases, the number of TIL used for clinical studies has ranged from approximately 1 x 10^{10} to 3 x 10^{11}. The critical factor in all studies has been to generate this therapeutic dose of TIL in as short a period of time as possible so the TIL can be administered to the patient before disease progresses. It is difficult to say which of the three techniques is best for the growth of TIL for clinical trials. There are advantages and disadvantages to each technique. The most common method and the one used in our studies at the National Cancer Institute from 1991-1995 involved culturing TIL from enzymatically digested single cell suspensions in a conventional cell culture system which included cell culture plates and Baxter/ Fenwal PL732 gas permeable culture bags [104]. This process, as initially described by Topalian et al. [89, 90], while requiring much time in preparing the sample for cell culture, actually provides the most consistent source of TIL. Although the tissue architecture is destroyed due to the enzyme process and lymphocytes are forced to re-establish spatial relationships with antigen presenting cells and other accessory cells in an artificial cell culture environment, the advantage is that lymphocytes are washed free of dead and necrotic tissue which may otherwise decrease TIL expansion. Using this technique, an average of greater than 1 x 10^{11} TIL were generated between 30-45 days from all histologies tested [104]. The remainder of the present chapter will focus on this methodology for the growth of TIL since it was successfully used for the expansion and characterization of 255 tumor biopsies including melanoma, renal cell cancer, breast cancer and colon cancer. Before we continue, however, the reader should be aware of the other techniques used to grow TIL. A second technique, originally described by Kradin et al. [49], and Maleckar et al. [55], utilized small tumor fragments or chunks for the initial culture of TIL. While this technique requires less initial preparation of the sample for culture (no enzymatic digestion and no Ficoll Hypaque separation), the technique requires a greater length of time for the expansion of TIL. Early studies showed a lag of about 10-14 days before a significant monolayer of TIL were present (Yannèlli, Unpublished observation). Thus, expansion to therapeutic levels took longer as documented by Dillman et al. [14] and Maleckar et al. [55] (79 days from chunks as opposed to 43 days from single cell suspensions, Yannelli et al. [104]).

The third technique used to expand TIL involves growth in the extracapillary space(EC) of a hollow fiber bioreactor (Knazek et al. [46]; Lewko et al. [50]; and Freedman et al. [22]). This technique involves the least manipulation of the single cell suspension. More importantly, the technique allows the continuous bathing of the TIL in fresh medium containing nutrients and IL-2, and at the same time provides continual waste removal. A major advantage of this technique is the expansion of cells in a small defined space eliminating the need for over 100 culture vessels and multiple incubators. The bioreactor requires less room in the laboratory, less manipulation of the cell product, and less medium to handle at harvest time. The disadvantages at the moment are the initial cost of the system, limited prior use by multiple investigators, and a relatively high cost to operate. However, weighing the advantages and disadvantages it seems that this technology should be further explored. This author feels it should be applied not only to TIL culture but also the expansion of tumor or viral peptide specific CTL which is currently on the near horizon.

GROWTH OF TIL USING CONVENTIONAL CELL CULTURE TECHNOLOGY

As mentioned, the following discussion will focus on the clinical expansion of TIL which occurred in the Surgery Branch of the NCI during the years 1991-1995. Once the tumor was removed from the cancer patient, every effort was made to maintain sterility in order to return a safe, microorganism free infusion product to the cancer patient. Tumor biopsies in our studies ranged in size from less than a gram to hundreds of grams. Tumors arrived in the lab shortly after surgery and were dissected in the presence of a pathologist. Tumor tissue was dissected away from normal and necrotic tissue using sterile scalpels and forceps under a laminar flow biological cabinet. Following dissection, the small tumor chunks (1-3mm^3 in size) were placed in RPMI-1640 containing the enzymes collagenase, hyaloronidase, and DNAase as well as antibiotics and fungizone [104]. The digestion was done overnight at room temperature to insure a complete digestion to a single cell suspension. Alternatively, the enzyme medium containing tumor chunks were placed in a 37°C incubator and the digestion sometimes occurred within 3-4 hrs. In either case, at the end of the digestion, the single cell suspensions were passed through a sterile wire grid in order to remove undigested tumor chunks. The single cell suspensions were washed 3 times in Ca++Mg++ free PBS at which point an initial cell count was done. Our results with melanoma biopsies indicated that cell yields up to 10^9 could be made erythrocyte (RBC) and dead cell free by using a conventional Ficoll Hypaque procedure (1ml packed cell volume per gradient; 1 ml packed cells resuspended in 30 ml of Ca++Mg++ free PBS and layered over 15 ml of Ficoll Hypaque in a 50 ml conical centrifuge tube; centrifuge at 400g for 20 minutes). This step was not necessary, however, if the total cell viability was greater than 60% and the ratio of RBC to WBC was less than 10: 1 (Unpublished data). These single cell populations were placed directly in culture with no adverse effects. In either case, it was important to wash the single cell suspensions extensively in Ca++Mg++ free PBS or HBSS before being placed in cell culture.

The washed single cell suspensions were placed in cell culture using a variety of different cell culture medium. During a five year period of time, we cultured TIL in either RPMI-1640 containing 10% human serum, AIMV serum free medium (Gibco, Grand Island New York) or a 50/50 mixture of the two medium formulations. No definitive advantage was observed using either of the formulations. However, serum free products reduce the risk of viral contaminants to the final TIL product. In place of AIMV serum free medium, many laboratories alternatively used the serum free product X-VIVO-10 or X-VIVO-15 produced by Whitaker Bioproducts (Walkersville, Maryland). The medium was further supplemented with antibiotics, fungizone, glutamine, and either a low or high concentration of Interleukin-2 (IL-2). It was our observation that TIL grew more consistently in the presence of high concentrations of IL-2 (1000 Cetus units/ml, 6000IU/ml) (Unpublished Observation). Speculating, the reason the low doses of IL-2 (120 IU/ml) did not work as consistently was due to the need for continued replenishing of the medium with IL-2. This required a rigid schedule of IL-2 dosing which could not always be accomplished. There was, however, always a desire to culture the TIL in low concentrations of IL-2 in order to make the TIL more physiologic and less IL-2 dependent following infusion of the TIL into cancer patients.

Additional cytokines were provided to TIL cultures in the form of supernatants obtained from standard LAK cultures. LAK supernatant appeared to have improved the probability of growing TIL with desired functional reactivities. The LAK supernatant was prepared by simply establishing LAK cultures by conventional methodology [60, 106]. Following 3-5 days of incubation, the cell culture medium was centrifuged and the supernatant removed and stored either in the refrigerator or freezer. When evaluated, we detected high levels of gamma interferon, IL-2, GMCSF, as well as other cytokines in the LAK supernatant[16]. The supernatants were stable for at least one year with storage in the cold at 4°C.

The enzymatically digested single cell suspensions were placed in culture in 24 well cluster plates at 1 x 10^6 total cells/well (5 x 10^5/ml, 2mls/well). Initially, culturing the cells at total cells/ml insured that no distinction needed to be made concerning the absolute lymphocyte count. The total number of lymphocytes in a tumor biopsy varied based on the tumor histology, anatomic site of the biopsy, age of the tumor and other yet defined factors. As mentioned, contained in a tumor biopsy, in addition to lymphocytes were tumor cells, fibroblasts, endothelial cells and macrophages. It will be advantageous at some point to understand more precisely what the optimum number and ratio of antigen presenting cells, tumor cells and precursor lymphocytes need to be for a more successful and consistent growth of TIL cultures.

In TIL cultures containing IL-2, clusters of lymphocytes (TIL) grew from the single cell suspension over the first 7-10 days. In medium lacking IL-2 and containing fetal bovine serum (FBS), we observed the outgrowth of fibroblasts and tumor cell colonies [15, 24, 51, 107]. The success rate at growing long term established tumor cell cultures was approximately 40% for melanoma and roughly less than 10% for colon, breast, lung, and other histologies. Melanoma cell lines could be initiated in medium containing 2-10% FBS. Often, the lower concentrations of FBS (2-5%) favored the growth of tumor cells while 10% FBS favored the growth of fibroblasts. In other histologies (breast, lung, and colon for instance), more specialized medium was required for the establishment of a stable tumor cell line. In some cases the cell lines required less serum to serum free conditions, and/or the addition of growth factors such as epidermal growth factor (EGF), insulin, selenium, and transferrin. Stable, long term tumor cell lines, once established and characterized, served a very useful function for the immunologic analysis of the T cells which grow from the tumor lesions. In addition, these long term stable tumor cell lines, particularly in melanoma, were instrumental in the identification of melanoma tumor associated antigens and have been used as immunogens in vaccine trials.

In the presence of IL-2 and either human or fetal bovine serum, the TIL often grew to confluency in 10 to 14 days. We observed successful growth of TIL to levels of 10^{10} or greater using the conditions described in this chapter 63% of the time (160/255 for all biopsies; 124/206 for melanoma, 16/23 for renal cell cancer, 10/14 for breast cancer, 10/12 for colon cancer) [104]. Once in a log phase of growth, TIL were transferred to increasingly larger culture vessels (24 well plates to 6 well plates). Upon reaching confluency in 6 well plates, the TIL were transferred to Fenwal PL732 plastic platelet storage bags. These bags had proven very useful for the activation of LAK cells [106] as well as useful for the expansion of TIL to therapeutic levels [89]. PL732 bags allow the free passage of oxygen and CO2 across the bags surface but not the passage of fluids. More importantly, for large scale expansions, these bags can be attached to larger bags containing medium and filled aseptically using a Baxter/ Fenwal solution transfer pump and sterile tubing kits. In addition, when ready for treatment, the bags can be attached to a harvesting machine (Manuscript in preparation, Yannelli et al.) designed for large scale harvesting. Each bag accommodates large volumes of medium containing cells (1 liter capacity bag, 500 ml of medium containing TIL at 5 x 10^5/ml; 3 liter capacity bag, 1500 ml of medium containing TIL at 5 x 10^5/ml). Using the PL732 cell culture bags resulted in a reduction in culture ware costs as well as a reduction in handling time by the technicians.

The manner in which the TIL were split for continued growth was critical. We found that it was important not to replace cell culture medium 100%, but rather, take advantage of the conditioned medium from the previous culture period. Thus, we performed a series of bag splitting procedures. We believed the carrying capacity of the TIL culture medium in static culture (conventional cell culture) was between 2 and 3 x 10^6 /ml. Metabolic waste products build up in static culture to a detrimental level(Unpublished data) faster than critical reagents such as serum components and IL-2 were exhausted by the TIL. Thus, the splitting procedures reduced the level of waste products to a manageable level and maintained usable concentrations of critical reagents which were supplemented further in the fresh medium added. The splitting procedure also maintained levels of cytokines produced by the activated lymphocytes during the previous culture period. Interestingly, similar culture medium used in hollow fiber bioreactors supported TIL expansion in excess of 100 x 10^6/ml [46, 50]. This further supported the idea that as long as wastes were removed, as they were in the hollow fiber bioreactor, the medium could support TIL growth far in excess of what was normally achieved in static culture.

Using bag splitting procedures, TIL double every 1.5 to three days. These procedures increased the number of culture bags proportionately. That is, bags containing cells at concentrations greater than 1.5 x 10^6/ml were split back to 5 x 10^5 TIL/ml by splitting 1: 3 (1.5 x 10^6/ml), 1: 4 (2 x 10^6/ml), or 1: 5 (>2.5 x 10^6/ml) by mixing 1 part old medium containing TIL with 2, 3, or 4 parts fresh medium respectively. In our experience at the NCI, cultures were maximally expanded to 108 bags. This was a convenient number since it involved routine splits of the bags from 3 to 12 to 36 to 108. The final split generally occurred between days 20 and 35 of cell culture. When cultures were initiated at 108 bags (5 x 10^5/ml), they contained approximately 8.1 x 10^{10} TIL and over the course of 4-7 days the cell number reached the therapeutic level desired (1.5 x 10^{11} to 3 x 10^{11}). The patients were routinely treated between 35 and 45 days from the beginning of TIL culture.

At the time of the final expansion of bags from 36 to 108, a series of steps were taken to insure that the infusion product would not compromise the patient in terms of bacterial, fungal, endotoxin, or tumor cell contamination. In general, 24 hrs after the split from 36 to 108 bags, 10% of the bags were randomly sampled and an aliquot of cell containing medium was sent to a certified microbiology lab. There the samples were monitored by routine culture techniques for the presence of bacteria and fungus. In addition, supernatants were tested by the LAL assay (limulus amoebocyte lysate, Whitaker Bioproducts, Walkersville Md) for the presence of endotoxin. In our experience, cultures routinely contained less than 1.0 endotoxin unit/ml with the average for 200 tests being 0.3 + 0.1 EU/ml. Finally, the cultures were monitored for the presence of residual tumor cells[62] by microscopic evaluation of Wright stained cytocentrifuge smears. In no case were tumor cells observed in TIL suspensions prepared for patient infusion. Knowledge of negative results of these tests were always known before final preparation of the cell product for reinfusion into the cancer patients.

Harvesting of the final TIL product presented a problem in most labs because volumes in the range of 162 liters of cell culture medium containing cells had to be reduced to a volume which could be safely infused into cancer patients. Both Baxter/Fenwal and Dupont developed special centrifuges which allow the harvesting of the TIL cells from the cell culture medium. In addition, techniques have been developed for the extensive washing of the final infusion product in sterile saline. The entire process resulted in a reduction in fluid volume from 162 liters of culture medium containing cells to approximately 300 mls of infusable saline containing TIL. To achieve this, the Fenwal PL732 cell culture plastic bags containing TIL were aseptically connected using sterile tubing kits which allowed the flow of medium containing cells into the centrifuge chamber of the Rapid cell harvester or the Dupont harvester. Using either machine, the cells were collected by standard centrifugation and the medium removed and discarded. The 162 liters of medium was processed at flow rates ranging from 100ml/minute to 1 liter a minute. The advantage of course of the faster speeds was to reduce the time the TIL spent in an environment of non-physiologic temperatures and at high cell densities (>1 x 10^8/ml). In our lab at the NCI, running the Baxter/Fenwal Rapid Cell Harvester at a flow rate of an average of 700ml/minute, a routine harvest of 162, 000 of medium containing cells took approximately 4 hrs.

Using the harvester, the final cell products were washed free of debris and reagents such as IL-2, amphotericin and antibiotics. The cell suspensions were washed in 1-4 liters of sterile saline. Following the wash, the TIL cell pellets were resuspended in a mixture of infusible saline and human albumin (25% V/V human albumin). The final volumes of TIL ranged from 300 to 500 mls. In earlier studies at Biotherapeutics Inc., the TIL harvested from over 100 culture bags were infused in a single infusion bag containing a small volume of 300-350 mls. In our trials at the Surgery Branch of the NCI, the TIL were infused over the course of 2 days (2 bags a day), up to 2 x 10^{11} TIL a day (1 x 10^{11} a bag). The author is aware of no adverse affects associated with either method of infusion. There is certainly an advantage to infusing the TIL as soon as possible in order to begin the IL-2 infusions. However, difficulties can be associated with large boluses of cells passing into the vasculature of the lungs at one time. The sheer size of the bolus and the cytokines released *in vivo* are potential areas of concern for clinical staff infusing the TIL.

Cryopreservation of TIL for clinical studies

TIL specimens can be cryopreserved both in small numbers or bulk frozen in larger numbers suitable for future clinical use. Upon thawing, the TIL most often retain growth characteristics and functional reactivity observed prior to cryopreservation. It is very common to cryopreserve small samples of TIL at various points of culture for future immunological study (cytotoxicity, cytokine release assays, cell surface phenotype assays). In our studies, TIL were frozen at cell densities ranging from 1 x 10^7 to 1.0 x 10^8 in a 1-1.5 ml volume. The TIL are frozen in a cryopreservation medium consisting of 90% serum (either human AB or FBS) and 10% DMSO (Dimethylsulfoxide, Sigma, St Louis, Mo). The vials of TIL were placed in a container specifically designed for vial cryopreservation. These containers were obtained from Fisher Scientific (Pittsburgh, Pa) and are called Nalgene cryogenic controlled rate freezing containers. The containers were filled with isopropanol which allows the container to chill to -70°C at 1° a minute. After 12-36 hrs at -70°C, the vials were transferred to liquid nitrogen to insure maintenance of cellular integrity. Alternatively, the vials containing cells were cryopreserved using a controlled rate freezer.

It was also advantageous to cryopreserve large portions of TIL for future clinical use. Situations arose where TIL were needed for additional courses of therapy. In addition, patients were sometimes not able to receive their treatment when the TIL were available. This varied depending upon patient clinical status and the status of other courses of therapy. In our studies we cryopreserved TIL in bone marrow cryopreservation bags (Baxter/Fenwal) between days 25 and 30 of cell culture. We routinely cryopreserved 1 x 10^{10} TIL per bag in a volume of 100 ml. The freeze medium consisted of 25% human serum albumin, 10% DMSO and 65% AIM V serum free medium. The bags were cryopreserved carefully in a controlled rate freezer designed for freezer bags (Cryoserve by Gordinier; Cryo Inc. Rockville Md). Once frozen, the bags were stored in liquid nitrogen until use. Bags were thawed after up to 3 years in liquid nitrogen and had growth and functional characteristics similar to when they were frozen. When therapy was needed, the bags were generally thawed 10-14 days before the treatment date. In that period of time, the 10^{10} aliquot of cells could expand to levels $>10^{11}$. There were instances in our studies at the NCI of thawed reinfused TIL, following long periods of time in liquid nitrogen, being responsible for clinical benefit.

FUNCTIONAL CHARACTERISTICS OF TIL

TIL derived from tumor biopsies of different histologies have been extensively studied for functional characteristics. These characteristics include: cell surface phenotype for T cell surface antigens, ability to lyse autologous and allogeneic fresh tumor cells and tumor cell lines, and the ability of the TIL to secrete various cytokines when stimulated with tumor cells. The functional reactivities can be classified as either none, nonspecific or LAK like activity (non MHC restricted lysis or cytokine release) or specific functional reactivity (lysis of or release of cytokines in response to autologous tumor and/or HLA matched fresh tumor or tumor cell lines of the same histology).

In general, TIL which grow from tumor biopsies are CD3+ T cells expressing the $\alpha\beta$ form of the T cell receptor. The subtype of lymphocyte, being CD4 or CD8, often depends upon the tumor histology from which it is derived. A variety of other T cell surface antigens have also been examined. For the most part, TIL populations uniformly express activation antigens such as HLA-DR and CD25. Finally, the observance of NK cells in tumor biopsies and the outgrowth of LAK cells, CD16+/CD56+ cells, was rare.

In terms of examining functional reactivity, most labs are concerned about cytotoxicity for predominantly CD8+ TIL populations and cytokine production for both CD8 and predominant CD4+ populations. In general, a mix of CD4 and CD8 cells grow out so most laboratories perform both assays. Cytotoxicity assays are short term 4 hr assays done by standard methodology. Cytokine assays are done as originally described by Hom and Schwartzentruber [30, 31, 79, 80]. Based on our studies, the following observations were made concerning TIL populations. In terms of cytotoxicity, young TIL cultures (<30 days old) were characterized by nonspecific lytic and cytokine producing activity which was not correlated with the presence of LAK cells (CD16+CD56+ cells). In some cases, as culture time passes, TIL populations become specific with a phenotypic shift toward more homogeneous CD3+/CD4+ or CD3+/CD8+ populations.

Specificity, or the ability to recognize tumor cells and not normal cells or tumor cells of other histologies, has been observed most consistently using TIL grown from melanoma lesions [1, 30, 31, 59, 61, 75, 79, 80, 91, 104, 105]. This is not to say that specific T cells have not been observed in other histologies. Rather, using the techniques described for the expansion of TIL from tumor biopsies, it has been less common to observe the outgrowth of specific T cells in other tumor histologies. Nonetheless, there are examples in the literature as illustrated by the following references: ovarian cancer [34, 63]; renal cell cancer [19, 40, 47, 77]; colon cancer [32]; breast cancer 4, 41, 52, 81, 96]; sarcoma [86] and head and neck cancer [108]. However, because of the extensive experience we gained in melanoma at the NCI between 1991 and 1995, the remainder of this chapter will focus on the functional reactivities of TIL derived from melanoma lesions.

TIL DERIVED FROM MELANOMA LESIONS

TIL can be derived from melanoma lesions and grown to therapeutic levels from a variety of anatomic sites including: subcutaneous sites (sc), tumor involved lymph nodes, lung, muscle, bowel, brain, spleen, adrenal gland, bone, and pleural fluid [104]. During the course of our study [104], 206 melanoma biopsies were processed from the 11 anatomic sites. Of 206 biopsies, 124 (60%) grew to therapeutic levels ($>10^{10}$) using the conditions described. In many of the other cultures the growth rate was too slow to reach a sufficient number of cells for therapy in a reasonable period of time (30-45 days). Eighty-nine TIL cultures were grown to levels of 10^{11} or greater. A number of the cultures which expanded to levels of 10^{10} were discontinued before reaching 10^{11} cells for various reasons ranging from the patient being too ill to receive therapy or the TIL were used for another protocol before 10^{11} cells were reached.

The cytolytic activity using 4 hour ^{51}chromium release cytotoxicity assays of the melanoma TIL cultures was evaluated in 115 of the 124 cultures grown to levels of 10^{10} or greater. This activity was normally measured between days 30 and 45 of TIL culture. Melanoma TIL from 78 (68%) of 115 cultures tested exhibited some cytolytic activity (>10% lysis) against tumor targets including in most cases: fresh autologous tumor, fresh allogeneic melanoma and/or allogeneic melanoma cell culture lines, K562 and Daudi. TIL from 57 (50%) of the cultures tested lysed autologous tumor at a level of 10% or greater. Furthermore, 43 (37%) of the cultures exhibited preferential lysis of autologous tumor, that is, the TIL lysed autologous tumor cells (>10%) with less than 10% lysis observed against the NK target K562, the LAK target Daudi, and <37> lysis against non-MHC matched melanomas. Thirty-seven TIL cultures had no cytolytic activity at all when tested.

We were most successful at growing TIL from subcutaneous lesions (62/84, 74%) compared to tumor involved lymph nodes (41/81, 50% $p<0.05$). Despite the small sample size, it appeared that TIL could be successfully grown from lung biopsies (7/9), and bowel biopsies (5/5). TIL from subcutaneous lesions had a greater tendency to lyse autologous tumor than TIL obtained from nodal sites. Out of 56 cases where cytotoxicity was measured from TIL obtained from subcutaneous tumor, 32 cultures (57%) contained TIL which could lyse autologous tumor (>10%) and 28 (50%) lysed autologous tumor preferentially. These numbers are in contrast to the cytolytic activity of the TIL derived from tumor involved lymph nodes. Of 39 evaluable cultures from nodal tumors, 15 (38%) were capable of lysing autologous tumor and significantly fewer ($P<0.05$), only 7 (18%), lysed autologous tumor preferentially. TIL which exhibited preferential lysis of autologous tumor were also obtained from tumors in lung (5/7, 71%) and bowel (3/4, 75%). TIL grown from muscle and sites listed as other (brain, pleural fluid, spleen, adrenal, retroperitoneal, bone, and pericardial fluid) did not give rise to TIL which lysed autologous tumor preferentially. In addition, only 9/27 (33%) of these TIL grew to therapeutic levels. TIL obtained from subcutaneous lesions and tumor involved lymph nodes (81 tested) were CD3+ (96%) and TIL from these cultures were predominantly CD8+ (69%) as opposed to CD4+ (31%). A high percentage of the cells were activated based on the expression of HLA-DR (82%) with 13% of the CD3+ lymphocytes co-expressing CD56.

CORRELATION OF CLINICAL RESPONSES AND *IN VITRO* FUNCTIONAL REACTIVITY

For a number of years, TIL populations from all histologies were grown and infused into cancer patients, regardless of the immunmologic properties of the lymphocyte populations. The question was often asked whether there was any relationship between *in vitro* function and clinical responses. In 1991, Aebersold et al. [1] were the first to report that there was a correlation between *in vitro* functional characteristics of melanoma derived TIL and clinical responses. Specifically, they reported that 1) the ability of melanoma derived TIL to lyse autologous tumor cells and 2) the age of the TIL (30-40 days old), generally correlated with clinical response. These findings were corroborated and extended in two reports using melanoma TIL by Schwartzentruber et al. [80] and Rosenberg et al. [75] in 1994. In addition, these studies showed that it was also important for the TIL to release cytokine, specifically GMCSF, when stimulated with autologous tumor cells. Finally, they reported that there was a correlation between the anatomic site TIL were derived from and clinical response. That is, infusion of TIL derived from extranodal sites were more likely to result in clinical responses than TIL derived from tumor involved lymph nodes. In retrospect, considering that the ability to generate TIL with the ability to lyse autologous tumor is only consistently found in melanoma, it suggests that until ways are devised to obtain functionally relevant cells in other histologies more regularly, that melanoma is the only histology which should be routinely treated with TIL. The clinical TIL trials at the NCI now focus on melanoma. This will probably change when functionally relevant lymphocytes are generated more frequently in the other histologies.

In 1994, we devised a clinical and laboratory scheme designed to take advantage of the correlates we found between functional reactivities of melanoma derived TIL and clinical responses. That is, we attempted to predict which populations of TIL would be most effective *in vivo* and use only those TIL for therapy. Through a process of *in vitro* screen techniques, only those patients were treated whose TIL fit certain criteria. Those criteria included: TIL derived from extranodal sites, young TIL cultures which could be infused no later than 30-35 days of cell culture, and TIL which demonstrated functional reactivity against autologous tumor as demonstrated by cytotoxicity or cytokine release. The screen process was performed between days 20 and 24 in order to learn whether the TIL therapeutic option was available. If not, patients could be moved to other available therapeutic options. Interestingly, we succeeded in being able to differentiate potentially efficacious populations of TIL from non-efficacious ones at the early time point. Clinical results were promising but unavailable at the time of the preparation of this chapter.

MELANOMA LYMPHOCYTE DEFINED TUMOR ASSOCIATED ANTIGENS

The identification of immunologically specific lymphocytes obtained from melanoma biopsies suggested the presence of tumor associated antigens. Thus, the search for the nature of lymphocyte defined tumor associated antigens began in a number of laboratories. Knowledge obtained from the structure and characteristics of the antigens would be invaluable to the field of immunotherapy considering their use in constructing vaccines and also their potential use *in vitro* in generating more efficiently, specific lymphocytes for clinical trials. The final section of this chapter will briefly introduce what has been learned to date about lymphocyte defined antigens in melanoma.

In humans, it has clearly been demonstrated that T cells, isolated from either tumor (TIL) [36, 59, 91, 105] or peripheral blood [13, 66, 88] can recognize specific antigens on melanoma tumor cells. Melanoma associated tumor antigens are recognized in an HLA restricted fashion, that is, antigen is recognized in context of the molecules encoded by the MHC [65, 109]. In addition, a number of these lymphocyte defined melanoma antigens are considered to be shared, that is, specific lymphocytes recognize tumor cells derived from different individuals as long as the tumor cells share the class I antigens responsible for presentation [30, 31, 91, 105]. The clinical relevance of at least two of these antigens has been verified when the lymphocytes recognizing the antigens were found to mediate tumor regression when adoptively transferred into patients [42, 67].

The molecular nature of CD8 lymphocyte defined antigens has been elucidated. CD8+ lymphocytes recognize tumor associated antigen derived peptides which are endogenously processed from full length molecules and are in turn presented to the T cell receptor in the context of HLA class I molecules [109]. The size of the peptides varies from 8 to 11 amino acids in length [65]. Certain amino acid residues are critical for the binding of the peptide to the class I molecule. These amino acids are termed anchor residues and are located at the second and the last positions in the peptide sequence [17]. The other amino acids in the peptide sequence help to form the three dimensional structure recognized by the T cell receptor.

CD4 + lymphocytes are also important in the tumor response. CD4+ cells provide help for B cells, activate macrophages and facilitate the activation and expansion of cytolytic T cells through the release of cytokines [102]. Tumor associated antigen derived peptides are presented by dendritic cells via class II molecules following uptake of antigens and processing through an endosomal pathway [110], although there is an indication that endogenous processing may also occur [7]. The length of class II presented peptides has been found to be more variable than class I peptides with the predominate size of peptides in the range of 13 to 25 amino acids [11].

There have been three approaches used in the identification of antigens recognized by tumor specific T cells in melanoma. These approaches include: 1) determine whether known proteins such as viral proteins, oncofetal products, oncogene products, tissue specific proteins and proteins recognized by antibodies were being recognized by T cells, 2) examine whether components derived from tumor cells contained in cell culture supernatants are targets for recognition by T cells and 3) DNA cloning technologies [43, 99]. The lymphocyte defined tumor associated antigens discovered to date using these techniques have been classified in three categories. This classification system is based on histologic expression of the genes. The first group are considered melanocyte lineage proteins and include gP100 [44], MART-1/Melan-A [12, 45], TRP-1 [100] and tyrosinase 9, 68, 93, 94, 95]. These antigens are expressed on tumor cells as well as normal melanoncytes. The second group of antigens include members of the MAGE gene family. These antigens are represented by MAGE-1 [97], MAGE 3 [10, 23], and BAGE [8]. These antigens are expressed not only in melanoma but also in normal testis as well as tumors of other histologies including breast, lung, bladder, and squamous carcinoma. The third group are the only 'tumor specific' antigens described to date. These antigens, β-Catenin [69] and p15 [70] contain epitopes probably resulting from certain defined mutations and appear to be restricted to tumor cells. For information on all of these antigens including their discovery, characterization and potential uses, the reader is urged to examine the following reviews [43, 99] as well as the listed primary references.

THE FUTURE OF CELLULAR IMMUNOTHERAPY

An attempt has been made in the current chapter to update the reader on where the field of cellular immunotherapy has come in the last five years and where it is potentially going. The recent discovery of tumor antigens is crucial to the rapid advancement of the field. Investigators can now use the knowledge of the antigens to design specific vaccines. These vaccines, while having exciting potential *in vivo*, can also be expected following immunization to provide increased numbers of tumor specific precursors in the peripheral blood. Upon removal of peripheral blood from the patients, one can expose the precursors *in vitro* to specific antigen using relevant antigen presenting cells. Potentially this could allow the clonal expansion of the most relevant tumor specific lymphocytes. Infusion of homogeneous populations of reactive lymphocytes might reduce the required number of cells needed for therapeutic responses, thus reducing laboratory costs and potential harm to patients caused by irrelevant cytokine producing cells. There are many other approaches which are being explored and are reviewed in references cited in this chapter [9, 100].

In summary, we now have the ability to routinely expand melanoma specific lymphocytes (both CD4+ and CD8+) to therapeutic levels. In addition, in some cases we know the antigens being recognized as well as the restriction elements responsible for the peptide presentation. This knowledge along with the finding that TIL can specifically traffic to tumor sites as demonstrated by ^{111}indium labeling [21, 26, 64], provides us with a very potent tool for tumor destruction *in vivo*. What remains is the refinement of this approach in melanoma and the broad application of this knowledge to the other tumor histologies responsible for the death of so many patients. It is hoped that over the next five years the same explosion in knowledge occurs in these other histologies. If this occurs, all cancer patients will have the same therapeutic options. In addition, we will move a few steps closer to the cure of cancer utilizing this fourth modality of cancer treatment.

REFERENCES

1. Aebersold P, Hyatt C, Johnson S, et al. Lysis of autologous melanoma cells by tumor-infiltrating lymphocytes: Association with clinical response. *J Natl Cancer Inst* 1991; 83: 932-937.
2. Aoki Y, Takakuwa K, Kodama S, et al. Use of adoptive transfer of tumor-infiltrating lymphocytes alone or in combination with cisplatin containing chemotherapy in patients with epithelial ovarian cancer. *Cancer Research* 1991; 51: 1934-1939.
3. Arienti F, Belli F, Rivoltini L, et al. Adoptive immunotherapy of advanced melanoma patients with interleukin-2 (IL-2) and tumor infiltrating lymphocytes selected in vitro with low doses of IL-2. *Cancer Immunol Immunother* 1993; 36: 315-322.
4. Baxevanis CN, Dedoussis GVZ, Papadopoulos NG, et al. Tumor specific cytolysis by tumor infiltrating lymphocytes in breast cancer. *Cancer* 1994; 74: 1275-1282.
5. Belldegrun A, Muul LM, Rosenberg SA. Interleukin 2 expanded tumor infiltrating lymphocytes in human renal cell cancer: Isolation, characterization, and anti-tumor activity. *Cancer Research* 1988; 48: 206-214.
6. Belldegrun A, Pierce W, Kaboo R, et al. Interferon-alpha primed tumor infiltrating lymphocytes combined with interleukin-2 and interferon-alpha as therapy for metastatic renal cell carcinoma. *J Urol* 1993; 150: 1384-1390.
7. Bodmer H, Viville S, Benoist C, et al. Diversity of endogenous epitopes bound to MHC class II molecules. *Science* 1994; 263: 1284-1286.
8. Boel P, Wildmann C, Sensi ML, et al. Bage: a new geneen-coding an antigen recognized on human melanomas by cytolytic T lymphocytes. *Immunity* 1995; 2: 167-174.
9. Brichard V, Van Pel A, Wolfel T, et al. The tyrosinase gene coded for an antigen recognized by autologous cytolytic T lymphocytes on HLA-A2+ melanoma. *J Exp Med* 1993; 178: 489-495.
10. Celis E, Tsai V, Crimi C, et al. Induction of anti-tumor cytotoxic T lymphocytes in normal humans using primary cultures and synthetic peptide epitopes. *Proc Natl Acad Sci* 1994; 91: 2105-2109.
11. Chicz RM, Urban RG, Lane WS, et al. Predominant naturally processed peptidesbound to HLA-DR1 are derived from MHC related molecules and are heterogeneous in size. *Nature* 1992; 358: 764-768.
12. Coulie PG, Brichard V, Van Pael A, et al. A new gene coding for a differentiation antigen recognized by autologous cytolytic T lymphocytes on HLA-A2 melanomas. *J Exp Med* 1994; 180: 35-42.
13. Crowley NJ, Slingluff CL, Darrow TL, Siegler H. Generation of human autologous melanoma specific cytotoxic T cells using HLA-A2 matched allogeneic melanomas. *Cancer Research* 1990; 50: 492-500.
14. Dillman RO, Oldham RK, Barth NM, et al. Continuous interleukin-2 and tumor infiltrating lymphocytes as treatment of advanced melanoma. A National Biotherapy Study Group Trial. *Cancer* 1991; 68: 1-14.
15. Dillman RO, Nayak SK, and Beutel L. Establishing in vitro cultures of autologous tumor cells for use in active specific immunotherapy. *J Immunotherapy* 1993; 14: 65-69.
16. Dupere S, Obiri N, Lackey A, et al. Patterns of cytokines released by peripheral blood leukocytes of normal donors and cancer patients during interleukin-2 activation in vitro. *J Biol Resp Modif* 1990; 9: 140-148.
17. Falk K, Rotzschke O, Stevanovic S, et al. Allele specific motifs revealed by sequencing of self peptides eluted from MHC molecules. *Nature* 1993; 351: 290-296.
18. Finke JH, Rayman P, Alexander J, et al. Characterization of the cytolytic activity of CD4+ and cytotoxic activity. *Int J of Cancer* 1990; 45: 119-124.
19. Finke JH, Rayman P, Edinger R, et al. Characterization of human renal cell carcinoma specific cytotoxic CD8+ T cell line. *J Immunother* 1992; 11: 1-11.
20. Finke JH, Zea AH, Stanley J, et al. Loss of T cell receptor ξ chain and p56^{lck} in T-cells infiltrating human renal cell carcinoma. *Cancer Research* 1993; 53: 5613-5616.
21. Fisher B, Packard BS, Read EJ, et al. Tumor localization of adoptively transferred indium-111 labeled tumor infiltrating lymphocytes in patients with metastatic melanoma. *J Clin Oncol* 1989; 7: 250-260.
22. Freedman RS, Edwards CL, Kavanagh JJ, et al. Intraperitoneal adoptive immunotherapy of ovarian carcinoma with tumor infiltrating lymphocytes and low-dose recombinant interleukin-2: A pilot study. *J Immunother* 1994; 16: 198-210.
23. Gaugler B, Van Den Eynde B, Van Der Bruggen P, et al. Human gene Mage-3 codes for an antigen recognized on a melanoma by autologous cytolytic T lymphocytes. *J Exp Med* 1994; 179: 921-927.
24. Gazdar AF, and Oie HK. Cell culture methods for human lung cancer. *Cancer Genet Cytogenet* 1986; 19: 5-10.
25. Gervois N, Heuze F, Diez E, and Jotereau F. Selective expansion of specific anti-tumor CD8+ cytotoxic T lymphocyte clone in the bulk culture of tumor infiltrating lymphocytes from a melanoma patient: cytotoxic activity and T cell receptor gene rearrangements. *Eur J Immunol* 1990; 20: 825-831.
26. Griffith KD, Read EJ, Carasquillo JA, et al. *In vivo* distribution of adoptively transferred Indium-111 labeled tumor infiltrating lymphocytes and peripheral blood lymphocytes in patients with metastatic melanoma. *J Natl Cancer Inst* 1989; 81: 1709-1717.

27. Haas GP, Solomon D, Rosenberg SA. Tumor infiltrating lymphocytes from nonrenal urological malignancies. *Cancer Immunol Immunother* 1990; 30: 342-350.
28. Hayakawa K, Salmeron MA, Parkinson DR, et al. Study of TIL for adoptive therapy of renal cell cancer and metastatic melanoma: Sequential proliferation of cytotoxic natural killer and noncytotoxic T cells in RCC. *J Immunother* 1991; 10: 313-325.
29. Heo DS, Whiteside TL, Johnson JT, et al. Long term interleukin-2 dependentgrowth and cytotoxic activity of tumor infiltrating lymphocytes from human squamous cell carcinomas of the head and neck. *Cancer Research* 1987; 47: 6353-6362.
30. Hom SS, Topalian SL, Simonis T, et al. Common expression of melanoma tumor-associated antigens recognized by human tumor infiltrating lymphocytes: Analysis by human lymphocyte antigen restriction. *J Immunother* 1991; 10: 153-164.
31. Hom SS, Schwartzentruber DJ, Rosenberg SA, Topalian SL. Specific release of cytokines by lymphocytes infiltrating human melanomas in response to shared melanoma tumor antigens. *J Immunother* 1993a; 13: 18-30.
32. Hom SS, Rosenberg SA, Topalian SL. Specific immune recognition of autologous tumor by lymphocytes infiltrating colon carcinomas: analysis by cytokine secretion. *Cancer Immunol Immunother* 1993b; 36: 1-8.
33. Ioannides CG, Freedman RS, Platsoucas CD, et al. Cytotoxic T cell clones isolated from ovarian tumor infiltrating lymphocytes recognize multiple antigenic epitopes on autologous tumor cells. *J Immunol* 1991; 146: 1700-1707.
34. Ionaaides CG, Fisk B, Jerome KR, et al. Cytotoxic T cells from ovarian malignant tumors can recognize polymorphic epithelial mucin core peptides. *J Immunol* 1993; 151: 3693-3703.
35. Itoh K, Tilden AB, Balch CM. Interleukin-2 activation of cytotoxic T lymphocytes infiltrating into human metastatic melanomas. *Cancer Res* 1986; 46: 3011-3017.
36. Itoh K, Platsoucas DC, Balch CM. Autologous tumor-specific cytotoxic T lymphocytes in the infiltrate of human metastatic melanomas: activation by interleukin-2 and autologous tumor tumor cells and involvement of the T cell receptor. *J Exp Med* 1988; 168: 1419-1441.
37. Itoh K, Balch CM, Murray JL, et al. Immunological properties of melanoma tumor-infiltrating lymphocytes before and after IL-2 based biotherapies. *In Vivo* 1991; 5: 647-654.
38. Itoh K, Hayakawa K, Salmeron MA, et al. Alterations in interactions between tumor infiltrating lymphocytes and tumor cells in human melanomas after chemotherapy or immunotherapy. *Cancer Immunol Immunother* 1991; 33: 238-246.
39. Jacob M-C, Piccinni M-P, Bonnefoix T, et al. T lymphocytes from invaded lymph nodes in patients with B-cell derived non-Hodgkins lymphoma: Reactivity toward the malignant clone. *Blood* 1990; 75: 1154-1160.
40. Jerome KR, Barnd DL, Bendt KM, et al. Cytotoxic T-Lymphocytes derived from patients with breast adenocarcinoma recognize an epitope present on the protein core of a mucin molecule preferentially expressed by malignant cells. *Cancer Research* 1991; 51: 2908-2916.
41. Jerome KR, Domenech N, Finn OJ. Tumor-specific cytotoxic T cell clones from patients with breast and pancreatic adenocarcinoma recognize EBV-immortalized B cellstransfected with polymporphic epithelial mucin complimentaryDNA. *J Immunology* 1993; 151: 1654-1662.
42. Kawakami Y, Eliyahu S, Delgado CH, et al. Identification of a human melanoma antigen recognized by tumor infiltrating lymphocytes associated with in vivo tumor rejection. *Proc Natl Acad Sci* 1994; 91: 6458-6462.
43. Kawakami Y, Robbins PF, Wang RF, Rosenberg SA. Identification of tumor regression antigens in melanoma. In: Biologic *Therapy of Cancer*, 2nd Edition, DeVita, VT, Hellman S, and Rosenberg SA, Eds. 1996; 3-21.
44. Kawakami Y, Eliyahu S, Delgado CH, et al. Identification of a human melanoma antigen recognized by tumor infiltrating lymphocytes associated with in vivo tumor rejection. *Proc Natl Acad Sci USA* 1994; 91: 6458-6462.
45. Kawakami Y, Eliyahu S, Delgado CH, et al. Cloning of the gene coding for a shared human melanoma antigen recognized by autologous T cells infiltrating into tumor. *Proc Natl Acad Sci USA* 1994; 3515-3519.
46. Knazek RA, Wu YW, Aebersold PA, Rosenberg SA. Culture of tumor infiltrating lymphocytes in hollow fiber bioreactors. *J Immunol Met* 1990; 127: 29-37.
47. Koo AS, Tso CL, Shimabukuro T, et al. Autologous tumor specific cytotoxicity of tumor infiltrating lymphocytes derived from human renal cell carcinoma. *J Immunother* 1991; 10: 347-354.
48. Kradin RL, Boyle LA, Preffer FI, et al. Tumor derived interleukin-2 dependent lymphocytes in adoptive immunotherapy of lung cancer. *Cancer Immunol Immunother* 1987; 24: 76-85.
49. Kradin RL, Kurnick JT, Lazarus DS, et al. Tumor infiltrating lymphocytes and interleukin-2 in treatment of advanced cancer. *Lancet* 1989; 1: 577-580.
50. Lewko WM, Good RW, Bowman D, et al. Growth of tumor derived activated cells for the treatment of cancer. *Cancer Biotherapy* 1994; 9: 211-224.
51. Lewko WM, Ladd P, Hubbard D, et al. Tumor acquisition, propagation and preservation: The culture of human colorectal cancer. *Cancer* 1989; 64: 1600-1612.
52. Linehan DC, Goedegebuure PS, Peoples GE, et al. Tumor specific and HLA-A2 restricted cytolysis by tumor associated lymphocytes in human metastatic breast cancer. *J Immunol* 1995; 155: 4486-4491.
53. Lopez M, Fechtenbaum J, David B, et al. Adoptive immunotherapy with activated macrophages grown in vitro fromblood monocytes in cancer patients: A pilot study. *J Immunother* 1992; 11: 209-217.
54. Luna-Fineman S, Lee JE, Wesley PK, et al. Human cytotoxic T lymphocytes specific for autologous follicular lymphoma recognize immunoglobulin in a major histocompatibility complex restricted fashion. *Cancer* 1992; 70: 2181-2191.
55. Maleckar JR, Friddell CS, Sferruzza A, et al. Activation and expansion of tumor derived activated cells for therapeutic use. *J Natl Cancer Inst* 1989; 81: 1655-1660.
56. Melioli G, Ratto G, Guastella M, et al. Isolation and in vitro expansion of lymphocytes infiltrating non-small cell lung carcinoma: Functional and molecular characterization for their use in adoptive immunotherapy. *Eur J of Cancer* 1994; 30: 97-102.
57. Miyatake SM, Hanada H, Yamishita J, et al. Induction of human glioma specific cytotoxic T lymphocyte lines by autologous tumor stimulation and interleukin-2. *J Neuro Oncol* 1986; 4: 55-64.
58. Morita T, Salmeron MA, Hayakawa K, et al. T cell

functions of IL-2 activated tumor infiltrating lymphocytes from renal cell carcinoma. *Regional Immunology* 1992; 4: 225-235.

59. Muul LM, Spiess PJ, Director EP, Rosenberg SA. Identification of specific cytolytic immune responses against autologous tumor in humans bearing malignant melanoma. *J Immunol* 1987a; 138: 989-995.
60. Muul LM, Director EP, Hyatt C, Rosenberg SA. Large scale production of human lymphokine activated killer cells for use in adoptive immunotherapy. *Jr Immunological Methods* 1986; 88: 265-273.
61. Nakashima M, Watanabe T, Koprowski H, et al. *In vitro* expansion of tumor specific, HLA restricted human CD8+ cytolytic T lymphocytes. *Cell Immunol* 1994; 155: 53-61.
62. Oliver G, Yannelli JR, Solomon D. Tumor infiltrating lymphocytes: A cytologic, phenotypic, and morphometric analysis. *Acta Cytologica* 1996; 40: 691-694.
63. Peoples GE, Gordegebuure PS, Andrews JVR, et al. HLA-A2 presents shared tumor associated antigens derived from endogenous proteins in ovarian cancer. *J Immunol* 1993; 151: 5481-5491.
64. Pockaj BA, Sherry RM, Wei JP, et al. Localization of 111 Indium-labeled tumor infiltrating lymphocytes to tumor in patients receiving adoptive immunotherapy. *Cancer* 1994; 73: 1731-1737.
65. Rammensee H-G, Falk K, Rotzschke O. Peptides naturally presented by MHC class I molecules. *Ann Rev Immunol* 1993; 11: 213-244.
66. Rivoltini L, Kawakami Y, Sakaguchi K, et al. Induction of tumor reactive CTL from peripheral blood and tumor infiltrating lymphocytes of melanoma patients by in vitro stimulation with an immunodominant peptide of the human melanoma antigen MART-1. *J Immunol* 1995; 154: 2257-2265.
67. Robbins PF, El-Gamil M, Kawakami Y, et al. Recognition of tyrosinase by tumor infiltrating lymphocytes from a patient responding to immunotherapy. *Cancer Res* 1994; 54: 3124-3126.
68. Robbins PF, El-Gamil M, Kawakami Y, et al. Recognition of tyrosinase by tumor infiltrating lymphocytes from a patient responding to immunotherapy. *Cancer Res* 1994; 54: 3124-3129.
69. Robbins PF, El Gamil M, Li YF, et al. A mutated β-catenin gene encodes a melanoma specific antigen recognized by tumor infiltrating lymphocytes. *J Exp Med* 1996; In Press.
70. Robbins PF, El Gamil M, Li YF. Cloning of a new geneencoding an antigen recognized by specific HLA-A24 restricted tumor infiltrating lymphocytes. *J Immunol* 1995; 154: 5944-5962.
71. Rosenberg SA, Lotze MT, Aebersold PM, et al. Prospective randomized trial of high dose interleukin-2 alone or with lymphokine activated killer cells for the treatment of patients with advanced cancer. *J Natl Cancer Inst* 1993; 85: 622-632.
72. Rosenberg SA. Cell transfer therapy: Clinical applications. In: Biologic *Therapy of Cancer.* Philadelphia: Lippincott, 1995: 487-506.
73. Rosenberg SA, Speiss P, Lafreniere R. A new approach to the adoptive immunotherapy of cancer with tumor infiltrating lymphocytes. *Science* 1986; 223: 1318-1321.
74. Rosenberg SA, Packard BS, Aebersold PA, et al. Use of tumor infiltrating lymphocytes and interleukin-2 in the immunotherapy of patients with metastatic melanoma. A preliminary report. *New Engl Jrn of Med* 1988; 319: 1676-1680.
75. Rosenberg SA, Yannelli JR, Yang JC, et al. Treatment of patients with metastatic melanoma with autologous tumor infiltrating lymphocytes and interleukin-2. *J Natl Cancer Inst* 1994; 86: 1159-1166.
76. Salmeron MA, Morita T, Seki H, et al. Lymphokine production by human melanoma tumor infiltrating lymphocytes. *Cancer Immunol Immunother* 1992; 35: 211-217.
77. Schendel DJ, Gansbacher B. Tumor specific lysis of human renal cell carcinomas by tumor infiltrating lymphocytes: Modulation of recognition through retrovirus transduction of tumor-cells with interleukin-2 complementaryDNA and exogenous alpha interferon treatment. *Cancer Research* 1993; 53: 4020-4025.
78. Schendel DJ, Gansbacher B, Oberneder R, et al. Tumor specific lysis of human renal cell carcinomas by tumor infiltrating lymphocytes. *J Immunol* 1993; 151: 4209-4220.
79. Schwartzentruber DJ, Topalian SL, Mancini M, Rosenberg SA. Specific release of granulocyte-macrophage colony stimulating factor, tumor necrosis factor α, and interferon-γ by human tumor infiltrating lymphocytes after autologous tumor stimulation. *J Immunology* 1991; 146: 3674-3681.
80. Schwartzentruber DL, Hom SS, Dadmarz R, et al. *In vitro* predictors of therapeutic response in melanoma patients receiving tumor infiltrating lymphocytes and interleukin-2. *J Clin Oncol* 1994; 12: 1475-1483.
81. Schwartzentruber DJ, Solomon D, Rosenberg SA, Topalian SL. Characterization of lymphocytes infiltrating human breast cancer: specific immune reactivitydetected by measuring cytokine secretion. *J Immunother* 1992; 12: 1-12.
82. Schwartzentruber DJ, Stetler-Stevenson M, Rosenberg SA, Topalian SL. Tumor-infiltrating lymphocytes derived from select B-cell lymphomas secrete granulocyte-macrophage colony stimulating factor and tumor necrosis factor-α in response to autologous tumor stimulation. *Blood* 1993; 82: 1204-1211.
83. Shi I, Bonnefoix T, Heuze-Le Vacon F, et al. Auto-tumor reactive T-cell clones among tumor infiltrating T lymphocytes in B-cell non-Hodgkin's lymphomas. *British Jrn of Haematology* 1995; 90: 837-843.
84. Shu S, Chou T, and Rosenberg SA. Generation from tumor bearing mice of lymphocytes with *in vitro* therapeutic efficacy. *J Immunol* 1987; 139: 295-304.
85. Sica D, Rayman P, Stanley J, et al. Interleukin-7 enhances the proliferation and effector function of tumor infiltrating lymphocytes from renal cell carcinoma. *Int J of Cancer* 1993; 53: 941-947.
86. Slovin SF, Lackman RD, Ferrone S, et al. Cellular immune response to human sarcoma: cytotoxic T cell clones reactive with autologous sarcomas. *J Immunol* 1986; 137: 3042-3048.
87. Somers SS, Guillou AJ. Isolation and expansion of lymphocytes from gastrointestinal tumor tissue. *Surgical Oncology* 1993; 2: 283-291.
88. Stevens EJ, Jacknin L, Robbins PF, et al. Generation of tumor specific CTLs from melanoma patients by using peripheral blood stimulated with allogeneic melanoma tumor cell lines: Fine specificity and MART-1 melanoma antigen recognition. *J Immunol* 1995; 154: 762-771.

89. Topalian SL, Muul LM, Solomon D, Rosenberg SA. Expansion of human tumor infiltrating lymphocytes for use in immunotherapy trials. *J Immunol Met* 1987; 102: 127-141.
90. Topalian SL, Solomon D, Avis FP, et al. Immunotherapy of patients with advanced cancer using tumor-infiltrating lymphocytes and recombinant interleukin-2: A pilot study. *Jrn Clin Oncol* 1988; 6: 839-853.
91. Topalian SL, Solomon D, Rosenberg SA. Tumor-specific cytolysis by lymphocytes infiltrating human melanomas. *J Immunol* 1989; 142: 3714-3732.
92. Topalian SL, Rivoltini L, Mancini M, et al. Melanoma-specific-CD4+ Tlymphocytes recognize human melanoma antigens processed and presented by epstein-Barr virus transformed B cells. *Int J Cancer* 1994; 58: 69-79.
93. Topalian SL, Rivoltini L, Mancini M, et al. Human CD4+ T cells specifically recognize a shared melanoma associated antigen encoded by the tyrosinase gene. *Proc Natl Acad Sci* 1994; 91: 9461-9465.
94. Topalian SL, Rivoltini L, Mancini M, et al. Melanoma specific CD4+ T lymphocytes recognize human melanoma antigens processed and presented by EBV transformed B cells. *Int J Cancer* 1994; 58: 69-79.
95. Topalian SL, Gonzales MI, Parkhurst M, et al. Melanoma specific CD4+ T cells recognize nonmutated HLA-DR-restricted tyrosinase epitopes. *J Exp Med* In Press 1996.
96. Toso JF, Oei C, Oshidari F, et al. MAGE-1 specific precursor cytotoxic T lymphocytes present among tumor infiltrating lymphocytes from a patient with breast cancer: Characterization and antigen specific activation. *Cancer Research* 1996; 56: 16-20.
97. Van der Bruggen P, Traversari C, Chomez P, et al. A gene encoding an antigen recognized by cytolytic T lymphocytes on human melanoma. *Science* 1991; 254: 1643-1647.
98. Vose BM, Gallagher P, Moore M, Schofield PF. Specific and non-specific lymphocyte cytotoxicity in colon carcinoma. *Br J Cancer* 1981; 44: 846-855.
99. Wang R-F, Rosenberg SA. Human tumor antigens recognized by T lymphocytes: implications for cancer therapy. *J Leukocyte Biol* 1996; 60: 296-309.
100. Wang RF, Robbins PF, Kawakami, et al. Identification of a gene encoding a melanoma antigen recognized by HLA-A31 restricted tumor infiltrating lymphocytes. *J Exp Med* 1995; 181: 799-804.
101. Weber F, Volgmann T, Menzel J. Tumor infiltrating lymphocytes in malignant brain tumors. *Arch Immunol Ther Exp* 1993; 41: 41-44.
102. Weiss A. T lymphocyte activation, In: Fundamental Immunology, 3rd Edition. Paul, W. Ed. 1993; 467-504.
103. Yannelli JR, Stevenson GW, Stevenson HC. Cancer adoptive cellular immunotherapy. In: *Principles of Cancer Biotherapy*. New York: Marcel Dekker, Inc, 1991: 503-523.
104. Yannelli JR, Hyatt C, McConnell S, et al. Growth of tumor infiltrating lymphocytes from human solid cancers: Summary of a 5-year experience. *Int J Of Cancer* 1996; 65: 413-421.
105. Yannelli JR, McConnell M, Parker L, et al. Melanoma TIL derived from 4 distinct anatomic sites obtained from a single patient: Comparison of functional reactivity and melanoma antigen recognition. *J Immunother* 1996; 18: 263-271.
106. Yannelli JR, Thurman GB, Dickerson SG, et al. An improved method for the generation of human lymphokine activated killer cells. *J Immunol Methods* 1987; 100: 137145.
107. Yannelli JR, Hyatt C, Johnson S, et al. Characterization of human tumor cell lines transduced with the CDNA encoding either tumor necrosis factor alpha (TNF-alpha) or interleukin-2 (IL-2). *J Immunol Meth* 1993; 161: 77-90.
108. Yasamura S, Weidman E, Hirabayashi H, HLA restriction and T cell receptor Vb gene expression of cytotoxic T lymphocytes reactive with human squamous cell carcinoma of the head and neck. *Int J of Cancer* 1994; 57: 297-305.
109. Yewdell JW, Bennink JR. Cell biology of antigen processing and presentation to major histocompatibility complex class I molecule restricted T lymphocytes. *Adv Immunol* 1992; 52: 1-123.
110. Yewdell JW, Bennink JR. The binary logic of antigen processing and presentation to T cells. *Cell* 1990; 62: 203-206.
111. Yoo YK, Heo DS, Hata K, et al. Tumor-infiltrating lymphocytes from human colon carcinomas. *Gastroenterology* 1990; 98: 259-268.
112. Yoshino I, Yano T, Murata M, et al. Tumor reactive T-cells accumulate in lung tissue but fail to respond due to tumor cell-derived factor. *Cancer Research* 1992; 52: 775-781.
113. Zocchi MR, Ferrarini M, Migone N, Casorati G. T-cell receptor Vδ gene usage by tumor reactive γδ T lymphocytes infiltrating human lung cancer. *Immunology* 1994; 81: 234-289.

GROWTH AND MATURATION FACTORS IN CANCER

ROBERT K. OLDHAM
Biological Therapy Institute Foundation, Franklin, Tennessee; and University of Missouri, Columbia, Missouri

The concept of biologic modification of cancer growth and differentiation has been based upon various observations suggesting that transformed leukemic stem cells may be induced to normality with respect to morphology, function, and regulation. This 'reversal of malignancy' in cancer and leukemia, while an attractive goal, is one that is rarely attainable in its entirety in clinical or experimental systems. What is more feasible, and has proved attainable, is removal of the maturation block in the leukemic lineage, with resulting development of varying but incomplete functional and phenotypic features of lineage-specific differentiation.

Another line of evidence suggesting that growth and maturation factors may be operative in some form of cancers is the observation that patients with neuroblastoma and germ cell tumors can show maturational effects in the tumor biopsies post treatment. It is not known whether this relates to the treatment since occasional spontaneous maturation had been seen prior to effective therapy for these cancers. The more recent evidence in promyelocytic leukemia shows that transretinoic acid can stimulate the leukemic cells to mature such that they are no longer capable of further division with the result being programmed cell death. These lines of evidence have led some researchers and clinicians to speculate that cancerous growth remains under some degree of control by differentiation and growth factors and that these processes might be augmented or altered therapeutically.

A major goal of current therapy in leukemia is the selective inhibition of leukemic cell proliferation relative to the proliferation of normal stem cells. Decades of chemotherapy research have defined several clinically effective agents. However, the 'toxic window' has proved too narrow for highly selective eradication of leukemic stem cells without substantial damage to the normal stem-cell compartment. Differentiation-inducing agents, while falling short in their ability to 'reverse' malignancy, can nevertheless prove highly effective in suppressing leukemic stem-cell self-renewal capacity by inducing 'death' by differentiation to a postmitotic stage. Reduction or elimination of leukemic stem-cell self-renewal, together with restoration of responsiveness to homeostatic control, may prove to be the most effective therapeutic strategy in myeloid leukemia, since the leukemic cells would lose their competitive advantage over normal stem cells and would no longer clonally dominate hematopoiesis.

In humans a number of observations suggest that differentiation of myeloid leukemic cells occurs *in vivo*. The most obvious example is chronic myeloid leukemia (CML), where glucose-6-phosphate dehydrogenase (G6PD) polymorphism revealed the derivation of mature granulocytes, red cells, and platelets from the leukemic clone. Similar analysis revealed differentiation of acute myeloid leukemia (AML) clones to red blood cells and platelets in some patients [84], and the presence of Auer rods in mature neutrophils of AML patients in remission and persistence of cytogenetic abnormalities in the absence of normal metaphases in patients with AML in clinical remission [25, 81].

DNA recombinant technology has also demonstrated leukemic cell differentiation in AML and preleukemia/ myelodysplastic syndrome (MDS). DNA restriction fragment-length polymorphism in heterozygous individuals has provided strong evidence for *in vivo* differentiation [84, 399]. HPRT gene analysis, quantitative analysis of chromosome 8 trisomy and chromosome 7 monosomy, and immunoglobin (Ig) gene rearrangement analysis showed that 5/6 patients with AML had maturation to mature granulocytes in the active phase of the disease even in aneuploid leukemia. Another approach has been to label myeloblasts *in vivo* with bromodeoxyuridine (BUdR), which allowed the demonstration of BUdR in mature granulocytes of AML patients [309].

Premature chromosome condensation has been used to detect the presence of abnormal cytogenetic clones in mature cells. Fusion of mitotic tissue culture cells with the mature cell in question (e.g., granulocytes) results in immediate chromosome condensation of the chromatin of interphase nuclei into discrete chromosomes. This permitted karyotype analysis of nondividing cells of 13 patients with CML, and with MDS or AML, after low-and high-dose chemotherapy [143]. Twelve of these cases showed evidence of maturation of cytogenetically abnormal leukemic clones *in vivo*.

Leukemic differentiation *in vitro* and *in vivo* can be mediated by a variety of agents. Indeed, over 80 distinct compounds (not including an even greater number of analogues) have been shown to induce differentiation of the HL-60 cell line (vide infra). Clearly, many of these

R.K. Oldham (ed.), Principles of Cancer Biotherapy. 3rd ed., 387–422.

agents operate via common pathways, but nevertheless a number of distinct categories of differentiation inducing agents can be recognized and will be reviewed. These include the following groups:

1. Vitamin A and D metabolites and analogues [e.g., 13-*cis*-retinoic acid, 1,25-$(OH)_2$ D_3]
2. Polar/planar compounds [e.g., dimethylsulfoxide (DMSO), hexamethylene bisacetamide (HMBA), *N*-methylformamide (NMF)]
3. Cytokines and hematopoietic growth factors (e.g., G-CSF, IL-1, IL-3, IL-6, LIF, TNF, TGFβ, IFNα, IFNβ, IFNγ)
4. Phorbol esters (e.g., phorbol myristate acetate)
5. Chemotherapeutic agents that interfere with DNA synthesis (e.g., cytosine arabinoside, tiazofurin, 6-thioguanine)
6. Chemotherapeutic agents that influence topoisomerase II
7. Chemotherapeutic agents that inhibit DNA methyltransferase (e.g., 5-azacytidine, 5-aza-2'-deoxycytidine).

HUMAN LEUKEMIC CELL LINES AS MODELS FOR DIFFERENTIATION THERAPY

Much of the history of the development of an effective chemotherapy for leukemia was based on the availability of cell lines, or transplantable leukemias, with sensitivity to cell cycle-specific agents. The development of biological response modification therapy and the recognition of leukemic cell differentiation as an obtainable goal led to the use of leukemic cell lines of myeloid lineage capable of terminal maturation.

The human myeloid leukemic cell lines HL-60 and U937 have been studied most extensively. HL-60 was isolated from a patient with acute promyelocytic leukemia, and it retains a promyelocytic morphology [99]. U937 was developed from the pleural fluid of a patient with true macrophage-type diffuse histiocytic lymphoma, and has an immature monoblast-macrophage morphology [346]. These lines are cloned, readily maintained in culture and, while resembling immature cells of their lineage, can be induced to terminal neutrophil, eosinophil, and macrophage (HL-60) or monocyte-macrophage (U937) differentiation.

The histochemistry and morphology of these cell lines mark them as immature cells of myelomonocytic lineage. The HL-60 cell line exists in many variants with differing doubling times and extents of spontaneous differentiation [99]. The cells weakly phagocytize latex particles or yeast in the uninduced state and possess low numbers of Fc C3b, insulin, and chemotactic fMLP receptors [4, 271], whose expression can be greatly enhanced following exposure to differentiation-inducing agents.

HL-60 cells are positive to myeloperoxidase, ASD chloracetate esterase, and Sudan black B, but unlike normal promyelocytes they do not stain for alkaline phosphatase, and unlike macrophages they are essentially acid phosphatase-negative [99, 391]. Activated forms of beta-glucuronidase, lysozyme, and G6PD, found at high levels in the granules of normal granulocytes, are present at low concentrations in HL-60 and are minimally involved in degranulation. It has been proposed that these enzymes are already synthesized in HL-60 and stored within the granules as zymogens, but are only converted to active enzymes upon stimulation [189, 405]. Uninduced HL-60 cells have a marginal capacity to produce H_2O_2 and O_2-, have a low level of HMPS activity [267], and have a greatly impaired ability to kill staphylococcus and other microorganisms [99].

The U937 cell line as originally reported grew slowly; however, later passages of the line have an accelerated population doubling of 20-48 h. The cells have a monoblastic morphology and histochemical profile (strong ANAE, NASDAE, and beta-glucuronidase positivity and weak acid and alkaline phosphatase) [346, 391]. U937 cells also secrete lysozyme, and neutral protease elastase is present within the cells; these are monocyte-specific characteristics [306, 346]. The cells bear few Fc, C3, and chemotactic peptide receptors when compared with normal monocytes, but histamine and insulin receptors are expressed [5, 346]. Only a small percentage of cells are phagocytic, and U937 only weakly produces H_2O_2 and O_2- and is incapable of killing microorganisms or tumor cells [189, 307, 336].

Upon induction of differentiation, morphological changes involve significant increases in substratum adherence. The HL-60 cell line changes morphology from promyelocytic to later stages of granulocyte degranule formation when treated with 1% DMSO and retinoic acid [34, 38, 99], whereas phorbol esters transform the cells to monocyte-macrophages with the disappearance of azurophilic granules and appearance of pseudopodia and a cerebriform nucleus [317]. There is evidence that these cells can differentiate to eosinophils spontaneously, and in response to stimulatory activities in human placenta-conditioned media [206]. U937 cells, under differentiation stimuli, increase in size and acquire lobated nuclei, and cytoplasmic granules are replaced by vacuoles, duplicating monoblast to monocyte transformation. Various granulocyte lysozyme, acid phosphatase, and beta-glucuronidase activities have been measured in induced cells; when HL-60 is induced with phorbol ester (TPA), the activity of these enzymes is increased up to 20-fold [317]. Similar increases in activity are usually seen after induction with all agents used for differentiation induction. The distinctive monocyte lysosomal enzyme, acid phosphatase, can be detected after exposure of HL-60 cells to phorbol ester for several days. The elaboration of this enzyme into surrounding media is also a monocyte-associated characteristic and accompanies the phorbol-induced maturation of these cells. Myeloperoxidase, an enzyme specific to the myelomonocytic lineage, is constitutively expressed in HL-60. However, activity is lost after induction with phorbol esters, lymphokines, or retinoic acid, but is unaffected when DMSO or cAMP-inducing agents are used [318].

Lactoferrin, a metal-binding glycoprotein, is present in normal granulocytes in the secondary (specific) granules and is one of the most specific markers for the neutrophil lineage. It has not been detected in HL-60 cells [267], nor in the segmented neutrophils of the majority of patients with leukemia [35]. Under normal conditions, lactoferrin is active as a suppressor molecule, and inhibits the production and/or release of granulocyte-macrophage colony-stimulating factors from monocytes and macrophages at concentrations as low as 10^{-15} *M. In vivo* lactoferrin inhibits myelopoiesis in mice at concentrations as low as 10^{-4} mg/mouse [32]. Therefore, detection of the synthesis of lactoferrin in HL-60 cells, even at low concentrations, would be of importance, especially if the synthesis could be increased by inducing agents and if the lactoferrin so induced was functionally active. We have detected lactoferrin in HL-60 cells at very low levels, using radioimmunoassay; in biosynthesis studies, using autoradiographic gel analysis, [^{3}H] leucine incorporated into material immunoprecipitated with lactoferrin antibody. Following induction of differentiation with DMSO or retinoic acid, a two- to fourfold increase in lactoferrin has been noted. This is still much lower than the 10^{-12} g per segmented neutrophil reported in normal peripheral blood, indicating a persisting abnormality in the differentiated HL-60 neutrophil, comparable to that noted in neutrophils of patients with leukemia [35].

The isozyme pattern of lactate dehydrogenase in uninduced HL-60 cells is reported to change after induction with DMSO; however, the resultant pattern is not characteristic of mature granulocytes or macrophages but rather of more immature stages [289]. Simultaneous expression of other granulocytic and monocytic specific markers may also be the result of incomplete or asynchronous maturation. Of particular interest is the observation that cell division is not required for the induction of many of these characteristics and may account for their uncoordinated expression [34].

Messenger RNA species have been isolated from HL-60 cells translated *in vitro* and analyzed by two-dimensional SDS-PAGE after phorbol ester or DMSO induction. The phorbol-induced protein pattern differed significantly from the DMSO pattern and was characterized as monocytoid rather than granulocytic [55]. Poly ADP-ribose metabolism has been linked to the maturation of granulocyte-macrophage progenitors. ADP-ribosyl transferase is a chromatin-bound enzyme catalyzing the transfer of ADP-ribose to chromatin proteins. The activity of this enzyme increases during the CSF-stimulated differentiation of marrow precursors to monocytes [93].

One of the most frequently employed and convenient qualitative measures of reactive oxygen intermediates as important microbicidal products or granulocytes of macrophages is the reduction of NBT to a black formizan precipitate. A variety of factors, both physiologic and pharmacologic, can induce HL-60 production of H_2O_2 [126, 105, 280]. The microbicidal capacity of granulocytes and HL-60 cells is metabolically linked to an increase in the hexose monophosphate shunt activity and consequent production of superoxide anion activity. Arachidonic acid metabolism has been analyzed after induction of maturation with several agents, and recent results suggest that there is enhanced synthesis and release of prostoglandins of the E and F2-alpha type [127].

Maturation of U937 cells is usually characterized by quantitative rather than qualitative changes, since the cells are constitutive producers of a variety of enzymes and growth factors. Because U937 cells are of monocytic derivation, agents that effect a maturational change may also be potent immunoadjuvants. Blood monocytes and U937 cells are characterized by their content of fluoride-inhabitable esterase, alkaline and acid phosphatase, and β-glucuronidase. These enzyme levels are elevated by exposure of normal or neoplastic cells to agents known to influence monocytic activation, such as vitamin D metabolites, phorbol esters, gamma-interferon, and lymphokines [126, 127, 131].

Other enzymatic activities that have been measured in U937 include elastase, collagenase, and plasminogen activator. U937 elastase is not released constitutively and is not readily modulated [272, 334].

The production of reactive oxygen species and the percentage of NBT-positive cells are increased in U937 cells by a variety of agents, such as phorbol esters, DMSO, lymphokines, α- and β-interferons, retinoic acids, 1,25-dihydroxy vitamin D3, prostaglandin (PG) E and other cAMP-inducing agents, cytosine arabinoside (ara-C), and protein DIFs [32, 126, 278, 279]. On a more quantitative basis, the activity of the hexose monophosphate shunt has been examined. Notably, db-cAMP and PGE are able to increase activity of the shunt, but cannot induce other characteristics of maturity in U937 [277]. Under certain conditions, U937 cells did not appear to produce prostaglandin E_2 in response to lipopolysaccharide (LPS), endotoxin, or concanavalin A (Con A) stimulation [186], and differed from peripheral blood monocytes and macrophages in this respect. However, if supplied with exogenous arachidonic acid, the cells can release PGE_2 [54]. The failure to release esterified arachidonic acid to the cyclooxygenase pathway was believed to be a property shared by U937 cells and certain macrophage subsets. It has been shown that U937 cells can be induced by certain agents, such as γ-interferon, to produce various arachidonate metabolites, both without stimulation and in response to Con A stimulation [186]. HL-60 cells constitutively produce a leukemia-associated inhibitor, which has been characterized as acidic isoferritin [32, 247]. This molecule is suppressive to normal, but not leukemic, marrow myelopoietic progenitors (CFU-GM, CFU-GEMM), reducing their proportion in the cell cycle [35, 276]. It has been proposed that release of these molecules by leukemic cells may be an important selective advantage, and may be responsible for the profound granulocytopenia seen in myeloid leukemia [35].

U937 is also a source of a variety of biologically active macromolecules. The monokine interleukin 1 (IL-1) (endogenous pyrogen, LAF) is constitutively released in small amounts. Production is increased by exposure of the cells to endotoxin or phorbol esters [288]. IL-2 is probably the factor released by U937 that increases the production of collagenase and PGE_2 in cultured synovial cells [8]. U937, like HL-60, secretes hematopoietic growth-stimulating factors that may act as autostimulatory growth factors [13]. The release of such factors can be suppressed, as in normal myelopoiesis, by agents such as lactoferrin [35]. U937 also produces the second component of complement, and the release of C2 can be augmented sevenfold by inducing maturation of U937 with phorbol ester or a lymphokine [288, 296]. U937 cells have also been demonstrated to produce an inhibitor of lymphocyte proliferation, characterized as being Con A-inducible, of molecular weight 65, 000, heat resistant, and distinct from lymphotoxin or interferons [385].

Modifications, both qualitative and quantitative, of the plasma membrane constituents of HL-60 and U937 have been associated with differentiation. Induction of HL-60 with DMSO or phorbol ester modifies the expression of 'fast-eluting' glycopeptides [368]. Comparison of the elution profiles of fucosyl-labeled glycopeptides with normal granulocytes and macrophages showed that HL-60 glycopeptides were larger and more complex than those on a normal band or polymorphonuclear neutrophils. DMSO or phorbol exposure of HL-60 did not induce a normalization of the elution profile to a mature conformation [366]. Induction of cell-surface glycoproteins on HL-60, particularly as seen in the time of appearance of gp130 following DMSO treatment, was concomitant with development of chemotactic ability [98]. In this context, patients with impaired granulocyte chemotaxis have greatly reduced amounts of GP130 in their granulocytes [322].

Cytoskeletal proteins of HL-60 have also been studied. During induced maturation, there is increased synthesis of vimentin and other structural proteins. As may be expected, the profiles of cytoskeletal proteins induced by DMSO resemble those of granulocytes and, following phorbol ester induction, resemble those of macrophages [26].

Modulation of expression of several cell surface antigens has been characterized by the use of monoclonal antibodies. In one study, two monoclonal antibodies, B9.8.1 (specific for monocytes and metamyelocytes), were used to characterize maturational changes [294]. Treatment of HL-60 with granulocyte- or macrophage-inducing agents resulted in enhanced antigen expression. In a similar study, reactivity with the monoclonal antibodies Mo1 and Mo2, recognizing determinants specific to the myelomonocytic lineage, could be induced with phorbol esters, as well as protein inducers of differentiation [63, 360].

HL-60 constitutively expresses HLA-A and -B antigens, and induction of HLA-DR determinants has been reported [63]. Normal myelomonocytic precursors express the DR antigens twice: transiently during early stages (CFU-GM) [87], and later as monocytes. HLA-DR determinants of HL-60 have been detected following treatment with inducers of monocyte macrophage differentiation, but not with agents that induce granulocyte maturation.

The expression of Fc and C3 receptors has been studied extensively in U937. The receptor for IgG1 can be induced by a variety of agents, both physiologic and pharmacologic [126, 186, 196]. The receptor for IgE is also present, but its modulation has not been studied. The C3B receptor (as recognized by EAC or Mac-1 monoclonal antibody) is inducible in a similar manner, as are Mac-1 and macrophage-restricted Mac-3 cell-surface antigens [308].

The chemotactic receptor for the potent chemotactic peptide fMLP is weakly expressed in U937 (7505 sites/cell). Within 3 days of exposure to phorbol esters, dexamethasone, and protein inducers of differentiation (excluding native or recombinant γ-interferon), up to fivefold increase in fMLP receptors is seen [127, 296]. U937 cells are generally considered devoid of any Ia antigen on their surface; however, small numbers of cells react with antibodies to HLA-DR and HLA-DS/CD molecules. It has proved possible to clone such Ia-positive cells and develop constitutively Ia antigen-positive variant lines of U937 [108]. Induction of HLA-DR determinants in response to treatment with gamma-interferon and PG has been reported [295]. $Beta_2$-microglobulin expression has also been shown to increase in response to protein inducers of differentiation [272]. Insulin may play an important role in the growth regulation of U937 cells, since the number of insulin receptors is reduced after incubation with differentiation-inducing agents, and this may have a causal role in the observed growth inhibition. The association between differentiation induction and growth inhibition of U937 and HL-60 cells may also be linked to the ability of potent inducers of macrophage differentiation, such as phorbol ester, to induce cellular production of the protein of molecular weight 17,000, termed tumor necrosis factor (TNF) [5, 293]. This activity is inhibitory to neoplastic cell proliferation, including that of leukemic cells and normal hematopoietic stem cells. The intriguing possibility of autoregulation of leukemic cells by production of an endogenous growth-inhibitory molecule (TNF) is suggested.

More than 80% of cells from a human promyelocytic leukemic cell line (HL-60) possess the capacity for self-renewal as evidenced by their ability to form large primary colonies in semisolid medium and the presence within these colonies of cells capable of subsequent colony formation. Colony development is independent of colony-stimulating factor. The observed autostimulation suggests the production of specific growth promoters by the cells. Differentiation, either to mature granulocytes or to macrophages, induced by various agents is associated with reduced cloning potential. Nevertheless, colonies containing differentiated cells can be developed either by cloning cells in the presence of suboptimal concentrations of inducer or by adding inducers to colonies developed in its absence. The loss of self-renewal was found to be one of the early properties that changed following the initiation of differentiation. The loss preceded not only the overt expression of maturation-specific functions but also cellular commitment to terminal differentiation; shorter contact with the inducer is required to cause loss of self-renewal than to induce an irreversible transition to differentiation. This results in cells that lose their self-renewal potential without being able to complete their program of differentiation [85]. Increased migration of tumor cells upon differentiation to form diffuse colonies may be the result of increased mobility and chemotactic responsiveness. In a modified chemotaxis assay, HL-60 cells increased their migration in response to fMLP after a 5-day induction with db-cAMP or DMF [88, 369].

Phagocytosis of latex beads or opsonized yeast and the capacity to kill microorganisms are readily induced by a wide variety of differentiation-inducing agents. Phagocytosis is one of the earliest acquired effector functions of both granulocytes and monocytes. Phorbol ester or DMSO-induced HL-60 cells effectively kill staphylococcus [177]. It has been demonstrated that differentiation-induced HL-60 cells can mediate monocyte ADCC-like reaction against antibody-coated chicken erythrocytes [63].

The U937 cell line is capable of being induced to mediate monocyte antibody-dependent cellular cytotoxicity (ADCC) effector function. First reports of ADCC capacity against tumor markers used lymphokine, interferon, and phorbol ester preparations to activate or 'induce' the cells [131, 307, 346]. ADCC activity of U937 cells against erythrocytes can be induced by as little as 10 units of γ-interferon and 300 units of α- and β-interferon associated with dexamethasone-resistant enhancement of Fc-R expression of Y29, 65H. U937 cells have been studied for their capacity to support the interacellular multiplication of *Toxoplasma gondii*. A small portion of U937 cells can spontaneously phagocytize these protozoans, and after 24 h those cells have either lysed or contain numerous trophozoites within their vacuoles. After a 3-day incubation with lymphokine preparations there is a significantly decreased number of organisms found within vacuoles in spite of a generalized increase in phagocytosis [388].

In the effort to analyze common pathways in differentiation of cell lines such as HL-60, many attempts have been made to select for sublines capable of sustaining exponential growth in the presence of a single inducer of differentiation but not in the presence of different, structurally unrelated inducers of differentiation. Neutrophilic granulocytic and monocyte/macrophage programs of HL-60 are mechanistically different and separable, and both agent-specific and common quantitative alterations contribute to the mechanism for resistance to granulocyte differentiation.

Numerous studies have demonstrated that the oncogene c-myc is amplified 20- to 40-fold in HL-60 cells compared with normal human DNA and is associated with an elevated level of cellular myc-mRNA, and a decrease in this mRNA follows chemically induced differentiation [34, 118]. Within 5 days of addition of DMSO or phorbol ester to HL-60 cultures, transcription of the c-myc gene was markedly reduced when compared with control cultures. This decrease was not accompanied by alteration in either the bulk rate of transcription or the c-myc copy number, suggesting that decreased cellular myc RNA levels are due to decreased transcription of the myc protooncogene [118]. The expression of c-myc in HL-60 does not correlate with the proportion of proliferating cells, and the kinetics of decrease upon DMSO induction is paralleled closely by an increasing proportion of histochemically detected, differentiated myeloid cells and by a decrease in clonogenic potential, but not by changes in the proportion of proliferating cells [86]. Changes in c-myc expression subsequent to differentiation of HL-60 can therefore be directly related to the differentiation process rather than to a cell cycle-related phenomenon. Gallagher observed little change or decrease in the amplification level of the known amplified c-myc gene in various drug-resistant sublines in comparison with wild-type HL-60 cells [101] and despite the existence of numerous double, minute chromosomes (indicators of amplified genes) in some drug-resistant sublines. Differential response to differentiation agents could still be related to amplification of genes other than c-myc; however, tests with several other oncogene probes, including N-ras, Ha-ras, Ki-ras, myb, and abl, showed no evidence of amplification or gross rearrangement of these genes in DNA in any HL-60 line or subline [59]. High levels of c-fos expression have been detected in macrophages, but not in uninduced HL-60 cells. However, when HL-60 cells were induced to macrophages, c-fos expression was readily detectable in the differentiated cells [254].

VITAMIN A ANALOGUES AS LEUKEMIA DIFFERENTIATION-INDUCING AGENTS

Vitamin A and its analogues (retinoids) affect proliferation and differentiation of normal and malignant hematopoietic cells. The most extensively studied system utilized HL-60 [118, 136, 149, 278, 289, 294]. Maximum differentiation (approximately 90% of cells) occurs with 1 μM retinoic acid, a concentration 500- to 160, 000-fold less than the concentration of butyrate and DMSO that promotes a similar increase in differentiation. Continuous exposure to retinoic acid is necessary for maximum differentiation, which occurs after 5 days of incubation. Retinol (vitamin A), retinal acetate, and retinal are approximately 1000-fold less potent than retinoic acid, which can induce some differentiation at concentrations as low as 1 nM.

The mode of action of retinoic acid has been extensively analyzed in HL-60 cells. A two-step model for induction of differentiation has been proposed where early events anteceding precommitment regulate growth arrest and late events, and subsequent to precommitment regulate the choice of a specific differentiation lineage [396]. Thus the lineage specificity of cells treated sequentially with two discrete exposures to alternative inducers depends on the order of exposure. Retinoic acid exposure of HL-60 for 24-72 h followed by phorbol ester treatment produces monocyte-macrophage differentiation, whereas reversing the order of treatment favors granulocyte differentiation [408]. The precommitment phase has a characteristic duration following retinoic acid exposure, persisting for several cell cycles despite removal of retinoic acid [120]. This precommitment is paralleled by elevations in c-myc. Other events associated with retinoid induction of differentiation involve elevation of tyrosine kinase activity [68] and a protein kinase C cascade system. Sphinganine, a potent inhibitor of PKC, enhances differentiation of HL-60 induced by retinoids, and the granulocytes produced are more fully differentiated as indicated by enhanced superoxide production in response to fMLP [344]. A role for topoisomerase II in retinoid-induced granulocytic differentiation has been suggested [91]. In HL-60 differentiation, retinoic acid stimulates transient relocation of DNA supercoiling, and this is associated with the formation of small numbers of protein-linked DNA breaks (a characteristic of topoisomerase reactions). Both events are perturbed by VP16, which inhibits differentiation [91].

Combinations of differentiation-inducing agents have been explored *in vitro* with retinoic acid. Twenty-two of 24 patients with ANLL showed differentiation of bone marrow in cultures with a combination of retinoic acid (10-6 *M*), aclacinomycin A (80 n*M*), and dimethylformamide (100 m*M*) [129]. Enhancement of differentiation was seen with retinoid combined with interferons α and β [183, 193], and γ [137, 364]. Tumor necrosis factor (TNF) at 2.5 U/ml inhibited growth and, synergistically with retinoic acid, induced differentiation in HL-60 and KG-1 cultures and in marrow cultures from 4/9 patients with ANLL [359]. Retinoic acid reversed TNF inhibition of normal marrow myeloid colonies and leukemic growth marrow cultures from 3/9 patients with ANLL.

In this context, leukemia differentiation-inducing factor (GM-DF) produced by mitogen-stimulated human leukocytes acted synergistically with retinoic acid in inducing maturation of the human leukemic lines U937 and HL-60 [278]. T-cell-derived GM-DF was subsequently shown to be due to the synergistic action of IFNγ, lymphotoxin, and GM-DSF [138]. Compounds elevating intracellular levels of cAMP, such as dibutryl cAMP, PGE, and choleratoxin, acted synergistically with retinoic acid to induce maturation of both cell lines. In contrast to the requirement for continuous presence of retinoic acid for up to 5 days in order to achieve terminal differentiation of HL-60 cells, differentiation proteins or cAMP-elevating compounds are active on leukemic cells primed with retinoic acid within 8-16 h [278].

Retinoid induction of myeloid leukemic differentiation is not a universal phenomenon. While the murine myelomonocytic leukemic cell line WEHI-3 can be induced to mature neutrophil differentiation [68] and retinoic acid induces the human malignant monoblast line U937 to monocyte-like cells with the capacity to reduce nitroblue tetrazolium [278], the human myeloid cell lines KG-1 and K562 cannot be induced to differentiate [71]. The mouse myeloid leukemia M1 can be induced to increased levels of lysomal enzyme production without induction of phagocytosis, locomotive activity, or morphological maturation. Indeed, retinoic acid was a potent inhibitor of induction of these latter differentiation-associated properties. Fresh leukemic cells from patients with various myeloid leukemias have also been exposed to retinoic acid in short-term primary suspension cultures, and morphological and functional maturation was observed only in cases of acute promyelocytic leukemia [102, 180]. The differential sensitivity of various leukemias to retinoic acid induction of terminal differentiation is probably not determined by the presence or absence of cellular retinoic acid binding protein [71, 351].

High-affinity retinoic acid receptors (RAR), predominantly alpha-type, were found in 12 leukemic cell lines and in marrow blasts from 32 patients with ANLL [188, 266, 375]. While some correlation was found between RAR expression and retinoid response with four leukemic cell lines [188], extensive analysis of marrow cultures from a large group of primary AML patients showed no correlation between receptor expression and ability of retinoic acid to inhibit colony formation or induce differentiation [375]. The potential for terminal differentiation may be irreversibly lost in many cases of acute myeloid leukemia, but this need not negate the therapeutic value of retinoic acid treatment in a wide range of leukemias, since considerable evidence has accumulated to suggest that retinoids can selectively inhibit leukemic cell self-renewal independently of activation of a differentiation program in the leukemic stem cell. Retinoic acid is a potent inhibitor of the clonal growth *in vitro* of myeloid leukemic cells, and a 50% growth inhibition of HL-60 was achieved by 2.4 n*M* retinoic acid. The human myeloid leukemic line KG-1, which is not inducible to differentiation, was nevertheless extremely sensitive to retinoic acid, with 50% of the colonies inhibited by 2.4 n*M* concentrations of the drug [71].

Retinoic acid inhibited colony formation by bone marrow from 10 patients in the blastic and accelerated phases of CML. Inhibition was seen with retinoic acid at 10^{-6}-10^{-7} *M* in marrow cultures from 17 of 35 cases of ANLL, but a striking stimulation of growth was seen in 10 cases [190].

The antiproliferative action of retinoids upon leukemic cells is more general than the incidence of induction of terminal differentiation, and is seen with retinoid concentrations readily attainable *in vivo*. The potential efficacy of retinoic acid in the treatment of human leukemia is further suggested by the observation that it enhances colony-stimulating factor (CSF) induced clonal growth of normal human myeloid and erythroid cells *in vitro* [72]. In long-term bone marrow culture it also enhanced progenitor cell production. Maximal stimulation occurred at a retinoic acid concentration of $3X10^{-7}$ *M* acid, which increased the mean number of colonies by 213 ± 8% over plates containing CSF alone [29]. Retinoic acid has no direct CSF activity, nor does it stimulate CSF production by the cultured bone marrow cells or marrow stroma. This stimulation may be mediated by increased responsiveness of the progenitor cells, possibly by increasing the number of growth factor receptors per cell. Retinoids are reported to enhance the binding of epidermal growth factor (EGF) to fibroblasts and epidermal cells by increasing the number of EGF receptors per cell [161]. Enhancement of normal myelopoiesis [29] and inhibition of myeloid leukemic cell proliferation by retinoic acid suggest that 13-*cis*-retinoic acid, which is significantly less toxic *in vivo* than retinoic acid, might be effective in the therapy of patients with myelodysplastic syndrome because of the possibility of prevention of progression to overt leukemia of these preleukemic patients, for whom no other effective treatment is currently available.

In a phase I clinical study of 19 patients with various myelodysplastic syndromes (MDS), including refractory anemias with or without excess of blasts and chronic myelomonocytic syndrome, dose-limiting hepatotoxicity was seen only at the 125 mg/m^2 level; the most common toxic manifestation was hyperkeratosis, which was mild and easily alleviated [112]. Of 16 evaluable patients, three were considered to have achieved a partial response, and three others showed improvement in one or more hematologic parameters.

Besa et al. [27] observed a 47% response including complete remissions in 17 patients with MDS receiving 100 mg/m^2 13-*cis*-retinoic acid with an improved survival in responders of 33 months versus 10 months in the nonresponders. No beneficial effects were reported with either retinoic acid or isoretinoin in two studies of 14 MDS patients [130, 148]. *N*-4-Hydroxyphenyl-retinamide (Fenretinide) lacked clinical effect in 15 MDS patients and in some may have enhanced leukemic progression [103]. In a double-blind, placebo-controlled trial of 13-*cis*-retinoic acid in 68 MDS patients with 100 mg/m^2 for 6 months, no significant differences were observed between treatment groups [182]. Approximately 30% of patients in both groups had progression of the disease and survival was virtually identical. Ninety percent of the treated patients developed mild to moderate skin toxicity.

In view of these generally negative results, MDS therapy with retinoic acid has been extended to combinations with other agents with potential differentiation-inducing capacity. In a comparative study of such combination therapy in 62 MDS patients, 50% response was seen with a combination of retinoic acid, 1,25$(OH)_2$ D_3, and interferon, a response rate comparable to that obtained with low-dose cytosine arabinoside [135]. Combining all four agents proved too toxic. Combining retinoic acid with low-dose ara-C produced favorable results in one study [92], but in another study of 14 MDS patients the response was no better than either agent alone [144]. Combining a tocopherol (800 mg/m^2) with retinoic acid (100 mg/m^2) produced a 62% response in 13 MDS patients and reduced the toxicity involving liver damage, hyperkeratosis, and mucositis [27].

In poor-prognosis acute nonlymphoblastic leukemia, 13-*cis*-retinoic acid has some efficacy on its own in one small study [148], and clinical improvements were seen using combinations with low-dose ara-C [330] or vincristine or 6-thioguanine [92]. Evidence of differentiation-induction was obtained in one case of a patient who achieved a complete remission with cytogenetic evidence of persistence of an abnormal clone in the marrow [330].

Acute promyelocytic leukemias almost uniformly respond to retinoic acid *in vitro*. *In vivo*, in a large study, all-*trans*-retinoic acid produced 82% complete remissions in 34 patients and a 60% remission in a further 10 patients when combined with low-dose ara-C [65, 154]. The value of retinoic acid maintenance therapy was clearly shown in a study in which retinoic acid (20 mg bid) was given for up to 2 years in patients achieving remission with high-dose ara-C alone or with daunomycin [62]. The duration of remission was significantly longer (10.4 months versus 5.5 months) at 24 months.

More recent results with acute promyelocytic leukemia have clarified the role of all-*trans*-retinoic acid (RA) in this disorder. In multiple studies [49, 82, 345, 378], it is now clear that a dose of 45 mg/m^2 per day given by mouth in one or two divided doses until complete remission followed by anthrocycline-based combination chemotherapy for consolidation, will induce a high response rate and improve survival in patients with APL. On the basis of these and other studies, RA has recently been approved by the FDA as standard treatment for APL.

Although *trans*-retinoic acid is effective in the treatment of APL, resistance is common with the return of leukemia cells shortly after treatment in the absence of effective programs of consolidation. The role of chemotherapy during induction treatment of APL is still unclear. European approaches have utilized high doses of chemotherapy including an anthracycline plus cytosine arabinoside in patients with white counts exceeding 10,000/m^2 at initiation of therapy. It is yet unclear whether the combination of chemotherapy with *trans*-retinoic acid is more effective than giving induction retinoid therapy plus follow-up consolidation chemotherapy. Clinical trials are underway to define the value of both approaches.

Trans-retinoic acid also has some significant toxicity. Leukocytosis with peripheral blood leukocyte counts in excess of 20,000 cells/ml is common in approximately 50% of APL patients treated with *trans*-retinoic acid.

About 20% of patients with APL when treated with *trans*-retinoic acid, develop a 'retinoic acid syndrome.' This is characterized by respiratory distress, pulmonary infiltrates, fever, sometimes with weight gain and effusions in the pleural or pericardial compartments. Autopsies on patients that die during this syndrome reveal infiltration of myeloid cells into lungs, kidneys, liver and skin and this is occasionally seen in association with the leukocytosis induced by *trans*-retinoic acid. Corticosteroids are effective in treatment of this phase and it is now felt that some combination of corticosteroids with *trans*-retinoic acid may be the best induction regimen for patients with APL [367].

No evidence of synergism of 13-*cis*-retinoic acid with chemotherapeutic agents was found in the treatment of patients with chronic myeloid leukemia. Based upon *in vitro* observations that retinoic acid significantly reduced the recloning capacity of bone marrow myeloid progenitors *in vitro* in certain cases of this disease, Arlin et al. [11] added retinoic acid to an intensive chemotherapy protocol including daunorubicin, cytosine arabinoside, and thioguanine, and in 17 evaluable patients did not observe any increase in the incidence and duration of true Ph chromosome-negative remission in the chronic phase of the disease.

The future of retinoid therapy resides in (a) development of analogues with enhanced differentiation inducing action with reduced toxicity, (b) developing combinations with either conventional chemotherapeutic drugs or other differentiation-inducing agents, (c) applying retinoids more extensively as a maintenance therapy, and (d) developing approaches to reduce toxicity such as tocopheral coadministration or use of liposome-encapsulated retinoic acid [219].

VITAMIN D METABOLITES AND ANALOGS AS LEUKEMIA DIFFERENTIATION-INDUCING AGENTS

The term vitamin D is generally used to describe a number of chemically related compounds having common anti-rachitic properties, but differing in the rapidity of their action and the conditions under which biologic activity is observed. In humans, cholecalciferol (D_3) produced in the skin and the fraction obtained from the diet undergo sequential hydroxylation reactions, first in the liver microsomes and then in the kidney mitochondira, resulting in the formation of 25-(OH) D_3 and 1,25-$(OH)_2$ D_3, respectively. The latter is thought to be the active form of D_3 in enhancing bone resorption mediated by osteoclasts and in enhancing absorption of calcium and phosphorus by the intestine. In addition, it appears to act on the kidney in concert with parathyroid hormone to promote calcium resorption. It was formerly believed that 1,25-$(OH)_2$ D_3 was synthesized in placenta and by calvarial cell suspension containing osteoclasts, osteoblasts, fibroblasts, and endothelial cells [366]. The local production of active metabolites of vitamin D by target organs such as bone raises interesting questions as to the role of these tissues in mediating vitamin D action, and may provide indications of a new dimension to local actions of vitamin D metabolites on normal or leukemic marrow cell function, as well as more conventional aspects of mineral metabolism. Interest in vitamin D action in hematopoiesis was prompted by the observations that osteoclasts originate by fusion of circulating mononuclear precursor cells and almost certainly represent one of the end-stage cells of mononuclear phagocyte differentiation [40, 163, 164, 357]. Like osteoclasts, other mature, nonproliferating phagocytic mononuclear cells, such as monocytes and macrophages, possess the capacity to attach to and degrade bone matrix [164]. Monocytes and macrophages possess receptors for 1,25-$(OH)_2$ D_3, and the culture of human monocytes with 10^{-8} M of this metabolite results in macrophage maturation [303]. In cultures of normal human bone marrow, 1,25-$(OH)_2$ D_3 induces extensive macrophage differentiation [217]. Long-term cultures of human cord blood myeloid cells also terminally differentiate to monocytes and macrophages with vitamin D [324]. Direct evidence of 1,25-$(OH)_2$ D_3 induction of osteoclast development has been reported by Abe et al. [2], who demonstrated that a 1.2 nM concentration of the metabolite induced extensive fusion of mouse alveolar macrophages, and that in the presence of the lymphokine macrophage fusion factor, as little as 0.012 nM was active in producing multinucleated giant cells. Multinucleated giant cell formation has also been observed when the HL-60 cell line and the mouse macrophage-like J774.2 cell line were exposed to 10^{-7-10} M 1,25-$(OH)_2$ D_3 for 24-72 h [21]. In this context, *in vivo* injection of 1,25-$(OH)_2$ D_3 into patients with malignant osteopetrosis corrected bone binding and resorptive deficiencies in the patients' monocytes [21].

Koeffler et al. [178] have shown that 10^{-7} to 10^{-9} M concentrations of either the active metabolite of vitamin D [1,25-$(OH)_2$ D_3] or certain fluorinated analogs of vitamin D can induce normal human myeloid progenitors (GM-CFC) in the presence of CSF to differentiate preferentially to macrophages *in vitro*. Marrow cultures exhibited an absolute, not just a proportional, increase in macrophage colonies, indicating that the action was not simply inhibition of granulopoiesis. The plasma concentration of 1,25-$(OH)_2$ D_3 in humans is approximately 7.7×10^{-11} M [132], and the concentration of 1,25-$(OH)_2$ D_3 inducing macrophage differentiation of progenitors *in vitro* is $>10^{-9}$ M, raising the question of physiologic relevance of this observation. Certainly, patients receiving superphysiologic doses of 1,25-$(OH)_2$ D_3 have not been reported to have monocytosis; likewise, patients with vitamin D-resistant rickets have not been reported to have low monocyte or macrophage levels. Nevertheless, the possibility of local production of the active form of vitamin D by cellular components of the marrow microenvironment [366], possibly even by tissue macrophages, raises the possibility of much higher local concentrations of 1,25-

$(OH)_2$ D_3 in the environment of the progenitor cells than plasma levels may suggest. Furthermore, recurrent infections, impaired phagocytic function, and decreased mobility of leukocytes have been shown in vitamin D-deficient states. This defect in phagocytic function has been reversed by *in vitro* culture of macrophages with 1,25-$(OH)_2$ D_3 [21, 314]. The immediate biological precursor of 1,25-$(OH)_2$ D_3, 25-(OH) D_3, is without biologic effect unless used at 10- to 100-fold higher concentrations than its hydroxylated metabolite. Thus, evidence that macrophages themselves have 1-hydroxylase activity and can synthesize 1,25-$(OH)_2$ D_3 from its precursor suggests that this molecule may also be a monokine with important local actions in recruitment and activation of macrophages [314] and of osteoclasts, with which they share a common derivation from a marrow hematopoietic progenitor.

ACTION OF VITAMIN D METABOLITES ON CANCER CELLS

The ability of 1,25-$(OH)_2$ D_3 to induce macrophage differentiation of myeloid leukemic cells was first established by Abe et al. [1], using the mouse myeloid leukemic cell line M1. Induction of phagocytes, lysozyme production, and locomotive activity were seen with concentrations as low as 10^{-10} *M* of the vitamin. The potency of this differentiation inducer was such that a 1000-fold higher concentration of the next most potent inducer of M1 differentiation, dexamethasone, was required to achieve a comparable level of maturation. Simultaneous treatment of M1 cells with low, physiologic concentrations of 1,25-$(OH)_2$ D_3 (0.12 n*M*) and dexamethasone (10 n*M*) induced a degree of differentiation equivalent to the response obtained with higher concentrations of either agent alone [230]. The isolation of two variant clones of M1, one resistant to dexamethasone and the other to 1,25-$(OH)_2$ D_3, strongly suggests that these differentiation-inducing agents act in different ways and that combination therapy with both steroids may be useful in reducing leukemogenicity [230].

The mouse myelomonocytic leukemic cell line WEHI-3 is also inducible to macrophage differentiation when exposed to 1,25-$(OH)_2$ D_3 in a clonal assay system. The differentiation-susceptible D^+ line was both growth-inhibited and macrophage-differentiated to the 50% level with 10^{-8}-10^{-10} *M* 1,25-$(OH)_2$ D_3. Of particular interest was the observation that a subline of WEHI-3 refractory to other differentiation-inducing agents was exquisitely sensitive to 1,25-$(OH)_2$ D_3, with 50% growth inhibition and macrophage differentiation seen with 10^{-13} *M* vitamin.

The first reports of the capacity of 1,25-$(OH)_2$ D_3 to induce differentiation of human leukemic cells indicated that HL-60 was growth-suppressed, and phagocytosis and C3-rosette formation were markedly induced in a dose-dependent manner over a range of 10^{-8} to 10^{-10} [229]. Unfortunately, these investigators concluded that HL-60 was induced to form granulocytes, as had previously been observed for retinoids and DMSO, rather than the uniform pattern of monocyte-macrophage differentiation reported in subsequent studies [176, 210, 215, 217, 257, 333, 337]. The range of monocyte-macrophage maturation features induced in HL-60 following exposure to 1,25-$(OH)_2$ D_3 is shown in Table 1. These maturation features were induced in a dose-dependent (10^{-11} to 10^{-7} *M*) and time-dependent (1-6 days) manner, and resulted in a functional phenotype and two-dimensional gel pattern of proteins close to, but not identical with, those of peripheral blood monocytes [232]. Cell division apparently is not required for expression of these differentiation features [83, 178].

The ability of low concentrations of 1,25-$(OH)_2$ D_3 to induce macrophage differentiation of HL-60 is similar to that reported for phorbol esters; however, this is not due to similar binding sites, since 1,25-$(OH)_2$ D_3 did not compete for phorbol diester binding sites as measured by [^{3}H]phorbol dibutyrate binding on HL-60 [257]. Variants of HL-60 have been developed which are resistant to differentiation induction by DMSO, retinoic acid, TPA, and 1,25-$(OH)_2$ D3. One variant resistant to phorbol esters was also resistant to 1,25-$(OH)_2$ D_3 [257], suggesting that mutants that cannot be induced to differentiate can involve common events following the receptor binding stage. The possibility of synergism between 1,25-$(OH)_2$ D_3 and phorbol esters or other differentiation inducers is definitely indicated in the case of HL-60, and has been reported with retinoic acid and with DMSO since low concentrations of 1,25-$(OH)_2$ D_3 in combination with DMSO produced cessation of proliferation of HL-60 cells within 2 days, as well as a greater expression of differentiation [333]. Simultaneous treatment of HL-60 with suboptimal concentrations of 1-a-25-$(OH)_2$ D_3 (0.12-1.2 n*M*) showed additive effects in reducing nitroblue tetra-

Table 1. Monocyte-macrophage differentiation markers induced in HL-60 promyelocytic leukemic cells following exposure to 10^{-8}-10^{-11} *M* 1,25-$(OH)_2$ D_3

Nonspecific esterase
Lysozyme
Monoclonal antibody to monocyte antigens
Adherence
Morphology
Phagocytosis
C_3 receptor
NBT reduction
Chemoattraction
Motility
Growth inhibition
Transferrin receptor
Bind to and degrade bone matrix
Two-dimensional gel monocyte-specific proteins

zolium, a common marker for monocyte-macrophage and granulocyte differentiation [231].

The human monocytoid cell line U937 is also induced to macrophage differentiation with loss of plating efficiency in the presence of 10^{-10} *M* 1,25-$(OH)_2$ D_3 [225, 279]. Differentiation involves development of adherence, macrophage morphology, lysozyme production, capacity to reduce NBT, expression of β-glucuronidase and alkaline phosphatase, Fc receptor expression, phagocytosis, and reactivity with antimonocyte-specific monoclonal antibodies [279]. As in the case of HL-60, the differentiation of U937 is not blocked by inhibitors of DNA synthesis, but is by the calcium ionophore A23187 [159]. The existence of synergism between 1,25-$(OH)_2$ D_3 and other biological response modifiers has been established with retinoic acid. U937 cells can be primed by short incubation with 1,25-$(OH)_2$ D_3 to respond by maturation to agents such as cAMP, PGE, and cholera toxin, which alone do not induce differentiation [279].

1,25-$(OH)_2$ D_3 or retinoic acid plus dibutyryl cAMP is effective in inducing a variety of differentiation markers in U937. Their actions on insulin receptors were the opposite, however. 1,25-$(OH)_2$ D_3 increased the binding, while retinoid decreased the binding. This effect was specific for insulin, since the transferrin receptors were reduced by both methods of differentiation [316]. Thus, changes in insulin receptors during maturation *in vitro* depend on the inducing agent and are not causally related to the differentiation process.

Other differentiation-inducing agents have been compared with 1,25-$(OH)_2$ D_3, which was the most effective. The polar/planar compound HMBA was most effective in reducing cell recovery, but did not induce cell maturation. Retinoic acid-reduced cell and total blast cell recovery with an increase in neutrophil differentiation. Protein inducers of differentiation, α- and γ-interferon, showed slight activity in reducing cell and blast recovery, whereas a murine serum source of differentiation factor (GM-DF) was highly effective in inducing macrophage differentiation and reduction in recovery of immature cells. 1,25$(OH)_2$ D_3 or IFN-γ decreased blast cells and increased macrophage differentiation in suspension cultures of marrow from patients with myelodysplastic syndrome [361, 401].

As an alternative to the suspension culture technique for monitoring differentiation induction of fresh leukemic marrow, an agar cloning assay has been used, in which colony or cluster incidence was measured in 7-day cultures of 10^5 leukemic marrow cells. Unlike the clonal assay for differentiation-induction of HL-60 or WEHI-3 cells, primary human leukemia cultures formed small clusters of 10-20 cells (microclusters), 20-40 cells (macroclusters), small colonies with an excess of clusters (microcolonies), or colonies of normal size with a normal cluster-to-colony ration [132, 178, 247]. In most cases, the clonal growth was diffuse and colonies or clusters failed to differentiate (with the exception of most patients with chronic myeloid leukemia and some patients with preleukemia) [231, 314, 316]. In view of this growth pattern, clonal differentiation can only be measured by isolation and staining of individual clones, a laborious and inexact procedure at best. As an alternative, 1,25-$(OH)_2$ D3-induced reduction of leukemic cloning capacity was used as an index of differentiation. The validity of this approach has been validated by studies showing that 50% growth inhibition of proliferation generally approximated to 50% growth inhibition when 1,25-$(OH)_2$ D_3 or its derivatives were used to induce differentiation. It should be stressed that this linkage between proliferation inhibition in clonal assay and differentiation induction generally does not hold true for other types of differentiation agents. For example, inhibition of the colony growth by most chemotherapeutic agents is not associated with differentiation, and protein sources of differentiation activity may not influence primary leukemic cloning capacity, but only recloning capacity.

In a more extensive analysis of heterogeneity of responsiveness to the growth-inhibitory/differentiation capacity of 1,25-$(OH)_2$ D_3, it was observed that preleukemic marrows exhibiting colony formation analogous to normal marrow were least responsive to 1,25-$(OH)_2$ D_3, whereas preleukemic marrows with cluster-forming acute myeloid leukemia-type clonal growth were most responsive, being comparable to the clinical observations. These observations suggest the interesting, perhaps surprising, conclusion that the more acute the leukemia the more it is responsive to 1,25-$(OH)_2$ D_3.

Koeffler et al. [178] have also shown that 1,25-$(OH)_2$ D_3 and two fluorinated analogs, 24, 24-F2-1,25-$(OH)_2$ D_3, inhibited colony formation of marrow from patients with ANLL (four cases) and chronic myeloid leukemia (four cases) at concentrations of 10^{-8} *M*, with 50-80% of leukemic colony-forming cells assuming a macrophage-like morphology. This result is comparable to the report of Moore et al. [247], with the exception that in the latter study more patients were investigated and the greater sensitivity seen in acute myeloid leukemia patients (50% inhibition at 4 x 10^{-12} *M*) may be explained by the use of total clonogenic units measured (i.e., colonies of >40 cells and clusters of 3-40 cells) rather than restricting inhibition analysis to colonies of >40 cells. The cells of the majority of patients with acute myeloid leukemia do not form colonies of 40 cells, and the leukemic cells in general form small clusters.

A variety of metabolites and analogs of vitamin D_3 have been developed and tested for biological activity and *in vivo* toxicity. Recent studies have extended biological screening to leukemia differentiation systems. HL-60 is induced to differentiate upon exposure to 10^{-7}-10^{-10} *M* 1,24-$(OH)_2$ D_3 or 1,24R-$(OH)_2$ D_3 in a fashion comparable to that with 1,25-$(OH)_2$ D_3. A different analog of 1,25-$(OH)_2$ D_3 has been found highly active in stimulating intestinal calcium transport and bone calcium mobilization in vitamin D-deficient rats [354]. This 24, 24-F_2-1,25-$(OH)_2$ is highly active in induction of WEHI-3 and HL-60 differentiation and growth inhibition, with 50%

activity at 10^{-14} *M*, thus making it the most active D_3 analog tested in the leukemic assay system [241]. Unfortunately, this analog is considerably more toxic *in vivo* than is 1,25-$(OH)_2$ D_3. These compounds showed the same relative activities, in that normal marrow was always least sensitive to growth inhibition and acute myeloid leukemia marrow most sensitive, with preleukemia and chronic myeloid leukemia occupying intermediate positions. Further, the D^- variants of HL-60 and WEHI-3 were considerably more sensitive to both compounds than were the D^+ lines (with the exception of the fluorinated analogs' action on HL-60).

24-Homo-, and 26-homo-1,25$(OH)_2$ D_3 and delta [39] analogues were 10-fold more potent than 1,25$(OH)_2$ D_3 in inducing differentiation of HL-60 [285]. The 24-homo-analogue was significantly less active in mobilizing calcium from bone.

It is obvious that more extensive screening must be undertaken to determine if the calcium-mobilizing activity and consequent toxicity as a feature of D_3 metabolites are invariably related to efficacy in induction of leukemic growth inhibition and differentiation. Obviously, as compared with a long *in vivo* half-life, low toxicity and retention of selective leukemia-cell differentiating activity would be highly desirable for clinical studies. Clinical trials with vitamin D have been limited because of intolerable hypercalcemia which often develops with this compound. Some responses have been seen in patients with myelodysplastic syndromes when treated at 2 mg per day [179]. With new analogues of vitamin D_3 now available, a separation of the effects of calcium metabolism and those on cell differentiation is now possible and clinical investigations are underway [287].

Receptors for vitamin D and its metabolites

The role of 1,25-$(OH)_2$ D_3 as an agent responsible for mineral homeostasis has been extensively studied. Its mechanisms of action within target cells is apparently steroid hormone-like in that 1,25-$(OH)_2$ D_3 first binds to a specific, high-affinity cytosolic receptor protein, which then translocates into the nucleus within 30-60 min, binds to chromatin, and consequently initiates genomic expression of the necessary mineral-regulating proteins. In support of this theory are the findings that all known 1,25-$(OH)_2$ D_3-responsive tissues, such as the intestine, bone, and kidney, contain cytosolic receptors. In addition, many other tissues and cultured cells have been shown to possess 1,25-$(OH)_2$ D_3 receptors, including some tumor cells. Breast cancer, melanoma, and osteogenic sarcoma cells possess a low density (8000-15, 000 per cell) of receptors with high affinity (K_d 10^{-10}-10^{-11} *M*) for 1,25-$(OH)_2$ D_3 [78, 89, 94, 211, 173]. Receptors with similar affinity and density have been reported on human monocytes, malignant B and T leukemic cell lines, activated T-cells, Epstein-Barr virus-transformed B-lymphocytes, and cell lines such as K562, HL-60 and U937 [210, 211, 303, 333]. Identification of 1,25-$(OH)_2$ D_3 receptors by specific immunochemical reactivity and selective chemical dissociation has shown that nuclear binding of the vitamin receptor is a rapid event (minutes) in HL-60, whereas the cellular differentiation response is delayed (6-7 days) [210]. This may be reconciled if the receptor must be maintained within the nucleus over the long term. A differentiation-noninducible variant of HL-60 has been reported to have only 8% of receptor copy numbers of the parent line, suggesting that assay of 1,25-$(OH)_2$ D_3 receptors in leukemic patients may be predictive of the ultimate response of the patient to adjunct therapy with 1,25-$(OH)_2$ D_3 [210]. This possibility is supported by the observation that the equilibrium dissociation constant of the 1,25-$(OH)_2$ D_3 receptor on HL-60 is close to the vitamin concentration, causing 50% of HL-60 cells to reduce NBT [176]. Against this view, there is the fact that the human myeloblastic leukemic cell line KG-1 has approximately the same number of 1,25-$(OH)_2$ D_3 receptors as HL-60, yet cannot be induced to differentiate by the vitamin [176].

There is extensive evidence for a classic steroid receptor-DNA interaction for the 1,25-$(OH)_2$ D_3 receptor, with selective binding of the receptor to A + T-rich segments of double-stranded DNA. Franceschi [90] demonstrated that the receptor can also interact with RNA as well as DNA. The physiologic significance of this observation remains obscure. However, in other steroid hormone systems, steroids can influence certain non-transcriptional processes, such as the stability of hormone-dependent mRNA, as well as posttranscriptional processing of secretory proteins, the regulation of 5S RNA synthesis, and the processing of heterogeneous nuclear RNAs.

Interaction of 1,25-$(OH)_2$ D_3 with receptors on normal or malignant target cells results in variable and complex changes in proliferation. A biphasic effect on the growth of breast tumor [104, 159] and osteosarcoma cells [211] has been reported, with physiologic concentrations of 1,25-$(OH)_2$ D_3 (10^{-10}-10^{-11} *M*) stimulating growth, and higher concentration (10^{-7}-10^{-8} *M*) inhibiting it. In contrast, a uniform pattern of growth inhibition is seen with the leukemic cell lines HL-60, U937 [280], M-1 and WEHI-3, and primary myeloid leukemia (Fig. 1) at concentrations as low as 10^{-12} *M*. No inhibition of normal marrow CFU-GM colony formation is seen with 1,25-$(OH)_2$ D_3 except at very high concentrations of 0.1-1 μg/ml; growth stimulation of normal mouse and human CFU-GM colony formation can be observed (Fig. 1).

Kuribayashi et al. [185] have reported on two variant clones of HL-60, resistant to differentiation and growth inhibition in the presence of 1,25-$(OH)_2$ D_3. One clone was also unresponsive to phorbol ester, actinomycin-D, and DMSO. The variant clones were found to possess reduced amounts of cytosol receptor protein, to which 1,25-$(OH)_2$ D_3 was specifically bound, but the hormone-receptor complex could be transferred to the chromatin acceptor site in both the wild-type and variant clones. This

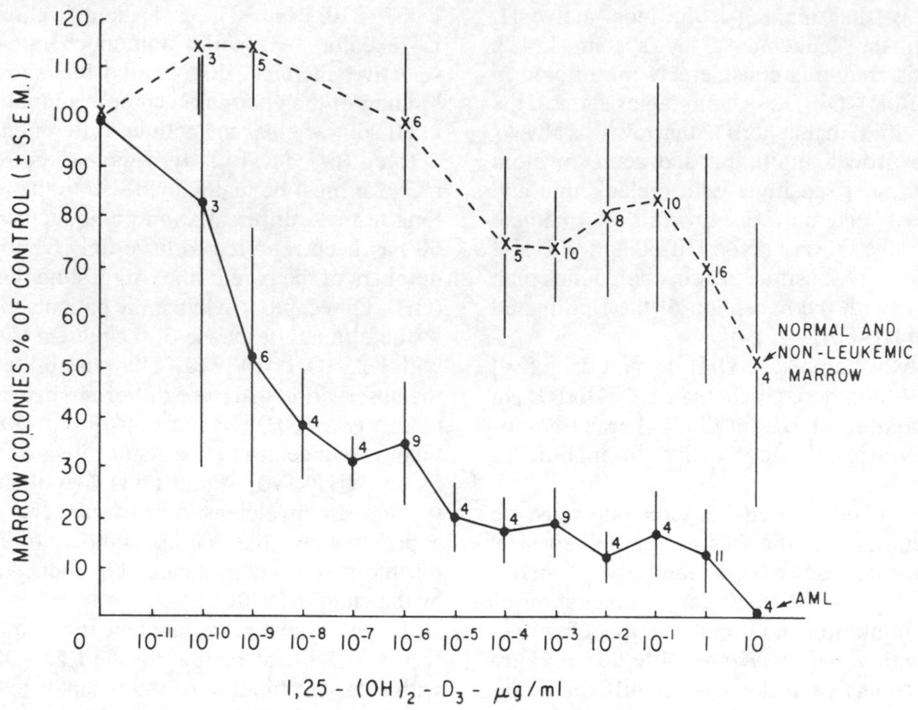

Figure 1. Action of varying concentrations of 1,25-$(OH)_2$ D_3 on the cloning capacity of 1 X 10^5 bone marrow cells of acute myeloid leukemic origin (untreated patients, •) or normal marrow and marrow from patients with nonhematopoietic tumors (X). Cultures were scored at day 7. Numbers indicate number of patients studied at each dosage point.

would indicate that 1,25-$(OH)_2$ D_3 resistance is due to a reduction in specific cytosol receptors.

Freake et al. [211] reported that whole chronic myeloid leukemic cells specifically took up 1,25-$(OH)_2$ D_3 with high affinity (K_d = 3.6 x 10^{-11} *M*) and low capacity. Subcellular fractionation of labeled cells showed that binding was restricted to cytosols and nuclei; however, chronic myeloid leukemic cells appeared to contain both the receptor for 1,25-$(OH)_2$ D_3 and an unknown substance that prevents its detection following the preparation of cytosol. Cells from patients in chronic phase specifically bound more vitamin (18 fmol/10^7 cells) than did those in the blastic phase (7 fmol/10^7 cells), or cells from patients with acute myeloid leukemia (2.6 fmol/10^7 cells). From observing that only cells from patients with chronic myeloid leukemia responded to 1,25-$(OH)_2$ D_3 by differentiation along the monocyte-macrophage pathway, it was concluded that differentiation induction was most likely dependent upon adequate levels of receptors, and that intact cells rather than cytosol preparations should be studied before cells of a particular tissue are designated as receptor negative. In view of the heterogeneity of the cellular composition of chronic myeloid leukemia and the heterogeneity of morphological type in blastic chronic myeloid leukemia (30% terminal transferase positive) and ANLL, general conclusions on receptor display with such small groups of patients should be treated with caution.

The HL-60 genome contains several different oncogenes, but only one, c-myc, is significantly amplified and transcribed at high levels (x20). Westin et al. [384] reported that myc on mRNA is no longer present in HL-60 cells induced to granulocytic differentiation by DMSO or retinoic acid. Reitsma et al. [312] have shown that 1,25-$(OH)_2$ D_3 reduced myc nRNA levels in HL-60 within 4 h of exposure to the vitamin/hormone, and this change preceded the onset of other measurable phenotypic changes by at least 8 h. It remains to be determined whether the altered transcription is the consequence of the hormone interaction with the c-myc promoter or a spectrum of promoters, each associated with a gene or gene cluster involved in determining cell phenotype.

Action of 1,25-$(OH)_2$ D_3 on other aspects of hematopoiesis

Myelofibrosis with myeloid metaplasia is considered a neoplastic disorder in which fibroblast proliferation and collagen synthesis in the marrow are increased by platelet-derived growth factor, or related substances, released by neoplastic megakaryocytes [45]. It has been postulated that 1,25-$(OH)_2$ D_3 may inhibit the formation of fibrous tissue (mainly collagen) in bone marrow and also may increase its degradation [218]. The hormone also inhibits the proliferation of megakaryocytes that normally promote collagen synthesis. Degradation of fibrous tissue is also mediated by monocytes and macrophages, and the number and activity of these cells are increased by 1,25-$(OH)_2$ D_3. Thus, the various actions of this vitamin contribute to a reduction in the collagen content; conversely, a deficiency of it may allow abnormal accumulation of collagen in the marrow. In this context, myelofibrosis in a rachitic infant regressed following vitamin D therapy [60], and a group of rachitic children with anemia and a blood picture typical of myelofibrosis also responded to vitamin D [397].

A novel immunoregulatory role has been proposed for 1,25-$(OH)_2$ D_3. Intracellular receptors that bind the vitamin and sediment at 3.35 were not detected in 'resting' T or B lymphocytes, but T cells activated by Epstein-Barr virus produced the receptor, and the amount of the macro-molecule induced was the same as in normal monocytes. Since the D_3-binding macro-molecule is seen in actively mitotic cells, it may exert an antiproliferative-differentiative influence in the immune system.

1,25-$(OH)_2$ D_3 at picomolar concentrations has also been shown to inhibit production of the T-lymphocyte growth-promoting lymphokine interleukin 2 (IL-2). Other metabolites of vitamin D_3 were less effective, and their order of potency corresponded to their respective affinity for the 1,25-$(OH)_2$ D_3 receptor, suggesting that suppression of T-cell production of IL-2 was mediated by this specific receptor [365]. 1,25-$(OH)_2$ D_3 may selectively inhibit the action of IL-1 in stimulation of thymocyte proliferation [255]. It also modulates GM-CSF production by T cells by posttranscriptional reduction in the half-life of GM-CSF, nRNA in mitogen-activated T cells and T-cell lines [358].

In view of the well-established calcium-mobilizing effect of 1,25-$(OH)_2$ D_3 in its classic target tissues [209], it is possible that the suppressive effect of this hormone on IL-2 is mediated by an influence on calcium translocation and again indicates a physiologic role of this hormone in immunoregulation.

In vivo effects of vitamin D metabolites

Sato et al. [328] have evaluated the effect of 1-α-(OH) D_3 on the growth of two solid tumors transplanted subcutaneously in mice. 1-α-(OH) D_3 administered orally by stomach tube at daily doses of 0.1 and 0.2 μg/kg body weight for 114 days suppressed sarcoma 180 tumor growth by 37 and 64% respectively, without significantly affecting serum calcium levels. Similar oral treatment with 0.1 and 0.2 μg/kg of 1-α-(OH) D_3 for 21 days resulted in a 75-80% decrease in pulmonary metastases in mice injected subcutaneously with Lewis lung carcinoma fragments. While the data illustrate a potential therapeutic anticarcinogenic effect of this metabolite, they should be considered as preliminary, since small numbers of mice (three to six) were tested in each treatment group.

1-α-(OH) D_3 and 1,25-$(OH)_2$ D_3 have marked effects on the growth and differentiation of cultured murine myeloid leukemia cells (M1 cells), established from an SL mouse with myeloid leukemia. These results, and the fact that syngeneic SL mice inoculated with M1 cells all die of leukemia, prompted a recent evaluation of the *in vivo* effects of 1-alpha-(OH) D_3 and 1,25-$(OH)_2$ D_3 by Honna et al. [150]. Thrice-weekly intraperitoneal injections of picomole amounts of 1-α-(OH) D_3 and 1,25-$(OH)_2$ D_3 considerably prolonged the survival time of syngeneic SL mice inoculated with M1 cells. A similar, marked prolongation of survival time was observed in athymic nude mice with M1 leukemia and treated intraperitoneally with 1-α-(OH) D_3. The results with the athymic mice suggested to the authors that T-lymphocyte-mediated immune responses were not directly involved in the effects of the vitamin D_3 metabolite. Serum levels of calcium and phosphorus were not significantly affected in the nude mice given M1 cells and 1-α-(OH) D_3 for 30 days, compared with mice given M1 cells alone.

Attempts to duplicate these observations in BALB/c mice inoculated with syngeneic WEHI-3 myelomonocytic leukemia cells proved unsuccessful [128]. Neither dexamethasone nor a combination of it with 1,25-$(OH)_2$ D_3 prolonged the survival of WEHI-3 tumor-bearing mice [128, 150]. The disparity between the *in vivo* observations with M1 and WEHI-3 leukemias could have a number of explanations, which require further testing before dismissing the therapeutic potential of vitamin D derivatives in leukemia. The WEHI-3B grows more rapidly than M1, and 10^5 cells generally result in 100% mortality within 21 days. However, treatment with conventional cytotoxic agents, such as Cytoxan, produces an increase in life span, even producing cures in a dose-dependent fashion [128]. In retrospect, however, the explanation may reside in the relative resistance of the WEHI-3D$^+$ line to 1,25-$(OH)_2$ D_3-induced growth inhibition (50% inhibition *in vitro* with 4 x 10^{-4} *M*), in contrast to the much greater sensitivity of the WEHI-3D$^-$, the HL-60, M1, and fresh acute myeloid leukemic cells (10^{-9}-10^{-12} *M*).

Potter and Moore [300] have extended *in vivo* studies with successful growth and maintenance of the human myeloid leukemia lines U937, KG-1, and K562, as subcutaneously induced granulocytic sarcomas in nude mice.

Studies involving routine and special histochemistry, enzyme histochemistry, immunocytochemistry, surface markers, cytogenetics, and electron microscopy have demonstrated virtual identity of cells from the induced granulocytic sarcomas in nude mice with respective cells from the cultured lines. The validity and reliability of the living model have thus been established. Using this *in vivo* model, preliminary experiments were undertaken to evaluate the effect(s) of 1,25-$(OH)_2$ D_3 on the development of these subcutaneous leukemic tumors induced on nude mice from cultured cells. Based on the work of Hartmann and Moore [128], a dosage of 1 μg/ml of 1,25-$(OH)_2$ D_3 was chosen as potentially the most effective, but least toxic. The method of administration involved subcutaneous implantation of an osmotic minipump (OMP) at a site remote from the concurrently inoculated tumorigenic cells. One group of mice received only washed cultured leukemic cells, another received cells and an OMP containing only solvent, and a third group of mice received leukemic cells and an OMP delivering 1 μg/ml of 1,25-$(OH)_2$ D_3. All mice were weighed on alternate days and observed for tumor development.

Of the mice receiving cultured K562 or HL-60 cells only, almost all developed granulocytic sarcomas within an average of 4-5 weeks after inoculation. A similar result was seen in mice inoculated with cultured cells from either of these lines that also bore implants of an OMP containing only solvent. Granulocytic sarcomas either failed to develop, or developed infrequently and (on the average) later in the group similarly inoculated with cultured cells from these lines, and bearing OMPs containing 1,25-$(OH)_2$ D3.

Since each mouse underwent the same priming and received the same number of cultured human leukemic cells, it appears that the absence of, or delay in the development of, induced granulocytic sarcomas may be attributable to the influence of the administered 1,25-$(OH)_2$ D_3 in the system. These results suggest that 1,25-$(OH)_2$ D_3 might have an inhibitory effect on the proliferative capacity of human leukemic cells *in vivo*. Whether the mechanism involves induction of terminal differentiation on the human tumor cell inoculum requires investigation. The involved mechanism(s) of inhibition are also of interest. In those few treated mice demonstrating proliferation of xenogenic (human) leukemic cells, the possibility of emergence of 1,25-$(OH)_2$ D_3-resistant clones should not be overlooked, and the availability of receptors for 1,25-$(OH)_2$ D_3 should be determined on cells derived from these tumors. Recently developed analogues of 1,25-$(OH)_2$ D_3 notably 1,25 (OH)2-16-ene-23-yne-D_3, were remarkably effective in 'curing' mice bearing the WEHI-3B + leukemia [30]. Differentiation was induced at dosages that did not produce hypercalcemia.

Translating these observations into a clinical application, it is clear that *in vitro* screening for response to 1,25-$(OH)_2$ D_3 can be used to identify resistant and susceptible patients with leukemia and preleukemia. While it is unlikely that the vitamin could prove effective on its own, it could be combined with conventional chemotherapy or used as maintenance therapy in patients achieving remission by conventional protocols. The toxicity of 1,25-$(OH)_2$ D_3 in mice at dosages unable to produce leukemic regression *in vivo* would require precise dose-response analysis in humans. In this regard, 1,25-$(OH)_2$ D_3 has been used effectively in patients with post-menopausal osteoporosis [58]. Short-term treatment (6-8 months) with 0.5 mg/day restored calcium absorption to normal, and calcium balance improved and the bone resorption rate decreased. With long-term therapy (2 years) both bone resorption and formation rates increased. The lack of side effects in long-term treatment with 1,25-$(OH)_2$ D_3 provides a dosage guideline for studies in leukemia [100].

Oral administration of 1-α-(OH) D_3 in two patients with AML and one with MDS was reported to reduce the number of leukemic cells in the marrow. In a study of 18 patients with MDS, 1,25-$(OH)_2$ D_3 produced a partial or minor response in blood in 8 cases but with no significant improvement in blood or marrow blasts [179]. Seven of the patients developed leukemia before or by 12 weeks of treatment and half the patients developed hypercalcemia. It was not possible to sustain serum levels of 1,25-$(OH)_2$ D_3 at levels necessary to induce differentiation or growth inhibition without producing unacceptable toxicity. Future clinical trials await the use of recently developed analogues with reduced calcium mobilizing action and enhanced differentiating activity [30]. A further rationale for therapy with 1,25-$(OH)_2$ D_3 and its analogues is provided by the observation that the metabolic pathway of 1,25-$(OH)_2$ D_3 is defective in patients with MDS or AML [28]. Bone marrow plasma levels of 1,25-$(OH)_2$ D_3, but not its immediate precursor 25-(OH) D3, was decreased significantly in 50% of MDS and 30% of AML patients.

POLAR-PLANAR COMPOUNDS AS DIFFERENTIATION INDUCERS

Differentiation-inducing activity has been reported for various polar-planar compounds, most particularly DMSO, hexamethylene bisacetamide (HMBA), and *N*-methylformamide [56, 57, 153]. The differentiation-inducing action has been most extensively analyzed in murine erythroleukemic (MEL) cells. Inducer-mediated differentiation is a multistep process characterized by a latent period when a number of changes occur [214, 329]. These include alterations in ion flux, increase in membrane bound PKC, appearance of CA^{2+} and phospholipid-independent PKC activity in the cytosol and modulation of the expression of genes such as c-myc, c-myb, c-fos and p53. Commitment to differentiation is seen within 12 h and increases stochastically over 48 h and is associated with suppression of c-myb expression and a 10- to 30-fold increase in globin gene expression [214, 313]. The levels of ornithine decarboxylase are also regulated by HMBA. HMBA induces a transient, genome-wide hypomethylation of DNA achieved by replacement of 5-methylcytosine with cytosine residues [310]. This may be a necessary but not sufficient step in triggering the whole program of differentiation. Superoxide dismutase activity is induced by HMBA in parallel with differentiation and enzyme levels are directly related to the degree of cytosolic hemoglobinization [290, 23]. Introduction of superoxide dismutase into MEL cells with liposomes induces differentiation as do other oxidative treatments (liposome amino acid oxidase, xanthine oxidase, potassium superoxide). In contrast, antioxidants inhibit HMBA-induced differentiation [23]. The induction of superoxide dismutase in MEL cells may also be a cellular response to oxidative stress from hemoglobin autooxidation.

Potential improvements in efficacy of HMBA may be accomplished by changes in the chemical structure of the inducing agents and by increasing the sensitivity of tumor cells to inducers of differentiation. MEL cell lines that have acquired low levels of resistance to vincristine display a markedly increased sensitivity to HMBA [213]. A series of hybrid increased polar/apolar compounds have been produced that in certain instances are more active than HMBA *in vitro* and whose chemical structure makes it likely that they have different pharmacokinetics [213].

The first Phase I trials of HMBA involved continuous infusion of escalating doses of HMBA for 5 or 10 days in patients with refractory solid tumors [10, 77, 197, 320]. Dose limiting toxicity, specifically thrombocytopenia, was observed at 20-40 g/m^2. The MTD of continuously infused HMBA was 28 g/m^2/day and acidosis and CNS dysfunction were toxicities, as well as hemorrhage related to thrombocytopenia. The plasma half-life was 2.5 h and plasma levels of 1.42 n*M* or higher could be achieved [402]. In Phase I trials nasogastric or oral administration of HMBA at 30-36 g/m^2/day was also associated with thrombocytopenia and neutrotoxicity. Attempts have been made to individualize patient dosage based on plasma levels and clearance rates of HMBA [58]. Plasma levels of 1.5-2.0 m*M* could be sustained but toxicity was seen. The cause of the thrombocytopenia is obscure but appears to be a production defect rather than a peripheral destruction or pooling of platelets. At the dosages of HMBA required to produce differentiation, significant inhibition of cloning of normal myeloid, erythroid, and megakaryocyte progenitors is seen *in vitro* in murine bone marrow culture. Fifty percent inhibition of cloning, and suppression myelopoiesis in long-term bone marrow cultures, are seen with doses of HMBA of 1.2 m*M* with an unusually steep dose response. This observation does not fully explain the observed clinical toxicity, since the thrombocytopenia was not usually associated with a neutropenia. The development of analogs of HMBA with differentiation-inducing capacity and reduced suppressive activity against myeloid progenitors is a like direction in development of an effective clinical differentiation protocol [213] that could be applied in leukemia and MDS as well as in a variety of solid tumor systems (colon, bladder, breast).

CHEMOTHERAPEUTIC AGENTS AS DIFFERENTIATION INDUCERS

It is becoming apparent that of the variety of agents utilized in cancer chemotherapy, some may be effective because of their capacity to induce, selectively, tumor cell differentiation, and this property may be more important than cytotoxic potential. After extensive screening [for reviews, see 153, 176, 323] a number of agents have been found to have differentiation capacity [57, 59, 153, 198, 226]: mitomycin, doxorubicin, bleomycin, daunomycin [153, 176, 198, 226], cytosine arabinoside [116, 151, 153, 176, 198, 256, 349], hypoxanthine [57], 3-deazauridine, 5-azacytidine, methotrexate [31, 332], 5-aza-2-deoxycytodine [52, 235, 297], aphidicolin [112], and adenine arabinoside [256].

In all the preceding cases the differentiation action was observed at concentrations either below cytotoxic levels or well below maximum growth inhibition in suspension or clonal assays of leukemic cells. Most compounds have been tested against murine (M1) and human (HL-60) myeloid leukemic cell lines, in which differentiation into macrophages and granulocytes is reported. When tested *in vitro* against leukemic blast cells from patients with acute myeloid leukemia, actinomycin D was reported effective in differentiation induction in all 14 cases studied [153]. In all three cases in another study [226], cytosine arabinoside [226] and 5-aza-2-deoxycytidine [297] were also effective in inducing macrophage differentiation of leukemic blast cells. In the absence of an *in vivo* measure of leukemogenicity, the ability of these agents to eliminate the proliferative potential of the leukemic clone must be measured indirectly. In recloning studies of primary human leukemias cultured in methylcellulose, a decrease self-renewal potential of clonogenic cells (plating efficiency 2, PE$_2$) can be observed with various chemotherapeutic agents, independent of their chemosuppressive action on primary leukemic cloning efficiency [38]. This action on PE$_2$ is a likely differentiation index, since more primitive leukemic stem cells with extensive proliferative potential are 'differentiated' into a non-self-renewing compartment. Furthermore, this PE$_2$ parameter correlated with clinical response [39]. The combination of low doses of the above-mentioned chemotherapeutic agents with other differentiation-inducing agents may prove effective when neither type of agent can induce differentiation directly. In this regard, differentiation-resistant clones of M1 (D$^-$) that failed to respond to protein differentiation factor or chemotherapeutic agents could be 'sensitized' by as little as 0.25 μg/ml of actinomycin D, daunomycin, mitomycin C, hydroxyurea, bleomycin, 5-fluorouracil, prednisone, or dexamethasone to terminal differentiation when combined with protein factor [133, 153].

Lotem et al. [203] report that *in vitro* screening for differentiation-inducing compounds and compounds that show toxicity to blast cells may be useful in selecting appropriate treatments. However, their results were ambiguous, in that with some patients studied both before and after *in vivo* chemotherapy there was a similar differentiation response, or an apparent loss, or a gain of response *in vitro* of the remaining leukemic cells tested. In further studies, using five compounds known to induce HL-60 differentiation [DMSO, hexamethylene bisacetamide (HMBA), hypoxanthine, actinomycin D, and 6-thioguanine], differentiation of fresh myelogenous leukemic cells was tested *in vitro* [179]. Of 12 patients studied, the blast cells in most cases showed little morphological, histological, or functional maturation after exposure to the various compounds, as compared with the blast cells cultured without the compound. Actinomycin D was the only agent capable of causing significant maturation. This study suggests that many compounds shown to differentiate HL-60 may not trigger differentiation of less mature myeloid leukemic cells.

Molecular mechanism implicated in leukemia cell differentiation

Cytosine arabinoside is one of the most effective single agents for the treatment of myeloid leukemia and is conventionally considered to act by incorporation into DNA and by inhibiting DNA replication through production poor primer termini. Cytosine arabinoside induces nonspecific esterase activity in HL-60 cells [96] and increases surface expression of the monocyte surface antigen MY-4. Aphidicolin, an analogue of deoxycytodine, also induces HL-60 differentiation and slows DNA synthesis, but, unlike cytosine arabinoside, it is not incorporated into DNA and acts as an inhibitor of DNA polymerase [116].

Using a purine rather than a pyrimidine antimetabolite-adenosinearabinoside, Monroe et al. [256] also observed differentiation of HL-60 that correlated with slowing of DNA synthesis by an agent known to act at the level of the DNA polymerase template complex. The relationship of differentiation to DNA synthesis is complicated by observations that terminal differentiation of HL-60 to macrophages induced by the tumor promoter TPA can occur in the absence of DNA synthesis [319] and that terminal differentiation to granulocytes without cell division is observed following treatment with actinomycin D, DMSO, and butyric acid [217].

Agents can, however, induce HL-60 differentiation without inhibiting cell proliferation [31], or inhibit proliferation without inducing differentiation [332]. Thus, it remains to be determined whether inhibition of DNA synthesis is causally or indirectly related to differentiation. Other mechanisms of action of chemotherapeutic agents directed toward differentiation induction may involve cell membrane effects. Anthracyclines may play a role in alteration of leukemic cell glycoproteins, and there is evidence that these drugs bind extensively to membrane-lipid domains, altering membrane fluidity and directly modifying the synthesis or expression of glycoproteins at the cell surface [331].

A more specific action has been suggested involving DNA methylation changes: for example, cytosine arabinoside may have a direct influence on methylation of the c-myc oncogene [116], the expression of which is considerably amplified in myeloid leukemic cells and rapidly reduced once the cells are exposed to differentiation-inducing agents [312, 384].

5-Azacytidine and the less toxic 2-deoxy derivatives are also interesting candidates for *in vivo* use in leukemia differentiation therapy. These compounds have been shown to trigger gene expression in several systems, including globin gene expression, when given *in vivo* to thalassemic and sickle-cell anemia patients [192]. The mechanism by which 5-aza-deoxycytidine induces leukemic cell differentiation most likely involves DNA hypomethylating ability [235, 297]. Synthesis of hypomethylated DNA takes place after incorporation of the drug into DNA and is due partially to the chemical structure of the compound and mainly to the trapping of DNA methyltransferases, thus blocking their action. The known differences regarding the molecular targets of the two drugs could account for the greater differentiation-inducing ability and lower toxicity of the 2-deoxy derivative. It is well known that 5-azacytidine is actively incorporated into mRNA and tRNA, thus producing its major toxic effects.

A cautionary note should be introduced in considering the potential therapeutic role of 5-azacytodine. Motojo et al. [253] exposed blast cells from patients with acute myeloid leukemia to 5-azacytidine, 6-azacytidine, and the 2-deoxy derivative. Simple negative exponential colony survival curves were obtained for the three drugs, with the 5-aza-2-deoxy compound being most toxic and the 6-aza least toxic. Although confirming other reports of increased expression of certain antigenically defined phenotypic markers of leukemic blast cell differentiation, colonies surviving drug exposure to 5-aza and 5-aza-2-deoxy compounds had increased secondary replating efficiency. This suggests that hypomethylation of DNA may promote leukemic cell self-renewal.

***In vivo* induction of differentiation with low-dose cytosine arabinoside or azocytidine in patients with ccute myeloid leukemia and myelodysplastic syndrome (MDS)**

The preceding *in vitro* observations provide a strong case for the efficacy of low doses of ara-C in induction of terminal differentiation of myeloid leukemic cell lines and fresh leukemic blast cells, this action being either direct or by synergy with endogenous differentiation-inducing factors. It was thus of interest to investigate the actions of low-dose ara-C in patients with acute myeloid leukemia and myelodysplastic refractory anemia with excess of blasts. Baccarani and Tura [16] reported the first remission in a patient with RAB and subsequently extended the study to 20 patients with myelodysplastic syndrome (MDS), observing one complete and two partial remissions. Complete or partial remissions in MDS have been reported by other groups [151 ,234, 301, 380, 389], but no response to low-dose-ara-C was observed in a large cooperative study of refractory anemia with excess of blasts [261]. In acute myeloid leukemia, Housset et al. [152] reported remission in all three patients, and Weh et al. [380] had seven complete and two partial remissions in 12 cases. Encouraging results have been obtained by others [234], but no response was reported by Hagenbeek et al. [122] in four acute myeloid leukemia patients treated with the same protocol that produced responses in other studies [152, 380]. The reasons for variable results are unclear, but the patient population, particularly the MDS cases, was heterogeneous, and the dosage and timing of drug administration in different studies varied between 10 and 30 mg/m^2, every 12 or 24 h, for 7-28 days. Indeed, the more encouraging results obtained by Housset et al. [152], compared with those of Baccarani et al. [15], may be due to the more frequent and longer duration of ara-C administration in the former study, thereby probably achieving a rather constant *in vivo* concentration of the drug.

In one series of 21 patient (five with refractory anemias with an excess of blasts and 16 with acute leukemias) treated with small doses of ara-C (10 mg/m^2/12 h for 15-21 days), improvement was noted in 15 cases (71%), and complete remission was observed in 12 (57%) [44]. Complete remission was obtained after one course of treatment in eight cases. The fact that these patients entered remission relatively slowly and did not suffer marrow aplasia suggests that low-dose ara-C was functioning by inducing differentiation. Generally, when clinical response has been obtained, the evidence points to a differentiating role for the drug rather than an antitumor effect, with progressive evolution of recovery, absence of aplasia, and the simultaneous presence of normal islets of promyelocytes and leukemic myeloblasts [152].

The availability of the *in vitro* assay for detection of leukemic cell responses to differentiation agents should mandate prescreening of patients for *in vitro* sensitivity before enrollment in a differentiation protocol such as low-dose ara-C. Toward this goal, leukemic marrow cultures were exposed to low doses of ara-C, and a reduction in blast cells and an increase in more mature granulocyte and macrophage elements were noted in two or three patients. Subsequent low-dose ara-C treatment *in vivo* resulted in complete remission in the two patients that showed a strong *in vitro* response [226].

In a large study of low-dose (10 mg/m^2) ara-C in poor-risk ANLL, overall survival was comparable to that observed following conventional therapy with high-dose (200 mg/m^2) ara-C and anthrocyclin [65]. While the high-dose regimen produced more complete remissions (55%) than the low dose (33%), there were more early deaths in the intensive therapy group. Very-low-dose (3 mg/m^2) ara-C produced hematologic improvement in the majority of patients in a study trial of 73 MDS patients [65]. In other recent studies of low-dose ara-C in 73 patients with ANLL and MDS [9] and 40 patients with ANLL and MDS, complete remission rates of 24-31% were reported with 35-45% responders. In these studies evidence for leukemic cell differentiation was obtained. Cytogenetic and morphologic studies suggested that cytotoxicity rather than differentiation was responsible for remissions observed in two other studies with low-dose ara-C in poor-risk ANLL [18, 46].

Low-dose 5-azacytodine has also proved effective in MDS, and in one study of 44 patients, 48% responded with 11% complete and 25% partial remissions [338]. The median duration of remission was 53 weeks. 5-Aza-2'-deoxycytidine in 134 patients with AML, CML in blastic crisis, and MDS produced two complete and four partial remissions. The drug appeared to modify the leukemic phenotype *in vivo* as well as producing a direct cytolytic effect [406].

Tiazofurin (2-beta-D-ribofuranosylthiazole-4-carboxamide) is an inhibitor of inosine^5-monophosphate (IMP) dehydrogenase and is the enzyme in the rate-limiting synthesis of guanylate [379]. Tiazofurin has both cytotoxic and cytodifferentiation activities and has been used to induce responses in patients with blast crisis in CML [363]. Toxicity has been severe with nausea, rash, myalgia and serositis. Given the high toxicity, further clinical trials to this approach must be conducted to determine optimal dose and schedule. Combinations of tiazofurin with other differentiations may be of interest to investigate in the near future.

CYTOKINES AND HEMATOPOIETIC GROWTH FACTORS ACTIVE IN REGULATING PROLIFERATION AND DIFFERENTIATION OF LEUKEMIC HEMATOPOIETIC CELLS

Recognition that physiologic inducers of differentiation of normal hematopoietic cells could also influence proliferation and differentiation of leukemic cell lines led to a series of studies over the last two decades involving characterization of hematopoietic growth factors, in many cases using leukemic cell lines as sources of growth factor and/or as target for growth factors in various bioassays. As discussed in other chapters, the genes for these factors have been cloned and recombinant factors have been tested *in vitro* and *in vivo* for biological activity. This large family of cytokines and polypeptides includes factors with pleotropic and overlapping activities, and additive or synergistic interactions are frequently observed [124].

CSF dependence of myeloid leukemic progenitors

The cloning of normal or leukemic human CFU-GM in either agar or methylcellulose has permitted analysis of both quantitative and qualitative changes in this cell compartment in leukemia and other myeloproliferative disorders. Changes observed include abnormalities in the maturation of leukemic cells *in vitro*, defective proliferation as measured by colon size or cluster-to-colony ratio, abnormalities in biophysical characteristics of leukemic GM-CFC, the existence of cytogenetic abnormalities *in vitro*, and regulatory defects in responsiveness to positive and negative feedback control mechanisms [for reviews, see refs. 236-238, 241, 243, 245-247]. Detection of this spectrum of abnormalities has proved to be of clinical use in diagnosis of leukemia and preleukemic states, in classification of leukemias, and in predicting remission in acute myeloid leukemia. Variation has been reported among different groups investigating the characteristics of human acute myeloid leukemia cells in culture. These differences reflect, in part, the heterogeneity of the disease as well as variation in the culture criteria, the source and activity of CSF, and the timing of the culture. The preceding studies indicated that leukemic cells from patients with acute or chronic myeloid leukemia or preleukemic states were absolutely dependent upon a source of stimulatory factors for their clonal proliferation in culture at low plating densities. Analysis of the dose response of myeloid leukemia CFU-GM indicates that in the majority of cases they do not differ markedly from normal in their responsiveness to various sources of CSF, although occasionally, hyperresponsiveness of leukemic cells is seen [236, 238, 241, 243, 245, 247].

In an analysis of growth-factor responsiveness in suspension cultures of leukemic marrow from 25 patients, Lowenberg et al. [204] showed that 17/25 cases exhibited spontaneous 'autocrine' proliferation, [342] and this was enhanced in 21 cases by IL-3, in 17 cases by GM-CSF of G-CSF, and in five cases by M-CSF. In four cases the cells responded to all factors and the remainder responded to three, two, or only one source of stimulus. As with normal progenitor assays, 'spontaneous' leukemic cloning is observed as the marrow cell or peripheral blood leukocyte plating density increases, owing to endogenous production of CSFs by accessory populations, which may be residual normal cells of T-cell lineage or leukemic cell subpopulations. The autocrine concept of malignant transformation proposes that cells become malignant by the endogenous production of polypeptide growth factors that act upon their producer cells through functional external receptors. Support for the concept has been obtained by studies on oncogene action, since oncogenes may confer growth-factor autonomy on cancer cells by coding directly for autocrine polypeptide growth factors or their receptors, or by amplifying the mitogenic signals generated as a consequence of growth factor-receptor interaction.

Strong evidence for an autocrine role for GM-CSF has been provided in a study of 22 cases of primary human acute myeloid leukemia in which Northern blot analysis revealed expression of the GM-CSF gene in 11 cases [403]. GM-CSF expression was not found in normal hematopoietic tissue, with the exception of activated T-cells, strongly indicating that the GM-CSF gene activation was intimately associated with the transformation event. Furthermore, in six cases, GM-CSF was secreted by leukemic cells of both early and late stages of differentiation, and activity was specifically neutralized by antiserum to GM-CSF.[115]

The paradox of CSF dependence of primary human myeloid leukemias in clonal assay, and the autocrine production of GM-CSF, can be answered in part by the concentration at which the cells are plated: at high concentrations, 'spontaneous' leukemic colony or cluster formation is the norm. In the study of Young et al. [403], 9 of 22 cases showed autonomous growth of leukemic clusters when cells were plated at $5x10^4$/ml, yet exogenous GM-CSF increased cloning number and clone size in 15 of 22 cases. It is possible that in some cases GM-CSF is not actually secreted by the leukemic cells, but is present in active form as a membrane-bound moiety. In this regard, Nara and McCulloch [264] showed that purified cell membranes from cells of some acute myeloid leukemia patients, but not normal bone marrow of ALL cells, could promote proliferation of other acute myeloid leukemic cells in short-term suspension culture, enhancing self-renewal.

A direct link between constitutive GM-CSF expression and leukemic transformation was provided by Lang et al. [187], who transfected the murine GM-CSF gene into CSF-dependent, nonleukemic, myeloid cell lines and produced leukemic cell lines that constitutively secreted GM-CSF. To date, no example of human myeloid leukemia constitutively producing and responding to IL-3 has been reported, but in the mouse system, the well-characterized spontaneous murine myelomonocytic leukemia WEHI-3 constitutively secretes IL-3, apparently because of insertion of retroviral sequences adjacent to the IL-3 gene [398].

Retroviral insertion of the IL-3 gene with a viral long terminal repeat promoter produces leukemic transformation [125]. The fact that insertion of G-CSF, GM-CSF, or IL-3 genes into normal hematopoietic stem cells or in transgenic mice did not lead to leukemia [220] suggests that autocrine induction of factor-independence is necessary, but not sufficient, for converting normal cells to a transformed state. Genetic alterations may predispose them to undergo leukemic transformation by an autocrine mechanism. In this context the murine factor-dependent cell line FDC-P1 develops into fully leukemic cells when transplanted into whole-body-irradiated mice associated with development of autocrine GM-CSF or IL-3 production [74, 75].

Expression of mRNA for GM-CSF, G-CSF and M-CSF is ubiquitous in the blast cells of AML but not CML [50, 376, 403, 404]. In a minority of these cases significant quantities of bioactive CSF were produced, sufficient to stimulate autocrine blast cell proliferation [311, 403]. The significance of these observations was questioned by studies showing that enhanced expression of the GM-CSF gene in ABL blast cells was a consequence of manipulations used to enrich blast cell populations [167, 348].

Constitutive expression of IL-1 on mRNA and bioactive protein production is a characteristic of the majority of AMLs and is not a consequence of manipulation of the cells. IN 10/17 cases of AML, IL-1β mRNA was identified [117], and this autocrine IL-1 can induce AML proliferation [228]. The proliferative effect of IL-1 on leukemic blast cells, like its action on normal cells, is mediated in synergy with growth factors such as IL-3, GM-CSF, and G-CSF [145, 146]. Since IL-1 induces G-CSF, GM-CSF, and M-CSF production by bone marrow stromal cells (endothelium, fibroblasts, macrophages; see Moore [242] for review), and these factors stimulate leukemic cell proliferation, a paracrine mode of stimulation of leukemic cell proliferation has been proposed for AML [117], and juvenile CML [17]. An IL-1-mediated autocrine growth stimulation was proposed in a study of 13 cases of AML [61]. In all cases, immunofluorescence showed that up to 80% of all fresh leukemic blast cells in all patients contained either the 33-kDa IL-1β propeptide or both the 33- and 17-dDa mature form. The bioactive IL-1a propeptide was also detected in all cases but was less frequently released. In six cases studied, anti-IL-1β and to a lesser extent anti-IL-1a inhibited spontaneous proliferation, and in 10/12 cases sufficient exogenous IL-1 was produced to stimulate significant proliferation. AML cells constitutively released as much IL-1 as did endotoxin-stimulated normal monocytes, and 2/12 patients that did not respond to exogenous IL-2 were both high endogenous producers and presumably were maximally stimulated. In most instances, exogenous IL-1 supported the establishment of continuous lines of AML cells that grew for > 2 months [61].

A more complex autocrine loop is suggested by the studies of Bradbury et al. [33]. AML cells at low cell density were stimulated independently by exogenous GM-CSF or IL-1, and the response to both factors was inhibited by antibody to GM-CSF. Antibody to IL-1 inhibited spontaneous proliferation of these cells, and endogenous GM-CSF could be detected. Thus, IL-1 is produced by the leukemic cells, particularly from the more differentiated cells, and this in turn induces GM-CSF production, which directly mediates autocrine proliferation. Autocrine IL-1 induction of GM-CSF may account for the appearance of GM-CSF mRNA in cultured rather than fresh AML blasts [167]. Therapeutic strategy in the face of IL-1-, GM-CSF-, or IL-3-dependent leukemogenesis, either autocrine or paracrine, would require intervention to block CSF or IL-1 production or action. High-affinity antibodies to the factor or its receptor, in the latter case coupled to some form of toxin, may be one possible strategy which is under active consideration as a therapy in the case of IL-2-dependent T-cell lymphoma (anti-IL-2 receptor antibody and IL-2 toxin conjugates). A second strategy envisages the use of GM-CSF to recruit resting leukemic stem cells into cell cycle and synchronize the population in S phase in conjunction with cycle-specific chemotherapy [80, 201, 305].

Colony-stimulating factors as leukemia differentiating agents

The G-CSF and GM-CSF induce granulocytic differentiation of HL-60 and WEHI-3B leukemic cell lines [24, 97, 270, 298], but leukemic blast-cell proliferation is the more general response in primary cultures of AML bone marrow. GM-CSF is a universal proliferative stimulus for AML cells, generally without differentiation, whereas G-CSF stimulates proliferation and in a proportion of cases granulocytic differentiation [66]. This area is reviewed elsewhere in this volume and the actions of G-CSF and GM-CSF in clinical trials in myelodysplastic syndrome and AML are discussed. M-CSF is also a proliferative stimulus for some AML cells, but in many instances it induces differentiation to adherent macrophages [376]. Most leukemic blast populations express the M-CSF receptor, fms, and M-CSF mRNA is found in about half the blast population. Marked heterogeneity of M-CSF response is seen with different patients, ranging from cases where blast populations were unresponsive to M-CSF, to examples where blast-cell self-renewal was stimulated, to instances where the major effect of M-CSF was the generation of terminally differentiated cells with monocyte-macrophage characteristics. This heterogeneity in proliferative versus differentiation responses of leukemic blasts to various CSF species in different patients indicates the necessity of prescreening for factor response on an individual patient basis.

Interleukin 1 and cell proliferation and differentiation

Interleukin 1 has been implicated in an autocrine or paracrine mode of stimulation of myeloid leukemic cells in synergy with GM-CSF [33, 61, 117, 145, 146, 228]. It has also been reported to inhibit proliferation of a human myelomonocytic leukemic cell in the presence of low to intermediate, but not high, levels of GM-CSF [327].

The IL-1 inhibition of tritiated thymidine incorporation into murine M1 cells was first reported by Onozaki et al. [281]. On its own, IL-1 did not induce differentiation, but both growth inhibition and macrophage differentiation were induced synergistically by IL-1 and LPS coadministration. In further studies these investigators reported that while IL-1α, TNF, and IFNβ1 all had antiproliferative, but not differentiation-inducing, action on M1 cells, as little as 1 unit of IL-1, in conjunction with TNF or IFNβ1, induced FcR, phagocytic activity, and morphological charge [283]. The differentiation induced by IL-1 plus TNF was inhibited by antibodies to IFNβ1, as was the antiproliferative effect of TNF (but not IL-1), indicating autocrine IFNβ1 is induced and mediates direct differentiation and antiproliferative effects. Thus IFNβ1 is one of two signals required for M1 differentiation, the other being IL-1, and the antiproliferative effect of IL-1 appeared to be a direct one. The differentiation-inducing factor for M1 cells in LPS-stimulated peritoneal macrophage conditioned medium was identified as TNF, synergistically active with IL-1 [352]. Interleukin 1 induction of another cytokine, MG1-2 or IL-6, has also been implicated in IL-1 induction of M1 differentiation. Lotem and Sachs [199, 200], in contrast to the results of Onozaki et al. [283], showed that IL-1 on its own induced M1 differentiation as measured by FcR and C3R induction, lysozyme secretion, and morphology. *In vitro*, and *in vivo* in diffusion chambers implanted in mice, IL-1 induced granulocytic differentiation of M1 cells. IL-1 also acted synergistically with GM-CSF to induce differentiation of a GM-CSF-responsive, IL-1-unresponsive clone of leukemic cells. The *in vivo* action of IL-1 was associated with rapid induction of elevated serum levels of MGI-

2/IL-6, but serum levels were not sufficiently elevated to account for the differentiation observed within the diffusion chamber. A more likely mechanism implicates IL-1 induction of autocrine production of IL-6 by leukemic cells, and this was observed within 6 h in IL-1-treated M1 cells, with production increasing by 2-3 days [199, 200]. The indirect differentiation induction mechanism was blocked using antibodies to IL-6. As with the autocrine IFNβ route for differentiation, the endogenous IL-6 may require a synergistic interaction with IL-1 to produce optimal differentiation. These results point to the importance of considering combinations of cytokines, both exogenous and endogenous, in designing optimal differentiation strategies.

The ability of IL-1 to induce certain leukemic cells to differentiate in association with growth inhibition involves synergistic interactions with other cytokines, some of which are produced by leukemic cells in response to IL-1. In normal hematopoiesis, IL-1 also induces a spectrum of hematopoietic growth factors (G-CSF, GM-CSF, M-CSF) by an action on endothelial cells, fibroblasts, and macrophages and acts synergistically with these and other (e.g., IL-3) hematopoietic growth factors to stimulate proliferation of early hematopoietic stem cells [59, 73, 244, 248]. *In vivo* IL-1 alone or in combination with G-CSF was particularly effective in accelerating myeloid regeneration following high-dose chemotherapy or radiation [240, 241, 244].

Interleukin 6 and leukemic cell proliferation and differentiation

Interleukin 6 promotes the terminal maturation of B cells to antibody-producing cells, augmenting IgM, IgG, and IgA production in stimulated B cells [171]. It was originally identified as novel fibroblast-type interferon (IFNβ2) and was found to be identical to a B-cell differentiation factor, BSF2 [142], a hybridoma/plasmacytoma growth factor [371], and a macrophage-granulocyte inducer of leukemic cell differentiation (MGI-2) [335]. Its action on normal hematopoiesis includes stimulation of multilineage blast cell colonies in synergy with IL-6 [156]. It may act to induce the entry of Go stem cells into cell cycle [184]. Interleukin 6 potentiates thrombocytosis [139, 158]. Chronic stimulation of B cells was achieved in transgenic mice carrying the human IL-6 gene conjugated with the Ig enhancer [171]. These mice developed polyclonal nontransplantable plasmocytomas. Freshly isolated human myeloma cells also produce and respond to IL-6, indicating an autocrine role of this molecule in the proliferation, but not differentiation, of certain malignant B cells [12, 407]. Dependence of myelomas on IL-6 may also involve a paracrine mechanism involving marrow stromal cell production of IL-6 in response to myeloma cells [174]. This could involve malignant B-cell production of IL-1, which is a potent inducer of IL-6 gene transcription and translation [242]. In contrast to its action on normal B cells, IL-6 does not augment Ig secretion in myeloma cells [353]. The IL-6-induced proliferation and autocrine IL-6 action have also been reported for certain human B-cell lymphomas, and elevated serum levels of IL-6 were found in 50% of patients with active lymphoma [395].

Interleukin 6 was found to be identical to a macrophage-granulocyte inducer (MGI-2A) that caused differentiation of myeloid leukemic cells but lacked the ability to stimulate colony formation [202, 335]. It was also identical to a differentiation factor (DIF or D Factor) produced by Krebs ascites tumor cells, although it should be noted that this source contains a second D-factor, which is leukemia inhibitory factor (LIF, see following section). IL-6 produces complete growth arrest of the murine myeloid leukemia M1 within 48 h, and this is associated with morphologic maturation of the blast cells to macrophages with upregulation of cfms, FcR, C3R, lysozyme secretion, and development of phagocytic capacity [221, 232, 233]. In clonogenic assay of M1 cells diffuse differentiated colonies develop within 48 h of addition of IL-6 and the number of colonies is reduced [221]. The murine myelomonocytic leukemic WEHI-3 (D^+ variant but not D^-) was also induced by IL-6 to macrophage differentiation with up-regulation of FcR and cfms [47, 220]. Interleukin 6 did not reduce the W3 leukemic clonogenic capacity.

Synergistic or additive interactions between IL-6 and other cytokines influence both proliferation and differentiation. The IL-6 and LIF or G-CSF have additive or supraadditive effects on M1 differentiation [220, 221, 232, 233]. The IL-1 and IL-6 were additive or synergistic in growth inhibition of U937, HL-60, and M1 [282, 299]. Interleukin 1 alone induced lysozyme production by M1 cells but had no direct effect on the expression of FcR or on morphology. Interleukin 6 independently induced FcR and lysozyme, but the combination triggered the entire sequence of differentiation markers [299]. The M-CSF also synergized with IL-6 to enhance differentiation of M1 cells but it counteracted the growth inhibition, resulting in increased size and number of macrophage colonies [220, 221]. The possibility existed that these interacting cytokines were in fact members of a cascade involving autocrine production of factors by leukemic cells. Interleukin 6, IL-1, LIF, and G-CSF are all differentiation-inducing factors, they are all endotoxin-inducible macrophage products, and they can be produced by myelomonocytic leukemic cells. The M1 cells produce IL-6, and levels are increased following LIF treatment [220, 221]; however, antibody to IL-6 does not block LIF induction of M1 cells. In U937 cells, IL-6 did not induce IL-1, nor did IL-1 induce IL-6, and both factors appear to provide distinct signals for differentiation of this neoplastic macrophage cell line [282].

The action of IL-6 on human acute myeloid leukemic blast cells is observed only when it is combined with GM-CSF or IL-3. A heterogeneous response is seen involving synergistic blast cell proliferation [117, 145, 146]. Like IL-1, IL-6 is secreted by most leukemic cells where there is evidence of monocytic differentiation (12/15 patients with ANLL: of FAB type M4 or M5) [370]. The significance of this potential autocrine look is uncertain.

Leukemia inhibitory factor

A spectrum of factors have been described that induce differentiation of the murine M1 myeloblastic leukemic line. This includes G-CSF, IL-1, IL-6, and TNF as well as a unique factor termed leukemia inhibitory factor (LIF) on the basis of its potent and selective inhibition of M1 cell proliferation in association with induction of macrophage differentiation [106]. This factor had earlier been characterized in the conditioned media of L929 cells and termed D-factor, inducing morphological maturation in M1 cells with the development of locomotor activity, phagocytic capacity, and upregulation of FcR, C3R, and prostaglandin E [362]. The factor was purified from Krebs II ascites conditioned medium as a 58-kDa glycoprotein [106] and from mouse Ehrlich ascites cells as a 40-kDa activity [205]. The native molecule of 179 amino acids [106] or 180 amino acids [205] has a molecular weight of 20 kDa with seven N-linked glycosylation sites. The human gene is located on human chromosome 22q11-q 12.2 [347]. The murine and human molecules are active across species and are 78% homologous at the amino acid level [114].

LIF was found to be identical to a variety of other cytokines that had been reported to possess diverse functions. Alloreactive human T cell clones obtained from rejected kidney, when stimulated with a specific antigen and IL-2, produced a factor that triggered the proliferation of a subline of the IL-3-sensitive murine factor-dependent cell line DA-1 [251, 252]. This factor, called HILDA (human interleukin DA), was a 38- to 41-kDa glycoprotein that was also reported to have eosinophil chemotactic and activating properties and erythroid burst-promoting activity [109]. In retrospect these latter activities were probably due to a minor contamination of the protein with GM-CSF and/or other lymphokines.

HILDA cDNA cloned from human lectin-stimulated T cells was shown to be identical to LIF [252]. A human macrophage differentiation-inducing factor (DIF) for M1 cells isolated from a human monocytic leukemia line, THP-1, was also shown by amino acid sequencing to be identical to LIF [3]. The growth of totipotential embryonic stem cells *in vitro* is sustained by a differentiation inhibitory activity (DIA) produced by a number of sources, including the 5637 human bladder carcinoma cell line. Purified DIA and LIF were very similar in biochemical features, and purified recombinant LIF can substitute for DIA in the maintenance of totipotent embryonic stem cells that retain the potential to form chimeric mice [386]. A factor constitutively produced by human squamous carcinoma cells stimulated hepatocytes to produce the same spectrum of acute phase proteins as IL-6 [22]. This hepatocyte stimulating factor III was distinct from IL-6 but was identical to LIF. Rat heart tissue produces a cholinergic differentiation factor that controls the phenotypic choice in neurons without affecting their survival or growth [392]. This factor was also identical to LIF and acted on postmitotic rat sympathetic neurons to specifically induce expression of acetylcholine synthesis and cholinergic function and suppress adrenergic function.

Receptor analysis with ^{125}LIF indicated that M1 cells possess a single class of high-affinity (K_d 100-200 p*M*) receptors of relatively low frequency (300-500 per cell) [140]. In bone marrow, spleen, and peritoneum, monocytes, macrophages, and their precursors were the most obvious cells binding LIF.

The *in vivo* action of LIF was revealed by studies in which mice were engrafted with cells of the murine hematopoietic cell line FDC-P1 multiply infected with a retroviral construct containing cDNA encoding LIF [222, 223]. The mice developed within 12-70 days a fatal syndrome characterized by cachexia, excess osteoblasts with new bone formation, calcification in heart and skeletal muscle, pancreatitis, thymus atrophy, and abnormalities in the adrenal cortex and ovarian corpora lutea. The development of this osteosclerotic syndrome, with marked increases in osteoblasts, indicates a role for LIF in osteoblast production and function and in regulation of bone formation and calcium metabolism. The presence of LIF receptors on osteoblasts further indicates the direct nature of the stimulation [222, 223].

The action of LIF on leukemic cells appears to be highly restricted, inducing M1 cell differentiation alone, or synergistically with G-CSF, IL-6, or M-CSF [224]. The growth inhibition and differentiation effect was rapid, being evident at 24 h and marked at 48 h. LIF was without effect on normal CFU-GM or WEHI-3 B myelomonocytic leukemic cells. Abe et al. [3] reported a direct differentiation-inducing, and proliferation-inhibiting, action on HL-60 and U937 cells. Maekawa and Metcalf [208] did not observe a direct action of LIF on HL-60 or U937 cells but reported clonal suppression of these leukemic cells by LIF in combination with GM-CSF or C-CSF. Sequential recloning of these cells was also suppressed by LIF-CSF combinations.

Despite the relatively weak action of LIF on human leukemic cells, LIF clearly is able to exhibit suppressive actions. This, coupled with its lack of suppressive effects on normal hematopoietic cells, suggests a role in suppressing human leukemias, possibly in combination with other hematopoietic factors.

Tumor necrosis factor (TNFα) and lymphotoxin (TNFβ)

Tumor necrosis factor was identified as a protein with antitumor activity in serum of mice infected with *Bacillus Calmette-Guerin* and treated with endotoxin [315]. TNFα has significant sequence homology to human lymphotoxin E and binds to the same receptor. The biological actions of TNF are multifaceted, involving both stimulatory and inhibitory actions depending upon the target cell population.

In normal human hematopoiesis TNFα was reported to inhibit CFU-GM day 7 (ED_{50} = 10 U) and CFU-GM on day 14, BFU-E, CFU-E, and CFU-GEMM (ED_{50} = 50 U) [36, 207, 291]. Even greater inhibition of BFU-E, CFU-GEMM and CFU-E was reported with both TNF alpha or β in other studies [258]. TNF inhibition was enhanced in a synergistic manner by interferon γ [36, 258, 291, 292]. TNF inhibition was reported to be nonreversible within 60 min, suggesting a cytotoxic mechanism [36], but others have reported either full reversibility following a 24 h preincubation [258] or partial reversibility [260]. The variable results can be attributed to the use of different sources of CSF and the variable presence of accessory cells in the preparation. With G-CSF as a stimulus, the (ED_{50} with TNFα or -β was 10 U whereas with a GM-CSF stimulus only a 20% inhibition was seen with 1000 U TNF [19]. Thus in normal marrow one cell in 500 will form a colony with G-CSF or GM-CSF, but with TNF only one cell in 100, 000 will respond to G-CSF, yet the frequency of cells responding to GM-CSF remains essentially unchanged [20, 181]. With highly purified marrow progenitors, the (ED_{50} for TNF was 5 U with G-CSF-stimulated colonies, and 500 U with GM-CSF stimulation [250]. Using CD34-positive selection for CFU-GM, G-CSF-stimulated colonies were strongly inhibited by TNF, but an actual enhancement of GM-CSF or IL-3-stimulated colonies was recently reported [325]. In murine serum-free bone marrow cultures the (ED_{50} for CFU-GM was 20-200 U or murine TNF and for BFU-E and CFU-GEMM it was 2000 U [79]. Using human TNF, a lower degree of inhibition is generally found. In most studies, human TNF does not inhibit at doses below 10, 000 U/ml, and indeed some slight potentiation of M-CSF stimulated colonies was reported [387].

In long-term murine or human bone marrow culture, TNF exhibits a dose-dependent (10-1000 U/ml) inhibition of CFU-GM production and neutrophil generation [79, 250]. The inhibition induced by TNF appears to be selective for neutrophil differentiation and is not manifest in reduction of eosinophils or monocyte/macrophages.

The interaction of TNF with leukemic cells is a complex one, variously resulting in differentiation, and growth inhibition or growth potentiation. A differentiating factor for HL-60 and ML-1 leukemic cells, produced by PHA-stimulated lymphocytes or the HUT 102 T cell line was shown to be TNF [350]. As little as 1, 10 U of TNF alone or in synergy with IFNγ promoted monocytic differentiation of HL-60, U937 and ML-1 [121, 181, 291, 327].

The action of TNF on fresh AML marrow cells has been investigated in clonogenic (PE_1) and recloning (PE_2) assays, and suspension culture. Early reports uniformly reported inhibition. In one study of 10 patients 50% inhibition was seen with 15 pM TNF and there was synergy with IFNγ [291]. Inhibition to a degree comparable to normal was reported in seven patients [36], and in 9/10 patients 75% inhibition of leukemic cell cloning was seen with 100 U TNF compared to 44-48% inhibition in remission marrow. Enhanced differentiation to monocyte macrophages with enhanced NBT-reducing activity was seen with TNF or TNF plus IFNγ in suspension cultures of marrow from 1 AML and 5 CML in blastic crisis [107]. Differentiated macrophages were observed with Auer rods, indicating their leukemic origin.

In other, more recent studies, a more complex picture emerges. Clonogenic assays stimulated with G-CSF or GM-CSF and exposed to high (1000 U) or low (100 U) doses of TNFβ showed four types of response in AML and preleukemic myelodysplastic syndrome: inhibition greater than normal or remission inhibition equivalent to normal, no response, and significant enhancement. This latter pattern, seen in 4/13 cases, involved a synergism with either G-CSF or GM-CSF and clonogeneic capacity increased up to 60-fold. Assessment of plating efficiency (PE_1, PE_2) using 5637 CM as a source of stimulus revealed three patterns of response with TNF [260]; (a) PE_1, PE_2, and suspension cell were inhibited 90-100% with 100-1000 U TNF; (b) PE_1 and PE_2 were not inhibited and possibly potentiated at low doses of TNF but suspension cells were markedly inhibited; and (c) marked inhibition of PE_1 and PE_2 but not of suspension cells. In no case was there evidence of TNF induction of differentiation. The nature of the stimulus may determine whether the TNF response is inhibitory or stimulatory. Proliferation of AML blast cells (10 patients), induced by G-CSF, was further stimulated by TNF, and clonogenic assays were potentiated 50-250% of maximum [147]. In contrast, IL-3- or G-CSF-stimulated cultures were inhibited 100% and 5637 CM-stimulated cultures by 30% with 600 p*M* of TNF.

Autocrine stimulation of AML cell proliferation seen at high cell densities was also enhanced by TNF, suggesting synergism with leukemia cell-derived GM-CSF. The mechanism of TNF potentiation is probably indirect and was inhibited by antibodies to I-1. Furthermore, IL-1 synergises with GM-CSF in stimulating leukemic blast cells [146], and TNF synergism was not seen in cultures in the presence of exogenous IL-1. IL-1 and TNF have been shown to be constitutive products of AML cells and production of bioactive IL-1 can be increased by TNF treatment [117, 147, 377]. The proliferative response of leukemic blast progenitors to TNF under conditions that favor autocrine stimulation may represent one property that allows leukemic cells to escape from negative regulation.

In the chronic phase of CML, TNF substantially inhibits DNA synthesis in cultures of purified progenitors and inhibits day 7 and day 14 CFU-GM at doses of 10-500 U [76, 181]. Some patient-to-patient variation is seen with inhibition in the normal to less-than-normal range. Antibodies to TNFα blocked the TNF inhibition and enhanced GM-CSF-stimulated colony formation twofold in cultures of accessory cell depleted progenitors [76]. Autocrine production of TNF by immature CML cells was confirmed by Northern analysis and ELISA assays. The quantities of TNF produced by leukemic cells were sufficient to inhibit normal hematopoiesis and may provide a selective advantage for leukemic clones if CML progenitors are less sensitive to TNF inhibition than normal. In this context TNF production by hairy-cell leukemic cells has been identified as the possible cause of myelosuppression and neutropenia seen in this cancer [195].

Transforming growth factor β

Transforming growth factor β (TGFβ) is a member of a group of polypeptide growth factors that regulate cell growth and differentiation. TGFβ exists as a 25-dK disulfide-linked dimer, and subtypes include TGFβ1, TGFβ2, TGFβ1, 2, existing in homodimer and heterodimer forms, and TGFβ3. The factor is produced by most normal cells and its pleiotropic actions include growth stimulation of fibroblasts and growth inhibition of epithelial cells, endothelial cells, and various malignant cells. It also affects differentiation of cells as varied as adipocytes, myoblasts, chondrocytes, and epithelium and is involved in production of extracellular matrix, bone remodeling, and repair. TGFβ acts as a modifier of the immune response and may play an important role in hematopoiesis. It is a potent monocyte chemoattractant and induces these cells to produce IL-1 and TNF [373].

In vitro, TGFβ1 and β2 (2-4 p*M*) inhibit megakaryocytopoiesis and CFU-MK [37, 157]. In both murine and human systems, pluripotential progenitors (high proliferative potential CFU, CFU-GEMM) and BFU-E are strongly inhibited [7, 123, 170, 286, 321, 339]. Erythropoietin-stimulated CFU-E are not inhibited [169, 170, 321]. The action of TGFβ on *in vitro* myelopoiesis is determined by the stage of differentiation of the progenitor the type of CSF used, and the species. In the murine and human systems, G-CSF and M-CSF stimulated colonies are not inhibited [123, 169, 170, 339]. The GM-CSF-stimulated murine colonies are variously reported to be resistant to TGFβ [169, 170] or inhibited, but to a lesser extent than earlier progenitors, at doses of 0.2-0.5 ng/ml [70, 123, 141, 274, 321]. Human day 7 CFU-GM (predominantly G-CSF responsive granulocyte-committed progenitors) were enhanced 150-175% by TGFβ1 or -β2 even in the presence of plateau concentrations of G-CSF, GM-CSF, or IL-3 [51, 286]. Day 14 CFU-GM were variously reported to be unaffected by TGFβ [7, 141], or inhibited to a lesser degree than earlier progenitors [170, 339]. Synergistic or additive interactions occur between TGFβ and other cytokines. BFU-E were synergistically inhibited by TGFβ plus TNFα, and these cytokines additively inhibited CFU-GEMM and CFU-GM [340]. Interferon gamma and TGFβ synergistically inhibited CFU-GM and additively inhibited BFU-E and CFU-GEMM.

In long-term bone marrow culture, TGFβ serves as a potent inhibitor of myelopoiesis, probably by inhibiting proliferation of early stem cells in the adherent stromal layer [43, 134]. Indeed, TGFβ production by marrow stromal cells may be an important negative regulator of steady-state hematopoiesis. Further evidence for a physiological role for TGFβ as negative regulator was provided in studies in which TGFβ1 (1-5 μg/mouse) was injected via the femoral artery into normal mice {110, 111]. The CFU-GEMM stimulated by IL-3 were completely inhibited in the femur, and CFU-GM were inhibited 50% by 24 h with reversal of inhibition at later times. This observation suggests that TGFβ, by reversibly inhibiting the cycling of early stem cells, may be effective in protecting such cells from damage inflicted by cell cycle-specific chemotherapy.

The action of TGFβ on myeloid leukemic cells generally involves potent growth inhibition; however, an influence on differentiation is seen in some systems. TGFβ alone induced monocyte-macrophage differentiation of the U937 and THP-1 cell lines but was only a weak inducer of HL-60 [165]. Synergism between TGFβ and TNFα, IFNγ, dexamethasone and phorbol esters is seen in differentiation induction of U937, THP-1, and ML-1 in human monocytic or myeloblastic leukemias [119, 165]. Low doses (0.5 ng) of TGFβ induced hemoglobinization of K562 with growth inhibition [48]. Inhibition of proliferation of M1 murine myeloid leukemic cells is produced by low doses of TGFβ with enhanced adherence, but differentiation-associated properties such as phagocytic activity, lysozyme secretion, and morphologic change were not induced [275]. Indeed, TGFβ inhibited the dexamethasone-induced differentiation of this cell line. Potent inhibition of proliferation was seen when TGFβ was added to a variety of factor-dependent cell lines (NFS-60, 32D, FDCP-1, B6 $S4_t$ A, DA-3) and to the IL-3-producing WEHI-3 myelomonocytic leukemic cell line [169]. Inhibition was also seen with the human leukemic cell lines U937, THP-1, and KG-1 but not with various other lines (e.g., HL-60, various T and B leukemias and lymphomas) [170]. The response of the cell lines to TGFβ appeared to correlate with the extent of display of TGFβ receptors.

In primary cultures of bone marrow from 15 patients with chronic myeloid leukemia, all showed TGFβ inhibition of D14 CFU=GM but only 4/15 showed the stimulation of D7 CFU-GM, which is the response seen with normal marrow, and in 11/15 TGFβ inhibited D7 CFU-GM [7]. Both TGFβ1 and -β2 inhibited 45% of CFU-GM stimulated by GM-CSF in marrow cultures from five CML patients but, in contrast to normal, G-CSF-stimulated colonies were also inhibited [339]. In studies of acute myeloid leukemia (18 patients), TGFβ suppressed both primary and secondary leukemic clonogenic capacity [265, 356]. These results showed that 1-10 ng/ml of TGFβ delayed progression of leukemic blast-cell progenitors from G1 to S phase in a cytostatic manner with no induction of differentiation.

It is now apparent that a large number of factors responsible for growth and differentiation have been identified. In addition, their receptors on normal and neoplastic cells are also being identified and investigated. It is clear that some of these factors are produced by tumor cells and represent autocrine growth factors. Obviously, the blockage of these growth factors by reducing their production or by blocking their attachment to receptors could be an effective strategy for cancer treatment. Likewise, the production of stimulatory factors for angiogenesis by tumor cells has now been well characterized and the blockage of their paracrine effect on adjacent blood vessels in normal tissue is another potential method of therapy. Some tumors produce a considerable quantity of growth factor proteins and peptides and others produced smaller amounts or a wider diversity of these factors. In some, factors which promote the growth of tumor cells clearly play a role in cancer growth and metastasis and the autonomy that cancer seems to enjoy. An interruption of this process will clearly lead to further approaches in cancer treatment.

A good example of the clinical significance of growth factors has been demonstrated in studies showing that approximately 50% of tumor tissue from breast cancer patients expresses epidermal growth factor receptor. These receptors appear to be inversely related to steroid receptors and therefore bring a poor prognosis to patients who are steroid-receptor negative and epidermal growth factor receptor positive. Since thousands of tumors have been studied with regard to this particular characteristic, it is abundantly clear that epidermal growth factor receptor should be explored as a target for cancer treatment. Monoclonal antibodies have been produced by various investigators which are being administered to patients with breast cancer in an attempt to block the epidermal growth factor receptor. Many of these studies are being done in association with chemotherapy to try to get an effective one-two punch in inhibiting tumor growth.

Oncogenes such as erb and v-cis are known to encode for growth factor receptors. Soluble receptors with high affinity binding might be useful in therapy to bind with growth factors and reduce their activities on membrane-bound receptors present in the tumor cell or adjacent blood vessel. Factors which are structurally similar to growth factors but are inactive in inducing receptor function (blockers) are also being explored as treatment strategies. Growth factor interaction can also be blocked by certain drugs such as Suramin. Suramin and its analogues are currently in clinical trials for these effects. Anti-angiogenesis factors have also been identified and these are also in clinical trials. In summary, the application of techniques to block growth factors and/or the transduction of biochemical effects from growth factor receptor stimulation represent advent technologies for the millennium. As more is known about autocrine and paracrine effects of growth factors, more can be done with respect to altering their effects on tumor cells and adjacent tissues. This approach, when employed in concert with the use of differentiation agents, may allow for the regulation and control of tumor growth in a manner very different than chemotherapy and radiation therapy. Perhaps one can regulate cancer in a manner similar to the use of insulin to regulate diabetes rather than attempting to destroy every last cancer cell with all the toxicity inherent in these historical approaches. For extensive reviews on the subject of growth factors and growth factor receptors, here are multiple recent reviews [175, 302, 304, 374, 409].

ACKNOWLEDGMENT

Dr. Malcolm A.S. Moore (Memorial Sloan-Kettering Cancer Center, New York, New York) contributed much of this chapter in the 2nd edition, but was unable to undertake the 3rd edition revisions.

REFERENCES

1. Abe E, Miyaura C, Sakagami H, et al. Differentiation of mouse myeloid leukemia cells induced by 1alpha, 25-dihydroxy-vitamin D_3. *Proc Natl Acad Sci USA* 1981; 78: 4990.
2. Abe E, Miyaura C, Tanaka H, et al. 1α25-Dihydroxy-vitamin D_3 promotes fusion of mouse alveolar macrophages both by a direct mechanism and by a spleen cell-mediated indirect mechanism. *Proc Natl Acad SCI USA* 1983; 80: 5583.
3. Abe T, Murakami M, Sato T, et al. Macrophage differentiation inducing factor from human monocytic cells is equivalent to murine leukemia inhibitory factor. *J Biol Chem* 1989; 264: 8941.
4. Abita J, Gauville C, Saal F. Characterization of insulin receptors in human promyelocytic leukemia cell HL-60. *Biochem Biophys Res Commun* 1982; 106: 574.
5. Abita JP, Gauville C, Baltrand N. Loss of insulin receptor during differentiation of U937 cells. *IRCS Med Sci* 1983; 11: 390.
6. Aggarwal PP, Kohr WJ, Hass PE, et al. Human tumor necrosis factor: Production, purification and characterization. *J Biol Chem* 1985; 260: 2345.
7. Aglietta M, Stacchini A, Severino A, et al. Interaction of transforming growth factor-beta 1 with hemopoietic growth factors in the regulation of human normal and leukemic myelopoiesis. *Exp Hematol* 1989; 17: 296.
8. Amento EP, Kurnick JT, Epstein A, et al. Modulation of synovial cell products by a factor from a human cell line: T lymphocyte induction of a mononuclear cell factor. *Proc Natl Acad Sci USA* 1982; 79: 5307.
9. Andreeff M, Kreis W, Miller W, et al. Low-dose cytosine-arabinoside (ARA-C) in acute non-lymphocytic leukemia (ANLL) and myelodysplastic syndromes (MDS): analysis of response and response mechanisms. *Proc Annu Meet Am Soc Clin Oncol* 1988; 7: A741.
10. Andreeff M, Stone R, Young C, et al. Treatment of myelodysplastic syndromes and acute myeloid leukemia with hexamethylene bisacetamide. *Blood* 1990. 76(Suppl.): 251a.
11. Arlin ZA, Mertelsman R, Berman E, et al. 13-*cis*-Retinoic acid does not increase the true remission (induced by cytotoxic chemotherapy) in patients with chronic phase chronic myelogenous leukemia. *J Clin Oncol* 1985; 3: 473.
12. Asaoku H, Kawano M, Kwato K, et al. Decrease in BSF-

2/IL-6 response in advanced cases of multiple myeloma. *Blood* 1988; 72: 429.

13. Ascencao J, Kay NE, Earenfight-Engler T, et al. Production of erythroid potentiating factor(s) by a human monocytic cell line. *Blood* 1981; 57: 170.
14. Auron PE, Webb AC, Rosenwasser LJ, et al. Nucleotide sequence of human monocyte interleukin-1 precursor cDNA. *Proc Natl Acad Sci USA* 1984; 81: 7907-7911.
15. Baccarani M, Zaccaria A, Bandini G, et al. Low dose arbinosyl cytosine for treatment of myelodysplastic syndromes and subacute myeloid leukemia. *Leuk Res* 1983; 7: 539.
16. Baccarin M, Tura S. Differentiation of myeloid leukaemic cells: new possibilities for therapy. *Br J Haematol* 1979; 42: 485.
17. Bagby GC, Dinarello CA, Neerhout RC, et al. Interleukin 1-dependent paracrine granulopoiesis in chronic granulocytic leukemia of the juvenile type. *J Clin Invest* 1988; 82: 1430.
18. Balaban EP, Cox JV, Schneider NR, et al. Treatment of 'poor risk' acute non-lymphocytic leukemia with continuously infused low-dose cytosine arabinoside. *Am J Hematol* 1988; 29: 79.
19. Barbar KE, Crosier PS, Gillis S, et al. Human granulocyte-macrophage progenitors and their sensitivity to cytotoxins: analysis by limiting dilution. *Blood* 1987; 70: 1773.
20. Barbar KE, Crosier PS, Watson JD. The differential inhibition of hemopoietic growth factor activity by cytotoxins and interferon-γ. *J Immunol* 1987; 139: 1108.
21. Bar-Shavit Z, Teitelbaum SL, Reitsma P, et al. Induction of monocyte differentiation and bone resorption by 1,25-dihydroxy-vitamin D3. *Proc Natl Acad Sci USA* 1983; 80: 5907.
22. Baumann H, Wong GG. Hepatocyte-stimulating factor III shares structural and functional identity with leukemia-inhibitory factor. *J Immunol* 1989; 143: 1163.
23. Beckman BS, Balin AK, Allen RG. Superoxide dismutase induces differentiation of Friend erythroleukemia cells. *J Cell Physiol* 1989; 139: 370.
24. Begley C, Metcalf D, Nicola N. Purified colony stimulating factors (G-CSF and GM-CSF) induce differentiation in human HL-60 leukemic cells with suppression of clonogenicity. *Int J Cancer* 1987; 39: 99.
25. Ben-Bassat I, Gale RP. New and evolving concepts in leukemia. *Leukemia* 1988; 2: 704.
26. Bernal S, Chen L. Induction of cytoskeleton-associated proteins during differentiation of human myeloid leukemic cell lines. *Cancer Res* 1982; 421: 5106.
27. Besa EC, Abraham JL, Nowell PC. Combinations of 13-cis-retinoic acid (RA) and alpha-tocopherol (AT) for the chronic phase and addition of alpha-interferon (IFN) for the transformed phase of myelodysplasia. *Third Int Conf Prev Hum Cancer* 1988: S4-13.
28. Blazsek I, Labat ML, Boule D, et al. Endocrine switch in myeloid neoplasia? *Proc Annu Meet Am Assoc Cancer Res* 1989; 30: A928.
29. Bleiberg I, Fabian I, Kantor S, et al. The effect of 13-*cis*-retinoic acid on hematopoiesis in human long-term bone marrow culture. *Leuk Res* 1988; 12: 545.
30. Bloch A, Koeffler HP, Pierce GB, et al. Meeting Report: Ninth Annual Sapporo Cancer Seminar on Cell Differentiation and Cancer Control. *Cancer Res* 1990; 50: 1346.
31. Bodner AJ, Ting RC, Gallo RC. Induction of differentiation of human promyelocytic leukemia cells (HL-60) by nucleosides and methotrexate. *J Natl Cancer Inst* 1981; 67: 1025.
32. Bougnoux P, Bovini E, Chang Z, et al. Effect of interferon on phospholipid methylation by peripheral blood mononuclear cells. *J Cell Biochem* 1983; 20: 215.
33. Bradbury D, Bowen G, Kozlowski R, et al. Endogenous interleukin-1 can regulate the autonomous growth of the blast cells of acute myeloblastic leukemia by inducing autocrine secretion of GM-CSF. *Leukemia* 1990; 4: 44.
34. Breitman T, Collins S, Keene B. Terminal differentiation of human promyelocytic leukemia cells in primary culture in response to retinoic acid. *Blood* 1981; 57: 1000.
35. Broxmeyer H, Gentile G, Bognacki J, et al. Lactoferrin, transferrin and acidic isoferritins: regulatory molecules with potential therapeutic value in leukemia. *Blood Cells* 1983; 9: 83.
36. Broxmeyer HE, Williams DE, Lu L, et al. The suppressive influence of human tumor necrosis factors on bone marrow hematopoietic progenitor cells from normal donors and patients with leukemia: synergism of tumor necrosis factor and interferon-γ. *J Immunol* 1986; 136: 4487.
37. Bruno E, Hoffman R. Interacting cytokines regulate human megakaryocytopoiesis. *Exp Hematol* 1988; 16: 505.
38. Buick RN, Till JE, McCulloch EA. Colony assay for proliferative blast cells circulating in myeloblastic leukemia. *Lancet* 1977; 1: 862.
39. Buick RN, Chang LJ-A, Curtis JE, et al. Self-renewal capacity of leukemic blast progenitor cells. *Cancer Res* 1981; 4: 4849.
40. Burger EH, Van Der Meer JWM, Van De Geuell JS, et al. *In vitro* formation of osteoclasts from long-term cultures of bone marrow mononuclear phagocytes. *J Exp Med* 1982; 156: 1604.
41. Burgess A, Camakaris J, Metcalf D. Purification and properties of colony stimulating factor from mouse lung-conditioned medium. *J Biol Chem* 1977; 252: 1998.
42. Burgess A, Metcalf D. The nature and action of granulocyte-macrophage colony stimulating factors. *Blood* 1980; 56: 947.
43. Cashman JD, Eaves AC, Raines EW, et al. Mechanisms that regulate the cell cycle status of very primitive hematopoietic cells in long-term marrow cultures. I. *Stimulatory role of a variety of mesenchymal cell activators and inhibitory role of TGF-β.* 1990; 75: 96.
44. Castaigne S, Daniel MT, Tilly H, et al. Does treatment with Ara-C in low dosage cause differentiation of leukemic cells? *Blood* 1983; 62: 85.
45. Castro-Malaspina H, Rabellino EM, Yen A, et al. Human megakaryocyte stimulation of proliferation of bone marrow fibroblasts. *Blood* 1981; 57: 781.
46. Chan CSP, Schechter GP. *In vitro* evidence for dose-dependent cytotoxicity as the predominant effect of low dose Ara-C on human leukemic and normal marrow cells. *Cancer Chemother Pharmacol* 1988; 23: 87.
47. Chen CP, Lee F. IL-6 is a differentiation factor for M1 and WEHI-3B myeloid leukemic cells. *J Immunol* 1989; 142: 1909.
48. Chen LL, Dean A, Jenkinson T, et al. Effect of transforming growth factor-β1 on proliferation and induction of hemoglobin accumulation in K-562 cells. *Blood* 1989; 74: 2368.
49. Chen ZX, Xue YQ, Zhang RI, et al. A clinical and experi-

mental study on all-*trans* retinoic acid-treated acute promyelocytic leukemia patients. *Blood* 1991; 78: 1413-1419.

50. Cheng GYM, Kelleher CA, Miyauchi J, et al. Structure and expression of genes of GM-CSF and G-CSF in blast cells from patients with acute myeloblastic leukemia. *Blood* 1988; 71: 204.
51. Chenu C, Pfeilschifter J, Mundy GR, et al. Transforming growth factor beta inhibits formation of osteoclast-like cells in long-term human marrow cultures. *Proc Natl Acad Sci USA* 1988; 85: 5683.
52. Christman JK, Mendelsohn N, Herzog D, et al. Effect of 5-azacytidine on differentiation and DNA methylation in human promyelocytic leukemia cells (HL 60). *Cancer Res* 1983; 43: 763.
53. Clark SC, Arya SK, Wong-Staal F, et al. Human T-cell growth factor: Partial amino acid sequence, cDNA cloning, and organization and expression in normal and leukemic cells. *Proc Natl Acad Sci USA* 1984; 81: 2543.
54. Cobb MA, Hseuh W, Pachman L, et al. Prostaglandin biosynthesis by a human macrophage-like cell line, U937. *J Reticuloendothel Soc* 1983; 33: 197.
55. Colbert D, Fontana J, Bode U, et al. Changes in the translational activity of polyadenylated messenger RNA of HL-60 promyelocytic leukemia cells associated with myeloid or macrophage differentiation. *Cancer Res* 1983; 43: 229.
56. Collins SJ, Ruscetti FW, Gallagher RE, et al. normal functional characteristics of cultured human promyelocytic leukemia cells (HL-60) after induction of differentiation by DMSO. *J Exp Med* 1979; 149: 969.
57. Collins S, Bodner A, et al. Induction of morphological and functional differentiation of human promyelocytic leukemia cells (HL-60) by compounds which induce differentiation of murine leukemia cells. *Int J Cancer* 1980; 25: 213.
58. Conley BA, Forrest A, Egorin MJ, et al. Phase I trial using adaptive control dosing of hexamethylene bisacetamide (NSC 95580). *Cancer Res* 1989; 49: 3436.
59. Cooper PC, Metcalf D, Burgess AW. Biochemical and functional characterization of mature progeny purified from a myelomonocytic leukemia. Leuk Res 1982; 6: 313.
60. Cooperberg AA, Singer OP. Reversible myelofibrosis due to vitamin D deficiency rickets *Can Med Assoc J* 1980; 94: 392.
61. Cozzolino F, Rubartelli A, Aldinucci D, et al. Interleukin 1 as an autocrine growth factor for acute myeloid leukemia cells. *Proc Natl Acad Sci USA* 1989; 86: 2369.
62. Curtis JE, Messner HA, Minden MD, et al. Improved maintenance therapy for acute myelogenous leukemia (AML) using 13-*cis*-retinoic acid-containing regimen. *Proc Annu Meet Am Assoc Cancer Res* 1989; 30: A1066.
63. Dayton ET, Perussia G, Trinchiere G. Correlation between differentiation, expression of monocyte-specific antigens, and cytotoxic functions in human promyelocytic cell lines treated with leukocyte conditioned media. *J Immunol* 1983; 3: 1120.
64. Das S, Stanley E. Structure-function studies of a colony stimulating factor (CSF-1). *J Biol Chem* 1982; 256: 13679.
65. Degos L, Castaigne S, Chomienne C, et al. Therapeutic trials of acute myeloid leukemia and of myelodysplastic syndromes by LD-ARA C and treatment of promyelocytic leukemia by retinoic acid. In: Waxman S, Ross GB, Takaku F, eds. *The status of differentiation therapy of cancer.* Serono Symposia, Publications from Raven Press, 1988; 45: 361.
66. Delwel R, Salem M, Pellens C, et al. Growth regulation of human acute myeloid leukemia: effects of five recombinant hematopoietic factors in a serum-free culture system. *Blood* 1988; 72: 1944.
67. Derynck R, Jarret JA, Chen EY, et al. Human transforming growth factor-β complementary DNA sequence and expression in normal and transformed cells. *Nature* 1985; 316: 701.
68. DiGiovanna MP, Sartorelli AC. Myeloid differentiation-associated protein tyrosine kinase activity in a murine monomyelocytic leukemia cell line. *Proc Annu Meet Am Assoc Cancer Res* 1989; 30: A212.
69. Dijke PT, Hansen P, Iwata KK, et al. Identification of another member of the transforming growth factor type β gene family. *Proc Natl Acad Sci USA* 1988; 85: 4715.
70. Dooley DC, Law P. Influence of transforming growth factor-beta one and T cells on human hematopoietic progenitor cells. *Exp Hematol* 1988; 16: 438.
71. Douer D, Koeffler HP. Retinoic acid inhibition of the clonal growth of human myeloid leukemia cells. *J Clin Invest* 1982; 69: 277.
72. Douer D, Koeffler HP. Retinoic acid enhances growth of human early erythroid progenitor cells *in vitro*. *J Clin Invest* 1982; 60: 1039.
73. Doyle M, Brindley L, Kawasaki E, et al. High level human interleukin 1 production by a hepatoma cell line. *Biochem Biophys Res Commun* 1985; 130: 768.
74. Duhrsen U. *In vitro* growth patterns and autocrine production of hemopoietic colony stimulating factors: analysis of leukemic populations arising in irradiated mice from cells of an injected factor-dependent continuous cell line. *Leukemia* 1988; 2: 334.
75. Duhrsen U, Metcalf D. A model system for leukemic transformation of immortalized hemopoietic cells in irradiated recipient mice. *Leukemia* 1988; 2: 329.
76. Duncombe AS, Heslop HE, Turner M, et al. Tumor necrosis factor mediates autocrine growth inhibition in a chronic leukemia. *J Immunol* 1989; 143: 3828.
77. Egorin MJ, Sigman LM, Van-Echo DA, et al. Phase I clinical and pharmacokinetic study of hexamethylene bisacetamide (NSC 95580) administered as a five-day continuous infusion. *Cancer Res* 1987; 47: 617.
78. Eisman JA, Martin TJ, MacIntyre I, et al. 1,25-Dihydroxyvitamin D_3 receptor in a cultured human breast cancer cell line (MCF 7 cells). *Biochem Biophys Res Commun* 1980; 93: 9.
79. Eliason JF, Vassalli P. Inhibition of hemopoiesis in murine marrow cell cultures by recombinant murine tumor necrosis factor γ: Evidence for long-term effects on stromal cells. *Blood Cells* 1988; 14: 339.
80. Estey E, Thall PF, Kantarijian H, et al. Treatment of newly diagnosed acute myelogenous leukemia with granulocyte-macrophage colony-stimulating factor (GM-CSF) before and during continuous infusion high-dose ara-C + daunorubicin: comparison to patients treated without GM-CSF. *Blood* 1992; 79: 2246.
81. Fearon ER, Burke PJ, Schiffer CA, et al. Differentiation of leukemic cells to polymorphonuclear leukocytes in patients with acute nonlymphocytic leukemia. *N Engl J Med* 315: 15.
82. Fenaux P, Le Dely MC, Castaigne S, et al. Effect of all-

trans retinoic acid in newly diagnosed acute promyelocytic leukemia: results of a multicenter randomized trial. *Blood* 1993; 82: 3241-3249.

83. Ferrero D, Tarella C, Gallo E, et al. Terminal differentiation of the human promyelocyte leukemia cell line, HL-60, in the absence of cell proliferation. *Cancer Res* 1982; 42: 4421.
84. Fialkow PJ, Singer JW, Adamson JW, et al. Acute nonlymphocytic leukemia: heterogeneity of stem cell origin. *Blood* 1981; 57: 1068.
85. Fibach E, Peled T, Rachmilewitz EA. Self-renewal and commitment to differentiation of human leukemic promyelocytic cells (HL-60). *J Cell Physiol* 1982; 113: 152.
86. Filmus J, Buick RN. Relationship of c-myc expression to differentiation and proliferation of HL-60 cells. *Cancer Res* 1985; 45: 822.
87. Fitchen J, LeFevre C, Ferrone S, et al. Expression of Ia-like and HLA-A, B, antigens on human multipotential hematopoietic progenitor cells. *Blood* 1982; 59: 188.
88. Fontana JA, Wright DG, Schifman E, et al. Development of chemotactic responsiveness in myeloid precursor cells: studies with a human leukemia cell line. *Proc Natl Acad Sci USA* 1980; 77: 3664.
89. Franpton RJ, Suva LJ, Eisman JA, et al. Presence of 1,25-dihydroxyvitamin D3 receptors in established human cancer cell lines in culture. *Cancer Res* 1982; 42: 1116.
90. Franceschi RT. Interaction of the 1-alpha, 25-dihydroxyvitamin D_3 receptor with RNA and synthetic polyribonucleotides. *Proc Natl Acad Sci USA* 1984; 81: 2337.
91. Francis GE, Berney JJ, North PS, et al. Evidence for the involvement of DNA topoisomerase II in neutrophil-granulocyte differentiation. *Leukemia* 1987; 1: 653.
92. Francis GE, Mufti GJ, Knowles SM, et al. Differentiation induction in myelodysplasia and acute myeloid leukemia: use of synergistic drug combinations. *Leuk Res* 1987; 11: 971.
93. Francis GE, Gray DA, Berney JJ, et al. Role of ADP-ribosyl transferase in the differentiation of human granulocyte-macrophage progenitors to the macrophage lineage. *Blood* 1983; 62: 1055.
94. Freake HC, Marcocci C, Iwasaki J, et al. 1,25-Dihydroxyvitamin D_3 specifically binds to a human breast cancer cell line (T47D) and stimulates growth. Biochem *Biophy Res Commun* 1981; 101: 1131.
95. Fung M, Hapel A, Ymer S, et al. Molecular cloning of cDNA for murine interleukin 3. *Nature* 1984; 307: 233.
96. Gabrilove JL, Welte K, Li L, et al. Constitutive production of a leukemia differentiation, colony stimulating, erythroid burst promoting and pluripoietic factor by a human hepatoma cell line: characterization of the leukemia differentiation factor. *Blood* 1985; 66: 407.
97. Gabrilove JL, Welte K, Harris P, et al. Pluripoietin alpha: A second human hematopoietic colony-stimulating factor produced by the human bladder carcinoma cell line 5637. *Proc Natl Acad Sci USA* 1986; 83: 2478.
98. Gahmberg CG, Nilsson K, Anderson LC. Specific changes in the surface of glycoprotein pattern of human promyelocytic leukemia cell line HL-60 during morphologic and functional differentiation. *Proc Natl Acad Sci USA* 1979; 76: 4087.
99. Gallagher R, Collins S, Trujillo J, et al. Characterization of the continuous, differentiating myeloid cell line (HL-60) from a patient with acute promyelocytic leukemia. *Blood* 1979; 54: 713.
100. Gallagher JC, Jerpbak CM, Jee WSS, et al. 1,25-Dihydroxyvitamin D3: short- and long-term effects on bone and calcium metabolism in patients with postmenopausal osteoporosis. *Proc Natl Acad Sci USA* 1982; 79: 3325.
101. Gallagher RE, Bilello PA, Ferrari AC, et al. Characterization of differentiation-inducer-resistant HL-60 cells. *Leuk Res* 1985; 9: 967.
102. Gallo RC, Breitman TR, Ruscelli FW. Proliferation and differentiation of human myeloid leukemia cell lines *in vitro*. In: Moore MAS, ed. *Maturation factors in cancer*. New York: Raven Press, 1987: 255.
103. Garewal HS, List A, Meyskens F, et al. Phase II trial of fenretinide [*N*-(4-hydroxyphenyl) retinamide] in myelodysplasia: possible retinoid-induced disease acceleration. *Leuk Res* 1989; 13: 339.
104. Gasson J, Weisbart R, Kaufman S, et al. Purified human granulocyte-macrophage colony-stimulating factor: direct action on neutrophils. *Science* 1984; 226: 1339.
105. Gately CL, Wahl SM, Oppenheim J. Characterization of a hydrogen peroxide-potentiating factor, a lymphokine that increases the capacity of human monocytes and monocyte-like cell lines to produce hydrogen peroxide. *J Immunol* 1983; 131: 2853.
106. Gearing DP, Gough NM, King JA. Molecular cloning and expression of cDNA encoding a murine myeloid leukaemia inhibitory factor (LIF). *EMBO J* 1987; 6: 3995.
107. Geissler K, Tricot G, Leemhus T, et al. Differentiation-inducing effect of recombinant human tumor necrosis factor α and γ-interferon *in vitro* on blast cells from patients with acute myeloid leukemia and myeloid blast crisis of chronic myeloid leukemia. *Cancer Res* 1989; 49: 3057.
108. Gitter BD, Finn OJ, Metzgar RS. Cytofluorometric isolation of I937, an Ia antigen-bearing variant of the Ia-negative human monocytic cell line U937. *J Immunol* 1985; 134: 280.
109. Godard A, Gascan H, Naulet J, et al. Biochemical characterization and purification of HILDA, a human lymphokine active on eosinophils and bone marrow cells. *Blood* 1988; 71: 1618.
110. Goey H, Keller JR, Jansen R, et al. Antiproliferative effects of transforming growth factor beta 1 for murine tumors and hematopoietic progenitor cells. *Proc Annu Meet Am Assoc Cancer Res* 1989; 30: A1295.
111. Goey H, Keller JR, Back T, et al. Inhibition of early murine hemopoietic progenitor cell proliferation after *in vivo* locoregional administration of transforming growth factor-β1. *J Immunol* 1989; 143: 877.
112. Gold EJ, Mertelsmann R, Itri LM, et al. Phase I clinical trial of 13-*cis*-retinoic acid in myelodysplastic syndrome. *Cancer Treat Rep* 1983; 11: 981.
113. Gough N, Gough J, Metcalf D, et al. Molecular cloning of cDNA encoding a murine haemopoietic growth regulator, granulocyte-macrophage colony stimulating factor GM-CSF. *Nature* 1984; 309: 763.
114. Gough NM, Gearing DP, King JA, et al. Molecular cloning and expression of the human homologue of the murine gene encoding myeloid leukemia-inhibitory factor. *Proc Natl Acad Sci USA* 1988; 85: 2623.
115. Griffin JD. Role of colony stimulating factors in the biology of leukemia. *Exp Hematol* 1988; 16: 417.
116. Griffin J, Munroe D, Major P, et al. Induction of differentiation of human myeloid leukemia cells by inhibitors of

DNA synthesis. *Exp Hematol* 1982; 9: 774.
117. Griffin JD, Rambaldi A, Vellenga E, et al. Secretion of interleukin-1 by acute myeloblastic leukemia cells *in vitro* induces endothelial cells to secrete colony stimulating factors. *Blood* 1987; 70: 1218.
118. Grosso LE, Pitot HC. Transcriptional regulation of c-myc during chemically induced differentiation of HL-60 cultures. *Cancer Res* 1985; 45: 847.
119. Guan XP, Fujii Y, Hromchak RA, et al. Synergistic induction of ML-1 human myeloblastic leukemia cell differentiation by combinations of 12-*O*-tetradecanoylphorbol 13-acetate (TPA) with transforming growth factor (TGF-beta) or with human tumor necrosis factor (TNF-alpha). *Proc Annu Meet Am Assoc Cancer Res* 1989; 30: A175.
120. Guernsey DL, Yen A. Retinoic-acid-induced modulation of c-myc not dependent on its continued presence: possible role in precommitment for HL-60 cells. *Int J Cancer* 1988; 42: 576.
121. Guyre PM, Morganelli PM, Miller R. Recombinant immune interferon increases IgG FcR receptors on cultured human mononuclear phagocytes. *J Clin Invest* 1983; 72: 393.
122. Hagenbeek A, Sizoo W, Lowenberg B. Treatment of acute myelocytic leukemia with low dose cytosine arabinoside: results of a pilot study in four patients. *Leuk Res* 1983; 7: 443.
123. Hampson J, Ponting ILO, Cook N, et al. The effects of TGF beta on haemopoietic cells. *Growth Factors* 1988; 1: 193.
124. Hansen F. Hemopoietic growth and inhibitory factors in treatment of malignancies. *Acta Oncologica* 1995; 34(4): 453-468.
125. Hapel AJ, Vande Woude G, Campbell HD, et al. Generation of an autocrine leukemia using a retroviral expression vector carrying the interleukin-3 gene. *Lymphokine Res* 1986; 5: 249.
126. Harris PE, Ralph P, Litcofsky P, et al. Distinct activities of interferon-gamma, lymphokine and cytokine differentiation inducing factors acting on the human monoblastic leukemia cell line U937. *Cancer Res* 1985; 45: 9.
127. Harris PE, Ralph P, Gabrilove J, et al. Broad spectrum induction by cytokine factors and limited induction by gamma interferon of differentiation in the human promyelocytic leukemia cell line HL-60. *Cancer Res* 1985; 45: 3090.
128. Hartman D, Sheridan AP, Moore MAS. *Effects of 1,25(OH)$_2$ D$_3$, dexamethasone and cytoxan on the survival of leukemic (WEHI-3B(D$^+$) Balb/c mice.* Unpublished observation, 1987.
129. Hassan HT, Rees JKH. Triple combination of retinoic acid + naclacinomycin A + dimethylformamide induces differentiation of human acute myeloid leukaemic blasts in primary culture. *Anticancer Res* 1989; 9: 647.
130. Hast R, Axdorph S, Lauren L, et al. Absent clinical effects of retinoic acid and isorethinoin treatment in the myelodysplastic syndrome. *Hematol Oncol* 1989; 7: 297.
131. Hattori T, Pack M, Bougnoux P, et al. Interferon-induced differentiation of U937 cells. *J Clin Invest* 1983; 72: 237.
132. Haussler MR, Baylink DJ, Hughes MR, et al. Assay of 1-alpha 25-dihydroxyvitamin D3: Physiological and pathological modulation of circulating hormone levels. *Clin Endocrinol* 1979; 5: 157.
133. Hayashi M, Okabe J, Hozumi M. Sensitization of resistant myeloid leukemia clone cells by anti-cancer drugs to factor-stimulating differentiation. *Gann* 1979; 70: 235.
134. Hayashi SI, Gimble JM, Henley A, et al. Differential effects of TGFβ1 on lympho-hemopoiesis in long-term bone marrow cultures. *Blood* 1989; 74: 1711.
135. Hellstrom E, Robert KH, Gahrton G, et al. Therapeutic effects of low-dose cytosine arabinoside, alpha-interferon, alpha-hydroxyvitamin D$_3$ and retinoic acid in acute leukemia and myelodysplastic syndromes. *Eur J Haematol* 1988; 40: 449.
136. Hemmi H, Breitman T. Induction by retinoic acid of NAD$^+$-glycohydrolase activity of myelomonocytic cell lines HL-60, THP-1 and U937 and human promyelocytic leukemia cells in primary culture. *Biochem Biophys Res Commun* 1982; 109: 669.
137. Hemmi H, Breitman TR. Combinations of recombinant human interferons and retinoic acid synergistically induce differentiation of the human promyelocytic leukemia cell line HL-60. *Blood* 1987; 69: 501.
138. Hemmi H, Nakamura T, Shimizu Y, et al. Identification of components of differentiation-inducing activity of human T-cell lymphoma cells by induction of differentiation in human myeloid leukemia cells. *J Natl Cancer Inst* 1989; 81: 952.
139. Hill R, Warren K, Stenberg P, et al. Purified human recombinant IL-6 stimulates murine megakaryocytopoiesis and increases platelet levels. *Blood* 1989; 74(suppl 1): 207 (abstr).
140. Hilton DJ, Nicola NA, Metcalf D. Specific binding of murine leukemia inhibitory factor to normal and leukemic monocytic cells. *Proc Natl Acad Sci USA* 1988; 85: 5971.
141. Hino M, Tojo A, Miyazono K, et al. Effects of type β transforming growth factors on haematopoietic progenitor cells. *Br J Haematol* 1988; 70: 143.
142. Hirano T, Yasukawa K, Harada H, et al. Complementary DNA for a novel human interleukin (BSF-2) that induces B lymphocytes to produce immunoglobulin. *Nature* 1986; 324: 73.
143. Hittelman WN, Agbor P, Petkovic I, et al. Detection of leukemic clone maturation *in vivo* by premature chromosome condensation. *Blood* 1988; 72: 1950.
144. Ho AD, Martin H, Knauf W, et al. Combination of low dose cytarabine and 13-*cis* retinoic acid in the treatment of myelodysplastic syndromes. *Leuk Res* 1987; 11: 1041.
145. Hoang T, Haman A, Goncalves O, et al. Interleukin-6 enhances growth factor-dependent proliferation of the blast cells of acute myeloblastic leukemia. *Blood* 1988; 72: 823.
146. Hoang T, Haman A, Goncalves O, et al. Interleukin 1 enhances growth factor dependent proliferation of the clonogenic cells in acute myeloblastic leukemia and of normal human primitive hemopoietic precursors. *J Exp Med* 1988; 168: 463.
147. Hoang T, Levy B, Onetto N, et al. Tumor necrosis factor a stimulates the growth of the clonogenic cells of acute myeloblastic leukemia in synergy with granulocyte-macrophage colony-stimulating factor. *J Exp Med* 1989; 170: 15.
148. Hoffman SJ, Robinson WA. Use of differentiation-inducing agents in the myelodysplastic syndrome and acute non-lymphocytic leukemia. *Am J Hematol* 1988; 28: 124.
149. Homma Y, Takenaga K, Kasukabe T, et al. Induction of differentiation of cultured human promyelocytic leukemia cells by retinoids. *Biochem Biophys Res Commun* 1980;

95: 507.
150. Homma Y, Hozumi M, Abe E, et al. 1,25-Dihydroxyvitamin D_3 prolong survival time of mice inoculated with myeloid leukemia cells. *Proc Natl Acad Sci USA* 1983; 80: 201.
151. Hossfeld DK, Weh H-J, Kleeberg UR. Low dose cytarabine: chromosomal findings suggesting its cytostatic as well as differentiating effect. *Leuk Res* 1985; 9: 329.
152. Housset M, Daniel MT, Degos L. Small doses of ARA-C in the treatment of acute myeloid leukaemia: differentiation of myeloid leukaemia cells? *Br J Haematol* 1982; 51: 125.
153. Hozumi M. Fundamentals of chemotherapy of myeloid leukemia by induction of leukemia cell differentiation. *Adv Cancer Res* 1983; 38: 121.
154. Huang ME, Ye YC, Chen SR. All-*trans* retinoic acid with or without low dose cytosine arabinoside in acute promyelocytic leukemia. Report of 6 cases. *Clin Med J* 1987; 100: 949.
155. Ihle J, Keller J, Henderson L, et al. Procedures for the purification of interleukin-3 to homogeneity. *J Immunol* 1982; 129: 2431.
156. Ikebuchi K, Ihle JN, Hirai Y, et al. Synergistic factors for stem cell proliferation: further studies of the target stem cells and the mechanism of stimulation by interleukin-1, interleukin-6, and granulocyte colony-stimulating factor. *Blood* 1988; 72: 2007.
157. Ishibashi T, Miller SL, Burstein SA. Type β transforming growth factor is a potent inhibitor of murine megakaryocytopoiesis *in vitro*. *Blood* 1987; 69: 1737.
158. Ishibashi T, Kimura H, Shkiama Y, et al. Thrombopoietic effect of interleukin 6 (IL-6) *in vivo* in mice: comparison of the action of erythropoietin (Epo) and granulocyte colony-stimulating factor (G-CSF) in combination with IL-6 on thrombocytopoiesis. *Blood* 1989; 74(suppl 1): 18 (abstr).
159. Iwasaki Y, Iwasaki J, Feake HC. Growth inhibition of human breast cancer cells induced by calcitonin. *Biochem Biophys Res Commun* 1983; 110: 235.
160. Jacobs K, Shoemaker C, Rudersdort R, et al. Isolation and characterization of genomic and cDNA clones of human erythropoietin. *Nature* 1985; 313: 806.
161. Jetten AM. Action of retinoids and phorbol esters on cell growth and the binding of epidermal growth factor. *Ann NY Acad Sci* 1981; 119: 200.
162. Jubinsky P, Stanley R. Purification of hemopoietin 1: a multilineage hemopoietic growth factor. *Proc Nat Acad Sci USA* 1985; 85: 2764.
163. Kahn AJ, Simmons DJ. Monocyte origin of osteoclasts. *Nature* 1975; 258: 325.
164. Kahn AJ, Stewart CC, Teitelbaum SL. Contact mediated bone resorption by human monocytes *in vitro*. *Science* 1978; 199: 988.
165. Kamijo R, Takeda K, Nagumo M, et al. Effects of combinations of transforming growth factor-β1 and tumor necrosis factor on induction of differentiation of human myelogenous leukemic cell lines. *J Immunol* 1990; 144: 1311.
166. Kashima N, Nishi-Takaoka C, Fujita T, et al. Unique structure of murine interleukin-2 as deduced from cloned cDNAs. *Nature* 1985; 131: 402.
167. Kaufman DC, Baer MR, Gao X, et al. Enhanced expression of the granulocyte-macrophage colony stimulating factor gene in acute myeloblastic leukemia cells following *in vitro* blast cell enrichment. *Blood* 1988; 72: 1329.
168. Kawasaki E, Ladner M, Wang A, et al. Molecular cloning of a complementary DNA encoding human macrophage-specific colony-stimulating factor (CSF-1). *Science* 1985; 230: 291.
169. Keller JR, Mantel C, Sing GK, et al. Transforming growth factor beta 1 selectively regulates early murine hematopoietic progenitors and inhibits the growth of IL-3-dependent myeloid leukemia cell lines. *J Exp Med* 1988; 168: 737.
170. Keller JR, Sing GK, Ellingsworth LR, et al. Transforming growth factor beta: possible roles in the regulation of normal and leukemic hematopoietic cell growth. *J Cell Biochem* 1989; 39: 175.
171. Kishimoto T. The biology of interleukin-6. *J Am Soc Hematol* 1989; 74: 1.
172. Kinashi T, Harada N, Severinson E, et al. Cloning of complementary DNA encoding T-cell replacing factor and identity with B-cell growth factor II. *Nature* 1986; 324: 70.
173. Kizaki M, Norman AW, Bishop JE, et al. 1,25-dihydroxyvitamin D_3 receptor RNA: Expression in hematopoietic cells. *Blood* 1991; 71: 1238-1247.
174. Klien B, Zhang XG, Jourdan M, et al. Paracrine rather than autocrine regulation of myeloma-cell growth and differentiation by interleukin-6. *Blood* 1989; 73: 517.
175. Klijn JGM, Berns PMJJ, Schmitz PIM, Foekens JA. The clinical significance of epidermal growth factor receptor (EGF-R) in human breast cancer: a review on 5232 patients. *Endocrine Reviews* 1992; 13: 3-17.
176. Koeffler HP. Induction of differentiation of human acute myelogenous leukemia cells: therapeutic implications. *Blood* 1983; 62: 709.
177. Koeffler H, Bar-Eli M, Territo M. Phorbol ester effect on differentiation of human myeloid leukemia cell lines blocked at different stages of maturation. *Cancer Res* 1981; 41: 919.
178. Koeffler HP, Amatruda T, Ikekawa N, et al. Induction of macrophage differentiation of human normal and leukemic myeloid stem cells by 1,25-dihydroxyvitamin D_3 and its fluorinated analogues. *Cancer Res* 1984; 44: 5624.
179. Koeffler HP, Kirfi K, Itri L. 1,25-dihydroxyvitamin D-3: *in vivo* and *in vitro* effects on human preleukemic and leukemic cells. *Cancer Treat Rep* 1985; 69: 1399.
180. Koeffler HP, Yelton L, Prokocimer L, et al. Study of the differentiation of fresh myelogenous leukemic cells by compounds that induce a human promyelocytic leukemic cell line (HL-60) to differentiate. *Leuk Res* 1985; 9: 73.
181. Koeffler HP, Tobler A, Munker R. Tumor necrosis factor: role in normal and abnormal hematopoiesis. In: Gale RP, Golde DW, eds. Recent advances in leukemia and lymphoma. *UCLA Symposia on Molecular and Cellular Biology*, New Series, 1987; 61: 433.
182. Koeffler HP, Heitjan D, Mertelsmann R, et al. Randomized study of 13-*cis*-retinoic acid v placebo in the myelodysplastic disorders. *Blood* 1988; 71: 703.
183. Kohlhepp EA, Condon ME, Hamburger AW. Recombinant human interferon alpha enhancement of retinoic-acid-induced differentiation of HL-60 cells. *Exp Hematol* 1987; 15: 414.
184. Koike K, Nakahata T, Takagi M, et al. Synergism of BSF-2/interleukin 6 and interleukin 3 on development of multipotential hemopoietic progenitors in serum-free

culture. *J Exp Med* 1988; 168: 879.

185. Kuribayashi T, Tanaka H, Abe E, et al. Functional defect of variant clones of a human myeloid leukemia cell line (HL-60) resistant to 1,25-dihydroxyvitamin D_3. *Endocrinology* 1983; 113: 1992.
186. Kurland JI, Pelus LM, Ralph P, et al. Induction of prostaglandin E synthesis in normal and neoplastic macrophages: role for colony-stimulating factor(s) distinct from myeloid progenitor cell proliferation. *Proc Natl Acad Sci USA* 1979; 76: 2326.
187. Lang R, Metcalf N, Gough N, et al. Expression of a hemopoietic growth factor cDNA in a factor-dependent cell line results in autonomous growth and tumorigenicity. *Cell* 1985; 43: 531.
188. Largman C, Detmer K, Corral JC, et al. Expression of retinoic acid receptor alpha MRNA in human leukemia cells. *Blood* 1989; 74: 99.
189. Larrick JW, Ficher DG, Anderson SJ, et al. Characterization of a human macrophage-like cell line stimulated *in vitro*: a model of macrophage functions. *J Immunol* 1980; 125: 6.
190. Lawrence HJ, Conner K, Kelly MA, et al. *cis*-Retinoic acid stimulates the clonal growth of some myeloid leukemia cells *in vitro*. *Blood* 1987; 69: 302.
191. Lee F, Yokota T, Otsuka T, et al. Isolation and characterization of a mouse interleukin cDNA clone that expresses B-cell stimulatory factor 1 activities and T cell and mast-cell-stimulating activities. *Proc Natl Acad Sci USA* 1986; 83: 2061.
192. Ley TJ, DeSimone J, Noguchi CT, et al. 5-Azacytidine increases γ globin synthesis and reduces the proportion of dense cells in patients with sickle-cell anemia. *Blood* 1983; 62: 370.
193. Lin J, Sartorelli AC. Stimulation by interferon of the differentiation of human promyelocytic leukemia (HL-60) cells produced by retinoid acid and actinomycin D. *J Interferon Res* 1987; 7: 379.
194. Lin FK, Suggs S, Lin C-H, et al. Cloning and expression of the human erythropoietin gene. *Proc Natl Acad Sci USA* 1985; 82: 7580-7584.
195. Lindemann W-D, Ludwig W, Oster R. High-level secretion of tumor necrosis factor-alpha contributes to hematopoietic failure in hairy cell leukemia. *Blood* 1989; 73: 880.
196. Littman B, Hall RE, *Muchmore A. Lymphokine and phorbol (PMA) regulation of complement (C2) synthesis using U937.*
197. Lombardo FA, Ward FT, Chun HG, et al. Phase I trial of oral hemamethylene bisacetamide (HMBA). *Proc Annu Meet Am Soc Clin Oncol* 1989; 8: A297.
198. Lotem J, Sachs L. Different blocks in the differentiation of myeloid leukemic cells. *Proc Natl Acad Sci USA* 1974; 71: 3507.
199. Lotem J, Sachs L. *In vivo* control of differentiation of myeloid leukemic cells by cyclosporine A and recombinant interleukin-1α. *Blood* 1988; 72: 1595.
200. Lotem J, Sachs L. Indirect induction of differentiation of normal and leukemic myeloid cells by recombinant interleukin 1. *Leuk Res* 1989; 13: 13.
201. Lotem J, Sachs L. Hematopoietic cytokines inhibit apoptosis induced by transforming growth factor β1 and cancer chemotherapy compounds in myeloid leukemic cells. *Blood* 1992; 80: 1750.
202. Lotem J, Lipton J, Sachs L. Separation of different molecular forms of macrophage- and granulocyte-inducing proteins for normal and leukemic myeloid cells. *Int J Cancer* 1980; 25: 763.
203. Lotem J, Berrebi A, Sachs L. Screening for induction of differentiation and toxicity to blast cells by chemotherapeutic compounds in human myeloid leukemia. *Leuk Res* 1985; 9: 249.
204. Lowenberg B, Salem M, Delwel R. Effects of recombinant multi-CSF, GM-CSF, G-CSF and M-CSF on the proliferation and maturation of human AML *in vitro*. *Blood Cells* 1988; 14: 539.
205. Lowe DG, Wylla N. Bombara M, et al. Genomic cloning and heterologous expression of human differentiation-stimulating factor. *DNA* 1989; 8: 351.
206. Lu L, Broxmeyer HE, Pelus LM, et al. Detection of Luxol-fast-blue positive cells in human promyelocytic leukemia cell line HL-60. *Exp Hematol* 1982; 9: 887.
207. Lu L, Welte K, Gabrilove JL, et al. Effects of recombinant human tumor necrosis factor a, recombinant human γ-interferon, and prostaglandin E on colony formation of human hematopoietic progenitor cells stimulated by natural human pluripotent colony-stimulating factor, pluripoietin a, and recombinant erythropoietin in serum-free cultures. *Cancer Resp* 1986; 46: 4357.
208. Maekawa T, Metcalf D. Clonal suppression of HL-60 and U937 cells by recombinant human leukemia inhibitory factor in combination with GM-CSF or G-CSF. *Leukemia* 1989; 3: 270.
209. Majeska RJ, Rodan GA. The effect of 1,25$(OH)_2$ D_3 on alkaline phosphatase in osteoblastic osteosarcoma cells. *J Biol Chem* 1982; 257: 3362.
210. Mangelsdorf DJ, Koeffler HP, Donaldson CA, et al. 1,25-Dihydroxyvitamin D3-induced differentiation in a human promyelocytic leukemia cell line (HL-60): receptor-mediated maturation to macrophage-like cells. *J Cell Biol* 1984; 98: 391.
211. Manloagas SC, Haussler MR, Deftos LJ. 1,25-Dihydroxyvitamin D_3 receptor-like macromolecule in rat osteogenic sarcoma cell lines. *J Biol Chem* 1980; 255: 4414.
212. March C, Mosley B, Larsen A, et al. Cloning, sequence and expression of two distinct human interleukin-1 complementary DNA. *Nature* 1985; 315: 641.
213. Marks PA, Breslow R, Rifkind RA, et al. Polar/apolar chemical inducers of differentiation of transformed cells: strategies to improve therapeutic potential. *Proc Natl Acad Sci USA* 1989; 86: 6358.
214. Marks PA, Rifkind RA. Hexamethylene bisacetamide-induced differentiation of transformed cells: molecular and cellular effects and therapeutic application. *Int J Cell Cloning* 988; 6: 230.
215. Matsui T, Nakao U, Kobayashi N, et al. Phenotypic differentiation-linked growth inhibition in human leukemia cells by active vitamin D_3 analogues. *Int J Cancer* 1984; 33: 193.
216. Matsushima K, Morishita K, Yoshimura T, et al. Molecular cloning of cDNA for a human monocyte derived neutrophil chemotactic factor (MDNCF) and the induction of MDNCF mRNA by interleukin 1 and tumor necrosis factor. *J Exp Med* 1988; 167: 1883-1890.
217. McCarthy DM, San Miguel JF, Freake HC, et al. 1,25-Dihydroxyvitamin D_3 inhibits proliferation of human promyelocytic leukaemia (HL-60) cells and induces monocyte-macrophage differentiation in HL-60 and normal human bone marrow cells. *Leuk Res* 1983; 7: 51.
218. McCarthy DM, Hibbins JA, Goldman JM. A role for 1,25-

dihydroxyvitamin D_3 in control of bone-marrow collagen deposition? *Lancet* 1984; 1: 78.

219. Mehta K, Pratt JA. Encapsulating all-trans-retinoic acid (RA) in liposomes reduces its toxic effects while maintaining its anti-tumor properties. *Proc Annu Meet Am Assoc Cancer Res* 1989; 30: A2408.
220. Metcalf D. The roles of stem cell-renewal and autocrine growth factor production in the biology of myeloid leukemia. *Cancer Res* 1989; 49: 2305.
221. Metcalf D. Actions and interactions of G-CSF, LIF, and IL-6 on normal and leukemic murine cells. *Leukemia* 1989; 3: 349.
222. Metcalf D, Gearing DP. A myelosclerotic syndrome in mice engrafted with cells producing high levels of leukemia inhibitory factor (LIF). *Leukemia* 1989; 3: 847.
223. Metcalf D, Gearing DP. Fatal syndrome in mice engrafted with cells producing high levels of the leukemia inhibitory factor. *Proc Natl Acad Sci USA* 1989; 86: 5948.
224. Metcalf D, Hilton DJ, Nicola NA. Clonal analysis of the actions of the murine leukemia inhibitory factor on leukemic and normal murine hemopoietic cells. *Leukemia* 1988; 2: 216.
225. Mezzetti G, Bagnara G, Monti MG, et al. 1,25-Dihydroxycholecalciferol and human histocytic lymphoma cell (U937): the presence of receptor and inhibition of proliferation. *Life Sci* 1984; 34: 2185.
226. Michaelewicz R, Lotem J, Sachs L. Cell differentiation and therapeutic effect of low doses of cytosine arabinoside in human myeloid leukemia. *Leuk Res* 1984; 8: 783.
227. Miyake T, Kung C, Goldwaser D. Purification of human erythropoietin. *J Biol Chem* 1977; 252: 5558.
228. Miyauchi J, Wang C, Kelleher CA, et al. The effects of recombinant CSF-1 on the blast cells of acute myeloblastic leukemia in suspension culture. *J Cell Physiol* 1988; 135: 55.
229. Miyaura C, Abe E, Kuribayashi T, et al. 1-α25-Dihydroxyvitamin D_3 induces differentiation of human myeloid leukemia cells. *Biochem Biophys Res Commun* 1981; 102: 937.
230. Miyaura C, Abe E, Honma Y, et al. Cooperative effect of 1,25-dihydroxyvitamin D_3 and dexamethasone in inducing differentiation of mouse myeloid leukemia cells. *Arch Biochem Biophys* 1983; 227: 397.
231. Miyaura C, Abe E, Suda T, et al. Alternative differentiation of human promyelocytic leukemia cells (HL-60) induced selectively by retinoic acid and 1,25-dihydroxyvitamin D3. *Cancer Res* 1985; 45; 4244.
232. Miyaura C, Onozaki K, Akiyama Y, et al. Recombinant human interleukin-6 (B-cell stimulatory factor 2) is a potent inducer of differentiation of mouse myeloid leukemia cells (M1). *FEBS Lett* 1988; 234: 17.
233. Miyaura C, Jin CH, Yamaguchi Y, et al. Production of interleukin 6 and its relation to the macrophage differentiation of mouse myeloid leukemia cells (M1) treated with differentiation-inducing factor and 1α, 25-dihydroxyvitamin D3. *Biochem Biophys Res Commun* 1989; 158: 660.
234. Moloney WC, Rosenthal DS. Treatment of early acute non-lymphatic leukemia with low dose cytosine arabinoside. *Haematol Blood Transfus* 1981; 26: 59.
235. Momparler RL, Bouchard J, Onetto N, et al. 5-Aza-2'-deoxycytidine therapy in patients with acute leukemia inhibits DNA methylation. *Leuk Res* 1984; 8: 181.
236. Moore M. Prediction of relapse and remission in AML by marrow culture criteria. *Blood Cells* 976; 2: 109.
237. Moore M. Agar culture in CML and blastic transformation. *Ser Haematol* 1977; 8: 11.
238. Moore M. Proliferation and differentiation control mechanisms in myeloid leukemia. In: Mehich H, ed. *Biological responses in cancer – progress toward potential applications*, vol. 2. New York: Plenum, 1984: 93.
239. Moore MAS. The use of hematopoietic growth and differentiation factors for bone marrow stimulation. In: Devita VT, Hellman S, Rosenberg SA, eds. *Important advances in oncology* 1988. Philadelphia: Lippincott, 1988: 31.
240. Moore MAS. Role of interleukin-1 in hematopoiesis. *Immunol Res* 1989; 8: 165.
241. Moore MAS. Interactions between hematopoietic growth factors in normal and leukemic stem cell differentiation. In: Diamond L, Wolman SR, eds. Viral oncogenesis and cell differentiation. *Ann NY Acad Sci* 1989; 567: 171.
242. Moore MAS. Coordinate actions of hematopoietic growth factors in stimulation of bone marrow function. In: Sporn MB, Roberts AB, eds. *Handbook of experimental pharmacology – peptide growth factors and their receptors.* 1990: Chap. 32 95 II: 299.
243. Moore M, Sheridan A. The role of proliferation and maturation factors in myeloid leukemia. In: Moore MAS, ed. *Maturation factors in cancer.* New York: Raven Press, 1982: 361.
244. Moore MAS, Warren DJ. Interleukin-1 and G-CSF synergism. *in vivo* stimulation of stem cell recovery and hematopoietic regeneration following 5-fluorouracil treatment in mice. *Proc Natl Acad Sci USA* 1987; 84: 7134.
245. Moore M, Williams N, Metcalf D. *In vitro* colony formation by normal and leukemic human hematopoietic cells: Characterization of the colony-forming cells. *J Natl Cancer Inst* 1973; 50: 603.
246. Moore M, Spitzer G, Williams N, et al. Agar culture studies in 127 cases of untreated acute leukemia. The prognostic value of reclassification of leukemia according to *in vitro* growth characteristics. *Blood* 1974; 44: 1.
247. Moore MAS, Gabrilove JL, Welte K, Platzer E. Maturational factors in leukemia. In: Reif AE, Mitchell MS, ed. *Immunity to cancer.* New York: Academic Press 1985: 513.
248. Moore MAS, Warren DJ, Souza L. Synergistic interaction between interleukin-1 and CSFs in hematopoiesis. In: Gale RP, Golde DW, eds. *UCLA symposium on leukemia, recent advances in leukemia and lymphoma*. New York: Alan R. Liss, 1987: 445.
249. Moore MAS, Muench MO, Warren DJ, et al. Cytokine networks involved in regulation of haemopoietic stem cell proliferation and differentiation. In: Molecular control of haemopoiesis. *CIBA Symposium No. 148.* 1990: 43.
250. Moore M, Welte K, Gabrilove J, et al. Biological activities of recombinant human granulocyte-colony stimulating factor (rhG-CSF) and tumor necrosis factor: *in vivo* and *in vitro* analysis. *Haematol Blood Transfus* 1987; 31: 210.
251. Moreau J-F, Bonneville M, Godard A, et al. Characterization of a factor produced by human T cell clones exhibiting eosinophil-activating and burst-promoting activities. *J Immunol* 1987; 138: 3844.
252. Moreau J-F, Donaldson DD, Bennett F, et al. Leukaemia inhibitory factor is identical to the myeloid growth factor human interleukin for DA cells. *Nature* 1988; 336: 690.
253. Motoji T, Hoang T, Tritchler D, McCulloch EA. The effect

of 5-aza-cytidine and its analogues on blast cell renewal in acute myeloblastic leukemia. *Blood* 1985; 65: 894.
254. Muller R, Muller D, Guilbert L. Differential expression of c-fos in hematopoietic cells: correlation with differentiation of myelomonocytic cells *in vitro*. *EMBO J* 1984; 3: 1887.
255. Muller K, Svenson M, Bendtzen K. 1-Alpha, 25-dihydroxyvitamin D_3 and a novel vitamin D analogue MC 903 are potent inhibitors of human interleukin 1 *in vitro*. *Immunol Lett* 1988; 17: 361.
256. Munroe E, Sugiura M, Griffin J, Kufe D. Effect of ara-A on differentiation and proliferation of HL-60 cells. *Leuk Res* 1984; 8: 355.
257. Murao S, Gemmell MA, Callaham MF, et al. Control of macrophage cell differentiation in human promyelocytic HL-60 leukemia cells by 1,25-dihydroxyvitamin D_3 and phorbol-12-myristate-13 acetate. *Cancer Res* 1983; 43: 4989.
258. Murphy M, Perussia B, Trinchieri G. Effects of recombinant tumor necrosis factor, lymphotoxin, and immune interferon on proliferation and differentiation of enriched hematopoietic precursor cells. *Exp Hematol* 1988; 16: 131.
259. Nagat S, Tsuchiya M, Asano S, et al. Molecular cloning and expression of cDNA for human granulocyte colony-stimulating factor. *Nature* 1986; 319: 415.
260. Nagata K, Tohda S, Suzuki T, et al. Effects of recombinant human tumor necrosis factor on the self-renewal capacity of leukemic blast progenitors in acute myeloblastic leukemia. *Leukemia* 1989; 3: 626.
261. Najean Y, Pecking A. Refractory anemia with excess of blast cells: prognostic factors and effect of treatment with androgens or cytosine arabinoside. *Cancer* 1976; 44: 345.
262. Namen AE, Lupton S, Hjerrild K, et al. Stimulation of B-cell progenitors by cloned murine interleukin-7. *Nature* 1988; 333: 571-573.
263. Namen AE, Schmierer AE, March CJ, et al. B cell precursor growth-promoting activity: purification and characterization of a growth factor active on lymphocyte precursors. *J Exp Med* 1988; 167: 988-1002.
264. Nara N, McCulloch E. Membranes replace irradiated blast cells as growth requirement for leukemic blast progenitors in suspension culture. *J Exp Med* 1985; 162: 1435.
265. Nara N, Tohda S, Nagata K, et al. Inhibition of the *in vitro* growth of blast progenitors from acute myeloblastic leukemia patients by transforming growth factor-beta (TGF-beta). *Leukemia* 1989; 3: 572.
266. Nervi C, Grippo JF, Sherman MI, et al. Identification and characterization of nuclear retinoic acid-binding activity in human myeloblastic leukemia HL-60 cells. *Proc Natl Acad Sci USA* 1989; 86: 5854.
267. Newburger PE, Chovaniec ME, Greenburger JS, Cohen H. Functional changes in human leukemic cell line HL-60. *J Cell Biol* 1979; 82: 315.
268. Nicola N, Metcalf D. Biochemical properties of differentiation factors for murine myelomonocytic leukemic cells in organ conditioned media separation from colony stimulating factor. *J Cell Physiol* 1981; 109: 253.
269. Nicola N, Metcalf C, Matsumoto M, Johnson GJ. Purification of a factor inducing differentiation in murine myelomonocytic leukemia cells: identification as granulocyte colony-stimulating factor G-CSF. *Biol Chem* 1983; 258: 9017.
270. Nicola N, Begley C, Metcalf D. Identification of the human analogue of a regulator that induces differentiation in murine leukaemia cells. *Nature* 1985; 316: 625.
271. Niedel J, Kahane I, Lachman L, Cuartrecassas P. A subpopulation of cultured human promyelocytic leukemia cells (HL-60) displays the formyl peptide chemotactic receptor. *Proc Natl Acad Sci USA* 1980; 77: 1000.
272. Nilsson K, Forsbeck K, Gidlund M, et al. Surface characteristics of the U937 histiocytic lymphoma cell line: specific changes during inducible morphologic and functional differentiation *in vitro*. In: Net R, Gallo R, Graf T, Mannweiler K, Winkler H, eds. *Haematology and blood transfusion*, vol. 26. Berlin: Springer-Verlag, 1981: 215.
273. Noma Y, Sideras P, Naito T, et al. Cloning of cDNA encoding the murine IgG1 induction factor by a novel strategy using SP6 promoter. *Nature* 1986; 319: 640.
274. Ohta M, Massague J, Anklesaria P, et al. Two forms of transforming growth factor-β distinguished by multipotential haematopoietic progenitor cells. *Nature* 1987; 329: 539.
275. Okabe-Kado J, Honma Y, Hayashi M, et al. Inhibitory action of transforming growth factor-β on induction of differentiation of myeloid leukemia cells. *Jpn J Cancer Res* 1989; 80: 228.
276. Olofsson T, Olsson I. Suppression of normal granulopoiesis *in vitro* by a leukemia associated inhibitor (LAI) derived from a human promyelocytic leukemia cell line (HL-60). *Leuk Res* 1980; 4: 437.
277. Olsson IL, Breitman T. Induction of differentiation of the human histiocytic lymphoma cell line U937 by retinoic acid and cyclic adenosine 3': 5'-monophosphate-inducing agents. *Cancer Res* 1982; 42: 3924.
278. Olsson IL, Breitman TR, Gallo RC. Priming of human myeloid leukemic cell lines HL-60 and U937 with retinoic acid for differentiation effects of cyclic adenosine 3': 5'-monophosphate-inducing agents and a T-lymphocyte-derived differentiation factor. *Cancer Res* 1982; 42: 3928.
279. Olsson I. Gullberg U, Ivhed I, et al. Induction of differentiation of the human histiocytic lymphoma cell line U937 by 1,25-dihydroxycholicalciferol. *Cancer Res* 1983; 43: 5862.
280. Olsson I, Sarngadharan MG, Breitman TR, Gallo R. Isolation and characterization of a T-lymphocyte-derived differentiation inducing factor for the myeloid leukemic cell line HL-60. *Blood* 1984; 63: 510.
281. Onozaki K, Tamatani T, Hashimoto T, et al. Growth inhibition and augmentation of mouse myeloid cell line differentiation by interleukin 1. *Cancer Res* 1987; 47: 2397.
282. Onozaki K, Akiyama Y, Okano A, et al. Synergistic regulatory effects of interleukin 6 and interleukin 1 on the growth and differentiation of human and mouse myeloid leukemic cell lines. *Cancer Res* 1989; 49: 3602.
283. Onozaki K, Urawa H, Tamatani T, et al. Synergistic interactions of interleukin 1, interferon-β and tumor necrosis factor in terminally differentiating mouse myeloid leukemic cell line (M1). *J Immunol* 1988; 140: 112.
284. Oppenheim J, Kovacs E, Matsushima K, Edurum S. There is more than one interleukin-1. *Immunol Today* 1986; 7: 45.
285. Ossenkoppele GJ, Wijermans PW, Nauta JJP, et al. Maturation induction in freshly isolated human myeloid leukemic cells, 1.25$(OH)_2$ vitamin D_3 being the most potent inducer. *Leuk Res* 1989; 13: 609.
286. Ottmann OG, Pelus LM. Differential proliferative effects

of transforming growth factor-β on human hematopoietic progenitor cells. *J Immunol* 1988; 140: 2661.
287. Pakkala S, de Vos S, Elstner E, et al. Antileukemic activities and effects on serum calcium of three novel vitamin D_3 analogs. *Blood* (Abstract) (Suppl.) 1993; 82: 255a.
288. Palacios R, Ivhed I, Sideras P, et al. Accessory function of human tumor cell lines I., production of interleukin 1 by the human histocytic lymphoma cell line U937. *Eur J Immunol* 1982; 12: 895.
289. Pantazis P, Lazarou S, Papadopoulos N. Isoenzymes of lactate dehydrogenase in human leukemic cells in culture treated with inducers of differentiation. *J Cell Biol* 1981; 90: 396.
290. Paoletti F, Mocali A. Changes in CuZn-superoxide dismutase during induced differentiation of murine erythroleukemia cells. *Cancer Res* 1988; 48: 6674.
291. Peetre C, Gullberg U, Nilsson E, et al. Effects of recombinant tumor necrosis factor on proliferation and differentiation of leukemic and normal hemopoietic cells *in vitro*. *J Clin Invest* 1986; 78: 1694.
292. Pelus LM, Ottmann OG, Nocka KH. Synergistic inhibition of human marrow granulocyte-macrophage progenitor cells by prostaglandin E and recombinant interferon-α, -β and -γ and an effect mediated by tumor necrosis factor. *J Immunol* 1988; 140: 479.
293. Pennica D, Nedwin GE, Hayflick JS, et al. Human tumor necrosis factor: precursor structure, expression and homology to lymphotoxin. *Nature* 1985; 312: 724.
294. Perussia B, Lebman D, Ip S, et al. Terminal differentiation surface antigens of myelomonocytic cells are expressed in human promyelocytic leukemia cells (HL-60) treated with chemical inducers. *Blood* 1981; 58: 836.
295. Piacibello W, Broxmeyer HE. Modulation of expression of Ia(HLA-DR)-antigens on human monocyte cell line U937 by gamma interferon and prostaglandin E and responsiveness of U937 colony forming cells to inhibition of lactoferrin, transferrin, acidic isoferritins and prostaglandin E. *Blood* 1983; (suppl. 1) 62: 86.
296. Pike MC, Fischer DG, Koren H, Snyderman R. Development of specific receptors for N-formylated chemotactic peptides in a human monocytic cell line stimulated with lymphokines. *J Exp Med* 1980; 152: 31.
297. Pinto A, Attadia V, Fusco A, et al. 5-Aza-2'-deoxycytidine induces terminal differentiation of leukemic blasts from patients with acute myeloid leukemias. *Blood* 1984; 64: 922.
298. Platzer E, Welte K, Gabrilove J, et al. Biological activities of human pluripotent hemopoietic colony stimulating factor on normal and leukemic cells. *J Exp Med* 1985; 162: 1788.
299. Pluznik DH. Synergistic activity of interleukin-1 alpha and interleukin-6 induces differentiation of myeloid cells into mature macrophages. *Exp Hematol* 1988; 16: 504.
300. Potter GK, Mohamed AN, Dracapoli NC, et al. The action of $1,25(OH)_2$ D_3 in nude mice bearing transplantable human myelogenous leukemic cell lines. *Exp Hematol* 1985; 13: 722.
301. Powell BL, Capizzi RL, Jackson DV, et al. Low dose ara-C for patients with myelodysplastic syndromes. *Leukemia* 1988; 2: 153.
302. Prigent SA, Lemoine NR. The type 1 (EGFR-related) family of growth factor receptors and their ligands. *Progress in Growth Factor Research* 1992; 4: 1-24.
303. Provendini DM, Tsoulas CD, Deftos LJ, Manolagas SC. 1,25-Dihydroxyvitamin D_3 receptors in human leukocytes. *Science* 1983; 221: 1181.
304. Pusztai L, Lewis CE, Lorenzen J, McGee JO'D. Growth factors: regulation of normal and neoplastic growth. *Journal of Pathology* 1993; 169: 191-201.
305. Raff MC. Social controls on cell survival and cell death. *Nature* 1992; 356: 397.
306. Ralph P, Moore MAS, Nilsson K. Lysozyme synthesis by established human and murine histiocytic cell lines. *J Exp Med* 1976; 143: 1528.
307. Ralph P, Williams N, Moore MAS, Litcofsky P. Induction of antibody-dependent and nonspecific tumor killing in human monocyte leukemic cells by nonlymphocyte factors and phorbol ester. *Cell Immunol* 1982; 71: 215.
308. Ralph P, Harris P, Punjabi CJ, et al. Lymphokine inducing 'terminal differentiation' of the human monoblast leukemia line U937: A role for gamma interferon. *Blood* 1983; 62: 1169.
309. Raza A, Preisler H. Evidence of *in vivo* differentiation in myeloblasts labeled with bromodeoxyuridine. *Cancer J* 1986; 1: 15.
310. Razin A, Levine A, Kafri T, et al. Relationship between transient DNA hypomethylation and erythroid differentiation of murine erythroleukemia cells. *Proc Natl Acad Sci USA* 1988; 85: 9003.
311. Reily IAG, Kozlowski R, Russell NH. Heterogenous mechanisms of autocrine growth of AML blasts. *Br J Haematol* 1989; 72: 363.
312. Reitsma PH, Rothberg PG, Astrin SM, et al. Regulation of myc gene expression in HL-60 leukemia cells by a vitamin D metabolite. *Nature* 1983; 306: 492.
313. Richon VM, Ramsay RG, Rifkind RA, et al. Modulation of the c-myb, c-myc and p42 on MRNA and protein levels during induced murine erythroleukemia cell differentiation. *Oncogene* 1989; 4: 165.
314. Rigby WFC, Shen L, Ball ED, et al. Differentiation of a human monocytic cell line by 1,25-dihydroxyvitamin D_3 (calcitriol): A morphological, phenotypic and functional analysis. *Blood* 1984; 64: 1110.
315. Rosenblum MG, Donato NJ. Tumor necrosis factor alpha: A multifaceted peptide hormone. *Crit Rev Immunol* 1989; 9: 21.
316. Rouis M, Thomopoulos P, Louache F, et al. Differentiation of U-937 human monocyte-like cell line by 1,25-dihydroxyvitamin D_3 or by retinoic acid. *Exp Cell Res* 1985; 157: 539.
317. Rovera G, O'Brien T, Diamond L. Induction of differentiation in human promyelocytic leukemia by tumor promoters. *Science* 1977; 204: 868.
318. Rovera G, Santoli D, Damsky C. Human promyelocytic leukemic cells in culture differentiate into macrophage-like cells when treated with a phorbol diester. *Proc Natl Acad Sci USA* 1979; 76: 2779.
319. Rovera G, Olashaw N, Meo P. Terminal differentiation in human promyelocytic leukemic cells *in vitro* by 6-thioguanine. *Cancer Lett* 1980; 10: 33.
320. Rowinsky EK, Ettinger DS, McGuire WP, et al. Prolonged infusion of hemaxamethylene bisacetamide: a phase I and pharmacological study. *Cancer Res* 1987; 47: 5788.
321. Ruscetti FW, Sing G, Ruscetti SK, et al. The role of transforming growth factor-beta in the regulation of normal and leukemic hematopoiesis. *Exp Hematol* 1988; 16: 417.
322. Ruutu P, Ruutu T, Vuopio P, et al. Defective chemotaxis in

monosomy-7. *Nature* 1977; 265: 146.
323. Sachs L. Control of normal cell differentiation and the phenotopic reversion of malignancy in myeloid leukemia. *Nature* 1978; 274: 535.
324. Salahuddin SZ, Markham PD, Ruscetti FW, Gallo RC. Long-term suspension cultures of human cord blood myeloid cells. *Blood* 1981; 58: 931.
325. Salem M, Delwel R, Touw I, et al. Modulation of colony stimulating factor-(CSF) dependent growth of acute myeloid leukemia by tumor necrosis factor. *Leukemia* 1990; 4: 37.
326. Sanderson C, O'Garra A, Warren D, Klaus G. Eosinophil differentiation factor also has B-cell growth factor activity: proposed name interleukin-4. *Proc Natl Acad Sci USA* 1986; 83: 437.
327. Santoli D, Yang Y-C, Steven CC, et al. Synergistic and antagonistic effects of recombinant human interleukin (IL) 3, IL-1a, granulocyte and macrophage colony-stimulating factors (G-CSF and M-CSF) on the growth of GM-CSF-dependent leukemic cell lines. *J Immunol* 1987; 139: 3348.
328. Sato T, Takusagawa K, Asso N, Konno K. Antitumor effect of 1 alpha-hydroxyvitamin D3. Tohoku *J Exp Med* 1982; 138: 445.
329. Sawyer S, Krantz S, Luna J. Identification of the receptor for erythropoietin by cross-linking to Friend virus-infected erythroid cells. *Proc Natl Acad Sci USA* 1987; 84: 3690.
330. Schif RD, Stuart RK. Treatment of myelodysplastic syndromes (MDS) and poor-prognosis acute myeloid leukemias (PP-AML) with low-dose cytarabine (LDS) plus 13-*cis*-retinoic acid (RA). *Proc Annu Meet Am Soc Clin Oncol* 1989; 8: A801.
331. Schwartz EL, Brown BJ, Nierenburg M, et al. Evaluation of marcellomycin using an *in vivo* model for studying drug-induced leukemia cell differentiation. *Proc Am Assoc Cancer Res* 1982; 23: 173.
332. Schwartz EL, Sartorelli AC. Structure-activity relationships for the induction of differentiation of HL-60 human acute promyelocytic leukemia cells by anthracyclines. *Cancer Res* 1982; 42: 2651.
333. Schwartz EL, Snoddy JR, Kreutter D, et al. Synergistic induction of HL-60 differentiation by 1alpha, 25-dihydroxyvitamin D_3 and dimethylsulfoxide (DMSO) (meeting abstract). *Proc Am Assoc Cancer Res* 1983; 23: 71.
334. Senior RM, Cambell EJ, Landis JA, et al. Elastase of U937 monocyte-like cells. *J Clin Invest* 1982; 69: 384.
335. Shabo Y, Lotem J, Rubinstein M, et al. The myeloid blood cell differentiation-inducing protein MGI-2A is interleukin-6. *Blood* 1988; 72: 2070.
336. Shen L, Guyre PM, Fanger MW. Direct stimulation of ADCC by cloned gamma interferon is not ablated by glucocorticoids: Studies using a human monocyte-like cell line (U937). *Mol Immunol* 1983; 21: 167.
337. Shiina Y, Abe E, Miyaura C, et al. Biological activity of 24, 24-difluoro-1alpha, 25-dihydroxyvitamin D_3 and 1-alpha, 25-dihydroxyvitamin D_3-26, 23-lactone in inducing differentiation of human myeloid leukemia cells. *Arch Biochem Biophys* 1983; 220: 90.
338. Silverman LR, Davis RB, Holland JF, et al. 5-Azacytidine (AZ) as a low dose continuous infusion is an effective therapy for patients with myelodysplastic syndromes (MDS). *Proc Annu Meet Soc Clin Oncol* 1989; 8: A768.
339. Sing GK, Keller JR, Ellingsworth LR, et al. Transforming growth factor beta selectively inhibits normal and leukemic human bone marrow cell growth *in vitro*. *Blood* 1988; 72: 1504.
340. Sing GK, Keller JR, Ellingsworth LR, et al. Transforming growth factor-β1 enhances the suppression of human hematopoiesis by tumor necrosis factor-α or recombinant interferon-α. *J Cell Biochem* 1989; 39: 107.
341. Souza L, Boone T, Gabrilove J, et al. Recombinant human granulocyte colony-stimulating factor: effects on normal and leukemic cells. *Science* 1986; 232: 61.
342. Sporn M, Todaro G. Autocrine secretion and malignant transformation of cells. *N Engl J Med* 1980; 303: 878.
343. Stanley E, Heard P. Factors regulating macrophage production and growth. Purification and some properties of the colony stimulating factor for medium conditioned by mouse L cells. *J Biol Chem* 1977; 252: 4045.
344. Stevens VL, Owens NE, Winton EF, et al. Modulation of retinoic acid-induced differentiation of human leukemia (HL-60) cells by serum factors and sphingamine. *Cancer Res* 1990; 50: 222.
345. Sun GL, Huang YG, Chang XF, Jiang GS, Zhang T. Clinical study on all-*trans* retinoic acid in treatment of 544 cass of acute promyelocytic leukemia treated. *Clin J Hematol* 1992; 13: 135-137.
346. Sundstrom C, Nilsson K. Establishment and characterization of a human histiocytic lymphoma cell line (U937). *Int J Cancer* 1976; 17: 565.
347. Sutherland GR, Baker E, Hyland VJ, et al. The gene for human leukemia inhibitory factor (LIF) maps to 22q12. *Leukemia* 1989; 3: 9.
348. Svet-Moldavskaya I, Arlin Z, Svet-Moldavskaya G. Induction by tumor-promoting phorbol diester of colony-stimulating activity in human myeloid leukemia cells transformed to macrophage-mimicking cells. *Cancer Res* 1981; 41: 4335.
349. Takeda K, Minowada J, Bloch A. Kinetics of appearance of differentiation-associated characteristics in ML-1, a line of human myeloblastic leukemia cells, after treatment with 12-O-tetradecanoylphorbol-13-acetate, dimethyl sulfoxide, or 1-β-D-arabinofuranosylcytosine. *Cancer Res* 1982; 42: 5152.
350. Takeda K, Iwamoto S, Sugimoto H, et al. Identity of differentiation inducing factor and tumour necrosis factor. *Nature* 1986; 323: 338.
351. Takenaga K, Hozumi M, Sakagami Y. Effect of retinoids on induction of differentiation of cultured mouse myeloid leukemia cells. *Cancer Res* 1980; 40: 914.
352. Tamatani T, Urawa H, Hashimoto T, et al. Tumor necrosis factor as an interleukin 1-dependent differentiation inducing factor (D-Factor) for mouse myeloid leukemic cells. *Biochem Biophys Res Commun* 1987; 143: 390.
353. Tanabe O, Kawano M, Tanaka H, et al. BSF-2/IL-6 does not augment Ig secretion but stimulates proliferation in myeloma cells. *Am J Hematol* 1989; 31: 258.
354. Tanaka Y, Deluca HF, Schnoes HK, et al. 24, 24-Difluoro-1.25-dihydroxyvitamin D3: *In vitro* production, isolation, and biological activity. *Arch Biochem Biophys* 1980; 199: 473.
355. Taniguchi T, Matsui H, Fujita T, et al. Structure and expression of a cloned cDNA for human interleukin-2. *Nature* 1983; 302: 305.
356. Tessier N, Hoang T. Transforming growth factor beta inhibits the proliferation of the blast cells of acute myeloblastic leukemia. *Blood* 1988; 72: 159.

357. Thesingh CW, Burger EH. Origin of osteoclast progenitor cells from central blood cell forming organs. *Calcif Tissue Int* 1981; 335: 108.
358. Tobler A, Gasson J, Reichel H, et al. Granulocyte-macrophage colony-stimulating factor. Sensitive and receptor-mediated regulation by 1,25-dihydroxyvitamin D_3 in normal human peripheral blood lymphocytes. *J Clin Invest* 1987; 79: 1700.
359. Tobler A, Munker R, Heitjan D, et al. *In vitro* interaction of recombinant tumor necrosis factor alpha and all-*trans*-retinoic acid with normal and leukemic hematopoietic cells. *Blood* 1987; 70: 1940.
360. Todd R III, Griffin J, Ritz J, et al. Expression of normal monocyte-macrophage differentiation antigens on HL-60 promyelocytes undergoing differentiation induced by leukocyte-conditioned medium or phorbol ester. *Leuk Res* 1981; 5: 491.
361. Tohyama K, Ohmori S, Ueda T, et al. Cooperative effects of gamma-interferon and 1 alpha, 25-dihydroxyvitamin D-3 on *in vitro* differentiation of the blast cells of RAEB and RAEB-T. *Blut* 1989; 58: 181.
362. Tomida M, Yamamoto-Yamaguchi Y, Hozumi M. Purification of a factor inducing differentiation of mouse myeloid leukemic M1 cells from conditioned medium of mouse fibroblast L929 cells. *J Biol Chem* 1984; 259: 10978.
363. Tricot G, Jayaram HN, Zhen W, et al. Biochemically directed therapy with tiazofurin of refractory leukemia and myeloid blast crisis of chronic granulocytic leukemia. *Proc Am Assoc Cancer Res* 1991; 32: 184.
364. Trinchieri G, Rosen M, Perussia B. Retinoic acid cooperates with tumor necrosis factor and immune interferon in inducing differentiation and growth inhibition of the human promyelocytic leukemic cell line HL-60. *Blood* 1987; 69: 1218.
365. Tsoukas C, Provvedine DM, Manolagas SV. 1,25-Dihydroxyvitamin D3: A novel immunoregulatory hormone. *Science* 1984; 224: 1438.
366. Turner RT, Puzas JE, Forte MD, et al. *In vitro* synthesis of 1,25$(OH)_2$ D_3 by isolated calvarial cells. *Proc Natl Acad Sci USA* 1980; 7i7: 5720.
367. Vadhat L, Eardley A, Heller G, Warrell RP Jr. Leukocytosis, the retinoic acid syndrome, and early mortality in acute promyelocytic leukemia: when is chemotherapy needed during remission induction with all-*trans* retinoic acid. *Blood (Suppl.)* 1993; 82: 192A.
368. Van Beek W, Tulp A, Egbers-Bogards M, et al. Continuous expression of cancer-related fucosyl glycopeptides on surface of human promyelocytic leukemic cells (HL-60) following terminal differentiation *in vitro*. *Cancer Res* 1982; 42: 5222.
369. Van Beek W, Tulp A, Bolscher J, et al. Transient versus permanent expression of cancer-related glycopeptides on normal versus leukemic myeloid cells coinciding with marrow egress. *Blood* 1984; 63: 170.
370. Van der Schoot CE, Jansen P, Porter M, et al. Interleukin-6 and interleukin-1 production in acute leukemia with monocytoid differentiation. *Blood* 1989; 74: 2081.
371. Van Snick J, Cayphas S, Szikora J-P, et al. cDNA cloning of murine interleukin-HP1: homology with human interleukin-6. *Eur J Immunol* 1988; 18: 193-197.
372. Van Snick J, Goethals A, Renauld JC, et al. Cloning and characterization of a cDNA for a new mouse T cell growth factor (P40). *J Exp Med* 1989; 169: 363.
373. Wahl SM, Hunt DA, Wakefield LM, et al. Transforming growth factor type beta induces monocyte chemotaxis and growth factor production. *Proc Natl Sci USA* 1987; 84: 5788.
374. Walsh JH, Karnes WE, Cuttitta F, Walker A. Autocrine growth factors and solid tumor malignancy: Conferences and Reviews. *The Western Journal of Medicine* 1991; 152.
375. Wang C, Curtis JE, Minden MD, et al. Expression of a retinoic acid receptor gene in myeloid leukemia cells. *Leukemia* 1989; 3: 264.
376. Wang C, Kelleher CA, Cheng GY, et al. Expression of the CSF-1 gene in the blast cells of acute myeloblastic leukemia: association with reduced growth capacity. *J Cell Physiol* 1988; 135: 133.
377. Wakamiya N, Stone R, Takeyama H, et al. Detection of tumor necrosis factor gene expression at a cellular level in human acute myeloid leukemias. *Leukemia* 1989; 3: 51.
378. Warrell RP Jr, Maslak P, Eardley A, et al. All-*trans* retinoic acid for treatment of acute promyelocytic leukemia: an update of the New York experience. *Leukemia* 1994; 8: 929-933.
379. Weber G. Biochemical strategy of cancer cells and the design of chemotherapy: G.H.A. Clowes Memorial Lecture. *Cancer Res* 1983; 43: 3466-3492.
380. Weh HZ, Zschaber R, Hossfeld DK. Low-dose cytosine-arabinoside in the treatment of acute myeloid leukemia (AML) and myelodysplastic syndrome (MDS). *Blut* 1984; 48: 239.
381. Wellstein A. Growth factor targeted and conventional therapy of breast cancer. *Breast Cancer Research and Treatment* 1994; 31: 141-152.
382. Welte K, Wang C, Mertelsmann R, et al. Purification of human interleukin-2 to apparent homogeneity and its molecular heterogeneity. *J Exp Med* 1982; 156: 454.
383. Welte K, Platzer E, Lu L, et al. Purification and biochemical characterization of human pluripotent hematopoietic colony-stimulating factor. *Proc Natl Acad Sci USA* 1985; 82: 1526.
384. Westin E, Wong-Staal F, Gelmann E, et al. Expressing cellular homologues of retroviral onc genes in human hematopoietic cells. *Proc Natl Acad Sci USA* 1982; 74: 2490.
385. Wilkins JA, Sigurdson SL, Rutherford W. The production of immunoregulatory factors by a human macrophage-like cell line, I. Characterization of an inhibitor of lymphocyte DNA synthesis. *Cell Immunol* 1983; 75: 328.
386. Williams RL, Hilton DJ, Pease S, et al. Myeloid leukaemia inhibitory factor maintains the developmental potential of embryonic stem cells. *Nature* 1988; 336: 684.
387. Williams DE, Cooper S, Broxmeyer HE. Effects of hematopoietic suppressor molecules on the *in vitro* proliferation of purified murine granulocyte-macrophage progenitor cells. *Cancer Res* 1988; 48: 1548.
388. Wing E, Koren H, Fischer D, Kelly V. Stimulation of a human macrophage-like cell line (U937) to inhibit the multiplication of an intracellular pathogen. *J Reticuloendothel Soc* 1981; 29: 321.
389. Wisch JS, Griffin JD, Dufe DW. Response of preleukemic syndromes to continuous infusion of low dose cytovabine. *N Engl J Med* 1985; 309.
390. Wong G, Witek J, Temple P, et al. Human GM-CSF: Molecular cloning of the complementary DNA and purification of the natural and recombinant proteins. *Science* 1985; 228: 810.
391. Yam LT, Li CY, Crosby WH. Cytochemical identification

of monocytes and granulocytes. *Am J Clin Pathol* 1971; 55: 283.

392. Yamamori T, Fukada K, Aebersold R, et al. The cholinergic neuronal differentiation factor from heart cells is identical to leukemia inhibitory factor. *Science* 1989; 246: 1412.
393. Yang Y, Ciarletta A, Temple P, et al. Human IL-2 (Multi-CSF): Identification by expression cloning of a novel hematopoietic growth factor related to murine IL-3. *Cell* 1986; 47: 3.
394. Yang YC, Ricciardi S, Ciarletta A, et al. Expression cloning of a cDNA encoding a novel human hematopoietic growth factor: human homologue of murine T cell growth factor P40. *Blood* 1989; 74: 1880.
395. Yee C, Biondi A, Wang XH, et al. A possible autocrine for interleukin-6 in two lymphoma cell lines. *Blood* 1989; 74: 798.
396. Yen A, Forbes M, DeGala G, et al. Control of HL-60 cell differentiation lineage specificity, a late event occurring after precommitment. *Cancer Res* 1987; 47: 129.
397. Yetgin S, Ozsoylu S. Myeloid metaplasia in vitamin D deficiency rickets. *Scand J Haematol* 1982; 28: 180.
398. Ymer S, Tucker Q, Sanderson C, et al. Constitutive synthesis of interleukin-3 by leukemia cell line WEHI-3B is due to retroviral insertion near the gene. *Nature* 1985; 317: 255.
399. Yoffe G, Spitzer G, Boggs BA. Determination of clonality in acute nonlymphocytic leukemia by restriction fragment length polymorphism and methylation analysis. *Leukemia* 1987; 1: 226.
400. Yokoto T, Otsuka T, Mosmann T, et al. Isolation and characterization of a human interleukin cDNA clone homologous to mouse B-cell stimulatory factor, that expresses B-cell and T-cell-stimulating activities. *Proc Natl Acad Sci USA* 1986; 83: 5894.
401. Yoshida Y, Tohyama K, Sakoda H, et al. *In vitro* and *in vivo* effects of interferon gamma and vitamin D3 in patient with RAEB. *Proc Annu Meet Jpn Cancer Assoc* 1987; 46: 168.
402. Young CW, Fanucci MP, Declan-Walsh T, et al. Phase I trial and clinical pharmacological evaluation of hexamethylene bisacetamide administration by ten-day continuous intravenous infusion at twenty-eight-day intervals. *Cancer Res* 1988; 48: 7304.
403. Young D, Wagner K, Griffin J. Constitutive expression of the granulocyte-macrophage colony stimulating factor gene in acute myeloblastic leukemia. *J Clin Invest* 1987; 79: 100.
404. Young DC, Demetri GD, Ernst TJ, et al. *In vitro* expression of colony-stimulating factor genes by human acute myeloblastic leukemia cells. *Exp Hematol* 1988; 16: 378.
405. Yourno J, Walsh J, Kornatowski G, et al. Nonspecific esterases of leukemia cell lines: evidence for activation of myeloid-associated zymogens in HL-60 by phorbol esters. *Blood* 1983; 63: 238.
406. Zagonel V, Pinto A, Attadia V, et al. Phase I-II clinical-biological study of 5-aza-2'-deoxycytidine (5AZACDR) as a differentiation inducer in acute myeloid leukemia (AML) and myelodysplastic syndromes (MDS) of elderly. *Proc Annu Meet Am Soc Clin Oncol* 1989; 8: A767.
407. Zhang XG, Klein B, Bataille R. Interleukin-6 is a potent myeloma-cell growth factor in patients with aggressive multiple myeloma. *Blood* 1989; 74: 11.
408. Zinzar S, Ohnuma T, Holland JF. Effects of simultaneous and sequential exposure to granulocytic and monocytic inducers on the choice of differentiation pathway in HL-60 promyelocytic leukemia cells. *Leuk Res* 1989; 13: 23.
409. Zumkeller W, Schofield PN. Growth factors, cytokines and soluble forms of receptor molecules in cancer patients. *Anticancer Res* 1995; 15: 343-348.

GRANULOCYTE COLONY-STIMULATING FACTOR: BIOLOGY AND CLINICAL POTENTIAL

GEORGE MORSTYN[1,2], MARYANN FOOTE[1], JEFFREY CRAWFORD[3], VERONIQUE TRILLET-LENOIR[4], DARRYL MAHER[5], DIANNE TOMITA[1], JAMES MATCHAM[6] and ROSEMARY MAZANET[1]

[1]*Amgen Inc., Thousand Oaks, California;* [2]*UCLA Medical School, Los Angeles, California;* [3]*Duke University Medical School, Durham, North Carolina;* [4]*Centre Hospitalier, Lyon Sud, France;* [5]*CSL Limited, Victoria, Australia;* [6]*Amgen Inc, Cambridge, UK*

INTRODUCTION

The study of hematopoiesis was greatly facilitated in the mid-1960s when techniques for studying hematopoietic cells in clonal culture were developed. Initially, serum or conditioned medium was added to cultures as a source of growth factors, the colony-stimulating factors (CSFs) [41]. Subsequently, four different CSFs that controlled the growth of granulocytes and macrophages were identified. In the early 1980s, the gene for granulocyte-macrophage colony-stimulating factor (GM-CSF) was cloned, and by the close of the decade, all four genes for the identified CSFs had been cloned for human and murine forms.

One of the factors that was isolated, purified, cloned, and produced in commercial quantities was granulocyte colony-stimulating factor (G-CSF), a protein that acts on the neutrophil lineage to stimulate the proliferation and differentiation of committed progenitor cells and activation of mature neutrophils. A property that distinguished G-CSF from other colony-stimulating factors and facilitated its purification, molecular cloning, and large-scale production in prokaryotic cells was its ability to induce terminal differentiation of a murine leukemic cell line (WEHI-3B). After observing that serum from endotoxin-treated mice was capable of causing the differentiation of a WEHI-3B myelomonocytic leukemic cell line Metcalf [40], named the activity GM-DF (granulocyte-macrophage differentiating factor). Further analysis showed that this serum contained G-CSF as well as GM-CSF. Nicola et al. [49] were able to further purify G-CSF from medium conditioned by lung tissue of endotoxin-treated mice. This G-CSF was able to stimulate WEHI-3B^{D+} cells as well as normal cells, supporting the formation of numerous, small, neutrophil-containing colonies at a concentration similar to that needed for WEHI-3B differentiation [50]. Subsequently, murine G-CSF was purified as a protein and was shown to have both differentiation-inducing activity for WEHI-3B^{D+} as well as granulocyte colony-stimulating activity in bone-marrow cells [49]. Other researchers, notably Asano et al. [1] and Welte et al. [73], found several human carcinoma cells that constitutively produce colony-stimulating factors, and one of these factors was purified to apparent homogeneity from the conditioned medium of bladder carcinoma 5637 cells [73] or squamous carcinoma CHU-2 [52]. As the purified CSF could stimulate specific neutrophilic granulocyte-colony formation from bone-marrow cells, it was concluded that this factor was the human counterpart to mouse G-CSF. The protein initially identified as G-CSF was also called CSF-β and Pluripoietin (pCSF).

The study of G-CSF progressed to the purification and molecular cloning of both murine and human forms and then to the first clinical trials of G-CSF in cancer patients [7, 18, 19, 45, 46, 47]. Because of its unique biological activities, recombinant human (rHu) G-CSF is used for the reversal or amelioration of neutropenias of various causes, for increasing cancer chemotherapy dose intensity, and for hematopoietic stem cell mobilization for transplantation.

Filgrastim, the non-glycosylated rHuG-CSF, was the first hematopoietic growth factor approved for commercial use (in 1991). Other forms of rHuG-CSF are lenograstim, a glycosylated rHuG-CSF; and marograstim, mutein rHuG-CSF, which has had limited clinical development to date.

Biochemistry and structure of granulocyte colony-stimulating factor

Native human G-CSF appears to exist in two forms. Type a has 177 amino acids and type b, presumably the more active form, has 174 amino acids [2, 56]. The gene for G-CSF is positioned at 17q21-22 [56].

The core protein of native human G-CSF has a molecular weight of 18.6 kilodaltons (KD) and 20 to 23.5 KD for the glycosylated protein [56]. Although marograstim has 174 amino acids as do the other two forms of rHuG-CSF, the molecule has been modified at the first, third, fourth, fifth, and seventeenth amino acids [51].

Native human G-CSF is glycosylated and crystallography studies of filgrastim have shown that the sugar chain is attached to the C-D loop, at a distance from the active biological sites [28, 53]. The actual glycosylation

R.K. Oldham (ed.), Principles of Cancer Biotherapy. 3rd ed., 423–431.

site is threonine 134 position. Although the glycosylation does not seem to have a role in the biological function of the molecule, it may partially protect the molecule from proteolytic degradation. The observation that a limited proteolytic degradation of filgrastim results in the cleavage of the molecule near threonine 134 points to a role of glycosylation for proteolytic protection, and that the residues along this portion of the protein structure may serve as handles for proteolytic degradation. The exact role of the carbohydrate group is unknown [56] and the presence and kind of glycosylation of the recombinant protein depend on the cellular source, eg, yeast, CHO, or *E. coli* [44]. It is possible that glycosylation influences the antigenicity of recombinant proteins [30].

Biology of granulocyte colony-stimulating factor

Native human G-CSF is produced by stromal cells, endothelial cells, fibroblasts, and monocytes [44, 56, 70]. Lipopolysaccharides induce monocytes and macrophages to release G-CSF [75].

The G-CSF receptor is expressed on cells of the neutrophil lineage from myeloblast to the mature neutrophil, as well as on a subset of cells of the monocyte lineage [42]. Studies in mice have shown that the number of G-CSF receptors increases as cells mature [50].

In vitro, G-CSF stimulates the proliferation, differentiation, and activation of committed progenitor cells of the neutrophil lineage and GM-CSF stimulates the proliferation, differentiation, and activation of committed progenitor cells of the monocyte/macrophage, neutrophil, and eosinophil lineages. G-CSF reduces neutrophil maturation time from 5 days to 1 day, leading to a rapid release of mature neutrophils from the bone marrow into the circulation [37, 38]. Neutrophils treated with G-CSF have at least normal survival [6, 37].

In the presence of G-CSF, neutrophils have enhanced superoxide production in response to chemoattractants [72]. G-CSF does not stimulate cytokine release, in contrast to the action of GM-CSF that stimulates the production of IL-1, IL-6, tumor necrosis factor (TNF), and other cytokines by mononuclear cells and neutrophils [57].

In vivo, in various animal species and in humans, G-CSF causes a dose-dependent increase in the number of neutrophils in the peripheral blood. This is due to decreased maturation time, increased number of cell divisions, and accelerated release into the peripheral blood. Its action on neutrophils causes rapid, dose-dependent increases while small or no effects are seen on monocytes and eosinophils, respectively [32, 36, 46].

Physiology of granulocyte colony-stimulating factor

In response to an infection or to neutropenia, the amount of circulating endogenous G-CSF in the blood increases [8], and this has been shown to increase in a variety of pathological conditions including exposure to endotoxin [8, 25, 41, 71]. The existing data suggest that within the human body, G-CSF is the primary factor for the up-regulation of neutrophils in infection and in various pathological conditions with decreased ANC levels [8]. One possible explanation for the importance of G-CSF is that G-CSF levels become elevated during bacterial infections and circulate in the blood, stimulating neutropoiesis in the marrow. GM-CSF appears to remain localized at the site of infection and may play a role in retaining and activating arriving cells [57]. In cases of Gram-negative and fungal infections, G-CSF, but not GM-CSF, levels are usually elevated in the blood [25]. The highest G-CSF levels have been found in neutropenic patients and febrile neutropenic patients [8].

G-CSF is an indispensable cytokine for normal murine myelopoiesis, as has been shown by knockout-mouse experiments [29]. Circulating neutrophil levels were reduced by 70% to 80% with less of a reduction in marrow stores of progenitors (50%) to those of normal mice. Despite appearing superficially healthy, these mice have a diminished ability to mount neutrophilia and monocytosis in response to infection and have a marked impairment in ability to control *Listeria* infections. The observations from this study indicate that G-CSF is required for maintaining the normal quantitative balance of neutrophil production during steady state granulopoiesis *in vivo*, and implicates rHuG-CSF in emergency granulopoiesis during infectious episodes.

Pharmacokinetics/Pharmacodynamics

Pharmacokinetic data from the different rHuG-CSF products are difficult to compare directly, as different study designs, doses, regimens, routes of administration, and populations were used.

Five normal male volunteers given single doses of 3.45 μg/kg filgrastim by 30-minute intravenous (IV) infusion had a mean serum concentration of 20.8 ng/mL 5 minutes after end of infusion. This is probably an underestimate of the peak concentration [3]. The mean (SD) elimination half-life was 163 (±7.4) minutes.

Cancer patients receiving filgrastim 11.5 μg/kg as a 30-minute IV infusion had a peak serum concentration of 384 ng/mL [18, 19].

When cancer patients received subcutaneous (SC) bolus or SC infusion doses, serum concentrations of filgrastim reflected rapid absorption [45].

With filgrastim, the maximum increase in ANC can be achieved by all routes of administration tested [45, 76].

Following single SC injections of lenograstim 10, 20, or 40 μg in healthy volunteers, C_{max} values were 0.09, 0.18, and 0.48 μg/L within 3.5 to 4.5 hours, peak serum concentrations were maintained for almost 4 hours, and lenograstim was almost eliminated from the serum by 48 hours [61].

The serum half-life of filgrastim has a $t_{1/2}$ of 3.5 hours; sargramostim (yeast-derived rHuGM-CSF), $t_{1/2}a$ 12 to 17 minutes; and molgramostim (*E. coli*-derived rHuGM-CSF) $t_{1/2}b$ 0.2 to 9.1 hours [30].

Adverse effects

Filgrastim does not produce dose-limiting side effects even at 115 μg/kg, a dose that can cause marked leukocytosis (50 x 10^9/L) [33]. The only commonly reported side effect of rHuG-CSF administration has been mild-to-moderate bone pain [16, 23]. Additional adverse events have been reported in patients with severe chronic neutropenia (SCN) receiving long-term rHuG-CSF therapy and have included splenomegaly (usually detected only on protocols requiring imaging studies), rash, and mild alopecia. Formation of antibodies to rHuG-CSF has not been reported [30].

Clinical implications

Chemotherapy

Reviews of clinical experience with rHuG-CSF can be found in several papers [23, 31, 65]. Phase III trials have demonstrated the beneficial effect of rHuG-CSF on neutropenia following standard-dose chemotherapy. Two randomized, placebo-controlled, double-blind studies involving more than 300 patients with small-cell lung cancer (SCLC) receiving cyclophosphamide, adriamycin, etoposide (CAE) chemotherapy showed that filgrastim significantly decreased the incidence, severity, and duration of severe neutropenia [12, 68] (reviewed in detail below). Crawford has recently reanalyzed the phase 3 trial conducted in the United States to assess for the incidence of mucositis, a secondary endpoint in the trial [10]. During the first cycle, 47% of the patients receiving placebo developed mucositis compared with 28% of patients receiving filgrastim ($p = 0.006$). Across all cycles of treatment, the crude relative risk of developing at least one episode of mucositis was 1.61 for the placebo group versus the filgrastim group.

In other randomized, placebo-controlled, double-blind trials, filgrastim allowed increases in dose intensity of doxorubicin [5] and cyclophosphamide, adriamycin, 5-fluorouracil (CAF) chemotherapy [15].

The two randomized, double-blind, placebo-controlled trials involved a total of 341 SCLC patients receiving CAE chemotherapy [12, 68]. Recombinant HuG-CSF (filgrastim) (230 μg/kg/day) was given SC beginning 24 hours after the last dose of chemotherapy and continuing for 14 days. These studies showed that filgrastim, compared with placebo, significantly reduced the incidence of febrile neutropenia as well as the duration of IV antibiotics and duration of hospitalization. Overall, the relative risk of infection was reduced by approximately 50% with filgrastim.

These two multicenter, randomized, double-blind, placebo-controlled trials of r-metHuG-CSF (filgrastim) as an adjunct to chemotherapy for SCLC were reanalyzed. The objective of both studies was to test the hypothesis that administration of filgrastim to patients with SCLC reduced the proportion of patients who experienced at least one febrile neutropenic episode during three cycles of CAE chemotherapy.

A total of 341 patients were randomized into the two studies and 321 were evaluable for analysis. Exclusion from analysis was primarily because of withdrawal before study treatment, not fulfilling entry criteria, and/or being febrile on day 1 of the first cycle of chemotherapy. All patients gave informed written consent before they were randomized to receive either CAE chemotherapy with filgrastim (n=155) or CAE chemotherapy with placebo (n=166). Although the treatments were given in a double-blind manner, patients in one study were unblinded before the start of the next cycle if they had experienced an episode of febrile neutropenia (ie, temperature ≥38.2° and absolute neutrophil count [ANC] $<0.5 \times 10^9$/L). These patients were then treated with open-label filgrastim. For this reason, only data from the first cycle of chemotherapy were used in the joint analysis. The patients in the two randomized treatment groups were similar in terms of disease status, ECOG status, bone-marrow involvement, age, weight, and sex.

Filgrastim was scheduled to be given at a dose of 230 or 240 μg/m^2. The first dose of study medication was given on day 4 of each cycle of chemotherapy and continued for a maximum of 14 consecutive days and could be discontinued if the ANC $>10 \times 10^9$/L after day 12. No dose escalation or reduction was permitted. Patients who developed an oral temperature ≥38.2°C and ANC $<1 \times 10^9$/L were hospitalized and treated with empiric IV antibiotics. The analyses were adjusted to account for the effects of center and disease.

The results of this study showed that the chances of a filgrastim-treated patient experiencing an episode of febrile neutropenia was 0.32 times lower than the same odds for a placebo-treated patient ($p<0.001$; CI = [0.19, 0.53]). Similarly, the odds of a filgrastim-treated patient experiencing an episode of fever was 0.41 times lower than the same odds for a placebo-treated patient ($p<0.001$). The reduction in odds was observed to be similar when the studies were analyzed individually also. This was due to a reduced incidence of both fever and febrile neutropenia (Table 1 and Table 2).

The use of Filgrastim translated into a reduction in the odds of requiring either IV antibiotics or hospitalization with evidence of infection (0.38 and 0.37 times lower, respectively; $p<0.001$ in each case) (Table 3 and Table 4). These reductions were observed also when the studies were analyzed separately.

The joint analysis demonstrated that the use of filgrastim significantly reduced the incidence of febrile neutropenia, fever, use of IV antibiotics, and hospitalization with evidence of infection.

In the Crawford et al. [12] and Trillet-Lenoir et al. [68] studies, it was shown that in the placebo or control group, many of the febrile neutropenic events occurred in the first cycle. Crawford et al. [11], in a follow-up study, showed that delaying filgrastim for 5 days after chemotherapy was inferior to initiating treatment 1 or 3 days

Table 1. Joint analysis for the incidence of fever in two studies of CAE chemotherapy for small-cell lung cancer

Study	Filgrastim or Placebo	Incidence	No incidence	Total	Adjusted Odds Ratio	Adjusted 95% CI	p value
Crawford	Filgrastim	35	58	93		(0.24,	
(1991)	Placebo	62	40	102	0.43	0.76)	0.004
Trillet-Lenoir	Filgrastim	18	44	62		(0.17,	
(1993)	Placebo	31	33	64	0.38	0.84)	0.017
	Filgrastim	53	102	155		(0.26,	
Total	Placebo	93	73	166	0.41	0.66)	<0.001

p value: Cochran-Mantel-Hanszel test.

Table 2. Joint analysis for the incidence of fever in two studies of CAE chemotherapy for small-cell lung cancer

Study	Filgrastim or Placebo	Incidence	No incidence	Total	Adjusted Odds Ratio	Adjusted 95% CI	p value
Crawford	Filgrastim	26	67	93		(0.17,	
(1991)	Placebo	58	44	102	0.31	0.57)	<0.001
Trillet-Lenoir	Filgrastim	10	52	62		(0.13,	
(1993)	Placebo	22	42	64	0.33	0.81)	0.016
	Filgrastim	36	119	155		(0.19,	
Total	Placebo	80	86	156	0.41	0.53)	<0.001

p value: Cochran-Mantel-Hanszel test.

Table 3. Joint analysis for the incidence of fever in two studies of CAE chemotherapy for small-cell lung cancer

Study	Filgrastim or Placebo	Incidence	No incidence	Total	Adjusted Odds Ratio	Adjusted 95% CI	p value
Crawford	Filgrastim	34	59	93		(0.21,	
(1991)	Placebo	62	40	102	0.37	0.68)	0.001
Trillet-Lenoir	Filgrastim	14	48	62		(0.17,	
(1993)	Placebo	26	38	64	0.39	0.91)	0.028
	Filgrastim	48	107	155		(0.23,	
Total	Placebo	88	78	166	0.38	0.62)	<0.001

p value: Cochran-Mantel-Hanszel test.

Table 4. Joint analysis for the incidence of hospitalization with evidence of infection in two studies of CAE chemotherapy for small-cell lung cancer

Study	Filgrastim or Placebo	Incidence	No incidence	Total	Adjusted Odds Ratio	Adjusted 95% CI	p value
Crawford	Filgrastim	33	60	93		(0.19,	
(1991)	Placebo	63	39	102	0.34	0.63)	<0.001
Trillet-Lenoir	Filgrastim	16	46	62		(0.19,	
(1993)	Placebo	27	37	64	0.43	0.98)	0.045
	Filgrastim	49	106	155		(0.23,	
Total	Placebo	90	76	166	0.38	0.60)	<0.001

p value: Cochran-Mantel-Hanszel test.

after chemotherapy. In this same study, patients with extensive SCLC were randomized to one of three filgrastim schedules following the same 3-day CAE chemotherapy regimen used in the initial US, randomized trial. Filgrastim was given SC at 5 μg/kg/day starting 1 day (day 4), 3 days (day 6), or 5 days (day 8) after completion of chemotherapy. Treatment with filgrastim continued through the neutrophil nadir until day 18 or until an ANC $>10 \times 10^9$/L was reached. During the first cycle of chemotherapy, the duration of neutropenia was similar for all three schedules, although the day-8 patients experienced a delayed neutrophil recovery compared with the other two groups. In subsequent cycles of treatment, delay of filgrastim was associated with suboptimal hematological recovery compared with patients who initiated filgrastim either 1 day or 3 days following chemotherapy. This study implies that the benefits of filgrastim are schedule dependent and caution must be used in empirically delaying the initiation of filgrastim for more than a few days following chemotherapy.

Filgrastim has a role as an adjunct to the use of antibiotics in the treatment of febrile neutropenia. Maher et al. (1994) performed a multicenter, randomized, placebo-controlled, double-blind study to determine if neutrophil and fever recovery were accelerated when filgrastim was started after the onset of chemotherapy-induced febrile neutropenia. Patients with solid tumors, lymphomas, or acute lymphoblastic leukemia were given filgrastim (109 patients) or placebo (107 patients) by SC infusion within 12 hours of a standard course of piperacillin and tobramycin. Treatment was continued until an ANC $> 0.5 \times 10^9$/L and four afebrile days (temperature <37.5°) had elapsed. The analyses were adjusted to account for baseline differences in ECOG performance status, tumor type, and number of days from the last day of chemotherapy to the onset of febrile neutropenia. The results of the study showed that Filgrastim reduced the mean days of neutropenia (3.3 vs 4.3 with ANC $<0.5 \times 10^9$/L), fever (4.1 vs 5.1 days), and febrile neutropenia (4.8 vs 6.3 days) (Table 5). The mean number of days hospitalized on study was reduced also from 10.0 to 8.7, although this was not statistically significant. Filgrastim was more beneficial, in general, for patients with culture-positive or clinically documented infections than for patients with possible or unlikely infections. The relative risk of prolonged hospitalization (fourth quartile, ie, >11 days) for the filgrastim group was half that of the placebo group. The use of filgrastim in this patient population with febrile neutropenia following chemotherapy resulted in accelerated recovery of neutrophil count and a decreased risk of prolonged hospitalization.

High-dose chemotherapy

In other studies, new chemotherapeutic concepts or new agents such as paclitaxel (Taxol®) have been tested with rHuG-CSF as a standard adjunct. Compared with previous experience without rHuG-CSF in a study of paclitaxel with filgrastim, the incidence, depth, and duration of neutropenia was reduced [58]. In a study to determine the maximum tolerated doses and principal toxicities of a combination of paclitaxel and cisplatin, doses of these drugs could be increased with the support of filgrastim, but severe peripheral neuropathy and/or severe myalgias became the predominant toxicities [59]. In a study undertaken to define and escalated dose schedule of MVAC (methotrexate, vinblastine, doxorubicin, and cisplatin) with the support of filgrastim, the delivered relative dose intensity was 33% higher than the previously reported one without hematopoietic support. Leukopenia and thrombocytopenia became dose limiting [60]. A randomized, phase 3 trial in patients with non-Hodgkin's lymphoma (NHL) showed that filgrastim significantly improved delivery of full-dose chemotherapy compared with control patients [55].

In the high-dose chemotherapy and autologous bone-marrow transplantation setting, use of filgrastim shortened the duration of severe neutropenia approximately 1 week compared with historical control patients [54, 64, 66]. An ANC recovery to $>0.5 \times 10^9$/L was achieved in 14 days or less in studies with rHuG-CSF.

The reduction in neutropenia was associated with a reduction in the number of days with fever and a shorter duration of parenteral antibiotic use post-transplantation [64]. In a 2-year, multicenter, randomized, vehicle-controlled, single-blind, dose-ranging trial lenograstim

Table 5. Intent-to-treat analysis of neutropenia, fever, febrile days, and days on study with filgrastim (Maher et al., 1994)

	Filgrastim		Placebo		P-value
Days of:	Mean	Median (range)	Mean	Median (range)	
ANC $<0.5 \times 10^9$/L	3.3	3.0 (0–12)	4.3	4.0 (0–15)	0.005
ANC $<1.0 \times 10^9$/L	3.9	3.0 (1–13)	4.6	5.0 (1–18)	0.001
Fever ≥37.5° C	4.1	3.0 (1–18)	5.1	3.0 (0–28)	0.12
Febrile neutropenia	4.8	4.0 (0–18)	6.3	5.0 (0–28)	0.001
Days on study	8.7	8.0 (1–20)	10.0	8.0 (3–28)	0.09

was administered SC in 121 patients with non-myeloid malignancies. A dose-response effect was apparent, and neutrophil recovery was significantly accelerated while infectious complications were reduced [21, 34, 35].

Recombinant HuG-CSF alone or in combination with chemotherapy is an effective agent for recruiting peripheral blood progenitor cells (PBPC) with long-term reconstituting ability [9, 17, 22, 26, 62, 63]. In an historically controlled study, filgrastim-generated PBPC, in conjunction with autologous bone-marrow transplantation and daily SC filgrastim, accelerated recovery of neutrophil and platelet count [62]. Use of filgrastim for mobilization resulted in a significantly accelerated time to recovery of granulocytes when compared with non-mobilized PBPC recipients in a study of 85 patients with relapsed (Hodgkin's disease (HD) [9]. The use of mobilized PBPC resulted in a significantly accelerated time to platelet engraftment when compared with non-mobilized PBPC recipients. There was a statistically significant reduction of costs in patients who received filgrastim-mobilized PBPC.

Marrow-failure states

Recombinant HuG-CSF has been shown to increase neutrophil counts in some patients with moderate aplastic anemia (AA) but, in general, patients with very severe hypoplasia do not respond to growth factors, and their use is still experimental [4, 27]. In a Japanese study with 20 children with severe or intermediate AA, a dose of 400 µg/m^2/day increased the neutrophil count in 12 patients. Increasing doses to as great as 1200 µg/m^2 were administered to five patients who did not respond to the initial dose, and three of the five then showed an increase in ANC [27].

Studies have been done in patients with myelodysplastic syndromes (MDS), and treatment with filgrastim has been associated with a sustained improvement in neutrophil function, but without increased adherence or impaired chemotaxis [48]. A phase 2 study showed the efficacy of lenograstim, with most patients responding to IV doses of 2 or 5 µg/kg/day [77]. In a phase 3 randomized study involving 102 patients with RAEB or RAEB-t subtypes of MDS, filgrastim was shown to be efficacious in increasing ANC [20], although imbalances in patient characteristics made the overall benefit, if any, of the use of rHuG-CSF in this setting difficult to define.

A phase 3 trial of filgrastim in SCN patients has shown long-term efficacy (>200 patient-years experience) and tolerance, and the hematologic and clinical benefits were sustained during maintenance treatment [13, 14]. In one study, when children with SCN did not respond to treatment with rHuGM-CSF, they were switched to treatment with filgrastim with a resulting increase in neutrophil counts [74].

Other myelosuppression

The potential of CSFs to ameliorate the myelosuppression of antiviral and anti-infective therapies has been investigated in uncontrolled studies. Filgrastim given for 2 weeks at doses of 0.3 to 3.6 µg/kg/day, increased neutrophil numbers 9-fold, and maintained this increase during concomitant therapy with recombinant human erythropoietin (rHuEPO) and zidovudine [43]. Use of filgrastim permitted some patients to receive full doses of antiviral therapy and these patients had preserved or improved neutrophil function. Filgrastim has been shown to improve tolerance to ganciclovir allowing delivery of full doses [24]. In a phase 1/2 trial, lenograstim 0.4 to 10 µg/kg/day SC at low doses was effective in ameliorating zidovudine-induced neutropenia [69]. Most patients required 2.0 µg/kg/day, and two of twelve patients required 0.4 µg/kg/day.

Current issues

The current issues being investigated include an evaluation of the cost benefit of using rHuG-CSF in various clinical settings. The American Society of Clinical Oncology (ASCO) reported guidelines on the appropriate usage in oncology. Studies are underway to investigate the impact on survival in dose-intensive chemotherapy with rHuG-CSF as an adjunct. The first results of a large, cooperative group trial in the United States are expected in 1997. New areas of research, including combining rHuG-CSF with thrombopoietic factors, started in 1995. It is already clear that the study of growing blood cells in culture more than 30 years ago established a scientific field from which many patients have already had great clinic benefits.

ACKNOWLEDGMENTS

Drs. Morstyn, Foote, and Mazanet, Ms Tomita, and Mr Matcham are employees of Amgen Inc., the manufacturer of filgrastim. The authors thank the patients and nursing staffs of the hospitals where the studies were done.

REFERENCES

1. Asano S, Sato N, Mori M, et al. Detection and assessment of human granulocyte-macrophage colony-stimulating factor (GM-CSF) producing tumours by heterotransplantation into nude mice. *Br J Cancer* 1980; 41: 689-694.
2. Asano S. Human granulocyte colony-stimulating factor: its basic aspects and clinical applications. *Am J Ped Hematol/Oncol* 1991; 13: 400-413.
3. Azuma J, Kurimoto T, Awata S, et al. Phase I study of KRN 8601 (rhG-CSF) in normal healthy volunteers: safety and pharmacokinetics in single subcutaneous administration. *Rinsho Iyaku* 1989; 5: 2231-2252.
4. Bessho M, Toyoda A, Itoh Y, et al. Trilineage recovery by

combination therapy with recombinant human granulocyte colony-stimulating factor (rhGCSF) and erythropoietin (rhEPO) in severe aplastic anemia. *Br J Haematol* 1992; 80: 409-411.

5. Bronchud MH, Howell A, Crother D, et al. Phase I/II study of recombinant human granulocyte colony-stimulating factor to increase the intensity of treatment with doxorubicin in patients with advanced breast and ovarian cancer. *Br J Cancer* 1989; 60: 121-128.
6. Bronchud MH, Potter MR, Morgenstern G, et al. *In vitro* and *in vivo* analysis of the effects of recombinant human granulocyte colony-stimulating factor in patients. *Br J Cancer* 1988; 58: 64-69.
7. Bronchud MH, Scarffe JH, Thatcher N, et al. Phase I/II study of recombinant human granulocyte colony-stimulating factor in patients receiving intensive chemotherapy for small cell lung cancer. *Br J Cancer* 1987; 56: 809-813.
8. Cebon JS, Layton JE, Maher D, Morstyn G. Endogenous haemopoietic growth factors in neutropenia and infection. *Br J Haematol* 1994; 86: 263-274.
9. Chao NJ, Schriber JR, Grimes K, et al. Granulocyte colony-stimulating factor 'mobilized' peripheral blood progenitor cells accelerate granulocyte and platelet recovery after high-dose chemotherapy. *Blood* 1993; 81: 2031-2035.
10. Crawford J, Glaspy J, Vincent M, Tomita D, Mazanet R. Effect of Filgrastim (r-metHuG-CSF) on oral mucositis patients with small cell lung cancer (SCLC) receiving chemotherapy (cyclophosphamide, doxorubicin and etoposide, CAE). *Proc ASCO* 1994; 13: 442 (abstract 1523).
11. Crawford J, Kreisman H, Garewal H, et al. A pharmacodynamic investigation of recombinant human granulocyte colony stimulating factor (r-metHuG-SCF) schedule variation in patients with small cell lung cancer (SCLC) given CAE chemotherapy. *J Clin Oncol* 1992; 11: 299 (abstract 1005).
12. Crawford J. Reduction by granulocyte colony-stimulating factor of fever and neutropenia induced by chemotherapy in patients with small-cell lung cancer. *N Eng J Med* 1991; 325: 164-170.
13. Dale DC, Bonilla MA, Davis MS, et al. A randomized controlled phase III trial of recombinant human granulocyte colony-stimulating factor (Filgrastim) for treatment of severe chronic neutropenia. *Blood* 1993; 81: 2496-2502.
14. Dale DC, Hammond WP, Gabrilove J, et al. Long term treatment of severe chronic neutropenia with recombinant human granulocyte colony-stimulating factor (r-metHuG-CSF). *Blood* 1990; 76: 139A (abstract 545).
15. Demetri G, Younger J, McGuire BW, et al. Recombinant methionyl granulocyte-CSF (r-metG-CSF) allows an increase in the dose intensity of cyclophosphamide / doxorubicin / 5-fluorouracil (CAF) in patients with advanced breast cancer. *Proc ASCO* 1991; 10: 70 (abstract 153).
16. Decoster G, Rich W, Brown SL. Safety profile of Filgrastim (r-metHuG-CSF). IN: *Filgrastim (r-metHuG-CSF) in Clinical Practice.* G Morstyn and TM Dexter, ed. Marcel Dekker, Inc. New York, NY. 1994; pages 267-290.
17. Dürhsen U, Villeval JL, Boyd J, Kannourakis G, Morstyn G, Metcalf D. Effects of recombinant human granulocyte colony-stimulating factor on hematopoietic progenitor cells in cancer patients. *Blood* 1988; 72: 2074-2081.
18. Gabrilove JL, Jakubowski A, Fain K, et al. Phase I study of granulocyte colony-stimulating factor in patients with transitional cell carcinoma of the urothelium. *J Clin Invest* 1988; 82: 1454-1461.
19. Gabrilove JL, Jakubowski A, Scher H, et al. Effect of granulocyte colony-stimulating factor on neutropenia and associated morbidity due to chemotherapy for transitional-cell carcinoma of the urothelium. *N Engl J Med* 1988; 318: 1414-1422.
20. Greenberg P, Taylor K, Larson R, et al. Phase III randomized multicenter trial of G-CSF vs observation for myelodysplastic syndromes (MDS). *Blood* 1993; 82: 196a (abstract768).
21. Harousseau JL. Lenograstim after bone marrow transplantation: results of a European multicenter randomised study in 315 patients. *Satellite Symposium to the 24th Congress of the ISH*; 1992.
22. Hohaus S, Goldschmidt H, Ehrhardt R, Haas R. Successful autografting following myeloablative conditioning therapy with blood stem cells mobilized by chemotherapy plus rhG-CSF. *Exp Hematol* 1993; 21: 508-514.
23. Hollingshead LM, Goa KL. Recombinant granulocyte colony-stimulating factor (rG-CSF). A review of its pharmacological properties and prospective role in neutropenic conditions. *Drug Evaluation* 1991; 42: 300-330.
24. Jacobsen MA, Stanley HD, Heard SE. Ganciclovir with recombinant methionyl human granulocyte colony-stimulating factor for treatment of cytomegalovirus disease in AIDS patients. *AIDS* 1992; 6: 515-517.
25. Kawakami M, Tsutsumi H, Kumakawa T, et al. Levels of serum granulocyte colony-stimulating factor in patients with infections. *Blood* 1990; 76: 1962-1964.
26. Kawano Y, Takaue Y, Watanabe T, et al. Effects of progenitor cell dose and preleukapheresis use of human recombinant granulocyte colony-stimulating factor on the recovery of hematopoiesis after blood stem cell autografting in children. *Exp Hematol* 1993; 21: 103-108.
27. Kojima S, Fukuda M, Miyajima Y, Matsuyama T, Horibe K. Treatment of aplastic anemia in children with recombinant human granulocyte colony-stimulating factor. *Blood* 1991; 77: 937-941.
28. Kuga T, Komatsu Y, Yamaski M, et al. Mutagenesis of human granulocyte colony stimulating factor. *Biochem Biophys Res Comm* 1989; 159: 103-111.
29. Lieschke GJ, Grail D, Hodgson G, et al. Mice lacking granulocyte colony-stimulating factor have chronic neutropenia, granulocyte and macrophage progenitor cell deficiency, and impaired neutrophil mobilization. *Blood.* 1994; 84: 1737-1746.
30. Lieschke GJ, Burgess AW. Granulocyte colony-stimulating factor and granulocyte-macrophage colony-stimulating factor (1). *N Engl J Med* 1992; 327: 28-35.
31. Lieschke GJ, Burgess AW. Granulocyte colony-stimulating factor and granulocyte-macrophage colony-stimulating factor (2). *N Engl J Med* 1992; 327: 99-016.
32. Lieschke GJ, Cebon J, Morstyn G. Characterization of the clinical effects after the first dose of bacterially synthesized recombinant human granulocyte-macrophage colony-stimulating factor. *Blood* 1989; 74A: 2634-2643.
33. Lieschke GJ, Morstyn G. Role of G-CSF and GM-CSF in the prevention of chemotherapy-induced neutropenia; IN: *Hematopoietic Growth Factors in Clinical Applications*; R Mertelsmann and F Herrmann, eds; 1990; pages 191-223.
34. Linch DC, Scarrffe H, Proctor S, et al. Randomised vehicle-controlled dose finding study of glycosylated recombinant human granulocyte colony-stimulating factor after bone marrow transplantation. *Bone Marrow Transplant* 1993; 11: 307-311.

35. Linch DC. Lenograstim, a new glycosylated rHuG-CSF: Pharmacology and clinical profile in bone marrow transplants. *Br J Haematol* 1992; 82: 274-275.
36. Lindemann A, Herrmann F, Oster W, et al. Hematologic effects of recombinant human granulocyte colony-stimulating factor in patients with malignancy. *Blood* 1989; 74: 2644-2651.
37. Lord BI, Bronchud MH, Owens S, et al. The kinetics of human granulopoiesis following treatment with granulocyte colony-stimulating factor. *Proc Natl Acad Sci USA* 1989; 86: 9499-9503.
38. Lord BI, Gurney H, Chang J, et al. Haemopoietic cell kinetics in humans treated with rGM-CSF. *Int J Cancer* 1992; 50: 26-31.
39. Maher DW, Lieschke GJ, Green M, et al. Filgrastim (r-metHuG-CSF) in patients with chemotherapy-induced febrile neutropenia. *Ann Int Med* 1994; 121: 492-501.
40. Metcalf D. Clonal extinction of myelomonocytic leukaemia cells by serum from mice injected with endotoxin. *Int J Cancer* 1980; 25: 225-233.
41. Metcalf D. *The Molecular Control of Blood Cells*. Harvard University Press. Cambridge, MS; 1988.
42. Metcalf D, Morstyn G. Colony Stimulating Factors: General Biology. IN: *Biologic Therapy of Cancer*; V De Vita, ed; Philadelphia, JB Lippincott; 1991; pages 417-444.
43. Miles SA, Mitsuyasu RT, Moreno J, et al. Combined therapy with recombinant granulocyte colony-stimulating factor and erythropoietin decreases hematologic toxicity from zidovudine. *Blood* 1991; 77: 2109-2117.
44. Morstyn G, Burgess AW. Hemopoietic growth factors: a review. *Cancer Res* 1988; 48: 5624-5637.
45. Morstyn G, Campbell L, Lieschke G, et al. Treatment of chemotherapy-induced neutropenia by subcutaneously administered granulocyte colony-stimulating factor with optimization of dose and duration of therapy. *J Clin Oncol* 1989; 7: 1554-1562.
46. Morstyn G, Campbell L, Souza LM, et al. Effect of granulocyte colony-stimulating factor on neutropenia induced by cytotoxic chemotherapy. *Lancet* 1988; 1: 667-672.
47. Morstyn G, Lieschke GJ, Cebon J, et al. Early clinical trials with colony-stimulating factors. *Cancer Invest* 1989b; 7: 443-456.
48. Negrin RS, Haeuber DH, Nagler A, et al. Maintenance treatment of patients with myelodysplastic syndromes using recombinant human granulocyte colony-stimulating factor. *Blood* 1990; 7: 36-43.
49. Nicola NA, Metcalf D, Matsumoto M, Johnson GR. Purification of a factor inducing differentiation in murine myelomonocytic leukaemia cells: identification as granulocyte colony-stimulating factor (G-CSF). *J Biol Chem* 1983; 258: 9017-9023.
50. Nicola NA. Hemopoietic cell growth factors and their receptors. *Annu Rev Biochem* 1989; 58: 45-77.
51. Nio Y, Shiraishi T, Tsubono M, et al. Comparative effects of a recombinant and a mutein type of granulocyte colony stimulating factor on the growth of Meth-A fibrosarcoma with 5-fluorouracil chemotherapy. *Biotherapy* 1992; 4: 81-86.
52. Nomura H, Imazeki I, Oheda M, et al. Purification and characterization of human granulocyte colony stimulating factor (G-CSF). *EMBO J* 1986; 5: 871-876.
53. Osslund T, Boone TC. Biochemistry and structure of Filgrastim (r-metHuG-CSF). IN: *Filgrastim (r-metHuG-CSF) in Clinical Practice*. G Morstyn and TM Dexter, ed. Marcel Dekker, Inc. New York, NY. 1994; pages 23-31.
54. Peters WP, Kurtzberg J, Atwater S, et al. Comparative effects of rHuG-CSF and rHuGM-CSF on hematopoietic reconstitution and granulocyte function following high dose chemotherapy and autologous bone marrow transplantation (ABMT). *Proc ASCO* 1989; 18: 18A.
55. Pettengell R, Gurney H, Radford J, et al. Granulocyte colony-stimulating factor to prevent dose-limiting neutropenia in non-Hodgkin's lymphoma: a randomized controlled trial. *Blood* 1992; 80: 1430-1436.
56. Platzer E. Human hemopoietic growth factors. *Eur J Haematol* 1989; 42: l-15.
57. Rapoport AP, Abboud CN, Di Persio JF. Granulocyte-macrophage colony-stimulating factor (GM-CSF) and granulocyte colony-stimulating factor (G-CSF): receptor biology, signal transduction, and neutrophil activation. *Blood Reviews* 1992; 6: 43-57.
58. Reichman BS, Seidman AD, Crown JP, et al. Paclitaxel and recombinant human granulocyte colony-stimulating factor as initial chemotherapy for metastatic breast cancer. *J Clin Oncol* 1993; 11: 1943-1951.
59. Rowinsky EK, Chaudhry V, Forastiere AA, et al. Phase I and pharmacologic study of paclitaxel and cisplatin with granulocyte colony stimulating factor: neuromuscular toxicity is dose-limiting. *J Clin Oncol* 1993; 11: 2010-2020.
60. Seidman AD, Scher HI, Gabrilove JL, et al. Dose-intensification of MVAC with recombinant granulocyte colony-stimulating factor in the treatment of advanced urothelial cancer. *J Clin Oncol* 1993; 11: 408-414.
61. Sekino H, Moriya K, Sugano T, Wakabayashi K, Okazaki A. Recombinant human G-CSF (rG-CSF). *Shinryo to Shinyaku* 1989; 26: 32-104.
62. Sheridan WP, Begley CG, Juttner CA, et al. Effect of peripheral-blood progenitor cells mobilised by filgrastim (G-CSF) on platelet recovery after high-dose chemotherapy. *Lancet* 1992; 339: 640-644.
63. Sheridan WP, Juttner C, Szer J, et al. Granulocyte colony-stimulating factor (G-CSF) in peripheral blood stem cell (PBSC) and bone marrow transplantation. *Blood* 1990; 76: S1.
64. Sheridan WP, Morstyn G, Wolf M, et al. Granulocyte colony-stimulating factor and neutrophil recovery after high-dose chemotherapy and autologous bone marrow transplantation. *Lancet* 1989; 2: 891-895.
65. Steward WP. Granulocyte and granulocyte-macrophage colony-stimulating factors. *Lancet* 1993; 342; 153-157.
66. Taylor KM, Jagganath S, Spitzer G, et al. Recombinant human granulocyte colony-stimulating factor hastens granulocyte recovery after high-dose chemotherapy and autologous bone marrow transplantation in Hodgkin's disease. *J Clin Oncol* 1989; 7: 1791-1799.
68. Trillet-Lenoir V, Green J, Manegold C, et al. Recombinant granulocyte colony stimulating factor reduces the infectious complications of cytotoxic chemotherapy. *Eur J Cancer* 1993; 29A: 319-324.
69. Van der Wouw PA, van Leeuwen R, van Oers RH, et al. Effects of recombinant human granulocyte colony-stimulating factor on leucopenia in zidovudine-treated patients with AIDS and AIDS related complex, a phase l/ll study. *Br J Haematol* 1991; 78: 319-324.
70. Vellenga E, Rambaldi A, Ernst TJ, Ostapovicz D, Griffin JD. Independent regulation of M-CSF and G-CSF gene

expression in human monocytes. *Blood* 1988; 71: 1529-1532.

71 Watari K, Asano S, Shirafuji N, et al. Serum granulocyte colony-stimulating factor levels in healthy volunteers and patients with various disorders as estimated by enzyme immunoassay. *Blood* 1989; 73: 117-122.

72. Weisbart RH, Golde DW. Physiology of granulocyte and macrophage colony-stimulating factors in host defense. *Hematol Oncol Clin of North Am* 1989; 3: 401-409.

73. Welte K, Platzer E, Lu L, et al. Purification and biochemical characterization of human pluripotent hematopoietic colony-stimulating factor. *Proc Natl Acad Sci USA* 1985; 82: 1526-1530.

74. Welte K, Ziedler C, Reiter A, et al. Differential effects of granulocyte colony-stimulating factor and granulocyte-macrophage colony-stimulating factor in children with severe congenital neutropenia. *Blood* 1990; 75: 1056-1063.

75. Wong GG, Witek JS, Temple PA, et al. Human GM-CSF: molecular cloning of the complementary DNA and purification of the natural and recombinant proteins. *Science* 1985; 228: 810-815.

76. Young JD, Cheung EN, Tanaka H, Hasibeder H, Asano K, Shimosaka A. Bioavailability of subcutaneously administered non-glycosylated recombinant hG-CSF (Filgrastim) in normal and neutropenic rats. *Proc ASCO* 1994; 13: 162 (abstract 443).

77. Yoshida Y, Hirashima K, Asano S, et al. A phase ll trial of recombinant human granulocyte colony-stimulating factor in the myelodysplastic syndromes. *Br J Haematol* 1991; 78: 378-384.

GRANULOCYTE-MACROPHAGE COLONY-STIMULATING FACTOR (GM-CSF): BIOLOGY AND CLINICAL STATUS

ANN JAKUBOWSKI
Memorial Sloan-Kettering Cancer Center, New York, New York

BIOCHEMICAL PURIFICATION AND MOLECULAR AND BIOLOGIC CHARACTERIZATION

Granulocyte-macrophage colony-stimulating factor (GM-CSF) is one of the naturally-occurring glycoprotein hormones which regulate hematopoietic precursors in the bone marrow and peripheral blood effector cells. It is one of the original 'colony-stimulating factors' whose name is derived from its major target cell lineages (Table 1). Although it was initially purified from media used to culture a monoclonal T-lymphoblastoid cell line (Mo) [50], it has also since been found to be produced by a variety of cell types including macrophages, endothelial cells and certain mesenchymal cells. There are no basal serum levels of GM-CSF in normal adults, but its production is readily inducible by many of the mediators of inflammation. The gene for GM-CSF was sequenced and cloned in 1985 [26, 151] and has been expressed in *E. coli*, chinese hamster ovary (CHO) cells and yeast resulting in the availability of large amounts of glycosylated and nonglycosylated material for clinical trials. The gene for GM-CSF encodes a protein of 127 amino acids whose molecular weight varies from 14-35,000 daltons depending upon the degree of glycosylation. It has been mapped to the long arm of chromosome 5 (5q21-32) [80] in the cluster region of genes for other growth factor proteins and their cell surface receptors, such as interleukin-3 [88], -4 [154], -5 [142] and macrophage colony stimulating factor, as well as its receptor – the c-fms proto-oncogene product [116] and the receptor for platelet-derived growth factor [153]. The growth factor produced by expression of the cDNA in bacteria is not glycosylated [21] but that expressed in mammalian cells and yeast demonstrates variable degrees of glycosylation [26]. Both the glycosylated and nonglycosylated forms are active *in vitro* or *in vivo* and are similar in activity to the natural form of the protein.

Table 1. Characteristics of human GM-CSF and its receptor

		Reference
	Gene location	
GM-CSF protein	5q23-31	(80)
GM-CSF receptor		
alpha subunit (low affinity)	X-Y pseudoautosomal region	(59)
beta subunit (high affinity)	22q.13.1	(137)
	Protein characteristics	
GM-CSF peptide	127 amino acids	(151)
M.W.	14.7 kD	
GM-CSF receptor		
alpha subunit	378 amino acids	(52)
M.W.	45 kD	
beta subunit	897 amino acids	(71)
rhGM-CSF proteins studied in clinical trials		
E. coli-derived	nonglycosylated	
yeast-derived	glycosylated	
CHO-derived	glycosylated	

GM-CSF generates predominantly granulocyte and monocyte colonies in semisolid culture systems [98, 132]. It acts as a potent stimulus for the growth of uncommitted and committed bone marrow progenitors including CFU-GEMM, CFU-GM, and CFU-E [98, 132] and human BFU-E in the presence of erythropoietin. As a growth factor for immature progenitors, it has greater activity than G-CSF, but less of a proliferative effect than IL-3. There is some evidence, *in vitro* and in animals that at low concentrations, GM-CSF stimulates proliferation only of macrophages while, as the concentration is increased, production of granulocytes is enhanced, followed by megakaryocytes and, at high concentrations, multilineage and erythroid precursors. Demonstration of such dose-related stimulation in humans has not been accomplished as yet.

At the level of mature cells, GM-CSF enhances the function of neutrophilic and eosinophilic granulocytes, and of monocyte/macrophages. Exposure of neutrophils to GM-CSF produces increased expression of cellular adhesion molecules [5, 32, 63] such as CD11b, an increased number of FMLP receptors [148], as well as increased FMLP- induced superoxide production [147], chemotaxis, antibody dependent cellular cytotoxicity (ADCC), phagocytosis and neutrophil viability. *In vitro*, it

R.K. Oldham (ed.), Principles of Cancer Biotherapy. 3rd ed., 432–446.

inhibits random neutrophil granulocyte migration [51] and *in vivo*, when administered by continuous infusion, prevents neutrophils from migrating into areas of inflammation [115]. Similarly, GM-CSF prolongs the survival of neutrophilic and eosinophilic granulocytes *in vitro* [94] and enhances their killing of parasites such as Schistosoma larvae, and their leukotriene synthesis [134]. Its effect on monocytes *in vitro* is to enhance ADCC, phagocytosis and microbicidal and tumoricidal activity [60, 69, 149] as well as the synthesis and secretion of other cytokines including TNF and IL-1 [25].

Granulocyte-macrophage colony-stimulating factor exerts its biologic activity by binding to specific transmembrane surface receptors on the target cells, which are subsequently internalized [34, 49]. They have been detected on neutrophils, monocytes, normal bone marrow progenitors, and fresh leukemic cells as well as leukemic cell lines [17, 18, 24, 111]. They are greatest in number on the most mature cells [24], and GM-CSF, itself, can downregulate these receptors on neutrophils, monocytes and normal bone marrow myeloid cells *in vitro* [24]. Although the signal transduction pathways remain somewhat obscure, and it is known that the receptor has no intrinsic tyrosine kinase activity, binding of GM-CSF does induce phosphorylation of a set of cytoplasmic phosphoproteins [81]. Crosslinking experiments have revealed molecular weights of 75-156 kD. There are now believed to be at least two types of GM-CSF receptors one higher affinity (approx. 20-100 pmol/L) and a second lower affinity (1 nmol/L), though one report has postulated as many as four types on AML cells [17]. There are two subunits (alpha and beta) which comprise the receptors; both have recently been cloned [52, 71]. Several studies have demonstrated that IL-3 receptors (also low and high affinity) which are coexpressed on many of the same cells as the GM-CSF receptors, competitively bind these two growth factor proteins [39, 55, 17]. Specifically IL-3 competes for the high affinity GM-CSF receptors. One proposed explanation for competitive binding is based on experiements in which the IL-3 high affinity receptor was reconstituted by combining the alpha-subunit of the IL-3 receptor with the beta-subunit of the GM-CSF receptor. These experiments suggested that IL-3 and GM-CSF receptor share a common beta-subunit, for which they compete when both proteins are present.

PATHOPHYSIOLOGIC ROLE OF rhGM-CSF IN HEALTH AND DISEASE

Basal serum levels of GM-CSF have not been detected in normal adults under physiologic conditions. *In vitro*, however, there appears to be an absolute requirement for such growth factors as GM-CSF for the survival and proliferation of hematopoietic progenitors, and it is possible that a similar requirement exists *in vivo*. In order to assimilate these facts, it has been suggested that GM-CSF may function locally at areas of production such as the bone marrow and/or that it is rapidly cleared from the circulation. Regulation of the production of growth factors like GM-CSF probably involves a complex network of positive and negative feedback mechanisms which incorporate other growth factors and cytokines especially those associated with inflammation.

As has been observed in studies of other hematopoietic growth factors such as G-CSF, IL-3 and M-CSF, mRNA for GM-CSF is produced by myeloblasts from some patients with acute myelogenous leukemia (AML) [155]. In addition, in clonogenic assay of fresh cells from patients with AML, GM-CSF was able to replace other exogenous growth factors required for maximum growth stimulation in the majority of cases studied [64]. Progenitors from patients with juvenile chronic myelogenous leukemia have also demonstrated increased sensitivity to stimulation by GM-CSF [40]. Similar studies of samples from patients with acute lymphocytic leukemia (ALL) have shown increased blast colony formation in approx. 40% of the 19 samples tested, and the presence of mRNA for GM-CSF or its receptor in 4 of 5 ALL cell lines studied [44]. Although the exact mechanisms and the signficance of these observations remains unclear, they do suggest a possible role for GM-CSF in the pathogenesis and/or management of acute leukemia. The issue of elevated serum growth factor levels overstimulating hematopoietic precursors and producing leukemia has been addressed by the transgenic mouse studies. Although these animals exhibit leukocyte hyperplasia, they do not develop a 'clonal' population of cells which would characterize a leukemia [86].

Since the focus of most hematopoietic growth factor clinical trials has been on bone marrow rescue following chemotherapy-treatment for solid tumors, the influence of these factors on the growth of such tumors has been of ongoing concern. Developmental similarities have been observed between blood and neural crest cells and, in fact, receptors for some hematopoietic growth factors have been detected on the normal counterparts of the neural crest tumors, i.e. high affinity GM-CSF receptors on microglia, astrocytes and oligodendrocytes from rats. The functionality of these receptors has been suggested by the report that the oligodendrocytes proliferate in the presence of GM-CSF [48]. Several laboratories have reported the expression of different types of GM-CSF receptors on a variety of cell lines and fresh tumor specimens. For example, while a high-affinity, functional GM-CSF receptor has been detected on small cell lung cancer cell lines [7, 125], a lower affinity receptor protein was found on melanoma cell lines and fresh melanoma tumor samples [9]. Studies of the growth response *in vitro*, as well as induction of early response genes on these melanoma tumors did not support the functionality of these receptors. The responsiveness to GM-CSF of osteogenic sarcoma, colon, breast and prostate cancer cell lines *in vitro* [11, 31, 43] as well as *in vitro* tumor cloning assays of a variety of tumor specimens from lung, breast, colon and ovarian cancer patients [43, 127] has shown variable response and there has even been a report of growth inhibition of a tumor cell line by GM-CSF [152]. The role of hematopoietic growth factors and more specifically GM-CSF in the growth *in vitro* of normal and malignant nonhematopoietic cells, thus, remains variable and in many cases ambiguous. Fortunately, despite its use *in vivo* for thousands of patients with tumors, stimulation of their solid tumors has not been reported.

CLINICAL APPLICATIONS

Both glycosylated and nonglycosylated forms of rhGM-CSF have undergone extensive clinical study. All three preparations of growth factor, *E. coli*-derived, CHO cell-derived and yeast-derived, and three possible routes of administration (short IV infusion, continuous IV infusion (CIV) and subcutaneous (SC)) have been studied. Although analysis and comparison of study results are therefore complex, a general overview will be presented. At the present time only glycosylated rhGM-CSF has received approval from the Food and Drug Administration (FDA) for use in patients. It has been approved for utilization in the setting of bone marrow transplantation for lymphoid malignancies, in bone marrow failure, and most recently following induction chemotherapy for patients with AML and in the generation of peripheral blood stem cells (Table 2).

In the classic phase I studies of rhGM-CSF in patients with normal hematologic profiles, the biologic effects and toxicities have frequently been dose-dependent. One exception to this is the rapid, transient neutropenia, which when produced by the IV route, has a maximum nadir at approx. 30 min [33, 75], and by SC administration at approx. 60 min [90]. The duration of these nadirs have been upto 2 and 4 hours, respectively, but the dose-dependence of this effect has been variable between studies [74, 90, 91]. The WBC recovers to baseline or above and may involve eosinophils and monocytes as well as neutrophils. Radiolabelling of leukocytes suggested that this transient leukopenia was due to sequestration of the cells within the lung [33]. *In vitro* and *in vivo* studies have suggested that this effect may be due to a change in cell surface adhesion molecules on the leukocytes such as those identified by CD11b [5, 136] which is upregulated on neutrophils, as well as LAM-1, which is down-regulated, and adherence to endothelial cells of the blood vessels [63].

Table 2. FDA approved indications for clinical use of rhGM-CSF

For acceleration of myeloid reconstitution in patients with non-Hodgkin's lymphoma, acute lymphoblastic leukemia and Hodgkin's disease undergoing autologous bone marrow transplantation
To promote engraftment when it is delayed or has failed in patients who have undergone allogeneic or autologous bone marrow transplantation
To accelerate myeloid recovery following induction chemotherapy in older adult patients with acute myelogenous leukemia
For use in mobilization and following transplantation of autologous peripheral blood progenitor cells.

The major effect of rhGM-CSF on hematopoiesis is the leukocytosis which has been reported to be dose-dependent in most of the early studies [3, 75, 90] when either glycosylated or nonglycosylated rhGM-CSF was administered daily by the SC route or by prolonged intravenous (IV) or SC infusions. Results from IV bolus administration were more variable [75, 91]. The pattern of the leukocytosis in many of these same trials frequently appeared as a biphasic response – an initial increase which frequently plateaued during the first few days of treatment, followed by a decline. With continued dosing, however, another increase in leukocytes, which often contained more immature myeloid cells such as myelocytes, promyelocytes and even myeloblasts was observed. Increases in leukocytes of up to 20-fold have been reported. Appearance of monocytes and eosinophils generally occurred later in the course of treatment and at higher doses of GM-CSF [75]. In comparing fold increases of neutrophils, monocytes and eosinophils for continuous SC to IV dosing on day 5 and day 10 [91] the results were greater for SC than IV. This is in agreement with the results of pharmacokinetic studies which usually demonstrated longer duration of serum levels for SC than IV administration at equivalent doses. In patients who had a history of extensive previous myelosuppressive therapy, or who had an altered hematologic profile, such as patients with AIDS, etc., the neutrophil response was frequently less than in the patients with 'healthier' bone marrows, and the increase in the WBC count was often comprised of greater numbers of immature myeloid cells as well as, in some cases, eosinophils and monocytes [2, 46, 65, 146]. Blood counts decreased to normal over a 1-2 week period after discontinuing the rhGM-CSF therapy. Over all of the phase I studies there was no consistent increase in platelets or reticulocytes. Morphologic changes in neutrophils included toxic granulation with an increase in leukocyte alkaline phosphatase, prominent Döhle bodies, cytoplasmic vacuolization and, at higher doses, increasing numbers of hypersegmented neutrophils [75]. In a variety of studies, including that of Bukowski et al. [19], there was no significant increase in NK or LAK activity in patients receiving rhGM-CSF. However, increased expresssion of HLA-DR and decreased expression of high affinity Fc receptors on monocytes, and transient increased expression of CD11b and CD16 on granulocytes has been observed [75, 137, 139]. At the higher doses of rhGM-CSF in patients with normal marrows, the cellularity of the bone marrow was increased with a ' left-shift' and an increase in the myeloid-to-erythroid ratio [3, 19, 75, 90, 139].

An important observation made during these early trials, which would later find significant clinical application, was the increase in peripheral blood erythroid and myeloid progenitors. This was noted to be dose dependent [75, 138, 139]. Bone marrow progenitors were found to be unchanged [75, 138] or decreased [139], probably somewhat dependent upon the degree of expansion of the non-colony forming myeloid mononuclear cells. Furthermore, kinetic studies of progenitors revealed that nonglycosylated rhGM-CSF given to patients produced a 32-79% increase in S-phase BFU-E, 43-82% increase in S-phase day14 CFU-GM and 41-56% increase in S-phase d7 CFU-GM in the bone marrow . The GM-CSF also decreased the duration of S-phase from 14.3 to 9.1 h and the cell cycle time from 86 to 26 h. Interestingly, within 24 h of discontinuing the GM-CSF, the proportion of BM cells in S-phase dropped to levels lower than those observed pretreatment and suggested a possible period of refractoriness to cycle specific drugs [1].

Pharmacokinetic studies have been conducted using both glycosylated and nonglycosylated rhGM-CSF by radioimmunoassay and by bioassay. Route of administration was reported to affect the peak serum concentration, area under the concentration-time curve, and the time during which GM-CSF was detectable in the serum. Cebon et al. [27], using their immunoassay, reported patient-to-patient variation in serum levels and rate of elimination, even for the same dose of nonglycosylated rhGM-CSF when it was administered by SC injection. The time during which the growth factor remained detectable was dose-dependent, and levels persisted for prolonged periods of time compared to those observed with IV dosing. When doses >10 mcg/kg were administered, serum levels of 1 ng/ml (that concentration *in vitro* required for near-maximal stimulation of colony formation) were detected for >12 h. In the patients who received IV bolus infusions, there appeared to be a two compartment model for this protein. The decrease in hGM-CSF levels occurred with a $T1/2\alpha < 5$ min, and a slower $T1/2\beta = 150$ min. For yeast=derived, glycosylated rhGM-CSF after IV bolus injection, the first phase of clearance was determined to be $T1/2 = 10 \pm 3$ min, that for the second phase was 85 ± 35 min, also by radioimmunassay [75].

CHEMOTHERAPY-INDUCED NEUTROPENIA

A number of phase I, I/II, II, and even III studies have been conducted in order to study the ability of both glycosylated and nonglycosylated rhGM-CSF to abrogate the hematologic toxicity of chemotherapy – standard and dose-intensified therapy – and following bone marrow transplantation. Most of these studies have been nonrandomized, have included relatively small numbers of patients, and have compared the results of cycles of chemotherapy given without growth factor to those given with growth factor, and cycles of chemotherapy given with growth factor compared to data of historical controls. Utilizing dose escalation regimens, or stable myelosuppressive doses of chemotherapy in combination with any of the preparations of rhGM-CSF, a number of observations have been reported. Results of studies have been published in patients with sarcoma [3, 144], ovarian cancer using IV [29, 36, 83, 126], SC [121] or intraperitoneal [96] chemotherapy, small cell [20, 95, 131] and non-small cell lung cancer [84], breast [56, 78, 110], bladder [93, 101], gastrointestinal [62, 140], head and neck [97], germ cell [6] cancers as well as those with 'advanced malignancies' [75, 100, 109, 118]. Hodgkin's [79] and non-Hodgkin's [53, 56, 77] lymphomas, and multiple myeloma [10]. In most of these studies, rhGM-CSF, like other growth factors, did not completely eliminate profound leukopenia. When the rhGM-CSF administration was initiated soon after the chemotherapy was completed, there was often a rise in the neutrophil count prior to its decline. In general, the neutrophil nadir occurred earlier in the courses of chemotherapy in which rhGM-CSF was administered than in the courses without. Higher doses of the growth factor in some studies resulted in lessening of the depth of the ANC nadir, and most frequently there was a shortening of the duration of neutropenia and time to an ANC of >1000 cells/μl at least during the first cycle of chemotherapy administered with the rhGM-CSF. The ability to reduce the morbidity (hematologic and in some cases the incidence of infection and mucositis) of dose intensification, i.e. to be able to dose more frequently or on schedule [79] or with higher doses of IV [36, 56, 84, 93, 97, 126] or intraperitoneal [96] chemotherapy, was demonstrated in several of these studies. In most cases, duration of neutropenia was reduced by the growth factor at least during the first cycle in which it was used. Its effect on the parameters of platelet count were variable. These ranged from reduced platelet transfusion requirements or improved platelet counts at least during the first cycle of chemotherapy [10, 29, 36, 56, 77, 140], to no difference between cycles with rhGM-CSF compared to those without [93, 144], to cumulative thrombocytopenia seen with >1 cycle which may even have been greater than that for controls [78, 84, 97, 101, 109] . It has been proposed that twice-a-day SC dosing of rhGM-CSF may be more beneficial to platelet counts than other schedules of administration [37, 126]. As a consequence, therefore, thrombocytopenia became dose limiting in several studies. Although dose intensification was feasible using rhGM-CSF, and some of the studies demonstrated increased tumor response, the issue of improved survival was not addressed in most. An interesting observation, made during some of these studies, was that the benefit in the neutrophil response with dose-intensified regimens was often not sustained with repeated cycles of chemotherapy and rhGM-CSF [6, 78, 101, 126, 131]. The incidence and severity of mucositis, and/or incidence of febrile neutropenia, and possible infection requring hospitalization with the use of antibiotics were described in a limited number of studies and

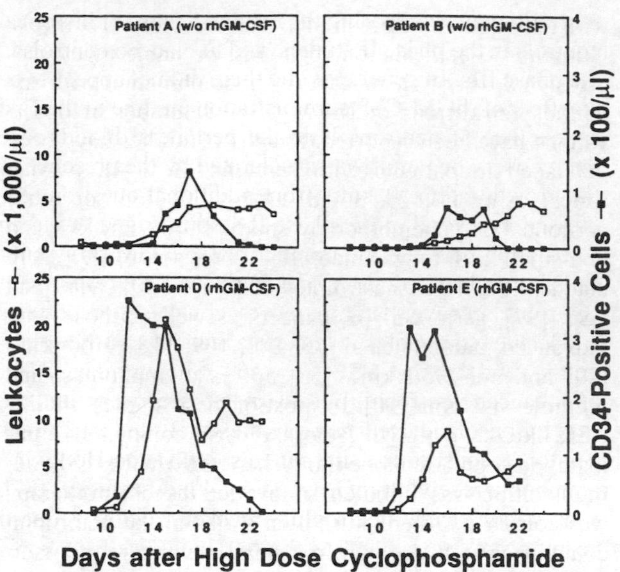

Figure 1.

were improved compared to control cycles of chemotherapy alone, for ≥ 1 cycle of therapy in some [53, 56, 76-78]. Unfortunately, fever, a known side effect of rhGM-CSF [114], may have contributed to the 'incidence' of 'febrile neutropenia' in some studies.

One important observation made during these earlier studies was the relationship of neutrophil response to dosing shedule. Figure 1 shows the leukocyte response of four patients with breast cancer and non-Hodgkin's lymphoma who received 7g/m² of cyclophosphamide. Patients A and B received no rhGM-CSF, D and E received it from day +1 to +14. Recovery of a patient, who received the rhGM-CSF from day +5 to +14, was reported to be essentially the same as that shown for patients A and B [133].

At least two reports have focussed attention on using novel scheduling of rhGM-CSF. In patients receiving oral daily etoposide with rhGM-CSF for five days prior to chemotherapy, or concurrently with the chemotherapy, the neutropenia and/or thrombocytopenia was increased compared to that of patients who received etoposide alone [129]. A second study reported enhanced myeloprotection and ability to dose-intensify the chemotherapy by shortening the duration of chemotherapy (CyADIC) from 5 to 3 days. Patients acted as their own controls by receiving the first course of chemotherapy without growth factor. After count recovery, a 14 day course of rhGM-CSF was administered and completed 1 week prior to the second course of chemotherapy [144]. The study design was also modified to 'compress' the duration of chemotherapy. Appropriate dose and scheduling of this growth factor, as with others, remains a common issue in clinical trials. There have been two randomized studies with larger numbers of patients published using rhGM-CSF in the post-chemotherapy setting [6, 53]. In one [53], a randomized, double-blind, placebo-controlled phase III trial, using a dose intensified regimen of COP-BLAM, there was a reduced frequency of clinically relevant infections, shorter periods of neutropenia, days with fever, and days of hospitalization for infection. In the second study [6] an open-labelled, randomized, crossover trial using a 5 day regimen of chemotherapy (VIP or VeIP), rhGM-CSF reduced the incidence of infections in the first cycle of chemotherapy, but not in subsequent cycles. This latter study again raises the possibility, as suggested prevously [144] that the prolonged duration of chemotherapy (and delay in starting treatment with the growth factor) may impact on the efficacy of the growth factor.

Despite all of the studies conducted with rhGM-CSF post-chemotherapy, and in spite of its clear effectiveness in elevating granulocyte counts in this setting, it has not been approved by the FDA for this indication and its use in this setting remains investigational.

PERIPHERAL BLOOD STEM CELLS

One of the more novel areas of research involving growth factors has been their use in generating peipheral blood stem cells (PBSC). Although it is difficult to collect stem cells from the peripheral blood of a patient who is in a hematologic 'steady-state', it has been known for some time that the number of circulating stem cells increases during blood count recovery after treatment with chemotherapy, especially cyclophosphamide. The phase I and I/II studies on hematopoietic growth factors, including rhGM-CSF, demonstrated that even when given alone they could increase the number of PBSC [138], and when administered after chemotherapy the number was enhanced even further [133]. Interestingly, however, the acceleration of neutrophil count recovery and increased number of CD34+ circulating cells was observed when the rhGM-CSF was administered on days 1-14, but not when the treatment was given on days 5-14 Figure 1. Immunologic phenotyping and *in vitro* growth characteristics of the CD34+ cells from peripheral blood and bone marrow were similar.

The PBSC harvested by leukopheresis during rhGM-CSF priming without chemotherapy, or while a patient is receiving growth factor to abrogate the myelosuppression of chemotherapy have been utilized to: 1) supplement bone marrow following autologous bone marrow transplantation [57], 2) support dose-intensified chemotherapy when growth factor alone is not adequate [130], and when autologous bone marrow was previously used for hematopoietic support [38, 68]. In these early studies, the standard criteria for days to engraftment, as well as number of days of antibiotic requirement, days of hospitalization and numbers of transfusions were determined for patients participating in these studies who received bone marrow alone, bone marrow plus rhGM-CSF, bone marrow plus rhGM-CSF-primed PBSC +/– rhGM-CSF, and/or rhGM-CSF-primed PBSC +/– rhGM-CSF. In many of these comparative trials, the use of rhGM-CSF-primed stem cells produced improved neutrophil recovery [38, 57, 113, 130]. In some studies, days to platelet engraftment, days of antibiotic use and hospitalization, and number of transfusions were also compared and shown to be improved by using the primed PBSC [38, 57, 130]. More recently, investigators at the University of Nebraska reported the results of PBSC transplantations in 144 patients, who had marrow defects that precluded autologous bone marrow transplantation [13]. Eighty-six patients had cells collected without mobilization, and fifty-eight received either 125 or 250 mcg/m^2 /day of rhGM-CSF by CI for mobilization. Results of these studies demonstrated: 1) that the number of aphereses required to collect the preestablished number of PBSC was significantly fewer in the rhGM-CSF mobilized patients than the unmobilized patients; 2) that the time to neutrophil recovery after transplant was significantly shorter for the mobilized groups; 3) that transplantation with mobilized stem cells resulted in a shorter time to platelet ($p = 0.04$) and red blood cells ($p = 0.01$) transfusion independence. As a consequence of these and similar studies, rhGM-CSF has not been approved by the FDA for use in mobilization and following transplantation of autologous PBSC. One important issue, in this area, which remains a focus of ongoing investigation is the possible contamination of PBSC by tumor cells [112, 123].

BONE MARROW TRANSPLANTATION

For autologous, allogeneic and syngeneic transplantation, rhGM-CSF has been administered after the conditioning regimen and reinfusion of bone marrow to shorten the duration and reduce the severity of neutropenia, and thus decrease the requirement for supportive care, and the duration of hospitalization.

The earliest study which utilized rhGM-CSF after autologous bone marrow reinfusion was conducted in 19 patients with breast cancer and melanoma using a CI of mammalian-derived rhGM-CSF [15]. The results in these patients were compared to historical controls and showed no statistically significant difference in days with ANC <1000 between the two groups, but did demonstrate faster recovery of WBC and higher day 14 counts in the grwoth factor-treated patients. There was no consistent effect noted on platelet counts. On the other hand, a phase I/II study utilizing yeast-derived rhGM-CSF as a 2 h IV infusion in patients with lymphoid malignancies found that, when compared to 86 disease-matched and treatment-matched historical controls, patients receiving ≥60 mcg/m^2/day rhGM-CSF recovered neutrophil and platelet counts more rapidly, had fewer days with fever, and were discharged from the hospital sooner [106]. Subsequent phase II, and III studies explored further the effect of rhGM-CSF on neutrophil recovery, incidence of fever and sepsis, duration of hospitalizations and in some cases mortality rate , comparing the results to those of historical controls in the phase II studies, and to placebo controls in the phase IIIs. In general, while there did not appear to be an effect of rhGM-CSF administration on time to the first appearance of neutrophils in the peripheral blood, once the recovery began, it was accelerated by the presence of the growth factor. Results from additional questions addressed in several of the phase II studies suggested a) an association between the number of CFU-GM progenitor cells infused per kilogram and an rhGM-CSF response in neutrophil recovery compared to controls, for patients with acute lymphoblastic leukemia receiving purged autografts and rhGM-CSF at ≥64 mcg/m^2/day [14]; b) enhanced neutrophil but not platelet recovery, and the suggestion of delayed marrow stem cell and early progenitor reconstitution in patients with non-Hodgkin's lymphoma receiving rhGM-CSF by 4 h IV infusion [87], and c) enhanced neutrophil recovery with reduced hospital stays in patients with non-Hodgkin's lymphoma receiving CI rhGM-CSF [108]. Toxicities were mild to moderate with the shorter infusions, and more severe with the CI method of administration. Subsequently, a number of prospective, randomized, placebo-controlled studies, with purged and unpurged bone marrow grafts were conducted using 2-6h or CIV of rhGM-CSF in patients with lymphoid malignancies, which confirmed the earlier phase II results [58, 67, 92, 104]. Studies conducted in patients with Hodgkin's [67] and lymphoid malignancies [104] using the shorter IV infusions (6 and 2 h, respectively) of rhGM-CSF demonstrated that the more rapid recovery of neutrophils, produced statistically significant fewer days of initial hospitalization, fewer infections and fewer days of antibiotics (in the latter study), with no difference in survival at 32 and 100/months, respectively, between controls and rhGM-CSF- treated patients. Although one study reported more rapid engraftment of platelets [67], in general, there was no consistent effect on red blood cells or platelets in the phase II and III studies. In addition, the study which demonstrated a platelet advantage also reported a cost benefit to the use of rhGM-CSF. The combined results of three studies in patients with lymphoid malignancies were instrumental in obtaining approval from the FDA for use of rhGM-CSF in such patients. The dose recommended for use following bone marrow transplantation is 250 mcg/m^2/day. Long-term follow-up of patients with lymphoid malignancies demonstrated no deleterious effects on bone marrow function, and disease-free and overall survival similar for the control and rhGM-CSF-treated groups [104, 120]. Furthermore, in an attempt to identify clinical variables which might predict for speed of neutrophil recovery, only previous exposure to stem cell toxins led to significant delays in neutrophil recovery, but even those patients benefited from the administration of rhGM-CSF [120].

Studies in patients undergoing allogeneic bone marrow transplantaion have been more limited. The earliest study reporting the use of rhGM-CSF in the allo-transplant setting was a double-blind, placebo-controlled trial conducted in patients with leukemia (AML, ALL, CML) receiving matched, sibling bone marrows. Glycosylated CHO-derived rhGM-CSF was administered at 8 mcg/kg/days as a CI for 14 days. With only 20 patients in each arm, the treated patients recovered an ANC of 500 only three days sooner than the controls (not significant), though the day 14 ANC was significantly higher in the former. Hemoglobin and platelet counts were lower in the rhGM-CSF treated group. There was no difference in relapse rate for the two groups [119]. A second, randomized, placebo-controlled multicenter study enrolled 57 patients with hematologic malignancies who received sibling-donor, T-cell-depleted grafts followed by a similar 14 day CI of glycosylated rhGM-CSF [30]. Earlier neutrophil engraftment was observed, with a significantly lower incidence of bronchopneumonias in the rhGM-CSF treated-group as well as a trend toward better overall disease-free survival at two years and lower relapse risk. There was no difference in incidence of graft-versus-host disease (GVHD) and transplant-related mortality between the rhGM-CSF-treated and placebo groups. Finally, the same investigators conducted a phase I/II trial in 47 patients undergoing allogeneic transplant from HLA-identical, sibling donors, and a phase II trial in 40 patients receiving transplants from unrelated donors for hematologic neoplasia or severe aplastic anemia, utilizing a 2–h IV infusion of glycosylated, yeast-derived rhGM-CSF for 20 or 27 days after bone marrow reinfusion. In the phase I/II study, the use of methotrexate GVHD prophylaxis appeared to influence the efficacy of the rhGM-CSF in facilitating neutrophil engraftment, i.e. without methotrexate prophylaxis there was a signficantly shorter time to ANC > 1000/µl compared to patients receiving methotrexate prophylaxis [103]. In the phase II study, prophylaxis included methotrexate, and neutrophils did not recover more rapidly than the historical controls. The results of the phase II study, however, suggested a decreased number of febrile days and septic episodes during the first 28 days in the rhGM-CSF-treated patients [102]. As in the randomized studies, there was no increase in the incidence of GVHD with growth factor treatment.

A second indication for which rhGM-CSF has been approved by the FDA is its use in patients with graft failure after bone marrow tranplantation (allogeneic, autologous or syngeneic). One early study [105] in this group of patients demonstrated >50% of patients achieving an ANC of ≥ 500/µl within two weeks of beginning rhGM-CSF therapy. Unfortunately, none of the patients who had received purged, autologous marrow grafts responded. Survival rates in the growth factor-treated group appeared significantly better than in the historical controls.

MYELODYSPLASIA

Granulocyte-macrophage colony-stimulating factor is one of the hematopoietic growth factors which has demonstrated multilineage activity, *in vitro* and somewhat more variably *in vivo*, stimulating the formation of granulocytes, macrophages, erythroid cells, and megakaryocytes. Furthermore, it has demonstrated an ability to enhance effector cell function, and to induce differentiation of some leukemic cell lines. Several investigators, therefore, studied its activity as therapy for patients with myelodysplastic syndrome, who frequently have bi- and often tri-lineage cytopenias, as well as dysfunctional granulocytes. The focus of most of these studies was improvement in blood counts, and determination of whether or not myeloblasts were stimulated; very little has been reported about changes in the incidence of infection and bleeding [2, 35, 47, 61, 73, 122, 128, 143, 146]. A wide range of doses were administered by a variety of dosing schedules for all of the preparations of rhGM-CSF. The reported studies have included relatively small numbers of patients, the majority of whom had been diagnosed with the poorer prognosis myelodysplastic FAB types: refractory anemia with excess of blasts (RAEB), refractory anemia with excess of blasts in transformation (RAEBT), and chronic myelomonocytic leukemia (CMMoL). In general these studies reported comparable increases in neutrophil counts but without consistent improvement in the other hematopoietic cell lines. An increase in bone marrow and peripheral blood myeloblasts and conversion to AML occurred more often in patients with RAEB and RAEBT, but in many cases, the number of myeloblasts decreased and/or returned to baseline upon discontinuation of the growth factor. In many patients the drug was discontinued due to progression of disease or to side effects. Two studies utilized rhGM-CSF + low dose cytosine arabinoside. One compared the use of rhGM-CSF to rhGM-CSF + low dose cytosine arabinoside [35] with the combined therapy producing partial short-term responses after three courses. The second study compared sequential vs. simultaneous use of the growth factor with the cytosine arabinoside [54]. The numbers of patients in each study were small, but there appeared to be no significant impact on the disease beyond what might have been expected from the low dose chemotherapy alone. Unfortunately, the results of the only phase III study have never been reported in detail [128]. Although the early report of this study noted improved neutrophil counts, similar to the smaller studies, none of the reports has demonstrated a significant improvement in the natural history of this disease or even a significant impact on its infectious or hemorrhagic complications.

ACUTE LEUKEMIA

Utilization of hematopoietic growth factors has taken a number of approaches in patients with acute leukemia: 1) for facilitating recovery from the myelosuppressive effects of induction and/or consolidation chemotherapy to reduce morbidity; 2) as a means of sensitizing myeloid leukemic cells to chemotherapy by recruitment of these cells into S-phase followed by treatment with a cycle specific drug, 3) for harvesting peripheral blood stem cells (following intensive chemotherapy) which may be used for stem cell support following bone marrow ablation; and 4) as differentiation/maturation therapy in myeloid leukemia. The appropriate concern about possibly stimulating the leukemic population, especially in AML, has resulted in the slow appearance of a limited number of studies in the literature.

The studies in which the rhGM-CSF was administered after chemotherapy to patients with AML included patients at high risk for early death during induction therapy, and older patients ≥ 55 years old who are believed to experience more complications associated with prolonged neutropenia than younger patients [16, 42, 124, 141]. Two studies [16, 124] administered the growth factor only after documenting successful ablation of leukemic myeloblasts in the bone marrow, two did not [42, 141]. Furthermore, chemotherapy varied widely among all of these studies and may have impacted on observations as suggested by a significantly improved rate of neutrophil recovery in patients receiving rhGM-CSF with the TAD9 regimen compared to those receiving the S-HAM regimen in the Buchner et al. trial. In the three earlier reports [16, 42, 141], there was no signficant difference in complete remission rate between control patients (randomized or historical) and growth factor-treated patients, though one of these did report a significantly improved 'early death rate' with rhGM-CSF treatment [16]. The phase III study, which randomized 124 patients in a double-blind, placebo-controlled trial, and monitored myeloablation prior to initiating rhGM-CSF treatment, demonstrated a significantly shortened median time to neutrophil recovery (13 v 17 days, $p = 0.001$), as well as reduced infectious toxicity ($p = 0.015$) on the rhGM-CSF arm. The median survival for the 60 patients on the rhGM-CSF arm was 10.6 v 4.8 months for the 57 patients on the placebo arm, attributable primarily to the difference in early mortality. Median disease-free survival was 8.5 v 9.6, respectively. Although 49 of the 61 patients who achieved remission received consolidation therapy (28 on rhGM-CSF and 21 on placebo), there was no significant difference in the neutrophil, platelet, or red blood cell recovery times. Based in large part on the results from this study, rhGM-CSF has been approved by the FDA for use following induction chemotherapy in older adult patients with AML to shorten time to neutrophil recovery and to reduce the incidence of severe and life-threatening infections.

The second approach taken in the use of myeloid growth factors in patients with AML has been an attempt to cycle activate leukemic cells, thus sensitizing them to cycle-specific chemotherapy, such as cytosine arabinoside, and potentially improve remission rates. Such a study design was incorporated into five clinical trials – once again some utilizing previously untreated patients, some relapsed/refractory patients, different chemotherapy regimens, and different doses and scheduling of the rhGM-CSF [4, 12, 23, 41, 72]. Overall, none of the studies demonstrated an absolute change of more than 15% in the S-phase fraction of cells during treatment with rhGM-CSF, and in general the percent change was small. When administered 24-48 h prior to and following induction chemotherapy, Bettelheim et al. [12] reported a shorter duration of neutropenia in the rhGM-CSF treated patients compared to historical controls (ANC <500, 22.5+/–3.4 v 25.2+/–3.7 days, $p<0.05$). On the other hand, a lower complete remission rate and lower survival probability was observed in a rhGM-CSF treated group of newly diagnosed patients with AML [41], and two additional studies [4, 72] reported no increased efficacy of treatment outcome in rhGM-CSF treated patients compared to controls. The marked variability in study designs, precludes any additional generalizations. Of note, however, is the observation of increased myeloblast +/– neutrophil counts in some patients who received rhGM-CSF prior to chemotherapy. Based on this and the lack of significant, demonstrable benefit, the use of rhGM-CSF in this type of study design should continue to be considered investigational.

The use of rhGM-CSF in acute lymphoblastic leukemia (ALL) has been less controversial but even fewer studies have been reported. The complex nature of most ALL chemotherapy regimens which include frequent dosing may have contributed to the limited number of reported studies. One of the early reports in patients with ALL described its use in treating two patients with profound neutropenia secondary to chemotherapy with life-threatening infections and in one case bleeding [135]. Subsequent studies, which have enrolled limited numbers of patients, have suggested reduced induction associated mortality [82], and more rapid ANC recovery [22, 70, 82]. None of the studies demonstrated an improved complete remission rate, however.

NONMALIGNANT DISEASE

Recombinant hGM-CSF has been employed in the treatment of a number of nonmalignant disorders with variable success. Numbers of patients have been limited and its use in the management of these patient populations is still considered investigational.

A handful of patients with chronic severe neutropenia have been treated with rhGM-CSF and their outcome reported . In one study [150], five children with severe congenital neutropenia were treated with rhGM-CSF at 3-30 mcg/kg/day IV. Four of these patients achieved a dose-dependent increase in granulocyte count which was comprised predominantly of eosinophils; in only one patient was it due to an increase in the neutrophil count. These responses were inferior to those observed when the same five patients received 3-15 mcg/kg/day of recombinant human granulocyte colony-stimulating factor after a one month rest period. With the rhG-CSF, all five patients demonstrated an increase in ANC to greater than 1000/µl. In a second study [45], the results were quite different. Four patients (1 congenital, 1 autoimmune, and 2 chronic idiopathic), two of whom had severe infections, were given 150-1000 mcg/m^2/day rhGM-CSF IV or SC for 12-14 days. In all of these patients, there was a marked improvement in the ANC with the therapy, which resulted in resolution of the infections in two of the patients. Finally, three patients with agranulocytosis were treated with rhGM-CSF on aplastic anemia studies [2, 28]. One demonstrated no improvement with therapy, and the other two were removed from study because of toxicity before they were able to show a response.

Clinical trials of rhGM-CSF in patients with moderate to severe aplastic anemia demonstated improvement in granulocyte and monocyte counts in at least half of the patients, but serious infections were observed even while patients were being treated in some of the studies [2, 28, 66, 107, 145]. Treatment was administered for only approx. 14 days at a time in most of the studies, and discontinuation usually resulted in an eventual return to baseline counts. Those patients with the greatest increments in white blood cell counts were those with the highest baseline counts and/or those with evidence of residual myelopoiesis. Generally, there were no consistent improvements in erythrocytes, platelets, or their transfusion requirements.

Finally, rhGM-CSF has been studied in patients with acquired immundeficiency syndrome (AIDS) and leukopenia. In fact, one of the earliest reported studies of rhGM-CSF *in vivo* was conducted in this patient population [65]. At least two studies have confirmed its efficacy in improving circulating granulocyte and monocyte counts [65, 99]. The neutrophils produced in one of these studies were found to have improved ADCC and phagocytosis properties [8]. Viral production was variable amongst these patients, and opportunistic infections continued to occur during the therapy. Subsequently, this growth factor was used to support neutrophil counts in patients with AIDS receiving azidothymidine and azidothymidine plus alpha-interferon [85, 89, 117].

ADVERSE EFFECTS

Adverse effects of rhGM-CSF have varied somewhat depending upon the expression system used to produce the protein and the method of administration. The signs and symptoms believed to be associated with the rhGM-CSF were most easily defined in the phase I and the non-chemotherapy portion of the phase I/II studies (Table 3).

Table 3. Adverse effects reported for any preparation of rhGM-CSF

- Fever
- Bone pain
- Rash
- Fluid retention
  - Peripheral edema
  - Pericardial and pleural effusions
- Local injection site reactions
- 'First dose reaction'
- Gastrointestinal symptoms
- Dyspnea
- Thrombus formation
- Pericarditis
- Elevations in serum bilirubin, alkaline phosphatase, liver enzymes, creatinine
- Arrhythmia
- Antibody formation

Most of the side effects resolved with cessation of therapy. Fever, which could be abrogated with ibuprofen [114], and bone pain are the most common side effects observed in patients treated with both glycosylated and non-glycosylated rhGM-CSF. In addition, myalgias, fatigue, rash, edema, facial flushing, and gastrointestinal symptoms, all mild, were reported in a variety of studies that employed glycosylated rhGM-CSF [3, 15, 74]. At the higher doses slight dyspnea, generalized edema, serositis, thrombus formation and hypotension have been described and were dose limiting for the CHO cell-derived glycosylated rhGM-CSF [3, 15]. The latter signs and symptoms were not observed with the yeast-derived glycosylated protein.

A reaction which has been referred to as 'the first dose effect' has been described in patients treated with the *E. coli*-derived, nonglycosylated rhGM-CSF. This syndrome, as well as a generalized rash, has been observed in higher incidence in the patients receiving IV as compared to equivalent sc dosing [91]. The 'first dose reaction', characterized by flushing, tachycardia, hypoxia, hypotension, syncope and leg spasm, generally occurred within 15-20 min of the first dose and was not dose-related. Although it did not recur with subsequent dosing during the same course of treatment, it often recurred with the first dose of the second course. Reaction at the injection site, and elevations in serum alkaline phosphatase and liver transaminases were more common with the SC dosing of nonglycoslylated rhGM-CSF [90]. Formation of neutralizing antibodies has been reported in small numbers of patients.

REFERENCES

1. Aglietta M, Piacibello W, Sanavio F, et al. Kinetics of human hemopoietic cells after *in vivo* administration of granulocyte-macrophage colony-stimulating factor. *J Clin Invest* 1989; 83: 551-557.
2. Antin JH, Smith BR, Holmes W, Rosenthal DS. Phase I/II study of recombinant human granulocyte-macrophage colony-stimulating factor in aplastic anemia and myelodysplastic syndrome. *Blood* 1988; 72: 705-713.
3. Antman KS, Griffin JD, Elias A, et al. Effect of recombinant human granulocyte-macrophage colony-stimulating factor on chemotherapy-induced myelosuppression. *N Engl J Med* 1988; 319: 593-598.
4. Archimbaud E, Fenaux P, Reiffers J, et al. Granulocyte-macrophage colony-stimulating factor in association to timed-sequential chemotherapy with mitoxantrone, etoposide, and cytarabine for refractory acute myelogenous leukemia. *Leukemia* 1993; 7: 372-377.
5. Arnout MA, Wang EA, Clark SC, Sieff CA. Human recombinant granulocyte-macrophage colony-stimulating factor increases cell-to-cell adhesion and surface expression of adhesion-promoting surface glycoproteins on mature granulocytes. *J Clin Invest* 1986; 78: 597-601.
6. Bajorin D, Nichols CR, Schmoll H-J, et al. Recombinant human granulocyte-macrophage colony-stimulating factor as an adjunct to conventional-dose ifosfamide-based chemotherapy for patients with advanced or relapsed germ cell tumors: A randomized trial. *J Clin Oncol* 1995; 13: 79-86.
7. Baldwin GC, Gasson JC, Kaufman SE, et al. Nonhematopoietic tumor cells express functional CSF receptors. *Blood* 1989; 73: 1033-1037.
8. Baldwin GC, Gasson JC, Quan SG, et al. Granulocyte-macrophage colony-stimulating factor enhances neutrophil function in acquired immunodeficiency syndrome patients. *Proc Natl Acad Sci USA* 1988; 856: 2763-2766.
9. Baldwin GC, Golde DW, Widhopf GF, et al. Identification and characterization of a low-affinity granulocyte-macrophage colony-stimulating factor receptor on primary and cultured human melanoma cells. *Blood* 1991; 78: 609-615.
10. Barlogie B, Jagannath S, Dixon DO, et al. High-dose melphalan and granulocyte-macrophage colony-stimulating factor for refractory multiple myeloma. *Blood* 1990; 76: 677-680.
11. Berdel WE, Danhauser-Riedel S, Steinhauser G, Winton EF. Various human hematopoietic growth factors (interleukin-3, GM-CSF, G-CSF) stimulate clonal growth of nonhematopoietic tumor cells. *Blood* 1989; 73: 80-83.
12. Bettelheim P, Valent P, Andreeff M, et al. Recombinant human granulocyte-macrophage colony-stimulating factor in combination with standard induction chemotherapy in de novo acute myeloid leukemia. *Blood* 1991; 77: 700-711.
13. Bishop MR, Anderson JR, Jackson JD, et al. High-dose therapy and peripheral blood progenitor cell transplantation: Effects of recombinant human granulocyte-macrophage colony-stimulating factor on the autograft. *Blood* 1994; 83: 610-616.
14. Blazar BR, Kersey JH, McGlave PB, et al. *In vivo* administration of recombinant human granulocyte/macrophage colony-stimulating factor in acute lymphoblastic leukemia patients receiving purged autografts. *Blood* 1989; 73: 849-857.
15. Brandt SJ, Peters WP, Atwater SK, et al. Effect of recombinant human granulocyte-macrophage colony-stimulating factor on hematopoietic reconstitution after high-dose chemotherapy and autologous bone marrow transplantation. *N Engl J Med* 1988; 318: 869-876.
16. Buchner T, Hiddemann W, Koenigsmann M, et al. Recombinant human granulocyte-macrophage colony-stimulating factor after chemotherapy in patients with acute myeloid leukemia at higher age or after relapse. *Blood* 1991; 78: 1190-1197.
17. Budel LM, Elbaz O, Hoogerbrugge H, et al. Common binding structure for granulocyte macrophage colony-stimulating factor and interleukin-3 on human acute myeloid leukemia cells and monocytes. *Blood* 1990; 75: 1439-1445.
18. Budel LM, Touw IP, Delwel R, Clark SC, Lowenberg B. Interleukin-3 and granulocyte-monocyte colony-stimulating factor receptors on human acute myelocytic leukemia cells and relationship the proliferative response. *Blood* 1989; 74: 565-571.
19. Bukowski RM, Murthy S, McLain D, et al. Phase I trial of recombinant granulocyte-macrophage colony-stimulating factor in patients with lung cancer. Clinical and immunologic effects. *J Immunother* 1993; 13: 267-274.
20. Bunn PA, Crowley J, Kelly K, et al. Chemoradiotherapy with or without granulocyte-macrophage colony-stimulating factor in the treatment of limited-stage small-cell lung cancer: A prospective phase III radomized study of the Southwest Oncology Group. *J Clin Oncol* 1995; 13: 1632-1641.
21. Burgess AW, Begley CG, Johnson GR, et al. Purification and properties of bacterially synthesized human granulocyte macrophage colony stimulating factor. *Blood* 1987; 69: 43-51.
22. Calderwood S, Rumeyer F, Freedman MH. GM-CSF in childhood acute lymphoblastic leukemia: Randomized double blind trial during intensification phase. *Blood* 1992; 80(supplement): 288a.
23. Cannistra SA, DiCarlo J, Groshek P, et al. Simultaneous administration of granulocyte-macrophage colony-stimulating factor and cytosine arabinoside for the treatment of relapsed acute myeloid leukemia. *Leukemia* 1991; 5: 230-238.
24. Cannistra SA, Groshek P, Garlick R, et al. Regulation of surface expression of the granulocyte/macrophage colony stimulating factor receptor in normal human myeloid cells. *Proc Natl Acad Sci USA* 1990; 87: 93-97.
25. Cannistra SA, Vallenga E, Groshek P, et al. Human granulocyte-monocyte colony-stimulating factor and interleukin 3 stimulate monocyte cytotoxicity through a tumor necrosis factor-dependent mechanism. *Blood* 1988; 71: 672-676.
26. Cantrell MA, Anderson D, Ceretti DP, et al. Cloning sequence and expression of human granulocyte/macrophage colony stimulating factor. *Proc Natl Acad Sci USA* 1985; 73: 6250-6254.
27. Cebon J, Dempsey P, Fox R, et al. Pharmacokinetics of human granulocyte-macrophage colony-stimulating factor using a sensitive immunoassay. *Blood* 1988; 72: 1340-1347.
28. Champlin RE, Nimer SD, Ireland P, et al. Treatment of refractory aplastic anemia with recombinant human granulocyte-macrophage colony-stimulating factor. *Blood* 1989; 73: 694-699.

29. de Vries EGE, Biesma B, Willemse PHB, et al. A double-blind placebo-controlled study with granulocyte-macrophage colony-stimulating factor during chemotherapy for ovarian carcinoma. *Cancer Res* 1991; 51: 116-122.
30. De Witte T, Gratwohl A, Van Der Lely N, et al. Recombinant human granulocyte-macrophage colony-stimulating factor accelerates neutrophil and monocyte recovery after allogeneic T-cell-depleted bone marrow transplantation. *Blood* 1992; 79: 1359-1365.
31. Dedhar S, Gaboury L, Galloway P, Eaves C. Human granulocyte-macrophage colony-stimulating factor is a growth factor active on a variety of cell types of nonhematopoietic origin. *Proc Natl Acad Sci USA* 1988; 85: 9253-9257.
32. Devereux S, Bull HA, Campos-Costa D, et al. Granulocyte macrophage colony stimulating factor induced changes in cellular adhesion molecule expression and adhesion to edothelium: *in-vitro* and *in-vivo* studies in man. *Br J Haemotol* 1989; 71: 323-330.
33. Devereux S, Linch DC, Campos-Costa D, et al. Transient leucopenia induced by granulocyte macrophage colony stimulating factor (Letter). *Lancet* 1987; ii: 1523-1524.
34. DiPersio J, Billing P, Kaufman S, et al. Characterization of the human granulocyte-macrophage colony-stimulating factor receptor. *J Biol Chem* 1988; 263: 1834-1841.
35. Economopoulos T, Papageorgiou E, Stathakis N, et al. Treatment of myelodysplastic syndromes with human granulocyte-macrophage colony-stimulating factor (GM-CSF) or GM-CSF combined with low-dose cytosine arabinoside. *Eur J Haematol* 1992; 49: 138-142.
36. Edmonson JH, Colon-Otero G, Long HG, et al. Granulocyte-macrophage `colony-stimulating factor (GM-CSF) permits escalation of carboplatin (CBDCA) doses. *Proc Am Soc Clin Oncol* 1990; 9: 330a.
37. Edmonson JH, Hartmann LC, Long HJ, et al. Granulocyte-macrophage colony-stimulating factor. Preliminary observations on the influences of dose, schedule, and route of administration in patients receiving cyclophosphamide and carboplatin. *Cancer* 1992; 70: 2529-2539.
38. Elias AD, Ayash L, Anderson KC, et al. Mobilization of peripheral blood progenitor cells by chemotherapy and granulocyte-macrophage colony-stimulating factor for hematologic support after high-dose intensification for breast cancer. *Blood* 1992; 79: 3036-3044.
39. Elliott MJ, Vadas MA, Eglinton JM, et al. Recombinant human interleukin-3 and granulocyte-macrophage colony-stimulating factor show common biological effects and binding characteristics on human monocytes. *Blood* 1989; 74: 2349-2359.
40. Emanuel PD, Bates LJ, Castleberry RP, et al. Selective hypersensitivity to granulocyte-macrophage colony-stimulating factor by juvenile chronic myeloid leukemia hematopoietic progenitors. *Blood* 1991; 77: 925-929.
41. Estey E, Thall PF, Kantarjian H, et al. Treatment of newly diagnosed acute myelogenous leukemia with granulocyte-macrophage colony-stimulating factor (GM-CSF) before and during continuous-infusion high-dose ara-C + daunorubicin: Comparison to patients treated without GM-CSF. *Blood* 1992; 79: 2246-2255.
42. Estey EH, Dixon D, Kantarjian HM, et al. Treatment of poor-prognosis, newly diagnosed acute myeloid leukemia with ara-C and recombinant human granulocyte-macrophage colony-stimulating factor. *Blood* 1990; 75: 1766-1769.
43. Foulke RS, Marshall MH, Trotta PP, von Hoff DD. *In vitro* assessment of the effects of granulocyte-macrophage colony-stimulating factor on primary human tumors and derived lines. *Cancer Res* 1990; 50: 6264-6267.
44. Freedman MJ, Grunberger T, Correa P, et al. Autocrine and paracrine growth control by granulocyte-monocyte colony-stimulating factor of acute lymphoblastic leukemia cells. *Blood* 1993; 81: 3068-3075.
45. Ganser A, Ottman OG, Erdmann H, et al. The effect of recombinant human granulocyte-macrophage colony-stimulating factor on neutropenia and related morbidity in chronic severe neutropenia. *Ann Intern Med* 1989; 111: 887-892.
47. Ganser A, Volkers B, Greher J, et al. Recombinant human granulocyte-macrophage colony-stimulating factor in patients with myelodysplastic syndromes-A phase I/II trial. *Blood* 1989; 73: 31-37.
48. Gasson JC. Hematopoietic growth factor receptors on solid tumors. Hematopoietic Therapy Index & Reviews 1993; II(1): 1.
49. Gasson JC, Kaufman SE, Weisbart RH, Tomonaga M, Golde DW. High-affinity binding of granulocyte-macrophage colony-stimulating factor to normal and leukemic human myeloid cells. *Proc Natl Acad Sci USA* 1986; 83: 669-673.
50. Gasson JC, Weisbart RH, Kaufman SE, et al. Purified human granulocyte-macrophage colony-stimulating factor: Direct action on neutrophils. *Science* 1984; 226: 1339-1342.
51. Gasson JC, Weissbart RH, Kaufman SE, et al. Purified human granulocyte-macrophage colony-stimulating factor: Direct action of neutrophils. *Science* 1984; 226: 1339-1342.
52. Gearing DP, King JA, Gough NM, Nicola NA. Expression cloning of a receptor for human granulocyte-macrophage colony-stimulating factor. *EMBO Journal* 1989; 8: 3667-3676.
53. Gerhartz HH, Engelhard M, Meusers P, et al. Randomized, double-blind, placebo-controlled, phase III study of recombinant human granulocyte-macrophage colony-stimulating factor as adjunct to induction treatment of high-grade malignant non-Hodgkin's lymphomas. *Blood* 1993; 82: 2329-2339.
54. Gerhartz HH, Marcus R, Delmer A, et al. A randomised phase II study of low-dose cytosine arabinoside plus GM-CSF in MDS with a high risk of developing leukemia. *Leukemia* 1994; 8: 16-23.
55. Gesner T, Mufson RA, Turner KJ, Clark SC. Identification through chemical cross-linking of distinct granulocyte-macrophage colony-stimulating factor and interleukin-3 receptors on myeloid leukemic cells, KG-1. *Blood* 1989; 74: 2652-2656.
56. Gianni AM, Bregni M, Siena S, et al. Recombinant human granulocyte-macrophage colony-stimulating factor reduces hematologic toxicity and widens clinical applicability of high-dose cyclophosphamide treatment in breast cancer and non-Hodgkin's lymphoma. *J Clin Oncol* 1990; 8: 768-778.
57. Gianni AM, Bregni M, Stern AC, et al. Granulocyte-macrophage colony-stimulating factor to harvest circulating haemopoietic stem cells for autotransplantation. *Lancet* 1989; ii: 580-584.
58. Gorin NC, Coiffier B, Hayat M, et al. Recombinant human granulocyte-macrophage colony-stimulating

factor after high-dose chemotherapy and autologous bone marrow transplantation with unpurged and purged marrow in non-Hodgkin's lymphoma: A double-blind placebo-controlled trial. *Blood* 1992; 80: 1149-1157.
59. Gough NM, Gearing DP, Nicola NA, et al. Localization of the human GM-CSF receptor gene to the X-Y pseudo-autosomal region. *Nature* 1990; 345: 734-736.
60. Grabstein KH, Urdal DL, Tushinski RJ, et al. Induction of macrophage tumoricidal activity by granulocyte-macrophage colony-stimulating fctor. *Science* 1986; 232: 506-508.
61. Gradishar W, Le Beau MM, O'Laughlin R, et al. Clinical and cytogenetic responses to GM-CSF in therapy-related myelodysplastic syndrome. *Blood* 1992; 80: 2463-2470.
62. Grem JL, McAtee N, Murphy RF, et al. Phase I and pharmacokinetic study of recombinant human granulocyte-macrophage colony-stimulating factor given in combination with fluorouracil plus calcium leucovorin in metastatic gastrointestinal adenocarcinoma. *J Clin Oncol* 1994; 12: 560-568.
63. Griffin JD, Spertini O, Ernst TJ, et al. Granulocyte-macrophage colony-stimulating factor and other cytokines regulate surface expression of the leukocyte adhesion molecule-1 on human neutrophils, monocytes, and their precursors. *J Immunol* 1990; 145: 576-584.
64. Griffin JD, Young D, Herrmann F, et al. Effects of recombinant human GM-CSF on proliferation of clonogenic cells in acute myeloblastic leukemia. *Blood* 1986; 67: 1448-1453.
65. Groopman JE, Mitsuyasu RT, De Leo MJ, et al. Effect of recombinant human granulocyte-macrophage colony-stimulating factor on myelopoiesis in the acquired immunodeficiency syndrome. *N Engl J Med* 1987; 317: 593-598.
66. Guinan EC, Sieff CA, Oette DH, et al. A phase I/II trial of recombinant granulocyte-macrophage colony-stimulating factor for children with aplastic anemia. *Blood* 1990; 76: 1077-1082.
67. Gulati S, Bennett CL. Granulocyte-macrophage colony-stimulating factor (GM-CSF) as adjunct therapy in relapsed Hodgkin's disease. *Ann Int Med* 1992; 116: 177-182.
68. Haas R, Ho AD, Bredthauer U, et al. Successful autologous transplanation of blood stem cells mobilized with recombinant human granulocyte-macrophage colony-stimulating factor. *Exp Hematol* 1990; 18: 94-98.
69. Handman E, Burgess AW. Stimulation by granulocyte-macrophage colony-stimulating factor of Leishmania tropica killing by macrophages. *J Immunol* 1979; 120: 1134-1137.
70. Harakati MS, Al-Momen A, Ajarim DS, et al. Granulocyte-macrophage colony-stimulating factor (GM-CSF) in adult patients with acute lymphoblastic leukemia treated with conventional chemotherapy. *Blood* 1994; 84(supplement): 582a.
71. Hayashida K, Kitamura T, Gorman DM, et al. Molecular cloning of a second subunit of the receptor for human granulocyte-macrophage colony-stimulating factor (GM-CSF): Reconsitution of a high-affinity GM-CSF receptor. *Proc Natl Acad Sci USA* 1990; 87: 9655-9659.
72. Heil G, Chadid L, Hoelzer D, et al. GM-CSF in a double-blind randomized, placebo controlled trial in therapy of adult patients with de novo acute myeloid leukemia (AML). *Leukemia* 1995; 9: 3-9.
73. Hermann F, Lindemann A, Klein H, et al. Effect of recombinant human granulocyte-macrophage colony-stimulating factor in patients with myelodysplastic syndrome with excess blasts. *Leukemia* 1989; 3: 335-338.
74. Herrmann F, Schulz G, Lindemann A, et al. Yeast-expressed granulocyte-macrophage colony-stimulating factor in cancer patients: A phase Ib clinical study. *Behring Inst Mitt* 1988; 83: 107-118.
75. Herrmann F, Schulz G, Lindemann A, et al. Hematopoietic responses in patients with advanced malignancy treated with recombinant human granulocyte-macrophage colony-stimulating factor. *J Clin Oncol* 1989; 7: 159-167.
76. Herrmann F, Wieser M, Kolbe K, et al. Effect of granulocyte-macrophage colony-stimulating factor on neutropenia and related morbidity induced by myelotoxic chemotherapy. *Amer J Med* 1990; 88: 619-624.
77. Ho AD, Del Valle F, Engelhard M, et al. Mitoxantrone/high-dose Ara-C and recombinant human GM-CSF in the treatment of refractory non-Hodgkin's lymphoma. *Cancer* 1990; 66: 423-430.
78. Hoekman K, Wagstaff J, van Groeningen CJ, et al. Effects of recombinant human granulocyte-macrophage colony-stimulating factor on myelosuppression induced by multiple cycles of high-dose chemotherapy in patients with advanced breast cancer. *J Natl Cancer Inst* 1991; 83: 1546-1553.
79. Hovgaard DJ, Nissen NI. Effect of recombinant human granulocyte-macrophage colony-stimulating factor in patients with Hodgkin's disease: A phase I/II study. *J Clin Oncol* 1992; 10: 390-397.
80. Huebner K, Isobe M, Croce CM, et al. The human gene encoding GM-CSF is at 5q21-q32, the chromosome region deleted in the 5q- anomaly. *Science* 1985; 230: 1282-1285.
81. Kanakura Y, Druker B, Cannistra SA, et al. Signal transduction of the human granulocyte-macrophage colony-stimulating factor and interleukin-3 receptors involves tyrosine phosphorylation of a common set of cytoplasmic proteins. *Blood* 1990; 76: 706-715.
82. Kantarjian HM, Estey EH, O'Brien S, et al. Intensive chemotherapy with mitoxantrone and high-dose cytosine arabinoside followed by granulocyte-macrophage colony-stimulating factor in the treatment of patients with acute lymphocytic leukemia. *Blood* 1992; 79: 876-881.
83. Kehoe S, Poole CJ, Stanely A, et al. A phase I/II trial of recombinant human granulocyte-macrophage colony-stimulating factor in the intensification of cisplatin and cyclophosphamide chemotherapy for advanced ovarian cancer. *Br J Cancer* 1994; 69: 537-540.
84. Krigel RL, Palackdharry CS, Padavic K, et al. Ifosfamide, carboplatin, and etoposide plus granulocyte-macrophage colony-stimulating factor: A phase I study with apparent activity in non-small-cell lung cancer. *J Clin Oncol* 1994; 12: 1251-1258.
85. Krown SE, Paredes J, Bundow D, et al. Interferon-a, zidovudine, and granulocyte-macrophage colony-stimulating factor: A phase I AIDS Clinical Trials Group study in patients with Kaposi's sarcoma associated with AIDS. *J Clin Oncol* 1992; 10: 1344-1351.
86. Lang RA, Metcalf D, Cuthbertson RA, et al. Transgenic mice expressing a hemopoietic growth factor gene (GM-CSF) develop accumulations of macrophages, blindness,

and a fatal syndrome of tissue damage. *Cell* 1987; 51: 675-686.

87. Lazarus HM, Andersen J, Chen MG, et al. Recombinant granulocyte-macrophage colony-stimulating factor after autologous bone marrow tramsplantation for relapsed non-Hodgkin's lymphoma: Blood and bone marrow progenitor growth studies. A phase II Eastern Cooperative Oncology Group trial. *Blood* 1991; 78: 830-837.
88. Le Beau MM, Epstein ND, O'Brien SJ, et al. The interleukin 3 gene is located on human chromosome 5 and is deleted in myeloid leukemias with a deletion of 5q. *Proc Natl Acad Sci USA* 1987; 84: 5913-5917.
89. Levine JD, Alan JD, Tessitore JH, et al. Recombinant human granulocyte-macrophage colony-stimulating factor ameliorates zidovudine-induced neutropenia in patients with acquired immunodeficiency syndrome (AIDS)/AIDS-related complex. *Blood* 1991; 78: 3148-3154.
90. Lieschke GJ, Maher D, Cebon J, et al. Effects of bacterially synthesized recombinant human granulocyte-macrophage colony-stimulating factor in patients with advanced malignancy. *Ann Int Med* 1989; 110: 357-364.
91. Lieschke GJ, Maher D, O'Connor M, et al. Phase I study of intravenously administered bacterially synthesized granulocyte-macrophage colony-stimulating factor and comparison with subcutaneous administration. *Cancer Res* 1990; 50: 606-614.
92. Link H, Boogaerts MA, Carella AM, et al. A controlled trial of recombinant human granulocyte-macrophage colony-stimulating factor after total body irradiation, high-dose chemotherapy, and autologous bone marrow transplantation for acute lymphoblastic leukemia or malignant lymphoma. *Blood* 1992; 80: 2188-2195.
93. Logothetis CJ, Dexeus FH, Sella A, et al. Escalated therapy for refractory urothelial tumors: Methotrexate-vinblastine-doxorubicin-cisplatin plus unglycosylated recombinant human granulocyte-macrophage colony-stimulating factor. *J Natl Cancer Inst* 1990; 82: 667-672.
94. Lopez AF, Williamson J, Gamble JR, et al. Recombinant human granulocyte-macrophage colony-stimulating factor stimulates *in vitro* mature human neutrophil and eosinophil function, surface receptor expression and survival. *J Clin Invest* 1986; 78: 1220-1228.
95. Luikart SD, MacDonald M, Huzar D, et al. Ability of daily or twice daily granulocyte-macrophage colony stimulating factor (GM-CSF) to support dose escalation of etoposide and carboplatin in extensive small cell lung cancer. *Proc Am Soc Clin Oncol* 1992; 10: 242a.
96. McClay EF, Braly PD, Kirmani S, et al. A phase I trial of intraperitoneal carboplatin and etoposide with granulocyte macrophage colony stimulating factor support in patients with intraabdominal malignancies. *Cancer* 1994; 74: 664-669.
97. Merlano M, Benasso M, Cavallari M, et al. Intensified chemotherapy with granulocyte-monocyte colony stimulating factor protection in advanced, relapsed squamous cell carcinoma of the head and neck. *Am J Clin Oncol* 1994; 17: 494-497.
98. Metcalf D, Begley CG, Johnson GR, et al. Biologic properties *in vitro* of a recombinant human granulocyte-macrophage colony stimulating factor. *Blood* 1986; 67: 37-45.
99. Mitsuyasu R, Levine J, Miles SA, et al. Effects of long term subcutaneous (SC) administration of recombinant granulocyte-macrophage colony-stimulating factor in patients with HIV-related leukopenia. *Blood* 1988; 72: 1297a.
100. Moore JDF, Pazdur R. Phase I study of 5-fluorouracil with folinic acid combined with recombinant human granulocyte-macrophage colony-stimulating factor. *Am J Clin Oncol* 1992; 15: 464-466.
101. Moore MJ, Iscoe N, Tannock IF. A phase II study of methotrexate, vinblastine, doxorubicin and cisplatin plus recombinant human granulocyte-macrophage colony stimulating factor in patients with advanced transitional cell carcinoma. *J Urol* 1993; 150: 1131-1134.
102. Nemunaitis J, Anasetti C, Storb R, et al. Phase II trial of recombinant human granulocyte-macrophage colony-stimulating factor in patients undergoing allogeneic bone marrow transplantation from unrelated donors. *Blood* 1992; 79: 2572-2577.
103. Nemunaitis J, Buckner CD, Appelbaum FR, et al. Phase I/II trial of recombinant human granulocyte-macrophage colony-stimulating factor following allogeneic bone marrow transplantation. *Blood* 1991; 77: 2065-2071.
104. Nemunaitis J, Rabinowe SN, Singer JW, et al. Recombinant granulocyte-macrophage colony-stimulating factor after autologous bone marrow transplantation for lymphoid cancer. *N Eng J Med* 1991; 324: 1773-1778.
105. Nemunaitis J, Singer J, Buckner CD, et al. Use of recombinant human granulocyte-macrophage colony-stimulating factor in graft failure after bone marrow transplantation. *Blood* 1990; 76: 245-253.
106. Nemunaitis J, Singer JW, Buckner CD, et al. Use of recombinant human granulocyte-macrophage colony-stimulating factor in autologous marrow transplantation for lymphoid malignancies. *Blood* 1988; 72: 834-836.
107. Nissen C, Tichelli A, Gratwohl A, et al. Failure of recombinant human granulocyte-macrophage colony-stimulating factor therapy in aplastic anemia patients with very severe neutropenia. *Blood* 1988; 72: 2045-2047.
108. O'Day SJ, Rabinowe SN, Neuberg D, et al. A phase II study of continuous infusion recombinant human granulocyte-macrophage colony-stimulating factor as an adjunct to autologous bone marrow transplantation for patients with non-Hodgkin's lymphoma in first remission. *Blood* 1994; 83: 2707-2714.
109. O'Dwyer PJ, LaCreta FP, Schilder R, et al. Phase I trial of thiotepa in combination with recombinant human granulocyte-macrophage colony-stimulating factor. *J Clin Oncol* 1992; 10: 1352-1358.
110. O'Reilly SE, Gelmon KA, Onetto N, et al. Phase I trial of recombinant human granulocyte-macrophage colony-stimulating factor derived from yeast in patients with breast cancer receiving cyclophosphamide, doxorubicin, and fluorouracil. *J Clin Oncol* 1993; 11: 2411-2416.
111. Onetto-Pothier N, Aumont N, Haman A, et al. Characterization of granulocyte-macrophage colony-stimulating factor receptor on the blast cells of acute myeloblastic leukemia. *Blood* 1990; 75: 59-66.
112. Passos-Coelho JL, Ross AA, Moss TJ, et al. Absence of breast cancer cells in a single-day peripheral blood progenitor cell collection after priming with cyclophosphamide and granulocyte-macrophage colony-stimulating factor. *Blood* 1995; 85: 1138-1143.
113. Peters WP, Rosner G, Ross M, et al. Comparative effects of granulocyte-macrophage colony-stimulating factor (GM-CSF) and granulocyte colony-stimulating factor (G-

CSF) on priming peripheral blood progenitor cells for use with autologous bone marrow after high-dose chemotherapy. *Blood* 1993; 81: 1709-1719.

114. Peters WP, Shogan J, Shpall EJ, et al. Recombinant human granulocyte-macrophage colony-stimulating factor produces fever. *Lancet* 1988; i: 950.

115. Peters WP, Stuart A, Affronti ML, et al. Neutrophil migration is defective during recombinant human granulocyte-macrophage colony-stimulating factor infusion after autologous bone marrow transplantation in humans. *Blood* 1988; 72: 1310-1315.

116. Pettenati MJ, Le Beau MM, Lemons RS, et al. Assignment of CSF-1 to 5q33.1: Evidence for the clustering of genes regulating hematopoiesis and for their involvement in the deletion of the long arm of chromosome 5 in myeloid disorders. *Proc Natl Acad Sci USA* 1987; 84: 2970-2974.

117. Pluda JM, Yarchoan R, Smith PD, et al. Subcutaneous recombinant granulocyte-macrophage colony-stimulating factor used as a single agent and in an alternating regimen with azidothymidine in leukopenic patients with severe human immunodeficiency virus infection. *Blood* 1990; 76: 463-472.

118. Poplin E, Smith H, Behrens B, et al. SWOG 8825: Melphalan GM-CSF: A phase I study. *Gynecol Oncol* 1992; 44: 66-70.

119. Powles R, Smith C, Milan S, et al. Human recombinant GM-CSF in allogeneic bone-marrow transplantation for leukaemia: double-blind, placebo-controlled trial. *Lancet* 1990; 336: 1417-1420.

120. Rabinowe SN, Neuberg D, Beirman PJ, et al. Long-term follow-up of a phase III study of recombinant human granulocyte-macrophage colony-stimulating factor after autologous bone marrow transplantation from lymphoid malignancies. *Blood* 1993; 81: 1903-1908.

121. Reed E, Janik J, Bookman MA, et al. High-dose carboplatin and recombinant granulocyte-macrophage colony-stimulating factor in advanced-stage recurrent ovarian cancer. *J Clin Oncol* 1993; 11: 2118-2126.

122. Rifkin RM, Hersh EM, Hultquist KN, et al. Therapy of the myelodysplastic syndrome (MDS) with subcutaneously (SC) administered recombinant human granulocyte-macrophage colony-stimulating factor. *Proc Am Soc Clin Oncol* 1989; 8: 178a.

123. Ross AA, Cooper BW, Lazarus HM, et al. Detection and viability of tumor cells in peripheral blood stem cell collections from breast cancer patients using immunocytochemical and clonogenic assay techniques. *Blood* 1993; 82: 2605-2610.

124. Rowe JM, Andersen JW, Mazza JJ, et al. A randomized placebo-controlled phase III study of granulocyte-macrophage colony-stimulating factor in adult patients (>55 to 70 years of age) with acute myelogenous leukemia: A study of the Eastern Cooperative Oncology Group (E1490). *Blood* 1995; 86: 457-462.

125. Ruff MR, et al. Interferon gamma and granulocyte-macrophage colony-stimulating factor inhibit growth and induce antigens characteristic of myeloid differentiation in small cell lung cancer cells. Proc Natl Acad Sci USA 1986; 83: 6613-6617.

126. Rusthoven J, Levin L, Esienhauer E, et al. Two phase I studies of carboplatin dose escalation in chemotherapy-naive ovarian cancer patients supported with granulocyte-macrophage colony-stimulating factor. *J Natl Cancer Inst* 1991; 83: 1748-1753.

127. Salmon SE, Liu R. Effects of granulocyte-macrophage colony-stimulating factor on *in vitro* growth of human solid tumors. *J Clin Oncol* 1989; 7: 1346-1350.

128. Schuster MW, Thompson JA, Larson R, et al. Randomized trial of subcutaneous granulocyte-macrophage colony-stimulating factor (GM-CSF) versus observation in patients (pts) with myelodysplastic syndrome (MDS) or aplastic anemia (AA). *Proc Amer Soc Clin Oncol* 1990; 9: 793a.

129. Shaffer DW, Smith LS, Burris HA, et al. A randomized phase I trial of chronic oral etoposide with or without granulocyte-macrophage colony-stimulating factor in patients with advanced malignancies. *Cancer Res* 1993; 53: 5929-5933.

130. Shea TC, Mason JR, Storniolo AM, et al. Sequential cycles of high-dose carboplatin administered with recombinant human granulocyte-macrophage colony-stimulating factor and repeated infusions of autologous peripheral-blood progenitor cells: A novel and effective method for delivering multiple courses of dose-intensive therapy. *J Clin Oncol* 1992; 10: 464-473.

131. Shepherd FA, Gross PE, Rusthoven J, Eisenhauer EA. Phase I trial of granulocyte-macrophage colony-stimulating factor with high-dose cisplatin and etoposide for treatment of small-cell lung cancer: A study of the National Cancer Institute of Canada Clinical Trials Group. *J Natl Cancer Inst* 1992; 84: 59-60.

132. Sieff C, Emerson SG, Donahue RE, et al. Human recombinant granulocyte-macrophage colony stimulating factor: a multi-lineage hematopoietin. *Science* 1985; 230: 1171-1173.

133. Siena S, Bregni M, Brando B, et al. Circulation of CD34+ hematopoietic stem cells in the peripheral blood of high-dose cyclophosphamide-treated patients: Enhancement by intravenous recombinant human granulocyte-macrophage colony-stimulating factor. *Blood* 1989; 74: 1905-1914.

134. Silberstein DS, Owen WF, Gasson JC, et al. Enhancement of human eosinophil cytotoxicity and leukotriene synthesis by biosynthetic (recombinant) granulocyte-macrophage colony-stimulating factor. *J Immunol* 1986; 137: 3290-3294.

135. Smith T. Successful use of granulocyte-macrophage colony-stimulating factor in patients with acute lymphocytic leukemia. *Am J Med* 1990; 89: 384-384.

136. Socinski MA, Cannistra SA, Sullivan R, et al. Human granulocyte-macrophage colony stimulating factor induces expression of the CD11b surface adhesion molecule on granulocytes *in vivo*. *Blood* 1988; 72: 691-697.

137. Takai S, Yamada K, Hirayama N, et al. Mapping of the human gene encoding the mutual signaltransducing subunit (β-chain) of granulocyte-macrophage colony-stimulating factor (GM-CSF), interleukin-3 (IL-3), and interleukin-5 (IL-5) receptor complexes to chromosome 22q113.1. *Hum Genet* 1994; 93: 198-200.

138. Socinski MA, Schnipper EA, et al. Granulocyte-macrophage colony-stimulating factor expands the circulating hemopoietic progenitor cell compartment in man. *Lancet* 1988; 1: 1194-1198.

139. Steis RG, VanderMolen LA, Longo DL, et al. Reombinant human granulocyte-macrophage colony-stimulating factor in patients with advanced malignancy: A phase Ib trial. *J Natl Cancer Inst* 1990; 82: 697-703.

140. Steward WP, Scarffe JH, Dirix LY, et al. Granulocyte-macrophage colony stimulating factor (GM-CSF) after high-dose melphalan in patients with advanced colon cancer. *Br J Cancer* 1990; 61: 749-754.
141. Stone R, George S, Berg D, et al. GM-CSF 'v' placebo during remission induction for patients >60 years old with de novo acute myeloid leukemia: CALGB study #8923. *Proc Amer Soc Clin Oncol* 1994; 13: 992a.
142. Sutherland GR, Baker E, Callen DF, et al. Interleukin-5 is at 5q31 and is deleted in the 5q- syndrome. *Blood* 1988; 71: 1150-1152.
143. Thompson JA, Lee DJ, Kidd P, et al. Subcutaneous granulocyte-macrophage colony-stimulating factor in patients with myelodysplastic syndromes: Toxicity, pharmacokinetics, and hematologic effects. *J Clin Oncol* 1989; 7: 629-637.
144. Vadhan-Raj S, Broxmeyer HE, Hittelman WN, et al. Abrogating chemotherapy-induced myelosuppression by recombinant granulocyte-macrophage colony-stimulating factor in patients with sarcoma: Protection at the progenitor cell level. *J Clin Oncol* 1992; 10: 1266-1277.
145. Vadhan-Raj S, Buescher S, Broxmeyer HE, et al. Stimulation of myelopoiesis in patient with aplastic anemia by recombinant human granulocyte-macrophage colony-stimulating factor. *N Engl J Med* 1988; 319: 1628-1634.
146. Vadhan-Raj S, Keating M, LeMaistre A, et al. Effects of recombinant human granulocyte-macrophage colony-stimulating factor in patients with myelodysplastic syndromes. *N Engl J Med* 1988; 317: 1545-1551.
147. Weisbart RH, Golde DW, Clark SC, et al. Human granulocyte-macrophage colony-stimulating factor is a neutrophil activator. *Nature* 1985; 314: 361-363.
148. Weisbart RH, Golde DW, Gasson JC. Biosynthetic human GM-CSF modulates the number and affinity of neutrophil f-met-leu-phe receptors. *J Immunol* 1986; 137: 3584-3587.
149. Weiser WY, Van Niel A, Clark SC, et al. Recombinant human granulocyte-macrophage colony-stimulating factor activates intracellular killing of Leishmania donovani by human monocyte-derived macrophage. *J Exp Med* 1987; 166: 1436-1446.
150. Welte K, Zeidler C, Reiter A, et al. Differential effects of granulocyte-macrophage colony stimulating factor in children with severe congenital neutropenia. *Blood* 1990; 75: 1056-1063.
151. Wong GG, Witek JS, Temple PA, et al. Human GM-CSF molecular cloning of the complementary DNA and purification of the natural and recombinant proteins. *Science* 1985; 228: 810-815.
152. Yamashita Y, Nara N, Nobuo A. Antiproliferative and differentiative effect of granulocyte-macrophage colony-stimulating factor on a variant human small cell lung cancer cell line. *Cancer Res* 1989; 49: 5334-5338.
153. Yarden Y, Escobedo JA, Kuang WJ. Structure of the receptor for platelet-derived growth factor helps define a family of closely related growth factor receptors. *Nature* 1986; 323: 226-232.
154. Yokota T, Arai N, De Vries V, et al. Molecular biology of interleukin 4 and interleukin 5 genes and biology of their products that stimulate B cells, T cells and hematopoietic cells. *Immunol Rev* 1988; 102: 137-187.
155. Young DC, Griffin JD. Autocrine secretion of GM-CSF in acute myeloblastic leukemia. *Blood* 1986; 68: 1178-1181.

CLINICAL APPROACHES TO CANCER GENE THERAPY

KATHARINE A. WHARTENBY[1], AIZEN J. MARROGI[2] and SCOTT M. FREEMAN[2]
[1]*Center for Biologics, Food and Drug Administration, Rockville, [2]Maryland, Department of Pathology, Tulane University Medical Center, New Orleans, Louisiana*

INTRODUCTION

Despite significant advances in standard therapy, many types of cancer currently have no effective treatment. The search for therapies that will be effective against tumors that are unresponsive to surgical removal, chemotherapy, and radiation therapy has led to a number of innovative approaches, including gene therapy, a form of cancer biotherapy. Many gene therapies have been designed to eliminate tumors through tumor-specific properties that are different from those targeted by conventional therapy. Thus, tumors that are resistant to conventional agents could be treatable through a separate mechanism. In addition, some types of gene therapies have been shown to enhance the effects of chemotherapy and other biotherapies such that they might serve as adjunct treatment in diseases for which no one therapy is curative. Clinical trials employing gene transfer for the treatment of cancer have been underway since 1989, when the first phase 1 trial was initiated [1].

Gene therapy trials have become a common experimental approach for may different types of cancer that have no available treatment. However, the novelty of this approach and concerns over potential safety of genetic modification of cells have led to the establishment of an additional regulatory process through which gene therapy proposals must pass. The National Institutes of Health Recombinant DNA Advisory Committee (RAC) was established to provide another level of review that these protocols must undergo in addition to the standard approvals required by the investigator's institutional review board and the U.S. Food and Drug Administration. RAC reviews are open to the public, and provide information on protocols as they are proposed, prior to the treatment of any patients. These regulatory processes emphasize the novelty of this type of therapy and concerns over potential safety of genetic modification of cells. As of mid-1995, seventy four protocols in six basic areas have received approval for the treatment of cancer (Table 1).

This review discusses approaches to cancer gene therapy in the context of current clinical protocols. The introduction covers background and methodology, and four additional sections are based on the types of therapeutic approaches. The first section discusses therapies related to altering oncogene and tumor suppressor gene function. The second section outlines the protocols based on immunotherapies. The third and fourth sections describe types of protocols that are based on altering phenotypes of cells to produce either drug sensitivities or drug resistance. The background and rationale for each of these approaches will be described.

Gene therapy can be defined as an alteration of the genetic material of a cell with resultant benefit to a patient [2]. Much of the early conceptualization of gene therapy

Table 1. Number of each type of cancer gene therapy protocols

Cytokines	Marker genes	MDR	HSV-T	Anti-ONC/ Tumor suppressor	Immunotherapy
24	22	4	11	6	7
Total cancer gene therapy protocol number: 74					

This table shows the number of protocols for cancer gene therapy that utilize the different approaches. Protocols listed under each column are defined as follows: 1) the cytokines column includes all protocols in which any cell type is modified to secrete a cytokine; 2) the marker genes column includes protocols designed only to label a cell to determine its fate–no therapeutic benefit is expected from these trials; 3) the MDR column refers to protocols employing the multidrug resistance gene–while most of these are currently intended to be marker studies, some therapeutic benefit may be derived; 4) the HSV-TK column includes the protocols in which the herpes simplex virus thymidine kinase gene is introduced into cells; 5) the anti-onc/tumor suppressor column refers to protocols using either anti-oncogenes or tumor suppressor genes to halt tumor growth; 6) the immunotherapy column includes trials designed to directly modify tumor cells to elicit an enhanced immune response.

R.K. Oldham (ed.), Principles of Cancer Biotherapy. 3rd ed., 447–462.

focused on genetic diseases in which a single gene was defective. A theoretically straightforward goal was to utilize gene transfer to replace the defective gene, thus curing the disease [8, 137, 99, 161]. Although application of this technique was first envisioned as a method to correct enzyme deficiencies of hereditary diseases, the first clinical protocol to receive RAC approval was for gene transfer in cancer patients. This trial, which will be discussed in section III, used gene transfer to label cells so that their fate could be followed. No benefit to the patient was expected from the modification of the cells. A number of other studies have since employed gene transfer for this purpose. These studies, known as marking studies, will be distinguished from therapeutic studies, in which the goal of genetic modification is to directly treat the patient for a specific disease.

Methodology

Gene transfer is accomplished through three major methods. Viral-based delivery systems carrying the gene of interest are the most commonly used mode of delivery. Other methods include lipid mediated transfer and mechanical injection of genes into cells. Viral vectors have predominated in clinical trials, and until recently, retroviral vectors were used almost exclusively (Table 2). Retroviral vectors are derived from wild type retroviruses but are modified genetically so that they are replication incompetent. These vectors are generated by removal of the structural genes of the wild type virus, including the gag, pol, and env genes which are then replaced with a gene of interest. Some regulatory sequences of the wild type virus are retained, including the LTR and psi sequences, which provide promoter, integration and packaging functions. Since the vector is defective and cannot replicate, it is dependent on externally provided helper functions for entrance into a cell. These functions are provided by specially designed packaging cells, which have the capability to generate empty viral particles, and once they are modified with a retroviral vector will produce particles containing that vector. Thus, packaging cells modified with a vector, termed producer cells, produce particles that contain the vector and can enter a cell through specific cell surface receptors to deliver the gene of interest. Since the integrating retroviral vector lacks the necessary genes to produce infective particles, they are replication incompetent [94, 95, 96].

Table 2. Number of cancer gene therapy protocols for vector types

Retroviral	Adenoviral	Lipid-mediated
57	7	10

This table shows the number of cancer gene therapy protocols that use each type of vector system. The first column shows the number of protocols using retrovirus-based vectors; the second column shows the number of protocols using adeno-virus based vectors; and the third column shows the number of protocols in which lipid-mediated transfer is utilized.

Retroviral vectors have been commonly used in clinical trials because of their high efficiency of transfer into cells and their persistence in the genome. A number of studies have been conducted to improve on the shortcomings of retroviruses. One major technical problem is that non-dividing cells are difficult to modify [97]. Additional safety concerns are that the viral sequences may insert next to an oncogene, thus activating it or that replication competent retroviruses (RCR) may be produced through a recombination event between sequences in the vector and in the packaging cell line. Although conflicting evidence exists regarding the significance of replication competent virus, one study demonstrated the development of a lymphoma in three of eight monkeys who were given RCR [33]. Alterations in vector and packaging line sequences have minimized the possibility of such a recombination event, and the viral stock must be extensively tested prior to use [87, 91, 92, 95, 96,]. No problems related to RCR have been reported in patients currently on clinical protocols [98].

Other viral vectors

Adenovirus is a non-enveloped DNA virus that infects a variety of cell types. As with the retroviral vectors, adenoviral vectors are generated by the deletion of specific genes, generally the E1 region, and a gene of interest is inserted [63]. Adenovirus-based vectors have been used more frequently in recent protocols, mostly in the context of gene delivery to the lung [133]. Adenovirus infects non-dividing cells efficiently [81] and is currently being tested in protocols as a delivery system for the cystic fibrosis transmembrane regulator gene (CFTR) [134, 129]. Two recent protocols have been RAC approved for cancer in which an adenoviral vector will be used to deliver the herpes simplex virus thymidine kinase gene for the treatment of cancer. These trials will be further discussed in section V. Adenoviral vectors have many of the same disadvantages of retroviral vectors in that they contain viral genes that may have undesired side effects on the host. In addition, they may produce replication competent particles and may be more toxic than retroviral vectors. In addition, adenoviral vectors do not integrate into the host's genome so that the vector will be lost as cells divide.

Other viral vectors that are being investigated in preclinical studies include herpes viruses, adeno-associated virus, poxvirus, and vaccinia virus. These vectors have not yet progressed to the clinic, but may offer advantages for certain indications.

Direct gene transfer: lipids

To avoid the pitfalls of viral vectors, other systems for direct delivery of a therapeutic gene are being developed.

One method currently being tried in the clinic is direct delivery of a gene to a tumor by complexing the DNA with a lipid for injection. The lipid fuses with cell membranes, delivers the DNA into the target cell, and then gets degraded by cellular enzymes because of hydrolyzable bonds in the particles [117, 166]. No significant toxicity has been observed in the first of these trials, which will be discussed in section III.

Other systems for direct entry of genes into cells include calcium phosphate co-precipitation and electroporation [75], but both of these methods are limited by their low efficiency and their technical difficulty in modifying large numbers of cells. Receptor mediated entry is being investigated in which the DNA is complexed with a ligand. Transferrin and asialoglycoprotein have been tested for use [29, 43, 163], but these studies are still preliminary.

The goal of direct DNA injection is to modify a tumor in situ such that only the tumor cells and not surrounding cells become modified. This approach is being developed in pre-clinical studies for melanoma. These studies were geared toward achieving tissue specific expression by modifying cells with a vector containing melanocyte-specific promoters. DNA directly injected into established B16 melanoma or Colo 26 tumors that were growing in syngeneic mice modified approximately 10% of cells. In addition, vector expression appeared to be melanoma-specific. Thus. this type of approach may have advantages in clinical applications [151].

Direct DNA injection has also been used to modify muscle cells for treatment of disease (74); for analyzing the functions of different genes [4, 126]; and for introducing a gene designed as a vaccine against influenza A [104].

ONCOGENES AND TUMOR SUPPRESSOR GENES

The discovery of oncogenes generated great excitement about the development of potential new cancer therapies. Oncogenes, which are normal cellular genes that when activated or overexpressed may lead to malignant transformation of cells [156], provided new information regarding possible mechanisms of tumorigenesis. Their discovery further validated the concept that some cancers may be genetic diseases. Cancers arising from oncogene action are likely candidates for gene therapy since the causative gene is identified and could be targeted.

Subsequent to the discovery of oncogenes, a separate class of genes involved in the development of cancer was identified that had the opposite effect from oncogenes. In their normal state, these tumor suppressor genes function to inhibit the malignant transformation of cells, and their deletion or mutation can thus lead to tumor formation [56, 80, 79, 76].

A number of animal models have shown that overexpression or mutation of an oncogene can lead to cancer. For example, studies in transgenic mice have shown that the introduction of an activated oncogene can lead to tumorigenesis [114]. In certain tumors, activation of multiple oncogenes may have a synergistic effect, suggesting that the mechanism of action of some oncogenes may be related [140]. Other studies have shown that decrease in oncogene expression can lead to differentiation of cells and slowing of malignant growth [37].

The role of tumor suppressor genes in the prevention of malignancy has been suggested by studies in which deletion of a tumor suppressor gene by homologous recombination has led to tumor formation [64]. The most widely studied tumor suppressor gene is p53, which has been analyzed in a number of different tumor types [5, 21, 19, 32, 83, 118, 143, 151, 159, 162] and is thought to act by inducing programmed cell death [90]. Some evidence suggests that tumor suppressor genes and certain oncogenes may be involved in tumorigenesis through similar mechanisms. Specifically, inactivation of p53 and activation of the bcl-2 oncogene led to lymphomas through the inhibition of apoptotic cell death [90]. Other studies showed that activation of the mdm-2 oncogene produced a protein that complexed with the p53 protein and inhibited its tumor suppressive activity [120, 103]. Thus, identification of all causative genes in a tumor may be necessary for effective therapy. In addition, another tumor suppressor gene was recently identified and termed the multiple tumor suppressor 1 gene (MTS-1). This gene is also thought to participate in the development of a number of different tumors [72].

Further evidence of the importance of these two types of genes in malignancy is provided by the statistics of altered oncogenes or tumor suppressor genes in human tumors: 25-40% of colon cancers contain mutations in the ras oncogene, and 30-50% of hepatocellular carcinomas contain mutations or deletions in the p53 tumor suppressor gene [41].

Oncogenes and antisense therapy

Although the approach of inhibiting expression of an oncogene seems straightforward, it has not been successful in a number of systems, and only one protocol has been approved using this approach. This protocol is for the treatment of breast cancers expressing c-fos or c-myc and proposes to utilize a retroviral vector to express anti-sense for either c-fos or c-myc. The vector will be introduced into the pleural or peritoneal space in patients with metastatic breast cancer with spread of the tumor into mesothelial lined spaces. The goal of this type of therapy is to introduce sufficient antisense message to inhibit the expression of the oncogene. Presumably, once expression of the oncogene is halted, the malignant growth will also be prevented. (Fig. 1) These investigators have previously shown that antisense therapy could inhibit oncogene expression and consequently cell growth in culture using antisense for both c-myc and c-fos [60-62].

Other studies suggest that antisense c-myc delivery

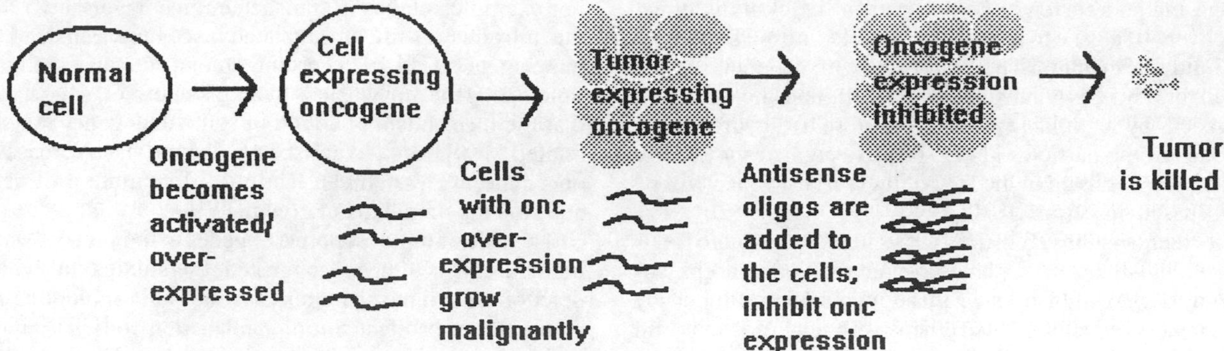

Figure 1. Approach to antisense therapy. If an oncogene in a normal cell becomes activated or overexpressed, its expression may lead to malignancy. If antisense oligonucleotides to the oncogene are added to the cells, the expression of the oncogene should be inhibited, and consequently, the tumor should not continue to grow.

may be useful as an adjunct therapy in tumors that overexpress this oncogene. In urinary bladder tumors that have been shown to be resistant to cisplatin because of c-myc expression, the addition of c-myc antisense increased their sensitivity to the drug [101].

Another protocol has been approved for the use of antisense therapy against insulin like growth factor type 1 (IGF-1). A number of brain tumors overexpress IGF-1 [136, 3], and preclinical studies showed that inhibition of its expression could cause tumor regression in rats. In this study, a plasmid vector is used to deliver the antisense to the brain. The mechanism of action of this therapy is thought to be mediated by generation of an immune response against the tumor, which IGF-1 expression had previously allowed the tumor cells to evade [152]. Although IGF-1 is not a classical oncoprotein, many oncogenes encode either growth factors or their receptors, so that this approach may be considered to be a subset of oncogene therapy.

Although oncogenes can function as specific targets for cancer therapy, improved delivery and expression will be necessary before this approach will be effective.

Tumor suppressor genes

The potential significance of the high percentage of tumors with defects in the p53 gene is underscored by the number of clinical protocols currently approved for this type of therapy. Of the six protocols approved for oncogene or tumor suppressor gene therapy, four utilize p53. These trials are designed to deliver the wild type p53 to the tumor with the goal of reversing the malignant phenotype by expression of the p53 within the tumor. (Fig. 2). Two of the four protocols are for treatment of non-small cell lung cancer, one is for head and neck squamous cell carcinoma, and one is for primary and metastatic malignant tumors of the liver.

Animal models and *in vitro* studies demonstrated that transfer of the p53 gene into tumor cells was possible. Preclinical studies have shown both transfer and expression of the p53 in the liver. These studies also showed no adverse effect on liver function by this modification [35]. Further, when the p53 gene was transferred into squamous cell cancer lines from cancers of the head and neck [82] or breast [17, 160] its expression correlated with

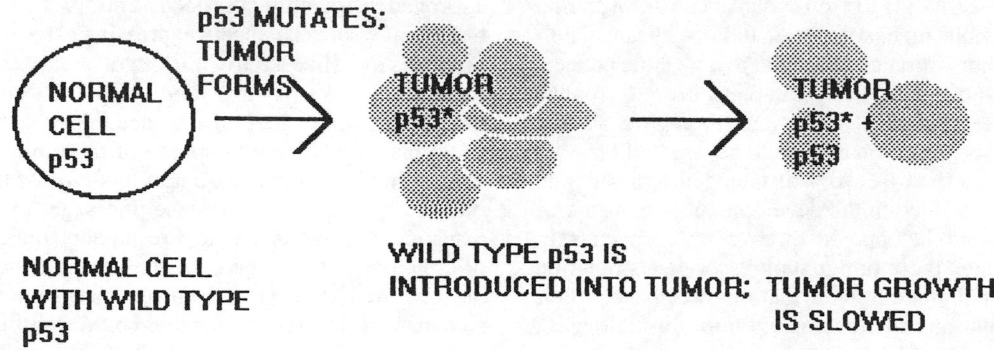

Figure 2. Approach to tumor suppressor gene therapy. If a tumor suppressor gene in a cell becomes mutated or deleted, its absence may lead to malignancy. If the function of the tumor suppressor gene is replaced, the tumor should not continue to grow.

a decrease in cell proliferation *in vitro.* Interestingly, an additional study showed that although tumorigenicity of cell lines was decreased by p53 expression, the overall growth rate was not changed, suggesting that other factors may need to be considered in the development of therapies [21].

One limitation of this type of therapy is that virtually all of the tumor cells must be modified to express the wild type p53 protein for the treatment to be effective. Recent developments in gene transfer technology have shown that adenoviral vectors are very efficient at transferring genes *in vivo* [165]. Unlike retroviral vectors, adenoviral vectors do not require actively dividing cells for efficient gene transfer to occur [81]. A number of investigators have shown the feasibility of using adenoviral vectors containing the p53 gene to alter tumor growth *in vivo* by injecting adenoviral vector into tumor nodules and demonstrating reduction of tumor growth in the treated tumors [35]. One shortcoming of the adenoviral system is that the genetic material remains episomal, and half of the progeny from dividing tumor cells lose the gene-altered phenotype as cell division occurs. Nevertheless, the most recent protocols to receive RAC approval have proposed an adenoviral system, suggesting that this approach may have some distinct advantages.

IMMUNOTHERAPY

The immune system is one of the first major defenses against the development of cancer, and a number of gene therapy protocols have been developed that attempt to capitalize on these properties. The concept of immunosurveillance was developed in the 1950s and refers to the immune system's recognition of tumor cells as foreign based on their expression of tumor associated antigens. Although this system is designed to recognize cancerous cells before they develop into a tumor, it also has the potential to attack a growing tumor. A recent study suggested that immunosurveillance may be functional in some spontaneously regressing tumors by demonstrating the presence of MHC-restricted CTL in a human melanoma that regressed [86]. Both immune cells themselves and the substances they secrete have been tested in clinical trials and will be discussed in this section. Since immune cells, cytokines, and other immunotherapeutic entities have overlapping uses, for purposes of clarification, each topic will be discussed in its own section but will be introduced as necessary into other sections.

The early immunotherapy protocols were based on the discovery that immune cells had natural anti-tumor properties that could be stimulated for cancer therapy. The first cells that were shown to have general (not tumor antigen specific) anti-tumor activity were lymphokine activated killer cells (LAK) and natural killer (NK) cells. Studies in tumor models in mice with pulmonary [110, 111] and hepatic [77, 78] metastases showed that LAK cells activated with IL-2 [53, 163, 84, 54] destroyed these tumors. Shortly after these studies were conducted, a separate subset of immune cells termed tumor infiltrating lymphocytes (TIL) was discovered and shown to have superior activity against tumors compared to the LAK cells. TIL are classic T lymphocytes that recognize the tumor from which they were derived specifically, presumably through recognition of tumor markers and MHC antigens [1, 93, 109, 115, 145, 149]. Tumor antigens include both Tumor Specific Transplantation Antigens (TSTA) and Tumor Associated Transplantation Antigens (TATA), which are generally processed in conjunction with Major Histocompatibility Complex (MHC) proteins. TATA are found on other tissues as well as the tumor while TSTA are specific to the tumor. The role of these antigens as anti-cancer agents will be discussed in greater detail in the Tumor Recognition Antigens section below. TIL are known to recognize TSTA and TATA, and have been shown to recognize melanoma cells bearing HLA-A24 but not normal cells with the same MHC [130]. A number of questions regarding the mechanism of action of TIL were raised, and the first gene transfer protocol to be conducted was designed to address some of these issues. In this protocol, the TIL were isolated from a patient and labeled with a marking gene, the neomycin resistance gene, so that the fate of the TIL could be followed after reintroduction to the patient. Prior attempts to label these cells were limited by ineffective or short term labels such as Indium 111 [44]. The gene marking protocol proposed to treat patients with advanced cancers with the labeled TIL as well as with more conventional therapy in an attempt to determine whether the TIL would return to the site of the tumor and exert any effect on the tumor. TIL were found in the circulation for up to 200 days and in the tumor for up to 64 days [132]. A major goal of this study was to determine whether any side effects would occur from delivering gene modified cells to the patients, and none has been reported.

Attempts to increase the natural anti-cancer properties of TIL have been made through their use as a gene delivery system. Since cytokines have a myriad of anti-tumor properties, which will be further discussed in the Cytokines Section, one extension of TIL therapy was to modify them to express a cytokine and reintroduce them to the patient. Ideally, the TIL would home to the site of the tumor and release high levels of the beneficial cytokine directly. This approach is being attempted in clinical trials where TIL are genetically modified to express the TNF-α gene. As is the case with many cytokines, the toxicity of TNF is its limiting factor for systemic use. Thus, this type of direct delivery system would allow for the necessary high local concentration of the cytokine while minimizing systemic exposure. However, technical complications have limited the effectiveness of this approach, since both the amount of TNF secreted by the cells and the duration of expression have been inadequate [67].

Cytokines

Cytokines comprise a significant part of the immune system's defense against tumors. These substances stimulate the immune cells to recognize and destroy tumor cells. Although many cytokines have shown great promise for eradicating tumors in preclinical studies, a common problem has been that significant toxicity has occurred at efficacious doses of the cytokine. Gene therapy trials have been undertaken in an attempt to directly deliver the cytokine to the tumor, as discussed in the previous example of TNF. (Fig. 3). Many other clinical protocols have been developed using additional cytokines.

IL-2 has significant anti-cancer activity, as demonstrated in preclinical and human studies. It has been shown to have a number of immunomodulatory properties, including stimulation of the immune defense against tumors [42, 153, 154, 155]. In addition to its *in vitro* activation of LAK cells, IL-2 can also stimulate a specific cytolytic T cell response against murine tumors [42]. Previous clinical studies using systemic IL-2 demonstrated some efficacy, but toxicity limited its usefulness. Thus, IL-2 was an ideal candidate for use in a direct delivery system. In this protocol, autologous tumor cells are modified with the IL-2 gene and returned to the patient. The theory of this approach was that the modified tumor cells would stimulate an enhanced tumor response that would kill unmodified tumor cells. An additional adoptive immunotherapeutic step was taken in which lymphocytes were taken from draining lymph nodes, grown *ex vivo*, and returned to the patient [131].

IL-4 also has been shown to be an effective stimulator of an anti-tumor response in preclinical studies and is currently being tested in three clinical trials. A number of preclinical studies demonstrated efficacy in animal models. For example, transfection of IL-4 into a mammary adenocarcinoma and a B cell lymphoma led to their regression [147, 148], which was likely to be mediated through the observed infiltration of immune cells, including macrophages, lymphocytes and eosinophils.

APPROACHES TO CYTOKINE GENE THERAPY

A. MODIFICATION OF AN EFFECTOR CELL, e.g., TIL

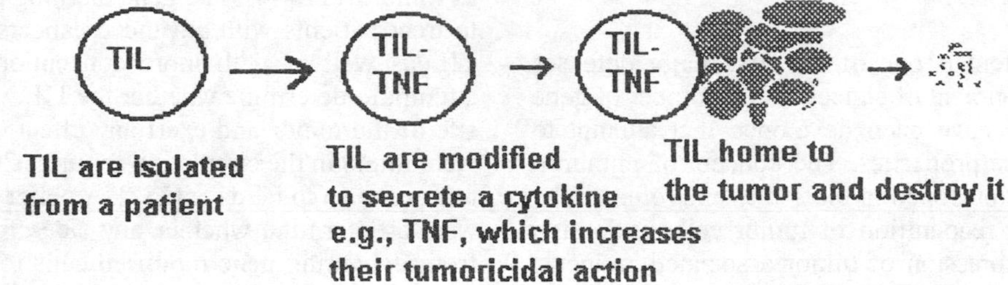

B. MODIFICATION OF CELLS FOR CYTOKINE DELIVERY TO TUMORS

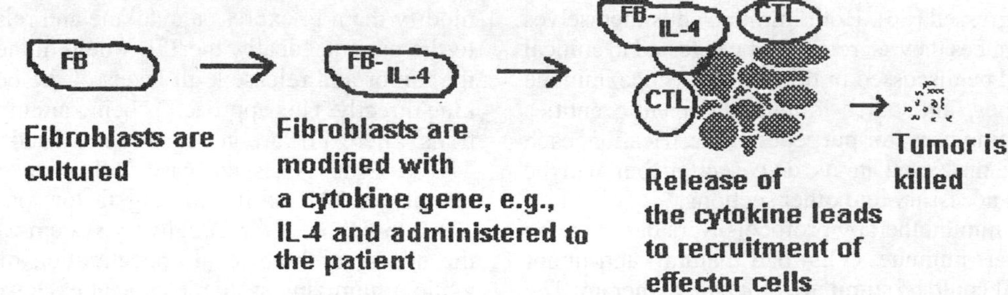

Figure 3. Approaches to cytokine gene therapy. *A.* Cytokines may be delivered to a tumor by modifying tumor infiltrating lymphocytes (TIL), which will home to the site of the tumor. Delivery of the cytokine enhances the efficacy of the TIL. *B.* An alternate method for delivering cytokines to the tumor is to modify autologous cells that are more easily obtained from a patient than TIL. One example is the use of fibroblasts, which have been modified to secrete IL-4. Delivery of the cytokine by injecting the gene-modified fibroblasts into the tumor leads to activation of the immune response, which kills the tumor.

Thus, IL-4 is likely to have a similar mechanism of action to IL-2. The first of the IL-4 clinical trials uses transduced irradiated autologous fibroblasts, which are mixed with irradiated autologous tumor, and then injected intradermally. Fibroblasts were selected because of the difficulty in growing tumor cells from a number of patients. Fibroblasts also have the advantage of rapid proliferation, which allows for higher levels of transduction efficiency. IL-2 will be administered systemically in this trial both to provide an additional therapy alone and to attempt to enhance any efficacy of the IL-4 transduced cells [85].

The second protocol also takes a tumor vaccine approach but with a different cell population being modified. In this protocol, allogeneic melanoma cells are modified with the IL-4 gene. The theory behind this procedure was that the allogeneic cells should stimulate an immune response that would react with the patient's own tumor, and the IL-4 would enhance that response. Use of the allogeneic cell line as a universal reagent simplified the procedure for multiple patients since a separate cell line would not need to be established for each patient. In addition, the allogeneic line selected expressed high levels of MHC class I antigens, which many patients' tumors do not. Expression of these antigens may be important in the immune system's recognition of tumor cells as foreign [16].

The third protocol is based on results of a tumor vaccine clinical study that demonstrated some efficacy in renal cancer patients in which the patients' tumor cells were isolated, irradiated, mixed with BCG adjuvant and injected near the lymph nodes, which were subsequently removed. This treatment was not successful in melanoma patients, so the protocol has been modified to include an additional step of modification of tumor cells with IL-4 in the hopes of increasing the immune reactivity of those cells. Thus, the tumor cells will be isolated, irradiated, and transduced, then co-injected with BCG. In addition, lymphocytes from the excised lymph nodes will be stimulated, expanded, and returned to the patient at the time of systemic IL-2 administration [18].

Gamma interferon is another cytokine whose immunostimulatory properties provide a mechanism for anti-tumor activity. It has been shown to increase expression of MHC class I molecules, β-2 microglobulin and intracellular adhesion molecule ICAM 1, and preclinical studies have demonstrated its efficacy at increasing a specific immune response to tumors [51, 52, 121, 127]. Two indications for IFN treatment are currently being tested in the clinic. Neuroblastoma was the first type of tumor to be tested, and there are currently two protocols with RAC approval for these patients. The design of these studies is similar to that of other cytokine protocols, in which autologous cells are modified and returned to the patients to generate a stronger immune response against the unmodified tumor cells. The second indication for IFN is for melanoma, and as before, autologous melanoma cells will be modified and returned to the patient [138].

Other cytokines with anti-tumor properties include IL-6 [89, 112], IL-7 [23, 68, 69], TNFα [9], β-interferon [100] and granulocyte – and granulocyte macrophage colony stimulating factor (CSF). G-CSF and GM-CSF have been used ex vivo to stimulate the growth and proliferation of bone marrow progenitor cells as a part of a number of gene therapy trials [10]. Some preclinical studies have demonstrated an anti-tumor response after GM-CSF administration [34, 135], and three trials have been approved for the treatment of cancer with GM-CSF. The first trial is for the treatment of metastatic renal cell cancer, the second is for prostate cancer, and the third is in melanoma.

Direct gene transfer

An increased local cytokine release has also been achieved through immunotherapy by modifying tumor cells with an allogeneic class I molecule, HLA-B7 In this direct gene transfer approach, the HLA-B7 molecule is delivered to the tumor through a DNA/lipid transfection. When the allogeneic MHC molecule is expressed on the surface of tumor cells, an immune response is stimulated, which recognizes both modified and unmodified tumor cells. These studies are currently underway in a phase I trial in which patients with malignant melanoma are given intratumoral injection of the HLA-B7/lipid complex [59, 116]. Two patients had an increase in the CTL response to tumor cells, and one partial remission has been observed. Based on these positive results, an additional protocol using the HLA-B7/lipid complex delivery system has been proposed with an improved lipid formulation. Patients with malignant melanoma and metastatic renal cell carcinoma will be treated in these trials. Since a functional MHC molecule consists of both the HLA gene product and β-2-microglobulin, other protocols have been proposed in which both genes are inserted together.

After the tumor has been recognized, lymphocytes must be activated to respond to the tumor cells. Lymphocyte activation requires two co-stimulatory signals, the CD28 receptor, which is present on T cells, and the B7 ligand, which is present on antigen presenting cells [20, 70]. Since T lymphocytes that encounter antigen in the absence of these co-stimulatory molecules become unresponsive or die, the success of an MHC-mediated cancer response depends on expression of these two molecules. Studies have been conducted with tumors that express class I antigens but lack the B7 protein, and shown that delivery of the B7 molecule led to regression of B7 negative tumors [150]. These and other studies have led to the development of a clinical protocol in which allogeneic melanoma cell lines are transduced with the B7 molecule in the hopes of generating an enhanced T cell response to melanoma antigens [144].

Tumor recognition antigens

Tumor antigens are now being utilized as immunotherapeutic agents for treatment of melanoma. One family of melanoma antigens, MAGE, has been found on a high percentage of melanomas analyzed [22]. This TATA is expressed on a variety of tumor types and normal cells. Three different genes have been isolated, termed MAGE1-3. MAGE 1 encodes an antigen known as MZ2E, which is being tested in Europe on melanoma patients with HLA-A1 haplotype. These patients are being vaccinated with irradiated allogeneic HLA-A1 tumor cells that express the MZ2E antigen [88].

The carcinoembryonic antigen (CEA) is another TATA found on different tumor types as well as normal cells and is also being developed for clinical trial use [24]. TSTA that are currently being developed for clinical use include the k-ras oncogene, which undergoes a point mutation that leads to production of an antigen that is recognizable by T cells [71, 124]. Although these studies have positive laboratory results, they have not yet progressed to the clinic.

DRUG SENSITIVITY/RESISTANCE

The phenotype of cells can be significantly altered using gene therapy technology. In these types of gene therapy, two different approaches exist for altering the phenotype of cells. In one approach, the goal is to modify normal cells, hematopoietic precursor cells, so that their resistance to toxic chemotherapeutic agents is increased. These protocols will be discussed under the stem cell marking and therapy section. In the second approach, tumor cells are modified to express a negative selectable gene, a gene that is toxic to a cell under specific conditions, such that the genetically modified cell becomes sensitive to an agent that is otherwise non-toxic to cells. These protocols will be discussed under the drug sensitivity section.

Hematopoietic stem cell marking and therapy

Stem cell marking

Bone marrow transplantation is crucial to a number of cancer therapies. Since an HLA matched donor may be difficult to locate, autologous bone marrow transplantation (ABMT) is often employed. Although autologous transplantation has some advantages over allogeneic, it carries a higher incidence of relapse. One explanation for this finding may be that the allogeneic graft recognizes and responds to leukemic cells that the patient's own cells do not. Another possibility is that residual leukemic cells are transplanted along with the patient's bone marrow. Determining the source of relapse in ABMT is critical to development of a regimen to prevent or treat the relapse. If the marrow is the source of tumor cells, then purging should decrease the incidence of relapse.

Gene transfer has been employed as a method to determine the source of relapse by using retroviral vectors to mark bone marrow cells prior to transplantation. A number of studies have been initiated using a vector containing the neo gene to mark the bone marrow [13, 14, 25, 31]. After administration of the marked marrow, the patient is followed and monitored for relapse. If relapse occurs, the malignant cells are analyzed for presence of the gene marker. If the marker is present in the tumor cells, then the bone marrow is the likely source for the relapse. One limitation of this study is that a number of unmarked bone marrow cells are returned along with the marked cells, which would not be detected.

A modification of this approach has been made in which peripheral blood stem cells are marked with a different, distinguishable vector from the one marking the bone marrow. In this type of study, the chances of detecting a marked gene are increased, since two separate populations of cells are monitored. It also provides a study design in which two different sources of stem cells are evaluated for their ability to repopulate the bone marrow and two different sources of relapse are considered.

Stem cell therapy

Marking studies in ABMT have been conducted with the multidrug resistance (MDR) gene, which also has the potential to be therapeutic. In the first phase of these studies, the MDR gene is introduced into the bone marrow in the same manner as the neo containing vectors. Marked cells can be identified by both the presence of the gene by DNA analysis and by function of the MDR gene product, which is a protein that confers a phenotype to cells of resistance to multiple agents often used in chemotherapy [141]. The initial phase of these studies has a similar design to the neo marking trials, but also has an additional phase if patients relapse. Bone marrow cells modified with the MDR gene are protected from the toxicity of a number of chemotherapeutic agents, which allows for treatment of the cancer patients with a higher and potentially more efficacious dose. Thus, if patients undergo additional cycles of chemotherapy after ABMT, the MDR gene should allow the labeled cells to survive the therapy [6, 30, 123]. One major shortcoming of this type of approach is that if residual malignant cells become modified with the MDR gene that they also would then be protected from chemotherapeutic agents. Procedural precautions are being taken in these studies to prevent this event from occurring, including evaluation of bone marrow samples for metastasis, but the risk cannot be fully eliminated.

Drug sensitivity: HSV-TK and the bystander effect

Negative selection

A different form of a drug delivery system is to deliver gene products directly to the tumor that will allow negative selection of malignant cells. There are three classes of negative selectable gene markers used for cancer gene therapy: antigenic modification with MHC genes, immune enhancement with cytokine genes, and conference of drug sensitivity with enzyme genes. The first two approaches require an action by the immune system to selectively kill the gene-modified cells. The third approach is to allow negative selection of tumor cells by transducing them with a gene encoding an enzyme that can metabolize a non-toxic pro-drug into its toxic form.

The herpes simplex virus thymidine kinase (HSV-TK) gene confers a drug sensitivity to cells, since the enzyme preferentially phosphorylates the antiviral agent acyclovir (ACV) and its derivative ganciclovir (GCV) into a monophosphate. Cellular enzymes can then di- and triphosphorylate the monophosphate ganciclovir into a compound that is highly toxic to cells. Cells that do not express the HSV-TK enzyme are minimally affected by GCV [38, 39].

Mosaic theory

Moolten and colleagues first used negative selectable marker genes to demonstrate that tumor cells genetically modified with the HSV-TK gene were killed by GCV both *in vitro* and *in vivo.* They developed the mosaic theory of cancer gene therapy, which is a prophylactic treatment designed to modify the cells such that they could be treated if a cancer developed. This anti-cancer approach was designed to generate a mosaicism within a tissue of an individual at high risk for developing cancer, by transducing the cells of an organ with the HSV-TK gene. If a tumor arose from one of the genetically modified cells, then the individual could be treated with GCV to eliminate it. Other negative selectable genes, such as cytosine deaminase, could also be used in this type of system. More important, the use of a number of negative selectable genes to transduce a tissue population would allow only a small percentage of normal cells to be susceptible to any one agent [104-106]. Thus, once a tumor develops and is determined to express a given negative selectable gene, a specific drug could be used to kill the tumor population while preserving cells that contain other negative selectable genes. The clinical use of this approach has been limited by practical difficulties, primarily that the treatment of pre-existing cancers would not be possible. Further, since individuals at high risk for developing cancer would need to have their cells modified prior to the onset of disease, long term expression of the gene in vivo would be required until the cancer developed. Unfortunately, gene transfer techniques have not allowed such long term expression, and the technology to genetically modify a large portion of a tissue is not yet available.

Therapeutic use of HSV-TK

For this system to be therapeutic, the HSV-TK gene must be delivered to pre-existing tumors. Studies by Freeman and colleagues demonstrated regression of a pre-existing tumor when tumor cells that were genetically modified to express the HSV-TK gene were injected into the peritoneal cavity of animals bearing peritoneal tumors, followed by treatment with GCV. These studies showed that HSV-TK expressing tumor cells are toxic to nearby unmodified tumors when exposed to ganciclovir. This killing of nearby unmodified tumor cells by the gene-modified HSV-TK tumor cells has been referred to as the 'bystander effect' [45, 46].

Ongoing studies have been analyzing the mechanism of bystander killing, since Freeman and colleagues presented the first gene therapy trial using HSV-TK [46]. It appears as though different mechanisms may be active *In vitro* from those active *in vivo,* which has implications for improving the *in vivo* bystander killing by enhancing the appropriate mechanism. *In vitro* studies have shown that the 'bystander effect' is likely to be mediated by the transfer of toxic ganciclovir metabolites from dying HSV-TK cells to nearby unmodified tumor cells [50]. Since the phosphorylated ganciclovir metabolites do not readily cross cell membranes, transfer of these compounds must involve cell to cell transfer. This mechanism was first suggested in studies showing that toxic ganciclovir metabolites were transferred from the HSV-TK gene-modified cells to nearby unmodified cells through apoptotic vesicles that were generated by the dying HSV-TK gene-modified cells [45]. Tumor cells have receptors to apoptotic vesicles since dying tumor cells within a growing tumor undergo apoptosis and nearby tumor cells engulf the apoptotic vesicles from the dying cells as a 'housekeeping function'. Stambrook and colleagues confirmed these initial findings by showing that toxic ganciclovir metabolites were transferred from the gene modified cells to nearby unmodified cells by using tritium labeled ganciclovir. They hypothesized that the transfer of the toxic metabolites was occurring through gap junctions [7, 125]. Further investigation is continuing in a number of laboratories to understand the *in vitro* bystander effect.

In vivo bystander effect

In vivo murine studies suggested that an additional or different mechanism is responsible for the bystander effect *in vivo.* Although the transfer of toxic metabolites may occur *in vivo,* it appears as though the immune system constitutes a significant element of this anti-tumor response. Freeman et al showed that bystander killing did not occur in immune compromised mice. Further, in immunocompetent mice, a hemorrhagic tumor necrosis occurred in animals within one day after receiving the

HSV-TK gene modified cells and GCV [46, 47]. A number of investigators observed that tumors would undergo a hemorrhagic necrosis following injection of HSV-TK tumor cells and ganciclovir [46, 50, 128]. Both the mechanism and the significance of the hemorrhagic necrosis may be different, depending on the animal model used. For example, Ram et al used a brain tumor animal model in which HSV-TK producer cells were injected into the tumor [12, 128, 119]. The observed hemorrhagic necrosis was hypothesized to be due to *in situ* transduction and killing of endothelial cells lining blood vessels in the tumor after ganciclovir therapy [128]. Alternatively, when Freeman et al injected gene-modified tumor cells that did not produce vectors, hemorrhagic necrosis occurred within 24 hours of intraperitoneal injection of HSV-TK tumor cells and ganciclovir into mice with an intraperitoneal tumor. Since the gene-modified cells in this case did not produce retroviral vectors and the hemorrhagic necrosis occurred rapidly, these investigators hypothesized that soluble factors were elicited or liberated by the gene-modified cells, causing the hemorrhagic necrosis [46, 48, 49].

Tumors were analyzed for cytokine production after injection of the HSV-TK expressing tumor cells and ganciclovir. A cytokine cascade developed in the intraperitoneal tumor after injection of the HSV-TK cells. To understand the mechanism of alteration of the tumor microenvironment by the injected gene-modified cells, a series of experiments was performed. Freeman and colleagues showed that ganciclovir exposure induced cytokine production in the HSV-TK gene-modified tumor cells and that these cytokine secreting gene-modified cells preferentially homed to the *in situ* tumor, thus stimulating the immune system at the tumor microenvironment [49] (Fig. 4). These findings led to the hypothesis that the *in vivo* 'bystander effect' is mediated through the release of soluble factors from the GCV exposed HSV-TK tumor cells. These GCV 'activated' gene-modified cells home to intraperitoneal (I.P.) tumor deposits when they are injected I.P. TNF, IL-1 and other cytokines are released within the tumor in response to the HSV-TK cells and induce a hemorrhagic tumor necrosis within twenty four hours of injection. This allows the influx of lymphoid cells that can adhere to the tumor because of upregulation of adhesion proteins on surface endothelial cells [48]. It is hypothesized that cytokines within the tumor can then activate lymphoid cells to kill the tumor.

The integral role of the immune/inflammatory system in the 'bystander effect' is highlighted not only by the cytokine cascade described above but also by experiments using immune compromised and immunized mice. Immunocompromised mice were shown to have a diminished or absent bystander killing effect [158]. This abrogation of the 'bystander effect' occurred even when all the tumor cells expressed the HSV-TK gene. Further, mice that were immunized with tumor cells prior to treatment with the HSV-TK tumor cells and ganciclovir survived longer than unimmunized mice. In addition, some differences were observed in the cytokines produced within the tumors of immunized and unimmunized mice. TNF and IL-6 were observed initially after the mice received the gene-modified cells. Although it would appear that stimulation of the immune system in conjunction with delivery of the HSV-TK gene-modified cells would enhance the effect, studies using a combination of IL-2 and HSV-TK transduced tumor cells to treat brain tumors [26] showed no increased killing of tumor cells by the addition of IL-2. Thus, the role of the immune system is complex, and further understanding of the mechanism of the 'bystander effect' is critical to developing more effective biotherapeutic approaches.

Other tumor types have also been shown to be killed by HSV-TK tumor cells in a 'bystander effect, ' including lung cancer cells [58], mesothelioma, glioblastoma, and hepatoma [15]. In these cases, tumor killing occurred when only a fraction of the tumor expressed the HSV-TK gene. Since the bystander effect appears to depend upon proximity of the modified and unmodified cells, ovarian cancer was selected as a model system for the first clinical trial, as stated above [48].

A number of methods have been used to effectively induce the expression of the HSV-TK gene in the tumor. As described above, the first studies used HSV-TK transduced tumor cells as delivery vehicles because they can effectively 'home' to *in situ* tumor deposits. However, *in vivo* gene transfer of the HSV-TK gene into the *in situ* tumor has gained widespread use. Retroviral vector producer cells have been used to deliver the HSV-TK gene directly to the tumor cell, using brain tumors as a model system. Short et al. [139] originally demonstrated that producer cell lines could directly deliver a marker gene, β-galactosidase, to brain tumors in rats. Ezzedine et al. [40] extended this system to deliver the HSV-TK gene to brain tumors. Tumor regression was observed following GCV treatment as described by Takayima et al. [146]. The brain provides an advantage since normal cells are not dividing, and genetic modification chiefly occurs in dividing cells, which are likely to be malignant. A clinical gene therapy protocol capitalizing on these results has been developed by Culver et al. [27] and Oldfield et al. [109], who have applied this technique to the experimental treatment of glioblastoma.

Some of the problems using retroviral vectors include their inability to transduce non-dividing cells and the low efficiency of *in vivo* transduction. Adenoviral vectors containing the HSV-TK gene have been recently used to genetically modify *in situ* tumor cells [11, 36, 55]. These studies have shown that prolonged survival in mice with glioblastomas and mesotheliomas can be achieved by injecting the adenoviral vectors into the tumors with subsequent GCV therapy. However, since adenoviral vectors transduce all cells, an effective method to control expression of the HSV-TK gene in tumors is being studied through tissue specific promoters [57, 66, 122].

The success of preclinical models using the HSV-TK gene has led to the search for other potential negative

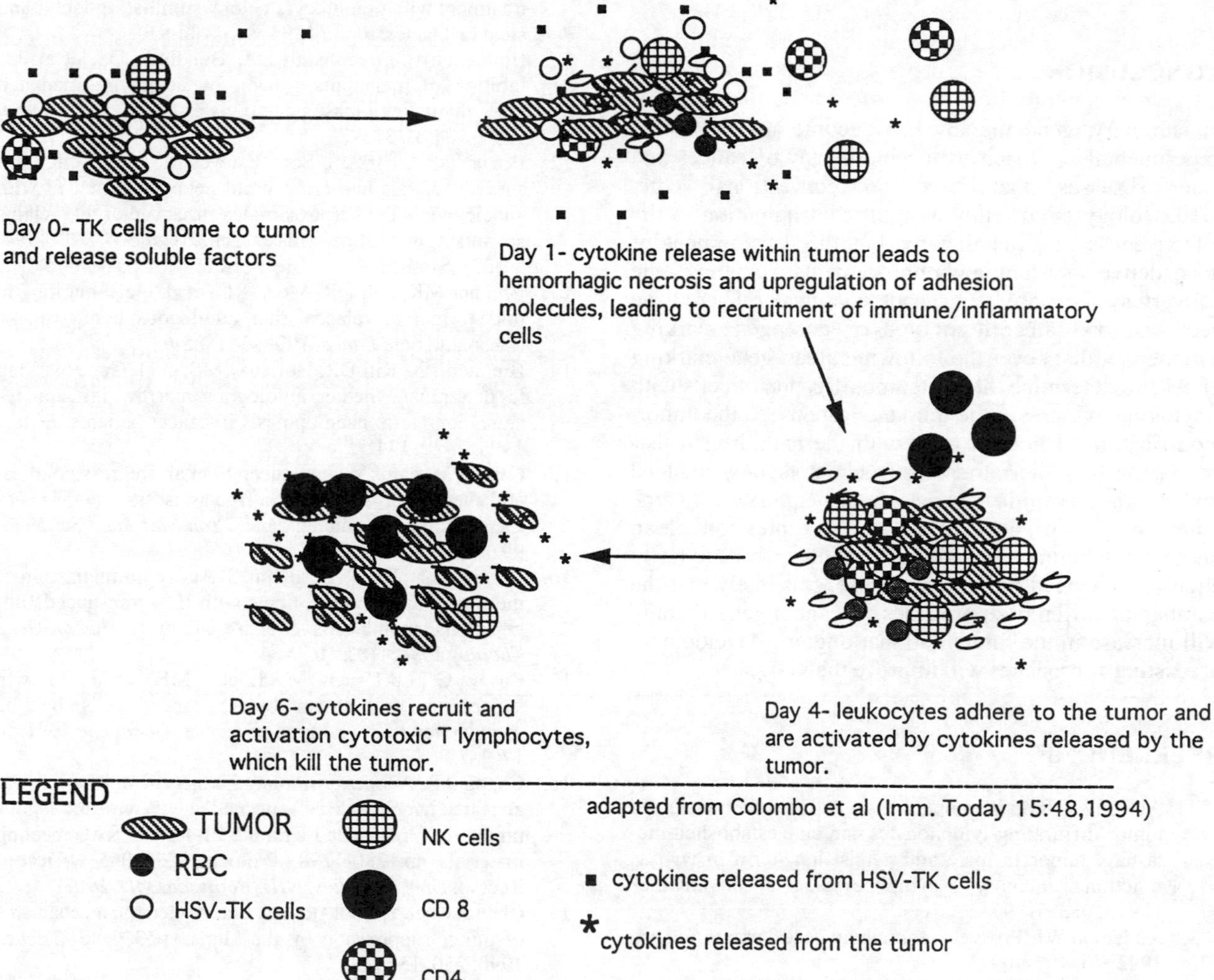

Figure 4. This figure is a schematic representation of the hypothesis by Freeman et al. on the mechanism of the 'bystander effect'. HSV-TK gene-modified tumors which have been injected intraperitoneally will migrate to an in situ tumor and become activated to produce soluble factors, such as cytokines, when exposed to GCV. These soluble factors will activate cells within the tumor to produce additional cytokines which leads to a hemorrhagic tumor necrosis and thus recruitment of leukocytes. These leukocytes adhere to and become activated by the tumor microenvironment due to upregulation of adhesion molecules and cytokines within the tumor microenvironment. The activated leukocytes will then kill the tumor.

selection systems for tumor cells. Although some have shown promise in animal studies, especially the cytosine deaminase (CD) gene, none has been introduced into clinical trials at this time. The CD gene, which is present in bacterial but not eukaryotic cells, encodes an enzyme that converts 5-fluorocytosine (5-FC) into its toxic metabolite, 5-fluorouracil (5-FU). Thus, modification of cells by this gene confers a sensitivity to 5-FC only in the cells expressing CD [113]. Any negative selection system requires a bystander effect, since it is not possible to modify all the tumor cells, and it appears that the CD gene elicits a potent one. Huber and colleagues [65] demonstrated an anti-tumor effect of cytosine deaminase expressing cells in a murine hepatoma model when animals were given 5-FC.

Other potential negative selectable markers include xanthine guaninephosphoribosyl transferase (XGPRT), which is encoded by the *E. coli* gpt gene, and purine nucleoside phosphorylase (PNP), which is encoded by the *E. coli* Deo D gene. These enzymes convert 6-thioxanthine and 6-methylpurine-2-deoxyribonucleoside, respectively, to toxic drugs [108, 142]. The ability to use negative selectable markers to treat cancer will depend on understanding the 'bystander effect' and developing methods to enhance the anti-tumor effect it produces.

CONCLUSION

In summary, gene therapy has become an established experimental approach to the biotherapy of cancer and other diseases that have no conventional cure. Methodology is currently a significant limitation to the effectiveness of gene therapy, but the development of novel delivery systems and improvements in existing gene delivery systems are being made continually. There have been six broad categories of types of cancer gene marking and therapy that cover the following areas: gene marking of cells to determine their fate; modification of cells with a cytokine to increase the immune response to the tumor; modification of normal cells with the multidrug resistance gene to protect them from chemotherapy-induced toxicity; modification of cells either to express a wild type tumor suppressor gene or to inhibit expression of an oncogene; and direct modification of tumor cells to try to elicit an enhanced immune response. It is likely that the number of different approaches to cancer gene therapy will increase in the future and that ongoing development of existing approaches will improve their efficacy.

REFERENCES

1. Alexander RB, Rosenberg SA. Adoptively transferred tumor infiltrating lymphocytes can cure established metastatic tumor in mice and persist long-term *in vivo* as functional memory T lymphocytes. *J of Immunother* 1991; 10: 387-397.
2. Anderson WF. Prospects for human gene therapy. *Science* 1992; 26: 401-409.
3. Antoniades HN, Galanopoulos T, Neville-Golden J, Maxwell M. Expression of insulin like growth factors I and II and their receptor mRNAs in primary human astrocytomas and meningiomas; *in vivo* studies using in situ hybridization and immunocytochemistry. *Int J Cancer* 1992; 50(2): 215-22.
4. Aoyagi T, Izumo S. Mapping of the pressure response element of the c-fos gene by direct DNA injection into beating hearts. *J Biol Chem* 1993; 268(36): 27176-9.
5. Baker SJ, Markowitz S, Fearon ER, et al. Suppression of human colorectal carcinoma cell growth by wild type p53. *Science* 1990; 249: 912-15.
6. Bank A. A phase I study of gene therapy for breast cancer. *Human Gene Therapy* 1994; 5(1): 102-6.
7. Bi WL, Parysek LM, Warnick R, Stambrook PJ. *In vitro* evidence that metabolic cooperation is responsible for the bystander effect observed with HSV tk retroviral gene therapy. *Human Gene Ther* 1993; 4: 725-31.
8. Blaese RM, Culver KW. Gene therapy for primary immunodeficiency disease. *Immunodefic Rev* 1992; 3(4): 329-49.
9. Blankenstein T, Qin Z, Uberla K, et al. Tumor suppression after tumor cell targeted tumor necrosis factor alpha gene transfer. *J. Exp. Med.* 1991; 173: 1047-1052.
10. Bodine DM, Seidel NE, Gale MS, et al. Efficient retrovirus transduction of mouse pluripotent hematopoietic stem cells mobilized into the peripheral blood by treatment with granulocyte colony stimulating factor and stem cell factor. *Blood* 1994; 84: 1482-91.
11. Bonnekoh B, Greenhalgh DA, Bundham DS, et al. Inhibition of melanoma growth by adenoviral-mediated HSV thymidine kinase gene transfer *in vivo*. *J Inv Derm* 1995; 104(3): 313-7.
12. Boviatsis EJ, Park JS, Sena-Esteves M, et al. Long term survival of rats harboring brain neoplasms treated with ganciclovir and a herpes simplex virus vector that retains an intact thymidine kinase gene. *Cancer Res* 1994; 54(22): 5754-51.
13. Brenner MK, Rill DR, Moen RC, et al. Gene marking to trace origin of relapse after autologous bone marrow transplantation. *Lancet* 1993; 341: 85-6.
14. Brenner MK, Rill DR, Holladay MS, et al. Gene marking to determine whether autologous marrow infusion restores long term haemopoiesis in cancer patients. *Lancet* 1993; 342: 1134-7.
15. Caruso M, Panis Y, Gagandeep S, et al. Regression of established macroscopic liver metastasesss after *in situ* transduction of a suicide gene. *Proc Natl Acad Sci* 1993; 90 (15): 7024-7028.
16. Cascinelli N, Foa R, Parmiani G. Active immunization of metastatic melanoma patients with IL-4 transduced allogeneic melanoma cells. A phase I-II study. *Human Gene Therapy* 1994; 5(8): 1059-64.
17. Casey G, Lo-Hsueh M, Lopez ME, et al. Growth suppression of human breast cancer cells by the introduction of a wild type p53 gene. *Oncogene* 1991; 6: 1791-7.
18. Chang AE. Adoptive immunotherapy of melanoma with activated lymph node cells primed *in vivo* with autologous tumor cells transduced with the IL-4 gene. RAC meeting materials pp.1280-1298. Protocol 9312-065 Office of Recom. *DNA Activities, NIH, Bethesda, MD*, 1993.
19. Chen P, Chen Y, Bookstein R, Lee W. Genetic mechanisms of tumor suppression by the human p53 gene. *Science* 1990; 250: 1576-80.
20. Chen L, Linsley PS, Hellstrom KE. Costimulation of T cells for tumor immunity. *Imm Today* 1993; 14: 483-486.
21. Chen Y, Chen P-L, Arnaiz N, et al. Expression of wild-type p53 in human A673 cells suppresses tumorigenicity but not growth rate. *Oncogene* 1991; 6: 1799-1805.
22. Chen Y-T, Stockert E, Chen Y, et al. Identification of the MAGE-1 gene product by monoclonal and polyclonal antibodies. *Proc Natl Acad Sci* 1994; 91: 1004-8.
23. Cohen PA, Kim H, Fowler DH, et al. Use of interlukin 7, IL-2, and gamma interferon to propagate CD4+ T cells in culture with maintained antigen specificity. *J Immunother* 1993; 14(3): 242-52.
24. Conry RM, LoBuglio AF, Kantor J, et al. Immune response to a carcinoembryonic polynucleotide vaccine. *Cancer Res* 1994; 54(5): 1164-8.
25. Cornetta K, Tricot G, Broun ER, et al. Retroviral mediated gene transfer of bone marrow cells during autologous bone marrow transplantation for acute leukemia. *Human Gene Therapy* 1992; 3(3): 305-18.
26. Culver KW, Blaese RM, Oldfield EH. In vivo transfer of the human interleukin-2 gene: negative tumoricidal results in experimental brain tumors. *J Neurosurg* 1994; 80(3): 535-40.

27. Culver KW, Ram Z, Wallbridge S, et al. *In vivo* gene transfer with retroviral vector-producer cells for treatment of experimental brain tumors. *Science* 1992; 256: 1550-1552.
28. Culver KW, Blaese RM, DeVroom HL, Anderson WF. Gene therapy for the treatment of brain tumors using intra-tumoral transduction with the thymidine kinase gene and intravenous ganciclovir. *Human Gene Therapy* 1993; 4(1): 39-69.
29. Curiel DT, Agarwal S, Romer MU, et al. Gene transfer to respiratory epithelial cells via the receptor mediated endocytosis pathway. *Am J Respir Cell Mol Biol* 1992; 6(3): 247-52.
30. Deisseroth AB. Use of safety-modified retroviruses to introduce chemotherapy resistance sequences into normal hematopoietic cells for chemoprotection during the therapy of ovarian cancer: a pilot trial. *Human Gene Therapy* 1994; 5(12): 1507-22.
31. Deisseroth AB, Zu Z, Claxton D, et al. Genetic marking shows that Ph+ cells present in autologous transplants of chronic myelogenous leukemia (CML) contribute to relapse after autologous bone marrow in CML. *Blood* 1994; 83(10): 3068-76.
32. Dobashi Y, Sugimura H, Sakamoto A, et al. Stepwise participation of p53 gene mutation during dedifferentiation of human thyroid carcinomas. *Diagn Mol Pathol* 1994; 3(1): 9-14.
33. Donahue RE, Kessler SW, Bodine D, et al. Helper virus induced T cell lymphoma in nonhuman primates after retroviral mediated gene transfer. *J Exp Med* 1992; 176: 1125-1135.
34. Dranoff G, Jaffee E, Lazenby A, et al. Vaccination with irradiated tumor cells engineered to secrete murine granulocyte-macrophage colony stimulating factor stimulates potent, specific, and long-lasting anti-tumor immunity. *Proc Nat Acad Sci* 1993; 90(8): 3539-43.
35. Drazan KE, Shen XD, Csete ME, et al. *In vivo* adenoviral mediated human p53 tumor suppressor gene transfer and expression in rat liver after resection. *Surgery* 1994: 116(2): 197-203.
36. Eck SJ, Wilson JM, Albelda SM. Successful adenovirus mediated gene transfer in an *in vivo* model of human malignant mesothelioma. *Annals Thor Surg* 1994; 57(6): 1395-1401.
37. Eckhardt SG, Dai A, Davidson KK. Induction of differentiation in HL60 cells by the reduction of extrachromosomally amplified c-myc. *Proc Natl Acad Sci* 1994; 91(14): 6674-8.
38. Elion GB. The chemotherapeutic exploitation of virus-specified enzymes. *Adv Enzyme Regul* 1980; 18: 53-60.
39. Elion GB, Furman PA, Fyfe JA, et al. Selectivity of action of an antiherpetic agent, 9-(2-hydroxyethoxy-methyl)-guanine. *Proc Natl Acad Sci* 1977; 74: 5716-5720.
40. Ezzedine ZD, Martuza RL, Platika D, et al. Selective killing of glioma cells in culture and *in vivo* by retrovirus transfer of the herpes simplex virus thymidine kinase gene. *New Biol* 1991; 3(6): 608-14.
41. Fearon ER and Vogelstein B. A genetic model for colorectal carcinogenesis. *Cell* 1990; 61: 759-767.
42. Fearon ER, Pardoll DM, Itaya T, et al. Interleukin 2 production by tumor cells bypasses T helper function in the generation of an antitumor response. *Cell* 1990; 60: 397-403.
43. Ferkol T, Lindberg GL, Chen J, et al. Regulation of the phosphoenolpuruvate carboxykinase/human factor IX gene introduced into the livers of adult rats by receptor mediated gene transfer. *FASEB J* 1993; 7(11): 1081-91.
44. Fisher B, Packard BS, Read EJ, et al. Tumor localization of adoptively transferred Indium-111 labeled tumor infiltrating lymphocytes in patients with metastatic melanoma. *J Clin Oncol* 1989; 7: 250-261.
45. Freeman SM, Abboud CN, Whartenby KA, et al. The bystander effect: tumor regression when a fraction of the tumor mass is genetically modified. *Cancer Res* 1993; 53: 5274-5283.
46. Freeman SM, McCune C, Angel C, et al. Treatment of ovarian cancer using HSV-TK gene-modified vaccine. *Human Gene Ther* 1992; 3: 342-9.159.
47. Freeman SM, Ramesh R, Shastri M, et al. The role of cytokines in mediating the bystander effect using HSV-TK xenogeneic cells. *Cancer Letters* (in press).
48. Freeman SM, Ramesh R, Marrogi AJ, *In vivo* studies on the mechanism of the bystander effect. *Cancer Gene Ther* 1994; 1: 326.
49. Freeman SM, Whartenby KA, Abboud CN, The use of *in situ* HSV-TK for cancer therapy. *Seminars in Oncology* (in press).
50. Freeman SM, Whartenby KA, Koeplin DS, et al. Tumor regression when a fraction of the tumor mass contains the HSV-TK gene. *J Cell Biol* 1992; 16F: 47.
51. Gastl G, Finstad CL, Guarini A, et al. Retroviral vector-mediated lymphokine gene transfer into human renal cancer cells. *Cancer Res* 1992; 52(22): 6229-36.
52. Gansbacher B, Bannerji R, Daniels B, et al. Retroviral vector-mediated gamma interferon gene transfer into tumor cells generates potent and long lasting antitumor immunity. *Cancer Res* 1990; 50: 7820-7825.
53. Grimm EA, Robb RJ, Roth JA, et al. Lymphokine activated killer cell phenomenon. III. Evidence that IL-2 is sufficient for direct activation of peripheral blood lymphocytes into lymphokine-activated killer cells. *J Exp Med* 1983; 158: 1356-1361.
54. Grimm EA, Mazumder ZA, Zhang HZ, and Rosenberg SA. Lymphokine activated kiler cell phenomenon. Lysis of natural killer-resistant fresh sholid tumor cells by interleukin 2-activated autologous human peripheral bloood lymphocytes. *J Exp Med* 1982; 155: 1823-1830.
55. Grossman RG, Woo SL. Gene therapy for brain tumors: regression of experimental gliomas by adenovirus mediated gene transfer *in vivo*. *Proc Natl Acad Sci* 1994; 91(8): 3054-7.
56. Harris CC, Hollstein M. Tumor suppressor genes. *PPO Updates* 1992; 6: 1-12.
57. Hart IR. Targeting of cytokine gene expression to malignant melanoma cells using tissue specific promoter sequences. *Ann Oncol* 1994; 5 Suppl4: 59-65.
58. Hasegawa Y, Emi N, Shimokata K, et al. Gene transfer of herpes simplex virus type I thymidine kinase gene as a drug sensitivity gene into human lung cancer cell lines using retroviral vectors. *Am J Respir Cell Mol Biol* 1993; 8(6): 655-61.
59. Hersh EM. Phase I study of immunotherapy of malignant melanoma by direct gene transfer. *Human Gene Therapy* 1994; 5: 1371-1384.
60. Holt JT, Redner RL, Nienhuis AW. (1988) An oligomer complementary to c-myc inhibits proliferation of HL60 promyelocytic cells and induces differentiation. *Mol Cell Biol* 1988; 8: 963-73.

61. Holt JT, Gopal TV, Moulton AD, Nienhuis AW. Inducible production of c-fos antisense RNA inhibits 3T3 cell proliferation. *Proc Natl Acad Sci* 1986; 83: 4794-99.
62. Holt JT. Antisense rescue defines specialized and generalized functions for c-fos protein during cell growth. *Mol Cel Biol* 1993; 13: 3821-30.
63. Horwitz MS. Adenoviridae and their replication. In: *Virology*, pp. 1679-1740, Fields, B.N., Knipe, D.M. (eds.) Raven Press, New York, 1990.
64. Huang H-JS, Yee J-K, Shew J-Y, Chen PL. Suppression of the neoplastic phenotype by replacement of the Rb gene in human cancer cells. *Science* 1988; 242: 1563-6.
65. Huber BE, Richards CA, Krenitsky TA. (1991) Retroviral-mediated gene therapy for the treatment of hepatocellular carcinoma: an innovative approach for cancer therapy. *Proc Natl Acad Sci* 1991; 88: 8039-8043.
66. Hurst H, Lemoine N. Therapeutic strategies using c-erb-B-2 promoter controlled drug activation. *Ann NY Acad Sci* 1994; 716: 115-24.
67. Hwu P, Yannelli J, Kriegler M, et al. Fumctional and molecular characterizartion of tumor infiltrating lymphocytes transduced with tumor necrosis factor alpha cDNA for the gene therapy of cancer in humans. *J Immunol* 1993; 150 (9): 4104-15.
68. Jicha DL, Mule JJ, Rosenberg SA. Interleukin 7 generates antitumor cytotoxic T lymphocytes against murine sarcomas with efficacy in cellular adoptive immunotherapy. *J Exp Med* 1991; 174(6): 1511-5.
69. Jicha DL, Schwarz S, Mule JJ, Rosenberg SA. Interleukin-7 mediates the generation and expansion of murine allosensitized and antitumor CTL. *Cell Immunol* 1992; 141(1): 71-83.
70. June CH, Bluestone JA, Nadler LM, Thompson CB. The B7 and CD28 receptor families. *Imm Today* 1994; 15: 321-31.
71. Jung S, Schluessner HJ. Human T lymphocytes recognize a peptide of single point-mutated oncogenic ras proteins. *J Exp Med* 1991; 173: 273-6.
72. Kamb A, Gruis NA, Weaver-Feldhaus J, et al. A cell cycle regulator potentially involved in genesis of many tumor types. *Science* 1994; 264: 436-40.
73. Kantoff PW, Kohn DB, Mitsuya H, et al. (1986) Correction of ADA deficiency in cultured human B and T cells by retroviral mediated gene transfer. *Proc Natl Acad Sci* 1986; 83(17): 6563-7.
74. Karpati G, Acsadi G.The potential for gene therapy in Duchenne muscular dystrophy and other genetic muscle diseases. *Muscle Nerve* 1993; 16(11): 1141-53.
75. Keating A., Toneguzzo F. Gene transfer by electroporation: a model for gene therapy. *Bone Marrow Purg and Proc* 1990: 491-498.
76. Klein G. The approaching era of the tumor suppressor gens. *Science* 1987; 238: 1539-1545.
77. Lafreniere R, Rosenberg SA. (1985) Succesful immunotherapy of murine experimental hepatic metastases with lymphokine-activated killer cells and recombinant interleukin 2. *Cancer Res* 1985; 45: 3735-3741.
78. Lafreniere R, Rosenberg SA. Adoptive immunothearpy of murine hepatic metastases with lymphokine activated killer cells and recombinant interleukin 2 can mediate the regression of both immunogenic and nonimmunogenic sarcomas and an adenocarcinoma. *J Imm* 1985; 135: 4273-4280.
79. Levine AJ, Momand J. Tumor suppressor genes, the p53 and retinblastoma sensitivity genes and gene products. *Biochim. Biophys Acta* 1990; 1032: 119-136.
80. Levine AJ. The tumor suppressor genes. *Annu Rev Biochem* 1993; 62: 623-51.
81. Levrero M, Barban S, Manteca S, et al. Defective and non-defective adenoviral vectors for expressing foreign genes *in vitro* and *in vivo*. *Gene* 1991; 101: 195-202.
82. Liu TJ, Zhang W-W, Taylor DL, et al. Growth suppression of human head and neck cancer cells by the introduction of a wild-type p53 gene via a recombinant adenovirus. *Cancer Res* 1994; 54(14): 3662-7.
83. Lohmann D, Ruhri C, Schmitt M, et al. Accumulation of p53 protein as an indicator for p53 gene mutation in breast cancer. *Diag Mol Pathol* 1993; 2: 36-41.
84. Lotze MT, Grimm EA, Mazumder A, et al. *In vitro* growth of cytotoxic human lymphocytes. IV. Lysis of fresh and cultured autologous tumor by lymphocytes cultured in T cell growth factor. *Cancer Res* 1981; 41: 4420-4425.
85. Lotze MT, Rubin JT. Gene therapy of cancer: a pilot study of IL-4 gene modified fibroblasts admixed with autologous tumor to elicit an immune response. *Human Gene Therapy* 1994; 5(1): 41-55.
86. Mackensen A, Carcelain G, Viel S, et al. Direct evidence to support the immunosurveillance concept in a human regressive melanoma. *J Clin Invest* 1994; 93(4): 1397-402.
87. Mann R and Baltimore D. Varying the position of a retroviral packaging sequence results in the encapsidation of both unspliced and spliced RNAs. *J Virol* 1985; 5 4: 401-407.
88. Marchand M, Brasseur F, vanderBruggen P, et al. Perspectives for immunization of HLA-A1 patients carrying a malignant melanoma expressing gene MAGE-1. *Dermatology* 1993; 186: 278-80.
89. Marcus SG, Perry-Lalley D, Mule JJ, et al. The use of interleukin-6 to generate tumor infiltrating lymphocytes with enhanced *in vivo* antitumor activity. *J Immunother Emphasis Tumor Immunol* 1994; 15(2): 105-12.
90. Marin MC, Hsu B, Meyn RE, et al. Evidence that p53 and bcl-2 are regulators of a common cell death pathway important for *in vivo* lymphomagenesis. *Oncogene* 1994; 9(11): 3107-12.
91. Markowitz D, Goff S, and Bank A. A safe packaging line for gene transfer: separating viral genes on two different plasmids. *J Virol* 1988; 62: 3725-3732.
92. Markowitz D, Goff S, Bank A. Construction and use of a safe and efficient amphotropic packaging cell line. *Virol* 1988; 167: 400-406.
93. Miescher S, Whiteside TL, Moretta L, Von Fliedner V. Clonal and frequency analyses of tumor infiltrating T lymphocytes from human solid tumors. *J Imm* 1987; 138: 4004-4011.
94. Miller AD, Bender MA, Harris EAS, et al. Design of retroviral vectors for transfer and expression of human beta globin gene. *J Virol* 1988; 62: 4337-4345.
95. Miller AD, Buttimore C. Redesign of retrovirus packaging cell lines to avoid recombination leading to helper virus production. *Mol Cell Biol* 1986; 6: 2895-2902.
96. Miller AD, Rossman GJ. Improved retroviral vectors for gene transfer and expression. *Biotechniques* 1989; 7: 980-990.
97. Miller DG, Adam MA, Miller AD. Gene transfer by retrovirus vectors occurs only in cells that are actively replicating at the time of infection. *Mol Cell Biol* 1990; 10(8): 4239-4242.

98. Miller AD. Human gene therapy comes of age. *Nature* 1992; 357: 455-460.
99. Mitani K, Wakamiya M, Caskey CT. Long term expression of retroviral transduced adenosine deaminase in human primitive hematopoietic progenitors. *Human Gene Therapy* 1993; 4(1): 9-16.
100. Mizuno M, Yoshida J, Sugita K, et al. (1990) Growth inhibition of glioma cells transfected with the human beta interferon gene by liposomes coupled with a monoclonal antibody. *Cancer Res* 1990; 50: 7826-7829.
101. Mizutani Y, Fukumoto M, Bonavida B, Yoshida O. Enhancement of sensitivity of urinary bladder tumor cells to cisplatin by c-myc antisense oligonucleotide. *Cancer* 1994; 74(9): 2546-54.
102. Montgomery DL, Shiver JW, Leander KR, et al. Heterologous and homologous protection against influenza A by DNA vaccination: optimization of DNA vectors. *DNA Cell Biol* 1993; 12(9): 777-83.
103. Momand J, Zambetti GP, Olson DC, The mdm-2 oncogene product forms a complex with the p53 protein and inhibits p53 mediated transactivation. *Cell* 1992; 69(7): 1237-45.
104. Moolten FL. Tumor chemosensitivity conferred by inserted herpes thymidine kinase genes: paradigm for a prospective cancer control strategy. *Canc Res* 1986; 46: 5276-5281.
105. Moolten FL. Mosaicism induced by gene insertion as a means of improving chemotherapeutic selectivity. *Crit Rev in Immunol* 1990; 10: 203-233.
106. Moolten FL and Wells JM. Curability of tumors bearing herpes thymidine kinase genes transferred by retroviral vectors. *J Natl Can Inst* 1990; 82: 297-300.
107. Morgan RA, Cornetta K, Anderson WF. Applications of the polymerase chain reaction in retroviral mediated gene transfer and the analysis of gene-marked human TIL cells. *Hum Gene Ther* 1990; 1: 135-49.145.
108. Mroz PJ, Moolten FL. Retrovirally transduced *E. coli* gpt genes combine selectability with chemosensitivity capable of mediating tumor eradication. *Human Gene Ther* 1993; 4: 589-595.
109. Mueller SN, Blaese RM, Oldfield EH. Intrathecal gene therapy for malignant leptomeningeal neoplasia. *Cancer Res* 1994; 54(8): 2141-5.
110. Mule JJ, Shu S, Schwarz SL, Rosenberg SA. Adoptive immunotherapy of established pulmonary metastases with LAK cells and recombinant interleukin 2. *Science* 1985; 225: 1487-1489.
111. Mule JJ, Shu S, Rosenberg SA. The anti-tumor efficacy of lymphokine activated killer cells and recombinant interleukin 2 *in vivo*. *J Immunol* 1985; 135: 646-652.
112. Mule JJ, Custer MC, Travis WD, and Rosenberg SA. Cellular mechanisms of the antitumor activity of recombinant IL-6 in mice. *J Imm* 1992; 148: 2622-2629.
113. Mullen CA, Kilstrup M, Blaese RM. Transfer of the bacterial gene for cytosine deaminase to mammalian cells confers lethal sensitivity to 5-fluorocytosine: a negative selection system. *Proc Natl Acad Sci* 1992; 89: 33-37.
114. Muller WJ, Sinn E, Pattengale PK, et al. Single step induction of mammary adenocarcinoma in trangenic mice bearing the activated c-neu oncogene. *Cell* 1988; 54: 105-15.
115. Muul LM, Spiess PJ, Director EP, Rosenberg SA. Identification of specific cytolytic immune responses against autologous tumor in humans bearing malignant melanoma. *J Imm* 1987; 138: 989-995.
116. Nabel GJ. Immunotherapy for cancer by direct gene transfer into tumors. *Human Gene Therapy* 1994; 5(1): 57-77.
117. Nabel GJ, Nabel EG, Yang ZY, et al. Direct gene transfer with DNA-liposome complexes in melanoma: expression, biologic activity, and lack of toxicity in humans. *Proc Natl Acad Sci* 1993; 90: 11307-11311.136.
118. Newcomb EW, Madonia WJ, Pisharody S, et al. A correlative study of p53 protein altertion and p53 gene mutation in glioblastoma multiforme. *Brain Pathol* 1993; 3(3): 229-35.
119. Oldfield EH, Ram Z, Culver KW, et al. Gene therapy for the treatment of brain tumors using intratumoral transduction with the thymidine kinase gene and intravenous ganciclovir. *Hum Gene Ther* 1993; 4(1): 39-69.
120. Olsen DC, Marechal V, Momand J, et al. Identification and characterization of multiple mdm-2 proteins and mdm-2-p53 protein complexes. *Oncogene* 1993; 8(9): 2353-60.
121. Ogasawara M, Rosenberg SA. Enhanced expression of HLA molecules and stimulation of autologous human tumor infiltrating lymphocytes following transduction of melanoma cells with gamma interferon genes. *Cancer Res* 1993; 53(15): 3561-8.
122. Osaki T, Tanio Y, Tachibana I, et al. Gene therapy for carcinoembryonic antigen producing human lung cancer cells by cell type specific expression of herpes simplex virus thymdine kinase gene. *Cancer Res* 1994; 54(20): 5258-61.
123. O'Shaughnessy JA, Cowan KH, Nienhuis AW, et al. Retroviral mediated transfer of the human multidrug resistance gene (MDR-1) into hematopoietic stem cells during autologous transplantation after intensive chemotherapy for metastatic breast cancer. *Human Gene Therapy* 1994; 5(7): 891-911.
124. Peace DJ, Smith JW, Disis ML, et al. Induction of T cells specific for the mutated segment of oncogneic p21 ras protein by immunization *in vivo* with the oncogenic protein. *J Immunother* 1993; 14: 110-4.
125. Pitts J. Cancer gene therapy: a bystander effect using the gap junctional pathway. Mol Carcin 1994; 11(3): 127-30.
126. Prigozy T, Dalrymple K, Kedes L, Shuler C. Direct DNA injection into mouse tongue muscle for analysis of promoter function *in vivo*. Somat. *Cell Mol Gemnnet* 1993; 19(2): 111-22.
127. Porgador A, Bannerji R, Watanabe Y, et al. Antimetastatic vaccination of tumor bearing mice with two types of IFN-gamma gene inserted tumor cells. *J Immunol* 1993; 150(4): 1458-70.
128. Ram Z, Walbridge S, Shawker T, et al. The effect of thymidine kinase transduction and ganciclovir therapy on tumor vasculature and growth of 9L glioma in rats. *J Neurosurg* 1994; 81(2): 256-60.
129. Rich DP, Couture M, Cardoza LM, et al. Development and analysis of recombinant adenovirus for gene therapy of cystic fibrosis. *Human Gene Therapy* 1993; 4: 461-76.
130. Rosenberg SA. Karnofsky Memorial Lecture. The immunotherapy and gene therapy of cancer. *J Clin Oncol* 1992; 10(2): 180-99.
131. Rosenberg SA. *Human Gene Therapy* 1992; 3(1): 75-90.
132. Rosenberg SA, Aebersold PM, Cornetta K, et al. Gene transfer into humans-immunotherapy of patients with advanced melanoma, using tumor-infiltrating lymphocytes modified by retroviral gene transduction. *New Engl J Med*

1990; 323: 570-578.
133. Rosenfeld MA, Siegfried W, Yoshimara K, et al. (1991) Adenovirus-mediated transfer of a recombinant alpha 1 antitrypsin gene to the lung epithelium *in vivo*. *Science* 1991; 252: 431-434.
134. Rosenfeld MA, Yoshimura K, Trapnell BC, et al. In vivo transfer of the human cystic fibrosis transmembrane conductance regulator gene to the airway epithelium. *Cell* 1992; 65: 183-185.
135. Sanda MG, Ayyagari SR, Jaffee EM, et al. (1994) Demonstration of a rational strategy for human prostate cancer gene therapy. *J Urol* 1994; 151(3): 622-8.
136. Sandberg-Nordqvist AC, Stahlbom PA, Reinecke M, et al. Characterization of insulin-like growth factor 1 in human primary brain tumors. *Cancer Res* 1993; 53(11): 2475-8.
137. Sawami H, Ito K, Norioka M, et al. Transfer of the adenosine deaminase gene of a B lymphoblastoid cell line to an ADA deficienct LCL by a microcell mediated chromosome transfer technique. *Nippon Ketsucki Gakkai Zasshi* 1989; 52(6): 1033-44.
138. Seigler HF, Darrow TL, Abdel-Waheb Z, et al. A phase I trial of human gamma interferon transduced autologous tumor cells in patients with disseminated malignant melanoma. *Human Gene Therapy* 1994; 5(6): 761-77.
139. Short MP, Choi B, Lee JK, Gene delivery to glioma cells in rat brain by grafting of a retrovirus packaging cell line. *J of Neurosci Res* 1990; 27: 427-433.
140. Sinn E, Muller W, Pattengale P, et al. Coexpression of MMTV/v-Ha-ras and MMTV/c-myc genes: synergistic actions of oncogenes *in vivo*. *Cell* 1987; 49: 465-74.
141. Sorrentino BP, Brandt SJ, Bodine D, et al. Selection of drug-resistant bone marrow cells *in vivo* after retroviral transfer of human MDR-1. *Science* 1992; 257: 99-103.
142. Sorscher EJ, Peng S, Bebok Z, et al. Tumor cell bystander killing in colonic carcinoma utilizing the *E. coli* DeoD gene to generate toxic purines. *Gene Ther* 1994; 1: 233-238.
143. Stuber G, Leder GH, Storkus WT, et al. Identification of wild type and mutant p53 peptids binding to HLA-A2 assessed by a peptide loading-deficient cell line assay and a novel major histocompatibility complex class I peptide binding assay. *Eur J Immunol* 1994; 24(3): 765-8.
144. Sznol M. A phase I trial of B7-transfected lethally irradiated allogeneic melanoma cell lines to induce cell mediated immunity against tumor associated antigens presented by HLA-A2 or HLA-A1 in patients with stage IV melanoma. RAC meeting materials pp.1505-37. Protocol 9312-065. Office of Recom. *DNA Activities, NIH, Bethesda, MD*, 1993.
145. Takagi S, Chen K, Schwarz R, et al. Functional and phenotypic analysis of tumor infiltrating lympocytes isolated from human primary and metastatic liver tumors and cultured in recombinant interleukin 2. *Cancer* 1989; 63: 102-111
146. Takamiya Y, Short MP, Moolten FL, et al. An experimental model of retrovirus gene therapy for malignant brain tumors. *J Neurosurg* 1993; 79(1): 104-110.
147. Tepper RI. The tumor-cytokine transplantation assay and the antitumor activity of interleukin-4. *Bone Marr Transp* 1992; 9S: 177-181.
148. Tepper RI, Pattengale PK, and Leder P. Murine interleukin 4 displays potent anti-tumor activity *in vivo*. *Cell* 1989; 57: 503-512.
149. Topalian SL, Solomon D, Rosenberg SA. Tumor-specific cytolysis by lymphcytes infiltrating human melanomas. *J Imm* 1989; 142: 3714-3725.
150. Townsend SE, Allison JP. Tumor rejection after direct costimulation of CD8+ T cells by B7-transfected melanoma cells. *Science* 1993; 259: 368-70.
151. Tripathy D, Benz CC. Activated oncogenes and putative tumor suppressor genes involved in human breast cancers. *Cancer Treat Res* 1992; 63: 15-60.
152. Trojan J, Johnson TR, Rudin SD, et al. Treatment and prevention of rat glioblastoma by immunogenic C6 cells expressing antisense insulin-like growth factor I *RNA*. *Science* 1993; 259(5091): 94-7.
153. Tohmatsu A, Okino T, Stabach P, et al. Analysis of cytolytic effector cell response *in vitro* against autologous human tumor cells genetically altered to synthesize interleukin-2. *Immunol Lett* 1993; 35(1): 51-7.
154. Tsai SC, Gansbacher B, Tait L, et al. Induction of antitumor immunity by interleukin-2 gene-transduced mouse mammary tumor cells versus transduced mammary stromal fibroblasts. *J Natl Cancer Inst* 1993; 85(7): 546-53.
155. Uchimaya A, Hoon DS, Morisaki T, et al. Transfection of interleukin 2 gene into human melanoma cells augments cellular immune response. *Cancer Res* 1993; 53(5): 949-52.
156. Varmus H. Oncogenes and the molecular origins of cancer. pp. 3-44. Cold Spring Harbor Press, New York, 1993.
157. Vile RG, Hart IR. *In vitro* and *in vivo* targetting of gene expression to melanoma cells. *Cancer Res* 1993; 53(5): 962-7.
158. Vile RG, Nelson JA, Castleden S, et al. Systemic gene therapy of murine melanoma using tissue specific expression of the HSVtk gene involves an immune component. *Cancer Research* 1994; 54(23): 6228-34.
159. Wang NP, Hoang T, Lee W-H, and Lee EY-HP. Tumor suppressor activity of Rb and p53 genes in human breast carcinoma cells. *Oncogene* 1993; 8: 279-88.
160. Wang NP, Hoang T, Lee W-H, Lee EY-HP. Tumor suppressor activity of Rb and p53 genes in human breast carcinoma cells. *Oncogene* 1993; 8: 279-88.
161. Wolff JA, Friedmann T. Approaches to gene therapy in disorders of purine metabolism. *Rheum Dis Clin North Am* 1988; 14(2): 459-77.
162. Wright C, Mellon K, Johnston P, et al. Expression of p53, c-erbB2 and the epidermal growth factor receptor in transitional cell carcinoma of the human urinary bladder. *Br J Cancer* 1991; 63: 967-70.
163. Wu GY, Wilson JM, Shalaby F, et al. Receptor mediated gene delivery *in vivo*. Partial correction of genetic analbuminemia in Nagase rats. *J Biol Chem* 1991; 266(22): 14338-42.
164. Yron I, Wood TA, Spiess PJ, Rosenberg SA. *In vitro* growth of murine T cells. V. The isolation and growth of lymphoid cell infiltrating syngeneic solid tumors. *J Immunol* 1980; 125: 238-241.
165. Zhang W-W, Fang X, Branch CD, et al. Generation and identification of recombinant adenovirus by liposome mediated transfection and PCR analyses. *Biotechniques* 1993; 15: 868-72.
166. Zhang W-W, Fang X, Mazur W, et al.High efficiency gene transfer and high level expression of wild type p53 in human lung cancer cells mediated by recombinant adenovirus. *Cancer Gene Therapy* 1994; 1: 5-13.

CANCER BIOTHERAPY: 1998 DISEASE-RELATED ACTIVITY

ROBERT K. OLDHAM[1], SCOTT EBBINGHAUS[2] and M. ERNEST MARSHALL[3]
[1] *Biological Therapy Institute Foundation, Franklin, Tennessee; and University of Missouri, Columbia, Missouri;*
[2] *University of Alabama at Birmingham, Birmingham, Alabama*
[3] *University of Texas, Galveston, Texas*

The 1990s will witness a burgeoning number of biologicals under clinical investigation, either singly or in combination with other biologicals or chemotherapeutic agents. Already, biotherapies have demonstrated efficacy against certain malignancies. It is expected that their assimilation into our standard anticancer armamentarium will continue to broaden in the 1990s, leading to the dominance of biotherapy in cancer treatment soon after the year 2000. This chapter will summarize disease-related activity for selected biotherapies as we complete the final decade of this millennium.

Historically, cancers have been classified by histopathological features, based on the pathologist's ability to discern similarities and differences among cancers by scrutinizing tissue sections under the microscope. Over 100 types of cancers have been so categorized. This disease-based classification scheme, upon which the previous standard modalities of cancer treatment – surgery, radiation therapy, and chemotherapy – were structured, has contributed to major advances in the treatment of selected malignancies.

As cancer biology becomes better understood, we may learn that the unregulated growth of tissues, the activation of oncogenes, the persistence of cells that normally become senescent, and maturational aberrations may segregate in patterns not amenable to simplistic histopathological classification. Early evidence of such categorizational conflict is provided by the presence of similar antigens on cancer cells arising from very different tissues. For example, antibodies have been described that react very clearly with breast cancer, colon cancer, and certain other adenocarcinomas. As such, these antibodies cross histopathological and anatomic borders. Similarly, there may be common reactivities among tumors of lymphoid origin, of squamous differentiation, and of mesenchymal derivation. A better understanding of oncogene activation and of normal and aberrant regulation of growth and differentiation may provide for a dynamic classification scheme rather than the static descriptive one we now use. As new approaches in biotherapy are tested, scientists and clinicians must be constantly aware that our current histological anatomic classification system is largely artificial and that clues to the clinical activity of biotherapy may allow us to reclassify neoplasms according to biological features and observations.

Such considerations transcend all aspects of classical developmental therapeutics, in which surgery, radiation therapy, and chemotherapy evolved along disease-specific and anatomic lines. Thus, although phase I toxicity trials are conducted across histological boundaries, phase II and III studies progress within a fairly rigid disease-specific format. As a consequence, antitumor activities in lung cancer, breast cancer, colon cancer, etc. are discussed and debated. While such a testing paradigm may have served oncologists well for protocol construction and for regulatory oversight, this mind set of classical disease oriented phase II-III studies may actually inhibit the development of biotherapy [245]. With this new modality, we must be open to the possibility that the biological activity of these agents and approaches may sort unpredictably and may require a more individualistic orientation. For example, it is abundantly clear that monoclonal antibody technology can allow for the precise description of an individual patient's cancer using panels of antibodies [10, 238, 239]. The use of the laboratory to develop patient-specific therapies may allow scientists and clinicians to approach the cancer problem from a completely different and more individualized perspective [240, 247].

Many biotherapies are supportive or ancillary to the antitumor activity of standard approaches such as chemotherapy. Use of colony-stimulating factors, erythropoietin, blood transfusions, marrow transplantation, etc. have broad application in oncology. These techniques were described in earlier chapters.

While recognizing the limitations of organ-specific categorization, it remains a standard and useful exercise to describe the clinical activities in biotherapy within such a historical framework. Therefore, in this chapter, a brief summary of the activity of various forms of biotherapy will be provided by cancer type. This chapter is designed to describe these activities briefly with references into 1996 and is for quick reference only. The reader is encouraged to refer to specific, subject-oriented chapters and references for detailed information on specific methods of cancer biotherapy.

R.K. Oldham (ed.), Principles of Cancer Biotherapy. 3rd ed., 463–492.

SOLID TUMORS

Melanoma

Melanoma is curable by surgery in early disease stages (stage I and some stage II). However, disseminated melanoma is refractory to current radiation therapy and chemotherapy. Although short term, palliative responses to chemotherapy are commonly seen, particularly in skin, lung and subcutaneous lesions, significant long-term benefit in visceral disease is infrequent.

Melanoma has long been known to be a tumor with unusual behavior in certain patients. Spontaneous complete regression is said to occur in one patient in 1000-10, 000 with lesser degrees of temporary spontaneous partial regression in as high as 0.5% of patients. Such observations indicate that the body has some inherent capacity to induce regression of this disease in selected instances. Despite considerable investigation, the mechanisms of such spontaneous regressions remain unclear. It is suspected that the immunological system plays a role in such occurrences, but this hypothesis lacks formal proof.

The biotherapy of malignant melanoma

Several features of malignant melanoma suggest that *in vivo* biological responses play a role in the progression and regression of this form of cancer. For this reason, melanoma is an attractive and well-examined model for the therapeutic use of biological agents. Histologically, primary skin melanomas and dysplastic nevi often reveal lymphoid infiltrates that suggest a host-defense response, and the degree of lymphocyte invasion is of prognostic significance [62, 134]. Furthermore, spontaneous regression of individual melanoma lesions is well described and has long been thought to represent an immune reaction to the melanoma cell. This phenomenon has recently been shown to involve cytolytic T-lymphocytes [91, 194, 195]. In addition, paraneoplastic depigmentation events, such as the development of vitiligo and 'halo' formation around primary skin melanomas and nevi are thought to indicate an immune mediated reaction against the pigmented cells in these lesions, and the development of vitiligo in malignant melanoma during biotherapy carries an improved prognosis.

In this light, many agents have been evaluated to enhance or mimic the host immune response against melanoma. These agents have included effector cells such as lymphocytes derived from resected tumors or the blood of melanoma patients; antibodies directed at various epitopes of the melanoma cell; vaccines composed of natural or synthetic components of the melanoma cell or derived from mimic 'anti-idiotype' antibodies; non-specific stimulators of the immune system such as BCG; and the cytokines. Of the numerous biological agents studied in the last two to three decades, only the cytokines have consistently shown clinical antitumor activity in melanoma, and two of these cytokines, interferon alpha and interleukin-2, have emerged as useful in clinical practice for the treatment of patients with malignant melanoma. The gene therapies for malignant melanoma are new topics of interest; in these strategies, a therapeutic gene is introduced into an effector cell or a gene encoding a strong antigen is introduced directly into the melanoma cell. Clinical trials with gene therapies are now underway.

Immunostimulation and vaccines

Attempts to augment native immunologic defenses using various non-specific immunostimulators, particularly *Bacillus Calmette-Guerin* (BCG), have been intensively studied in melanoma. Up to 90% of melanoma nodules injected intralesionally with BCG will demonstrate regression in immunocompetent patients. In 15-20% of such patients, associated distant shrinkage of nodules may be seen [218]. Preparations of cellular constituents, such as cell-wall skeleton, may also serve as effective adjuvants [366]. Systemic effects have been demonstrated by the emergence of antimelanoma antibodies and by lymphocytic infiltration of regressing noninjected lesions [218]. Allogeneic melanoma cells have also been infused intralymphatically; in one report, nine of 34 patients so treated, who had not received prior chemotherapy, responded. Patients previously exposed to chemotherapy did not respond. Interestingly, effects were not limited to regional lymph nodes; systemic responses were seen [378]. While encouraging, these immunomodulating efforts have not significantly improved the survival of melanoma patients. However, immunizing melanoma patients with a pure G_{m2} ganglioside, known to be on melanoma cell membranes, has induced circulating IgG and IgM antibodies. The induction of such antibodies has been reported to be accompanied by prolonged survival [189].

More recent studies using genetically engineered vaccines have been performed. Details can be found in the chapter on vaccines and the chapter on gene therapy. This work was prompted by previous studies using partially purified tumor vaccines (Table 1).

More recent studies have used highly purified or genetically engineered vaccines with a variety of antigens and adjuvants which are immunogenic in humans (Table 2 and 3).

Clinical trials with purified genetically engineered vaccines are ongoing and while there is evidence of stimulation of cytotoxic T cells, enhancement of antibody titers and augmentation of DTH responses, the clinical activities of these vaccines in phase I/II studies remain to be reported.

Interferon

In phase I trials with alpha-interferon, an occasional melanoma patient experienced objective tumor regression. Subsequent phase II studies using partially purified human leukocyte or lymphoblastoid alpha-interferon showed response rates as high as 12% [108, 285]. The

Table 1. Tumor antigen vaccine trials

Stage of disease	No. of patients	Vaccine preparation	Adjuvant	Controls	Results	Ref
Resected II	25	Autologous soluble membrane extract	BCG	Historical	Improved survival over historical growth	162
Disseminated	56	Specific TAA	Freund's complete	None	Regression seen in approximately 25% of patients	137
Disseminated	13	Polyvalent TAA	None	None	CR 1 of 13 PR 1 of 13	36
Resected Stage II	94	Polyvalent melanoma-tumor antigen vaccine	40 pts-Alum 17 pts-Cytoxan	Historical	Improved survival over historical controls	38

Table 2. Adjuvants: effects on immunogenicity

Approach	Mechanism of action: Depot effect	Macrophage	CD4+ T Cell and B cell	CTL
Conjugate vaccines	+	–	++	–
Recombinant vector vaccines				
BCG	+	+	+	++
Vaccinia	+	–	+	++
Immunological adjuvants				
Alum or oil (squalene)	+	–	–	–
BCG or BCG CWS	+	+	+	–
Endotoxin (Lipid A)	–	++	+	–
Liposomes	+	–	–	+
MDP derivatives	–	+	+	+

Table 3. Clinical trials with immunogenic antigens

Antigen	Vaccine	# Patients responding	Reference
GM2	BCG	50/58	37
GM2	KLH	30/30	131,217
GD2	KLH	4/6	""
Mage 1	–	Ongoing trial	361
Mage 3	–	Ongoing trial	106
Tyrosinase	–	Ongoing trial	29

composite experience using recombinant alpha-interferon has yielded a response rate of approximately 20% [158, 234]. On occasion, these responses have been complete, but activity in visceral disease has been infrequent. Perhaps as many as 30% of patients achieving a complete response enjoy an enduring remission. Studies using alpha-interferon in the adjuvant surgical setting demonstrated a reduced recurrence rate with substantial doses of interferon. This study lead to approval of interferon for the treatment of melanoma. Beta and gamma interferon are also being evaluated in melanoma. A suggested potentiation by cimetidine of human leukocyte interferon activity in malignant melanoma [26, 136] has not been confirmed by later studies using natural or recombinant alpha-interferon [158, 188, 326].

Studies of interferon alpha in metastatic melanoma patients have shown response rates ranging from 0-30% with an overall average of 16% [49, 56, 58, 77, 82, 134, 157, 178, 293, 322, 338]. As such, about 1 in 6 patients with metastatic melanoma will benefit from interferon alpha therapy. However, it is notable that a small percentage of the total group responding to this treatment will achieve a complete response, and occasionally, long remissions have been observed. It is important to compare these responses to those observed for single agent chemotherapy (also in the 15-20% range). Higher response rates were seen with drug combinations and the best three drug combinations report responses in the 30-40% range and generally include cisplatin and dacarbazine. However, even the best chemotherapy combinations have failed to demonstrate a survival advantage, and the duration of response is usually less than six months [180]. The combination of interferon alpha with chemotherapy met with early encouragement. Several phase II studies showed the combination of dacarbazine and alpha interferon to induce responses in 25-30% of patients with metastatic melanoma [13, 88, 135, 271]. In randomized studies comparing the combination to single agent dacarbazine, two showed superior activity for the two drugs [88, 323] while a third showed no improvement over dacarbazine alone [353]. It is difficult to extrapolate the optimal dose and frequency of administration of interferon alpha from the available data; a very wide range of doses and frequencies have been evaluated in the reported clinical trials (Table 4 and 5). It is also not clear that a strong dose-response relationship exists for interferon alpha in malignant melanoma.

Table 4. Clinical trials with recombinant interferon

Study	Dose (MU) route/schedule	Evaluable patients	Response CR/PR (%)
Creagan [56]	12/M² IM 3 times per week	30	20
Creagan [58]	50/M² IM 3 times per week	31	23
Coates [49]	20/M² IV daily x 5	15	0
Hersey [134]	50/M² IM 3 times per week	18	11
Legha [178]	3-36 IM daily or 3 times per week	62	8

Table 5. Biochemotherapy treatment programs

Study	Evaluable patients	CR/PR (%)
Interferon + DTIC		
Kirkwood [159]	23	4
Gundersen [124]	15	20
Mulder [220]	31	35
Thompson [354]	86	21
Sertoli [322]	72	26
Interferon + Platinum/combinations		
Hamblin [130]	12	83%
Richards [286]	74	57
Legha [179]	30	56
Pyrhonen [271]	45	53
Richner [288]	20	35

Interleukin 2/lymphokine-activated killer (LAK) cells

Interleukin-2/lymphokine activated killer (LAK) cells have been reported to provide a response rate of 50% for patients with advanced metastatic melanoma [297, 381] (Table 6). Most of these responses have been partial and of only several months duration, although occasional patients do experience complete responses. Subsequent studies with interleukin 2/LAK cells and studies using interleukin 2 in combination with interferon continue to demonstrate that melanoma is a neoplasm sensitive to these kinds of biological approaches [32, 75, 76, 177, 300, 330, 363]. Overall, response rates have been in the 20-30% range. Responses continue to be most frequent in patients with skin, lymph node, and lung metastasis and less frequent with abdominal and bony metastasis. The propensity of melanoma to metastasize to the brain has been a limiting factor, since many of these patients have responded peripherally only to relapse and die with central nervous metastases. The major challenge from these studies using interleukin-2-based biotherapies is to determine why one patient will respond with a complete remission and another patient will not respond at all. Is this related to the state of immunological activation inherent to the patient or the state achieved by these biotherapies or does it somehow relate to the sensitivity of the melanoma cells to biotherapy?

If it is possible to summarize all the available data into a single response rate by combining a very heterogenous group of clinical trials, IL-2 would appear to benefit about 1 melanoma patient out of every 5 treated with an overall response rate of 18% (Table 7). Complete responses with long-term remissions, rare in chemotherapy treated patients, are occasionally seen with IL-2. Many studies showing a high percentage of responders have used high dose IV bolus IL-2 that requires intensive support (and expense). Similar to the situation with the alpha-2 interferons, the optimal dose and schedule of admin-

Table 6. Interleukin 2/LAK for melanoma

Study	Evaluable patients	CR/PR (%)
Rosenberg [65]	48	21
West [381]	10	50
Paciucci [255]	6	20
Hawkins [132]	32	19
Dutcher [80]	33	3

Table 7. The activity of IL-2 in malignant melanoma

First author	Year	LAK	# Patients evaluable	CR + PR
Rosenberg [301]	1989	yes in some	90	22%(20)
Rosenberg [302]	1993	yes in some	55	22%(12)
Dutcher [79]	1989	yes	36	17%(6)
Parkinson [258]	1990	no	47	21%(10)
McCabe [202]	1991	yes in some	94	12%(11)
Sparano [331]	1993	no	44	5%(2)

istration have not been determined, and a clear dose-response relationship has not been demonstrated. IL-2 has been used alone or in combination with lymphokine-activated killer ('LAK') cells. The addition of LAK cells, while of historical importance in the original description of IL-2 therapy for advanced malignancies, provides, at best, marginal improvement over IL-2 alone [202, 301, 302]. Good preclinical models support the combination of IL-2 and interferon alpha, but studies, both phase II and randomized trials, showed no benefit for this combination in metastatic melanoma [331]. However, interferon alpha in addition to IL-2 and chemotherapy may provide some additional benefit.

Of great current interest is the combination of chemotherapy and IL-2. Although the clinical trials combining single agent dacarbazine with IL-2 did not demonstrate a benefit for combining these modalities (Table 8) [73, 93, 96, 256, 341], cisplatin based regimens have recently shown remarkable results [7, 21, 63, 130, 155, 181, 287]. Four trials with cisplatin and IL-2 have shown overall response rates in excess of 50%, and all of these also included alpha interferon. Randomized studies will be needed to confirm these data and the role of alpha interferon as well as determine the optimal schedule, combination, and dose of IL-2 with the chemotherapeutic agents.

Interleukin 2/T Cells

As further evidence for the interleukin-2 mediated effect on melanoma, Rosenberg et al. recently reported a 50% response rate using T-cells isolated from melanoma nodules and grown to large numbers *in vitro*, another example of adoptive immunotherapy of cancer [299]. These tumor-infiltrating lymphocytes (TIL) appear to have a higher level of specific activity and, in large part, are MHC-restricted T cells specifically reactive with the individual's melanoma from whom the T cells were derived. Concomitant studies by Dillman and Oldham [74, 250, 251, 381] have confirmed the feasibility of this approach using tumor-derived activated cells (TDAC) although with much lower response rates. This approach of growing T cells from the tumor and/or draining lymph nodes is technologically demanding and very expensive [241, 251]. To date, the results are not clearly superior to the use of interleukin 2 alone or interleukin with peripheral blood cells (LAK) activated *in vitro*. On the other hand, these cells are exquisitely more specific for the melanoma cells. Clearly, this approach validates the belief of many investigators that specific T-cell reactivity occurs in advanced cancer and demonstrates the feasibility of applying such approaches as a clinical biotherapy [72, 249, 299].

Table 8. The activity of combined IL-2 + chemotherapy in malignant melanoma

First author	Year	Chemotherapy	Other therapy	# Patients	CR + PR
Papadopoulos [256]	1990	DTIC		30	33%(10)
Flaherty [96]	1990	DTIC		32	22%(7)
Dillman [70]	1990	DTIC		27	26%(7)
Stoter [341]	1991	DTIC		25	24%(6)
Fiedler [93]	1992	DTIC		16	13%(2)
Blair [21]	1991	CDDP, DTIC		28	43%(12)
Demchak [63]	1991	CDDP		27	37%(10)
Hamblin [130]	1991	CDDP, DTIC	IFN	12	83%(10)
Richards [286]	1992	CDDP, BCNU	IFN, TAM	74	57%(40)
Legha [179]	1992	CDDP, DTIC, VLB	IFN	30	56%(17)
Khayat [155]	1993	CDDP	IFN	39	54%(21)
Atkins [7]	1994	CDDP, DTIC	TAM	38	42%(16)

Rosenberg has pioneered the use of TIL cells plus interleukin-2 in the treatment of cancer utilizing IL-2/TIL with and without Cytoxan and in various schedules and doses in several clinical trials. In summary, approximately 86 patients were treated; 28 of whom had had prior IL-2 and 58 had no prior IL-2. A 34% response rate was seen for the total group of patients with the same response rates in the both the IL-2 pretreated patients and the IL-2 naive patients. Both the response rate and duration of response were equivalent in the two groups and some of the remissions were of very long duration.

^{111}In labeled TIL cells were given to selected patients and with nuclear imaging the presence of these labeled cells in tumor tissue was verified. Thus, both based on the *in vitro* studies showing enhanced killing by T cells compared to LAK cells and in studies using TIL cells clinically where a higher response rate was seen, the evidence is accumulating that these more specific T cells are more powerful when used with interleukin-2 in the treatment of advanced melanoma. It's of particular interest to note that patients resistant to interleukin-2 respond to interleukin-2 plus TIL cells, indicating a role for the cells alone as a therapeutic approach in treating advanced melanoma. Curiously, no one has performed the kind of T cell dose response studies normally done with drugs in patients with advanced cancer. The major question that remains is what would be the effect of giving repeated massive doses of activated T cells to patients with advanced melanoma? What would be the influence of dose, schedule, type of T cell, etc.? These studies need to be done before conclusions on the efficacy of T cell therapy are drawn.

A new category of biological therapy has become recognized, utilizing gene engineered cells. By definition, gene therapy is the introduction of genetic material into cells for therapeutic purposes. The gene therapy of cancer has used advanced melanoma as a model for the development of this new therapeutic approach. The first patient treated on an approved gene therapy protocol was a patient with malignant melanoma who on May 22, 1989, received an infusion of tumor infiltrating lymphocytes (TILs) marked with the neomycin phosphotransferase gene (a gene which carries neomycin resistance in bacteria). While this gene transfer was not designed for the therapeutic enhancement of TIL activity, the ten melanoma patients who consented to this gene 'therapy' demonstrated that foreign genes could be effectively and safely transferred into human cells and administered to patients without apparent adverse effects on the patient nor risk to the caregivers or public [303]. This study also confirmed that the engineered T cells 'trafficked' to the melanoma nodules. These results allowed Rosenberg and colleagues to proceed to alter the TILs with therapeutic intent. On January 29, 1991, the first patient treated on a true gene therapy protocol was an advanced melanoma patient who received an infusion of TILs that contained the gene for tumor necrosis factor (TNF). Several metastatic melanoma and other advanced cancer patients have been treated in this early study. Although the final results remain unpublished at the time of this writing, responses have been observed [304]. The rationale for this strategy is to provide high local concentrations of TNF at tumor sites. TNF is quite toxic when systemically administered, but presumably the TILs provide sufficient local concentrations of TNF for an antitumor effect while sparing systemic toxicity. Another gene therapy approach described by Nabel and colleagues is to introduce the HLA B-7 gene directly into cutaneous melanomas of non-HLA B-7 patients with metastatic disease. The concept is to induce a cytotoxic immune response against a foreign major histocompatibility complex (MHC) class I antigen. Hopefully, the recognition of the cutaneous melanoma cell as foreign will lead to immune attack of distant sites of metastatic melanoma as well. The five patients treated on this protocol all showed evidence of safe and successful gene transfer. Cytotoxic T-lymphocytes were shown to invade the lesions, and one patient showed tumor regression not only of the lesion that had the HLA B7 gene delivery but also of distant cutaneous and pulmonary metastases [222].

Other genes under evaluation include granulocyte macrophage colony stimulating factor (GM-CSF) and B2-microglobin, whose gene products will induce an antitumor immune response when inactivated autologous tumor cells are reinfused into the patient. The cytokine gene therapy concept has been expanded in other clinical trials that will evaluate the feasibility of genes for IL-2, gamma interferon, TNF, and IL-4 transduced into autologous tumor cells or fibroblasts to produce active cytokines effective in the treatment of melanoma and other cancers [60].

Antibodies

Relatively specific visualization of tumor nodules with radiolabeled antibody has been reported [41] and antibody given intravenously can subsequently be demonstrated on the melanoma cell surface by histopathologic techniques [236, 314, 315]. However, only minor clinical activity has been observed with either unconjugated antibody or with preparations of radiolabeled, drug-conjugated, or toxin-conjugated anti-melanoma monoclonal antibodies [173, 243]. Thus far, only murine monoclonal antibody preparations have been extensively studied in clinical studies.

The 9.2.27 antimelanoma monoclonal antibody recognizes a melanoma-associated antigen (a 250-kD chondroitin sulfate proteoglycan core glycoprotein) that is found on 90% of melanoma cells and relatively few nonmelanomatous cells [236]. Oldham et al. reported the selective targeting of this antibody to biopsied melanoma nodules in eight patients [236]. The 9.2.27 antibody does not activate complement, poorly activates ADCC, but may have application because its target antigen modulates very little. Their studies suggest that quantities on the order of 0.5 to several grams of antibody are necessary for saturation of target antigens *in vivo*. Schroff et al. have observed that an interrupted infusional schedule appears to compromise the *in vivo* localization of antibody to tumor, presumably by the development of human anti-murine antibodies (HAMA), which impede antibody localization and accelerate clearance [315]. Goodman et al. later administered MAb96.5 and MAb48.7 to four patients and MAb96.5 alone to a fifth patient. MAb96.5 is an IgG2a immunoglobulin that recognizes p97, a transferrin-like cell surface glycoprotein of 97 kD [114]. MAb48.7 is an IgG1 immunoglobulin recognizing a melanoma-associated cell surface proteoglycan. Although the infusion of antibody was well tolerated, there were no objective remissions nor histopathologic changes found in biopsied tissue, although impressive antibody binding to melanoma cells was observed. Perhaps the lack of activity reflected the lack of *in vitro* activation of human complement and very modest ADCC.

Studies by Vadhan-Raj et al. [360] are of interest in that the IgG3 anti-GD3 mouse monoclonal antibody R24, directed against the sialoganglioside membrane antigen GD3, appears to have induced clinical responses (four partial and two minor responses among 21 patients) using unconjugated antibody [360]. These studies are in contrast to previous studies using other antimelanoma antibodies. MAb R24 provoked a clear inflammatory reaction with increased number of mast cells with evidence of their degranulation, an influx of polymorphonuclear cells, complement deposition, particularly C3, C5, and C9, and infiltration with T3+/T8+/Ia+ lymphocytes [142, 360]. More recently, MAb R24 has been studied in conjunction with other biological modalities such as IL-2 [14], interferon-alfa-2a, with total lymphoid irradiation (which did not interdict the human antimurine antibody response as had been hoped) [143] and by novel routes of administration (e.g., isolated limb perfusion) [51]. Cheung et al. have studied another IgG3 anti-ganglioside MAb, 3F8, in a phase I trial [46]. Two of nine patients with metastatic malignant melanoma achieved partial responses, one lasting 22 weeks and the other continuing at 56 weeks. The most prominent toxicities consisted of severe pain, hypertension, and focal urticaria; a decrease in serum complement activity was observed when dosages equaled or exceeded 20 mg/m^2. Houghton reported that the combination of MAb R24 and MAb 3F8 yielded one complete remission among 13 patients with melanoma [142]. Goodman et al. observed no antitumor activity among eight patients given MAb MG-21, another antibody recognizing a GD3 surface antigen commonly displayed by human melanoma cells [115]. In an intriguing report, Lichtin and associates reported one complete response among 13 patients with metastatic malignant melanoma who received murine IgG2a MAb ME-36.1, which recognizes the melanoma-associated gangliosides GD2 and GD3 [187]. This patient's post-treatment B lymphocytes, when stimulated with polyclonal goat anti-idiotypic ME-36.1, were found to synthesize human antibodies preferentially and specifically recognizing GD2, suggesting to the researchers that the induction of human antimelanoma ganglioside antibodies provoked by ME-36.1 may have mediated the observed clinical response. These observations that murine monoclonal antibodies can induce complement activation, active antibody-dependent cellular cytotoxicity, and generate human antimelanoma antibodies may support a further role for the investigation of unconjugated antibody in malignant melanoma.

A murine monoclonal antimelanoma antibody-ricin A chain immunotoxin (XOMAZYME-MEL) has been studied in several clinical trials to date, since the initial report of its use in 22 patients in early 1987 [190, 332]. The monoclonal antibody moiety of this immunotoxin is an IgG2A antibody recognizing melanoma-associated proteoglycan membrane antigens of 220 kD and greater than 500 kD. One patient demonstrated complete disappearance of detectable melanoma (a retrocardiac pulmonary metastasis)over an 8-month period following a single infusion of immunotoxin, with maintenance of a complete remission for greater than 2 years until relapse occurred in the brain. However, no major responses were seen in the remaining 21 patients. The treatment was accompanied by a transient reduction of serum albumin with associated fluid retention and weight gain, alopecia, fever, fatigue, and malaise, with mild allergic reactions occurring in three patients. In a phase II trial with this immunotoxin, three partial responses were observed among 43 patients, these responses lasting for 10+, 13+, and 15+ months [332]. Current trials are addressing the problem of anti-immunotoxin antibody responses by efforts at immunosuppression utilizing cyclophosphamide, prednisone, and azathioprine in varying combinations [190]. Oratz et al. have recently reported that cyclophosphamide at a dose of 1 g/m^2 administered following the infusion of immunotoxin has not inhibited the generation of host immune responses directed against the immunotoxin preparation [253].

Given the studies by various investigators using unlabeled antibodies, which have been marginally useful in the treatment of melanoma, several investigators have pursued studies using antibody in combination with cytokines [15, 59, 336] with no evidence of activity over and above using the cytokines alone. Similarly, early trials with radiolabeled antibodies for therapy of melanoma have not proven useful [174, 227].

Since antibodies can induce inflammatory infiltrates and activities around melanoma nodules, further work is ongoing with regard to using these antibodies to produce inflammatory effects and combining these effects with cytokines and chemotherapy. Engineered subfragments of antibody as well as humanized antibodies are currently in clinical trials and it is felt some of these improved molecules may improve the delivery of immunotoxins and/or radionuclides to melanoma deposits. This is an area of continuing investigation and the literature must be watched on an ongoing basis for evidence of clinical activity with regard to monoclonal antibody immunoconjugates in melanoma.

These early results do show evidence of selective localization of antibody on melanoma cells and modest clinical activity. Future trials with unconjugated and conjugated antibodies are expected to better define the activity of these approaches in melanoma [71, 246].

GENITOURINARY CANCERS

Renal cell carcinomas

Immunostimulation

Renal-cell carcinoma, like melanoma, would appear to constitute an ideal human tumor system for biotherapy given the occasional (less than 1%) reported incidence of spontaneous regression [87, 252, 365]. Several studies have evaluated the use of a variety of active specific immunization techniques. Tykka, in 1974, reported a 17% complete response rate of pulmonary metastatic lesions in patients receiving a monthly vaccine composed of homogenized tumor plus either tuberculin or *Candida* every 4 weeks [358]. Subsequently, three separate trials using either tumor homogenate plus tuberculin, enzymatically digested tumor tissue plus *Corynebacterium parvum*, or whole tumor cells plus attached dimethyldioctadecyl ammonium bromide (DDA) as vaccine have all reported responses in 15-25% of patients [204, 226, 265]. Furthermore, immune RNA has been extracted from lymphocytes of guinea pigs specifically immunized with renal tumor cells and coincubated with autologous lymphocytes; these reinfused lymphocytes induced a response in three of six patients [335]. The area of immune RNA therapy has been reviewed [257]. Thymosin fraction V, a partially purified extract of calf thymus glands, has induced objective responses in approximately 15% of advanced renal cancer patients [316].

Embolization of the renal artery has induced subsequent objective responses in metastatic disease. A recent study has demonstrated that renal artery embolization will significantly augment NK activation 48-96 hours later, suggesting a possible immunologic role in its mechanism of action [16].

There have been no definitive studies on the use of vaccines in renal cancer. Only preliminary studies were done and these have been largely inconclusive [2, 204, 281]. Different tumor cell preparations, different adjuvants, diverse routes of administrations and concomitant therapy make all of these studies difficult to analyze. However, objective tumor regressions were noted in these three studies and while infrequent, it points to a rationale for continuing studies with vaccines in patients with renal cancer.

Interferon

Alpha-interferon is active against metastatic renal cell carcinoma [163, 234, 275, 276]. Response rates as high as 27% have been reported [227]. The mean time to response may be as long as 3-4 months [227]. It can be argued that an *optimal* dose and schedule for alpha-interferon has never been defined for renal cell carcinoma. The antitumor activity of interferon can be attributed to either its ability to modulate cellular immunity or to its direct (non-immunologically mediated) antiproliferative activity. It is not clear that *both* of these properties of interferon can be evoked optimally simultaneously from a single dose and schedule of interferon *in vivo*. Some data appear to demonstrate a dose-response relationship for interferon, suggesting that the clinical responses induced by interferon are likely to be due to its known antiproliferative activity rather than to immunomodulation. Quesada et al., using recombinant alpha-interferon, observed no responses among patients treated with 'low-dose' interferon (2 million units/m^2 intramuscularly daily), whereas 12 of 41 patients treated with a 'high-dose' regimen (20 million units/m^2 intramuscularly daily) did respond [276].

Evidence for a dose-response relationship for interferon has not been consistently observed among investigators. While some toxicities from interferon do appear to be dose-related, not all antitumor responses appear to be dose-related. Creagan et al. [57, 58], in separate phase II trials for the treatment of malignant melanoma, found similar response rates for 'high' (50 million units/m^2 three times weekly) and 'low' (12 million units/m^2 three times weekly) dose regimens of alpha-interferon. The inherent weakness of these observations is that they were made from sequential studies rather than from randomized trials. From his extensive review of the literature relating to the treatment of renal cell carcinoma with interferon, Muss [221] concluded that toxicity from interferon was dose-related and that the highest therapeutic index for interferon occurred at doses ranging from 5-10 million units/m^2.

Kirkwood et al. [156] conducted a randomized trial for the treatment of renal cell carcinoma in which patients were randomized prospectively to receive a 'low' or 'high' dose of alpha-interferon. Patients randomized to the low dose received interferon 1 million units intramuscularly daily (as opposed to the traditional three times weekly schedule used with higher doses). Patients randomized to the higher dose received 10 million units daily. Patients were treated for 28 days. At the end of 28 days, patients who were stable were treated for an additional month. Among the 30 patients treated on this study it was found that both doses were well tolerated. Six of the seven responses observed occurred at the higher dose but the difference in response rate between the two dose levels was not statistically significant.

Marshall et al. [198] conducted a single-armed pilot study of 'low' dose interferon for the treatment of advanced renal cell carcinoma in which patients received 1 million units subcutaneously daily continually. This differed from the trial of Kirkwood et al. [156] in that the interferon was given subcutaneously instead of intramuscularly and it was given continually instead of for a short course of one to two months. Because the mean time to response for interferon tends to be long (several months), it was thought that the ability to continue the low dose regimen over many months might have a higher likelihood of rendering objective responses than a short course especially if it could be done with acceptable cumulative toxicity. Of 17 patients treated on this regimen, 16 were evaluable for tumor response. At the time of report, there were 4 partial responses (25%) and 5 patients with stable disease (31%). Subsequently, 2 of the partial responses developed into complete responses (unpublished data). One of these complete responses occurred in a patient with pulmonary metastases and one occurred in patients with bone metastases. Both of these complete responses were durable. In this pilot study, treatment at this low daily dose for many months was tolerated very well with no patient withdrawing from treatment because of toxicity. These pilot data served as the basis for a single-arm phase II trial conducted by the Southwest Oncology Group [198], in which previously untreated patients with advanced renal cell carcinoma were treated with alpha-interferon 1 million units subcutaneously daily continually until there was evidence of disease progression. Among 40 patients who were *fully evaluable* for response, there were 6 responses (response rate, 15%; 95% confidence interval, 5.7-30%). More toxicity was encountered in this trial than was seen in the pilot study of Marshall et al. [198] but treatment was tolerated generally well with only two patients withdrawing from treatment because of toxicity. These two separate reports indicate that very low doses of interferon can have activity against renal cell carcinoma. Further trials randomizing patients to the daily low dose regimen versus traditional high dose regimens given three times weekly would be needed in order to draw firm conclusions about dosing and scheduling of interferon. While the response rates for any of the regimens may be too low to warrant such trials they would be interesting because they would address directly some important issues with regard to dosing and scheduling of biotherapies.

The role of beta-interferon in the treatment of renal-cell carcinoma remains to be established. A trial of combination interleukin-2 and beta-interferon evoked objective responses in 6 of 22 evaluable patients, with one complete remission and five partial remissions. Two of these responses lasted for almost 2 years [163]. Although this 27% overall response rate is similar to that achieved with interleukin-2 and lymphokine-activated killer (LAK) cell therapy and to higher doses of single agent interleukin-2, the contribution of beta-interferon is uncertain.

Early experience with gamma-interferon suggested little if any activity [24, 274, 290]. Gamma-interferon is a product of activated T cells and is unique in its ability to stimulate macrophages. Although approved for chronic granulomatous disease, it has demonstrated some activity in metastatic renal cancer and in one study using a low-dose weekly subcutaneous injection of 100 mg, a 30% response rate was observed in patients with metastatic renal cancer [8]. A second study reported a 15% response rate [81]. These studies should be confirmed and the use of gamma-interferon in combination with other interferons or other treatment modalities would be of interest given the low toxicity of gamma-interferon in these doses and schedules. Combinations of alpha and gamma-interferon have shown additive toxicities without added therapeutic benefit [273]. An effort to improve response by combining alpha-interferon and gamma-interferon failed to achieve this intent, perhaps attributable to additive toxicities and inability to suitably escalate dosages [99]. Some of the same principles regarding dose and schedule of alpha-interferon, discussed above, pertain to gamma-interferon. A dose-response relationship for gamma-interferon may not be straightforward. Brown et al. [31] conducted a phase I trial of gamma-interferon in which antitumor responses were observed. However, the responses occurred at the lowest doses tested. The authors suggested that, in an attempt to improve the therapeutic index for gamma-interferon, phase II trials should include low doses of the drug.

IFN plus IL-2 also gives significant responses. Some have been complete and durable in patients with advanced renal cancer [300]. Other studies have been less encouraging [95, 382]. The optimal doses and schedule needs further study and may produce even better results.

Interleukin-2/Lymphokine-activated killer (LAK) cells

Interleukin-2/lymphokine-activated killer (LAK) cells are effective in the treatment of metastatic renal-cell cancer [297, 298, 381]. An initial response rate in excess of 75% was reported [298], but broader studies suggest a true response rate of less than 30%. Moreover, most of these responses have been partial and transient, typically lasting no more than several months. However, 5-10% have a complete response, and durations as long as 5 years have been reported.

Interleukin-2/Tumor-infiltrating lymphocytes (TIL)/Tumor-derived activated cells (TDAC)

IL-2 with TIL/TDAC would also seem to be a promising approach, but with less specificity for the expanded T cells than has been seen in melanoma [242, 249, 299]. Sufficient studies utilizing acceptable doses of Interleukin-2 along with escalating doses of activated cells have not been done. Perhaps the most extensive studies have been accomplished by Oldham and co-workers [251] in utilizing as many as 10 doses of activated T cells in treatment of patients with advanced malignancy. With regard to patients with renal cancer, only 4 doses have been used, giving total cell doses up to 2 x 10^{11} cells. Responses have been seen, sometimes with dramatic shrinkage of tumor, in patients with advanced renal cancer. Unfortunately, these responses have only been seen in 5 to 10% of the patients and it is yet unclear whether the response rate can be increased by changing the dose and schedule of Interleukin-2 or by preparing and administering more of the activated cells. These studies continue and will be of major interest with regard to the biotherapy of metastatic renal cancer. The optimal doses and schedule needs further study and may provide even better results.

Antibodies

Antibody MAb F23 is an IgG2a murine monoclonal antibody that recognizes a surface glycoprotein of 140 kD expressed by 7 of 10 hypernephroma cell lines and reacts with a high percentage of fresh frozen sections from specimens of renal cell carcinoma, as well as with proximal tubules and connective tissue. Real et al. studied 29 patients with metastatic renal cell carcinoma with either radiolabeled F23 or unlabeled F23; one partial response was seen among the nine patients who received six iv injections over a 2-week period of the unlabeled preparation [283]. MAb A6H also recognizes renal cancer cells. A phase I-II imaging and therapy trial of 15 patients receiving MAb A6H has been reported [364]. No striking clinical responses have been seen in these very preliminary studies.

Bladder

Several recent trials have demonstrated both objective responses and prolongation of disease-free interval following the intravesical installation of BCG for superficial stage A bladder carcinoma [172, 216, 263]. The mechanism of action remains unknown, although a nonspecific inflammatory response has been postulated. These studies led to FDA approval of BCG as a standard intravesical treatment of bladder cancer.

Intravesical interferon has also been reported to be effective [356, 357]. Torti has demonstrated that intravesical BCG and interferon have levels of activity comparable to those of cytotoxic agents. Systemically administered interferon has been reported to improve the disease-free interval and induce responses in patients with multiple papillomas of the bladder [317]. The use of biotherapy in early-stage bladder cancer warrants more intensive investigation.

Murine monoclonal antibodies have been developed against transitional-cell carcinomas of the urinary bladder; to date, however, no clinical trials have been reported. Preclinical testing of anti-epidermal growth factor receptor antibodies is also underway.

Although systemic chemotherapy using regimens such as MVAC remains the standard for treating advanced bladder cancer, at least one trial utilizing alpha-interferon plus 5-fluorouracil gave a response rate of 30% in 32 patients who had not responded to previous platinum-based regimens [192]. These studies and others that are underway indicate the importance of looking at combined protocols of biochemotherapy in advanced bladder cancer.

Prostate

Twenty-five patients with stage D2 prostate cancer have undergone radioimmunoimaging analysis by means of an antiprostatic acid phosphatase MAb (indium-labeled PAY276) [11]. The detection of metastatic sites improved as the quantity of unlabeled MAb increased; at a dose of 80 mg, 101 of 134 metastatic sites demonstrated localization, with a false negative rate of 24.6% and a false positive rate of 2.3%. Other monoclonal antibodies against prostatic acid phosphatase, as well as prostate-specific antigen, have been generated for purpose of radioimmunolocalization and toxicity evaluation [129]. Trials of IL-2/IFN are underway with some preliminary data showing responses in refractory prostate cancer. Multiple vaccine trials are also underway.

Gastrointestinal cancer

Immunostimulation

Trials of immunotherapy with irradiated autologous tumor cells and BCG are being pursued. Reduced recurrence rates in Dukes B and Dukes C colon cancers have been reported [139]. This trial is more fully described in Chapter 8.

Levamisole, which may act as a biological response modifier (BRM), reduces recurrence rates for Dukes C colon cancer when used with adjuvant 5-fluorouracil (5-FU). This approach is now widely used since levamisole has been approved for human use. The exact mechanism of action of 5-FU plus levamisole is unknown.

Interferon

Many studies have evaluated alpha-interferon in colorectal carcinoma. As a single agent, alpha-interferon has very little activity against colorectal cancer [23, 225]. 5-fluorouracil (5-FU) remains the single most active chemotherapy drug for the treatment of colon cancer. Objective response rates for 5-FU range from 3-25% [213]. Although responses are seen with 5-FU, complete responses are rare and the duration of response tends to be relatively short. Further, 5-FU has not produced improvements in survival among patients with metastatic colorectal cancer. Because combination chemotherapy regimens containing 5-FU have not produced results which are superior to 5-FU alone, attempts have been made to improve upon the results of 5-FU alone by modulating the activity of 5-FU. Modulation of the activity of 5-FU has been accomplished by combining it with leucovorin. This has resulted in improved response rates and some improvement in survival when compared to the results obtained with 5-FU alone [84, 262, 264]. While alpha-interferon alone has no appreciable activity against colorectal carcinoma, there is a separate body of evidence which has demonstrated that alpha-interferon is capable of modulating the antitumor activity of 5-FU and that it does so through a mechanism which is different from that of leucovorin [224, 369]. An early clinical trial which combined 5-FU with alpha-interferon for the treatment of advanced colorectal carcinoma reported a 75% objective response rate among patients who had not been treated previously with chemotherapy [367, 368]. None of the previously treated patients responded to this regimen. While these early results were very promising, subsequent trials of 5-FU and interferon for colorectal carcinoma resulted in response rates which were much lower. Response rates have been reported over the range of 24-76% [153, 259, 260, 306, 370, 373]. Subsequently, attempts were made to improve upon the results obtained with 5-FU and leucovorin or 5-FU and interferon through the strategy of *double modulation* – i.e., combining 5-FU with leucovorin *and* interferon. Such attempts, however, have not resulted in higher response rates. Presently, the practice of combining 5-FU with interferon cannot be recommended as standard therapy for colorectal cancer. Such efforts should be restricted to formal clinical trials designed to find ways to take advantage of the *in vitro* observations of interferon's chemomodulatory activity.

Follow-up studies using alpha-interferon with 5-FU in a variety of doses and schedules have recently been reported [64, 117, 145, 153, 260, 270, 370] and can be summarized as demonstrating that interferon does appear to add marginally to the activity of 5-FU or 5-FU plus folinic acid in patients with advanced colorectal cancer. Response rates have varied from 20% to 65% with some evidence of marginally increased survival measured in periods of approximately six months. Further studies are certainly indicated since the monetary cost and toxic cost are somewhat greater in trials combining interferon with 5-fluorouracil.

There were no responses seen in a study of 14 patients with gastric adenocarcinoma treated with alpha-interferon [234]. Similar studies in cancer of the esophagus have not been encouraging.

Antibodies

A variety of murine monoclonal antibodies are now available that react with adenocarcinomas of the colon and rectum. There appears to be considerable cross-reactivity between breast and colon adenocarcinomas, and antibodies that have been generated to each have often been cross-reactive.

Sears et al. have reported their experience using antibody 17-1A, an IgG2a mouse antibody, in the treatment of 62 patients with advanced gastrointestinal malignancies. No convincing responses solely attributable to antibody were seen [318-320]. Studies are now underway using this same antibody for radioimmunolocalization and radioimmunotherapy. It is also anticipated that trials of drug and toxin immunoconjugates will be forthcoming. One attempt to enhance antibody-dependent monocyte cytotoxicity by pretreatment with gamma-interferon prior to antibody 17-1A administration failed to induce any objective response in 27 patients [374, 375, 377].

Goldenberg and co-workers have performed a series of clinical studies using anti-CEA antibody to demonstrate that such antibodies can target colon cancer and metastases therefrom [111]. Dillman et al. administered a variety of anti-CEA mouse monoclonal antibodies to 30 patients with colorectal cancer; there were no antitumor responses [68, 71]. A similar lack of therapeutic efficacy has been reported by others [183]. A major difficulty with these studies has been the sea of antigen that is often present with circulating CEA.

Investigators at the National Cancer Institute have extensively studied monoclonal antibody B72.3, which recognizes a high-molecular-weight glycoprotein (labeled TAG-72), which reacts to a majority of primary and metastatic adenocarcinomas of colorectal, breast, ovarian, lung, gastric, and endometrial origin. MAb B72.3 had previously been demonstrated to localize to deposits of tumor [85]. These earlier studies demonstrated a 3-fold to 40-fold concentration of antibody in tumor versus normal tissues in 70% of the tumor samples studied. The antibody appears to be well tolerated by patients. These investigators have also shown that the intracavitary administration of B72.3 may better traffic to peritoneal implants, whereas the intravenous infusion of this antibody more efficiently targets local, nodal, and hepatic metastases [52]. The clinical application of two human immunoglobulins, both of the IgM class, have recently been described [334]. These human monoclonal antibodies, MAbs 16.88 and 28A32, were obtained from patients following immunization with irradiated autologous tumor cells intermixed with *Bacillus Calmette-Guerin* (BCG). Peripheral blood mononuclear cells were then obtained and either transformed by Epstein-Barr virus (EBV) or fused to form a human-mouse heterohybridoma to produce MAb16.88 or MAb28A32, respectively. No clinical responses were observed in 26 patients treated with one or both antibodies, although the MAbs were seen to localize to tumor deposits, to be relatively well tolerated, and to be poorly immunogenic.

A recent adjuvant study in Germany evaluated the 17-1A murine monoclonal antibody in 189 patients with resected colon cancer assigned to receive the antibody treatment versus a control arm. With a median follow-up of 5 years, the antibody therapy reduced the death rate by about 30% and the recurrence rate by slightly less. There was little in the way of toxicity and this study would point to the need to compare such adjuvant treatments to other active adjuvant treatments, such as levamisole and 5-FU, in patients with resectable colon cancer. It is interesting to note that this antibody trial was positive in the adjuvant setting in spite of minimal evidence of activity in advanced disease, using the same antibody.

Order has reported responses and, in some patients, prolongation of survival with radiolabeled antiferritin polyclonal antibody in phase I/II studies of hepatocellular carcinoma. Results of a phase III clinical trial are anticipated [86, 254]. Chimeric antibodies, such as chimeric 17-1A, should be much more interesting than murine antibodies. Not only do the chimerics often have high ADCC capabilities, they are less immunogenic and have very much longer plasma half-lives, as described by LoBuglio et al. in their experience in 10 patients with metastatic colon cancer [191].

A large number of antibodies suitable for testing in gastrointestinal malignancies is now available. Clinical trials are expanding [71, 208].

Interleukin-2/Lymphokine-activated killer (LAK) cells

Interleukin-2/lymphokine-activated killer (LAK) cells have not been highly effective as systemic treatment for colorectal cancer, although occasional minor responses have been seen [298]. The direct infusion of LAK cells into the liver harboring metastases in patients receiving systemic interleukin-2 has been beneficial [244].

Breast cancer

The immunobiology of adenocarcinoma of the breast remains to be fully elucidated. Several studies have established that patients with carcinoma of the breast remain reasonably immunocompetent throughout the natural history of their disease [165, 372]. Antitumor immunity is demonstrable in patients by a number of techniques. An *in vitro* immune reaction to tumor-associated antigens, using the leukocyte migration inhibition (LMI) and the leukocyte adherence inhibition (LAI) assays, has been demonstrated using as stimulants tumor cell extracts, soluble membrane extracts of MCF-7 cells (a breast cancer cell line), and soluble membrane extracts of biopsy-derived tumor tissue [39, 104, 308]. Several of these studies demonstrated blocking factors, presumably immune complexes, in the serum [348]. The T-antigen, a precursor of the M and N blood group antigens whose expression is masked on normal tissue, is expressed on nearly all breast carcinoma tissue. Patients also mount a strong cellular immune reaction to this antigen as demonstrated by both delayed hypersensitivity and *in vitro* LMI [333]. The demonstration of delayed hypersensitivity to tumor-associated antigens has not been particularly useful clinically, but the use of crude membrane extracts prepared from cultured breast tumor cells (MCF-7) previously infected with vesicular stomatitis virus enhanced reactivity. Eighty-five percent of patients reacted to a skin test using this augmented antigen [9].

Immunostimulation

Nonspecific immunotherapy in the form of BCG [35, 203, 321], levamisole [127, 160, 295, 327, 339], and poly A: U has been evaluated in a number of studies. In three of eight studies involving the use of BCG or levamisole, benefit was reported. Poly A: U, an interferon inducer and stimulator of natural killer cytotoxicity, has been evaluated in a randomized adjuvant study (not incorporating chemotherapy) in patients with stage II carcinoma of the breast, all of whom had previously undergone mastectomy. Patients receiving poly A: U had a better overall survival than those not receiving this polynucleotide. This benefit was comparable to other studies using adjuvant chemotherapy in breast cancer. Benefit was essentially limited to patients with one to three involved lymph nodes and could be correlated with natural killer cytotoxicity augmentation and 2', 5'-A synthetase production (an indicator of interferon induction) [170, 171].

Immunoactivation/absorption/ultrafiltration

Protein A is a polypeptide (molecular weight 42, 000) that has a high affinity for the Fc portion of mammalian IgG. A number of studies have demonstrated therapeutic efficacy in animal models (spontaneous mammary carcinoma of dogs; a chemically induced mammary carcinoma of rats) following the exposure of plasma to staphylococcal protein A [138, 282, 330, 350]. It was postulated that the removal of immune complexes, which had been immunosuppressive in some way, allowed tumor cytotoxic antibodies to become effective. In a pilot study of five patients with advanced carcinoma of the breast, a significant antitumor effect was induced following repeated exposure of plasma to protein A imbedded in a colloidal charcoal mixture [351]. Several attempts to confirm these results have failed to reproduce the earlier responses [89, 90]. These observations remain under investigation [235].

A protein A/silica device (Prosorba) that has recently been approved for the treatment of immune-mediated thrombocytopenia is undergoing both on-line and off-line investigation in cancer treatment, particularly that of breast cancer [133]. Evidence is mounting that there is antitumor activity in the serum that can be augmented by passing a cancer patient's serum over such columns. While many of these studies have focused on breast cancer, there is the possibility that this device may be active more broadly in other malignancies. Studies are underway to further elucidate the mechanisms of action of protein A.

A related approach, pursued by Lentz, uses ultrafiltration to remove suppressive factors (or induce activation), with a net effect of tumor regression [185]. Attempts by others to confirm this early report have been unsuccessful.

Interferon

Early studies investigating leukocyte-derived alpha-interferon reported response rates of about 25-30% [25, 125]. However, subsequent studies using either lymphoblastoid [176] or recombinant alpha-interferon [325] showed no significant efficacy. Since there are over 12 alpha-interferon molecules in the human-derived leukocyte interferon preparation by the Cantell method, at least eight in the lymphoblastoid product, but only one in each recombinant interferon product, it is possible that one or more of these substituent molecules present in the natural product is important for antitumor effect. However, an analysis of many reported studies would suggests that the antitumor activity of alpha-interferons in breast cancer is clearly marginal, tempering enthusiasm for further phase II or phase III trials [234]. Synergy with cytotoxic agents has been shown in animal models and *in vitro*, but to date combination drug/interferon studies in breast cancer have not been reported in humans. Homogenates of breast cancer cells exposed to interferon express increased levels of estrogen receptor protein [67]; the clinical relevance of this observation warrants study [23].

Antibodies

Several laboratories have recently produced monoclonal antibodies to a variety of breast-cancer-associated antigens. Ceriani and others originally produced polyclonal heterologous antisera to human milk fat globules [43, 44]. As milk is secreted, the breast epithelial cell encases the fat globule in the plasma membrane. Thus, using milk fat globules as immunogens, antibody formation is also directed against antigens on the plasma membrane component. Three such antigenic structures have been demonstrated (MW 150K, 75K, 45K). These antigens circulate in most patients with breast cancer, an observation that may be useful diagnostically [43, 44]. More recently, murine monoclonal antibodies have been induced by these antigens [349]. Vitetta and associates, using the cultured breast cancer cell line MCF-7 as an immunogen, have induced murine monoclonal antibody formation [22], have tagged them with the toxin ricin, and have observed the induction of *in vitro* cytotoxicity [164]. Schlom and co-workers [311] have induced human monoclonal antibody formation to breast cancer antigens by hybridizing lymphocytes from axillary lymph nodes of patients with breast cancer with a murine myeloma cell line [309]. They have also used metastatic breast cancer cells as immunogens and produced a number of murine monoclonal antibodies, many of which are selective for tumor-associated antigens found on a variety of adenocarcinomas [53]. One of these antibodies has been evaluated in a nude mouse xenograft system; localization to breast cancer cells was demonstrated [54].

Clinical trials with monoclonal antibodies are just beginning. Many of these early trials were focused on radioimmunolocalization of labeled antibody in breast cancer tissue [85]. Oldham and co-workers have been able to specifically design antibody cocktails (containing two to six antibodies per patient) chosen from *in vitro* specificity data. These cocktails have been used as chemotherapy immunoconjugates to direct drug (Adriamycin and Mitomycin-C) to tumor cell sites. Preliminary results indicate an attenuated pattern of toxicity of chemotherapy directed by this method, some selective targeting of drug to metastatic sites of breast cancer, but no major clinical responses. A more definitive analysis awaits further accumulation of patients, but the trafficking of the chemotherapy-directed conjugates was encouraging [238-240]. Winer and his colleagues have investigated a ricin-A immunotoxin (260F9) directed against a 50-kD target by one hour infusion daily for 6-8 days; there was considerable toxicity, including fluid overload and incapacitating sensorimotor neuropathies [376].

More recent studies using antibody and antibody conjugates in advanced breast cancer have been summarized by Goldenberg [110] and Reiley [284]. While many of these studies focused on other adenocarcinomas, such as ovarian and colorectal cancer, patients with breast cancer have been assessed both in radioimaging and antibody therapy. For example, Goodman and colleagues have studied antibody L6 in patients with advanced breast cancer, demonstrating some evidence of localization of the antibody in the tumor [116]. Studies continue to be performed using a variety of monoclonal antibodies in breast cancer for imaging and therapy.

Lung cancer

Immunomodulation

The observation that the inadvertent development of postsurgical empyema in patients undergoing thoracotomy for lung cancer improved survival [307, 345] prompted clinical trials of intrapleural BCG following resection. Although initial results were promising [206], a more recent American trial showed no effect [105], and the European experience suggests deleterious rather than salutary effects. Bakker and associates report diminished disease-free survival in stage I and II squamous-cell carcinoma at both 2 and 5 years among patients receiving BCG compared to untreated controls [17].

An initial trial demonstrating benefit of thymosin fraction V in small-cell carcinoma of the lung was not confirmed on further investigation [50, 324].

Interferon

Alpha-interferon does not appear to have any meaningful activity against non-small-cell carcinoma of the lung [94, 166, 234, 257]. There is a suggestion that alpha-interferon might delay metastatic dissemination in small-cell carcinoma of the lung; however, there also appears to be concomitant increased radiation toxicity to normal tissues as well as tumor [201]. Interferon may inhibit repair of sublethal damage induced by radiation [23].

A marked decreased expression of HLA class I antigens has been described in small cell carcinoma of the lung [78]. Interferon had previously been observed to augment the expression of class I HLA antigens. These contradictory observations have stimulated further investigation.

Interleukin-2/Lymphokine-activated killer (LAK) cells

There is evidence of some modest activity of interleukin-2/lymphokine-activated killer (LAK) cells in non-small-cell carcinoma of the lung. Rosenberg et al. have seen responses in one of four such patients, and experience elsewhere is comparable [297, 363, 376]. There are no significant data regarding the use of interleukin-2/LAK cells in small-cell carcinoma of the lung.

Antibodies

The early experience using both unconjugated antibody and antibody conjugated with methotrexate in the treatment of non-small-cell carcinoma of the lung demonstrated no convincing responses [355]. Various other antibodies against non-small-cell lung cancer are available for clinical trials [337]. Bombesin is an autocrine growth factor for small-cell carcinomas of the lung; a monoclonal antibody preparation to bombesin has been tested both *in vitro* and in animal studies with encouraging antitumor activity [61].

GYNECOLOGICAL CANCER

Ovarian cancer

Immunomodulation

The intraperitoneal administration of *Corynebacterium parvum* following combination chemotherapy in patients with minimal residual diseases has been reported to yield objective responses confirmed by surgical examination. Enhancement of both natural killer and antibody-dependent cell-mediated cytotoxicity within the peritoneal cavity was observed [20, 186].

Interferon

Leukocyte-derived alpha-interferon has shown modest activity in the treatment of advanced ovarian cancer [19, 103]. A recent phase II trial using human recombinant interferon-gamma demonstrated four responses among 14 patients with relapsing ovarian cancer so treated [379]. Further studies with interferon seem warranted in this disease.

Interferon has also been administered intraperitoneally in the treatment of ovarian cancer. The experience is still too early to permit a meaningful clinic evaluation, but there is evidence of augmentation of natural killer cytotoxicity [20, 186].

Interleukin-2/Lymphokine-activated killer (LAK) cells

Lymphokine-activated killer cells have been administered intraperitoneally in association with systemic interleukin-2 to patients with ovarian cancer [244]. A toxicity study of intraperitoneal interleukin-2 without activated cells has recently been reported; enhancement of peripheral natural killer cells and lymphokine activated killer cell activities was observed [45]. A full discussion of this approach can be found in Chapter 17.

Antibody

A large number of studies using radiolabeled antibodies have been performed in ovarian cancer [110]. These include using studies using radioimaging with antibodies selective for ovarian cancers [284]. Some predictive value has been noted when radiolabeled antibodies have been used prior to a second surgery for ovarian cancer in terms of detecting occult peritoneal disease. Perhaps the most studied area is the use of radioisotope antibody conjugates intraperitoneally in ovarian cancer [83] with evidence that a relatively high dose of radioactive iodine could induce regression with intraperitoneal ovarian cancer. For example, studies using rhenium-186 and yttrium-90 conjugated to radioactive isotopes have demonstrated the ability to induce partial response and relief of ascites in patients with advanced ovarian cancer [148, 305, 380].

Cancer of the uterine cervix

In the treatment of cancer of the uterine cervix, no responses were seen in one study of 18 patients administered human leukocyte alpha-interferon [234].

Endocrine cancers

The biotherapy of malignancies arising from endocrine organs has been little studied. Human leukocyte interferon at doses of 3-6 million units per day has produced encouraging objective and subjective responses in patients with malignant carcinoid tumors [229]. Seventeen of 36 patients experienced objective responses, and two achieved a complete remission. In many instances interferon reduced urinary 5-hydroxyindoleacetic acid secretion by the tumor and thus provided palliative benefit as well. The median duration of response was in excess of 2-1/2 years. Several hormonal agents/analogues such as somatostatin are active in suppressing the manifestations of endocrine tumors. These are not directly cytotoxic or antiproliferative and are beyond the scope of this book. In contrast, a more recent report from the Mayo Clinic cites a lower incidence of objective regression (20%) and, noting the very transitory benefit, disputes the routine use of alpha-interferon for either carcinoid tumor or syndrome [212].

Tumors of the nervous system

Interferon

Human lymphoblastoid interferon induced a greater than 50% reduction in tumor mass or degree of computed tomography (CT) scan enhancement of six of 19 patients with recurrent glioma (five with glioblastoma multiforme, one with oligodendroglioma) failing radiation therapy and, in all but three, failing chemotherapy as well [196]. In another study, recombinant and natural preparations of interferon achieved an overall response rate of 27%, with natural beta-interferon exhibiting the highest efficacy [223]. Beta-interferon may also improve response rates when added to radiation therapy and nitrosoureas following surgery. Takakura has reported a 42% response rate with the three-pronged regime, compared to a response rate of only 17% with radiation and a nitrosourea alone [344].

Interleukin-2/Activated killer cells

Ingram et al. have reported phase I trials of interleukin-2/activated killer cell suspensions placed intralesionally in patients with incompletely resected gliomas; toxicity has been minimal [144]. Phase II trials are planned.

Antibodies

In 1984 Melino et al. reported their experience using heterologous human monoclonal antibodies conjugated with daunorubicin or chlorambucil in 12 pediatric patients over 2 years of age with disseminated neuroblastoma. Nine of these patients exhibited major antitumor responses, and three were reported to be free of disease more than 3 years later [207]. An updated analysis of these observations is long overdue. Cheung et al. have evaluated an IgG3 mouse monoclonal antibody directed against GD2, a ganglioside membrane constituent of human neuroblastoma cells, among others; complete and partial responses in a limited experience have been observed [46]. Other investigators are exploring the use of radiolabeled monoclonal antibody to the epidermal growth factor receptor in patients with high-grade astrocytomas [28] and to human glioma extracellular matrix antigen [219], with evidence of preferential uptake by tumor. Some antitumor activity has been reported, and continued patient accrual is anticipated. Lashford and her co-investigators have instilled intrathecally radiolabeled monoclonal antibodies selected on the basis of tissue typing from a panel of available antibodies [175]. In a small pilot study, five patients with refractory leptomeningeal tumors received three differing antibodies tagged with 11-40 mCi of radioactive I^{131} by direct lumbar puncture or by means of a lumbar reservoir. Four of these five patients enjoyed clinical improvement (improved sensorium, diminished pain, weight gain) and objective benefit (normalization of CSF cell count and protein, CT scan improvement) lasting from 7 months to 2 years without evidence of undue toxicity.

Sarcomas

Interferon

The initial emphasis on interferon came from the studies of Strander and colleagues in Sweden, who, aware of interferon's *in vitro* antiproliferative activity, used interferon in the adjuvant treatment of osteogenic sarcoma [342]. Unfortunately, while these studies prompted much interest in Cantell interferon, activity remained unconfirmed in subsequent trials, and it is now clear the activity of interferon in advanced sarcoma is either minimal or absent [23].

The emergence of the acquired immune deficiency syndrome (AIDS) as a major public health problem has provided the opportunity to evaluate interferon in the treatment of a frequent malignant concomitant of this disease, Kaposi's sarcoma. Studies have suggested response rates of roughly 30%; in addition, there appears to be a dose-response relationship in this entity [168, 169]. High dose interferon therapy was recently approved by the FDA as standard therapy for Kaposi's sarcoma. Improvement of natural killer cell activity and helper-suppressor T-cell ratios does not appear to be necessary for responses to occur; interferon has not been shown to reduce opportunistic infections nor prolong survival among AIDS patients [23].

Interleukin-2/Activated killer cells

The composite available experience in the treatment of patients with sarcoma with interleukin-2/activated killer cells is not encouraging; there have been no responses in the few patients studied [297].

Antibodies

Antigens common to both sarcoma and melanoma cells have recently been described [46]. These reports have prompted further investigation with monoclonal antibodies and antibody-based immunoconjugates for the treatment of sarcoma. It will be of interest to see whether future studies confirm cross-reactivity between melanoma and sarcoma and whether similar therapeutic approaches may be useful in these two groups of diseases, which have previously been separated by histologic criteria.

HEMATOPOIETIC MALIGNANCIES

Lymphoma/Leukemia

Immunomodulation

Reports of prolongation of survival among children with acute lymphocytic leukemia (ALL) following repetitive administration of BCG rekindled interest in nonspecific immunotherapy in the late 1960s [200]. Later, Clarkson et al. reported similar therapeutic benefit in adult acute myelogenous leukemia (AML) patients receiving a heptavalent Pseudomonas vaccine [48]. However, a broader experience, accumulated in the 1970s, did not substantiate improved response rates nor duration of response from nonspecific immunotherapy, but did suggest a possible 6-month survival advantage after first relapse [97].

Interferon

Leukocyte interferon has been extensively tested in patients with a variety of leukemias and lymphomas [98, 99, 234, 237]. The early studies with Cantell preparations revealed an occasional partial response in patients with leukemia. Phase II trials in acute leukemia documented the ability of leukocyte interferon to decrease the circulating cell count, but prolonged remissions in acute leukemia were not seen [294]. The capacity of gamma-interferon, but not alpha- or beta-interferon, to induce *in vitro* the terminal differentiation of leukemic cells of myelocytic, monocytic, and B-lymphocytic origin should prompt clinical trials [4, 24, 152, 279].

Responses to interferon in lymphoma have been more encouraging. While the aggressive lymphomas have been relatively unresponsive, the favorable histology lymphomas have responded quite well to leukocyte interferon preparations with response rates of approximately 50% [98, 100, 230, 234]. These responses have occurred in drug and radiation resistant patients with bulky advanced disease. The median duration of response has been in excess of 6 months. It appears that higher doses of interferon induce a higher response rate and may salvage patients failing interferon at lower doses, suggesting an antiproliferative effect, although modulation of immune responses may also pertain [100, 340]. Alpha-interferon has previously demonstrated activity against mycosis fungoides and the Sezary syndrome [33, 237]. A recent high-dose but intermittent interferon regimen has been shown to be better tolerated and to preserve antitumor efficacy; an overall response rate of 29% in 24 patients has recently been reported [161].

More recent trials in lymphoma have focused on combining interferon with chemotherapy that is known to be effective in the low-grade lymphomas. For example, when CHOP was compared to CHOP plus interferon a longer remission duration was noted although the response rates were not different [328]. In a European study, supportive data was noted with a survival advantage on the interferon arm versus interferon plus chemotherapy [329]. However, a recently completed ECOG study showed no evidence that interferon added to Cytoxan improved response rate, remission duration or total survival [261]. Studies using interferon as maintenance therapy have been reported in low-grade lymphoma with evidence that maintenance post chemotherapy [126, 205, 269]. These studies are still being designed and conducted by various cooperative groups since the dose and schedule of interferon as well as the dose and schedules of the chemotherapy drugs utilized in these studies can vary widely. There does appear to be effect of interferon when added to chemotherapy in these low-grade lymphomas and studies are ongoing to better define the capacity of this biological to extend survival in patients with lymphoma.

Trials in chronic lymphocytic leukemia have been less rewarding, with decrements in circulating cell counts and occasional transient antitumor responses in enlarged organs and lymph nodes [98]. Interferon has been little studied in the treatment of refractory Hodgkin's disease [234].

Antibodies

Numerous trials of monoclonal antibodies in leukemia and lymphoma have been described [69, 71, 101, 209, 210, 242, 243]. The T-101 antibody against the T-65 antigen has been used in the treatment of chronic lymphocytic leukemia; these studies have documented the ability of unconjugated monoclonal antibodies to decrease the circulating cell count rather dramatically, but, with modulation of the antigen from the cell surface, the circulating count often rises back to baseline levels within 24 h. The T-101 antibody, as well as the Leu-1 antibody, has also been used in the treatment of cutaneous T-cell lymphoma, often with clearing of the skin and regression of lymph node masses. Some of these responses have been maintained for 1-4 months with continued antibody therapy. Indium-111-labeled T-101 antibody has demonstrated localization within involved organs [40]; these observations suggested the feasibility of radioisotope-tagged antibody for therapeutic purpose. Rosen and associates administered radiolabeled T-101 to six patients with cutaneous T-cell lymphoma with therapeutic intent. Five patients received between 9, 9 and 16.9 mg of antibody conjugated to 100.5 to 150.1 mCi ^{131}I, with transient responses being seen in all patients as characterized by regression of cutaneous lesions and peripheral lymphadenopathy, as well as relief of pruritis. Responses, however, were transient, from 3 weeks to 3 months; myelosuppression was significant and likely to be dose-limiting [296]. Monoclonal antibodies directed against the common ALL antigen (CALLA) in acute lymphoblastic leukemia (ALL) and against myeloid differentiation antigens in acute myelogenous leukemia (AML) have likewise shown transient and incomplete responses [18, 291, 292]. Studies employing the anti-TAC antibody in adult T-cell leukemia/lymphoma have yielded only marginal results, although a clinical complete remission endured for five months [371]. Such preliminary trials have not revealed striking evidence of prolonged therapeutic response.

Very preliminary information is available utilizing anti-idiotypic antibodies for the treatment of lymphomas [211, 232]. In these disorders, the malignant clone can be distinguished by the presence of a specific immunoglobulin on the cell surface. It is to this idiotype that monoclonal antibody has been produced. It has been postulated that the antibody can incite a localized cellular attack. Of the patients treated, a very small percentage have enjoyed complete responses. More frequently, patients have had meaningful partial responses with this therapy. Prompted by observations in animal models of synergy between anti-idiotypic antibodies and alpha-interferon, as well as by the demonstrated independent activity of alpha-interferon against low-grade malignant lymphomas, Brown and her colleagues studied the use of anti-idiotypic antibodies alone versus its combination with alpha-interferon in patients who initially had presented with follicular lymphoma. However, patient numbers were insufficient to demonstrate whether or not alpha-interferon added to responses achieved. The observation of idiotype-negative cells within tumor specimens at the time of disease progression would appear to support the need for multiple agents each with antilymphomatous activity [30]. Given the low response rate and rare complete responses seen with unconjugated antibody, trials with conjugated anti-idiotypic antibodies are underway and their therapeutic effects may be significantly greater [243]. Radiolabeled anti-idiotypic antibody is also being evaluated; one patient so treated did demonstrate a regression of bulky tumor for greater than 3 months, but did require autologous bone marrow because of myelosuppression [12].

Antigenic modulation may provide for entry of the attached toxic substance into the intracellular space where its toxic effects can be exerted. Idiotype variants have been reported after immunotoxin treatment of leukemia [107]. In an attempt to circumvent modulation, which may be disadvantageous for radiolabeled antibody, as is circulating free antigen, weak host effector mechanisms, emergence of idiotype variants and poor tissue penetration, Press et al. have developed an antibody against a nonmodulating pan-B-cell antigen, which has been safely administered at high dose and with penetration of peripheral tissues [266]. The unconjugated anti-CD20 antibody produced a 50% response rate in multicenter studies which recently (1997) led to approval by the FDA.

Several recent studies have reported striking responses in selected patients with lymphoma using radiolabeled antibody targeting cluster differentiation (CD) antigens [54, 296]. Press and colleagues have investigated a radiolabeled anti-CD37 antibody MB-1, an IgG1 murine immunoglobulin that has high immunoreactivity (ranging from 80 to 92%), avidity, and reactivity with 90% of B cell lymphomas. Although there is minor binding to platelets, granulocytes, and T cells, this antibody binds preferentially to B cells and to B-cell malignancies. Nine patients with advanced, low- or intermediate-grade non-Hodgkin's lymphomas refractory to conventional therapy received escalating dosages of ^{131}I-labeled antibody. Five of these patients on entry biodistribution studies were found to have an excessive tumor burden that prevented selective radioactive exposure to tumor as opposed to normal organs, and these patients were not treated with therapeutic intent. All four patients having tumor burdens less than 0.5 kg did show preferential localization and retention of the antibody, and these patients attained a complete remission (lasting 4, 6, 11+, and 8+ months). A fifth patient was treated similarly but with an anti-CD20 monoclonal antibody 1F5 and achieved a partial response (this patient's lymphoma did not express the CD37 antigen). Two patients required reinfusion of previously stored autologous purged bone marrow. Further dose-escalation studies are underway with favorable responses being reported [109, 147, 266, 267, 268]. These studies may be uniquely positive in these lymphomas, due to their radiosensitivity [71].

Clinical trials are now underway investigating immunotoxins (specifically, an Fab fragment conjugated to deglycolysated ricin A-chain) directed against CD-22 in lymphoproliferative disorders [359]. A monoclonal antibody conjugated to whole ricin was used in 25 patients with B-cell malignancies with the finding of a single complete response and 2 partial responses [120]. A similar conjugate was used in 6 CLL patients with 1 partial response [119]. In another very interesting study, the ligand IL-2 was conjugated to a modified diphtheria toxin (DAB486) and patients with CLL were treated with the finding of at least 1 response [182]. These innovative studies using antibodies or cytokines linked to toxic substances continued to be encouraging and point to new directions in the use of antibodies and/or biological substances linked to toxic entities for cancer therapy.

Studies by Vitetta et al. using deglycolysated A-chain ricin conjugated to Fab' fraction of RFB4 antibody were done in 15 patients with indolent lymphomas. Although these were primarily phase I studies, 5 of 15 showed some evidence of responsiveness [362]. In the second study with the same conjugate using the whole antibody RFB4, there was an increased serum half-life but no increased response rate [6]. Follow-up studies to these using antibody immunotoxins in lymphoma have been conducted by a variety of investigators [121, 122, 123, 310]. These studies consistently demonstrated responses in the patients that appear to be related to dose and schedule of the antibody immunotoxin as well as the bulk of disease in the patients. Trials using these immunotoxins in association with bone marrow transplantation and chemotherapy are underway in an attempt to reduce tumor bulk and to make these agents more effective. This is an area of an intense interest that must be followed closely in the current literature.

A pan T-cell monoclonal antibody has been used *in vitro* to eradicate bone marrow of malignant T cells [146]. Despite fears of damaging pluripotential stem cells, an anti-HLA-DR antibody (AB4) has been used for immunomagnetic bone marrow purging without compromise to engraftment [151]. Studies investigating such bone marrow purging are continuing. In addition, monoclonal antibodies directed against T cells are being used in allogeneic bone marrow transplantation in both leukemia and lymphoma to abrogate graft versus host disease [54].

Hale and colleagues have administered a chimeric monoclonal antibody, CAM-PATH-1H, to two patients with refractory malignant lymphoma with impressive, if transient, results [128]. These investigators had previously treated patients with lymphoid malignancies with a rat monoclonal antibody but had been concerned about the limitations on therapy imposed by the human antiglobulin response. Therefore, they fashioned a chimeric antibody by transplanting genes for the hypervariable region of the rat antibody into the corresponding region of the human immunoglobulin gene [289]. IgG1 was selected for its relatively greater capacity to activate, complement and mediate antibody-dependent cellular cytotoxicity. One patient with bone marrow involvement and splenomegaly enjoyed clearance of lymphoma from the marrow and an eight-fold reduction in splenic size; however, by day 100, lymphoma cells were again detectable in the blood, and the spleen had begun to enlarge; she was retreated with disappearance of tumor from the blood stream and reduction of splenic size (to be followed after the second treatment by splenectomy). A second patient enjoyed a similar response to therapy. Production obstacles and the company decision to discontinue trials have been disappointing.

Studies continue with radiolabeled antiferritin polyclonal antibody in the treatment of refractory Hodgkin's disease [184].

Interleukin-2/Activated killer cells

There are anecdotal reports of a small number of patients with both low grade non-Hodgkin's lymphomas and refractory Hodgkin's disease exhibiting encouraging early responses to interleukin-2/activated killer cell therapy [248]. The experience is still quite small and broad assessment is not yet possible.

Myeloproliferative syndromes

Interferon

Hematologic remission has been achieved with alpha-interferon in a high percentage of patients in chronic-phase chronic myelogenous leukemia (CML). Using a daily induction dose of 5 million units/m^2 of intramuscular interferon alfa-2a, with subsequent dose modification based upon toxicity and response, Talpaz et al. observed complete normalization of peripheral blood counts in 13 of 17 patients [346]. Disappearance of the Philadelphia chromosome was observed on at least one occasion in six of these patients. These same investigators have recently updated their experience in CML with dosages of alpha-interferon from 3 million units every other day to 9 million units daily; in this latest reported series of 51 patients, 36 (or 71%) achieved a complete hematologic remission, but complete suppression of the Philadelphia chromosome was infrequent [347]. Niederle et al. have reported a similar experience in 15 patients treated with interferon alfa-2b [228]. Using an induction dose of 4 million units per day, they observed hematologic remission in 12 of these 15 patients at a median of 6 weeks into treatment, with a range of 3-20 weeks. More recent studies continue to show high response rates and significant numbers of complete responses with conversion to Ph1 chromosome negativity. A recent summary of information from M.D. Anderson, which has pioneered the studies of alpha-interferon in patients with chronic myelogenous leukemia report on 274 patients so treated; 80% of these individuals achieved a complete response with nearly half having major cytogenetic responses (disappearance of the Philadelphia chromosome). It is apparent from these studies that a major cytogenetic response is associated with improved survival although patients with complete responses with residual Ph1-positive cells also enjoy a prolonged survival compared to historical controls [149].

Unlike many other types of cancer, there does seem to be a fairly strong response curve for alpha-interferon in CML. Doses above 5 million units/m^2 per day are necessary to achieve optimal responses [313, 352] and randomized studies have indicated that lower doses are less effective than higher doses [5]. There is some controversy here with regard to dose since one recent study did show very little difference between lower and higher dose regimens [313]. From all of these studies it is apparent that interferon has major activity in CML. It appears to be most active in early phase disease and may be useful in conjunction with inductive chemotherapy and/or bone marrow transplantation. These studies should be the prelude to highly effective combination programs of biotherapy and chemotherapy in AML.

Hairy-Cell Leukemia

Interferon

The treatment of hairy-cell leukemia with alpha-interferon represents one of only four approved oncologic uses of this recombinant interferon (the others being CML, melanoma and Kaposi's sarcoma). First recognized as a distinct clinical entity in 1958 [27], hairy-cell leukemia is a chronic lymphoproliferative disorder of B cells with associated cytopenias. Until recently, the standard initial mode of therapy has been splenectomy (which can often restore hematologic parameters to normal for an extended period of time), followed by various chemotherapeutic agents. Quesada et al. reported the earliest success with partially purified interferon in 1984, stimulating considerable further clinical investigation [277]. Recent trials with recombinant alpha-interferon have shown hematologic response rates in excess of 80%, although stringently scored pathologic complete remissions are much less frequent [102, 118, 278, 280]. Improvement was observed in all three hematologic cell lines, often demonstrated earliest in the platelet count. Correction of neutropenia may take 2-3 months, with resolution of anemia occurring over perhaps as long as 9 months. In addition to these objective responses, the incidence of serious infection also diminishes. Most trials using interferon alfa-2a have incorporated a regimen of 3 million units/m^2 daily; most studies investigating interferon alfa-2b have employed a dose of 2 million units/m^2 three times a week. A low-dose interferon alfa-2b regimen of 200, 000 units/m^2 three times a week produced an unacceptably low response rate and cannot be recommended [215].

Alpha-interferon is not curative in this illness. The exact mode of action is unclear. Evidence of enhanced natural killer cell activity has been reported [102]. Other proposed mechanisms of action include a direct anti-proliferative effect and induction of differentiation [118]. Issues of duration of interferon treatment, durability of response after discontinuation of interferon, the proper sequencing of splenectomy and interferon, and the use of combined interferon and chemotherapy remain under current study. Some have recommended that alpha-interferon therapy be discontinued after one year in responding asymptomatic patients, in an effort to balance depth of response with the countervailing toxicity of excessive fatigue [112]. Alpha-interferon is usually able to reactivate an earlier response upon its reintroduction. It has also been noted that the discontinuation of alpha-interferon does not eventuate in rapid recrudescence of disease [113]. Comparative studies with another effective agent, the adenosine deaminase inhibitor, 2-deoxy-coformycin, are ongoing as well. A combined trial of 2-deoxycoformycin and alpha-interferon, alternating monthly, yielded responses similar to those previously reported with 2-deoxycoformycin alone [199]. Recent news reports on 'one-shot' therapy with a chloro derivative of 2-deoxycoformycin in the induction of CR make this leukemia a likely candidate to be rather easily cured with combination chemo-biotherapy.

MULTIPLE MYELOMA

Interferon

Several studies have demonstrated response rates of about 20% in patients with refractory multiple myeloma treated with recombinant alpha-interferon [42, 55, 231]. An attempt to augment this response experience by using high dose induction schedules, often with the addition of Prednisone, did not result in enhanced response [42]. Anecdotal observations have suggested possible synergism between the interferons and cytotoxic drugs [47, 92]. Because of response rates of 50% in untreated patients [272], studies are underway evaluating the combination of interferon with standard chemotherapeutic regimens as initial therapy for multiple myeloma. Preliminary interpretation has suggested that the duration of initial response may be extended with the addition of alpha-interferon [197]. Interesting observations on the induction of stability in myeloma will require prolonged studies. Perhaps interferon will be most effective in stabilizing the disease rather than eradicating the myeloma cell population.

Antibodies

Plasma cells produce myeloma protein (antibody), giving ready availability of a secreted protein target for antibody induction. However, this very characteristic makes it unlikely that antibody therapy will be useful in myeloma, at least not with the myeloma protein as target, since the therapeutic antibody would be totally absorbed in the vascular and extracellular pool. Anti-CEA studies in colon cancer suggest this is not a rational approach to follow, but targeting myeloma cell membrane proteins (nonsecreted) could be attempted. No major clinical studies of antibody against other plasma cell membrane targets have been reported.

CONCLUSION

Encouraging reports on cancers responding to various forms of biotherapy are appearing almost daily. This chapter brings the clinician up to 1996, but within the span of a few months, many of the recommendations in this chapter will be outdated. *Principles of Cancer Biotherapy* will be revised every few years in an attempt to stay current with this rapidly evolving area. Clinicians are advised to carefully follow the literature if they wish to stay abreast of the latest developments in biotherapy and combination modality treatment using biotherapy. It is apparent that biotherapy has already provided major benefit in areas of hairy-cell leukemia, chronic myelogenous leukemia, lymphoma, Kaposi's sarcoma, renal cancer, and melanoma. It is anticipated that this modality will be broadly useful in the treatment of a wide variety of human cancers. It has only been 17 years since the development of the first cloned biological for cancer therapy, which marked the beginning of cancer biotherapy. Clearly, these cloned gene products are already producing a major impact in cancer and other diseases, and the clinician would be well advised to undergo continued medical education yearly in this rapidly evolving field. It is the belief of the authors of this textbook that these approaches in biotherapy will soon dominate the field of clinical oncology.

REFERENCES

1. Abrams DI, Volberding PA. Alpha interferon therapy of AIDS-associated Kaposi's sarcoma. *Semin Oncol* 1986; 13(3, 2): 43-47.
2. Adler A, Gillon G, Lurie H, et al. Active specific immunotherapy of renal cell carcinoma patients: A prospective

randomized study of hormono-immuno-versus hormonotherapy. Preliminary report of immunological and clinical aspects. *J Biol Response* Mod 1987; 6: 610-624.

3. Ajani JA, Rios AA, Ende K, et al. Phase I and II studies of the combination of recombinant human interferon-gamma and 5-fluorouracil in patients with advanced colorectal carcinoma. *J Biol Response* Modif 1989; 8: 140-146.
4. Al-Kativ A, Wang CY, Koziner V. Gamma interferon (IFN-gamma)-induced phenotypic changes of chronic lymphocytic leukemia (CLL) and non-Hodgkin's lymphoma (NHL) cells. *Proc AACR* 1984; 25: 235.
5. Alimena G, Morra E, Lazzarino M, et al. Interferon-α2b as therapy for Ph[1]-positive chronic myelogenous leukemia: A study of 82 patients treated with intermittent or daily administration. *Blood* 1988; 72: 642-647.
6. Amlot PL, Stone MJ, Cunningham D, et al. A phase I study of an anti-CD22-deglycosylated ricin A chain immunotoxin in the treatment of B-cell lymphomas resistant to conventional therapy. *Blood* 1993; 82: 2624-2633.
7. Atkins MB, O'Boyle KR, Sosman JA. Multiinstitutional phase II trial of intensive combination chemoimmunotherapy for metastatic melanoma. *J Clin Oncol* 1994; 12: 1553-1560.
8. Aulitzky W, Gastl G, Aulitzky WE, et al. Successful treatment of metastatic renal cell carcinoma with a biologically active dose of recombinant interferon-gamma. *J Clin Oncol* 1989; 7: 1875-1884.
9. Austin FC, Boone CW, Levin DL, et al. Breast cancer skin test antigens of increased sensitivity prepared from vesicular stomatitis virus infected tumor cells. *Cancer* 1982; 49: 2034-2042.
10. Avner BP, Liao SK, Avner B, et al. Therapeutic murine monoclonal antibodies developed for individual cancer patients. *J Biol Response Modif* 1989; 8(1): 25-36.
11. Babaian RJ, Murray JL, Lamkie LM, et al. Radioimmunological imaging of metastatic prostatic cancer with 111 indium-labeled monoclonal antibody PAY 276. *J Urol* 1987; 137(3): 439-43.
12. Badger. *Proc AACR* 1987; 28: 338.
13. Bajetta E, Negretti E, Giannotti B. Phase II study of interferon alpha 2a and dacarbazine in advanced melanoma. *Am J Clin Oncol* 1990; 13: 405-409.
14. Bajorin D, Chapman P, Kunicka J, et al. Phase I trial of a combination of R24 mouse monoclonal antibody and recombinant interleukin-2 in patients with melanoma. *Proc ASCO* 1987; 6: 210.
15. Bajorin DF, Chapman PB, Dimaggio J, et al. Phase I evaluation of a combination of monoclonal antibody R24 and interleukin 2 in patients with metastatic melanoma. *Cancer Res* 1990; 50: 7490-7495.
16. Bakke A, Gothlin JH, Haukaas SA, Kalland T. Augmentation of natural killer cell activity after arterial embolization of renal carcinomas. *Cancer Res* 1982; 42: 3880-3883.
17. Bakker W, Nijhuis-Heddes JMA, van der Velde EA. Postoperative intrapleural BCG in lung cancer: a 5-year follow-up report. *Cancer Immunol Immunother* 1986; 22: 155-159.
18. Ball ED, Bernier GM, Cornwell GG. Monoclonal antibodies to myeloid differentiation antigens: *in vivo* studies of three patients with acute myelogenous leukemia. *Blood* 1983; 62: 1203-1210.
19. Berek JS, Hacker NF, Lichtenstein A. Intraperitoneal recombinant alpha-interferon for 'salvage' immunotherapy in stage III epithelial ovarian cancer: a Gynecologic Oncology Group Study. *Semin Oncol* 1986; XIII (3, suppl. 2): 61-71.
20. Berek JS, Knapp R, Hacker N. Intraperitoneal immunotherapy of human ovarian carcinoma with *Corynebacterium parvum*. *Proc ASCO* 1984; 3: 173.
21. Blair S, Flaherty L. Valdivieso M. Comparison of high dose interleukin 2 with combined chemotherapy and low dose IL2 in metastatic malignant melanoma. *Proc Am Soc Clin Oncol* 1991; 10: 294 (abstract).
22. Yuan D, Handler FJ, Vitetta ES. Characterization of a monoclonal antibody reactive with a subset of human breast tumors. *J Natl Cancer Inst* 1982; 68: 719-728.
23. Bonnem EM, Spiegel RJ. Interferon-alpha: current status and future promise. *J Biol Response Modif* 1984; 3(6): 580-598.
24. Bonnem E, Oldham RK. Gamma interferon physiology and potential role in cancer therapy. *J Biol Response Modif* 1987; 6: 275-301.
25. Borden EC, Holland JF, Dao TL, et al. Leukocyte derived interferon (alpha) in human breast carcinoma. *Ann Intern Med* 1982; 97: 1-6.
26. Borgstrom S, von Eyben FE, Flodgren P, et al. Human leukocyte interferon and cimetidine for metastatic melanoma. *N Engl J Med* 1982; 307: 1080-1081.
27. Bouroncle BA, Wiseman BK, Doak CA. Leukemic reticuloendotheliosis. *Blood* 1958; 13: 609-629.
28. Brady LW, Woo DV, Karlsson U, et al. Radioimmunotherapy of human gliomas using I-125 labeled monoclonal antibody to epidermal growth factor receptor. *Proc ASCO* 1988; 7: 83.
29. Brichard V, Van Pel A, Wolfel T, et al. The tyrosinase gene codes for an antigen recognized by autologous cytolytic T lymphocytes on HLA-A2 melanomas. *J Exp Med* 1993; 178: 489-495.
30. Brown SL, Miller RA, Horning SJ. Treatment of B cell lymphomas with anti-idiotype antibodies alone and in combination with alpha interferon. *Blood* 1989; 73(3): 651-661.
31. Brown TD, Koeller J, Beougher K, et al. A phase I clinical trial of recombinant DNA gamma interferon. *J Clin Oncol* 1987; 5: 790-798.
32. Budd GT, Osgood B, Barna B, et al. Phase I clinical trial of interleukin-2 and alpha-interferon: toxicity and immunologic effects. *Cancer Res* 1989; 49: 6432-6436.
33. Bunn PA, Ihde DC, Foon KA. The role of recombinant interferon alpha-2A in the therapy of cutaneous T cell lymphomas. *Cancer* 1986; 57: 1689-1695.
34. Buzaid AC, Todd MB. Therapeutic options in renal cell carcinoma. *Semin Oncol* 1989; 16(1 suppl 1): 12-19.
35. Buzdar AU, Blumenschein GR, Hortovagyi GN, et al. Adjuvant chemotherapy with 4-fluorouracil, doxorubicin (Adriamycin) and cyclophosphamide, with or without BCG immunotherapy in state II or stage III breast cancer. In: Terry WD, Rosenberg SA, eds. Immunotherapy of human cancer. New York: Elsevier North Holland, 1982: 175-181.
36. Bystryn J-C, Jacobsen S, Harris MN, et al. Preparation and characterization of a polyvalent human melanoma antigen vaccine. *J Biol Resp Modif* 1986; 5: 221-224.
37. Bystryn J-C, Miller K, Cui J, Oratz R. Identification of candidate antigens for construction of melanoma vaccines. *Clin Res* 1993; 41(2): 489A.

38. Bystryn J-C, Oratz R, Roses DF, et al. Improved survival of melanoma patients with delayed type hypersensitivity response to melanoma vaccine immunization. *Clin Res* 1991; 39: 503A.
39. Cannon GB, McCoy JL, Connor RJ, et al. Use of the leukocyte migration inhibition assay to evaluate antigenic differences in human breast cancers in melanoma. *J Natl Cancer Inst* 1978; 60: 969-978.
40. Carrasquillo JA, Bunn PA Jr, Kennan AM, et al. Radioimmunodetection of cutaneous T-cell lymphoma with ^{111}In-T101 monoclonal antibody. *N Engl J Med* 1986; 315: 673-680.
41. Carrasquillo JA, Abrams PG, Schroff R, et al. Effect of antibody dose on the imaging and biodistribution of indium-111 0.2.27 anti-melanoma monoclonal antibody. *J Nucl Med* 1988; 29(1): 39-47.
42. Case DC Jr, Sonneborn HL, Paul SD. Phase II study of rDNA alpha II interferon (Intron-A) in patients with multiple myeloma utilizing an escalating induction phase. *Cancer Treat Rep* 1986; 70(11): 1251-1254.
43. Ceriani RL, Thompson K, Pesterson JA, Abraham S. Surface differentiation antigens of human mammary epithelial cells carried on the human milk fat globule. *Proc Natl Acad Sci USA* 1977; 74: 582-586.
44. Ceriani RL, Saki M, Sussman H, et al. Circulating human mammary epithelial antigens in breast cancer. *Proc Natl Acad Sci USA* 1982; 79: 5420-5424.
45. Chapman PV, Hakes T, Gabrilove JL. A phase I pilot study of intraperitoneal (I.P.) rIL-2 in ovarian cancer. *Proc ASCO* 1986; 5: 231.
46. Cheung N-KV, Lazarus H, Miraldi FD, et al. Ganglioside GD2 specific monoclonal antibody 3F8: a phase I study in patients with neuroblastoma and malignant melanoma. *J Clin Oncol* 1987; 5: 1430-1440.
47. Clark RH, Dimitrov NV, Axelson JA, Charmella LJ. Leukocyte interferon as a biological response modifier in lymphoproliferative diseases resistant to standard therapy. *Am Soc Hematol* 1983; 62: 188a.
48. Clarkson VD, Dowling MD, Gee TS, et al. Treatment of acute leukemia. *Cancer* 1975; 36: 775.
49. Coates A, Rallings M, Hersey P, et al. Phase II study of recombinant alpha 2-interferon in advanced malignant melanoma. *J Interferon Res* 1986; 6: 1-4.
50. Cohen MH, Chreten PB, Ihde DC, et al. Thymosin fraction V prolongs the survival of lung cancer patients treated with intensive combination chemotherapy. *J Am Med Assoc* 1979; 245: 1813-1815.
51. Coit D, Houghton A, Corden-Cardo C, et al. Isolation limb perfusion with monoclonal antibody R24 in patients with malignant lymphoma. *Proc ASCO* 1988; 7: 248.
52. Colcher D, Esteban J, Carrasquillo JA. Complementation of intracavity and intravenous administration of a monoclonal antibody (B72.3) in patients with carcinoma. *Cancer Res* 1987; 47: 4218-4224.
53. Colcher D, Horan-Hand P, Nuti M, Scholm J. A spectrum of monoclonal antibodies reactive with human mammary tumor cells. *Proc Natl Acad Sci USA* 1981; 78: 3199-3203.
54. Colcher D, Zalutsky M, Kaplan W, et al. Radiolocalization of human mammary tumors in athymic mice by a monoclonal antibody. *Cancer Res* 1983; 43: 736-742.
55. Cooper MR. Interferons in the treatment of multiple myeloma. *Semin Oncol* 1986; 13(3, 2): 13-20.
56. Creagan ET, Ahmann DL, Green SJ, et al. Phase II study of recombinant leukocyte A interferon (rIFN-αA) in disseminated malignant melanoma. *Cancer* 1984; 54(12): 2844-2849.
57. Creagan ET, Ahmann DL, Green SJ, et al. Phase II study of recombinant leukocyte A interferon (rIFN-aA) in disseminated malignant melanoma. *Cancer* 1984; 54(12): 2844-2849.
58. Creagan ET, Ahmann DL, Green SJ, et al. Phase II study of low-dose recombinant leukocyte A interferon in disseminated malignant melanoma. *J Clin Oncol* 1984; 2: 1002-1005.
59. Creekmore S, Urba W, Koop W, et al. Phase IB/II trial of R24 antibody and interleukin-2 (IL2) in melanoma. *Proc Am Soc Clin Oncol* 1992; 1886: 345 (abstract).
60. Culver KW, Blaese RM. Gene therapy for cancer. [review]. *Trends Genet* 1994; 10: 174-178.
61. Cuttitta F, Carney DN, Mulshine J, et al. Bombesin-like peptides can function as autocrine growth factors in human small cell lung cancer. *Nature* 1985; 316: 823-826.
62. Day CL, Lew RA, Mihm MC, Sober AJ. A multivariate analysis of prognostic factors for melanoma patients with lesions >3.65 mm in thickness. The importance of revealing alternative cox models. *Ann Surg* 1982; 195: 44-49.
63. Demchak PA, Mier JW, Robert NJ. Interleukin-2 and high dose cisplatin in patients with metastatic melanoma: a pilot study. *J Clin Oncol* 1991; 9: 1821-1830.
64. Diaz RE, Jimeno J, Camps C, et al. Treatment of advanced colorectal cancer with recombinant interferon alpha and fluorouracil: activity in liver metastasis. *Cancer Invest* 1992; 10: 259-264.
65. DeVita VT Jr, Hellman S, Rosenberg SA. Cell transfer therapy: Clinical applications. In: *Biologic Therapy of Cancer*, 2nd Edition. DeVita VT Jr, Hellman S, Rosenberg SA eds. J.B. Lippincott Company, Philadelphia, 1995: 489.
66. DeVita VT Jr, Hellman S, Rosenberg SA. Cell transfer therapy: Clinical applications. In: *Biologic Therapy of Cancer*, 2nd Edition. DeVita VT Jr, Hellman S, Rosenberg SA eds. J.B. Lippincott Company, Philadelphia, 1995: 501.
67. Dimitrov NV, Myer C, Einhorn S, et al. Interferon as modifiers of estrogen receptors in cancer tissues. Proc ASCO 1982; 23: 240.
68. Dillman RO, Beauregard JC, Shawler DL, et al. In: Peters H, ed. *Protides of the biological fluids*. New York: Pergamon Press, 1983: 353-358.
69. Dillman RO, Shawler DL, Sobol RE, et al. Murine monoclonal antibody therapy in 2 patients with lymphocytic leukemia. *Blood* 1982; 59: 1036-1045.
70. Dillman RO, Oldham RK, Barth NM, et al. Continuous interleukin-2 and lymphokine activated killer cells alternated with DTIC as treatment of advanced melanoma. *J Natl Cancer Inst* 1990.
71. Dillman RO. Monoclonal antibodies for treating cancer. *Ann Intern Med* 1989; 111: 592-603.
72. Dillman RO, Oldham RK, Barth NM, et al. Continuous interleukin-2 and tumor derived activated cells as treatment of advanced melanoma. *J Clin Oncol* 1990.
73. Dillman RO, Oldham RK, Barth NM. Recombinant interleukin-2 and adoptive immunotherapy alternated with dacarbazine therapy in melanoma: a national biotherapy study group trial. *J Natl Cancer Inst* 190; 82: 1345-1349.
74. Dillman RO, Oldham RK, Barth NM, et al. Continuous

interleukin-2 and tumor infiltrating lymphocytes as treatment of advanced melanoma. *Cancer* 1991; 68(1): 1-8.

75. Dillman RO, Oldham RK, Tauer KW, et al. Continuous interleukin-2 and lymphokine activated killer cells for advanced cancer: an NBSG trial. *J Clin Oncol* 1991; 9: 1233-1240.
76. Dillman RO, Church C, Oldham RK, et al. Inpatient continuous infusion interleukin-2 in 788 cancer patients: the NBSG experience. *Cancer* 1993; 71: 2358-2370.
77. Dorval T, Palangie T, Jouve M, et al. Clinical phase II trial of recombinant DNA interferon (interferon alfa 2b) in patients with metastatic malignant melanoma. *Cancer* 1986; 58: 215-218.
78. Doyle A, Martin J, Funa K, et al. Markedly decreased expression of class I histocompatibility antigens, protein and mRNA in human small cell lung cancer. *J Exp Med* 1985; 161: 1135-1151.
79. Dutcher JP, Creekmore S, Weiss GR. Phase II study of high-dose interleukin-2 and lymphokine-activated killer cells. *J Clin Oncol* 1989; 7: 477-485.
80. Dutcher JP, Gaynor ER, Boldt DH, et al. A phase II study of high dose continuous infusion interleukin-2 with lymphokine activated killer cells: Not the optimal schedule for metastatic melanoma. *J Clin Oncol* 1991; 9: 641-648.
81. Ellerhorst J, Jones E, Kilbourn R, et al. Fixed low dose gamma interferon is active against metastatic renal cell carcinoma (abstract). *Proc Am Soc Clin Oncol* 1992; 11: 220.
82. Elsasser-Beile U, Drews H. Interferon in the treatment of malignant melanoma. Results of clinical studies. *Fortschr Med* 1987; 105: 401.
83. Epenetos AA, Munro AJ, Stewart S, et al. Antibody-guided irradiation of advanced ovarian cancer with intraperitoneally administered radiolabeled monoclonal antibodies. *J Clin Oncol* 1987; 5: 1890-1899.
84. Erlichman C, Fine S, Wong A, Elhakim T. A randomized trial of fluorouracil and folinic acid in patients with metastatic colorectal carcinoma. *J Clin Oncol* 1988; 6: 469-475.
85. Esteban JM, Colcher D, Sugerbaker P, et al. Quantitative and qualitative aspects of radiolocalization in colon cancer patients of intravenously administered MAb B72.3. *Int J Cancer* 1987; 39: 50-59.
86. Ettinger DS, Order SE, Wharam MD, et al. Phase I-II study of isotopic immunoglobulin therapy for primary liver cancer. *Cancer Treat Rep* 1982; 66: 289-297.
87. Fairlaub DJ. Spontaneous regression of metastasis of renal cancer. *Cancer* 1981; 47: 2102-2106.
88. Falkson CI, Falkson G, Falkson HC. Improved results with the addition of interferon alpha 2b to dacarbazine in the treatment of patients with metastatic malignant melanoma. *J Clin Oncol* 1991; 9: 1403-1408.
89. Fer MF, Oldham RK. Protein A immunoadsorption/immunoactivation: a critical review. In: Salinas FA, Hanna MG, eds. Immune complexes and human cancer. Contemporary topics in immunobiology, vol. 15. New York: *Plenum Publishing*, 1985: 257-276.
90. Fer MF, Beman J, Stevenson HC. A trial of autologous plasma perfusion over protein A in patients with breast cancer. *J Biol Response Modif* 1984; 3: 352-358.
91. Ferradini L, Mackenson A, Genevee C, et al. Analysis of T cell receptor variability in tumor-infiltrating lymphocytes from a human regressive melanoma. *J Clin Invest* 1993; 91: 1183-1190.
92. Ferraresi R, Rudnick SA, Bonnem EM, et al. Enhanced response to chemotherapy after treatment with DNA alpha-2 interferon. *Am Soc Hematol* 1983; 62: 212a.
93. Fiedler W, Jasmin C, DeMulder PHM. A phase II study of sequential recombinant interleukin-2 followed by dacarbazine in metastatic melanoma. *Eur J Cancer* 1992; 28: 443-446.
94. Figlin RA, Sarna GP. Human leukocyte interferon (alpha IFN): phase II trial in non-small cell lung cancer and adenocarcinoma of the lung. *Proc ASCO* 1983; 2: 45.
95. Figlin RA, Belldegrun A, Moldaver N, et al. Concomitant administration of recombinant human interleukin-2 and recombinant interferon alfa-2A: An active outpatient regimen in metastatic renal cell carcinoma. *J Clin Oncol* 1992; 10: 414-421.
96. Flaherty LE, Redman BG, Chabot GG. A Phase I-II study of dacarbazine in combination with outpatient interleukin-2 in metastatic malignant melanoma. *Cancer* 1990; 65: 2471-2477.
97. Foon KA, Smalley RV, Riggs CW, et al. The role of immunotherapy in acute myelogenous leukemia. *Am Arch Intern Med* 1983; 143: 1726-1731.
98. Foon KA, Bottino GC, Abrams PG, et al. Phase II trial recombinant leukocyte A interferon in patients with advanced chronic lymphocytic leukemia. *Am J Med* 1985; 78: 216-220.
99. Foon KA, Doroshow J, Bonnem E, et al. A prospective randomized trial of alpha-2b-interferon/gamma interferon or the combination in advanced metastatic renal cell carcinoma. *J Biol Response Modif* 1988; 7: 540-545.
100. Foon KA, Sherwin SA, Abrams PG, et al. Treatment of advanced non-Hodgkin's lymphoma with recombinant leukocyte A interferon. *N Engl J Med* 1984; 311: 1148-1152.
101. Foon KA, Schroff RW, Bunn PA, et al. Effects of monoclonal antibody therapy in patients with chronic lymphocytic leukemia. *Blood* 1984; 64(5): 1085-1093.
102. Foon KA, Maluish AE, Abrams PG. Recombinant leukocyte A interferon therapy for advanced hairy cell leukemia: therapeutic and immunologic results. *Am J Med* 1986; 80: 351-356.
103. Freedman RS, Gutterman JU, Wharton JT, Rutledge RN. Leukocyte interferon (IFN alpha) in patients with epithelial ovarian carcinoma. *J Biol Response Modif* 1983; 2: 133-138.
104. Fujisawa T, Waldman SR, Yonemoto RH. Leukocyte adherence inhibition by soluble tumor antigens and breast cancer patients. *Cancer* 1977; 39: 506-513.
105. Gail MH, Eagan RT, Feld R, et al. Prognostic factors in patients with resected stage I non-small cell lung cancer; a report from the Lung Cancer Study Group. *Cancer* 1984; 54: 1802-1813.
106. Gaugler B, Van den Eynde B, van der Bruggen P, et al. Human gene MAGE-3 codes for an antigen recognized on a melanoma by autologous cytolytic T lymphocytes. *J Exp Med* 1994; 179: 921-930.
107. Glennie J, et al. Emergents of immunoglobulin variants following treatment of a B cell leukemia with an immunotoxin composed of anti-idiotypic antibody and saporin. *J Exp Med* 1987; 166: 43-62,
108. Goldberg R, Silgals R, Ayoob M, et al. A phase II trial of lymphoblastoid interferon (IF) in malignant melanoma.

Proc ASCO 1984; 3: 49.

109. Goldenberg DM, Horowitz JA, Sharkey RM, et al. Targeting, dosimetry, and radioimmunotherapy of B-cell lymphomas with iodine-131-labeled LL2 monoclonal antibody. *J Clin Oncol* 1991; 9: 548-564.
110. Goldenberg DM. Monoclonal antibodies in cancer detection and therapy. *Am J of Med* 1993; 94: 297-312.
111. Goldenberg DM, DeLand FH. History and status of tumor imaging with radiolabeled antibodies. *J Biol Response Modif* 1982; 1: 121-136.
112. Golomb HM, Ratain MJ, Fefer A, et al. Randomized study of the duration of treatment with interferon alpha-2b in patients with hairy cell leukemia. *J Natl Cancer Inst* 1988; 80: 359-373.
113. Golomb HM. The treatment of hairy cell leukemia. *Blood* 1987; 69(4): 979-983.
114. Goodman GE, Beaumier P, Hellstrom I, et al. Pilot trial of murine monoclonal antibodies in patients with advanced melanoma. *J Clin Oncol* 1985; 3: 340-352.
115. Goodman GE, Hellstrom I, Hummel D, et al. Phase I trial of monoclonal antibody MG-21 directed against a melanoma-associated GD3 ganglioside antigen. *Proc ASCO* 1987; 6: 209.
116. Goodman GE, Hellstrom I, Brodzinsky L, et al. Phase I trial of murine monoclonal antibody L6 in breast, colon, ovarian, and lung cancer. *J Clin Oncol* 1990; 8: 1083-1092.
117. Grem JL, Jordan E, Robson ME, et al. Phase II study of fluorouracil, leucovorin and interferon-alfa-2a in metastatic colorectal carcinoma. *J Clin Oncol* 1993; 11: 1737-1745.
118. Groopman JE. Therapeutic options and hairy cell leukemia. *Semin Oncol* 1985; 12(4, 5): 30-34.
119. Grossbard ML, Nadler LM. Immunotoxin therapy of malignancy, in DeVita VT Jr, Hellman S, Rosenberg SA (eds): *Important Advances in Oncology* pp 11-135. Philadelphia, JP Lippincott, 1992.
120. Grossbard ML, Freedman AS, Ritz J, et al. Serotherapy of B-cell neoplasms with anti-B4-blocked ricin: A phase I trial of daily bolus infusion. *Blood* 1992; 79: 576.
121. Grossbard ML, Lambert JM, Goldmacher VS, et al. Anti-B4-blocked ricin: A phase I trial of 7-day continuous infusion in patients with B-cell neoplasms. *J Clin Oncol* 1993; 11: 726-737.
122. Grossbard ML, Gribben JG, Freedman AS, et al. Adjuvant immunotoxin therapy with anti-B4-blocked ricin after autologous bone marrow transplantation for patients with B-cell non-Hodgkin's lymphoma. *Blood* 1993; 81: 2262-2271.
123. Grossbard ML, O'Day S, Gribben JG, et al. A phase II study of anti-B4-blocked ricin (Anti-B4-bR) therapy following autologous bone marrow transplantation (ABMT) for B-cell non-Hodgkin's lymphoma. *Proc ASCO* 1994; 13: 293.
124. Gundersen S, Flokkmann A. Interferon plus dacarbazine in advanced malignant melanoma: A phase I-II study. *Eur J Cancer* 1991; 27(2): 220-221.
125. Gutterman JU, Blumenschein GR, Alexanian R, et al. Leukocyte interferon induced tumor regression in human metastatic breast cancer, multiple myeloma, and malignant lymphoma. *Ann Intern Med* 1980; 93: 399-406.
126. Hagenbeek A, Van Hoof A, Conde P, et al. Interferon-alpha 2b vs control as maintenance therapy for low-grade non-Hodgkin's lymphoma: Results from a prospective randomized clinical trial on behalf of the EORTC Lymphoma Cooperative Group. *Proc ASCO* 1995; 14: 386.
127. Hakes TB, Currie VE, Kaufman RG, et al. CMF +/- levamisole breast adjuvant chemotherapy: 5 year analysis. *Proc ASCO* 1982; 1: 83.
128. Hale G, Clark MR, Marcus R, et al. Remission induction in non-Hodgkin's lymphoma with reshaped human monoclonal antibody CAMPATH-1H. *Lancet* 1988; ii: 1394-1399.
129. Halpern SE, Dillman RO. Radioimmunodetection with monoclonal antibodies against prostatic acid phosphatase. In: Winkler C, ed. *Nuclear medicine in clinical oncology.* Berlin: Springer Verlag, Heidelberg, 1986: 164-170.
130. Hamblin TJ, Davies B, Sadullah S, et al. A Phase II study of the treatment of metastatic malignant melanoma with a combination of dacarbazine, cisplatin, interleukin-2 (IL-2) and alfa-interferon (IFN). *Proc ASCO* 1991; 10: 294 (abstract).
131. Hanna MG Jr, Ransom JH, Pomato N, et al. Active specific immunotherapy of human colorectal carcinoma with an autologous tumor cell/bacillus calmette-guerin vaccine. *Ann NY Acad Sci* 1993; 690: 135-146.
132. Hawkins MJ. PPO Updates IL-2/LAK. *Princ Prac Oncol* 1989; 3(8): 1-14.
133. Henry DH, et al. Phase I clinical trial of Prosorba(tm) Protein A columns in malignancy: report on toxicity. *Proc ASCO* 1986; 5: 227.
134. Hersey P, Hasic E, MacDonald M, et al. Effects of recombinant leukocyte interferon (rIFN-αA) on tumour growth and immune responses in patients with metastatic melanoma. *Br J Cancer* 1985; 51: (6): 815-826.
135. Hersey P, McLeod GRC, Thompson DB. Treatment of advanced malignant melanoma with recombinant interferon alpha 2a in combination with DTIC: long term follow-up of two phase II studies. *Br J Haematol* 1991; 79: 60-66.
136. Hill NO, Pardue A, Khan A, et al. Interferon and cimetidine for malignant melanoma. *N Engl J Med* 1983; 308: 286.
137. Hollinshead A, Arlen M, Yonemoto R, et al. Pilot studies using melanoma tumor-associated antigens (TAA) in specific-active immunotherapy of malignant melanoma. *Cancer* 1982; 49: 1387.
138. Holohan TV, Phillips TM, Bowles C, Deissertroh A. Regression of canine mammary carcinoma after immunoadsorption therapy. *Cancer Res* 1982; 42: 3663-3668.
139. Hoover HC Jr, Surdyke MG, Dangel RB, et al. Prospectively randomized trial of adjuvant active specific immunotherapy for human colorectal cancer. *Cancer* 1985; 55: 1236.
140. Houghton AN, Mintzer D, Cordon-Cardo C, et al. Mouse monoclonal antibody detecting GD3 ganglioside: a phase I trial in patients with malignant melanoma. *Proc Natl Acad Sci USA* 1985; 82: 1242-1246.
141. Houghton AN, Scheinberg DA. Monoclonal antibodies: potential applications to the treatment of cancer. *Semin Oncol* 1986; 13(2): 165-179.
142. Houghton A. Passive immunotherapy: monoclonal antibodies along as therapy (presentation). *Williamsburg Conference*, 1987.
143. Houghton A. Treatment of malignant melanoma with monoclonal antibodies (presentation). The significance of human response to monoclonal antibodies, *Williamsburg Conference*, 1987.
144. Ingram M, Sheldon CH, Jacques S. Development and

preliminary clinical trial of immunotherapy for malignant glioma. *J Biol Response Modif* 1987; 6(5): 489-498.

145. John WJ, Neefe JR, Macdonald JS, et al. 5-fluorouracil and interferon-alpha-2a in advanced colorectal cancer: results of two treatment schedules. *Cancer* 1993; 72: 191-195.
146. Kaizer H, Levy R, Vorvall C. Autologous bone marrow transplantation in T-cell malignancies: a case report involving *in vitro* treatment of marrow with a pan T-cell of monoclonal antibody. *J Biol Response Modif* 1982; 1(3): 233-243.
147. Kaminski MS, Fig LM, Zasadny KR, et al. Imaging, dosimetry, and radioimmunotherapy with iodine 131-labeled anti-CD37 antibody in B-cell lymphoma. *J Clin Oncol* 1992; 10: 1696-1711.
148. Kavanagh JJ, Kudelka AP, Freedman R, et al. The amelioration of toxicity of intraperitoneal monoclonal Ab 90y-B72.3 with EDTA: A phase I study in refractory ovarian cancer. *Proc Am Assoc Cancer Res* 1993; 34: 223.
149. Kantarjian HM, Deisseroth A, Kurzrock R, et al. Chronic myelogenous leukemia: A concise update. *Blood* 1993; 82: 691-703.
150. Kantarjian HM, Smith TL, O'Brien S, et al. Prolonged survival following achievement of a cytogenetic response with alpha interferon therapy in chronic myelogenous leukemia. *Ann Intern Med* 1995; 122: 254-261.
151. Kbalheim G, Funderud S, Kbaloy S. Successful clinical use of an anti-HLA-DR monoclonal antibody for autologous bone marrow transplantation. *J Natl Cancer Inst* 1988; 80(16): 1322-1325.
152. Kelley VE, Fers W, Strom TB. Cloned human interferon-gamma, but not interferon-alpha or -beta, induces expression of HLA-DR determinants by fetal monocytes and myeloid leukemic cell lines. *J Immunol* 1984; 132: 240-245.
153. Kemeny N, Younes A. Alfa-2a interferon and 5-fluorouracil for advanced colorectal carcinoma: the Memorial Sloan-Kettering experience. *Sem Oncol* 1992; 19(2 suppl 3): 171-175.
154. Kempf RA, Grunberg SM, Daniels JR, et al. Recombinant interferon alpha-2 (Intron A) in a phase II study of renal cell carcinoma. *J Biol Resp Modif* 1986; 5(1): 27-35.
155. Khayat D, Borel C, Tourani JM. Sequential chemo-immunotherapy with cisplatin, interleukin-2, and interferon alfa-2a for metastatic melanoma. *J Clin Oncol* 1993; 12: 2173-2180.
156. Kirkwood JM, Harris JE, Vera R, et al. A randomized study of low and high doses of leukocyte a-interferon in metastatic renal cell carcinoma: the American Cancer Society Collaborative Trial. *Cancer Res* 1985; 45: 863-871.
157. Kirkwood JM, Ernstoff MS, Davis CA, et al. Comparison of intramuscular and intravenous recombinant alpha-2 interferon in melanoma and other cancers. *Ann Int Med* 1985; 103: 32-36.
158. Kirkwood JM, Ernstoff M. Potential applications of the interferons in oncology: lessons drawn from studies of human melanoma. *Semin Oncol* 1986; 13(3, 2): 48-56.
159. Kirkwood JM, Ernstoff MS, Giuliano AE, et al. Interferon α-2a and dacarbazine in melanoma. *J Natl Cancer Inst* 1990; 82: 1062-1063.
160. Klefstrom T, Holsti P, Grohn P, Heinonen E. Combination of levamisole immunotherapy with conventional treatments in breast cancer. In: Terry WD, Rosenberg SA, eds. *Immunotherapy of human cancer*. New York: Elsevier North Holland, 1982: 187-194.
161. Kohn EC, Steis RG, Sausbille EA, et al. Phase II trial of intermittent high dose recombinant interferon alpha-2A and mycosis fungoides and the Sezary syndrome. *J Clin Oncol* 1990; 8: 155-160.
162. Kokoschka EM, Micksche M. Active specific immunotherapy as adjuvant treatment for stage II malignant melanoma. *Pigment Cell* 1979; 5: 111.
163. Krigel RL, Padavic-Shaller KA, Rudolph AR, et al. Renal cell carcinoma: treatment with recombinant interleukin-2 plus beta interferon. *J Clin Oncol* 1990; 8: 460-467.
164. Krolick KA, Yaun D, Vitetta ES. Specific killing of a human breast carcinoma cell line by a monoclonal antibody coupled to the A-chain of ricin. *Cancer Immunol Immunother* 1981; 12: 39-41.
165. Krown SE, Pinsky CM, Wanebo HJ, et al. Immunologic reactivity and prognosis in breast cancer. *Cancer* 1980; 46: 1746-1752.
166. Krown SE, Stoopler MB, Gralla RJ, et al. Phase II trial of human leukocyte interferon in non-small cell lung cancer: preliminary results. In: Jerry WD, Rosenberg SA, eds. *Immunotherapy of human cancer*. New York: Elsevier-North Holland, 1982: 397-405.
167. Krown SE. Interferons and interferon inducers in cancer treatment. *Semin Oncol* 1986; 13(2): 207-217.
168. Krown SE, Real FX, Vadhan Raj S, et al. Kaposi's sarcoma and the acquired immune deficiency syndrome: treatment with recombinant interferon alpha and analysis of prognostic factors. *Cancer* 1986; 57(8 suppl): 1662-1665.
169. Krown SE. The role of interferon in the therapy of epidemic Kaposi's sarcoma. *Semin Oncol* 1987; 14(2 suppl 3): 27-33.
170. Lacour J, Lacour F, Spira A, et al. Adjuvant treatment with polyadenylic-polyuridylic acid in operable breast cancer: updated results of a randomized trial. *Br Med J* 1984; 288: 589-592.
171. Lacour J, Lacour F, Spira A, et al. Adjuvant immunotherapy with polyadenylic-polyuridylic acid in operable breast cancer. In: Terry WD, Rosenberg SA, eds. *Immunotherapy of human cancer*. New York: Elsevier North Holland, 1982: 183-187.
172. Lamm DL, Stogvill VD, Redwin HM. BCG immunotherapy of transitional cell carcinoma of the bladder. *Proc ASCO* 1983; 2: 55.
173. Larson SM, Carrasquillo JA, Krohn KA. Radiotherapy with 'anti-p97' iodinated monoclonal antibodies in melanoma. In: Raymond C, ed. Proc World Congr *Nuclear Medicine and Biology*. New York: Pergamon Press, 1982: 3666-3669.
174. Larson SM, Carasquillo JA, Krohn KA, et al. Localization of p97 specific Fab fragments in human melanoma as a basis for immunotherapy. *J Clin Invest* 1983; 72: 2101-2114.
175. Lashford LS, Davies AG, Richardson RV, et al. A pilot study of I-131 monoclonal antibodies in the therapy of leptomeningeal tumors. *Cancer* 1988; 61: 857-868.
176. Laszlo J, Hood L, Cox E, Goodwin V. A randomized trial of low doses of alpha interferon in patients with breast cancer. *J Biol Resp Modif* 1986; 5: 206-210.
177. Lee KH, Talpaz M, Rothberg JM, et al. Concomitant administration of recombinant human interleukin-2 and recombinant interferon alpha-2A in cancer patients: a

phase I study. *J Clin Oncol* 1989; 7(11): 1726-1732.

178. Legha SS, Papadopoulos NEJ, Plager C, et al. Clinical evaluation of recombinant interferon alfa-2a (roferon-a) in metastatic melanoma using two different schedules. *J Clin Oncol* 1987; 5: 1240-1246.

179. Legha S, Plager C, Ring S, et al. A phase II study of biochemotherapy using interleukin-2 (IL-2) + interferon alfa 2A (IFN) in combination with cisplatin (C) Vinblastine (V) and DTIC (D) in patients with metastatic melanoma. *Proc ASCO* 1992; 11: 343 (abstract) and 1179 (abstract).

180. Legha SS. Current therapy for malignant melanoma. *Semin Oncol* 1989; 16: 34-44.

181. Legha SS, Buzaid AC. Role of recombinant interleukin-2 in combination with interferon-alpha and chemotherapy in the treatment of advanced melanoma. *Semin Oncol* 1993; 20 (suppl 9): 27-32.

182. LeMaistre C, Rosenblum MG, Reuben JM, et al. Therapeutic effects of genetically engineered toxin (DAB486-IL-2) in patients with chronic lymphocytic leukemia. *Lancet* 1991; 337: 1124.

183. Lemkin S, Tokita K, Sherman G. Phase I-II study of monoclonal antibodies (MCA) in gastrointestinal cancer. *Proc ASCO* 1984; 3: 47.

184. Lenhard RE, Order SE, Spunberg JJ, et al. Isotopic immunoglobulin: a new systemic therapy for advanced Hodgkin's disease. *J Clin Oncol* 1985; 3: 1296-1300.

185. Lentz MR. Continuous whole blood ultrapheresis procedure in patients with metastatic cancer. *J Biol Resp Modif* 1989; 8(5): 511-527.

186. Lichtenstein A, Spina C, Berek JS, et al. Intraperitoneal administration of human recombinant interferon-alpha in patients with ovarian cancer: effects on lymphocyte phenotype and cytotoxicity. *Cancer Res* 1988; 48: 5853-5859.

187. Lichtin A, Iliopoulos D, Guerry D. Therapy of melanoma with an anti-melanoma ganglioside monoclonal antibody (a possible mechanism of a complete response). *Proc ASCO* 1988; 7: 247.

188. Lipton A, Harvey HA, Simmonds MA, et al. Lack of enhanced activity of systemic interferon by cimetidine in malignant melanoma. *Proc ASCO Oncol* 1984; 3: 56.

189. Livingston PO, Ritter G, Srivastava P, et al. Characterization of IgG and IgM antibodies induced in melanoma patients by immunization with purified Gm2 ganglioside. *Cancer Res* 1989; 49: 7045-7050.

190. LoBuglio AF, Khazaeli MV, Lee J, et al. Pharmacokinetics and immune response to XOMAZYME-MEL in melanoma patients. *Antibody Immunoconj Radiopharm* 1988; 1(4): 305-310.

191. LoBuglio AF, Wheeler R, Leavitt RD, et al. Pharmacokinetics and immune response to chimeric mouse/human monoclonal antibody (CH17-1A) in man (Abstr). *Proc ASCO* 1988; 7: 111.

192. Logothetis CJ, Hossan E, Sella A, et al. Fluorouracil and recombinant human interferon alpha-2a in the treatment of metastatic chemotherapy-refractory urothelial tumors. *J Natl Cancer Inst* 1991; 83: 285-288.

193. Lotze MT, Carrasquillo JA, Weinstein JN, et al. Monoclonal antibody imaging of human melanoma. Radioimmunodetection by subcutaneous or system injection. *Ann Surg* 1986; 204: 223-235.

194. Mackenson A, Ferradini L, Carcelain G, et al. Evidence for in situ amplification of cytolytic T-lymphocytes with antitumor activity in a human regressive melanoma. *Cancer Res* 1993; 53: 3569-3573.

195. Mackenson A, Carcelain G, Viels S, et al. Direct evidence to support the immunosurveillance concept in a regressive melanoma. *J Clin Invest* 1994; 93: 1397-1402.

196. Mahaley M, Urso M, Whaley R. Malignant glioma treatment with interferon. *Proc ASCO* 1984; 3: 65.

197. Mandell F, Tribalto M, Cantonetti M, et al. Recombinant alpha-2b interferon as maintenance therapy in responding multiple myeloma patients. *Blood* 1987; 70(suppl 1): 247a.

198. Marshall ME, Simpson W, Butler K, et al. Treatment of renal cell carcinoma with daily low-dose alpha-interferon. *J Biol Resp Mod* 1989; 8: 453-461.

199. Martin A, Nerenstone S, Urba WJ, et al. Treatment of hairy cell leukemia with alternating cycles of pentostatin and recombinant leukocyte A interferon: results of a phase II study. *J Clin Oncol* 1990; 8: 721-730.

200. Mathe G, Amiel JL, Schwarzenberg L, et al. Active immunotherapy for acute lymphoblastic leukemia. *Lancet* 1969; 1: 697-699.

201. Mattson K, Holsti LR, Niiranen A. et al. Human leukocyte interferon as part of a combined treatment for previously untreated small cell lung cancer. *J Biol Resp Modif* 1985; 4(1): 8-17.

202. McCabe MS, Stablein D, Hawkins MJ. The modified group C experience–phase III randomized trials of IL-2 vs IL-2/LAK in advanced renal cell carcinoma and advanced melanoma. *Proc ASCO* 1991; 10: 213 (abstract).

203. McCulloch PB, Poon M, Dent PB, Dawson P. A stratified randomized trial of 5-fluorouracil, doxorubicin (Adriamycin) and cyclophosphamide alone or with BCG in stage IV breast cancer. In: Terry WD, Rosenberg SA, eds. *Immunotherapy of human cancer*. New York: Elsevier North Holland, 1982: 183-186.

204. McCune CS, Schapira DV, Henshaw EC. Specific immunotherapy of advanced renal carcinoma: evidence for the polyclonality of metastases. *Cancer* 1981; 47: 1984-1987.

205. McLaughlin P, Cabanillias F, Hagemeister F, et al. CHOP-Bleo plus interferon for stage IV low-grade lymphoma. *Am J Oncol* 1993; 4: 205-211.

206. McKneally MF, Maver C, Kausel HW, Alley RD. Regional immunotherapy with intrapleural BCG for lung cancer. *J Thorac Cardiovasc Surg* 1976; 72: 333.

207. Melino G, Elliott P, Cooke KB, et al. Allogeneic antibodies (Abs) for drug targeting to human neuroblastoma. (Nb). *Proc ASCO* 1984; 3: 47.

208. Mellstedt H, Frodin JE, Masucci G. Clinical status of monoclonal antibodies in the treatment of colorectal carcinoma. *Oncology* 1989; 25-32.

209. Miller RA, Maloney DJ, McKillop J, et al. *In vivo* effects of murine hybridoma monoclonal antibody in a patient with T-cell leukemia. *Blood* 1981; 68: 78-86.

210. Miller RA, Levy R. Response of cutaneous B-cell lymphoma to therapy with hybridoma monoclonal antibody. *Lancet* 1981; 2: 226-230.

211. Miller RA, Maloney DJ, Warnke R, et al. Treatment of B-cell lymphoma with monoclonal anti-idiotype antibody. N *Engl J Med* 1982; 306: 517-522.

212. Moertel CG, Rubin J, Kbols LK. Therapy of metastatic carcinoid tumor and the malignant carcinoid syndrome with recombinant leukocyte A interferon. *J Clin Oncol* 1989; 7: 865-868.

213. Moertel CG, Reitemeier RJ. *Advances in Gastrointestinal*

Cancer: Clinical Management and Chemotherapy. New York, NY, Harper and Row, 1989: 86-107.

214. Molinolo A, Simpson JF, Thor A, Schlom J. Enhanced tumor binding using immunohistochemical analyses by second generation anti-tumor-associated glycoprotein 72 monoclonal antibodies versus monoclonal antibody B72.3 in human tissue. *Cancer Res* 1990; 50: 1291-1298.
215. Moormeier JA, Ratain MJ, Westbrook CA, et al. Low-dose interferon alpha-2b in the treatment of hairy cell leukemia. *J Natl Cancer Inst* 1989; 81: 1172-1174.
216. Morales A, Ersil A. Adjuvant BCG immunotherapy in the prophylaxis and treatment of non-invasive bladder cancer. In: Terry WD, Rosenberg SA, eds. *Immunotherapy of human cancer*. New York: Elsevier North Holland, 1982: 301-307.
217. Morton D, Hoon D, Nizze J, et al. Polyvalent vaccine improves survival of patients with metastatic melanoma. *Ann Surg* 1992; 216(4): 463-482.
218. Morton DL. Active immunotherapy against cancer: present status. *Semin Oncol* 1986; 13(2): 180-185.
219. Moseley R, Zalutsky MR, Coakham HB, et al. Distribution of I-131 81C6 monoclonal antibody administered via carotid artery in patients with glioma. *J Nucl Med* 1987; 28(4): 603-604.
220. Mulder NH, deVries EGE, Sleifjer DTh, et al. Dacarbazine (dtic), human recombinant interferon alpha 2a (roferon) and 5-fluorouracil for disseminated malignant melanoma. *Br J Cancer* 1992; 65: 303-304.
221. Muss HB. Interferon therapy for renal cell carcinoma. *Semin Oncol* 1987; 14 (Suppl.2): 36-42.
222. Nabel GJ, Nabel EG, Yang ZY, et al. Direct gene transfer with dna-liposome complexes in melanoma: expression, biologic activity, and lack of toxicity in humans. *Proc Natl Acad Sci USA* 1993; 90: 11307-11311.
223. Nagai M, Watanabe K. Treatment of malignant brain tumors with interferons – special reference to the combination therapy and maintenance therapy. *J Interferon Res* 1988; 8: S21.
224. Namba M, Miyoshi T, Kanamori T, et al. Combined effects of 5-fluorouracil and interferon on proliferation of human neoplastic cells in culture. *Jpn J Cancer Res* 1982; 73: 819-824.
225. Neefe JR, Silgals R, Ayoob M, Schein PS. Minimal activity of recombinant clone A interferon in metastatic colon cancer. *J Biol Resp Modif* 1984; 3(4): 366-370.
226. Neidhart JA, Murphy SG, Hennick LA, Wise HA. Active specific immunotherapy of stage IV renal carcinoma with aggregated tumor antigen adjuvant. *Cancer* 1980; 46: 1128-1134.
227. Neidhart JA. Interferon therapy for the treatment of renal cancer. *Cancer* 1986; 57: 1696-1699.
228. Niederle N, Doberauer C, Kloke O. Treatment of chronic myelogenous leukemia with recombinant interferon-alpha (IFN-2b). *Proc ASCO* 1986; 5: 236.
229. Oberg K, Norheim I, Lind E. Treatment of malignant carcinoid tumors with human leukocyte interferon: long term results. *Cancer Treat Rep* 1986; 70(11): 1297-1304.
230. O'Connell MJ, Colgan JP, Oken MM, et al. Clinical trial of recombinant leukocyte A interferon as initial therapy for favorable histology non-Hodgkin's lymphomas and chronic lymphocytic leukemia: an Eastern Cooperative Oncology Group Pilot Study. *J Clin Oncol* 1986; 4: 128-136.
231. Ohno R, Kimura K. Treatment of multiple myeloma with recombinant interferon alpha-2a. *Cancer* 1986; 57: 1685-1688.
232. Oldham RK. Monoclonal antibodies in cancer therapy. *J Clin Oncol* 1983; 1(9): 582-590.
233. Oldham RK. Antibody-drug and antibody toxin conjugates. In: Reif AE, Mitchell MS, eds. *Immunity to cancer*. New York: Academic Press, 1985: 575-586.
234. Oldham RK. Biologicals for cancer treatment: interferons. *Hosp Pract* 1985; 20: 72-91.
235. Oldham RK, ed. Symposium on *ex vivo* plasma immunoabsorption and protein A in cancer therapy. *J Biol Resp Modif* 1984; 3(3): 229-230.
236. Oldham RK, Foon KA, Morgan AC, et al. Monoclonal antibody therapy of malignant melanoma: *in vivo* localization in cutaneous metastasis after intravenous administration. *J Clin Oncol* 1984; 2(11): 1235-1244.
237. Oldham RK, Smalley RV. The role of interferon in the treatment of cancer. In: Zoon KC, Noguchi PC, Lui TY, eds. *Interferon: research, clinical application, and regulatory consideration*. Amsterdam: Elsevier Science, 1984: 191-205.
238. Oldham RK, Lewis M, Orr DW, et al. Adriamycin custom-tailored immunoconjugates in the treatment of human malignancies. *Mol Biother* 1988; 1(2): 103-113.
239. Orr DW, Oldham RK, Lewis M, et al. Phase I trial of mitomycin-c immunoconjugate cocktails in human malignancies. *Mol Biother* 1989; 1(4): 229-240.
240. Oldham RK. Custom tailored drug immunoconjugates in cancer therapy. *Mol Biother* 1991; (3): 148-162.
241. Oldham RK. Cancer cures: by the people, for the people at what cost? *Mol Biother* 1990; 2(1): 2-3.
242. Oldham RK. IL-2 activated tumor derived activated cells. In: Hiddleman, ed. *Oncologic dialogue*, 1990.
243. Oldham RK. Monoclonal antibody therapy. In: Chiao JW, ed. *Biological response modifiers and cancer research*, vol. 40. New York: Marcel Dekker, 1988: 3-16.
244. Oldham RK, Bartal AH, Yannelli JR, et al. Intra-arterial and intracavitary administration with advanced cancer: feasibility and laboratory results. *Proc AACR* 1988.
245. Oldham RK. Biologicals and biological response modifiers: the design of clinical trials. *J Biol Resp Modif* 1985; 4: 117-128.
246. Oldham RK. Monoclonal antibodies. In: Nathanson L, ed. Management of advanced melanoma. Contemporary issues in clinical oncology. New York: Churchill Livingstone, 1986: 195-207.
247. Oldham RK. Patients as research partners. In: *The privatization of cancer research*. City Club of Cleveland, Cleveland, OH. Vital speeches of the day. October 1, 1987: 763-766.
248. Oldham RK. Interferon treatment of non-Hodgkin's lymphoma and myeloma: a model for biotherapy. In: Revel M, ed. *Clinical aspects of interferons*. Boston: Kluwer Academia, 1988: 109-120.
249. Oldham RK, Maleckar JR, Friddell CS, et al. Tumor-derived activated cells: preliminary laboratory and clinical results. *Clin Chem* 1989; 35(8): 1576-1580.
250. Oldham RK, Dillman RO, Yannelli JR, et al. Continuous infusion interleukin-2 and tumor derived activated cells as treatment of advanced solid tumors: An NBSG trial. *Molecular Biotherapy* 1991; 3(2): 68-73.
251. Oldham RK, Lewko W, Good R, et al. Growth of tumor derived activated T cells for the treatment of cancer. *Cancer Biotherapy* 1994; 9(3): 211-224.

252. Oliver RTD, Mehta A, Miller RM, Barnett MJ. Unexplained spontaneous regression of renal cell carcinoma. *J Biol Resp Modif* 1987.
253. Oratz et al. *Society for Biological Therapy meeting*, Berkeley, CA; November 1988.
254. Order SE, Stillwagon GB, Klein JL, et al. Iodine 131 antiferritin, a new treatment modality in hepatoma: a Radiation Therapy Oncology Group Study. *J Clin Oncol* 1985; 3(12): 1573-1582.
255. Paciucci PA, Holland JF, Glidewell O, et al. Recombinant interleukin-2 continuous infusion and adoptive transfer of recombinant interleukin-2 activated cells in patients with advanced cancer. *JCO* 1989; 7: 869-878.
256. Papadopoulos NEJ, Howard JG, Murray JL. Phase II DTIC and interleukin 2 (IL-2) trial for metastatic malignant melanoma. *Proc Am Soc Clin Oncol* 1990; 9: 277 (abstract).
257. Paque RE. RNA as a biological response modifier: a reassessment. *J Biol Resp Modif* 1983; 2: 563-576.
258. Parkinson DR, Abrams JS, Wiernik PH. Interleukin-2 therapy in patients with metastatic malignant melanoma: a phase II study. *J Clin Oncol* 1990; 8: 1650-1656.
259. Pazdur R, Bready B, Moore DF Jr. Clinical trials of fluorouracil with alpha-interferon in advanced colorectal carcinomas. *Semin Oncol* 1991; 18 (Suppl.7): 67-70.
260. Pazdur R, Moore DF Jr, Bready B. Modulation of fluorouracil with recombinant alfa interferon: M.D. Anderson Clinical Trial. *Semin Oncol* 1992; 19 (Suppl.3): 176-179.
261. Peterson BA, O M, Ozer H, et al. Cyclophosphamide vs cyclophosphamide and interferon alpha 2b in follicular low grade lymphoma: A preliminary report of an intergroup trial (CAL GB 869 & EST 7486) *Proc ASCO* 1993; 12: 1240-1241.
262. Petrelli N, Douglass HO, Herrera L, et al. The modulation of fluorouracil with leucovorin in metastatic colorectal carcinoma: A prospective randomized phase III trial. *J Clin Oncol* 1989; 7: 1419-1426.
263. Pinsky C, Camcko F, Kerr D, et al. Treatment of superficial bladder cancer with intravesical BCG. *Proc ASCO* 1983; 2: 57.
264. Poon MA, O'Connell MJ, Moertel CG, et al. Biochemical modulation of fluorouracil: Evidence of significant improvement of survival and quality of life in patients with advanced colorectal carcinoma. *J Clin Oncol* 1989; 7: 1407-1418.
265. Prager MD, Baechtel FS, Peters PC, et al. Specific immunotherapy of human metastatic renal cell carcinoma. *Proc AACR* 1981; 22: 163.
266. Press O, Applebaum F, Ledbetter J. Serotherapy of malignant B-cell lymphomas with monoclonal antibody 1F5 (anti-CD20). *Proc ASCO* 1986; 5: 221.
267. Press O, Applebaum F, Ledbetter J. Serotherapy of malignant B-cell lymphomas with monoclonal antibody 1F5 (anti-CD20). *Proc ASCO* 1986; 5: 221.
268. Press OW, Eary JF, Appelbaum FR, et al. Radiolabeled-antibody therapy of B-cell lymphoma with autologous bone marrow support. *N Engl J Med* 1993; 329: 1219-1224 and 1265-1268.
269. Price CG, Rohatiner A, Lister TA, et al. Interferon-alpha 2b in addition to chlorambucil in the treatment of follicular lymphoma: Preliminary results of a randomized trial. *Eur J Cancer* 1991; 27(4): S34-36.
270. Punt CJ, Burhouts JT, Croles JJ, et al. Continuous infusion of high-dose 5-fluorouracil in combination with leucovorin and recombinant interferon-alpha-2b in patients with advanced colorectal cancer. *A multicenter phase II study. Cancer* 1993; 72: 2107-2111.
271. Pyrhonen S, Hahka-Kemppinen M, Muhonen T. A promising interferon plus four-drug chemotherapy regimen for metastatic melanoma. *J Clin Oncol* 1993; 10: 1919-1926.
272. Quesada JR, Alexanian R, Hawkins M, et al. Treatment of multiple myeloma with recombinant alpha-interferon. *Blood* 1986; 67: 275-278.
273. Quesada JR, Evans L, Saks SR, Gutterman JU. Recombinant interferon alpha and gamma in combination as treatment for metastatic renal cell carcinoma. *J Biol Resp Modif* 1988; 7; 234-239.
274. Quesada JR, Kurzrock R, Sherwin SA, et al. Phase II studies of recombinant human interferon gamma in metastatic renal cell carcinoma. *J Biol Resp Modif* 1987; 6: 20-27.
275. Quesada JR, Swanson DA, Trindade A, Gutterman JR. Renal cell carcinoma: antitumor effects of leukocyte interferon. *Cancer Res* 1983; 43: 940-947.
276. Quesada JR, Rio A, Swanson D, et al. Antitumor activity of recombinant-derived interferon alpha in metastatic renal cell carcinoma. *J Clin Oncol* 1985; 3(11): 1522-1528.
277. Quesada JR, Reuben JR, Manning JT, et al. Alpha interferon for the induction of remission in hairy cell leukemia. *N Engl J Med* 1984; 310: 15-18.
278. Quesada JR, Gutterman JU, Hersh EM. Treatment of hairy cell leukemia with alpha interferons. *Cancer* 1986; 57: 1678-1680.
279. Ralph P, Harris PE, Punjabi CG, et al. Lymphokine and using 'terminal' differentiation of the human monoblast leukemia line U937: a role for gamma interferon. *Blood* 1983; 62: 1169-1175.
280. Ratain MJ, Vardiman JW, Golomv HM. The role of interferon and the treatment of hairy cell leukemia. *Semin Oncol* 1986; 13(3, 2): 21-28.
281. Rauschmeier HA. Immunotherapy of metastatic renal cancer. *Semin Surg Oncol* 1988; 4: 169-173.
282. Ray PK, Raychaudhuri S, Allen P. Mechanism of regression of mammary adenocarcinomas in rats following plasma absorption over protein A-containing Staphylococcus aureus. *Cancer Res* 1982; 42: 4970-4974.
283. Real FX, Bander NH, Yeh S, et al. Monoclonal antibody F23: radiolocalization in phase I study in patients with renal cell carcinoma. *Proc ASCO* 1987; 6: 240.
284. Reily RM. Immunoscintigraphy of tumours using $^{99}Tc^{m}$-labelled monoclonal antibodies: a review. *Nucl Med Commun* 1993; 14: 347-359.
285. Retsas S, Preistman TJ, Newton KA, et al. Evaluation of human lymphoblastoid interferon in advanced malignant melanoma. *Cancer* 1983; 51: 273-276.
286. Richards JM, Mehta N, Ramming K, et al. Sequential chemoimmunotherapy in the treatment of metastatic melanoma. *J Clin Oncol* 1992; 8: 1338-1343.
287. Richards JM, Mehta N, Schroeder L. Sequential chemotherapy/immunotherapy for metastatic melanoma. *Proc Am Soc Clin Oncol* 1992; 11: 346 (abstract).
288. Richner J, Joss RA, Goldhirsch A, Brunner KW. Phase II study of continuous subcutaneous interferon-alfa combined with cisplatin in advanced malignant melanoma. *Eur J Cancer* 1992; 28A: 1044-1047.
289. Riechman L, Clark MR, Waldmann H, Winter G. Reshaping human antibodies with therapy. *Nature* 1989;

332: 323-327.

290. Rinehart JJ, Malspeis L, Young D, Neidhart JA. Phase I/II trial of human recombinant interferon gamma and renal cell carcinoma. *J Biol Resp Modif* 1986; 5(4): 300-308.
291. Ritz J, Pesando JM, Sallan SE, et al. Serotherapy of acute lymphoblastic leukemia with monoclonal antibody. *Blood* 1981; 58: 141-152.
292. Ritz J, Schlossman SF. Utilization of monoclonal antibodies in treatment of leukemia and lymphoma. *Blood* 1982; 59: 1-11.
293. Robinson WA, Mughal TI, Johnson M, Spiegel RJ. Treatment of metastatic malignant melanoma with recombinant interferon alpha 2. *Immunobiol* 1986; 172: 275-282.
294. Rohatiner AZS, Balkwill FR, Malpas JS, et al. Experience with human lymphoblastoid interferon and acute myelogenous leukemia (AML). *Cancer Chemother Pharmacol* 1983; 11: 56-58.
295. Rojas AF, Firestein JN, Mickiewicz E, et al. Levamisole in advanced breast cancer. *Lancet* 1976; 1: 211-215.
296. Rosen ST, Zimmer AM, Goldman-Leikin R, et al. Radioimmunodetection and radioimmunotherapy of cutaneous T cell lymphoma using an ^{131}I-labeled monoclonal antibody: an Illinois Cancer Council Study. *J Clin Oncol* 1987; 5(4): 562-573.
297. Rosenberg SA. The adoptive immunotherapy of cancer using the transfer of activated lymphoid cells and interleukin-2. *Semin Oncol* 1986; 13(2): 200-206.
298. Rosenberg SA, Lotze MT, Muul LM, et al. Observations on the systemic administration of autologous lymphokine-activated killer cells and recombinant interleukin-2 to patients with metastatic cancer. *N Engl J Med* 1985; 313(23): 1485-1492.
299. Rosenberg SA, Packard BS, Aebersold PM, et al. Use of tumor-infiltrating lymphocytes and interleukin-2 in the immunotherapy of patients with metastatic melanoma, special report. *N Engl J Med* 1988; 319: 1676-1680.
300. Rosenberg SA, Lotze MT, Yang JC, et al. Combination therapy with interleukin-2 and alpha-interferon for the treatment of patients with advanced cancer. *J Clin Oncol* 1989; 17(12): 1863-1874.
301. Rosenberg SA, Lotze MT, Yang JC. Experience with the use of high-dose interleukin-2 in the treatment of 652 cancer patients. *Ann Surg* 1989; 210: 474-485.
302. Rosenberg SA, Lotze MT, Yang JC. Prospective randomized trial of high-dose interleukin-2 alone or in conjunction with lymphokine-activated killer cells for the treatment of patients with advanced cancer. *J Natl Cancer* Inst 1993; 85: 622-632.
303. Rosenberg SA, Aebersold P, Cornetta K. Gene transfer into humans–immunotherapy of patients with advanced melanoma, using tumor-infiltrating lymphocytes modified by retroviral gene transduction. *NEJM* 1990; 323: 570-578.
304. Rosenberg SA. The immunotherapy and gene therapy of cancer. *J Clin Oncol* 1992; 10: 180-199.
305. Rubin SC. Monoclonal antibodies in the management of ovarian cancer. *Cancer* 1993; 71(4 suppl): 1602-1612.
306. Rubio ED, Jimeno J, Camps C, et al. Treatment of advanced colorectal cancer with recombinant interferon alpha and fluorouracil: Activity in liver metastasis. *Cancer Invest* 1992; 10: 259-264.
307. Ruckdeschel JC, Codish SD, Stranahan A, McKneally MF. Postoperative empyema improved survival in lung cancer. *N Engl J Med* 1972; 287: 1013.
308. Rudczynski AB, Dyer CA, Mortensen RF. Detection of cell-mediated immune reactivity of breast cancer patients by the leukocyte adherence inhibition response to MCF-7 extracts. *Cancer Res* 1978; 38: 3590-3594.
309. Sarna J, Figlin R, Callaghan M. Alpha (human leukocyte)-interferon as treatment for non-small cell carcinoma of the lung: a phase II trial. *J Biol Resp Modif* 1983; 2(4): 343-347.
310. Scadden DT, Doweiko J, Schenkein D, et al. A Phase I/II trial of combined immunoconjugate and chemotherapy for AIDS-related lymphoma. *Blood* 1993; 82(suppl 1): 386a.
311. Schlom J, Wunderlich D, Teramoto YA. Generation of human monoclonal antibodies reactive with human mammary carcinoma cells. *Proc Natl Acad Sci USA* 1980; 77: 6841-6845.
312. Schnall SF, Davis C, Ziyadeh T, et al. Treatment of metastatic renal cell carcinoma (RCC) with intramuscular (IM) recombinant interferon alpha (aIFN, Hoffman-LaRoche). *Proc ASCO* 1986; 5: 227.
313. Schofield JR, Robinson WA, Murphy JR, et al. Low doses of interferon-α are as effective as higher doses in inducing remissions and prolonging survival in chronic myeloid leukemia. *Ann Intern Med* 1994; 121: 736-744.
314. Schroff RW, Woodhouse CS, Foon KA, et al. Intratumor localization of monoclonal antibody in patients with melanoma treated with antibody to a 250K dalton melanoma associated antigen. *J Natl Cancer Inst* 1985; 74: 299-306.
315. Schrof RW, Morgan AC Jr, Woodhouse CS, et al. Monoclonal antibody therapy in malignant melanoma: factors effecting *in vivo* localization. *J Biol Resp Modif* 1987; 6: 457-472.
316. Schulof RS, Lloyd MJ, Ueno WM, et al. Phase II trial of thymosin fraction 5 in advanced renal cancer. *J Biol Resp Modif* 1984; 3: 151-159.
317. Scorticatti CH, DeLaPena NC, Vellora OG, et al. Systemic interferon IFN-alpha treatment of multiple bladder papilloma grade I or II patients: pilot study. *J Interferon Res* 1982; 2: 339-343.
318. Sears HF, Herlyn D, Steplewski Z, Kropowski H. Effects of monoclonal antibody immunotherapy on patients with gastrointestinal adenocarcinoma. *J Biol Resp Modif* 1984; 3: 138-150.
319. Sears HF, Atkinson B, Mattis J, et al. Phase I clinical trial of monoclonal antibody in treatment of gastrointestinal tumors. *Lancet* 1982; 1: 762-765.
320. Sears HF, Herlyn D, Steplewski Z, Koprowski H. Phase II clinical trial of a murine monoclonal antibody cytotoxic for gastrointestinal adenocarcinoma. *Cancer Res* 1985; 45: 5910-5913.
321. Serrou B, Sancho-Garnier H, Cappelaere P, et al. Inefficacy of post radiotherapeutic BCG immunotherapy in T3-T4 breast cancer patients: a randomized trial. In: Terry WD, Rosenberg SA, eds. *Immunotherapy of human cancer*. New York: Elsevier North Holland, 1982: 195-198.
322. Sertoli MR, Bernengo MG, Ardizzoni A, et al. Phase II trial of recombinant alpha-2b interferon in the treatment of metastatic skin melanoma. *Oncology* 1989; 46: 96-98.
323. Sertoli MR, Queirolo P, Bajetta E. Dacarbazine (DTIC) with or without recombinant interferon alpha 2a at different dosages in the treatment of stage IV melanoma

patient: preliminary results of a randomized trial. *Proc ASCO* 1992; 11: 345 (abstract).

324. Sher H, Chapman R, Shack B, et al. Combination chemotherapy and radiotherapy with and without thymosin in small cell lung cancer. *Proc Third World Conf on Lung Cancer*, Abstr, Jpn, 1982: 155.

325. Sherwin SA, Mayer D, Ochs JJ, et al. Recombinant leukocyte A interferon in advanced breast cancer. *Ann Intern Med* 1983; 98: 598-602.

326. Slater DE, Krown SE, Pinsky CM, et al. Human leukocyte (alpha) interferon (HuIFN-(Le)) and cimetidine in malignant melanoma. *Proc ASCO* 1984; 3: 54.

327. Smalley RV, Bartolucci AA, Moore MA, et al. Southeastern Cancer Study Group Breast Cancer Studies 1971-1981. *Int J Rad Oncol Biol Phys* 1983; 9: 1867-1874.

328. Smalley R, Andersen J, et al. Interferon-alpha combined with cytotoxic chemotherapy for patients with non-Hodgkin's lymphoma. *N Engl J Med* 1984; 311: 1148.

329. Solal-Celigney P. Recombinant interleukin alpha 2b combined with a regimen containing doxorubicin in patients with advanced follicular lymphoma. Groupe d'Etude des Lymphomes l'Adulte. *N Engl J Med* 1993; 329: 1108-1114.

330. Sosman JA, Hank JA, Sondel PM. *In vivo* activation of lymphokine-activated killer activity with interleukin-2: prospects for combination therapies. *Semin Oncol* 1990; 17(1): 22-30.

331. Sparano JA, Fisher RI, Sunderland M. Randomized phase III trial of treatment with high-dose interleukin-2 either alone or in combination with interferon alpha 2a in patients with advanced melanoma. *J Clin Oncol* 1993; 11: 1969-1977.

332. Spitler LE, Wussow P, Carey RW, et al. Phase II trial of a monoclonal antimelanoma antibody ricin a chain immunotoxin in therapy of malignant melanoma. *J Clin Oncol* 1990.

333. Springer GF, Murphy S, Desai PR, Scanlon EF. Breast cancer patient's cell-mediated immune response to Thomsen-Friedenreich (T) antigen. *Cancer* 1980; 45: 2949-2954.

334. Steis RG, Carrasquillo JA, McCabe R, et al. Toxicity, immunogenicity, and tumor radioimmunodetecting ability of two human monoclonal antibodies in patients with metastatic colorectal carcinoma. *J Clin Oncol* 1990; 8: 476-490.

335. Steele G Jr, Wang BS, Richie GP, et al. Results of xenogeneic I-RNA therapy in patients with metastatic renal cell carcinoma. *Cancer* 981; 47: 1286-1288.

336. Steffens TA, Bajorin DF, Williams LJ, et al. A phase I trial of R24 monoclonal antibody and recombinant human macrophage colony stimulating factor (rhM-CSF) in patients with advanced melanoma. *Proc ASCO* 1992; 1182: 344(abstract).

337. Stein R, Chen S, Sharkey RM, Goldenberg DM. Murine monoclonal antibodies raised against human non-small cell carcinoma of the lung: specificity and tumor targeting. *Cancer Res* 1990; 50: 1330-1336.

338. Steiner A, Wolf C, Pehamberger H. Comparison of the effects of three different treatment regimens of recombinant interferons in disseminated malignant melanoma. *J Cancer Res Clin Oncol* 1987; 113: 459-465.

339. Stephens EGW, Wood HF, Mason V. The influence of levamisole on the survival of patients with disseminated mammary carcinoma treated with chemotherapy. In: Terry WD, Rosenberg SA, eds. *Immunotherapy of human cancer*. New York: Elsevier North Holland, 1982: 199-204.

340. Stevenson HC, Ochs JJ, Halvorson L, et al. Recombinant alpha interferon in treatment of 2 patients with pulmonary lymphoma: dramatic responses with resolution of pulmonary complications. *Am J Med* 1984; 77: 355-358.

341. Stoter G, Aamdal S, Rodenhius S. Sequential administration of recombinant human interleukin-2 and dacarbazine in metastatic melanoma: a multicenter phase II study. *J Clin Oncol* 1991; 9: 1687-1691.

342. Strander H, Canctell K, Jacobsson PA, et al. Exogenous interferon therapy in osteogenic sarcoma. *Acta Orthop Scand* 1974; 45: 958.

343. Sukumar S, Zbar B, Tereta N, et al. Plasma therapy of primary rat mammary carcinoma: antitumor activity of tumor-bearer plasma adsorbed against inactivated CNBr sepharose or protein A-sepharose. *J Biol Resp Modif* 1984; 3(3): 303-315.

344. Takakura K. Effect of combined treatment with Interferon-B and chemoradiotherapy for malignant gliomas. *J Interferon Res* 1988; 8: S20(abstr).

345. Takita H. Effect of postoperative empyema in survival of patients with bronchogenic carcinoma. *J Thorac Cardiovasc Surg* 1970; 59: 642.

346. Talpas M, Kantarjian HM, McCredie K, et al. Hematologic remission and cytogenetic improvement induced by recombinant human interferon alpha-A in chronic myelogenous leukemia. *N Engl J Med* 1986; 314(17): 1065-1069.

347. Talpaz M, Kantarjian HM, McCredie KB, et al. Clinical investigation of human alpha interferon and chronic myelogenous leukemia. *Blood* 1987; 69(5): 1280-1288.

348. Tanaka F, Yonemoto RH, Waldman S. Blocking factors in sera of breast cancer patients. *Cancer* 1979; 43: 838-847.

349. Taylor-Papadimitriou J, Peterson JA, Arklie J, et al. Monoclonal antibodies to epithelium-specific components of the human milk fat globule membrane: production and reaction with cells in culture. *Int J Cancer* 1981; 28: 17-21.

350. Terman DS, Yamamoto T, Mattioli M, et al. Extensive necrosis of spontaneous canine mammary adenocarcinoma after extracorporeal perfusion over *Staphylococcus aureas* Cowans I. *J Immunol* 1980; 124: 795-805.

351. Terman DS, Young JB, Shearer WT, et al. Preliminary observations of the effects on breast adenocarcinoma of plasma perfused over immobilized protein *A. N Engl J Med* 1981; 305: 1195-1200.

352. The Italian Cooperative Study Group on Chronic Myelogenous Leukemia: Interferon-α2a compared with conventional chemotherapy for the treatment of chronic myeloid leukemia. *N Engl J Med* 1994; 330: 820-825.

353. Thompson D, Adena M, McLeod GRC. Interferon alpha 2a does not improve response or survival when added to dacarbazine (DTIC) in metastatic melanoma: results of a multi-institutional Australian randomized trial QMP8704. *Proc ASCO* 1992; 11: 343 (abstract).

354. Thompson JA, Shulman KL, Benyunes MC, et al. Prolonged continuous intravenous infusion interleukin-2 and lymphokine-activated killer-cell therapy for metastatic renal cell carcinoma. *J Clin Oncol* 1992; 10(6): 960-968.

355. Timms RM, Walker LE, Hirschowitz L, et al. Human lung cancer KS1/4-methotrexate phase I (abstr). In: Dillman

RO, Royston I, eds. Proc 2nd Annual Int Conf on Monoclonal *Antibody Immunoconjugates for Cancer*. San Diego, 28, 1987.

356. Torti FM, Lum BL. Superficial carcinoma of the bladder: natural history and the role of interferons. *Semin Oncol* 1986; 13(3, 2): 57-60.
357. Torti FM, Chotliffe LD, Williams RD, et al. Superficial bladder cancers are responsive to alpha 2 interferon administered intravesically. *Proc ASCO* 1984; 3: 160.
358. Tykka RF, Hjelt L, Orauisto KG, et al. Disappearance of lung metastases during immunotherapy in 5 patients suffering from renal carcinoma. *Scand J Respir Dis* 1974; 89: 123-134.
359. Uhr J, *Monoclonal antibodies as carriers for toxins*. Williamsburg Conference, November 1987.
360. Vadhan-Raj S, Cordon-Cardo C, Carswell E, et al. Phase I trial of a mouse monoclonal antibody against GD3 ganglioside in patients with melanoma: induction of inflammatory responses at tumor sites. *J Clin Oncol* 1988; 6(10): 1636-1648.
361. Van Der Bruggen P, Traversari C, Chomez P, et al. A gene encoding an antigen recognized by cytolytic T lymphocytes on a human melanoma. *Science* 1991; 254: 1643-1647.
362. Vitetta ES, Stone M, Amlot P, et al. Phase I immunotoxin trial in patients with B-cell lymphoma. *Cancer Res* 1991; 51: 4052-4058.
363. West WH, Tauer KW, Orr DW, et al. Continuous infusion recombinant interleukin-2 in adoptive immunotherapy of advanced cancer: results of a multi-centered trial. *J Clin Oncol* 1990.
364. Vessela RL, Chiou RK, Grund FM, et al. Renal cell carcinoma (RCC) phase I-II trials with ^{131}I-labeled monoclonal antibody A6H: imaging and pharmacokinetic studies. *Proc AACR* 1987; 28: 385.
365. Vigel M, Oster MW, Austin JHM. Spontaneous regression of a pulmonary metastasis after nephrectomy for renal cell carcinoma. *J Surg Oncol* 1979; 12: 175.
366. Vosika GJ. Clinical immunotherapy trials of bacterial components derived from mycobacteria and nocardia. *J Biol Response Modif* 1983; 2(4): 321-342.
367. Wadler S, Schwartz EL, Goldman M, et al. Fluorouracil and recombinant alpha-2a interferon: an active regimen against advanced colorectal carcinoma. *J Clin Oncol* 1989; 7: 1769-1775.
368. Wadler S, Wiernik PH. Clinical update on the role of fluorouracil and recombinant interferon alpha-2a in the treatment of colorectal carcinoma. *Semin Oncol* 1990; 17(1): 16-21.
369. Wadler S, Wersto R, Weinberg V, et al. Interaction of fluorouracil and interferon in human colon cancer cell lines: Cytotoxic and cytokinetic effects. *Cancer Res* 1990; 50: 5735-5739.
370. Wadler S, Lembersky B, Atkins M, et al. Phase II trial of fluorouracil and recombinant interferon alfa-2a in patients with advanced colorectal carcinoma: An Eastern Cooperative Oncology Group Study. *J Clin Oncol* 1991; 9: 1806-1810.
371. Waldman TA, Goldman CK, Bongiovanni KF. Therapy of patients with human T-cell lymphotrophic (sic) virus I-induced adult T-cell leukemia with anti-Tac, a monoclonal antibody to the receptor for interleukin-2. *Blood* 1988; 72(5): 1805-1816.
372. Weese JL, Oldham RK, Tormey DC, et al. Immunologic monitoring in carcinoma of the breast. *Surg Gynecol Obstet* 1977; 145: 208-218.
373. Weh HJ, Platz D, Braumann D, et al. Treatment of metastatic colorectal carcinoma with a combination of fluorouracil and recombinant interferon alfa-2b: Preliminary data of a phase II study. *Semin Oncol* 1992; 19 (Suppl.3): 180-184.
374. Weiner LM, Comis RL. Phase I trial of murine monoclonal antibody administration preceded by recombinant gamma interferon therapy in patients with advanced gastrointestinal carcinoma. *Proc ASCO* 1986; 5: 225.
375. Weiner LM, Moldofsky PJ, Gatenby RA, et al. Antibody delivery and effector cell activation in a Phase II trial of recombinant gamma interferon and the murine monoclonal antibody O17-1A in advanced colorectal carcinoma. *Cancer Res* 1988; 48: 2568-2573.
376. Weiner LM, O'Dwyer J, Kitson J, et al. A phase I evaluation of the ricin A chain anti-breast carcinoma immunoconjugate 260F9-MAb-rRa. Society for Biological Therapy Meeting Abstracts, 1988. *J Biol Response Modif* 1989; 8(3): 311.
377. Weiner LM, Steplewski Z, Koprowski H, et al. Biologic effects of gamma interferon pre-treatment followed by monoclonal antibody 17-1A administration in patients with gastrointestinal carcinoma. *Hybridoma* 1986; 5(suppl 1): 565-577.
378. Weisenburger TH, Jones PC, Oahn SS, et al. Active specific intralymphatic immunotherapy in metastatic malignant melanoma: evidence of clinical response. *J Biol Resp Modif* 1982; 1(1): 57-66.
379. Welander C, Homesley H, Levin E, Reich S. Phase II trial of the efficacy of human recombinant interferon gamma (rIFN gamma) in recurrent ovarian adenocarcinomas. *Proc ASCO* 1986; 5: 221.
380. Wessels BW, Rogus RD. Radionuclide selection and model absorbed dose calculations for radiolabeled tumor antibodies. *Med Phys* 1984; 11: 638-645.
381. West WH. Constant infusion recombinant interleukin-2 in adoptive immunotherapy of advanced cancer. *N Engl J Med* 1987; 316(15): 898-905.
382. Wirth MP. Immunotherapy for metastatic renal cell carcinoma. *Urol Clin North Am* 1993; 20: 283-295.

SPECULATIONS FOR 2000 AND BEYOND

ROBERT K. OLDHAM
Biological Therapy Institute Foundation, Franklin, Tennessee; and University of Missouri, Columbia, Missouri

It is now apparent that the genomic capacity of mammalian cells to produce biological substances that have medicinal value is enormous. Only the first few lymphokines/cytokines, growth and maturation factors, cellular therapies, and antibody-based approaches are being explored. Even now, there is clear evidence of clinical activity with respect to colony stimulating factors (CSF), interferon (IF), interleukin 2 (IL-2), activated cells, vaccines, monoclonal antibodies, and their immunoconjugates. If one analyzes the current level of clinical activity for biotherapy in the historical context of chemotherapy, it is obvious that much more rapid progress is being made in biotherapy, leading to development of improved and more selective forms of treatment. From the earliest days of chemotherapy, massive searches were done among tens of thousands of chemical compounds, searching for the one right drug that might have antitumor activity without excessive toxicity for the patient. The successes were few. From analyzing nearly 1 million chemical structures, less than 60 anticancer drugs have come to the clinic, and no more than 20 of these can be considered even moderately active.

This is not to say that the drug development paradigm has not had some success. However, the search has been arduous, complex, expensive, and almost wholly based on the process of random screening of large numbers of compounds to find the rare active chemical. By contrast, the first genetically engineered biological to be approved as an anticancer agent, alpha-interferon, has been an unqualified success in the clinic. It is a drug of choice for the treatment of hairy-cell leukemia and chronic myelogenous leukemia and is moderately active in other forms of leukemia and lymphoma. Substantial activity has been reported in renal cancer, melanoma, and selected other tumors. Promising combination studies are showing high response rates with interferon, IL-2 and combinations with chemotherapy. Compared with its chemotherapeutic brethren, interferon certainly ranks within the top ten of our active systemic approaches in cancer treatment.

IL-2 is now approved for renal cancer and as its broader clinical applications become validated, a second approved biotherapy will be widely utilized. Thus, biotherapy can claim a high success rate in terms of new substances that have come through the complete testing program with approval for clinical use.

The process of drug development was historically based on the idea that sufficient random testing would identify those active substances that could selectively kill cancer cells. Ancillary was the hope that specific processes, unique to cancer cells, would be identified that might allow chemicals to be selectively active on those cells. A secondary hypothesis that rational drug development could be based on structure-function relationships, receptor information, or analog development has proven equally difficult. These concepts have been difficult to validate and the level of selectivity for chemotherapy is very low. In fact, for every chemotherapeutic agent, there are normal tissues that are probably more affected by the drug than the cancer in which the drug is active. While there is still hope for the discovery of some unique drug that is selectively active against cancer, this goal seems much less likely to be achieved than it was a decade ago.

In contrast, biotherapy works through physiologic molecules for which the body has receptors and known mechanisms of action. These substances are often used in huge amounts pharmacologically, but they are message molecules known to our cellular systems. Emerging evidence in laboratory animal model systems raises the hope that cancer cells are not completely without the ability to be controlled by appropriate growth, differentiation, and antiproliferative influences. Most of the early data for interferon supports an antiproliferative activity on cancer cells, in that higher doses have generally been more effective, and tumors resistant to lower doses sometimes respond to an increased dose. In addition, the doses active in many cancers are well above the level where interferon is most active as an immunomodulator. If interferon is acting primarily as an antiproliferative substance, this opens up the possibility that one or more analogs of interferon or one or more biological molecules still to be identified might have a much more powerful antiproliferative effect on cancer cells through the exploitation of what might be a residual physiologic mechanism for growth control of the cancer.

As the process of developmental therapeutics for biotherapy is expanded, there is a great need for all those involved to remain open-minded with respect to new paradigms for drug development. Simply to presume that biologicals must fit into the mold used for chemotherapy

R.K. Oldham (ed.), Principles of Cancer Biotherapy. 3rd ed., 493–497.

drug development would be a major error, since the process of developmental therapeutics for biologics is very different from that for drugs. Even in the preclinical screening programs now in use for biologicals, the process is more one of rational selection than of random screening – the need is to exploit the activities of known molecules rather than to search among the thousands for the singular active substance. As the information base in cancer biology grows, it will become increasingly important to exploit what we know of the power of biological molecules rather than to search among unknown chemicals for active substances.

BEYOND INTERFERON

Alpha-interferon is an approved agent for hairy-cell leukemia, chronic myelogenous leukemia, Kaposi's sarcoma and melanoma; it is also active against a variety of other cancers. Beta- and gamma-interferon are both now approved for clinical use. Beyond these three interferons, the process of genetic engineering is bringing forth a huge number of interferon molecules for testing. Given any small protein of 140-160 amino acids, the possibility now exists for making an infinite number of molecules simply altering portions of the amino acid chain. This process is underway for the interferons, and will demonstrate whether more active interferons can be developed to enhance the immunomodulatory, antiviral or antiproliferative activity of the natural molecules.

LYMPHOKINES/CYTOKINES

Interleukin 2 came into the clinic in the mid 1980s by way of a process that used a growth factor to activate lymphocytes that could subsequently be used therapeutically as effector cells in patients. The cancer-killing capacity of these activated cells was apparent from their *in vitro* activity, and the major questions related to their *in vivo* use, distribution, and anticancer activity. Interleukin 2 is being used in amounts far in excess of its normal physiologic role, and toxicities are the natural result. This particular approach is very intensive; it requires hospitalization and truly enormous doses of both IL-2 and the activated cells. The future may bring a better strategy for using this approach in patients, whereby repeated treatment may become less toxic and more active than the current intensive regimens. Outpatient regimens that are much less toxic are now being actively explored.

Interleukin 2 is part of a broad cascade of biological molecules that have activities in cellular activation and the control of cellular proliferation. These molecules include IL-1-18 and beyond. The future may allow the use of these components in combination or sequence to strengthen what are natural but ineffective bodily responses to the problem of cancer growth and metastasis. Although induction of such a cascade by one particular substance may not be feasible, the artificial programming and the medicinal use of these lymphokines are now both feasible and practical. As the process of administration of biotherapy becomes better defined, so will the programmability of therapeutic regimens using these substances. One can envision pre-programmed infusions of combinations of lymphokines designed for maximal exploitation of their biologic activities.

ANTIGEN-SPECIFIC LYMPHOKINES

Over and above the use of lymphokines in a more general sense, as just described, there is evidence that certain lymphokines act in antigen-specific ways. As the proteins constituting tumor-associated antigens become more thoroughly characterized, as a result of monoclonal antibody technology and genetic engineering, one can envision the use of specific antigens with specific lymphokines, thus allowing oncologists to mount antigen-specific, and perhaps cancer-specific, immunologic responses in individual patients. It is likely that these antigen-specific lymphokines will have to be used in ways that are selected specifically for individual patients. If, as will be reasoned below, the array of tumor-associated antigens present on the tumor cells of each individual is slightly different from the array present on cancers of a like type in other individuals, the use of antigen-specific lymphokines with specific antigenic preparations will of necessity be unique to each individual. Parallels for the clinic are already being explored in animal models for transplantation and other specific immune responses. The application of this technology to human therapeutics will occur in the not-too-distant future.

GROWTH AND DIFFERENTIATION FACTORS

Cancer might be likened to a juvenile delinquent: a derivative of one's own self but without the controls necessary for appropriate socialization. If cancer cells were to have only a limited spread and growth and if subsequent therapeutic approaches could simply limit further growth, there would be no need to eradicate the cancer cells completely. Such an approach has an obvious parallel in the use of physiologic mediators for endocrinopathies. For example, diabetes did not disappear by virtue of the discovery of insulin. The genetic anomaly continues to exist, and diabetes has become a more frequent clinical problem in our society. However, insulin has been used to control the pathologic manifestations of this disorder. Is it possible there are growth and differentiation factors, coded for by the mammalian genome, that could be used similarly on treating cancer? There is early evidence of such mediators *in vitro* and in animal models. The control of growth in certain cellular systems and the use of growth factors, as well as agonists and antibodies to those factors, provide substance to the argument that molecular manipulation of growth and differentiation is a major area for developmental therapeutics for cancer.

If one takes the growth and differentiation of cells *in vitro* as a model, the use of epidermal growth factor, nerve growth factor, insulin, and other hormones has a profound effect on both the rate of replication and the degree of deviance of replicating cells from their 'normal' counterparts. Similarly, cancer growth, proliferation, and spread may be controllable by manipulation of growth factors made by normal tissues and/or by the cancer cells themselves.

These approaches will be available in the clinic early in the new millennium. Rudimentary attempts, using certain chemicals that cause *in vitro* differentiation, have had interesting effects on cell lines and experimental models; however, the use of retinoids, butyrates, and other factors that might regulate growth and differentiation are just reaching the point of clinical exploitation. With the almost daily discovery of substances that support growth of cancer cells *in vitro*, one might imagine that the antithesis of such factors might also be developed, exploited, and utilized for clinical therapeutics. In biology as in physics, there seems to be a reaction for every action. For many of the molecules that support growth, experimental data also indicates that other molecules exist to offset that increased growth. As these molecules are isolated and characterized, and subsequently produced by genetic engineering, they will broaden our potential arsenal for cancer biotherapy.

MONOCLONAL ANTIBODIES

The current evidence to support the therapeutic use of monoclonal antibodies and their immunoconjugates has been presented in earlier chapters. While it is early in the clinical application of this biotherapeutic approach, it is already apparent that monoclonal antibodies offer the probability of selective cancer treatment that has never before been available.

The search for the perfect 'magic bullet' is probably futile. With the exception of anti-idiotypic antibodies, which can be quite specific for the clone that has deviated and become a malignant lymphoma or leukemia, it seems unlikely that such specific antigens are represented on all cancers. Rather, the evidence seems to support a bewildering array of cancer-associated antigens present in different quantitics on cancers from different individuals.

Data are accumulating concerning the use of typing panels of monoclonal antibodies. They indicate that one can assess the antigenic array on each individual's tumor cells and decide which antibodies should compose a cocktail to cover the available specificities of that cancer. This testing mechanism reveals cancer to be individualistic. It is different for every patient and perhaps even among the clones of cancer present within an individual patient. This should not be surprising, since the genetic apparatus that governs each of us is individualistic. With the exception of identical twins, no two humans are exactly alike, and one would be amazed if cancers were exactly alike. Unless a specific genetic lesion is identified as the cause of each histological type of cancer, each malignancy in each patient may be an individual problem in biology. It is possible a singular change leads to all forms of lung cancer, or all forms of breast cancer, or all forms of colon cancer. It is also possible that genetic change will result in specific markers for each of those cancers, which can be exploited in treatment. However, it is perfectly obvious that the cells in which those changes occur are genetically distinct from one person to another. Many genetic alterations, caused by the same chemical or physical carcinogen, result in the outgrowth of cells that markedly differ from each other. If such is the case, one might postulate that cancer in each patient is the individualistic expression of a response to that multistep, complex carcinogenic impulse, thereby embodying the genetic characteristics of both the host and the carcinogenic influence. If such is the case, then the actual problem in developmental therapeutics will be individualistic and each patient will have to be analyzed as an individual problem in cancer biology.

This concept of individuality of cancers has been difficult for many cancer biologists and clinicians to accept. We have learned, and grown up with, the histological classification systems embodied in the minds of pathologists and transmitted through the textbooks of medicine. These concepts classify cancers categorically according to tissue of origin and histological features. In spite of the clinical and laboratory observations that phenotypic analysis and even 'genotype' in cancer biology confer great diversity within cancers of the same histological type, we continue to develop therapeutics as if all breast cancer, all lung cancer, and all colon cancer are replicates. This is the simplest system to teach, the simplest to learn, and the simplest to practice. However, it appears to be fundamentally and biologically incorrect.

Heretofore, there has never been a technology that allows cancer biologists to understand cancer on an individualistic basis. Monoclonal antibody technology represents what may be the solution to the problem. If cancer is indeed diverse and individualistic, might not the immune system, itself individualistic and diverse, be able to solve the problem? Each person's immune system has the ability to produce several hundred thousand to several million different antibody molecules. Taken together, the diversity of the immune system from the broader perspective of a population of individuals is gigantic. By the use of *in vitro* techniques and the cellular diversity inherent in the immune system, it is probable that the response capabilities in antibody technology exceed the diversity implicit in cancer. It may well be postulated that each cancer in each patient presents with an individual array of antigens. If such is the case, it might be possible to generate antibodies and/or type tumors with a multiphasic approach, leading to the generation of cocktails of antibody to respond to the diversity inherent in cancer biology.

CANCER TREATMENT 1998

It has been categorically stated by various authorities that cancer is a problem that should be largely solved or under control before the end of the century. The National Cancer Institute has set a national priority of reducing the cancer death rate by at least 50% by the year 2000. These projections were certainly optimistic, and they will not be achieved. On the horizon for surgery, radiotherapy, and chemotherapy, there seems little to support the goal of reducing the cancer death rate by 50% by 2000. Although it is doubtful that the cancer death rate can easily be reduced by this magnitude, it is likely that the approaches available through biotherapy will play a major role in developmental therapeutics in the next decade. If the field is allowed to progress by using the best minds of science rather than proceeding in an overly structured and rigidified way, new paradigms for developmental therapeutics may allow for greater strides to be made using biotherapy.

End-point reductions in cancer death rates are difficult to achieve, or even to detect, because of time factors. To know that the death rate from breast cancer has been reduced by 50%, one would have to have at least a 5-year followup of the patients at risk since the recurrence rate, although highest in the first 2 years, continues to be significant for several years after diagnosis. For colon cancer and lung cancer, the problem is somewhat more straightforward, in that end points of an effective change in therapeutics can be discerned within 3-5 years. Breast, colon, and lung cancers being the most common malignancies, the reduction of death rate by 50% in these three tumors by the year 2000 would require that the actual change would have to have occurred between 1990 and 1995. This simply did not occur. Although biotherapy is likely to play an increasingly important role within the next decade, it is doubtful that changes of such magnitude can be produced in the near term. Rather, it seems more likely that the decade of the 1990s will be one in which the early phases of such changes may occur, and the actual end point for death-rate reduction will then fall well after the year 2000.

It is 1996. Interferon, interleukin 1-18, growth and maturation factors, tumor necrosis factor, colony stimulating factor, activated cells, monoclonal antibodies, and immunoconjugates are clinical realities – but they are all in an early phase of developmental therapeutics. If developed as drugs have been tested in the past, the average time to take these from the laboratory to an approved therapeutic is 10 years, at a cost of over $400, 000, 000 each. If we are to move forward in developmental therapeutics for biologicals, we cannot take 10 years to develop each approach individually. Certainly, it is impossible to image a series of events that will allow an end-point reduction of 50% by the year 2000 or even 2050 if each biopharmaceutical takes 10 years to be brought from concept to widespread clinical use.

BIOTHERAPY IS NOT JUST IMMUNOTHERAPY

This fourth modality of cancer treatment is constituted more broadly to include all of the factors described in this book [3]. To take maximum advantage of the opportunities available through biotherapy, major structural changes are necessary in our system of translation of developmental therapeutics from concept to the laboratory and then to the clinic [2]. We cannot afford to develop biologicals in the protracted, expensive unidimensional manner of drug development. We have a huge number of new biological substances, and the current system of access and opportunity for patients, the system of funding of research, our method of government regulation, and our reimbursement system for developmental therapeutics must undergo major change [4-11, 15, 18, 19, 21-27, 29-32]. We are now faced with the reality of many more opportunities for effective cancer therapy than mechanisms by which these opportunities can be brought to clinical reality.

For more than two decades, cancer research and treatment have operated on the 'kill and cure' hypothesis. Developmental therapeutic programs have functioned under a format where a new drug is brought to the clinic tested in phase I for toxicity and phase II for activity with the presumption that short-term effects on cancer (response rates) will ultimately lead, if positive, to survival benefit. While this paradigm has been useful in developing cytoxic drugs, there is much to suggest that we should now broaden our concept of developmental therapeutics, as cancer biotherapy comes to the fore, to include the idea of cancer control. Much as one treats diabetes with insulin, it may soon be possible through the use of growth and maturation factors and other forms of cancer biotherapy to arrest the growth and spread of cancer and thus make these diseases more amenable to long-term control even in the absence of tumor eradication. The implications in terms of cost and reimbursement for clinical services are obvious. We cannot afford to pay for developmental therapeutics as we have in the past. How is society going to pay for the very long-term clinical trials, perhaps constituted over a 3- to 5-year period, to test the various hypotheses for cancer control. Witness the difficulty in establishing clinical trials for cancer prevention and the high cost intrinsic to these programs as examples of the difficulty in envisioning clinical research for long-term cancer control projects. Obviously, this is going to require a major restructuring of developmental therapeutics if society is to take advantage of these opportunities [8-10, 12, 13].

For more than two decades the major factors slowing developmental therapeutics have been the regulations promulgated by Congress and the Food and Drug Administration (FDA) for the development of new drugs [14]. These regulations have resulted in a system of drug development costing more than $400 million per new drug taken through to commercial availability. In the last 10 years it has become apparent that the funding for clinical research is becoming less available. Much of the funding was derived from insurance reimbursement for clinical trials, and with the current pressure on insurers to reduce costs, at the behest of employers and patients who pay for their insurance premiums, it is becoming increasingly difficult to fund clinical research through third-party reimbursement. Thus, while the regulation and the intrinsic cost were the major impediments to rapid drug development in the 1980s, reimbursement for clinical trials and even reimbursement for the 'off-label' use of new forms of therapy has become the major limiting factor in the 1990s. We are now faced with the probability that cancer cures are being developed that will not be reimbursed by government or private insurance programs [13, 16, 17, 20].

With our current reimbursement system, autologous bone marrow transplantation for certain forms of cancer has reached a level of cure of 20% of patients with selected neoplasms at a cost of $100,000-150,000 per procedure. Thus, the upper limit of the price for a human life is becoming more clear. New technology tends to be expensive early and to become less expensive later. However, we now face the probability that certain new technologies will be available and highly effective while still very expensive [20]. Society must decide how much life is worth and what percentage of the gross national product should be allocated to health care. This is an area that needs public debate and should not be simply left to 'social planners and thought leaders.'

Therefore, it is apparent that cancer biotherapy brings cancer research and developmental therapeutics to a crossroad. In the next millennium, we will not be limited by our ability to conceptualize and develop highly effective approaches to cancer treatment. We will be limited by broader social considerations of who shall pay for such approaches and how much each life is worth [20, 28].

Thus, it is apparent that the many opportunities biotherapy brings to scientists and clinician will have to be moved at a much faster rate from laboratory to clinic if our patients are to derive benefit from these new approaches. Perhaps the use of the laboratory in conjunction with the clinical practice of medicine, as suggested by Dr. Peter Medawar, is the true 'break-through' in the developmental therapeutics of cancer [1]:

'The cure of cancer is never going to be found. It is far more likely that each tumor in each patient is going to present a unique research problem for which laboratory workers and clinicians between them will have to work out a unique solution'.

REFERENCES

1. Medawar P, ed. *The life sciences*. New York: Harper & Row, 1977.
2. Oldham RK. Biologicals: new horizons in pharmaceutical development. *J Biol Response Modif* 1983; 2: 199-206.
3. Oldham RK. Biologicals and biological response modifiers: the fourth modality of cancer treatment. *Cancer Treat Rep* 1984; 68: 221-232.
4. Oldham RK. The cure for cancer. *J Biol Response Modif* 1985; 4: 111-116.
5. Oldham RK. Whose rights come first? *J Biol Response Modif* 1985; 4: 211-212.
6. Oldham RK. The government-academic 'industrial' complex. *J Biol Response Modif* 1986; 5: 109-111.
7. Oldham RK. Profits: who benefits? *J Biol Response Modif* 1986; 5: 203-205.
8. Oldham RK. Patient-funded cancer research. *N Engl J Med* 1987; 316: 46-47.
9. Oldham RK. Drug development: who foots the bill? *Bio/technology* 1987; 5: 648.
10. Oldham RK. False hope vs. opportunity. *Cope* 1987; April: 66.
11. Oldham RK. Whose life is it anyway? *Wall Street Journal* April 24, 1987.
12. Oldham RK. Letter to the Editor: Patient-funded cancer research. *N Engl J Med* 1987; July 16: 172.
13. Oldham RK. Who pays for new drugs? *Nature* 1988; 332(28): 795.
14. Oldham RK. Regulatory hierarchies (editorial). *Mol Biother* 1988; 1(1): 3-6.
15. Oldham RK. Fundamentally flawed? *Mol Biother* 1988; 1(2): 58-60.
16. Oldham RK. Why deny health care? *The Freeman* 1989; March: 94-95.
17. Oldham RK. Clinical research in cancer: a time for consensus. *Pharm Exec* 1989; July: 23-24.
18. Oldham RK, Avent RA. Clinical research: who pays the bill? *Oncology Issues* 19889; 4(2): 13-14.
19. Oldham RK. Clinical research in cancer: a time for consensus. *Mol Biother* 1989; 1(5): 242-243.
20. Oldham RK. Cancer cures. By the people, for the people, at what cost? (editorial). *Mol Biother* 1990; 2: 2-3.
21. Oldham RK. Cancer and diabetes: are there similarities? *Mol Biother* 1990; 2(3): 130-131.
22. Oldham RK. Whose rights come first? *Mol Biother* 1991; 3(2): 58-59.
23. Oldham RK. Cancer research: a public trust. *BioPharm* 1991; 4(3): 8-9.
24. Oldham RK. Is informed consent a function of why pays? *Mol Biother* 1991; 3(1): 2-5.
25. Oldham RK. The rights and wrongs of national health care. *Pharm Exec* 1991; 11(4): 92-93.
26. Oldham RK. Cancer research for whom? *Bio/Technology* 1991; 9: 772.
27. Oldham RK. Peer Review. Mol Biother 1992; 4: 2-3.
28. Oldham RK. BioEthics: Opportunities, risks and ethics: the privatization of cancer research. *Media America, Franklin, TN*, 1992.
29. Oldham RK. Fundamentally flawed. *Cancer Biotherapy* 1993; 8(2): 111-114.
30. Oldham RK. What's the score? *Cancer Biotherapy* 1993; 8(3): 187-188.
31. Oldham RK. Cancer research: does it deliver for the patient? *Cancer Biotherapy* 1994; 9(2): 99-102.
32. Oldham RK. The war on cancer: new battle plan needed. *Cancer Biotherapy* 1994; 9(4): 289-290.

ABOUT THE EDITOR

Robert K. Oldham is the Founder and Director of the Biological Therapy Institute Foundation, Franklin, Tennessee. He is a Clinical Professor of Medicine in Hematology/Oncology at the University of Missouri and Assistant Professor of Medicine at The University of Kentucky. The author of over 400 scientific papers and 13 books, Dr. Oldham is the Founder and former Editor-in-Chief of the *Journal of Biological Response Modifiers* (now *Journal of Immunotherapy*) and was the Editor-in-Chief of *Molecular Biotherapy*. He is the Founder and Editor-in-Chief of *Cancer Biotherapy* which recently merged with *Antibody, Immunoconjugates and Radiopharmaceuticals* where he now serves as Co-Editor-in-Chief for *Cancer Biotherapy and Radiopharmaceuticals*. One of the discoverers of natural killer cells and a developer of improved therapy for small cell lung cancer and of biologicals and biological response modifiers for cancer treatment, he is noted for using cryopreserved cells for immunological standardization and applying monoclonal antibodies and immunoconjugates in cancer treatment.

Dr. Oldham is a Diplomate of the National Board of Medical Examiners and American Board of Internal Medicine; a Fellow of the American College of Physicians; and a member of the American Association of Immunologists, American Association of Cancer Research, American Federation for Clinical Research, and American Society for Clinical Oncology, among others. He is board certified in medical oncology and internal medicine. He received the M.D. degree (1968) from the University of Missouri, Columbia and did subsequent training at Vanderbilt and the National Cancer Institute. He served as Founding Director of Medical Oncology at Vanderbilt and Founding Director of the NCI Biological Response Modifiers Program. He is currently Director, Biological Therapy Institute Foundation, and President of American Patient Services and Cancer Therapeutics Inc.

INDEX

R.K. Oldham (ed.), Principles of Cancer Biotherapy. 3rd ed., 499–502.